Jim
Pats

Molecular Pathology
of
Lung Diseases

MOLECULAR PATHOLOGY LIBRARY SERIES
Philip T. Cagle, MD, Series Editor

1. D.S. Zander, H.H. Popper, J. Jagirdar, A.K. Haque, P.T. Cagle, R. Barrios:
   ISBN 978-0-387-72429-4
   Molecular Pathology of Lung Diseases. 2008

Molecular Pathology
of
Lung Diseases

Edited by

Dani S. Zander, MD
Penn State Milton S. Hershey Medical Center,
Hershey, Pennsylvania

Helmut H. Popper, MD
Institute of Pathology, Laboratories for Molecular Cytogenetics,
Environmental and Respiratory Pathology,
Medical University of Graz, Graz, Austria

Jaishree Jagirdar, MD
University of Texas Health Science Center at San Antonio,
San Antonio, Texas

Abida K. Haque, MD
Weill Medical College of Cornell University, New York;
San Jacinto Methodist Hospital, Baytown, Texas

Philip T. Cagle, MD
Weill Medical College of Cornell University, New York;
The Methodist Hospital, Houston, Texas

Roberto Barrios, MD
Weill Medical College of Cornell University, New York;
The Methodist Hospital, Houston, Texas

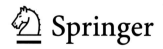 Springer

Dani S. Zander, MD
Department of Pathology
Penn State Milton S. Hershey Medical Center
Hershey, PA
USA

Helmut H. Popper, MD
Institute of Pathology
Laboratories for Molecular Cytogenetics
Medical University of Graz
Graz, Austria

Jaishree Jagirdar, MD
Department of Pathology
University of Texas Health Science Center
San Antonio, TX
USA

Abida K. Haque, MD
Weill Medical College of Cornell University
New York, NY
San Jacinto Methodist Hospital
Department of Pathology
Baytown, TX
USA

Philip T. Cagle, MD
Pathology and Laboratory Medicine
Weill Medical College of Cornell University
New York, NY
The Methodist Hospital
Houston, TX
USA

Roberto Barrios, MD
Pathology and Laboratory Medicine
Weill Medical College of Cornell University
New York, NY
The Methodist Hospital
Houston, TX
USA

Series Editor:
Philip T. Cagle, MD
Pathology and Laboratory Medicine
Weill Medical College of Cornell University
New York, NY
The Methodist Hospital
Houston, Texas
USA

Library of Congress Control Number: 2007928822

ISBN: 978-0-387-72429-4   e-ISBN: 978-0-387-72430-0

Printed on acid-free paper.

9 8 7 6 5 4 3 2 1

springer.com

Series Preface

The past two decades have seen an ever-accelerating growth in knowledge about molecular pathology of human diseases, which received a large boost with the sequencing of the human genome in 2003. Molecular diagnostics, molecular targeted therapy, and genetic therapy are now routine in many medical centers. The molecular field now impacts every field in medicine, whether clinical research or routine patient care. There is a great need for basic researchers to understand the potential clinical implications of their research, whereas private practice clinicians of all types (general internal medicine and internal medicine specialists, medical oncologists, radiation oncologists, surgeons, pediatricians, and family practitioners), clinical investigators, pathologists, and medical laboratory directors and radiologists require a basic understanding of the fundamentals of molecular pathogenesis, diagnosis, and treatment for their patients.

Traditional textbooks in molecular biology deal with basic science and are not readily applicable to the medical setting. Most medical textbooks that include a mention of molecular pathology in the clinical setting are limited in scope and assume that the reader already has a working knowledge of the basic science of molecular biology. Other texts emphasize technology and testing procedures without integrating the clinical perspective. There is an urgent need for a text that fills the gap between basic science books and clinical practice.

In the *Molecular Pathology Library Series* the basic science and the technology is integrated with the medical perspective and clinical application. Each book in the series is divided according to neoplastic and nonneoplastic diseases for each of the organ systems traditionally associated with medical subspecialties.

Each book in the series is organized to provide (1) a succinct background of the essential terminology, concepts; and technology of molecular biology; (2) an overview of the broad application of molecular biology principles to disease; and (3) specific application of molecular pathology to the pathogenesis, diagnosis, and treatment of neoplastic and nonneoplastic diseases specific to each organ system. These broad section topics are broken down into succinct chapters, averaging about 15 to 20 pages each, to cover a very specific disease entity. The chapters are written by established authorities on the specific topic from academic centers around the world. In one book, diverse subjects are included that the reader would have to pursue from multiple sources in order to have a clear understanding of the molecular pathogenesis, diagnosis, and treatment of specific diseases. Attempting to hunt for the full information from basic concept to specific applications for a disease from the varied sources is time consuming and frustrating. By providing this quick and user-friendly reference, understanding and application of this rapidly growing field are made more accessible to both expert and generalist alike.

As books that bridge the gap between basic science and clinical understanding and practice, the *Molecular Pathology Library Series* serves the basic scientist, the clinical researcher, and the practicing physician or other health care provider who require more understanding of the application of basic research to patient care, from "bench to bedside." This series is unique and an invaluable resource to those who need to know about molecular pathology from a clinical, disease-oriented perspective. These books will be indispensable to physicians and health care providers in multiple disciplines as noted above, to residents and fellows in these multiple disciplines as well as their teaching institutions, and to researchers who increasingly must justify the clinical implications of their research.

Philip T. Cagle, MD
Series Editor

Preface

Molecular Pathology of Lung Diseases is the first volume in the *Molecular Pathology Library Series* by Springer Science+Business Media. Molecular pathology is rapidly becoming part of everyday medical practice from targeted molecular therapy to molecular imaging, and it is no longer limited to the basic research bench. Knowledge in this field is increasingly essential to those who provide patient care, and they are unlikely to find the perspective they need in traditional basic science textbooks. Because the goal of *Molecular Pathology of Lung Diseases* is to provide a bridge between clinical pulmonary pathology and basic molecular science, selection of chapter topics and approaches to the material were based largely on the needs of the practicing pathologist or other health care provider. As a result, this book has a very unique perspective compared with the more traditional molecular genetics textbooks or molecular laboratory procedure manuals. This alternative perspective is also valuable to the clinical and translational researchers who must think in terms of clinical objectives for their investigations.

Clinical pulmonary pathology is extensive and complex, including an intimidating list of environmental, hereditary, immunologic, and idiopathic diseases, both neoplastic and nonneoplastic. The first two sections of *Molecular Pathology of Lung Diseases* briefly familiarize the reader with general concepts, terminology, and procedures in molecular pathology. Subsequent to the introductory sections, this book is broadly subdivided into neoplastic and nonneoplastic lung diseases. Following discussion of general molecular pathologic principles of lung and pleural diseases under each of these two broad categories, separate chapters detail the current molecular pathologies of specific diseases. This design approximates the approach to lung disease that is most familiar to pathologists, pulmonologists, thoracic surgeons, and other health care providers; to medical students, residents, and fellows; and to those involved in clinical investigations or translational research.

The unique format of this book results in multiple relatively short chapters that can serve as a ready reference to specific medical topics. No other book currently provides the practical disease-based overview that is found in *Molecular Pathology of Lung Diseases.*

Philip T. Cagle, MD

Contents

**Section 3   Molecular Pathology of Pulmonary and Pleural
                Neoplasms: General Principles**

Contributors

Jeffrey K. Actor, PhD
Associate Professor, Department of Pathology and Laboratory Medicine, University of Texas–Houston Medical School, Houston, TX, USA

Timothy Craig Allen, MD, JD
Department of Pathology, University of Texas Health Center at Tyler, Tyler, TX, USA

Sadir Alrawi, MD, FRCS
Assistant Professor, Department of Surgery, University of Florida, Jacksonville, FL, USA

Jeffrey J. Atkinson, MD
Assistant Professor, Department of Internal Medicine/Pulmonary and Critical Care, Washington University School of Medicine, St. Louis, MO, USA

Roberto Barrios, MD
Professor, Department of Pathology and Laboratory Medicine, Weill Medical College of Cornell University, New York, NY; Methodist Hospital, Houston, TX, USA

Cindy Noel Berthelot, MD
Department of Internal Medicine, University of Texas Houston Health Science Center, Houston, TX, USA

Candice C. Black, DO
Assistant Professor, Department of Pathology, Dartmouth Medical School, Dartmouth Hitchcock Medical Center, Lebanon, NH, USA

Gregory L. Blakey, MD
Assistant Professor, Department of Pathology, University of Oklahoma Health Sciences Center, Oklahoma City, OK, USA

Steven R. Blumen, MS
Graduate Student, Department of Pathology, University of Vermont, Burlington, VT, USA

Tracey L. Bonfield, PhD
Department of Pediatric Pulmonary, Case Western Reserve University School of Medicine, Cleveland, OH

Alain C. Borczuk, MD
Associate Professor, Department of Pathology, Columbia University Medical Center, New York, NY, USA

Elisabeth Brambilla, MD
Department of Pathology, CHU de Grenoble Albert Michallon, Lung Cancer Research Group, INSERM U578, Grenoble, France

Steven L. Brody, MD
Associate Professor, Division of Pulmonary and Critical Care Medicine, Department of Internal Medicine, Washington University School of Medicine, St. Louis, MO, USA

Philip T. Cagle, MD
Professor, Pathology and Laboratory Medicine, Weill Medical College of Cornell University, New York, NY; Director Pulmonary Pathology, The Methodist Hospital, Houston, TX, USA

Marco Chilosi, MD
Professor, Department of Pathology, University of Verona, Verona, Italy

Annick Clement, MD, PhD
Pediatric Pulmonology Department, Hopital d'enfants Armand Trousseau, Paris, France

William B. Coleman, BS, PhD
Associate Professor, Department of Pathology and Laboratory Medicine, University of North Carolina School of Medicine, Chapel Hill, NC, USA

David B. Corry, MD
Associate Professor, Department of Medicine and Immunology, Baylor College of Medicine, Houston, TX, USA

Harriet Corvol, MD, PhD
Department of Pediatric Pulmonology, Hopital d'enfants Armand Trousseau, Paris, France

Manuel G. Cosio, MD
Professor, Department of Medicine, McGill University, Royal Victoria Hospital, Montreal, QB, Canada

Sanja Dacic, MD, PhD
Assistant Professor, Department of Pathology, University of Pittsburgh Medical Center, Pittsburgh, PA, USA

J. Stephen Dumler, MD
Professor, Division of Medical Microbiology, Department of Pathology, Johns Hopkins University School of Medicine, Baltimore, MD, USA

Aamir Ehsan, MD
Associate Professor, Department of Pathology, Director of Molecular Diagnostics and Flow Cytometry, University of Texas Health Science Center at San Antonio and Audie L. Murphy VA Medical Center, San Antonio, TX, USA

Jennifer A. Eleazar, MD
Assistant Professor, Department of Clinical Pathology, Columbia University Medical Center, New York, NY, USA

Steven N. Emancipator, MD
Professor, Department of Pathology, Case Western Reserve University, Louis Stokes Cleveland VA Medical Center, University Hospitals of Cleveland, Cleveland, OH, USA

Daniel H. Farkas, PhD, HCLD
Executive Director, Center for Molecular Medicine, Grand Rapids, MI, USA

Carol Farver, MD
Director, Pulmonary Pathology, Department of Anatomic Pathology, Cleveland Clinic Foundation, Cleveland, OH, USA

Brigitte Fauroux, MD, PhD
Department of Pediatric Pulmonology, Hopital d'enfants Armand Trousseau, Paris, France

Larry Fowler, MD
Professor, Department of Pathology, University of Texas Health Science Center at San Antonio, San Antonio, TX, USA

Armando E. Fraire, MD
Professor, Department of Pathology, University of Massachusetts Medical School, Worchester, MA, USA

Wieslaw Furmaga, MD
Assistant Professor, Department of Pathology, University of Texas Health Science Center at San Antonio, San Antonio, TX, USA

Françoise Galateau-Sallé, MD
Professor, Department of Pathology, INSERM ERI 3, CHU Caen, Caen, Calvados, France

Armond S. Goldman, MD
Emeritus Professor, Department of Pediatrics, University of Texas Medical Branch, Galveston, TX, USA

Thomas Goodwin, PhD
Department of Biomedical Research and Operations Branch, NASA/Johnson Space Center, Houston, TX, USA

Kevin C. Halling, MD, PhD
Co-Director of Molecular Cytology and Imaging Laboratory, Department of Laboratory Medicine and Pathology, Mayo Clinic, Rochester, MN, USA

Abida K. Haque, MD
Professor, Pathology and Laboratory Medicine, Weill Medical College of Cornell University, New York, NY; Chair and Director of Medical Laboratories, Department of Pathology, San Jacinto Methodist Hospital, Baytown, TX, USA

Josefine M. Heim-Hall, MD
Associate Professor, Department of Pathology, University of Texas Health Science Center at San Antonio, San Antonio, TX, USA

Jennifer L. Herrick, MD
Hematopathology Fellow, Department of Pathology, University of Texas Health
Science Center at San Antonio, San Antonio, TX, USA

Jennifer L. Hunt, MD, MEd
Head Section, Surgical Pathology, Director, Head and Neck/Endocrine Pathology,
Director, AP Molecular Diagnostics Unit, Department of Anatomic Pathology,
Cleveland Clinic, Cleveland, OH, USA

Robert L. Hunter, Jr., MD, PhD
Professor and Chairman, Department of Pathology and Laboratory Medicine, University of Texas–Houston Medical School, Houston, TX, USA

Chinnaswamy Jagannath, PhD
Associate Professor, Department of Pathology and Laboratory Medicine, University of Texas–Houston Medical School, Houston, TX, USA

Jaishree Jagirdar, MD
Professor, Department of Pathology, Director of Anatomic Pathology,
University of Texas Health Science Center at San Antonio, San Antonio, TX,
USA

Jeffrey M. Jordan, BS
Department of Pathology, University of Texas Medical Branch, Galveston, TX,
USA

Soon-Hee Jung, MD, PhD
Professor, Department of Pathology, Yonsei University/Wonju Christian Hospital,
Wonju, Kangwon-Do, Korea

Rekha Kar, MS
Graduate Student, Department of Pathology and Biochemistry, University of Texas
Health Science Center at San Antonio, San Antonio, TX, USA

Michael P. Keane, MD
Associate Professor, Department of Pulmonary and Critical Care Medicine, David
Geffen School of Medicine at UCLA, Los Angeles, CA, USA

Farrah Kheradmand, MD
Associate Professor, Department of Medicine and Immunology, Baylor College of
Medicine, Houston, TX, USA

Geoffrey A. Land, BS, MS, PhD
Professor, Department of Clinical Pathology and Laboratory Medicine, Director
of Histocompatibility, Transplant Immunology, and Microbiology, Methodist
Hospital/Weill-Cornell Medical College, Houston, TX, USA

Norman B. Levy, MD
Associate Professor, Department of Pathology, Dartmouth Hitchcock Medical
Center, Lebanon, NH, USA

Hanzhong Liu, MD, PhD
Scientist, Department of Pediatrics, Children's Hospital of Philadelphia, Philadelphia, PA, USA

Li Mao, MD
Professor, Department of Thoracic and Head and Neck Medical Oncology, University of Texas MD Anderson Cancer Center, Houston, TX, USA

Michael R. McGinnis, PhD
Professor, Department of Pathology, University of Texas Medical Branch, Galveston, TX, USA

Brooke T. Mossman, PhD
Professor, Department of Pathology, University of Vermont, Burlington, VT, USA

John S. Munger, MD
Assistant Professor, Department of Medicine and Cell Biology, New York University School of Medicine, New York, NY, USA

Bruno Murer, MD
Department of Anatomic Pathology, Regional Hospital, Mestre-Venice, Italy

Lawrence M. Nogee, MD
Associate Professor, Department of Pediatrics, Johns Hopkins University School of Medicine, Baltimore, MD, USA

Juan P. Olano, MD
Associate Professor, Department of Pathology, University of Texas Medical Branch, Galveston, TX, USA

Dwight Oliver, MD
Assistant Professor, Department of Pathology and Laboratory Medicine, University of Texas–Houston Medical School, Houston, TX, USA

Venerino Poletti, MD, FCCP
Professor, Department of Diseases of the Thorax, Ospedale GB Morgagni, Forli, Italy

Helmut H. Popper, MD
Institute of Pathology, Laboratories for Molecular Cytogenetics, Environmental and Respiratory Pathology, Medical University of Graz, Graz, Austria

Sharon C. Presnell, PhD
Director, Cell and Tissue Technologies, Becton Dickinson, Research Triangle Park, NC, USA

Gary W. Procop, MD
Section Head, Clinical Microbiology, Department of Clinical Pathology, Cleveland Clinic, Cleveland, OH, USA

Jae Y. Ro, MD, PhD
Professor, Department of Pathology, Cornell University/Methodist Hospital and University of Texas MD Anderson Cancer Center, Houston, TX, USA

William N. Rom, MD, MPH
Sol and Judith Bergstein Professor, Department of Medicine and Environmental Medicine, New York University School of Medicine, New York, NY, USA

Jack A. Roth, MD, FACS
Professor and Bud Johnson Clinical Distinguished Chair, Professor of Molecular and Cellular Oncology, Director, WM Keck Center for Innovative Cancer Therapies, Chief, Section of Thoracic Molecular Oncology, Department of Thoracic and Cardiovascular Surgery, University of Texas MD Anderson Cancer Center, Houston, TX, USA

Pothana Saikumar, PhD
Associate Professor, Department of Pathology, University of Texas Health Science Center at San Antonio, San Antonio, TX, USA

Frank C. Schmalstieg, MD, PhD
Professor, Department of Pediatrics, University of Texas Medical Branch, Galveston, TX, USA

Nabin K. Shrestha, MD
Associate Staff Physician, Department of Infectious Diseases, Cleveland Clinic, Cleveland, OH, USA

Anna Sienko, MD
Department of Pathology, Methodist Hospital, Houston, TX, USA

Richard N. Sifers, PhD
Associate Professor, Department of Pathology, Baylor College of Medicine, Houston, TX, USA

Michael B. Smith, MD
Department of Pathology, University of Texas Medical Branch, Galveston, TX, USA

Arwen A. Stelter, BS
Graduate Assistant, Department of Pharmacology and Toxicology, University of Texas Medical Branch, Galveston, TX, USA

Robert M. Strieter, MD
Henry B. Mulholland Professor and Chair, Department of Medicine, University of Virginia School of Medicine, Charlottesville, VA, USA

Dongfeng Tan, MD
Associate Professor, Department of Pathology, University of Texas MD Anderson Cancer Center, Houston, TX, USA

Wim Timens, MD, PhD
Professor, Department of Pathology, University Medical Center Groningen, Groningen, The Netherlands

Gregory J. Tsongalis, PhD
Director, Department of Molecular Pathology, Associate Professor, Department of Pathology, Dartmouth Medical School, Dartmouth Hitchcock Medical Center, and Norris Cotton Cancer Center, Lebanon, NH, USA

Stephen K. Tyring, MD, PhD, MBA
Professor, Department of Dermatology, Microbiology/Molecular Genetics, and Internal Medicine, University of Texas Health Science Center, Houston, TX, USA

Reinhard Ullmann, PhD
Department of Human Molecular Genetics, Max Planck Institute for Molecular Genetics, Berlin, Germany

Roger A. Vertrees, PhD
Department of Surgery, University of Texas Medical Branch, Galveston, TX, USA

Jean Michel Vignaud, MD
Department of Pathology (Mesopath Group) and INSERM ER3, CHU Caen, France

Gary A. Visner, DO
Associate Professor, Department of Pediatrics, University of Pennsylvania, Children's Hospital of Philadelphia, Philadelphia, PA, USA

Guoping Wang, MD, PhD
Professor, Department of Pathology, Tongji Medical College, Huazhong University of Science and Technology, Wuhan, China

Amy J. Wendel, SCT, MP, HT(ASCP)CM
Education Coordinator, Department of Laboratory Medicine and Pathology, Mayo Clinic, Rochester, MN, USA

Susan E. Wert, PhD
Associate Professor, Department of Pediatrics, Division of Neonatology and Pulmonary Biology, The University of Cincinnati College of Medicine and Cincinnati Children's Hospital Medical Center, Cincinnati, OH, USA

Jingwu Xie, PhD
Associate Professor, Department of Pharmacology and Toxicology, University of Texas Medical Branch, Galveston, TX, USA

Dani S. Zander, MD
Professor and Chair, Department of Pathology, Penn State Milton S. Hershey Medical Center, Hershey, PA, USA

Bihong Zhao, MD, PhD
Fellow, Department of Pathology, Methodist Hospital, Weill Medical College, Cornell University, Houston, TX, USA

Joseph B. Zwischenberger, MD
Department of Surgery, University of Texas Medical Branch, Galveston, TX, USA

Section 1
Basic Concepts of Molecular Pathology

1
Genes, Gene Products, and Transcription Factors

Philip T. Cagle

Introduction

Molecular pathology employs an ever-expanding array of special techniques to study nucleic acids, genes, gene products, receptors, signaling pathways, the cell cycle, and mutations. This chapter and the others in this section provide a quick review of basic terminology and concepts for the understanding of subsequent chapters.

Nucleic Acids, Genes, and Gene Products

Genes are the bits of information that code for the proteins that are necessary for structure and metabolic reactions in living tissues. Genes and the molecules that construct their protein products using the blueprints or genetic code in the genes are composed of nucleic acids. Nucleotides are the building blocks of the nucleic acids, deoxyribonucleic acid (DNA) and ribonucleic acid (RNA), the essential compounds that make up genes and transcribe the genetic code into proteins, respectively. Nucleotides are basic compounds composed of a sugar-phosphate backbone and a nitrogenous base. Nucleotides consist of two types of bases: purines and pyrimidines. In DNA, there are two purines (adenine, abbreviated as A, and guanine, abbreviated as G) and two pyrimidines (thymine, abbreviated as T, and cytosine, abbreviated as C). In RNA, there are also two purines (A and G) and two pyrimidines (uracil, abbreviated as U, replaces T and C). DNA is typically double stranded, with the nucleotide bases paired together as described below, and RNA is typically single stranded. When nucleotides are assembled together in a nucleic acid, formation of covalent phosphodiester bonds results in a free 5′ phosphate at the origin of the nucleic acid and a free 3′ hydroxyl at the end (terminus) of the nucleic acid. For this reason, the synthesis of the nucleic acid is said to occur in a 5′ to 3′ direction (see below).[1–9]

DNA is composed of nucleotides arranged sequentially in a deliberate order that encodes as genes for a matching sequential order of amino acids that will form proteins, as further discussed below. The nucleotides in genes are arranged in a double-stranded right-handed helix in the cell nucleus so that the purine A always binds with the pyrimidine T and the purine G always binds with the pyrimidine C in base pairs. As a result, the DNA in a double helix is arranged in complementary strands: the sequence of nucleotides in one strand of DNA is a "mirror image" of the nucleotide sequence in the other DNA strand. Groups of DNA base pairs are wrapped around small proteins called *histones* forming arrangements of DNA called *nucleosomes*, allowing the DNA to fit within the cell nucleus. Genes are located on chromosomes that consist of DNA packaged with histone and nonhistone proteins. There are 23 pairs of chromosomes in the human for a total of 46. Each gene is located at a specific site or locus on a specific pair of chromosomes. Because the chromosomes are in pairs and each chromosome has a locus for each gene, the genes occur as two copies or alleles, one copy or allele on each of the members of the chromosome pair. Chromosomes are ordinarily indistinct in the nuclear chromatin but are discreet during mitosis or cell division.[1–14]

The genome is the entirety of the DNA sequence or chromosomes of an organism or its "complete genetic complement." Genomics is the sequencing and study of genomes and cytogenetics is the study of chromosomes, traditionally through visualization of the karyotype or set of chromosomes of an organism. The somatic cells are diploid with a pair of each of the chromosomes and, therefore, two copies or alleles of each gene, one allele at the equivalent locus on each paired chromosome. The gametes are haploid, which means that these cells have only one set of each of the chromosomes with only one allele of each gene. During fertilization, the nuclear material of the two gametes combine, restoring the diploid number of chromosomes and alleles to the diploid number in the fertilized egg.[1-9]

The genotype is the genetic information in an individual's DNA, and the phenotype is how the genotype is manifested or expressed. Genotype and phenotype can differ. If two alleles are the same in one individual, they are said to be homozygous, and if the two alleles are different, they are said to be heterozygous. If a person is heterozygous for a gene, one allele may be expressed preferentially over the other allele in which case the former allele is considered dominant and the latter allele is considered recessive. In this situation, the dominant allele codes for features that mask the features coded for by the recessive allele so that the phenotype is different from the genotype. For example, a person is heterozygous for eye color and has an allele for brown eyes on one chromosome and an allele for blue eyes on the other member of that pair of chromosomes. That person will have brown eyes (the phenotype) because the allele for brown eyes is dominant over the allele for blue eyes. On the other hand, if the person is homozygous and has two recessive alleles for blue eyes, that person will have blue eyes.[1-9]

Single nucleotide polymorphisms, or SNPs (pronounced "snips") are inherited, naturally occurring variations in one base between the DNA sequences in the same gene in two individuals and account for most of the genetic variation between individuals. Alleles or SNPs that are in close proximity on a chromosome are often inherited together as a haplotype. Polymorphisms are differences in DNA between individuals, and the most simple polymorphism is the SNP.[1-9]

Prior to cell division, new DNA must be synthesized from an existing strand of DNA, a process called *replication*. The synthesis of new DNA is a tightly controlled phase of the cell cycle (the S phase). The cell cycle is described in greater detail in Chapter 2. Prior to initiation of DNA replication, a prereplicative complex is constructed. This prereplicative complex is composed of the minichromosome maintenance protein complex (MCM), the origin recognition complex (ORC), and Cdc6/Cdc18. The S phase kinases Cdc7 and Cdk (cyclin-dependent kinase) activate the prereplicative complex to yield an initiation complex at the origin with binding of Cdc45 to MCM. Replication is initiated at specific points in the DNA referred to as *origins of replication*, and this creates a Y-shaped replication fork where the parental DNA duplex splits into two daughter DNA duplexes. As further described below, the duplex DNA is unwound with the assistance of special enzymes called topoisomerases, and then replication proteins, including DNA polymerases, bind to the unwound DNA.[15-60]

The synthesis of RNA, including messenger RNA (mRNA), from a strand of DNA (referred to as the *DNA template*) is known as *transcription* and is a fundamental step in the formation of the protein for which the DNA or gene codes. Condensed, inactive DNA at the periphery of the nucleus is called *heterochromatin*, and less condensed DNA available for transcription is referred to as *euchromatin*, which is generally found in the central part of the nucleus.[1-9]

DNA polymerase is an enzyme that synthesizes DNA using single-stranded DNA as a substrate and requires a small segment of double-stranded DNA to initiate new DNA synthesis. RNA polymerase is an enzyme that synthesizes an RNA transcript from a DNA template during transcription. RNA polymerase first binds to a section of bases on the DNA called the *transcription initiation site* (TIS) or promoter "upstream" of the gene that is being transcribed. RNA polymerase I transcribes genes encoding for ribosomal RNAs (rRNAs), RNA polymerase II transcribes genes encoding for mRNAs (mRNAs), and RNA polymerase III transcribes genes encoding for transfer RNAs (tRNAs).[61-66]

The double-stranded helix of DNA must be unraveled and separated into single strands of DNA before it can undergo either transcription or replication. Topoisomerases are enzymes that break or "nick" a DNA strand, releasing the tension of the coiled helix and allowing the DNA to unwind. Transient DNA single-strand breaks are induced by topoisomerase I, and transient DNA double-strand breaks are induced by topoisomerase II. Once the DNA is separated into single strands, the DNA strand that serves as the template for the mRNA during transcription is referred to as *antisense*, and the complimentary DNA strand that has the identical sequence of bases as the mRNA (except that U replaces T) is referred to as *sense*.[67-78]

During transcription, base pairs are matched with the single strand of antisense DNA template to form a strand of mRNA. The resulting mRNA strand is a "mirror image" of the DNA template except that uracil replaces thymine such that a DNA template with nucleotide sequence AGTC results in a strand of mRNA nucleotide sequence UCAG.[1-9]

A codon is a series of three base pair nucleotides in a gene that codes for a specific amino acid, and a series of base pair codons codes for a precise sequence of specific amino acids resulting in the synthesis of a specific protein. The gene product is the final molecule, usually a protein, for which the gene codes that generates the effect of the gene. During translation, the mRNA, derived from the DNA template through transcription, is used as a template for the assembly of the protein product. The assembly of the protein product occurs in association with ribosomes, a component of which are rRNAs, and tRNAs add the amino acids to the protein under assembly. Each tRNA has a specific acceptor arm that attaches a specific amino acid. The tRNA ensures that the amino acid is added to the protein in the correct sequence based on the mRNA template, because the tRNA also has a specific anticodon that binds to the corresponding specific codon in the mRNA. The assembly of the protein product via mRNA is referred to as *gene expression*. Most gene expression is controlled at the level of transcription.[79–81]

Genes are made up of DNA segments called *exons* and *introns*. Exons are translated into the gene product, and introns are intervening DNA segments that are believed to play a regulatory role or serve as "punctuation" in the gene. As such, introns are spliced out of the sequence at the mRNA level, and the splice junction is the site between an exon and an intron where the splicing occurs.[1–9] A short tandem repeat (STR) consists of a sequence of two to five nucleotides that are repeated in tandem, frequently dozens of times, in introns.[82] These STRs are found in microsatellite DNA, which is important in certain types of cancers such as colon cancer, although not significant in lung cancer.[83–99]

The end regions of chromosomes are composed of the nucleotide sequence TTAGGG repeated hundreds of times and are called *telomeres*. Telomere sequences are lost each time that a cell replicates until the cell loses its ability to divide as part of the aging process. Telomerase is a specialized DNA polymerase that replaces the DNA sequences at the telomeres of the chromosomes. Telomerase allows cells to divide indefinitely, a factor that can be important in cancer.[100–115]

Posttranslational Modifications of Gene Products

The specific sequence of amino acids in a protein imparts unique physicochemical properties that cause the polypeptide chain to fold into a tertiary structure that gives the protein its three-dimensional functional form. Domains are compact, spherical units of the three-dimensional tertiary structure.[1–9]

Dimerization is the binding of two proteins together. Binding of proteins to other proteins can enhance or inhibit their function. Dimers are frequently encountered, but trimers (three proteins), tetramers (four proteins), or other combinations can occur. Homodimers consist of two identical proteins bound together, and heterodimers consist of two different proteins bound together.[1–9]

Many proteins present in a cell are inert until they are activated by posttranslational modifications such as proteolytic cleavage or phosphorylation and become functional. The activation and inactivation of proteins by posttranslational modifications is essential in control of receptors, signaling pathways, transcription factors, and the cell cycle.

Phosphorylation and Acetylation

Phosphorylation is the addition of a phosphate group to a protein that is catalyzed by enzymes called *kinases*. Dephosphorylation is removal of a phosphate group from a protein that is catalyzed by enzymes called *phosphatases*. Many of the proteins in signaling pathways, including transcription factors, and the cell cycle are activated or inactivated by kinases and phosphatases. Depending on the domain that is phosphorylated, phosphorylation causes varying effects to a transcription factor. Phosphorylation can cause translocation (movement of a protein from the cytosol into the nucleus) and transactivation of genes or inhibit binding proteins from binding to DNA.[116–120]

Acetylation is the addition of an acetyl group to a protein that is catalyzed by acetyltransferases, and deacetylation is the removal of an acetyl group from a protein that is catalyzed by deacetylases. Similar to kinases and phosphatases, acetyltransferases and deacetylases activate and inactivate proteins involved in various molecular events.[121]

Protein Degradation and Ubiquitinylation

To limit signaling proteins and remove damaged or abnormal proteins, protein degradation is necessary. Ubiquitinylation or polyubiquitinylation (the ubiquitin-proteasome pathway) is the rapid degradation of proteins by reversible cross-linkage to a polypeptide called *ubiquitin*. Ubiquitin-activating enzyme (E1) activates ubiquitin, and the activated ubiquitin is transferred to a ubiquitin-conjugating enzyme (E2). The activated ubiquitin is transferred to the specific target protein by ubiquitin ligase (E3). Multiple ubiquitins are added to the protein, resulting in a polyubiquinated protein that is degraded by a large protease complex known as the *proteasome*. During this process, the ubiquitin is released to participate in more cycles of ubiquitinylation. Ubiquitinylation rapidly removes cell cycle regulators and signaling proteins, including those involved in cell survival and cell death (apoptosis).[122]

Transcription Factors

Gene expression is primarily controlled at the level of transcription initiation. The transcriptional unit of DNA starts with the 5′ regulatory sequences and ends with the 3′ terminator signal of the gene. Gene-activating proteins are blocked from DNA by the tight binding of histone proteins to the DNA blocks. Histone acetyltransferases acetylate histones, which allows the gene-activating proteins to bind to the DNA. By blocking this process, histone deacetylases silence gene transcription.[123-133]

Transcription factors, also called *trans-acting factors* or *transactivators*, are proteins that bind to DNA and regulate the activity of RNA polymerase. Transcription factors affect gene expression directly by induction or activation of the gene or by reducing transcription levels causing silencing or inhibition of the gene.[134-141]

Transcription factors that stimulate transcription or the synthesis of an RNA molecule from a DNA template are called *transcriptional activators*. In most cases, transcriptional activators have two domains: the DNA binding domain recognizes and binds to a specific DNA sequence, and the transactivation domain interacts with the transcriptional machinery to induce transcription. Transcription factors can be categorized into families according to their DNA binding domains; for example, zinc finger, leucine zipper, copper fist, basic helix-loop-helix, helix-turn-helix, and bZIP.[142-148]

Trans-acting DNA sequences encode for diffusible transcription factors that bind to distant cis-acting DNA regulatory sequences but may sometimes bind to other proteins that, in turn, bind to DNA or the transcription machinery. There are two categories of diffusible transcription factors that bind to DNA: (1) General transcription factors are part of the basic transcription machinery by directly interacting with the RNA polymerase complex. Cis-acting DNA sequences that bind general transcription factors and function in all genes are called *promoters*. (2) Regulatory transcription factors activate or inactivate specific genes. Cis-acting DNA sequences that bind regulatory transcription factors to induce specific genes are called *enhancers*.[134-148]

The initiation of transcription by RNA polymerase requires general transcription factors. A cis-acting DNA regulatory sequence that contains adenine-thymidine–rich nucleotide sequences, referred to as a *TATA box*, is found in the promoters of many genes. The TATA binding protein (TBP) and TBP-associated factors bind to form the general transcription factor TFIID. This transcription factor combined with other general transcription factors (TFIIB, TFIIF, TFIIE, and TFIIH) initiate transcription by binding RNA polymerase II to the promoter. A transcription bubble is formed when the transcriptional preinitiation complex binds to a specific sequence of nucleotides and there is separation or melting of the double-stranded DNA in conjunction with histone acetylation. After separation from the preinitiation complex, the transcribing enzyme moves down the DNA template along the reading frame. During transcription elongation, the transcription bubble moves down the DNA template in a 5′ to 3′ direction (as noted earlier). Once transcription is terminated, the resultant mRNA is freed and processed before it is actively transported into the cytoplasm.

In the cytoplasm, the mRNA enters the ribosome for translation of the protein product.[149-161]

Loops in the DNA bring enhancers into proximity of the transcription initiation sites even when they are located a distance away in sequence. This allows the enhancers to interact with general transcription factors or RNA polymerase complexes at the promoter, allowing enhancers to stimulate gene transcription above the basal level.

An example of transcription factors is the Myc/Max/Mad network of transcription factors that regulate cell growth and death. The Myc family includes N-myc, c-myc, and L-myc. The Mad family includes Mad1, Mxi1, Mad3, Mad4, Mnt, and Mga. The Mad family functions in part as antagonists of the Myc family. These proteins form heterodimers that determine their effect. Myc/Max heterodimers activate transcription causing cell growth, proliferation, and death. Mad/Max heterodimers competitively inhibit the Myc/Max-induced transcription, causing differentiation, cell survival, and inhibition of growth and proliferation.[162-172]

References

1. Coleman WB, Tsongalis GJ, eds. The Molecular Basis of Human Cancer. Totowa, NJ: Humana Press; 2002.
2. Watson JD, Baker TA, Bell SP, Gann A, Levine M, Losick R, eds. Molecular Biology of the Gene, 5th ed. Menlo Park, CA: Benjamin Cummings; 2003.
3. Epstein RJ, ed. Human Molecular Biology: An Introduction to the Molecular Basis of Health and Disease. Cambridge UK: Cambridge University Press; 2003.
4. Strachan T, Read A, eds. Human Molecular Genetics, 3rd ed. New York: Garland Science/Taylor and Francis Group; 2003.
5. Swansbury J, ed. Cancer Cytogenetics: Methods and Protocols. Totowa, NJ: Humana Press; 2003.
6. Cooper GM, Hausman RE, eds. The Cell: A Molecular Approach, 3rd ed. Washington, DC: ASM Press/Sunderland, MA: Sinauer Associates; 2004.
7. Farkas DH, ed. DNA from A to Z. Washington, DC: AACC Press; 2004.
8. Killeen AA, ed. Principles of Molecular Pathology. Totowa, NJ: Humana Press; 2004.
9. Leonard DGB, Bagg A, Caliendo A, et al., eds. Molecular Pathology in Clinical Practice. New York: Springer-Verlag; 2005.
10. Watson JD, Crick FH. Molecular structure of nucleic acids: a structure for deoxyribose nucleic acid. Nature 1953;171:737–738.
11. Thoma F, Koller T. Influence of histone H1 on chromatin structure. Cell 1977;12:101–107.
12. Varshavsky AJ, Bakayev VV, Nedospasov SA, Georgiev GP. On the structure of eukaryotic, prokaryotic, and viral chromatin. Cold Spring Harb Symp Quant Biol 1978;42 Pt 1:457–473.
13. Tyler-Smith C, Willard HF. Mammalian chromosome structure. Curr Opin Genet Dev 1993;3:390–397.

14. Lamond AI, Earnshaw WC. Structure and function in the nucleus. Science 1998;280:547–553.
15. Blow JJ, Laskey RA. A role for the nuclear envelope in controlling DNA replication within the cell cycle. Nature 1988;332:546–548.
16. Nishitani H, Nurse P. p65cdc18 plays a major role controlling the initiation of DNA replication in fission yeast. Cell 1995;83:397–405.
17. Cocker JH, Piatti S, Santocanale C, et al. An essential role for the Cdc6 protein in forming the pre-replicative complexes of budding yeast. Nature 1996;379:180–182.
18. Coleman TR, Carpenter PB, Dunphy WG. The *Xenopus* Cdc6 protein is essential for the initiation of a single round of DNA replication in cell-free extracts. Cell 1996;87:53–63.
19. Muzi Falconi M, Brown GW, Kelly TJ. cdc18+ regulates initiation of DNA replication in *Schizosaccharomyces pombe*. Proc Natl Acad Sci USA 1996;93:1566–1570.
20. Owens JC, Detweiler CS, Li JJ. CDC45 is required in conjunction with CDC7/DBF4 to trigger the initiation of DNA replication. Proc Natl Acad Sci USA 1997;94:12521–12526.
21. Tanaka T, Knapp D, Nasmyth K. Loading of an Mcm protein onto DNA replication origins is regulated by Cdc6p and CDKs. Cell 1997;90:649–660.
22. Williams RS, Shohet RV, Stillman B. A human protein related to yeast Cdc6p. Proc Natl Acad Sci USA 1997;94:142–147.
23. Hateboer G, Wobst A, Petersen BO, et al. Cell cycle-regulated expression of mammalian CDC6 is dependent on E2F. Mol Cell Biol 1998;18:6679–6697.
24. Hua XH, Newport J. Identification of a preinitiation step in DNA replication that is independent of origin recognition complex and cdc6, but dependent on cdk2. J Cell Biol 1998;140:271–281.
25. Leatherwood J. Emerging mechanisms of eukaryotic DNA replication initiation. Curr Opin Cell Biol 1998;10:742–748.
26. McGarry TJ, Kirschner MW. Geminin, an inhibitor of DNA replication, is degraded during mitosis. Cell 1998;93:1043–1053.
27. Mimura S, Takisawa H. *Xenopus* Cdc45-dependent loading of DNA polymerase onto chromatin under the control of S-phase Cdk. EMBO J 1998;17:5699–5707.
28. Saha P, Chen J, Thome KC, et al. Human CDC6/Cdc18 associates with Orc1 and cyclin-cdk and is selectively eliminated from the nucleus at the onset of S phase. Mol Cell Biol 1998;18:2758–2767.
29. Williams GH, Romanowski P, Morris L, et al. Improved cervical smear assessment using antibodies against proteins that regulate DNA replication. Proc Natl Acad Sci USA 1998;95:14932–14937.
30. Yan Z, DeGregori J, Shohet R, et al. Cdc6 is regulated by E2F and is essential for DNA replication in mammalian cells. Proc Natl Acad Sci USA 1998;95:3603–3608.
31. Zou L, Stillman B. Formation of a preinitiation complex by S-phase cyclin CDK-dependent loading of Cdc45p onto chromatin. Science 1998;280:593–596.
32. Donaldson AD, Blow JJ. The regulation of replication origin activation. Curr Opin Genet Dev 1999;9:62–68.
33. Fujita M, Yamada C, Goto H, et al. Cell cycle regulation of human CDC6 protein. Intracellular localization, interaction with the human mcm complex, and CDC2 kinase-mediated hyperphosphorylation. J Biol Chem 1999;274:25927–25932.
34. Masai H, Sato N, Takeda T, Arai K. CDC7 kinase complex as a molecular switch for DNA replication. Front Biosci 1999;4:D834–D840.
35. Petersen BO, Lukas J, Sorensen CS, et al. Phosphorylation of mammalian CDC6 by cyclin A/CDK2 regulates its subcellular localization. EMBO J 1999;18:396–410.
36. Coverley D, Pelizon C, Trewick S, Laskey RA. Chromatin-bound Cdc6 persists in S and G2 phases in human cells, while soluble Cdc6 is destroyed in a cyclin A-cdk2 dependent process. J Cell Sci 2000;113:1929–1938.
37. Homesley L, Lei M, Kawasaki Y, et al. Mcm10 and the MCM2–7 complex interact to initiate DNA synthesis and to release replication factors from origins. Genes Dev 2000;14:913–926.
38. Maiorano D, Moreau J, Mechali M. XCDT1 is required for the assembly of pre-replicative complexes in *Xenopus laevis*. Nature 2000;404:622–625.
39. Nishitani H, Lygerou Z, Nishimoto T, Nurse P. The Cdt1 protein is required to license DNA for replication in fission yeast. Nature 2000;404:625–628.
40. Petersen BO, Wagener C, Marinoni F, et al. Cell cycle- and cell growth-regulated proteolysis of mammalian CDC6 is dependent on APC-CDH1. Genes Dev 2000;14:2330–2343.
41. Takisawa H, Mimura S, Kubota Y. Eukaryotic DNA replication: from pre-replication complex to initiation complex. Curr Opin Cell Biol 2000;12:690–696.
42. Whittaker AJ, Royzman I, Orr-Weaver TL. *Drosophila* double parked: a conserved, essential replication protein that colocalizes with the origin recognition complex and links DNA replication with mitosis and the down-regulation of S phase transcripts. Genes Dev 2000;14:1765–1776.
43. Wohlschlegel JA, Dwyer BT, Dhar SK, et al. Inhibition of eukaryotic DNA replication by geminin binding to Cdt1. Science 2000;290:2309–2312.
44. Diffley JF. DNA replication: building the perfect switch. Curr Biol 2001;11:R367–R370.
45. Lei M, Tye BK. Initiating DNA synthesis: from recruiting to activating the MCM complex. J Cell Sci 2001;114:1447–1454.
46. Nishitani H, Taraviras S, Lygerou Z, Nishimoto T. The human licensing factor for DNA replication Cdt1 accumulates in G1 and is destabilized after initiation of S-phase. J Biol Chem 2001;276:44905–44911.
47. Tada S, Li A, Maiorano D, et al. Repression of origin assembly in metaphase depends on inhibition of RLF-B/Cdt1 by geminin. Nat Cell Biol 2001;3:107–113.
48. Yanow SK, Lygerou Z, Nurse P. Expression of Cdc18/Cdc6 and Cdt1 during G2 phase induces initiation of DNA replication. EMBO J 2001;20:4648–4656.
49. Arentson E, Faloon P, Seo J, et al. Oncogenic potential of the DNA replication licensing protein CDT1. Oncogene 2002;21:1150–1158.

50. Bell SP, Dutta A. DNA replication in eukaryotic cells. Annu Rev Biochem 2002;71:333–374.

51. Bermejo R, Vilaboa N, Cales C. Regulation of CDC6, geminin, and CDT1 in human cells that undergo poly-ploidization. Mol Biol Cell 2002;13:3989–4000.

52. Bonds L, Baker P, Gup C, Shroyer KR. Immunohisto-chemical localization of cdc6 in squamous and glandular neoplasia of the uterine cervix. Arch Pathol Lab Med 2002;26:1164–1168.

53. Mihaylov IS, Kondo T, Jones L, et al. Control of DNA replication and chromosome ploidy by geminin and cyclin A. Mol Cell Biol 2002;22:1868–1880.

54. Nishitani H, Lygerou Z. Control of DNA replication licensing in a cell cycle. Genes Cells 2002;7:523–534.

55. Robles LD, Frost AR, Davila M, et al. Down-regulation of Cdc6, a cell cycle regulatory gene, in prostate cancer. J Biol Chem 2002;277:25431–2538.

56. Shreeram S, Sparks A, Lane DP, Blow JJ. Cell type-specific responses of human cells to inhibition of replication licens-ing. Oncogene 2002;21:6624–6632.

57. Wohlschlegel JA, Kutok JL, Weng AP, Dutta A. Expression of geminin as a marker of cell proliferation in normal tissues and malignancies. Am J Pathol 2002;161:267–273.

58. Li X, Zhao Q, Liao R, et al. The SCF(Skp2) ubiquitin ligase complex interacts with the human replication licensing factor Cdt1 and regulates Cdt1 degradation. J Biol Chem 2003;278:30854–30858.

59. Vaziri C, Saxena S, Jeon Y, et al. A p53-dependent check-point pathway pre prevents rereplication. Mol Cell 2003; 11:997–1008.

60. Yoshida K, Inoue I. Regulation of geminin and Cdt1 expression by E2F transcription factors. Oncogene 2004;23: 3802–3812.

61. Krieg PA, Melton DA. In vitro RNA synthesis with SP6 RNA polymerase. Methods Enzymol 1987;155:397–415.

62. Lawyer FC, Stoffel S, Saiki RK, et al. Isolation, character-ization, and expression in Escherichia coli of the DNA polymerase gene from Thermus aquaticus. J Biol Chem 1989;264:6427–6437.

63. Studier FW, Rosenberg AH, Dunn JJ, Dubendorff JW. Use of T7 RNA polymerase to direct expression of cloned genes. Methods Enzymol 1990;185:60–89.

64. Kollmar R, Farnham PJ. Site-specific initiation of transcrip-tion by RNA polymerase II. Proc Soc Exp Biol Med 1993;203:127–139.

65. Chou KC, Kezdy FJ, Reusser F. Kinetics of processive nucleic acid polymerases and nucleases. Anal Biochem 1994;221:217–230.

66. Tabor S, Richardson CC. A single residue in DNA poly-merases of the Escherichia coli DNA polymerase I family is critical for distinguishing between deoxy- and dideoxy-ribonucleotides. Proc Natl Acad Sci USA 1995; 92:6339–6343.

67. Goldberg S, Schwartz H, Darnell JE Jr. Evidence from UV transcription mapping in HeLa cells that heterogeneous nuclear RNA is the messenger RNA precursor. Proc Natl Acad Sci USA 1977;74:4520–4523.

68. Hoffmann-Berling H. DNA unwinding enzymes. Prog Clin Biol Res 1982;102 Pt C:89–98.

69. Wang JC. DNA topoisomerases: why so many? J Biol Chem 1991;266:6659–6662.

70. Anderson HJ, Roberge M. DNA topoisomerase II: a review of its involvement in chromosome structure, DNA replication, transcription and mitosis. Cell Biol Int Rep 1992;16:717–724.

71. Gasser SM, Walter R, Dang Q, Cardenas ME. Topoisom-erase II: its functions and phosphorylation. Antonie Van Leeuwenhoek 1992;62:15–24.

72. D'Incalci M. DNA-topoisomerase inhibitors. Curr Opin Oncol 1993;5:1023–1028.

73. Ferguson LR, Baguley BC. Topoisomerase II enzymes and mutagenicity. Environ Mol Mutagen 1994;24:245–261.

74. Larsen AK, Skladanowski A, Bojanowski K. The roles of DNA topoisomerase II during the cell cycle. Prog Cell Cycle Res 1996;2:229–239.

75. Kato S, Kikuchi A. DNA topoisomerase: the key enzyme that regulates DNA super structure. Nagoya J Med Sci 1998;61:11–26.

76. Wang JC. Cellular roles of DNA topoisomerases: a molec-ular perspective. Nat Rev Mol Cell Biol 2002;3:430–440.

77. Gimenez-Abian JF, Clarke DJ. Replication-coupled topoi-somerase II templates the mitotic chromosome scaffold? Cell Cycle 2003;2:230–232.

78. Leppard JB, Champoux JJ. Human DNA topoisomerase I: relaxation, roles, and damage control. Chromosoma 2005; 114:75–85.

79. Sharp SJ, Schaack J, Cooley L, et al. Structure and tran-scription of eukaryotic tRNA genes. CRC Crit Rev Biochem 1985;19:107–144.

80. Persson BC. Modification of tRNA as a regulatory device. Mol Microbiol 1993;8:1011–1016.

81. Green R, Noller HF. Ribosomes and translation. Annu Rev Biochem 1997;66:679–716.

82. Sutherland GR, Richards RI. Simple tandem DNA repeats and human genetic disease. Proc Natl Acad Sci USA 1995;92:3636–3641.

83. Horii A, Han HJ, Shimada M, et al. Frequent replication errors at microsatellite loci in tumors of patients with mul-tiple primary cancers. Cancer Res 1994;54:3373–3375.

84. Loeb LA. Microsatellite instability: marker of a mutator phenotype in cancer. Cancer Res 1994;54:5059–5063.

85. Mao L, Lee DJ, Tockman MS, et al. Microsatellite altera-tions as clonal markers for the detection of human cancer. Proc Natl Acad Sci USA 1994;91:9871–9875.

86. Merlo A, Mabry M, Gabrielson E, et al. Frequent micro-satellite instability in primary small cell lung cancer. Cancer Res 1994;54:2098–2101.

87. Wooster R, Cleton-Jansen AM, Collins N, et al. Instability of short tandem repeats (microsatellites) in human cancers. Nat Genet 1994;6:152–156.

88. Fong KM, Zimmerman PV, Smith PJ. Microsatellite insta-bility and other molecular abnormalities in non–small cell lung cancer. Cancer Res 1995;55:28–30.

89. Miozzo M, Sozzi G, Musso K, et al. Microsatellite altera-tions in bronchial and sputum specimens of lung cancer patients. Cancer Res 1996;56:2285–2288.

90. Bocker T, Diermann J, Friedl W, et al. Microsatellite insta-bility analysis: a multicenter study for reliability and quality control. Cancer Res 1997;57:4739–4743.

91. Dietmaier W, Wallinger S, Bocker T, et al. Diagnostic microsatellite instability: definition and correlation with mismatch repair protein expression. Cancer Res 1997; 57:4749–56.

92. Lothe RA. Microsatellite instability in human solid tumors. Mol Med Today 1997;3:61–68.

93. Arzimanoglou II, Gilbert F, Barber HR. Microsatellite instability in human solid tumors. Cancer 1998;82: 1808–1820.

94. Boland CR, Thibodeau SN, Hamilton SR, et al. A National Cancer Institute Workshop on Microsatellite Instability for cancer detection and familial predisposition: development of international criteria for the determination of microsatellite instability in colorectal cancer. Cancer Res 1998;58:5248–5257.

95. Boyer JC, Farber RA. Mutation rate of a microsatellite sequence in normal human fibroblasts. Cancer Res 1998;58:3946–3949.

96. Hanford MG, Rushton BC, Gowen LC, Farber RA. Microsatellite mutation rates in cancer cell lines deficient or proficient in mismatch repair. Oncogene 1998;16: 2389–2393.

97. Jackson AL, Chen R, Loeb LA. Induction of microsatellite instability by oxidative DNA damage. Proc Natl Acad Sci USA 1998;95:12468–12473.

98. Johannsdottir JT, Jonasson JG, Bergthorsson JT, et al. The effect of mismatch repair deficiency on tumourigenesis; microsatellite instability affecting genes containing short repeated sequences. Int J Oncol 2000;16:133–139.

99. Kim WS, Park C, Hong SK, et al. Microsatellite instability(MSI) in non–small cell lung cancer (NSCLC) is highly associated with transforming growth factor-beta type II receptor(TGF-beta RII) frameshift mutation. Anticancer Res 2000;20:1499–1502.

100. Biessmann H, Mason JM. Telomeric repeat sequences. Chromosoma 1994;103:154–161.

101. Feng J, Funk WD, Wang SS, et al. The RNA component of human telomerase. Science 1995;269:1236–1241.

102. Counter CM. The roles of telomeres and telomerase in cell life span. Mutat Res 1996;366:45–63.

103. Wellinger RJ, Sen D. The DNA structures at the ends of eukaryotic chromosomes. Eur J Cancer 1997;33: 735–749.

104. Chakhparonian M, Wellinger RJ. Telomere maintenance and DNA replication: how closely are these two connected? Trends Genet 2003;19:439–446.

105. Bayne S, Liu JP. Hormones and growth factors regulate telomerase activity in ageing and cancer. Mol Cell Endocrinol 2005;240:11–22.

106. Blackburn EH. Telomeres and telomerase: their mechanisms of action and the effects of altering their functions. FEBS Lett 2005;579:859–862.

107. Blasco MA. Telomeres and human disease: ageing, cancer and beyond. Nat Rev Genet 2005;6:611–622.

108. Boukamp P, Popp S, Krunic D. Telomere-dependent chromosomal instability. J Invest Dermatol Symp Proc 2005; 10:89–94.

109. Brunori M, Luciano P, Gilson E, Geli V. The telomerase cycle: normal and pathological aspects. J Mol Med 2005;83: 244–257.

110. Dong CK, Masutomi K, Hahn WC. Telomerase: regulation, function and transformation. Crit Rev Oncol Hematol 2005;54:85–93.

111. Jacobs JJ, de Lange T. p16INK4a as a second effector of the telomere damage pathway. Cell Cycle 2005;4:1364–1368.

112. Opitz OG. Telomeres, telomerase and malignant transformation. Curr Mol Med 2005;5:219–226.

113. Viscardi V, Clerici M, Cartagena-Lirola H, Longhese MP. Telomeres and DNA damage checkpoints. Biochimie 2005;87:613–624.

114. Autexier C, Lue NF. The structure and function of telomerase reverse transcriptase. Annu Rev Biochem 2006;75: 493–517.

115. Bhattacharyya MK, Lustig AJ. Telomere dynamics in genome stability. Trends Biochem Sci 2006;31:114–122.

116. Pallen CJ, Tan YH, Guy GR. Protein phosphatases in cell signaling. Curr Opin Cell Biol 1992;4:1000–1007.

117. Boulikas T. Control of DNA replication by protein phosphorylation. Anticancer Res 1994;14:2465–2472.

118. Berndt N. Protein dephosphorylation and the intracellular control of the cell number. Front Biosci 1999;4:D22–D42.

119. Appella E, Anderson CW. Post-translational modifications and activation of p53 by genotoxic stresses. Eur J Biochem 2001;268:2764–2772.

120. Obaya AJ, Sedivy JM. Regulation of cyclin-Cdk activity in mammalian cells. Cell Mol Life Sci 2002;59:126–142.

121. Fu M, Wang C, Wang J, et al. Acetylation in hormone signaling and the cell cycle. Cytokine Growth Factor Rev 2002;13:259–276.

122. Haglund K, Dikic I. Ubiquitylation and cell signaling. EMBO J 2005;24:3353–3359.

123. Legube G, Trouche D. Regulating histone acetyltransferases and deacetylases. EMBO Rep 2003;4:944–947.

124. Marmorstein R. Structural and chemical basis of histone acetylation. Novartis Found Symp 2004;259:78–98.

125. Moore JD, Krebs JE. Histone modifications and DNA double-strand break repair. Biochem Cell Biol 2004; 82:446–452.

126. Peterson CL, Laniel MA. Histones and histone modifications. Curr Biol 2004;14:R546–R551.

127. Quivy V, Calomme C, Dekoninck A, et al. Gene activation and gene silencing: a subtle equilibrium. Cloning Stem Cells 2004;6:140–149.

128. Wang Y, Fischle W, Cheung W, et al. Beyond the double helix: writing and reading the histone code. Novartis Found Symp 2004;259:3–17.

129. Fraga MF, Esteller M. Towards the human cancer epigenome: a first draft of histone modifications. Cell Cycle 2005;4:1377–1381.

130. Khan AU, Krishnamurthy S. Histone modifications as key regulators of transcription. Front Biosci 2005;10: 866–872.

131. Verdone L, Caserta M, Di Mauro E. Role of histone acetylation in the control of gene expression. Biochem Cell Biol 2005;83:344–353.

132. Yu Y, Waters R. Histone acetylation, chromatin remodelling and nucleotide excision repair: hint from the study on MFA2 in Saccharomyces cerevisiae. Cell Cycle 2005; 4:1043–1045.

133. Verdone L, Agricola E, Caserta M, Di Mauro E. Histone acetylation in gene regulation. Brief Funct Genomic Proteomic 2006;5:209–221.

134. Haura EB, Turkson J, Jove R. Mechanisms of disease: insights into the emerging role of signal transducers and activators of transcription in cancer. Nat Clin Pract Oncol 2005;2:315–324.

135. Wang JC. Finding primary targets of transcriptional regulators. Cell Cycle 2005;4:356–358.

136. Wittenberg C, Reed SI. Cell cycle–dependent transcription in yeast: promoters, transcription factors, and transcriptomes. Oncogene 2005;24:2746–2755.

137. Zaidi SK, Young DW, Choi JY, et al. The dynamic organization of gene-regulatory machinery in nuclear microenvironments. EMBO Rep 2005;6:128–133.

138. Barrera LO, Ren B. The transcriptional regulatory code of eukaryotic cells—insights from genome-wide analysis of chromatin organization and transcription factor binding. Curr Opin Cell Biol 2006;18:291–298.

139. Dillon N. Gene regulation and large-scale chromatin organization in the nucleus. Chromosome Res 2006;14:117–126.

140. Maston GA, Evans SK, Green MR. Transcriptional regulatory elements in the human genome. Annu Rev Genomics Hum Genet 2006;7:29–59.

141. Thomas MC, Chiang CM. The general transcription machinery and general cofactors. Crit Rev Biochem Mol Biol 2006;41:105–178.

142. Engelkamp D, van Heyningen V. Transcription factors in disease. Curr Opin Genet Dev 1996;6:334–342.

143. Tamura T, Konishi Y, Makino Y, Mikoshiba K. Mechanisms of transcriptional regulation and neural gene expression. Neurochem Int 1996;29:573–581.

144. Bieker JJ, Ouyang L, Chen X. Transcriptional factors for specific globin genes. Ann NY Acad Sci 1998;850:64–69.

143. Hertel KJ, Lynch KW, Maniatis T. Common themes in the function of transcription and splicing enhancers. Curr Opin Cell Biol 1997;9:350–357.

146. Arnosti DN. Analysis and function of transcriptional regulatory elements: insights from *Drosophila*. Annu Rev Entomol 2003;48:579–602.

147. Scannell DR, Wolfe K. Rewiring the transcriptional regulatory circuits of cells. Genome Biol 2004;5:206.

148. Villard J. Transcription regulation and human diseases. Swiss Med Wkly 2004;134:571–579.

149. Hampsey M. Molecular genetics of the RNA polymerase II general transcriptional machinery. Microbiol Mol Biol Rev 1998;62:465–503.

150. Berk AJ. Activation of RNA polymerase II transcription. Curr Opin Cell Biol 1999;11:330–335.

151. Berk AJ. TBP-like factors come into focus. Cell 2000;103:5–8.

152. Green MR. TBP-associated factors (TAFIIs): multiple, selective transcriptional mediators in common complexes. Trends Biochem Sci 2000;25:59–63.

153. Pugh BF. Control of gene expression through regulation of the TATA-binding protein. Gene 2000;255:1–14.

154. Burley SK, Kamada K. Transcription factor complexes. Curr Opin Struct Biol 2002;12:225–230.

155. Featherstone M. Coactivators in transcription initiation: here are your orders. Curr Opin Genet Dev 2002;12:149–155.

156. Davidson I. The genetics of TBP and TBP-related factors. Trends Biochem Sci 2003;28:391–398.

157. Hochheimer A, Tjian R. Diversified transcription initiation complexes expand promoter selectivity and tissue-specific gene expression. Genes Dev 2003;17:1309–1320.

158. Asturias FJ. RNA polymerase II structure and organization of the preinitiation complex. Curr Opin Struct Biol 2004;14:121–129.

159. Matangkasombut O, Auty R, Buratowski S. Structure and function of the TFIID complex. Adv Protein Chem 2004;67:67–92.

160. Brady J, Kashanchi F. Tat gets the "green" light on transcription initiation. Retrovirology 2005;2:69.

161. Thomas MC, Chiang CM. The general transcription machinery and general cofactors. Crit Rev Biochem Mol Biol 2006;41:105–178.

162. Dang CV, Resar LM, Emison E, et al. Function of the c-Myc oncogenic transcription factor. Exp Cell Res 1999;253:63–77.

163. Kuramoto N, Ogita K, Yoneda Y. Gene transcription through Myc family members in eukaryotic cells. Jpn J Pharmacol 1999;80:103–109.

164. Grandori C, Cowley SM, James LP, Eisenman RN. The Myc/Max/Mad network and the transcriptional control of cell behavior. Annu Rev Cell Dev Biol 2000;16:653–699.

165. Baudino TA, Cleveland JL. The Max network gone mad. Mol Cell Biol 2001;21:691–702.

166. Eisenman RN. The Max network: coordinated transcriptional regulation of cell growth and proliferation. Harvey Lect 2000–2001;96:1–32.

167. Luscher B. Function and regulation of the transcription factors of the Myc/Max/Mad network. Gene 2001;277:1–14.

168. Zhou ZQ, Hurlin PJ. The interplay between Mad and Myc in proliferation and differentiation. Trends Cell Biol 2001;11:S10–S14.

169. Lee LA, Dang CV. Myc target transcriptomes. Curr Top Microbiol Immunol 2006;302:145–167.

170. Nair SK, Burley SK. Structural aspects of interactions within the Myc/Max/Mad network. Curr Top Microbiol Immunol 2006;302:123–143.

171. Pirity M, Blanck JK, Schreiber-Agus N. Lessons learned from Myc/Max/Mad knockout mice. Curr Top Microbiol Immunol 2006;302:205–234.

172. Rottmann S, Luscher B. The Mad side of the Max network: antagonizing the function of Myc and more. Curr Top Microbiol Immunol. 2006;302:63–122.

2
Receptors, Signaling Pathways, Cell Cycle, and DNA Damage Repair

Philip T. Cagle

Cell Surface Receptors and Signal Transduction

Ligands are extracellular messenger molecules such as growth factors, inflammatory cytokines, and hormones that bind to specific receptors on the cell surface (i.e., growth factor receptors, cytokine receptors, and hormone receptors). Binding of the ligands to their receptors causes activation of second messengers in the cytosol and eventually activation of nuclear transcription factors (Transcription factors are discussed in Chapter 1.) The transcription factors then direct the transcription of a gene product as a result of the extracellular message (e.g., a growth factor may stimulate a growth factor receptor on the cell surface, causing activation of second messengers that eventually cause a transcription factor to cause transcription of a protein involved in cell growth). This cascade or activation and inactivation of protein messengers from the cell surface receptors through proteins in the cytosol to the transcription factors in the nucleus is known as *signal transduction*. The series of steps that occurs during this process is called the *signal transduction pathway* or *signaling pathway*. Much of the activation and inactivation of proteins in signaling pathways occurs through reversible phosphorylation of tyrosine, serine, or threonine in the pathway proteins (see Chapter 1). Phosphorylation is accomplished by tyrosine kinases and serine/threonine kinases with phosphates donated from adenosine triphosphate or guanosine triphosphate (GTP). Tyrosine kinases are much more common in signaling pathways than are serine/threonine kinases.[1-10] This discussion focuses on growth factor receptors and cytokine receptors and their associated signaling pathways.

Growth factor receptors are a common type of cell surface receptor. Polypeptide growth factors such as epidermal growth factor (EGF) serve as ligands that bind to cell surface receptor protein-tyrosine kinases, which causes activation of the receptor by dimerization result-

ing in autophosphorylation. The activated receptor binds other proteins within the cell, leading to their phosphorylation and activation of their enzyme activity as part of the signaling pathway. The type I growth factor receptor tyrosine kinase family consists of epidermal growth factor receptor (EGFR), and ErbB1, ErbB2, ErbB3, and ErbB4 make up the type I growth factor receptor tyrosine kinase family. In addition to EGF, EGFR has multiple ligands, including transforming growth factor-α (TGF-α).[11-16] These receptors and ligands and their associated signaling pathways are involved in many lung diseases.

Signaling Pathways

Several signaling pathways are well studied and important to disease, including neoplastic and nonneoplastic lung disease. Signaling pathways transmit the "message" from extracellular ligands such as growth factors, cytokines, and steroid hormones. Signaling pathways are involved in regulation of cell proliferation, cell differentiation, cell death or apoptosis, and cell survival. Some of the more noteworthy and established pathways are briefly reviewed. Most signaling pathways have multiple complex interactions and "cross-talk" with other pathways, so discussion of specific pathways is limited here to an abbreviated overview.

The mitogen-activated protein kinase (MAPK) family is involved in multiple signaling pathways influencing cell growth, differentiation, and apoptosis, including the Ras/Raf-1/MAPK pathway mentioned later. The MAPK family includes the extracellular signal-regulated kinases (ERK1 and ERK2); the c-Jun NH2-terminal kinases (JNK1, JNK2, and JNK3), and p38 (p38 MAP kinases α, β, γ, and δ). The MAP kinase kinase kinases (MKKK) are activated by a wide range of agents, including growth factors, oxidative stress, inflammatory cytokines, and ultraviolet radiation. Activated MKKK activate the MAP kinase kinases (MKK), which subsequently activate the

MAP kinases. Examples of MKKK include Raf-1, TGF-β—activated kinase (TAK), apoptosis signal-regulating kinase 1 (ASK1), MAP/ERK kinase kinases (MEKK), germinal center kinase (GCK), and p21-activated kinase (PAK). The ERKs have about 160 substrates and are antiapoptotic and involved in cell proliferation, cellular differentiation, and cell cycle progression. On the other hand, JNK and p38 are usually, but not exclusively, pro-apoptotic and have many complex effects on different cells and on the cell cycle.[17–25]

The Ras/Raf-1/MAPK pathway is significant in carcinogenesis. H-Ras, K-Ras, and N-Ras are members of the Ras family, a class of *small GTP binding proteins* that are downstream targets of receptor tyrosine kinases. Ras is located at the plasma membrane inner surface. Activation of growth factor receptors converts Ras from its inactive guanosine diphosphate (GDP)-bound state to its active GTP-bound state. Activated Ras recruits Raf protein–serine/threonine kinase from the cytosol to the plasma membrane where kinases activate Raf. ERK, a member of the MAPK family, is activated by Raf through MAP/ERK kinase (MEK). In turn, the activated ERK phosphorylates and activates multiple other proteins, including other protein kinases. Activated ERK also translocates into the nucleus where it phosphorylates and activates transcription factors including Elk-1. Guanosine triphosphate hydrolysis by GTPase-activating proteins (GAPs) inactivates Ras. Ras is involved in many pathways, and epithelial cell proliferation is one of several possible results of Ras activation.[26–41]

The JAK/STAT pathway is linked with cytokine receptors. When ligands stimulate cytokine receptors, the signal transducers and activators of transcription (STAT) proteins associate with the activated cytokine receptors. The STATs are phosphorylated by the JAK nonreceptor protein tyrosine kinases that are members of the Janus kinase (JAK) family, undergo dimerization, and translocate into the nucleus where they function as transcription factors for their target genes. The STAT proteins can also be activated in growth factor receptor pathways.[42–49]

In the TGF-β/Smad pathway, cytokines in the transforming growth factor-β (TGF-β) superfamily inhibit the growth of many types of epithelial cells by formation of a complex of TGF-β type II and type I serine/threonine kinase receptors (TβRI and TβRII). The TGF-β1 ligand binds to TβRII, which subsequently phosphorylates and activates TβRI. Next, TRβI phosphorylates the receptor-regulated Smads (R-Smads) Smad2 and Smad3. Activated Smad2/3 complex with Smad4 (Co-Smad), translocate into the nucleus and function as transcriptional modulators of TGF-1–regulated genes. On the other hand, the inhibitory Smads, Smad6 and Smad7, inhibit TGF-β1 signaling. The inhibitory Smads bind to Smad4 to prevent it from complexing with Smad2/3 or by binding to TRβI, blocking phosphorylation of Smad2 and Smad3.[50–59]

The Wnt/B/catenin pathway involves Wnt ("Wingless," derived from fruit fly studies), which binds to Frizzled cell surface receptors. Signaling from Frizzled phosphorylates and activates Disheveled, which, in turn, inhibits the protein kinase glycogen synthase kinase-3 (GSK-3). β-Catenin phosphorylated by GSK-3 forms a complex with the adenomatous polyposis coli (APC) protein and the axin protein, restricting the quantity of free β-catenin in the cytosol. When activated Disheveled inhibits GSK-3, dephosphorylated β-catenin is freed from the APC–axin complex. This pathway is the classic Wnt signaling pathway, known as the *canonical Wnt signaling pathway*, and there are noncanonical Wnt signaling pathways not discussed here. β-Catenin associates with the TCF/LEF transcription factors, converting them to gene activators from gene repressors and, after translocation into the nucleus, binds to transcription factor TCF4 which induces Myc.[60–81] β-Catenin also has roles in cell adhesion, which is discussed in Chapter 3.

The PI3K/Akt/mTOR pathway regulates cell survival. Akt is a protein serine/threonine kinase. Cell membrane phosphatidylinositol 4,5-biphosphate in the cell is phosphorylated by phosphatidylinositol 3-kinase (PI3K), resulting in inositol 1,4,5-triphophate (PIP_3). The PIP_3 binds to the protein serine/threonine kinase Akt and recruits it to the inner surface of the cell membrane. At the inner surface of the cell membrane, Akt is phosphorylated and activated. Activated Akt phosphorylates proteins directly involved in cell survival as well as transcription factors and other protein kinases.[82–90]

The nuclear factor-κB (NF-κB) transcription factor and NF-κB signaling pathways regulate many proteins of the immune system, proteins that inhibit apoptosis and proteins that promote cell survival and proliferation. Nuclear factor-κB consists of various dimers of the Rel protein family: Rel (c-Rel), RelA (p65), RelB, NF-κB1 (p50 and its precursor p105), and NF-κB2 (p52 and its precursor p100), of which the p50–p65 dimer is the most common. NF-κB complexes bind to promoters to assist transcription in the majority of situations but homodimer complexes of p50 or p52 may inhibit transcription. Nuclear factor-κB proteins are maintained in the cytoplasm in resting cells by associating with members of the inhibitory IκB family (IκB-α, IκB-β and IκB-ε).[91–100]

Inhibitory-κB must be degraded for NF-κB to be activated. Inhibitory-κB kinases (IKKs) are activated by MAPKKK or by ligands for Toll-like receptors (TLRs), interleukin (IL)-1/IL-18 receptors, the TNF receptor superfamily, and B- and T-cell receptors. Activated IKKs phosphorylate IκB, which is subsequently bound by E3[IκB] ubiquitin ligase complex-TrCP-SCF, which ubiquinylates IκB. The 26S proteasome degrades the ubiquinylated IκB, releasing NF-κB complex to translocate into the nucleus where it binds to specific κB sites on DNA. The NF-κB complex is a transcription factor that regulates expression of proinflammatory cytokines, chemokines, adhesion molecules, cycloxygenase-2, inducible nitric oxide synthase, major histocompatibility complex, IL-2, IL-12, and interferon-γ in addition to antiapoptotic and apoptotic genes.[101-107] Apoptosis is discussed in Chapter 4.

In the Hedgehog-Patched-Smoothened signaling pathway, after attachment of a lipid, Sonic Hedgehog (Shh) polypeptide binds to Patched on the cell surface that prevents inhibition of Smoothened (Smo), a G protein–coupled receptor, by Patched. Smoothened activates the serine/threonine kinase Fused and the zinc finger transcription factor Gli (first detected in gliomas as a mutation), which induces Wnt signaling.[108-116]

Notch is a receptor for direct cell to cell signaling. Delta binds to Notch, resulting in proteolytic cleavage of Notch. The intracellular domain of Notch is released and translocates into the nucleus, where it interacts with a transcription factor.[117-122]

The Cell Cycle

The cell cycle is the tightly regulated, sequential series of events or phases that govern cell proliferation, including preparation for DNA replication, DNA replication (see Chapter 1), preparation for cell division, cell division, and cell rest. The cell cycle provides orderly control of DNA replication and cell division in response to external and internal stimuli. The cell cycle is divided into several phases: G0 (cell at rest), G1 (preparation for DNA synthesis), S (DNA synthesis or replication), G2, and M (mitosis with nuclear and cellular division). Progression through the series of steps in the cell cycle is tightly regulated by cyclin-dependent kinases (Cdks) after they form complexes with proteins called *cyclins*. These complexes activate and inactivate proteins by phosphorylation, including proteins that otherwise act as "brakes" on progression through the cell cycle and the proliferation process. There are many interacting pathways and positive and negative feedback loops that control passage through the cell cycle. The cell cycle may be stimulated appropriately or inappropriately in various inflammatory diseases, and loss of cell cycle regulation is a very important step in uncontrolled cell proliferation during carcinogenesis.

Checkpoints in the cell cycle ordinarily prevent the passage of damaged DNA to daughter cells. Checkpoints temporarily arrest the cell cycle at specific steps in the cell cycle to allow repair of damaged DNA or programmed cell death or apoptosis if the damage is to severe to be repaired (discussed in Chapter 4). The major checkpoint in the cell cycle is the restriction point where "commitment" to the cell cycle occurs in G1 as further discussed below. In addition to the G1–S checkpoint, there are an S phase checkpoint and a G2–M checkpoint.[123-142]

The Rad9–Rad1–Hus1 heterotrimer complex (9-1-1 complex) and the Rad17–RFC complex are damage sensor proteins that detect DNA damage at the checkpoints. The 9–1–1 complex is loaded around DNA by the Rad17–RFC complex. The ATR (ataxia-telangiectasia-mutated [ATM] and Rad3-related protein kinase)–mediated and ATM-mediated phosphorylation and activation of Chk1 and Chk2 follow, and ATM and Chk2 phosphorylate and stabilize p53. Cyclin-dependent kinases are inactivated by the regulation of Cdc25, Wee1, and p53, which causes cell cycle arrest. DNA damage repair is discussed later.[143-146] After DNA damage repair, the DNA damage checkpoint is silenced, and the cell cycle restarts in a process called *recovery* involving polo-like kinase (Plk1).[147,148]

Growth factor signaling initiates the cell cycle and maintains the transition through the G1 phase. When the cell passes through the restriction point of the cell cycle, the cell no longer requires growth factor signaling to complete the cell cycle, and the cell is "committed" to the cell cycle. Passage through the restriction point depends on phosphorylation of the retinoblastoma (Rb) gene product, pRb. The Rb product governs progression past the restriction point of the cell cycle and governs the expression of genes involved in DNA synthesis.[149-152] Activation of cyclin D is necessary for progression of the cell cycle.[153-159]

In response to stimuli for mitosis, such as growth factor signaling, complexes of cyclin D with Cdk4 and Cdk6 phosphorylate pRB during G1 in response to stimuli for mitosis. In addition, cyclin E–Cdk2 complexes phosphorylate pRb just prior to the S phase. Families of Cdk inhibitors (the INK4 family, including p16^{INK4}, and the p21$^{WAF1/Cip1}$/p27^{Kip1}/p57^{Kip2} family) control these cyclin–Cdk complexes.[160-171] Phosphorylation inactivates pRb in G1, releasing E2F transcription factors[172-182] that activate transcription of numerous genes involved in DNA replication, such as c-Myc,[183-187] initiating the S phase. As complexes with Cdks, cyclin A functions in both G1/S phase transition and in mitosis[188] and cyclin B is involved in entry into mitosis.[189]

One of the primary roles of p53, the product of the *TP53* gene, is to "protect" the DNA through the arrest of the cell cycle at checkpoints in response to DNA damage or to help induce apoptosis when damage is beyond repair. Because of these roles, p53 has been referred to as the guardian of the genome. Part of the p53 arrest of the cell cycle is by activation of p21^{WAF1}, which blocks cyclin–Cdk complexes necessary for cell cycle progression.[190-196] A member of the TGF-β superfamily of cytokines, TGF-β1, is involved in inhibition of cell cycle progression.[197,198]

It is apparent that Rb and p53 play very crucial roles in the management of the cell cycle. Abnormalities of Rb and p53 are the most common abnormalities associated with the cell cycle dysregulation of malignancy. However, because there are so many redundancies, interacting pathways, and positive and negative feedback loops, there are many other abnormalities that can produce effects similar to the direct loss of Rb or p53.

The *CDKN2A* gene encodes for two completely unrelated protein products, p16[INK4A], the Cdk inhibitor mentioned earlier,[199–204] and p14[ARF].[205–209] Both of these proteins are transcribed from different exons of the *CDKN2A* gene. Abnormalities of either of these genes or their products can produce effects similar to abnormalities of the *Rb* or *p53* genes themselves. By inhibiting Cdk4/6 kinase, p16 blocks phosphorylation and inactivation of pRb. Loss of p16 function results in loss of *Rb* function because Cdk4/6 kinase inactivation of pRb is not blocked. The other *CDKN2A* product, p14, destabilizes the MDM2 protein, which binds and degrades p53. Excessive levels of MDM2 resulting from loss of p14 function causes excess degradation of p53 and loss of p53 function. Abnormalities of *CDKN2A*, p16, p14, and MDM2 and other genes and their products upstream or downstream of *Rb* and *p53* can produce loss of control of the cell cycle similar to the direct loss of *Rb* and *p53*.

DNA Damage Repair

DNA is regularly damaged by endogenous factors (such as oxygen radicals), extracellular factors (such as chemicals, radiation, ultraviolet light), and errors in replication (such as stalled replication forks). As a result of exposure to these harmful agents, DNA undergoes depurination, deamination, hydrolysis, and nonenzymatic methylation (alkylation), which attach chemical groups called *adducts* to the DNA. DNA damage repair during cell cycle checkpoints typically involves excision of the damaged DNA and filling of the resultant gap by newly synthesized DNA using the undamaged complementary DNA strand as template. Depending on the type of damage, there are several DNA repair pathways. The DNA damage repair pathways are important in individual susceptibility to lung cancer (see Chapter 17) and in response to therapy (see Chapter 22).

The base excision repair (BER) pathway repairs small lesions such as oxidized or reduced single bases and fragmented or nonbulky adducts. In the BER pathway, a single damaged base is excised by base-specific DNA glycosylases (e.g., oxidized 8-oxoguanine is excised by 8-oxoguanine DNA glycosylase or OGG1). Some glycosylates are bifunctional and have an apurinic/apyrimidinic lyase activity to incise the phosphodiester bond of the intact apurinic/apyrimidinic site. An apurinic/apyrimidinic endonuclease (APE1/APEX1) is required by monofunctional glycosylates to incise the apurinic/apyrimidinic site. DNA polymerase-fills in the single nucleo-

tide gap[210–216] and a DNA ligase III/x-ray repair cross-complementing group 1 (XRCC1) complex seals the nick.[217–222]

The nucleotide excision repair (NER) repairs lesions large enough to deform the DNA helical structure, such as pyrimidine dimers, bulky chemical adducts, and crosslinks, by excising damaged bases as part of an oligonucleotide. Xeroderma pigmentosum (XP) proteins are an important part of the NER pathway. A protein complex including xeroderma pigmentosum group C protein (XPC) and hHR23B recognizes helical distortion by bulky chemical adducts. TFIIH is composed of nine protein subunits, including p62, p52, p44, p34, Cdk7, cyclin H, MAT1, and the two DNA helicases XPD (xeroderma pigmentosum group D protein), also known as ERCC2 (excision repair cross-complementation group 2), and XPB (xeroderma pigmentosum group B protein), also known as ERCC3 (excision repair cross-complementation group 3). TFIIH, xeroderma pigmentosum group A protein (XPA), and replication protein A (RPA) accumulate at the damage site, and the XPD and XPB helicases of TFIIH unwind the DNA double helix. This permits excision of the damaged single-stranded DNA fragment (usually about 27–30 bp) by a complex that includes ERCC1 and xeroderma pigmentosum group F protein (XPF). DNA polymerases synthesize a new strand of DNA using the undamaged complementary DNA strand as template to complete the repair process.[223–226]

Mismatch repair genes (*MMR*) participate in an excision repair pathway by scanning newly replicated DNA for mismatched base pairs such as deamination of a nucleotide into a different nucleotide. Heterodimers from *MMR* (including MLH1, MSH2, PMS1, and PMS2) cause cell cycle arrest, permitting DNA repair.[227–239]

The enzyme O^6-meG–DNA methyltransferase (MGMT/AGT) repairs O^6-meG and other alkylated bases in the direct damage reversal (DR) pathway.[240–249] O^6-Methylguanine (O^6-meG) formed by alkylating compounds in tobacco smoke may mismatch with thymine during DNA replication if not repaired.

The DNA damage response or DSB repair (double-strand break repair) pathway (or during the S-phase checkpoint, the DNA replication stress response pathway) occurs in response to DSB DNA damage. The DSB repair pathway includes a cascade of events: sensing of the DNA damage and transduction of the damage signal to multiple pathways (cell cycle checkpoints, DNA repair, responses to telomere maintenance, and apoptosis (see Chapter 4). The DSB repair process involves many genes and their products, including the MRE11–Rad50–NBS1 complex (MRN); x-ray repair cross complementing (XRCC); the PI3K-like protein kinases (PIKKs) DNA-PKcs, ATM (mutated in ataxia telangiectasia), and ATR (ATM–Rad3-related); and ATM substrates NBS1 (Nijmegen breakage syndrome protein 1), SMC1 (structural maintenance of chromosomes 1), Chk1, Chk2, MRE11, p53, MDM2, BRCA1 (BReast CAncer protein 1), BRCA2/FANCD1 (BReast CAncer protein 2/Fanconi anemia protein D1), and FANCD2 (Fanconi anemia protein D2).[250-269]

The ATM pathway reacts to DSBs in all phases of the cell cycle. The ATR pathway reacts to DSBs more slowly than ATM and reacts to factors that impede the function of replication forks. The ATM pathway activates many downstream proteins of the ATR pathway. In response to replication stress, ATM and ATR activate members of the Chk kinase family. The ATM phosphorylates Chk2 which, in turn, phosphorylates p53 and Cdc25A, blocking Cdk2.[250-269]

References

1. Williams LT, Escobedo JA, Fantl WJ, et al. Interactions of growth factor receptors with cytoplasmic signaling molecules. Cold Spring Harb Symp Quant Biol 1991;56: 243–250.
2. Fantl WJ, Escobedo JA, Martin GA, et al. Distinct phosphotyrosines on a growth factor receptor bind to specific molecules that mediate different signaling pathways. Cell 1992;69:413–423.
3. Hunter T, Lindberg RA, Middlemas DS, et al. Receptor protein tyrosine kinases and phosphatases. Cold Spring Harb Symp Quant Biol 1992;57:25–41.
4. Fantl WJ, Johnson DE, Williams LT. Signalling by receptor tyrosine kinases. Annu Rev Biochem 1993;62:453–481.
5. Johnson GL, Vaillancourt RR. Sequential protein kinase reactions controlling cell growth and differentiation. Curr Opin Cell Biol 1994;6:230–238.
6. van der Geer P, Hunter T, Lindberg RA. Receptor protein-tyrosine kinases and their signal transduction pathways. Annu Rev Cell Biol 1994;10:251–337.
7. Schlessinger J. Cell signaling by receptor tyrosine kinases. Cell 2000;103:211–225.
8. Gavi S, Shumay E, Wang HY, Malbon CC. G-protein–coupled receptors and tyrosine kinases: crossroads in cell signaling and regulation. Trends Endocrinol Metab 2006; 17:48–54.
9. Li E, Hristova K. Role of receptor tyrosine kinase transmembrane domains in cell signaling and human pathologies. Biochemistry 2006;45:6241–6251.
10. Perona R. Cell signalling: growth factors and tyrosine kinase receptors. Clin Transl Oncol 2006;8:77–82.
11. Tiganis T. Protein tyrosine phosphatases: dephosphorylating the epidermal growth factor receptor. IUBMB Life 2002;53:3–14.
12. Jorissen RN, Walker F, Pouliot N, et al. Epidermal growth factor receptor: mechanisms of activation and signalling. Exp Cell Res 2003;284:31–53.
13. Bazley LA, Gullick WJ. The epidermal growth factor receptor family. Endocr Relat Cancer 2005;12 Suppl 1: S17–S27.
14. Normanno N, Bianco C, Strizzi L, et al. The ErbB receptors and their ligands in cancer: an overview. Curr Drug Targets 2005;6:243–257.
15. Zaczek A, Brandt B, Bielawski KP. The diverse signaling network of EGFR, HER2, HER3 and HER4 tyrosine kinase receptors and the consequences for therapeutic approaches. Histol Histopathol 2005;20:1005–1015.
16. Warren CM, Landgraf R. Signaling through ERBB receptors: multiple layers of diversity and control. Cell Signal 2006;18:923–933.
17. Bagrodia S, Derijard B, Davis RJ, Cerione RA. Cdc42 and PAKmediated signaling leads to Jun kinase and p38 mitogen-activated protein kinase activation. J Biol Chem 1995;270:27995–27998.
18. Xia Z, Dickens M, Raingeaud J, et al. Opposing effects of ERK and JNKp38 MAP kinases on apoptosis. Science 1995;270:1326–1331.
19. Ichijo H, Nishida E, Irie K, et al. Induction of apoptosis by ASK1, a mammalian MAPKKK that activates SAPK/JNK and p38 signaling pathways. Science 1997;275:90–94.
20. Wilkinson MG, Millar JB. SAPKs and transcription factors do the nucleocytoplasmic tango. Genes Dev 1998;12:1391–1397.
21. Davis RJ. Signal transduction by the JNK group of MAP kinases. Cell 2000;103:239–252.
22. Wada T, Penninger JM. Mitogen-activated protein kinases in apoptosis regulation. Oncogene 2004;23:2838–2849.
23. Bradham C, McClay DR. p38 MAPK in Development and Cancer. Cell Cycle 2006;5:824–828.
24. MacCorkle RA, Tan TH. Mitogen-activated protein kinases in cell-cycle control. Cell Biochem Biophys 2005;43: 451–461.
25. Yoon S, Seger R. The extracellular signal-regulated kinase: multiple substrates regulate diverse cellular functions. Growth Factors 2006;24:21–44.
26. Magnuson NS, Beck T, Vahidi H, et al. The Raf-1 serine/threonine protein kinase. Semin Cancer Biol 1994;5:247–253.
27. Williams NG, Roberts TM. Signal transduction pathways involving the Raf proto-oncogene. Cancer Metastasis Rev 1994;13:105–116.
28. Burgering BM, Bos JL. Regulation of Ras-mediated signalling: more than one way to skin a cat. Trends Biochem Sci 1995;20:18–22.
29. Morrison DK. Mechanisms regulating Raf-1 activity in signal transduction pathways. Mol Reprod Dev 1995;42:507–514.
30. Morrison DK, Cutler RE. The complexity of Raf-1 regulation. Curr Opin Cell Biol 1997;9:174–179.
31. Dhillon AS, Kolch W. Untying the regulation of the Raf-1 kinase. Arch Biochem Biophys 2002;404:3–9.
32. Bernards A, Settleman J. GAP control: regulating the regulators of small GTPases. Trends Cell Biol 2004;14: 377–385.
33. Bernards A, Settleman J. GAPs in growth factor signalling. Growth Factors 2005;23:143–149.
34. Chan A. Teaching resources. Ras-MAPK pathways. Sci STKE 2005;2005(271):tr5.
35. Hancock JF, Parton RG. Ras plasma membrane signalling platforms. Biochem J 2005;389(Pt 1):1–11.
36. Kranenburg O. The KRAS oncogene: past, present, and future. Biochim Biophys Acta 2005;1756:81–82.

37. McCudden CR, Hains MD, Kimple RJ, et al. G-protein signaling: back to the future. Cell Mol Life Sci 2005;62: 551–577.

38. Mitin N, Rossman KL, Der CJ. Signaling interplay in Ras superfamily function. Curr Biol 2005;15:R563–574.

39. Philips MR. Compartmentalized signalling of Ras. Biochem Soc Trans 2005;33(Pt 4):657–661.

40. Wennerberg K, Rossman KL, Der CJ. The Ras superfamily at a glance. J Cell Sci 2005;118(Pt 5):843–846.

41. Mor A, Philips MR. Compartmentalized Ras/MAPK signaling. Annu Rev Immunol 2006;24:771–800.

42. Pellegrini S, Dusanter-Fourt I. The structure, regulation and function of the Janus kinases (JAKs) and the signal transducers and activators of transcription (STATs). Eur J Biochem 1997;248:615–633.

43. Liu KD, Gaffen SL, Goldsmith MA. JAK/STAT signaling by cytokine receptors. Curr Opin Immunol 1998;10:271–278.

44. Shuai K. The STAT family of proteins in cytokine signaling. Prog Biophys Mol Biol 1999;71:405–422.

45. Boudny V, Kovarik J. JAK/STAT signaling pathways and cancer. Janus kinases/signal transducers and activators of transcription. Neoplasma 2002;49:349–355.

46. Kisseleva T, Bhattacharya S, Braunstein J, Schindler CW. Signaling through the JAK/STAT pathway, recent advances and future challenges. Gene 2002;285:1–24.

47. O'Shea JJ, Gadina M, Schreiber RD. Cytokine signaling in 2002: new surprises in the Jak/Stat pathway. Cell 2002;109 Suppl:S121–S131.

48. Rawlings JS, Rosler KM, Harrison DA. The JAK/STAT signaling pathway. J Cell Sci 2004;117(Pt 8):1281–1283.

49. Hebenstreit D, Horejs-Hoeck J, Duschl A. JAK/STAT-dependent gene regulation by cytokines. Drug News Perspect 2005;18:243–249.

50. Lutz M, Knaus P. Integration of the TGF-beta pathway into the cellular signalling network. Cell Signal 2002;14:977–988.

51. Mehra A, Wrana JL. TGF-beta and the Smad signal transduction pathway. Biochem Cell Biol 2002;80:605–622.

52. Cohen MM Jr. TGF beta/Smad signaling system and its pathologic correlates. Am J Med Genet A 2003;116:1–10.

53. Derynck R, Zhang YE. Smad-dependent and Smad-independent pathways in TGF-beta family signalling. Nature 2003;425:577–584.

54. Chin D, Boyle GM, Parsons PG, Coman WB. What is transforming growth factor-beta (TGF-beta)? Br J Plast Surg 2004;57:215–221.

55. ten Dijke P, Hill CS. New insights into TGF-beta-Smad signalling. Trends Biochem Sci 2004;29:265–273.

56. Feng XH, Derynck R. Specificity and versatility in tgf-beta signaling through Smads. Annu Rev Cell Dev Biol 2005;21:659–693.

57. Park SH. Fine tuning and cross-talking of TGF-beta signal by inhibitory Smads. J Biochem Mol Biol 2005;38:9–16.

58. Massague J, Seoane J, Wotton D. Smad transcription factors. Genes Dev 2005;19:2783–2810.

59. Massague J, Gomis RR. The logic of TGFbeta signaling. FEBS Lett 2006;580:2811–2820.

60. Gumbiner BM. Signal transduction of beta-catenin. Curr Opin Cell Biol 1995;7:634–640.

61. Shimizu H, Julius MA, Giarre M, et al. Transformation by Wnt family proteins correlates with regulation of beta-catenin. Cell Growth Differ 1997;8:1349–1358.

62. Boutros M, Mlodzik M. Dishevelled: at the crossroads of divergent intracellular signaling pathways. Mech Dev 1999;83:27–37.

63. Miller JR, Hocking AM, Brown JD, Moon RT. Mechanism and function of signal transduction by the Wnt/beta-catenin and Wnt/Ca²⁺ pathways. Oncogene 1999;18:7860–7872.

64. Hinoi T, Yamamoto H, Kishida M, et al. Complex formation of adenomatous polyposis coli gene product and axin facilitates glycogen synthase kinase-3 beta-dependent phosphorylation of beta-catenin and downregulates beta-catenin. J Biol Chem 2000;275:34399–34406.

65. Polakis P. Wnt signaling and cancer. Genes Dev 2000;14:1837–1851.

66. Doble BW, Woodgett JR. GSK-3: tricks of the trade for a multi-tasking kinase. J Cell Sci 2003;116:1175–1186.

67. Lee E, Salic A, Kruger R, et al. The roles of APC and Axin derived from experimental and theoretical analysis of the Wnt pathway. PLoS Biol 2003;1:E10.

68. van Es JH, Barker N, Clevers H. You Wnt some, you lose some: oncogenes in the Wnt signaling pathway. Curr Opin Genet Dev 2003;13:28–33.

69. Veeman MT, Axelrod JD, Moon RT. A second canon. Functions and mechanisms of beta-catenin–independent Wnt signaling. Dev Cell 2003;5:367–377.

70. Logan CY, Nusse R. The Wnt signaling pathway in development and disease. Annu Rev Cell Dev Biol 2004;20:781–810.

71. Malbon CC. Frizzleds: new members of the superfamily of G-protein–coupled receptors. Front Biosci 2004;9:1048–1058.

72. Nelson WJ, Nusse R. Convergence of Wnt, beta-catenin, and cadherin pathways. Science 2004;303:1483–1487.

73. Tolwinski NS, Wieschaus E. Rethinking WNT signaling. Trends Genet 2004;20:177–181.

74. Bejsovec A. Wnt pathway activation: new relations and locations. Cell 2005;120:11–14.

75. Senda T, Shimomura A, Iizuka-Kogo A. Adenomatous polyposis coli (Apc) tumor suppressor gene as a multifunctional gene. Anat Sci Int 2005;80:121–131.

76. Takada R, Hijikata H, Kondoh H, Takada S. Analysis of combinatorial effects of Wnts and Frizzleds on beta-catenin/armadillo stabilization and Dishevelled 77 phosphorylation. Genes Cells 2005;10:919–928.

77. Cadigan KM, Liu YI. Wnt signaling: complexity at the surface. J Cell Sci 2006;119:395–402.

78. Kikuchi A, Kishida S, Yamamoto H. Regulation of Wnt signaling by protein–protein interaction and post-translational modifications. Exp Mol Med 2006;38:1–10.

79. Malbon CC, Wang HY. Dishevelled: a mobile scaffold catalyzing development. Curr Top Dev Biol 2006;72:153–166.

80. Pongracz JE, Stockley RA. Wnt signalling in lung development and diseases. Respir Res 2006;7:15.

81. Tian Q. Proteomic exploration of the Wnt/beta-catenin pathway. Curr Opin Mol Ther 2006;8:191–197

82. Franke TF, Kaplan DR, Cantley LC. PI3K: downstream AKTion blocks apoptosis. Cell 1997;88:435–437.

83. Wymann MP, Pirola L. Structure and function of phosphoinositide 3-kinases. Biochim Biophys Acta 1998;1436: 127–150.
84. Krasilnikov MA. Phosphatidylinositol-3 kinase dependent pathways: the role in control of cell growth, survival, and malignant transformation. Biochemistry (Mosc) 2000;65: 59–67.
85. Cantley LC. The phosphoinositide 3-kinase pathway. Science 2002;296:1655–1657.
86. Franke TF, Hornik CP, Segev L, et al. PI3K/Akt and apoptosis: size matters. Oncogene 2003;22:8983–8998.
87. Liang J, Slingerland JM. Multiple roles of the PI3K/PKB (Akt) pathway in cell cycle progression. Cell Cycle 2003;2:339–345.
88. Asnaghi L, Bruno P, Priulla M, Nicolin A. mTOR: a protein kinase switching between life and death. Pharmacol Res 2004;50:545–549.
89. Osaki M, Oshimura M, Ito H. PI3K-Akt pathway: its functions and alterations in human cancer. Apoptosis 2004; 9:667–676.
90. Henson ES, Gibson SB. Surviving cell death through epidermal growth factor (EGF) signal transduction pathways: Implications for cancer therapy. Cell Signal 2006 May 24; [Epub ahead of print].
90. Liang Y, Zhou Y, Shen P. NF-kappaB and its regulation on the immune system. Cell Mol Immunol 2004;1:343–350.
92. Xiao W. Advances in NF-kappaB signaling transduction and transcription. Cell Mol Immunol 2004;1:425–435.
93. Courtois G. The NF-kappaB signaling pathway in human genetic diseases. Cell Mol Life Sci 2005;62:1682–1691.
94. Moynagh PN. The NF-kappaB pathway. J Cell Sci 2005; 118(Pt 20):4589–4592.
95. Zingarelli B. Nuclear factor-kappaB. Crit Care Med 2005;33(12 Suppl):S414–S416.
96. Bubici C, Papa S, Pham CG, et al. The NF-kappaB–mediated control of ROS and JNK signaling. Histol Histopathol 2006;21:69–80.
97. Campbell KJ, Perkins ND. Regulation of NF-kappaB function. Biochem Soc Symp 2006;(73):165–180.
98. Hoffmann A, Baltimore D. Circuitry of nuclear factor kappaB signaling. Immunol Rev 2006;210:171–186.
99. Piva R, Belardo G, Santoro MG. NF-kappaB: a stress-regulated switch for cell survival. Antioxid Redox Signal 2006;8:478–486.
100. Vermeulen L, Vanden Berghe W, Haegeman G. Regulation of NF-kappaB transcriptional activity. Cancer Treat Res 2006;130:89–102.
101. Karin M. The beginning of the end: IkappaB kinase (IKK) and NF-kappaB activation. J Biol Chem 1999;274:27339–27342.
102. Karin M. How NF-kappaB is activated: the role of the IkappaB kinase (IKK) complex. Oncogene 1999;18:6867–6874.
103. Rothwarf DM, Karin M. The NF-kappa B activation pathway: a paradigm in information transfer from membrane to nucleus. Sci STKE 1999;1999:RE1.
104. Senftleben U, Karin M. The IKK/NF-kappa B pathway. Crit Care Med 2002;30(1 Suppl):S18–S26.
105. Hayden MS, Ghosh S. Signaling to NF-kappaB. Genes Dev 2004;18:2195–2224.
106. Viatour P, Merville MP, Bours V, Chariot A. Phosphorylation of NF-kappaB and IkappaB proteins: implications in cancer and inflammation. Trends Biochem Sci 2005;30: 43–52.
107. Gloire G, Dejardin E, Piette J. Extending the nuclear roles of IkappaB kinase subunits. Biochem Pharmacol 2006 Jul 15; [Epub ahead of print].
108. Kalderon D. Similarities between the Hedgehog and Wnt signaling pathways. Trends Cell Biol 2002;12:523–531.
109. Mullor JL, Sanchez P, Altaba AR. Pathways and consequences: Hedgehog signaling in human disease. Trends Cell Biol 2002;12:562–569.
110. Cohen MM Jr. The hedgehog signaling network. Am J Med Genet A 2003;123:5–28.
111. McMahon AP, Ingham PW, Tabin CJ. Developmental roles and clinical significance of hedgehog signaling. Curr Top Dev Biol 2003;53:1–114.
112. Wetmore C. Sonic hedgehog in normal and neoplastic proliferation: insight gained from human tumors and animal models. Curr Opin Genet Dev 2003;13:34–42.
113. Lum L, Beachy PA. The Hedgehog response network: sensors, switches, and routers. Science 2004;304:1755–1759.
114. Ogden SK, Ascano M Jr, Stegman MA, Robbins DJ. Regulation of Hedgehog signaling: a complex story. Biochem Pharmacol 2004;67:805–814.
115. Yu TC, Miller SJ. The hedgehog pathway: revisited. Dermatol Surg 2004;30:583–584.
116. Neumann CJ. Hedgehogs as negative regulators of the cell cycle. Cell Cycle 2005;4:1139–1140.
117. Baron M, Aslam H, Flasza M, et al. Multiple levels of Notch signal regulation (review). Mol Membr Biol 2002;19: 27–38.
118. Baron M. An overview of the Notch signalling pathway. Semin Cell Dev Biol 2003;14:113–119.
119. Collins BJ, Kleeberger W, Ball DW. Notch in lung development and lung cancer. Semin Cancer Biol 2004;14:357–364.
120. Hansson EM, Lendahl U, Chapman G. Notch signaling in development and disease. Semin Cancer Biol 2004;14: 320–328.
121. Bianchi S, Dotti MT, Federico A. Physiology and pathology of notch signalling system. J Cell Physiol 2006;207:300–308.
122. Wilson A, Radtke F. Multiple functions of Notch signaling in self-renewing organs and cancer. FEBS Lett 2006; 580:2860–2868.
123. Hartwell LH, Weinert TA. Checkpoints: controls that ensure the order of cell cycle events. Science 1989;246: 629–634.
124. Pardee AB. G1 events and regulation of cell proliferation. Science 1989;246:603–608.
125. Kastan MB, Kuerbitz SJ. Control of G1 arrest after DNA damage. Environ Health Perspect 1993;101 Suppl 5:55–58.
126. Sherr CJ. G1 phase progression: cycling on cue. Cell 1994;79:551–555.
127. Elledge SJ. Cell cycle checkpoints: preventing an identity crisis. Science 1996;274:1664–1672.
128. Sanchez I, Dynlacht BD. Transcriptional control of the cell cycle. Curr Opin Cell Biol 1996;8:318–324.

129. O'Connor PM. Mammalian G1 and G2 phase checkpoints. Cancer Surv 1997;29:151–182.

130. Mercer WE. Checking on the cell cycle. J Cell Biochem Suppl 1998;30–31:50–4.

131. Weinert T. DNA damage checkpoints update: getting molecular. Curr Opin Genet Dev 1998;8:185–193.

132. Johnson DG, Walker CL. Cyclins and cell cycle checkpoints. Annu Rev Pharmacol Toxicol 1999;39:295–312.

133. Clarke DJ, Gimenez-Abian JF. Checkpoints controlling mitosis. Bioessays 2000;22:351–363.

134. Nyberg KA, Michelson RJ, Putnam CW, Weinert TA. Toward maintaining the genome: DNA damage and replication checkpoints. Annu Rev Genet 2002;36:617–656.

135. Shreeram S, Blow JJ. The role of the replication licensing system in cell proliferation and cancer. Prog Cell Cycle Res 2003;5:287–293.

136. Lisby M, Rothstein R. DNA damage checkpoint and repair centers. Curr Opin Cell Biol 2004;16:328–334.

137. Lukas J, Lukas C, Bartek J. Mammalian cell cycle checkpoints: signalling pathways and their organization in space and time. DNA Repair (Amst) 2004;3:997–1007.

138. Stark GR, Taylor WR. Analyzing the G2/M checkpoint. Methods Mol Biol 2004;280:51–82.

139. Branzei D, Foiani M. The DNA damage response during DNA replication. Curr Opin Cell Biol 2005;17:568–575.

140. Macaluso M, Montanari M, Cinti C, Giordano A. Modulation of cell cycle components by epigenetic and genetic events. Semin Oncol 2005;32:452–457.

141. Musgrove EA. Cyclins: roles in mitogenic signaling and oncogenic transformation. Growth Factors 2006;24:13–19.

142. Niida H, Nakanishi M. DNA damage checkpoints in mammals. Mutagenesis 2006;21:3–9.

143. Burtelow MA, Roos-Mattjus PM, Rauen M, et al. Reconstitution and molecular analysis of the hRad9-hHus1-hRad1 (9-1-1) DNA damage responsive checkpoint complex. J Biol Chem 2001;276:25903–25909.

144. Bao S, Lu T, Wang X, et al. Disruption of the Rad9/Rad1/Hus1 (9-1-1) complex leads to checkpoint signaling and replication defects. Oncogene 2004;23:5586–5593.

145. Parrilla-Castellar ER, Arlander SJ, Karnitz L. Dial 9-1-1 for DNA damage: the Rad9-Hus1-Rad1 (9-1-1) clamp complex. DNA Repair (Amst) 2004;3:1009–1014.

146. Majka J, Burgers PM. unction of Rad17/Mec3/Ddc1 and its partial complexes in the DNA damage checkpoint. DNA Repair (Amst) 2005;4:1189–1194.

147. van Vugt MA, Medema RH. Checkpoint adaptation and recovery: back with Polo after the break. Cell Cycle 2004;3:1383–1386.

148. van Vugt MA, Bras A, Medema RH. Restarting the cell cycle when the checkpoint comes to a halt. Cancer Res 2005;65:7037–7040.

149. Pardee AB. A restriction point for control of normal animal cell proliferation. Proc Natl Acad Sci USA 1974;71:1286–1290.

150. Campisi J, Medrano EE, Morro G, Pardee AB. Restriction point control of cell growth by a labile protein: evidence for increased stability in transformed cells. Proc Natl Acad Sci USA 1982;79:436–440.

151. Blagosklonny MV, Pardee AB. The restriction point of the cell cycle. Cell Cycle 2002;1:103–110.

152. Boonstra J. Progression through the G1-phase of the on-going cell cycle. J Cell Biochem 2003;90:244–252.

153. Baldin V, Lukas J, Marcote MJ, et al. Cyclin D1 is a nuclear protein required for cell cycle progression in G1. Genes Dev 1993;7:812–821.

154. Dowdy SF, Hinds PW, Louie K, et al. Physical interaction of the retinoblastoma protein with human D cyclins. Cell 1993;73:499–511.

155. Kato J, Matsushime H, Hiebert SW, et al. Direct binding of cyclin D to the retinoblastoma gene product (pRb) and pRb phosphorylation by the cyclin D–dependent kinase CDK4. Genes Dev 1993;7:331–342.

156. Sewing A, Burger C, Brusselbach S, et al. Human cyclin D1 encodes a labile nuclear protein whose synthesis is directly induced by growth factors and suppressed by cyclic AMP. J Cell Sci 1993;104:545–555.

157. Lukas J, Muller H, Bartkova J, et al. DNA tumor virus oncoproteins and retinoblastoma gene mutations share the ability to relieve the cell's requirement for cyclin D1 function in G1. J Cell Biol 1994;125:625–638.

158. Xiao ZX, Ginsberg D, Ewen M, Livingston DM. Regulation of the retinoblastoma protein-related protein p107 by G_1 cyclin-associated kinases. Proc Natl Acad Sci USA 1996;93:4633–4637.

159. Ortega S, Malumbres M, Barbacid M. Cyclin D–dependent kinases, INK4 inhibitors and cancer. Biochim Biophys Acta 2002;1602:73–87.

160. El-Deiry WS, Tokino T, Velculescu VE, et al. WAF1, a potential mediator of p53 tumor suppression. Cell 1993;75:817–825.

161. Polyak K, Kato JY, Solomon MJ, et al. p27Kip1, a cyclin-Cdk inhibitor, links transforming growth factor-beta and contact inhibition to cell cycle arrest. Genes Dev 1994;8:9–22.

162. Biggs JR, Kraft AS. Inhibitors of cyclin-dependent kinase and cancer. J Mol Med 1995;73:509–514.

163. Datto MB, Li Y, Panus JF, et al. Transforming growth factor beta induces the cyclin-dependent kinase inhibitor p21 through a p53-independent mechanism. Proc Natl Acad Sci USA 1995;92:5545–5549.

164. Datto MB, Yu Y, Wang XF. Functional analysis of the transforming growth factor beta responsive elements in the WAF1/Cip1/p21 promoter. J Biol Chem 1995;270:28623–28628.

165. Quelle DE, Zindy F, Ashmun RA, Sherr CJ. Alternative reading frames of the INK4a tumor suppressor gene encode two unrelated proteins capable of inducing cell cycle arrest. Cell 1995;83:993–1000.

166. Yeudall WA, Jakus J. Cyclin kinase inhibitors add a new dimension to cell cycle control. Eur J Cancer B Oral Oncol 1995;31B:291–298.

167. Serrano M, Lee H, Chin L, et al. Role of the INK4a locus in tumor suppression and cell mortality. Cell 1996;85:27–37.

168. Craig C, Kim M, Ohri E, et al. Effects of adenovirus-mediated p16INK4A expression on cell cycle arrest are determined by endogenous p16 and Rb status in human cancer cells. Oncogene 1998;16:265–272.

169. Niculescu AB 3rd, Chen X, Smeets M, et al. Effects of p21(Cip1/Waf1) at both the G1/S and the G2/M cell cycle

transitions: pRb is a critical determinant in blocking DNA replication and in preventing endoreduplication. Mol Cell Biol 1998;18:629–643.

170. Sherr CJ, Roberts JM. CDK inhibitors: positive and negative regulators of G1-phase progression. Genes Dev 1999;13:1501–1512.

171. Ohtani N, Yamakoshi K, Takahashi A, Hara E. The p16INK4a-RB pathway: molecular link between cellular senescence and tumor suppression. J Med Invest 2004;51:146–153.

172. Chellapan SP. The E2F transcription factor: role in cell cycle regulation and differentiation. Mol Cell Diff 1994;2:201–220.

173. Schwarz JK, Bassing CH, Kovesdi I, et al. Expression of the E2F1 transcription factor overcomes type beta transforming growth factor–mediated growth suppression. Proc Natl Acad Sci USA 1995;92:483–487.

174. Hurford RK, Jr., Cobrinik D, Lee MH, Dyson N. pRB and p107/p130 are required for the regulated expression of different sets of E2F responsive genes. Genes Dev 1997;11:1447–1463.

175. Ohtani K. Implication of transcription factor E2F in regulation of DNA replication. Front Biosci 1999;4:D793–D804.

176. Humbert PO, Verona R, Trimarchi JM, et al. E2f3 is critical for normal cellular proliferation. Genes Dev 2000;14:690–703.

177. Ren B, Cam H, Takahashi Y, et al. E2F integrates cell cycle progression with DNA repair, replication, and G(2)/M checkpoints. Genes Dev 2002, 16:245–256.

178. Schlisio S, Halperin T, Vidal M, Nevins JR. Interaction of YY1 with E2Fs, mediated by RYBP, provides a mechanism for specificity of E2F function. EMBO J 2002;21:5775–5786.

179. Stevaux O, Dyson NJ. A revised picture of the E2F transcriptional network and RB function. Curr Opin Cell Biol 2002;14:684–691.

180. Mundle SD, Saberwal G. Evolving intricacies and implications of E2F-1 regulation. EMBO J 2003;17:569–574.

181. Rogoff HA, Kowalik TF. Life, death and E2F: linking proliferation control and DNA damage signaling via E2F1. Cell Cycle 2004;3:845–846.

182. Korenjak M, Brehm A. E2F–Rb complexes regulating transcription of genes important for differentiation and development. Curr Opin Genet Dev 2005;15:520–527.

183. Henriksson M, Luscher B. Proteins of the Myc network: essential regulators of cell growth and differentiation. Adv Cancer Res 1996;68:109–182.

184. Schmidt EV. MYC family ties. Nature Genet 1996;14:8–10.

185. Amati B, Alevizopoulos K, Vlach J. Myc and the cell cycle. Front Biosci 1998;3:D250–D268.

186. Burgin A, Bouchard C, Eilers M. Control of cell proliferation by Myc proteins. Results Probl Cell Differ 1998;22:181–197.

187. Matsumura I, Tanaka H, Kanakura Y. E2F1 and c-Myc in cell growth and death. Cell Cycle 2003;2:333–338.

188. Yam CH, Fung TK, Poon RY. Cyclin A in cell cycle control and cancer. Cell Mol Life Sci 2002;59:1317–1326.

189. Porter LA, Donoghue DJ. Cyclin B1 and CDK1: nuclear localization and upstream regulators. Prog Cell Cycle Res 2003;5:335–347.

190. Livingstone LR, White A, Sprouse J, et al. Altered cell cycle arrest and gene amplification potential accompany loss of wild-type p53. Cell 1992;70:923–935.

191. Harper JW, Adami GR, Wei N, et al. The p21 cdk-interacting protein Cip1 is a potent inhibitor of G_1 cyclin-dependent kinases. Cell 1993;75:805–816.

192. Xiong Y, Hannon GJ, Zhang H, et al. p21 is a universal inhibitor of cyclin kinases. Nature 1993;366:701–704.

193. Chen CY, Oliner JD, Zhan Q, et al. Interactions between p53 and MDM2 in a mammalian cell cycle checkpoint pathway. Proc Natl Acad Sci USA 1994;91:2684–2688.

194. El-Deiry WS, Harper JW, O'Connor PM, et al. WAF1/CIP1 is induced in p53-mediated G_1 arrest and apoptosis. Cancer Res 1994;54:1169–1174.

195. Chen X, Bargonetti J, Prives C. p53, through p21 (WAF1/CIP1), induces cyclin D1 synthesis. Cancer Res 1995;55:4257–4263.

196. Del Sal G, Murphy M, Ruaro E, et al. Cyclin D1 and p21/waf1 are both involved in p53 growth suppression. Oncogene 1996;12:177–185.

197. Laiho M, DeCaprio JA, Ludlow JW, et al. Growth inhibition by TGF-beta linked to suppression of retinoblastoma protein phosphorylation. Cell 1990;62:175–185.

198. Ewen ME, Sluss HK, Whitehouse LL, Livingston DM. TGF beta inhibition of Cdk4 synthesis is linked to cell cycle arrest. Cell 1993;74:1009–1020.

199. Foulkes WD, Flanders TY, Pollock PM, Hayward NK. The CDKN2A (p16) gene and human cancer. Mol Med 1997;3:5–20.

200. Serrano M. The tumor suppressor protein p16INK4a. Exp Cell Res 1997;237:7–13.

201. Carnero A, Hannon GJ. The INK4 family of CDK inhibitors. Curr Top Microbiol Immunol 1998;227:43–55.

202. Huschtscha LI, Reddel RR. p16(INK4a) and the control of cellular proliferative life span. Carcinogenesis 1999;20:921–926.

203. Roussel MF. The INK4 family of cell cycle inhibitors in cancer. Oncogene 1999;18:5311–5317.

204. Shapiro GI, Edwards CD, Rollins BJ. The physiology of p16(INK4A)-mediated G1 proliferative arrest. Cell Biochem Biophys 2000;33:189–197.

205. Chin L, Pomerantz J, DePinho RA. The INK4a/ARF tumor suppressor: one gene—two products—two pathways. Trends Biochem Sci 1998;23:291–296.

206. Stott FJ, Bates S, James MC, et al. The alternative product from the human CDKN2A locus, p14(ARF), participates in a regulatory feedback loop with p53 and MDM2. EMBO J 1998;17:5001–5014.

207. James MC, Peters G. Alternative product of the p16/CKDN2A locus connects the Rb and p53 tumor suppressors. Prog Cell Cycle Res 2000;4:71–81.

208. Weber HO, Samuel T, Rauch P, Funk JO. Human p14(ARF)-mediated cell cycle arrest strictly depends on intact p53 signaling pathways. Oncogene 2002;21:3207–12.

209. Satyanarayana A, Rudolph KL. p16 and ARF: activation of teenage proteins in old age. J Clin Invest 2004;114:1237–1240.

210. Laval J, Jurado J, Saparbaev M, Sidorkina O. Antimutagenic role of base-excision repair enzymes upon free radical-induced DNA damage. Mutat Res 1998;402:93–102.

211. Boiteux S, Radicella JP. Base excision repair of 8-hydroxyguanine protects DNA from endogenous oxidative stress. Biochimie 1999;81:59–67.

212. Boiteux S, Radicella JP. The human OGG1 gene: structure, functions, and its implication in the process of carcinogenesis. Arch Biochem Biophys 2000;377:1–8.

213. Nishimura S. Mammalian Ogg1/Mmh gene plays a major role in repair of the 8-hydroxyguanine lesion in DNA. Prog Nucleic Acid Res Mol Biol 2001;68:107–123.

214. Nishimura S. Involvement of mammalian OGG1(MMH) in excision of the 8-hydroxyguanine residue in DNA. Free Radic Biol Med 2002;32:813–821.

215. Fortini P, Pascucci B, Parlanti E, et al. 8-Oxoguanine DNA damage: at the crossroad of alternative repair pathways. Mutat Res 2003;531:127–139.

216. Nakabeppu Y, Tsuchimoto D, Furuichi M, Sakumi K. The defense mechanisms in mammalian cells against oxidative damage in nucleic acids and their involvement in the suppression of mutagenesis and cell death. Free Radic Res 2004;38:423–429.

217. Thompson LH, West MG. XRCC1 keeps DNA from getting stranded. Mutat Res 2000;459:1–18.

218. Tomkinson AE, Chen L, Dong Z, et al. Completion of base excision repair by mammalian DNA ligases. Prog Nucleic Acid Res Mol Biol 2001;68:151–164.

219. Caldecott KW. XRCC1 and DNA strand break repair. DNA Repair (Amst) 2003;2:955–969.

220. Dianov GL, Sleeth KM, Dianova II, Allinson SL. Repair of abasic sites in DNA. Mutat Res 2003;531:157–163.

221. Malanga M, Althaus FR. The role of poly(ADP-ribose) in the DNA damage signaling network. Biochem Cell Biol 2005;83:354–364.

222. Williams RS, Bernstein N, Lee MS, et al. Structural basis for phosphorylation-dependent signaling in the DNA-damage response. Biochem Cell Biol 2005;83:721–727.

223. Johnson RT, Squires S. The XPD complementation group. Insights into xeroderma pigmentosum, Cockayne's syndrome and trichothiodystrophy. Mutat Res 1992;273:97–118.

224. Wood RD. DNA damage recognition during nucleotide excision repair in mammalian cells. Biochimie 1999;81:39–44.

225. Bernstein C, Bernstein H, Payne CM, Garewal H. DNA repair/pro-apoptotic dual-role proteins in five major DNA repair pathways: fail-safe protection against carcinogenesis. Mutat Res 2002;511:145–178.

226. Chen J, Suter B. Xpd, a structural bridge and a functional link. Cell Cycle 2003;2:503–506.

227. MacPhee DG. Mismatch repair as a source of mutations in non-dividing cells. Genetica 1996;97:183–195.

228. Peltomaki P. DNA mismatch repair gene mutations in human cancer. Environ Health Perspect 1997;105(Suppl 4):775–780.

229. Kirkpatrick DT. Roles of the DNA mismatch repair and nucleotide excision repair proteins during meiosis. Cell Mol Life Sci 1999;55:437–449.

230. Kolodner RD, Marsischky GT. Eukaryotic DNA mismatch repair. Curr Opin Genet Dev 1999;9:89–96.

231. Harfe BD, Jinks-Robertson S. Mismatch repair proteins and mitotic genome stability. Mutat Res 2000;451:151–167.

232. Harfe BD, Jinks-Robertson S. DNA mismatch repair and genetic instability. Annu Rev Genet 2000;34:359–399.

233. Aquilina G, Bignami M. Mismatch repair in correction of replication errors and processing of DNA damage. J Cell Physiol 2001;187:145–154.

234. Hsieh P. Molecular mechanisms of DNA mismatch repair. Mutat Res 2001;486:71–87.

235. Schofield MJ, Hsieh P. DNA mismatch repair: molecular mechanisms and biological function. Annu Rev Microbiol 2003;57:579–608.

236. Isaacs RJ, Spielmann HP. A model for initial DNA lesion recognition by NER and MMR based on local conformational flexibility. DNA Repair (Amst) 2004;3:455–464.

237. Stojic L, Brun R, Jiricny J. Mismatch repair and DNA damage signalling. DNA Repair (Amst) 2004;3:1091–1101.

238. Kunkel TA, Erie DA. DNA mismatch repair. Annu Rev Biochem 2005;74:681–710.

239. Jun SH, Kim TG, Ban C. DNA mismatch repair system. Classical and fresh roles. FEBS J 2006;273:1609–1619.

240. Montesano R, Becker R, Hall J, et al. Repair of DNA alkylation adducts in mammalian cells. Biochimie 1985;67:919–928.

241. D'Incalci M, Citti L, Taverna P, Catapano CV. Importance of the DNA repair enzyme O6-alkyl guanine alkyltransferase (AT) in cancer chemotherapy. Cancer Treat Rev 1988;15:279–292.

242. Pegg AE, Byers TL. Repair of DNA containing O6-alkylguanine. FASEB J 1992;6:2302–2310.

243. Sekiguchi M, Nakabeppu Y, Sakumi K, Tuzuki T. DNA-repair methyltransferase as a molecular device for preventing mutation and cancer. J Cancer Res Clin Oncol 1996;122:199–206.

244. Pieper RO. Understanding and manipulating O6-methylguanine-DNA methyltransferase expression. Pharmacol Ther 1997;74:285–297.

245. Sekiguchi M, Sakumi K. Roles of DNA repair methyltransferase in mutagenesis and carcinogenesis. Jpn J Hum Genet 1997;42:389–399.

246. Yu Z, Chen J, Ford BN, et al. Human DNA repair systems: an overview. Environ Mol Mutagen 1999;33:3–20.

247. Kaina B, Ochs K, Grosch S, et al. BER, MGMT, and MMR in defense against alkylation-induced genotoxicity and apoptosis. Prog Nucleic Acid Res Mol Biol 2001;68:41–54.

248. Drablos F, Feyzi E, Aas PA, et al. Alkylation damage in DNA and RNA—repair mechanisms and medical significance. DNA Repair (Amst) 2004;3:1389–1407.

249. Gerson SL. MGMT: its role in cancer aetiology and cancer therapeutics. Nat Rev Cancer 2004;4:296–307.

250. Varon R, Vissinga C, Platzer M, et al. Nibrin, a novel DNA double-strand break repair protein, is mutated in Nijmegen breakage syndrome. Cell 1998;93:467–476.

251. Buscemi G, Savio C, Zannini L, et al. CHK2 activation dependence on NBS1 after DNA damage. Mol Cell Biol 2001;21:5214–5222.

252. Xu B, Kim S, Kastan MB. Involvement of BRCA1 in S-phase and G(2)-phase checkpoints after ionizing irradiation. Mol Cell Biol 2001;21:3445–3450.
253. D'Amours D, Jackson SP. The MRE11 complex: At the crossroads of DNA repair and checkpoint signalling. Nat Rev Mol Cell Biol 2002;3:317–327.
254. Girard PM, Riballo E, Begg AC, et al. NBS1 promotes ATM dependent phosphorylation events including those required for G1/S arrest. Oncogene 2002;21:4191–4199.
255. Huang J, Dynan WS. Reconstitution of the mammalian DNA double-strand break end-joining reaction reveals a requirement for an MRE11/RAD50/NBS1-containing fraction. Nucleic Acids Res 2002;30:667–674.
256. Nakanishi K, Taniguchi T, Ranganathan V, et al. Interaction of FANCD2 and NBS1 in the DNA damage response. Nat Cell Biol 2002;4:913–920.
257. Osborn AJ, Elledge SJ, Zou L. Checking on the fork: the DNA-replication stress-response pathway. Trends Cell Biol 2002;12:509–516.
258. Yazdi PT, Wang Y, Zhao S, et al. SMC1 is a downstream effector in the ATM/NBS1 branch of the human S-phase checkpoint. Genes Dev 2002;16:571–582.
259. Carson CT, Schwartz RA, Stracker TH, et al. The MRE11 complex is required for ATM activation and the G2/M checkpoint. EMBO J 2003;22:6610–6620.
260. Goodarzi AA, Block WD, Lees-Miller SP. The role of ATM and ATR in DNA damage-induced cell cycle control. Prog Cell Cycle Res 2003;5:393–411.
261. Shiloh Y. ATM and related protein kinases: safeguarding genome integrity. Nat Rev Cancer 2003;3:155–168.
262. Uziel T, Lerenthal Y, Moyal L, et al. Requirement of the MRN complex for ATM activation by DNA damage. EMBO J 2003;22:5612–5621.
263. Abraham RT. PI 3-kinase related kinases: "big" players in stress-induced signaling pathways. DNA Repair (Amst) 2004;3:883–887.
264. Lee JH, Paull TT. Direct activation of the ATM protein kinase by the MRE11/RAD50/NBS1 complex. Science 2004;304:93–96.
265. Matsuura S, Kobayashi J, Tauchi H, Komatsu K. Nijmegen breakage syndrome and DNA double strand break repair by NBS1 complex. Adv Biophys 2004;38:65–80.
266. Lavin MF, Birrell G, Chen P, et al. ATM signaling and genomic stability in response to DNA damage. Mutat Res 2005;569:123–132.
267. Lee JH, Paull TT. ATM activation by DNA double-strand breaks through the MRE11-RAD50-NBS1 complex. Science 2005;308:551–554.
268. O'Driscoll M, Jeggo PA. The role of double-strand break repair—insights from human genetics. Nat Rev Genet 2006;7:45–54.
269. Zhang Y, Zhou J, Lim CU. The role of NBS1 in DNA double strand break repair, telomere stability, and cell cycle checkpoint control. Cell Res 2006;16:45–54.

3
Cell Adhesion Molecules

Timothy Craig Allen and Philip T. Cagle

Introduction

Cell adhesion molecules, also termed *cell adhesion receptors*, are one of three classes of macromolecules—along with extracellular matrix molecules and adhesion plaque proteins—that mediate cell adhesion, an activity that is critical for the commencement and maintenance of the three-dimensional structure and normal function of tissues.[1,2] Cell adhesion molecules are predominantly transmembrane glycoproteins that mediate binding to extracellular matrix molecules or to associated receptors on other cells in a manner that determines the specificity of cell–cell or cell–extracellular matrix interactions.[1] There are five families of adhesion receptors—integrins, cadherins, immunoglobulin cell adhesion molecules (IgCAMs), selectins, and CD44.[1,3–7] Complexes formed by cell adhesion receptors are not static, but are dynamic units capable of obtaining and incorporating extracellular environmental signals and are indeed the foundation of two-way signaling between the cell and its external environment.[1,8] These cell adhesion molecule families are also involved in cell motility, migration, signaling, differentiation, apoptosis, and gene transcription.[5]

The intricate processes involved in cancer invasion and metastasis require tumor cell detachment from the primary tumor, then tumor cell entry and exit from the lymphatic or vascular systems in turn, culminating in tumor cell growth at distant tissue sites.[5,9] These steps can only take place with the dysregulation of normal cell–cell adhesion and cell–matrix interactions that are mediated by the cell adhesion receptor families.[5] These families of cell adhesion molecules play a role in both non–small cell lung cancers (NSCLCs) and small cell lung cancers (SCLCs). Integrins, selectins, and cadherins have been relatively widely studied and IgCAMs and CD44 less so.

Integrins

The integrin superfamily is one of the cellular adhesion molecule superfamilies that has been, and continues to be, relatively widely studied as it relates to lung cancer. Integrins are transmembrane glycoproteins that form heterodimers consisting of one α-subunit and one β-subunit.[3] The specific combination of the subunits determines the ligand binding specificity, and various specific combinations of α- and β-subunits exhibit binding specificity for collagen receptors, fibronectin receptors, laminin receptors, vitronectin receptors, and other integrin receptors.[3] Most integrins are substrate adhesion molecules that mediate interactions between cells and extracellular matrix components; however, some integrins are cell–cell adhesion molecules.[3] Lymphocytes express integrins that mediate heterotypic cell–cell adhesion, binding some IgCAMs.[3] The integrin receptor family plays a critical role in complex cellular events such as cellular differentiation, proliferation, and migration and is involved in biologic processes related to organogenesis, wound healing, and the altered adhesive and invasive properties of tumor cells.[10–12] Integrins transmit signals bidirectionally across plasma membranes.[13] Alterations in integrin secretion or functional activity may regulate the development and progression of cancers, and changes in integrins in vivo leading to more aggressive tumor behavior have been identified in cancers of the lung, breast, colon, prostate, stomach, pancreas, liver, kidney, ovary, skin, and endometrium.[3,14–24] β-Integrins have been associated with tumor cell migration in cell lines including fibrosarcoma, bladder cancer, and colon cancer.[3,25] Integrin subunits have been identified immunohistochemically in bronchial epithelium, endothelium, and smooth muscle.[3] Although integrins have been shown to be active in normal lung development, host defense to lung infection, and development of acute respiratory distress syndrome, research regarding the importance of integrins in lung cancer cell migration is ongoing.[3,26] In squamous cell NSCLCs, for example, increased $\alpha_1\beta_1$- and $\alpha_2\beta_1$-integrin expression has been related to increased metastatic ability.[3,27]

$\alpha_3\beta_1$-Integrin and Small Cell Lung Carcinoma

$\alpha_3\beta_1$-Integrin, critical for lung development, is the primary laminin binding integrin, anchoring alveolar and bronchial epithelial cells to the basement membrane during fetal development through adulthood.[3,28] A stepwise reduction in the expression of integrins, including $\alpha_3\beta_1$-integrin, occurs from normal epithelium, with the greatest amount to NSCLC and finally to SCLC with the least amount.[3,29,30] The reduced expression of $\alpha_3\beta_1$-integrin in SCLC has been attributed to that cancer's aggressiveness.[3] Also, $\alpha_3\beta_1$-integrin has been found to be significantly reduced in poorly differentiated NSCLCs.[3,29] However, Bartolazzi et al. noted that 82% of NSCLC patients studied expressed integrins, with no association found with type and degree of differentiation.[3,31] Furthermore, Bartolazzi et al. found that only 13% of SCLCs expressed $\alpha_3\beta_1$-integrin in their series.[3,31] Using an SCLC cell line, Barr et al. found that decreased $\alpha_3\beta_1$-integrin expression correlated with highly invasive behavior and metastatic behavior in SCLCs.[3,32] c-Myc expression reportedly leads to reduced $\alpha_3\beta_1$-integrin expression, and $\alpha_3\beta_1$-integrin is thought to mediate the homotypic adhesion of SCLC cells.[3] Unengaged $\alpha_3\beta_1$-integrin may suppress the growth of disaggregated SCLC cells; and the downregulation of the α_3-subunit might contribute to enhanced tumorgenicity of c-Myc–overexpressing SCLCs by allowing growth of tumor cells that have reduced contact with ligand-expressing substratum or cells, a condition occurring during primary tumor growth, tumor invasion, and tumor metastases.[3]

CXCR4 Chemokine Receptors

As mentioned earlier, cancer cells must pass through blood or lymphatic circulation and through the vessel walls in order to metastasize. Metastatic tumor cells are thought to coopt signals normally controlling leukocyte movement, such as chemokine-mediated cell migration.[33] Emigration from vessels is regulated by a sequence of distinct molecular signals, one of which involves chemokines that activate integrins and direct migration of leukocytes.[33] The chemokine stromal cell–derived factor-1 (SDF-1/CXCL12) is a CXC chemokine expressed in bone marrow stromal cells.[33] CXCR4, the receptor for CXCL12, has a critical role for the homing of hematopoietic stem cells in the bone marrow microenvironment.[33] The CXCR4/CXCL12 axis may regulate migration and metastasis of several cancers, and the neutralization of the CXCR4/CXCL12 axis has been shown in vivo to inhibit or attenuate metastases of breast cancer.[33] Using a murine model, Phillips et al. reported similar findings with regard to NSCLC and concluded that the CXCL12/CXCR4 axis is involved in regulating NSCLC metastases.[33,34] As SCLC has a propensity to metastasize to the bone marrow, Hartmann, et al., using three SCLC cell lines, examined the signaling mechanisms that regulate CXCL12-influenced adhesion of SCLC cells to fibronectin, collagen, and stromal cells.[33] The authors found that CXCL12-induced integrin activation resulted in increased adhesion of SCLC cells to fibronectin and collagen and mediated α_2-, α_4-, α_5-, and β_1-integrins as well as CXCR4 activation—able to be inhibited by CXCR4 antagonists.[33] The authors further noted that stromal cells protected SCLC cells from chemotherapy-induced apoptosis—a protection that could also be antagonized by CXCR4 inhibitors.[33] Hartmann et al. concluded that activation of integrins and CXCR4 chemokine receptors cooperate in mediating adhesion and survival signals from the tumor microenvironment to SCLC cells and that CXCR4 antagonists in combination with cytotoxic drugs should be considered as potential therapy in SCLCs to overcome CXCL12-mediated adhesion and survival signals in the tumor microenvironment.[33]

Cyclooxygenase-2

Cyclooxygenase (COX-2) expression in tumor cells has been shown to play a key role in lung cancer progression, and nonsteroidal antiinflammatory drug inhibition of COX-2 has been shown to reduce cancer risk in human beings and to suppress cancer growth in animal models. Cyclooxygenase-2 inhibitors may also be a useful adjunct to standard chemotherapy protocols in treating NSCLC patients.[10,35–39] Inhibition of COX-2 activity, with subsequent inhibition of prostaglandin synthesis, is generally considered the mechanism involved in inhibition, but some studies suggest that other mechanisms may be involved, such as cell cycle progression, induction of apoptosis, and inhibition of angiogenesis.[10,40,41] $\alpha_5\beta_1$-Integrin is a fibronectin receptor, and its interaction is important for cell adhesion and migration, matrix assembly, cytoskeletal organization, and tumor development.[10,42,43] The $\alpha_5\beta_1$-integrin ligand fibronectin stimulates lung cancer cells, an effect mediated by $\alpha_5\beta_1$-integrin signals. The α_5-integrin subunit is typically absent in normal lung but has been shown to be significantly expressed in lung cancer cells, and NSCLC patients overexpressing the subunit have significantly decreased overall survival compared with patients with normal expression of that subunit.[10,44] Han and Roman, examining human NSCLC cell lines, explored the link between COX-2 inhibitor anticancer effects and $\alpha_5\beta_1$-integrin expression and found that COX-2 inhibitors suppress α_5

gene expression in human NSCLC cells, mediated by increased Sp1 protein and Sp1–DNA binding, along with an associated decrease in c-Jun and AP-1–DNA binding in the α_5 gene promoter.[10] Activation of Sp1 and the ERK signaling pathway contribute to α_5 gene downregulation in the presence of COX-2 inhibitors.[10] Further research into this mechanism of action against NSCLC—involving COX-2 inhibitors relating to α5 gene expression and consequently tumor cell recognition of extracellular matrixes such as fibronectin—may allow for better future therapies for NSCLC patients.

Focal Adhesion Kinase

As integrin receptors are not catalytically active, they must recruit and activate other signaling molecules. Focal adhesion kinase, a nonreceptor tyrosine kinase enriched in focal adhesions and ubiquitously expressed during development, plays a key role in cell migration, proliferation, and survival.[13] Focal adhesion kinase may be a critical mediator of integrin signaling and has been linked to the integrin and growth factor receptor–signaling pathways that regulate several biologic processes concerning neoplastic transformation, invasion, and metastasis, including cell adhesion, migration, and apoptosis.[13,45–47] Focal adhesion kinase phosphorylation and kinase activity are regulated by integrin-mediated and matrix-dependent cell adhesion in tumor cells of many cancers.[13,48,49] Focal adhesion kinase overexpression and phosphorylation are related to increased cell tumor cell motility, invasion, and cytoskeleton alteration.[13] Carelli et al., examining 60 NSCLCs and surrounding nonneoplastic lung parenchyma, as well as 5 normal lungs, found focal adhesion kinase to be weakly expressed in nonneoplastic lung parenchyma and upregulated in NSCLC.[47] The authors also found focal adhesion kinase upregulation to be significantly related to higher disease stage, suggesting focal adhesion kinase upregulation in NSCLCs is potentially involved with NSCLC progression.[47] Mukhopadhyay et al., examining a squamous cell NSCLC cell line, Calu-1, found that tumor cells from the cell line bound collagen type IV through β_1-integrin and resulted in focal adhesion kinase phosphorylation.[13,50] In a later study, Mukhopadhyay et al., studying potential mechanisms of focal adhesion kinase activation and regulation in human NSCLC cell line Calu-1 cells, found multiple and potentially parallel collagen type IV/β1 integrin-mediated signaling events in the tumor cells, involving focal adhesion kinase, extracellular signal regulating kinases, and protein kinase C.[13] Future studies defining focal adhesion kinase regulation and signaling, and the relationship between focal adhesion kinase and β_1-integrin may enable researchers to identify molecular targets to block the process of NSCLC metastasis.

Other Integrin-Related Research

Recent research into a variety of aspects of integrin molecular biology has opened up new avenues of investigation for new prognostic markers and therapies for lung cancer. Targeted therapy is becoming a realistic approach to NSCLC treatment. Gefitinib and erlontinib, epidermal growth factor receptor (EGFR) inhibitors, are being used to treat patients with NSCLC refractory to standard chemotherapy.[51–53] Integrin has been proposed as another potential target for molecular therapy.[51,54] In a 2006 article, Lau et al. identified a peptide ligand, cNGXGXXc, that targets $\alpha_3\beta_1$-integrin, an integrin that promotes adhesion that is overexpressed in NSCLC.[51] Using a technique allowing tumor cell growth on beads, the authors captured cancer cells in pleural fluid.[51] Such a technique using the novel peptide ligand might be developed to produce target-specific diagnostic and therapeutic agents for NSCLC treatment.[51]

$\alpha_5\beta_3$-Integrin and $\alpha_5\beta_5$-integrin have been shown to be critical for tumor growth and angiogenesis.[55] In 2006, Albert et al. studied the effect of the integrin antagonist cilengitide (EMD 121974) and ionizing radiation on human umbilical vein endothelial cell line cells and human NSCLC cell line cells and found that irradiation induces expression of $\alpha_5\beta_3$-integrin in all cell lines examined.[55] The authors found an increased rate of apoptosis and decreased endothelial tubule formation after combination treatment and an increase in detached cells after cilengitide treatment.[55] These findings suggest a potential benefit of therapy regimens incorporating integrin antagonists for NSCLC patients.

Lack of cellular adhesion may be important in the metastatic potency of NSCLC.[56] Examining eight NSCLCs and eight normal bronchi from the respective patients, Boelens et al. in 2006 identified 43 cancer-related genes, 5 of which are related to epithelial adhesion, including α_3-integrin and β_4-integrin.[56] α_3-Integrin was found to be upregulated in adenocarcinoma, and β_4-integrin was found to be upregulated in squamous cell carcinoma, leading authors to conclude that their role in cellular adhesion affects the metastatic potential of NSCLC.[56]

Addressing the problem of chemotherapy resistance in SCLC in 2006, Hodkinson found that extracellular matrix activates phosphatidylinositol-3 kinase (PI3K) signaling in SCLC cells, preventing etoposide-induced caspase-3 activation and subsequent β_1-integrin/PI3K-dependent apoptosis.[57] By β1-integrin/PI3K activation, extracellular matrix overrides treatment-induced cell cycle arrest and apoptosis, allowing SCLC cells to survive with persistent DNA damage, thereby accounting for the acquisition of drug resistance in these tumor cells.[57] The authors note that this chemoprotective effect is not mediated by altered SCLC cell proliferation or by DNA repair.[57]

In 2004, Oshita et al., examining 72 patients with pathologic stage I adenocarcinomas less than 2 cm in diameter, studied the effect of surviving, cyclin D1, vascular endothelial growth factor (VEGF), and β_1-integrin and found that overall survival of patients expressing surviving, cyclin D1, and β_1-integrin was significantly worse for patients not expressing each gene.[58] Furthermore, while no individual gene expression independently predicted poor prognosis, overall survival was significantly worse when two or more genes were positive than in patients with no or one gene overexpressed.[58] The authors found that only having two or more genes positive was a significant independent prognostic factor for poor prognosis in these patients with early stage small adenocarcinomas.[58]

Nicotine increases DNA synthesis and proliferation of vascular endothelial cells in vitro.[59,60] Endothelial cells express nonneuronal nicotinic receptors and $\alpha_5\beta_3$-integrin receptors.[59,61,62] In 2006, Mousa and Mousa used human cancer cell line cells to study the effect and mechanism of nicotine on angiogenesis and various angiogenesis-mediated processes and found the proangiogenesis effect of nicotine to be mediated by the nonneuronal nicotinic receptor and the $\alpha_5\beta_3$-integrin receptors on endothelia cell surfaces, mediated through intracellular signaling involving mitogen-activated protein kinase (ERK1/2).[59] Nicotine has endothelial cell–stimulating effects causing increased angiogenesis similar to the effects of a standard growth factor such as basic fibroblast growth factor.[59] The authors conclude that nicotine's proangiogenesis effects may promote tumor cell growth.[59] The continuing research into the various aspects of the molecular interactions of integrins in lung cancer patients may one day yield more effective therapeutic regimens and prognostic indicators for lung cancer patients.

Cadherins

Similar to integrins, the cadherin family of cellular adhesion molecules has been, and continues to be, widely studied as it relates to lung cancer. The cadherin family consists of calcium-dependent cell–cell adhesion molecules that are highly conserved transmembrane glycoproteins with similar domains for homophilic binding, calcium binding, and interaction with intracellular proteins.[6,63,64] The cytoplasmic domain of cadherins interacts with catenins (α-catenin, β-catenin, γ-catenin) and the resulting complexes associate with cortical actin filaments.[6,65] The cadherin–catenin interaction is necessary for cadherin-mediated adhesion and association of the complexes with the cytoskeleton.[6,66] The cadherin family contains 16 members, of which the most significant is E-cadherin (epithelial cadherin), which is found in epithelial tissues and involved in formation and maintenance of cell histoarchitecture.[6] Other important cadherins include N-cadherin (neural cadherin), found in neural and muscle tissues, P-cadherin (placental cadherin), R-cadherin (retinal cadherin), and VE-cadherin (vascular endothelial cadherin).[6,67] Loss of function or secretion of the E-cadherin–catenin complex, or any of its components, eliminates a cell's capacity to adhere, with resulting loss of normal tissue architecture.[6] Altered or absent E-cadherin expression has been identified in various cancers, including stomach, head and neck, bladder, prostate, breast, and colon.[6,68–72] α-Catenin absence or alteration has been identified in breast, gastric, and esophageal cancers,[6,73,74] and alteration of β-catenin expression or phosphorylation has been found in cancers of the esophagus, stomach, and colon.[6,75] Reduced E-cadherin expression has also been identified in lung cancer.[6,76]

E-Cadherin

Cadherins are essential for tight junctions between cells, and E-cadherin is the cadherin most strongly expressed in epithelial cells.[63,77,78] Cadherins form a complex with cytoplasmic proteins known as catenins, and the resulting complex, along with other cytoskeletal components such as actin, constitutes the intercellular adherence junction.[63,65,77,79] Cadherin-mediated cell adhesion suppresses invasion of cancer cells in vitro, and dysfunction of the E-cadherin system correlates with cancer invasion in human cancers.[77,80–84] There are two groups of catenins—α-catenins and β-catenins.[77] The human lung cancer cell line PC9 expresses an aberrant α-catenin messenger RNA and the cells have very loose cell–cell associations.[77,85,86] α-Cadherin is considered by some authors to be indispensable for cadherin-mediated cell–cell adhesion.[77] Researchers have identified reduced or heterogeneous E-cadherin expression and/or α-catenin expression in undifferentiated invasive cancers, and impaired expression of E-cadherin and α-catenin has been associated with increased lymph node metastases in breast, esophageal, and head and neck cancers.[69,72,73,77,87–90] The prognostic value of reduced E-cadherin expression in cancer patients has not been widely studied.[68,70,77,91–93]

The relationship between E-cadherin and α-catenin is mediated by β-catenin, and β-catenin in turn mediates the interactions of the cadherin–catenin complex with the c-ErbB2 gene product and EGFR.[77,94–97] Adenomatous polyposis coli protein, a tumor suppressor gene product, interacts with β-catenin and plakoglobin and is important in the E-cadherin–mediated cell adhesion system, influencing tumor invasion and metastasis.[77]

Kato et al., studying 84 cases of intrabronchial precancerous lesions, including squamous metaplasia, squamous metaplasia with atypia, and dysplasia, 21 cases of in situ carcinoma, 4 cases of tumor microinvasion of the bronchial wall, and 32 cases of stage I well-differentiated squamous cell NSCLC, noted that downregulation of

E-cadherin and/or catenins was associated with squamous metaplasia with atypia in intrabronchial lesions.[77] The authors concluded that downregulation of α-catenin and/or β-catenin, possibly reflecting a dysfunctional cadherin-mediated cell–cell adhesion system, is a marker for atypia during bronchial epithelium carcinogenesis.[77]

Cadherins and Cyclooxygenase-2

Cyclooxygenase-2 and its metabolite prostaglandin E_2 (PGE_2) are critical for regulating diverse cellular functions under both physiologic and pathologic conditions.[98–101] Cyclooxygenase-2 is overexpressed in human NSCLC, and its inhibition causes tumor reduction in vivo in murine lung cancer models.[98,102] Cyclooxygenase-2 activity is identified throughout the progression of a premalignant lesion to the metastatic phenotype.[98,103] Higher COX-2 expression has been identified in lung adenocarcinoma lymph node metastases.[98,103] Cyclooxygenase-2 overexpression has been associated with angiogenesis, decreased host immunity, and enhanced invasion and metastasis, and therefore COX-2 has been considered to have an important role in multiple pathways in lung cancer carcinogenesis, suggesting it has a multifaceted role in conferring malignant and metastatic phenotypes.[98,104–108] Cyclooxygenase-2 may be a central element in orchestrating the multiple genetic alterations required for lung cancer invasion and metastasis.[98,108] Cyclooxygenase-2–dependent invasive capacity in NSCLC is due to PGE_2-mediated regulation of CD44 and matrix metalloproteinase-2.[98]

Normal cell–cell adhesion disruption leads to enhanced tumor cell migration and proliferation, with resulting invasion and metastasis.[98,109,110] Downregulating the cadherin family or catenin family members, or activation of signaling pathways that prevent cell–cell cadherin junction assembly, can cause this disruption.[98,109] As such, extracellular matrix and cell–cell adhesion are significant barriers to tumor metastasis.[98,109] The E-cadherin–catenin complex is required for intercellular adhesiveness and normal tissue architecture maintenance.[98,109] E-cadherin reduction has been likened to tumor invasion, metastasis, and poor prognosis.[98,111] E-cadherin loss, along with increased COX-2 expression, has been identified in familial adenomatous polyposis; however, pathways of COX-2 regulation of E-cadherin in NSCLC have not been extensively studied.[98,107] Dohadwala et al., studying NSCLC cells and cell lines including human lung adenocarcinoma and human lung squamous cell carcinoma, COX-2-sense, and COX-2-antisense cells, recently identified a pathway whereby $COX-2/PGE_2$ contribute to the regulation of E-cadherin expression in NSCLC.[98]

The authors made several observations that lead them to conclude that PGE_2 functions in an autocrine or paracrine fashion to modulate transcriptional repressors of E-cadherin, thus regulating COX-2–dependent E-cadherin expression in NSCLC, and that therefore the inhibition or blockage of PGE_2 production or activity might play a role in NSCLC prevention and treatment.[98] Those observations include the following: (1) Genetically modified COX-2-sense NSCLC cells express low levels of E-cadherin and show reduced capacity for cellular aggregation, and genetic or pharmacologic inhibition of tumor COX-2 led to increased E-cadherin expression and to augmented homotypic cellular aggregation by NSCLC cells in vitro, with an inverse relationship between COX-2 and E-cadherin identified in situ by double immunohistochemical staining of human lung adenocarcinoma tissue. (2) Non–small cell lung carcinoma cell treatment with exogenous PGE_2 markedly decreased E-cadherin expression, while COX-2-sense cell treatment with celecoxib resulted in increased expression of E-cadherin. (3) The transcriptional E-cadherin suppressors ZEB1 and Snail were upregulated in COX-2-sense cells and PGE_2-treated NSCLC cells but were decreased in COX-2-antisense cells. Furthermore, PGE_2 exposure caused enhanced ZEB1 and Snail binding at the chromatin level, with Small interfering RNA-mediated knockdown of ZEB-1 or Snail interrupting PGE_2's capacity to downregulate E-cadherin. (4) An inverse relationship between E-cadherin and ZEB1 and a direct relationship between COX-2 and ZEB were identified by immunohistochemical staining of human lung adenocarcinoma tissue.[98]

Cadherins and Epidermal Growth Factor Receptor

Epidermal growth factor receptor is overexpressed in many NSCLCs, and treatment with the EGFR tyrosine kinase inhibitors gefitinib and erlotinib has shown improved survival in some chemotherapy-resistant NSCLC patients.[112–115] Nonetheless, about half of these NSCLC patients have tumor progression within 8 months and show no treatment benefit.[112] Activating mutations in the EGFR tyrosine kinase domain have been shown to increase EGFR copy number and/or expression of EGFR protein, correlating with response and survival after EGFR tyrosine kinase inhibitor therapy.[112,116,117]

Epidermal growth factor receptor's activation and signaling through its downstream targets is modulated by E-cadherin; specifically, E-cadherin inhibits EGFR ligand activation and enhances Akt activation in neighboring cells.[112,114–117] High phosphorylated Akt levels may predict tumor response to EGFR tyrosine kinase inhibitors.[114,118] In lung cancer cell lines, E-cadherin expression is regulated by β-catenin signaling and by zinc finger proteins, including the Slug/Snail family, SIP1, and ZEB1.[112,119] These transcription factors regulate gene expression by interaction with two 5′-CACCTG (E-box) promoter sequences.[112,120] This regulation is facilitated by interaction with the transcriptional corepressor CtBP, which recruits histone deacetylase (HDAC), causing chromatin condensation and gene silencing.[112,121] Inhibiting HDACs using trichostatin A in lung cancer cell lines reactivates E-cadherin expression.[112,119] Histone deacetylase inhibitors are potential therapeutic agents that promote differentiation and apoptosis in hematologic and solid malignancies through chromatin remodeling and regulation of gene expression.[112,122] A benzamide HDAC inhibitor, MS-275, is being investigated in hematologic and solid cancers and causes changes in histone acetylation that last for several weeks after being administered.[112,123] Witta et al., examining cell cultures, investigated E-cadherin expression in response to EGFR tyrosine kinase inhibitors and found a significant correlation between NSCLC cell line cell sensitivity to gefitinib and E-cadherin expression, as well as ZEB1.[112] The authors suggest that E-cadherin and ZEB1 have predictive value for EGFR tyrosine kinase inhibitor responsiveness.[112] Furthermore, the authors noted that E-cadherin transfection into a gefitinib-resistant cell line increased the cell line cells' sensitivity to gefitinib and that pretreating resistant cell lines with the HDAC inhibitor MS-275 induced E-cadherin as well as EGFR, leading to a growth inhibitory and apoptotic effect of gefitinib similar to that found in gefitinib-sensitive NSCLC cell lines, including those with EGFR mutations.[112] The authors concluded that combined HDAC inhibitor and gefitinib therapy may be a new treatment regimen that to overcome NSCLC tumor cell resistance to EGFR inhibitors.[112]

Deeb et al. immunohistochemically evaluated 130 resectable NSCLCs for E-cadherin and EGFR and found no significant association between E-cadherin expression and EGFR expression except that patients exhibiting E-cadherin negativity and EGFR positivity in tumor cells had a worse prognosis than those patients with tumor cells showing E-cadherin positivity and EGFR negativity ($p = 0.026$).[124] Future studies continuing to examine the relationship between EGFR and E-cadherin may provide information valuable for the development of prognostic indicators as well as for lung cancer therapy. In 2002, Al Moustafa et al., after examining human lung cancer cell lines, reported that EGFR modulation regulated the E-cadherin–catenin complex and cell motility of the lung cancer cells. They concluded that restoration of the cadherin–catenin complex with EGFR inhibitors might be beneficial in treating NSCLC patients.[125]

H-Cadherin

The H-cadherin gene, a cadherin superfamily member that has been isolated and mapped to 16q24, lacks the cytoplasmic domain, unlike E-cadherin, P-cadherin, and N-cadherin.[126] Genetic abnormalities in the H-cadherin gene have been identified in human cancer cell lines and

in lung, stomach, and ovarian cancers.[126] Takeuchi et al. noted that expression of H-cadherin downregulated surfactant protein D in bronchoalveolar cells.[127] Evaluating the role of H-cadherin in NSCLC, Zhong et al. examined 6 NSCLC cell lines and 35 pairs of primary NSCLC tumors and nonmalignant lung tissue. They noted that H-cadherin loss was related to more advanced local tumor growth, although the result did not reach statistical significance.[126] The authors concluded that H-cadherin loss occurs often in NSCLC patients and that the loss might facilitate tumor cell implantation and local growth in NSCLC.[126] Toyooka et al., noting that H-cadherin might be a tumor suppressor gene, examined the methylation status of H-cadherin promoter in breast and lung cancers and correlated it with mRNA expression.[128] The authors noted that frequent aberrant methylation of H-cadherin in breast and lung cancers was due to loss of gene expression, but expression might occasionally be lost by other mechanisms.[128]

Other Cadherin-Related Research

Bremnes et al., reported on 193 NSCLC patients with stages I to III disease in a 2002 article. They determined that reduced E-cadherin and catenin expression was associated with tumor cell dedifferentiation, local tumor invasion, regional metastasis, and reduced survival in NSCLC. They concluded that E-cadherin is an independent prognostic factor in NSCLC patients.[129]

α-1,6-Fucosyltransferase catalyzes core fucosylation by transferring a fucosyl residue from GDP-fucose to the asparagine-linked GlcNAC residue of complex N-glycans by α-16 linkage, a process important in posttranslational glycoprotein modification and functional regulation.[130] Normally, core fucosylated N-linked oligosaccharide content is low, but there are markedly increased levels found in lung, stomach, and liver tumorigenesis.[130] The calcium-dependent transmembrane glycoprotein E-cadherin, with five-repeated extracellular domains, performs homotypic cell–cell adhesion by the clustering of symmetric cis dimers of N-terminal domains, an event necessary for regulating cell growth and migration.[130] The N-terminal extracellular domain CAD1, containing a histidine-alanine-valine sequence necessary for cell–cell adhesion, is critical for cell–cell contact.[130] Because reduced E-cadherin levels are related to increased tumor invasiveness in some cancers, and because bisected high mannose type N-linked glycan has been identified on E-cadherin, Geng et al. examined the biologic function of core fucosylation on E-cadherin in human NSCLC cells.[130] They noted that α-1,6-fucosyltransferase regulates E-cadherin–mediated cell adhesion and as such might be important in tumor development and progression.[130] The authors further hypothesized that core fucosylation of E-cadherin might impair N-glycan three-dimensional architecture, with resulting conformational asymmetry that suppresses E-cadherin function.[130] The demonstration of core fucosylated E-cadherin might be an important prognostic factor in NSCLC.[130]

In 2003, Choi et al., studying 141 pathologic stage I NSCLC patients without preoperative chemotherapy or radiotherapy, found that decreased E-cadherin and β-catenin expression was correlated in stage I NSCLC, indicating tumor cell dedifferentiation.[110] Furthermore, the authors found that reduced β-catenin expression correlated with poor recurrence-free survival in stage I adenocarcinomas.[110]

Nakashima et al., examining 150 NSCLC patients, found that E-cadherin expression and tumor vascularity were significant prognostic factors.[131] The authors also noted that N-cadherin expression was associated with tumor angiogenesis and that its expression was a prognostic factor in large cell NSCLC patients.[131]

Bremnes et al., reviewing the medical literature for the relevance of the E-cadherin–catenin adhesion complex in malignancy, concluded that inactivation of the complex, induced by genetic and epigenetic events, was important for multistage carcinogenesis, and it appeared to be associated with dedifferentiation, local invasion, regional metastases, and reduced survival in NSCLC patients.[132]

In a 2005 article reporting on mRNA expression and genetic structural analyses of the E-cadherin and *nm23* genes in 54 NSCLC patients and 46 normal lung controls, Chen et al. did not identify any E-cadherin or *nm23* genetic mutation; however, the authors noted that E-cadherin and *nm23* mRNA reduction was related to poor histologic differentiation, increased tumor stage, and increased lymph node metastases.[133] They concluded that E-cadherin and *nm23* dysfunction are important in NSCLC progression and that further understanding of their expression may provide information important for future treatment of NSCLC.[133]

Herbst et al. examined 60 stage I NSCLC cases for expression of E-cadherin, type IV collagenase (matrix metalloproteinase [MMP]-2 and MMP-9), the angiogenic molecules basic fibroblast growth factor VEGF/vascular permeability factor, and interleukin (IL)-8 by colorimetric in situ mRNA hybridization. They found higher ratios of type IV collagenase expression to E-cadherin expression (the MMP:E-cadherin ratio) in NSCLC patients with tumor recurrence versus patients who remained disease-free ($p = 0.00003$).[134] They also found that lower MMP:E-cadherin ratios (<2) were related to longer patient survival ($p = 0.0002$) and to a reduced rate of disease recurrence ($p = 0.0001$) and that the MMP:E-cadherin ratio was a significant prognostic factor when corrected for age ($p = 0.0001$).[134]

Kimura et al. studied the expression of S100A4 (a member of the S100 family that has been associated with a malignant phenotype, including cell motility), E-

cadherin, α-catenin, and β-catenin in 135 NSCLC cases.[135] The authors found that (1) S100A4 correlated with tumor progression ($p = <0.001$) and with lymph node metastases ($p = <0.05$);(2) E-cadherin expression was closely related to tumor differentiation and inversely associated with S100A4 expression;(3) α-catenin expression was related to lymph node metastases and decreased patient survival; and (4) patients with S100A4 positive/α-catenin negative tumor cell expression had significantly shorter survival than patients with S100A4 negative/α-catenin positive tumor cell expression.[135] They concluded that both S100A4 and α-catenin are important in NSCLC progression and metastasis, and their immunohistochemical detection may be helpful in defining a subpopulation of NSCLC patients with a poor prognosis.[135]

To determine the value of VEGF in NSCLC and its association with vascularity and E-cadherin expression, Stefanou et al. in 2003 examined 88 NSCLC cases and found that the simultaneous high VEGF expression and reduced E-cadherin expression correlated with tumor dedifferentiation and that reduced E-cadherin expression was associated with poor tumor differentiation.[136] The authors concluded that VEGF and E-cadherin evaluation may be helpful in determining the biologic behavior of NSCLC and provide therapeutically useful information.[136]

Shimamoto et al. examined 45 NSCLC patients for methylation status of p16[INK4a] and E-cadherin genes by methylation-specific PCR.[137] They found that E-cadherin gene inactivation by promoter methylation occurs in some epithelial cancers. Seventy-six percent of NSCLC patients had an abnormal methylation pattern in at least one gene. Although the authors identified no difference in overall patient survival between methylated and unmethylated p16[INK4a] patients, NSCLC patients with hypermethylation of both genes (concordant pattern) had a significantly better prognosis.[137] In contrast, NSCLC patients with hypermethylated p16[INK4a] but an unmethylated E-cadherin gene (discordant pattern) had a significantly worse prognosis.[137] The authors concluded that the methylation pattern of p16[INK4a] and E-cadherin may be of prognostic benefit for NSCLC patients.[137]

In a 2005 article, Tang et al., after examining 112 NSCLC cases and 30 benign pulmonary lesions immunohistochemically for *nm23*, E-cadherin, and β-catenin expression, found that downregulation of *nm23*, E-cadherin, and β-catenin was related to NSCLC metastases.[138] Qiao et al. examined 365 NSCLC cases via tissue microarray in 2005. They found that reduced E-cadherin expression was significantly related to lymph node metastases ($p = 0.001$), histologic dedifferentiation ($p = 0.010$), advanced clinical stage ($p = 0.024$), and poor prognosis ($p = 0.0001$). They concluded that E-cadherin dysfunction is important in lung cancer progression and that E-cadherin expression is an independent prognostic factor for NSCLC patients.[139]

Charalabopoulos et al. studied serum levels of soluble E-cadherin in 20 newly diagnosed NSCLC patients and 29 healthy volunteers and found that NSCLC patients had significantly increased circulating levels of soluble E-cadherin compared with healthy volunteers ($p = 0.001$).[140] The authors identified an association between serum soluble E-cadherin levels and distant metastases but not between increased levels and histologic type, gender, or smoking history.[140] The NSCLC patients in the study with increased soluble E-cadherin levels had a worse outcome, but the increased levels did not statistically represent an independent prognostic factor.[140] Continuing research regarding cadherins and their relationships to primary and metastatic lung cancer may allow for newer prognostic and therapeutic modalities for the treatment of NSCLC and SCLC.

Selectins

Although research regarding selectins and lung cancer is ongoing, the majority of the research has been performed in the realm of their activity in leukocytes. The selectin family of adhesion molecules, consisting of L-, E-, and P-selectin, has been studied predominantly by examination of the recruitment of leukocytes from the circulation.[4] Adhesion with selectins is calcium dependent, and the ligands are cell surface glycans possessing a specific sialyl-Lewis X–type structure also found in blood group antigens.[1,4] P-selectin binds to P-selectin glycoprotein ligand-1 (PSGL-1), L-selectin interacts with glycosylation-dependent cell adhesion molecule-1 and CD34, and E-selectin possibly reacts with E-selectin ligand-1.[4] Selectins, similar to IgCAMs, are expressed on cell surfaces in low levels.[4] P-selectin is recruited from storage in Weibel-Palade bodies to the cell surface after inflammatory stimuli activate cells, and E-selectin is synthesized and transported to the cell surface upon exposure to inflammatory mediators.[4,141] L-selectin, present on leukocyte surfaces, is shed from the cell surface into circulation.[4,142] Enhanced cell surface selectin expression is related to slowing and rolling of leukocytes at the endothelial cell wall.[4,143] Targeted disruption of P-selectin in mice confirms that the selectin–ligand interaction is vital for leukocyte recruitment from the circulation, and this step has been examined for possible therapeutic intervention for inflammatory diseases, with antibodies against selectins and against carbohydrate moieties used to block inflammatory cell recruitment in animal models.[4,143,144]

The selectin family of cell adhesion molecules interacts with their cognate glycoprotein ligands to mediate tethering, rolling, and weak adhesion.[145] The integrin family of cell adhesion molecules interacts with their ligands of the IgCAM superfamily to mediate firm adhesion and signal transduction, eventually triggering shape changes in the adherent leukocytes and transendothelial migration.[145] P-selectin rapidly translocates to the cell surface by exocytosis and mediates leukocyte rolling to the activated endothelial cells and heterotypic aggregation of activated platelets to leukocytes upon thrombogenic and inflammatory challenges.[145,146] P-selectin interacts with the leukocyte surface sialomucin PSGL-1, which is expressed on a variety of human leukocytes.[145] P-selectin has been found to bind to several human cancers and cancer cell lines, including NSCLC and SCLC, colon cancer, breast cancer, malignant melanoma, gastric cancer, and neuroblastoma.[145,147–149] Cells from the human malignant melanoma cell line NKI-4 bind P-selectin and express glycoprotein ligands for P-selectin that are functionally and structurally distinct from leukocyte PSGL-1.[145,149]

Research regarding lung cancer and selectins is limited compared to that relating to integrins and cadherins, but P Selectin has been shown to stain tissue section of human lung cancer.[145] Also, platelets attach in a P Selectin-dependent manner to NCI-H345 cells, a human SCLC cell line.[145,147] P selectin antibodies, but not E selectin antibodies, inhibit adhesion of human SCLC cells to activated human umbilical vein endothelial cells.[145,147] P selectin specifically mediates adhesion of NCI-H345 cells by interaction with glycoprotein ligands distinct from PSGL-1.[145]

Sialyl-Lewis X (sLe-X) and sialyl-Lewis A (sLe-A) are cancer-associated carbohydrate antigens involved in metastasis.[150] Both serve as ligands for P-, I-, and E-selectin that are found on the surfaces of platelets, leukocytes, and endothelial cells, and both mediate adhesion of tumor cells to endothelial cells.[150,151] Their importance in tumor metastasis is supported by the findings that (1) their antibodies block tumor cell adhesion on endothelial cells in vitro, (2) their expression is associated with an increased metastatic potential of tumor cells, and (3) their antibodies have inhibitory effects on angiogenesis.[150,152] Increased sLe-X and sLe-A antigen expression is often found in cancers, including lung cancer; however, despite correlations between their expression and poor prognosis in breast and colon cancers, such a prognostic correlation with lung cancer is controversial.[150,153]

Lung cancers that overexpress sialomucins (highly sialylated mucins) have been found to have an increased risk of recurrence and metastasis, and patients with sialomucin-expressing tumors tend to have postoperative relapses and poor prognosis despite attempted curative resection.[150,154] Sialomucin overexpression correlates with at least one mucin core peptide, MUC5AC apomucin, and its overexpression in cancer cells may guide the cancer cell's pattern of glycosylation and generate specific sialylated carbohydrate antigens, such as sLe-X and sLe-A, that mediate the cancer cell's metastatic or invasive behavior.[150,155] Yu et al., examining 61 stages I and II NSCLC patients immunohistochemically for sLe-X, sLe-A, and MUC5AC, found that expressions of sLe-X and MUC5AC were both associated with adenocarcinoma subtype and that NSCLCs with sLe-X and/or MUC5AC expression had an increased risk of postoperative distant metastases.[150] They also found that NSCLC patients with sLe-X expression or MUC5AC expression had overall survival. The authors concluded that sLe-X expression was related to MUC5AC protein and the expression was associated with worse survival.[150]

CD24, a ligand of P-selectin, is a gene that is expressed in developing and regenerating tissue, as well as leukocytes, keratinocytes, and renal tubules.[156] It is expressed in cancers not only in hematologic malignancies but also in a variety of solid tumors, including renal cell cancer, SCLC, nasopharyngeal cancer, liver cancer, urinary bladder cancer, glioma, breast cancer, and ovarian cancer.[156] Investigating the status of *CD24* in NSCLC patients, Kristiansen et al. examined 89 NSCLC patients immunohistochemically with monoclonal CD24 antibody and found that high *CD24* expression in NSCLC correlated with significantly shorter survival ($p = 0.033$) and that *CD24* expression and tumor stage and grade were independent prognostic factors for NSCLC patients.[156] The authors concluded that the decreased survival of NSCLC patients with strong CD24 tumor cell positivity may be related to an enhanced propensity for P-selectin–mediated hematogenous metastasis formation.[156]

E-selectin is the endothelial ligand for sialyl carbohydrate antigens expressed on the surface of tumor cells.[157] Its secretion is reportedly stimulated by tumor cells, and serum titers have correlated with prognosis in breast cancer patients and, in a limited number of studies, in NSCLC patients.[157–159] D'Amico et al. studied preoperative and postoperative serum levels of E-selectin, CD44, basic epidermal growth factor, hepatocyte growth factor, basic fibroblast growth factor, urokinase plasminogen activator, and urokinase plasminogen activator receptor by enzyme-linked immunosorbent assay.[157] The authors found that decreasing serum E-selectin levels and increasing CD44 and urokinase plasminogen activator receptor levels were significantly associated with increased recurrence risk.[157] CD44 is further discussed later.

P-selectin, present on activated platelets and endothelial cells after thrombogenic and inflammatory challenges, interacts with cancer cells in a manner that promotes tumor metastasis.[160,161] Although P selectin has several roles in tumor metastasis, its role in the initial step of metastasis, compared with other adhesion molecules, is singular and necessary for the metastatic process.[160,162] As such, interference with the P-selectin–tumor cell interaction may attenuate the ability for long-term organ colonization with tumor cells.[160] Heparin, aside from its anticoagulant effects, interferes with tumor cell–platelet association via antiplatelet agents targeted to P-selectin–mediated interaction has been shown to potentially

inhibit both spontaneous and experimental metastasis in vivo; however, the bleeding risk from heparin administration is significant.[160] Modified heparins, with diminished anticoagulant activity but with retained antimetastatic properties, have recently been developed; however, their evaluation with respect to NSCLC is limited.[160] Gao et al., using a large cell NSCLC cell line, NCI H460, and a lung adenocarcinoma cell line, SPC-A-1, examined the interaction of NSCLC cells with P-selectin and modified heparins and found that the administration of modified heparin can reduce P-selectin binding with NSCLC cells with a capacity similar to that of heparin.[160] The P-selectin binding with NSCLC cells involved heparin sulfate-like proteoglycans on the tumor cell surfaces.[160] The authors concluded that modified heparins may be of potential antimetastatic value for P-selectin–mediated NSCLC metastasis.[160] Although research regarding selectins and lung cancer is relatively limited compared with the cadherins and integrins, continued study of the selectins and their interactions with primary and metastatic lung cancers could provide insight into potentially more effective lung cancer therapies.

Immunoglobulin-Like Cell Adhesion Molecules

Less research has been performed regarding IgCAMs and lung cancer than regarding the more widely studied cellular adhesion molecule superfamilies such as integrins and cadherins. The IgCAMs are a superfamily of cell adhesion molecules that have diverse structures and functions but that all contain one or more of a common Ig-like repeat characterized by two cysteines separated by 55 to 75 amino acids.[4,163] The Ig-like domains are expressed on the extracellular domain of the protein, and typically these molecules span the cell membrane and contain only a short cytoplasmic tail.[4,163] The molecules are important in nervous system development, embryonic development, and immune and inflammatory responses.[4,163,164]

Neural cell adhesion molecules (NCAM) are critical for the preservation and integrity of the nervous system.[4,164] The IgCAM intercellular cell adhesion molecules (ICAMs) are important for cellular adhesion in the immune system. The ICAMs, including vascular cell adhesion molecule-1 (VCAM-1) and mucosal addressin cell adhesion molecule-1 (MAdCAM-1) serve as ligands for integrins.[4,142,143] Platelet-endothelial cell adhesion molecule (PECAM), another IgCAM, is vital for leukocyte adhesion and is important in cell–cell contact to promote adhesion between endothelial cells and leukocytes.[4] Modulation in ICAM expression may help regulate the type of leukocyte recruited to an area of inflammation and the temporal pattern of leukocyte recruitment.[4,142]

Alveolar macrophages may be important in the immune response to lung cancer.[165] Some authors have found NSCLC-associated alveolar macrophages to correlate positively with tumor regression, whereas other authors have found the presence of NSCLC-associated alveolar macrophages to be related to increased microvessel counts and a poorer prognosis.[165,166] Pouniotis et al. examined bronchoalveolar lavage specimens from NSCLC and SCLC patients and controls. They found that ICAM-1 surface expression was decreased on alveolar macrophages in NSCLC and SCLC patients, except for adenocarcinoma patients, and concluded that there are type-specific alterations in uptake ability, cytokine secretion, and phenotype in alveolar macrophages from lung cancer patients that may cause an inability to stimulate antitumor immunity.[165]

Intercellular cell adhesion molecule-3, found on leukocytes and endothelial cells, interacts with lymphocyte function-associated antigen-1 and is involved in leukocyte intercellular adhesion.[167] It may also be important for angiogenesis and may play a role in tumor progression, as studies have shown a relationship between ICAM-3 and some diseases.[167,168] Radiation-resistant cervical cancer cases have shown increased ICAM-3 expression in tumor stromal endothelial cells and lymphocytes.[167,169] Kim et al., examining H1299 human lung cancer cell line cells in an attempt to determine the ICAM-3–activated downstream pathway in the cells, found that ICAM-3 expression induces cancer cell proliferation, and an increased ICAM-3 expression contributes to cancer progression.[167]

Some adhesion molecules serve not only as adhesion substances but also as regulators of other cell functions by influencing signaling, a process termed "outside-to-in signaling."[170] β_1-Integrins, β_2-integrins, and CD28 induce costimulatory signals in the binding of T cells to antigen-presenting cells via multiple cellular signaling molecules, including focal adhesion kinases, causing cell activation and cytokine production.[170,171] Adhesion molecules are regulated by intracellular signaling induced by various cellular stimuli in the process termed "inside-to-out signaling."[170] Intercellular cell adhesion molecule-3 expression is highly regulated by locally produced inflammatory cytokines such as IL-1β, tumor necrosis factor-α, IL-6, and interferon-γ.[170,172] The ICAM-1/leukocyte function–associated antigen-1 pathway regulates important cell–cell interactions such as leukocyte adhesion and migration, including tumor cell killing by natural killer cells and cytotoxic T lymphocytes.[170,173] Although several tumor cells highly express ICAM-1, a potent ligand for leukocyte function–associated antigen-1 on cytotoxic T lymphocytes in vitro, many tumor cells remain viable against killing by cytotoxic T lymphocytes in vivo.[170] Examining 11 human lung cancer cell lines, Yasuda et al. hypothesized that β_1-integrin engagement by matrix proteins

potentially occurs in lung cancer cells in vivo and that continuous β_1-integrin stimulation reduces ICAM-1 expression, ICAM-1–mediated adhesion of cancer cells to cytotoxic T lymphocytes, and cytotoxic T-lymphocyte killing of those cancer cells.[170] Furthermore, such processes may lead to escape of lung cancer cells in vivo from immunologic surveillance.[170] The authors based their hypothesis on the findings that (1) β_1-integrin engagement on certain lung cancer cells by a specific antibody or by ligand matrixes such as fibronectin or collagen—extracellular matrix proteins that surround cancer cells, including lung cancer cells—markedly reduced ICAM-1 expression on the cell surface and induced soluble ICAM-1;(2) ICAM-1 downregulation by β_1-integrin stimulation was abrogated by tyrosine kinase inhibitors or by transfection of dominant negative truncations of focal adhesion kinase;(3) β_1-integrin stimulation reduced ICAM-1–dependent adhesion of lung cancer cells to T cells, a process completely inhibited by tyrosine kinase inhibitors and by transfection of dominant negative forms of focal adhesion kinase; and (4) β_1-integrin stimulation prevented lung cancer cell killing by autologous cytotoxic T lymphocytes.[170]

Human Vα24+Vβ11+natural killer T cell (Vα cell) activation induces effective antitumor responses with secondary immune effects via activation of natural killer cells and conventional T cells.[174] Konishi et al., in a 2004 study analyzing the characteristics of human natural killer T cells in lung cancer patients, found that ICAM-1 expression on tumor cells is associated with Vα cell cytotoxicity, suggesting that Vα cells may be important in antitumor response to lung cancer.[174]

Zhang et al. examined VEGF expression and ICAM-1 expression in 86 NSCLC patients and found that positive VEGF expression was significantly positively related, and ICAM-1 expression was significantly negatively related, to lymph node metastases, tumor stage, prognosis, and hematogenous tumor metastases.[175] Patients with both positive VEGF expression and negative ICAM-1 expression had the lowest 5-year survival rates of the patients.[175] The authors concluded that VEGF and ICAM-1 expressions correlate with malignant behavior in NSCLC and that they may be important in NSCLC development and metastases.[175]

Noting that ICAM-1 expression has been identified in colon cancer, lung cancer, bladder cancer, melanoma, pancreatic cancer, and hepatocellular cancer, Shin et al. in a 2004 study examined serum ICAM-1 in 84 NSCLC patients and identified no difference in serum ICAM-1 concentrations in different stages of lung cancer and no difference among the histologic types of NSCLC.[176] They found that overall survival times of NSCLC patients with low (<306 ng/mL) concentrations of serum ICAM-1 tended to be longer than those of patients with higher serum ICAM-1 concentrations and concluded that high serum ICAM-1 levels portended a poor prognosis for NSCLC patients.[176]

Osaki et al. measured serum concentrations of soluble ICAM-1 in 80 NSCLC patients and found that the concentrations were significantly positively correlated with tumor size ($p = 0.002$) and that overall patient survival tended to be longer for patients with low (<306 ng/mL) serum concentrations of ICAM-1.[177] The authors concluded that serum ICAM-1 might be a useful diagnostic marker or monitoring marker for NSCLC patients.[177]

Impairment of alveolar macrophages in vitro cytotoxicity and tumoricidal function in lung cancer patients has been reported in several studies.[178] Dabrowska et al. cultured cells from 13 NSCLC patients, 6 patients with nonmalignant pulmonary disease, and 6 healthy volunteers to evaluate the expression of ICAM-1 by flow cytometry on alveolar macrophages after interferon-γ stimulation. They found that interferon-γ increased alveolar macrophage ICAM-1 expression in all patient groups ($p = 0.05$).[178] The degree of increase in alveolar macrophage ICAM-1 expression was significantly lower in NSCLC patients ($p = 0.002$) than in other patients ($p = 0.022$) and healthy volunteers ($p = 0.002$).[178] The authors hypothesized that the impaired reactivity of alveolar macrophage ICAM-1 expression after interferon-γ stimulation in NSCLC patients might be associated with functional defects in alveolar macrophages in those patients.[178] Ongoing research into the IgCAMs and their associations with other molecular pathway components such as VGFR and focal adhesion kinase, as well as their interactions with T lymphocytes, alveolar macrophages, and other immune system components, may one day lead to the development of better prognostic markers and targeted therapies for lung cancer patients.

CD44

CD44 is a relatively recent addition to the cellular adhesion molecule superfamily, and research regarding CD44 and lung cancer is limited. CD44, a transmembrane protein on cell surfaces, is distributed extensively and can be detected on lymphocytes and fibroblasts.[179] CD44 is a principal cell surface receptor for hyaluronan, a major extracellular matrix component, and it communicates cell–matrix interactions into cells via "outside-in signaling."[180] CD44 assists in cell–cell interactions and cell–matrix interactions. It has been identified in several isoforms on tumor cells, and serum levels have been shown to be prognostically relevant in stomach cancer patients.[157,181] Tumor expression of CD44 has been found to be an independent predictor of cancer recurrence with both colorectal cancer and NSCLC.[157,182] Several isoforms are expressed by tumor cells, and serum levels have been reported to have prognostic significance in gastric

cancer.[157] CD44v expression, related to tumor progression, metastasis, and prognosis, has been detected in cancers of the lung, colon, esophagus, liver, cervix, and kidney, as well as reticulosarcoma.[179]

The secretion of E-selectin, an endothelial ligand for sialyl carbohydrate antigens expressed on the surface of tumor cells, is reportedly stimulated by tumor cells, and serum E-selectin titers have reportedly correlated with prognosis in breast cancer and, in a few small studies, in NSCLC.[157] D'Amico et al. examined serial serum samples from 196 stage I NSCLC patients and found that decreasing serum E-selectin levels ($p = 0.002$), increasing serum C44 levels ($p = 0.001$), and increasing serum urokinase plasminogen activator receptor ($p = 0.003$) predicted NSCLC recurrence before clinical or radiographic determination.[157] Future research regarding such markers might one day allow for the prediction of NSCLC recurrence in patients who have undergone resection therapy so that earlier and improved systemic therapy might be provided.

Noting that surgical manipulation of lung cancers may increase circulating tumor cells and contribute to metastatic recurrence after resection, and that COX-2 is overexpressed in most NSCLCs and upregulated the cell adhesion receptor CD44, Backhus et al. examined human NSCLC cells with a murine model of tumor metastasis to determine the effects of perioperative COX blockade on the metastatic potential of circulating tumor cells, CD44 expression, and cancer cell adhesion to extracellular matrix.[183] The authors found that the COX inhibitor celecoxib significantly reduced establishment of metastases by circulating tumor cells in the murine model and also inhibited CD44 expression and extracellular matrix adhesion in vitro. These results suggest that perioperative modulation of COX-2 may minimize the risk of perioperative circulating tumor cell metastases.[183]

Lee et al. studied 52 NSCLCs and found that lung adenocarcinoma recurrence was associated with negative expression of CD44v6–10 or CD44v3–10 mRNA and with low-level expression of CD44v6 or CD44v3 by immunohistochemistry.[184] Furthermore, negative CD44v6 mRNA expression and reduced CD44v6 protein expression were associated with decreased disease-free and overall survival rates for NSCLC patients, suggesting that CD44 splicing pattern is associated with lung adenocarcinoma disease progression.[184]

Tumor cells are surrounded in vivo by, and encounter, extracellular matrix components such as hyaluronan primarily through CD44 on the cell surface, indicating that engagement of CD44 by extracellular matrix always occurs on tumor cells.[185] CD44 is a transmembrane glycoprotein involved in various cell adhesion events, including lymphocyte migration, early hematopoiesis, and tumor metastasis.[185,186] Many primary carcinoma tissues express CD44 at high levels.[185] Studying 11 lung cancer cell lines,

Yasuda et al. identified CD44 at high levels of expression in lung cancer cells and found that engagement of CD44 by a specific antibody or potent ligand hyaluronan reduced Fas expression and Fas-mediated apoptosis of lung cancer cells. These results suggest that continuous stimulation of tumor cells by hyaluronan—abundantly present around tumor cells in vivo—primarily by CD44, leads to immune escape from cytotoxic T-lymphocyte–dependent killing in vivo.[185]

Noting that CD44 expression has been shown to be important for tumor progression in human breast cancer, colon cancer, melanoma, lymphoma, gastric cancer, and lung cancer, Suzuki and Yamashiro studied 93 Japanese lung adenocarcinoma patients and found that reduced expression of CD44v3 and CD44v6 were associated with invasion in lung adenocarcinoma.[187]

CD44, expressed in a large number of normal and malignant tissues, interacts with its ligands hyaluronate and osteopontin and is involved in lymphocyte homing, as well as T-lymphocyte activation and tumor metastasis.[188] Several CD44 isoforms have been identified, arising from mRNA alternative spicing, with CD44s, also termed CD44h, being the isoform expressed with hematopoietic cells, fibroblasts, glial cells, and melanoma cells.[188] The isoform generally identified on epithelial cells and epithelial tumor cells is high-molecular-weight CD44, containing one or more alternatively spliced exons.[188] CD44 isoform alterations are associated with the transformation of normal cells into cancer cells.[188] CD44 isoforms, including high-molecular-weight CD44 isoforms such as CD44v6, have been shown to be overexpressed in NSCLC.[188] CD44 isoform function in tumors varies with the organ involved.[188] CD44s overexpression in melanoma and lymphoma enhances tumorigenicity, whereas upregulation of CD44s in colon cancer reduces tumorigenicity.[188] CD44 expression reduction in NSCLC has been shown to be associated with lymph node metastases and shortened disease-free survival.[188]

Takahashi et al., investigating the role of CD44s downregulation in NSCLC cell culture cells, found that enhanced susceptibility of the cells to activated macrophage toxicity was mediated by the interaction between CD44s expression on the tumor cells and osteopontin produced by activated alveolar macrophages.[188] The authors concluded that the CD44s isoform is significantly downregulated in NSCLC compared with normal lung tissue and may confer a protective advantage to NSCLC cells by allowing escape from tumoricidal effector cells, including activated alveolar macrophages.[188] Continuing research concerning the interactions between CD44 and alveolar macrophages might give insights for newer therapeutic regimens to enhance patient alveolar macrophage response to lung cancer.

The interplay between CD44 and extracellular matrix proteins such as osteopontin may regulate osteoclastic motility, responsible for osteolytic metastases.[189] In a 2006 study, Li et al., using human SCLC cells injected into nude mice and examining them for metastatic lesions, concluded that osteoclasts play an important role in degrading unmineralized extracellular matrixes in lung cancer cell bone metastases. They also found that osteopontin may facilitate osteoclastic migration in the metastasis by mediating its affinity to CD44 on the osteoclast cell membrane, leading to immediate osteolysis.[189] Further research regarding the association between CD44 and osteolysis might be valuable in providing improved therapies targeted toward metastatic disease in SCLC and other lung cancers.

Conclusion

Research continues regarding the various mechanisms of action of each of the cell adhesion molecules, and their interactions with other molecular pathways, in the development and spread of lung cancer. New and effective prognostic markers and therapeutic regimens to benefit lung cancer patients will hopefully result from this work.

References

1. Aplin AE, Howe A, Alahari SK, Juliano RL. Signal transduction and signal modulation by cell adhesion receptors: the role of integrins, cadherins, immunoglobulin-cell adhesion molecules, and selectins. Pharmacol Rev 1998; 50:197–263.
2. Gumbiner BM. Cell adhesion: the molecular basis of tissue architecture and morphogenesis. Cell 1996;84:345–357.
3. Gogali A, Charalabopoulos K, Constantopoulos S. Integrin receptors in primary lung cancer. Exp Oncol 2004; 26:106–110.
4. Petruzzelli L, Takami M, Humes HD. Structure and function of cell adhesion molecules. Am J Med 1999;106:467–476.
5. Nair KS, Naidoo R, Chetty R. Expression of cell adhesion molecules in oesophageal carcinoma and its prognostic value. J Clin Pathol 2005;58:343–351.
6. Charalabopoulos K, Gogali A, Kostoula OK, Constantopoulos SH. Cadherin superfamily of adhesion molecules in primary lung cancer. Exp Oncol 2004;26:256–260.
7. Meyer T, Hart IR. Mechanisms of tumour metastasis. Eur J Cancer 1998;34:214–221.
8. Rosales C, O'Brian V, Kornberg L, Juliano RL. Signal transduction by cell adhesion receptors. Biochim Biophys Acta 1995;1242:77–98.
9. Nicolson GL. Cancer metastasis: tumor cell and host organ properties important in metastasis to specific secondary sites. Biochim Biophys Acta 1988;948:175–224.
10. Han SW, Roman J. COX-2 inhibitors suppress integrin $\alpha 5$ expression in human lung carcinoma cells through activation of Erk: Involvement of Sp1 and AP-1 sites. Int J Cancer 2005;116:536–546.

11. Watt FM. Role of integrins in regulating epidermal adhesion, growth and differentiation. EMBO J 2002;21: 3919–3926.

12. Okegawa T, Li Y, Pong RC, Hsieh JT. Cell adhesion proteins as tumor suppressors. J Urol 2002;167:1836–1843.

13. Mukhopadhyay NK, Gordon GJ, Chen CJ, et al. Activation of focal adhesion kinase in human lung cancer cells involves multiple and potentially parallel signaling events. J Cell Mol Med 2005;9:387–397.

14. Damjanovich L, Albelda SM, Mette SA. Distribution of integrin cell adhesion receptors in normal and malignant lung tissue. Am J Respir Cell Mol Biol 1992;6:197–206.

15. Hanby AN, Gilet CE, Pignatelli M, Stamp GW. Beta1 and beta4 integrin expression in metacarn and formalin fixed material from in situ ductal carcinoma of the breast. J Pathol 1993;171:257–262.

16. Kitayama J, Nayawa H, Nakayama H, et al. Functional expression of beta1 and beta2 integrins on tumor infiltrating lymphocytes (TILs) in colorectal cancer. J Gastroenterol 1999;34:327–333.

17. Bankhof H, Stein V, Remberger K. differential expression of a6 and a2 very late-antigen integrins in the normal, hyperplastic and neoplastic prostate. Hum Pathol 1993;24: 243–248.

18. Damkisson YP, Wilding JC, Filipe M, Hall PA, Pignatelli M. Cell–matrix interactions in gastric carcinoma. J Pathol 1993;169:120.

19. Elenrieder V, Alder G, Gress TM. Invasion and metastasis in pancreatic cancer. Ann Oncol 1999;4:46–50.

20. Volpes R, Van der Oord J, Pesmet VJ. Distribution of the VLA family of integrins in normal and pathological human liver tissue. Gastroenterology 1991;101:200–206.

21. Bichler KH, Wechsel HW. The problematic nature of metastasized cell carcinoma. Anticancer Res 1999;19: 1463–1466.

22. Stamb GW, Pignatelli M. Distribution of β1, α1, α2 and α3 integrin chains in basal cell carcinomas. J Pathol 1991;103: 307–313.

23. Strobel T, Cannisha SA. Beta-1 integrins partly mediate binding of ovarian cancer cells to perimetral mesothelium in vitro. Gynecol Oncol 1999;73:362–367.

24. Vessey BA, Albelda S, Buck CA, et al. distribution of integrin cell adhesion molecules in endometrial cancer. Am J Pathol 1995;146:717–726.

25. Yamada KM, Kennedy DW, Yamada SS, et al. Monoclonal antibody and synthetic peptide inhibitors of human tumor cell migration. Cancer Res 1990;50:4485–4496.

26. Rostagno C, Felini M, Gensimn GF. Hemostatic vascular interactives in the pathogenesis and the treatment of adult respiratory distress syndrome. Ann Hal Med Int 1994;9: 236–232.

27. Chen FA, Alosco T, Croy BA, et al. Clones of tumor cells derived from single primary human lung tumor reveal different patterns of beta1 integrin expression. Cell Adhes Commun 1994;2:345–357.

28. Virtanen I, Laitinen A, Tani T, et al. Differential expression of laminins and their integrin receptors in developing and adult human lung. Am J Respir Cell Mol Biol 1996;15:184–196.

29. Smythe WR, LeBel E, Bavaria JE, et al. Integrin expression in non small cell carcinoma of the lung. Cancer Metastasis Rev 1995;14:229–239.

30. Bredin CG, Sundqvist KG, Hauzenberger D, Klominek J. Integrin dependent migration of lung cancer cells to extracellular matrix components. Eur Respir J 1998;11:400–407.

31. Bartolazzi A, Cerboni C, Flammini G, et al. Expression of α3β1 integrin receptor and its ligands in human lung tumors. Int J Cancer 1995;64:248–252.

32. Barr L, Campbell S, Bochner B, Dang C. Association of the decreased expression of the α3β1 integrin with the altered cell: environmental interactions and enhanced soft agar cloning ability of c-myc–overexpressing small cell lung cancers. Cancer Res 1998;58:5537–5545.

33. Hartmann TJ, Burger JA, Gloded A, Fujii N, Burger M. CXCR4 chemokine receptor and integrin signaling cooperate in mediating adhesion and chemoresistance in small cell lung cancer (SCLC) cells. Oncogene 2005;24:4462–4471.

34. Phillips RJ, Burdick MD, Lutz M, et al. The stromal derived factor-1/CXCL12–CXC chemokine receptor 4 biological axis in non–small cell lung cancer metastases. Am J Respir Crit Care Med 2003;15:1676–1686.

35. Laga AC, Zander DS, Cagle PT. Prognostic significance of cyclooxygenase 2 expression in 259 cases of non–small cell lung cancer. Arch Pathol Lab Med 2005;129:1113–1117.

36. Castelao JE, Bard FD III, DiPerna CA, Sievers EM, Bremner RM. Lung cancer and cyclooxygenase-2. Ann Thorac Surg 2003;76:1327–1335.

37. Liao Z, Komaki R, Mason KA, Milas L. Role of cyclooxygenase-2 inhibitors in combination with radiation therapy in lung cancer. Clin Lung Cancer 2003;4:356–365.

38. Masferrer JL, Leahy KM, Koki AT, et al. Antiangiogenic and antitumor activities of cyclooxygenase-2 inhibitors. Cancer Res 2000;60:1306–1311.

39. Aktorki NK, Keresztes RS, Port JL, et al. Celecoxib, a selective cyclo-oxygenase-2 inhibitor, enhances the response to preoperative paclitaxel and carboplatin in early-stage non–small-cell lung cancer. J Clin Oncol 2003;21:2645–2650.

40. Jendrosek V, Handrick R, Belka C. Celecoxib activates a novel mitochondrial apoptosis signaling pathway. FASEB J 2003;17:1547–1549.

41. Wong BC, Jiang XH, Lin MC, et al. Cyclooxygenase-2 inhibitor (SC-236) suppresses activator protein-1 through c-Jun NH2-terminal kinase. Gastroenterology 2004;126: 136–147.

42. Rajeswari J, Pande G. The significance of alpha 5 beta 1 integrin dependent and independent actin cytoskeleton organization in cell transformation and survival. Cell Biol Int 2002;26:1043–1055.

43. Tani N, Higashiyama S, Kawaguchi N, et al. Expression level of integrin alpha 5 on tumour cells affects the rate of metastasis to the kidney. Br J Cancer 2003;88:327–333.

44. Adachi M, Taki T, Higashiyama M, et al. Significance of integrin alpha5 gene expression as a prognostic factor in node-negative non–small cell lung cancer. Clin Cancer Res 2000;6:96–101.

45. Liotta LA, Stetler-Stevenson WG. Tumor invasion and metastasis: an imbalance of positive and negative regulation. Cancer Res 1991;51:5054–5049.

46. Furuta SM, Ilic D, Kanazawa S, et al. Mesodermal defect in late phase of gastrulation by a targeted mutation of focal adhesion kinase FAK. Oncogene 1995;11:1989–1995.

47. Carelli S, Zadra G, Vaira V, et al. Up-regulation of focal adhesion kinase in non–small cell lung cancer. Lung Cancer 2006;53:263–271.

48. Sanders MA, Basson MD. Collagen IV–dependent ERK activation in human Caco-2 intestinal epithelial cells requires focal adhesion kinase. J Biol Chem 2000;275:38040–38047.

49. Guan JL, Shalloway D. Regulation of pp1256FAK both by cellular adhesion and by oncogenic transformation. Nature 1992;358:690–692.

50. Mukhopadhyay NK, Gillchrist D, Gordon JG, et al. Integrin dependent tyrosine phosphorylation is a key regulatory event in collagen IV mediated adhesion and proliferation of human lung cancer cell line Calu-1. Ann Thorac Surg 2004;78:450–457.

51. Lau D, Guo L, Liu R, Marik J, Lam K. Peptide ligands targeting integrin α3β1 in non–small cell lung cancer. Lung Cancer 2006;52:291–297.

52. Lynch T, Bell D, Sordella R, et al. Activating mutations in the epidermal growth factor receptor underlying responsiveness of non–small-cell lung cancer to gefitinib. N Engl J Med 2004;350:2129–2139.

53. Shepherd FA, Pereira JR, Ciuleanu T, et al. Erlotinib in previously treated non–small-cell lung cancer. N Engl J Med 2005;353:123–132.

54. Giancotti FG, Rouslahti E. Integrin signaling. Science 1999;285:1028–1032.

55. Albert JM, Cao C, Geng L, et al. Integrin alpha(v)beta(3) antagonist cilengitide enhances efficacy of radiotherapy in endothelial cell and non–small-cell lung cancer models. Int J Radiat Oncol Biol Phys 2006;65:1536–1543.

56. Boelens MC, van den Berg A, Vogelzang I, et al. Differential expression and distribution of epithelial adhesion molecules in non–small cell lung cancer and normal bronchus. J Clin Pathol 2006 Feb 17; [Epub ahead of print].

57. Hodkinson PS, Elliott T, Wong WS, et al. ECM overrides DNA damage-induced cell cycle arrest and apoptosis in small Erlotinib cell lung cancer cells through beta1 integrin Erlotinib dependent activation of PI3-kinase. Cell Death Differ 2006;Jan 27; [Epub ahead of print].

58. Oshita F, Ito H, Idehara M, et al. Prognostic impact of survivin, cyclin D1, integrin beta1, and VEGF in patients with small adenocarcinoma of stage I lung cancer. Am J Clin Oncol 2004;27:425–428.

59. Mousa S, Mousa SA. Cellular and molecular mechanisms of nicotine's pro-angiogenesis activity and its potential impact on cancer. J Cell Biochem 2006;97:1370–1378.

60. Villablanca AC. Nicotine stimulates DNA synthesis and proliferation in vascular endothelial cells in vitro. J Appl Physiol 1998;84:2089–2098.

61. Macklin KD, Maus AD, Pereira EF, Albuquerque EX, Conti-Fine BM. Human vascular endothelial cells express functional nicotinic acetylcholine receptors. J Pharmacol Exp Ther 1998;287:435–439.

62. Ruegg C, Mariotti A. Vascular integrins: pleiotropic adhesion and signaling molecules in vascular homeostasis and angiogenesis. Cell Mol Life Sci 2003;60:1135–1157.

63. Takeichi M. Cadherin cell adhesion receptors as morphogenetic regulator. Science 1991;251:1451–1459.

64. Kemler R. From cadherins to catenins: cytoplasmic protein interactions and regulation of cell adhesion. Trends Genet 1993;9:317–321.

65. Ozawa M, Baribault H, Kemler R. The cytoplasmic domain of the cell adhesion molecule uvamorulin associates with three independent proteins structurally related in different species. EMBO J 1989;8:1711–1717.

66. Hirano S, Kinoto N, Shimoyama Y, Hirohashi S, Takeichi M. Identification of a neural α-catenin as a key regulator of cadherin function and multicellular organization. Cell 1992;70:293–301.

67. Breier G, Breviario F, Caveda L, et al. Molecular cloning and expression of murine vascular endothelial cadherin in early stage development of cardiovascular system. Blood 1996;87:630–641.

68. Mayer B, Johnson JP, Leitl F, et al. E-cadherin expression in primary and metastatic gastric cancer: down-regulation correlates with cellular dedifferentiation and glandular disintegration. Cancer Res 1993;53:1690–1695.

69. Schipper JH, Frixen UH, Behrens J, et al. E-cadherin expression in squamous cell carcinomas of head and neck: inverse correlation with tumor dedifferentiation and lymph node metastasis. Cancer Res 1991;51:6328–6337.

70. Bringuier PP, Umbas R, Schaafsma HE, et al. Decreased E-cadherin immunoreactivity correlates with poor survival in patients with bladder tumors. Cancer Res 1993;53:2341–2345.

71. Dorudi S, Sheffield JP, Poulsom R, Northover JM, Hart IR. E-cadherin expression in colorectal cancer. An immunocytochemical and in situ hybridization study. Am J Pathol 1993;142:981–986.

72. Oka H, Shiozaki H, Kobayashi K, et al. Expression of E-cadherin cell adhesion molecules in human breast cancer tissues and its relationship to metastasis. Cancer Res 1993;53:1696–1701.

73. Ochiai A, Akimoto S, Shimoyama Y, et al. Frequent loss of α-catenin expression in scirrhous carcinomas with scattered cell growth. Jpn J Cancer Res 1994;85:266–273.

74. Kadowaki T, Shiozaki H, Inoue M, et al. E-cadherin and α-catenin expression in human esophageal cancer. Cancer Res 1994;54:291–296.

75. Takayama T, Shinozaki H, Shibamoto S, et al. β-Catenin expression in human cancer. Am J Pathol 1996;148:39–46.

76. Nawrocki-Raby B, Gilles C, Polette M, et al. Upregulation of MMPs by soluble E-cadherin in human lung tumor cells. Int J Cancer 2003;105:790–795.

77. Kato Y, Hirano T, Yoshida K, et al. Frequent loss of E-cadherin and/or catenins in intrabronchial lesions during carcinogenesis of the bronchial epithelium. Lung Cancer 2005;48:323–330.

78. Takeichi M. Functional correlation between cell adhesive properties and some cell surface proteins. J Cell Biol 1997;75:464–474.

79. Hirano S, Nose A, Hatta K, et al. Calcium dependent cell–cell adhesion molecules (cadherins). J Cell Biol 1987;105:2501–2510.

80. Behrens J, Mareel MM, Van Roy FM, Birchmeier W. Dissecting tumor cell invasion: epithelial cells acquire invasive properties after the loss of uvomorulin-mediated cell–cell adhesion. J Cell Biol 1989;108:2435–2447.

81. Frixen UH, Behrens J, Sachs M, Et al. E-cadherin–mediated cell–cell adhesion prevents invasiveness of human carcinoma cells. J Cell Biol 1991;113:173–185.

82. Vleminckx K, Vakaet Jr L, Mareel M, Fiers W, Van Roy F. Genetic manipulation of E-cadherin expression by epithelial tumor cells reveals an invasion suppressor role. Cell 1991;66:107–119.

83. Hirohashi S. Inactivation of the E-cadherin–mediated cell adhesion system in human cancers. Am J Pathol 1998;153:333–339.

84. Akimoto S, Ochiai A, Inomata M, Hirohashi S. Expression of cadherin–catenin cell adhesion molecules, phosphorylated tyrosine residues and growth factor receptor–tyrosine kinases in gastric cancer. Jpn J Cancer Res 1998;89:829–836.

85. Shimoyama Y, Nagafuchi A, Fujita S, et al. Cadherin dysfunction in a human cancer line: possible involvement of loss of α-catenin expression in reduced cell–cell adhesiveness. Cancer Res 1992;52:5770–5774.

86. Oda T, Kanai Y, Shimoyama Y, et al. Cloning of the human α-catenin cDNA and its aberrant mRNA in a human cancer cell line. Biochem Biophys Res Commun 1993;193:897–904.

87. Shimoyama Y, Hirohashi S, Hirano S, et al. Cadherin cell-adhesion molecules in human epithelial tissue and carcinomas. Cancer Res 1989;49:2128–2133.

88. Shimoyama Y, Hirohashi S. Cadherin intercellular adhesion molecule in hepatocellular carcinomas: loss of E-cadherin expression in an undifferentiated carcinoma. Cancer Lett 1991;57:131–135.

89. Shimoyama Y, Hirohashi S. Expression of E- and P-cadherin in gastric carcinomas. Cancer Res 1991;51:2185–2192.

90. Kadowaki T, Shiozaki H, Inoue M, et al. E-cadherin and α-catenin expression in human esophageal cancer. Cancer Res 1994;54:291–296.

91. Mattijssen V, Peters HM, Schalwijk L, et al. E-cadherin expression in head and neck squamous-cell carcinoma is associated with clinical outcome. Int J Cancer 1993;55:580–585.

92. Umbas R, Isaacs WB, Bringuier PP, et al. Decreased E-cadherin expression is associated with poor prognosis in prostate cancer. Cancer Res 1994;15:3929–3933.

93. Nakanishi Y, Ochiai A, Akimoto S, et al. Expression of E-cadherin, α-catenin, β-catenin, and plakoglobin in esophageal carcinomas and its prognostic significance: immunohistochemical analysis of 96 lesions. Oncology 1997;54:158–165.

94. Oyama T, Kanai Y, Ochiai A, et al. A truncated β-catenin disrupts the interaction between E-cadherin and α-catenin: a cause of loss of intercellular adhesiveness in human cancer cell lines. Cancer Res 1994;54:6282–6287.

95. Hoschuetzky H, Aberle H, Kemler R. β-Catenin mediates the interaction of the cadherin–catenin complex with epidermal growth factor receptor. J Cell Biol 1994;127:1375–1380.

96. Ochiai A, Akimoto S, Kanai Y, et al. c-erbB-2 gene product associates with catenins in human cancer cells. Biochem Biophys Res Commun 1994;205:73–78.

97. Kanai Y, Ochiai A, Shibata T, et al. c-erbB-2 gene product directly associates with β-catenin and plakoglobin. Biochem Biophys Res Commun 1995;208:1067–1072.

98. Dohadwala M, Yan SC, Luo J, et al. Cyclooxygenase-2–dependent regulation of E-cadherin: prostaglandin E2 induces transcriptional repressors ZEB1 and Snail in non–small cell lung cancer. Cancer Res 2006;66:5338–5345.

99. Brown JR, DuBois RN. Cyclooxygenase as a target in lung cancer. Clin Cancer Res 2004;10:4266–4269s.

100. Dubinett SM, Sharma S, Huang M, et al. Cyclooxygenase-2 in lung cancer. Prog Exp Tumor Res 2003;37:138–162.

101. Dannenberg AJ, Zakim D. Chemoprevention of colorectal cancer through inhibition of cyclooxygenase-2. Semin Oncol 1999;26:499–504.

102. Pold M, Zhu L, Sharma S, et al. Cyclooxygenase-2-dependent expression of angiogenic CXC chemokines ENA-78/CXC ligand (CXCL) 5 and interleukin8/CXCL8 in human non–small cell lung cancer. Cancer Res 2004;64:1853–1860.

103. Hilda T, Yatabe Y, Achiwa H, et al. Increased expression of cyclooxygenase 2 occurs frequently in human lung cancers, specifically in adenocarcinomas. Cancer Res 1998;58:3761–3764.

104. Huang M, Stolina M, Sharma S, et al. Non–small cell lung cancer cyclooxygenase-2 dependent regulation of cytokine balance in lymphocytes and macrophages: up-regulation of interleukin 10 and down-regulation of interleukin 12 production. Cancer Res 1998;58;1208–1216.

105. Sharma S, Yang SC, Zhu L, et al. Tumor cyclooxygenase-2/prostaglanding E2–dependent promotion of FOXP3-expression and CD4+ CD25+ T regulatory cell activities in lung cancer. Cancer Res 2005;65:5211–5220.

106. Sharma S, Zhu L, Yang SC, et al. Cyclooxygenase 2 inhibition promotes IFN-γ–dependent enhancement of antitumor responses. J Immunol 2005;175:813–819.

107. Jungck M, Grunhage F, Spengler U, et al. E-cadherin expression is homogeneously reduced in adenoma from patients with familial adenomatous polyposis: an immunohistochemical study of E-cadherin, β-catenin and cyclooxygenase-2 expression. Int J Colorectal Dis 2004;19:438–445.

108. Riedl K, Krysan K, Pold M, et al. Multifaceted roles of cyclooxygenase-2 in lung cancer. Drug Resist Update 2004;7:169–184.

109. Cavallaro U, Christofori G. Cell adhesion and signaling by cadherins and Ig-CAMs in cancer. Natl Rev Cancer 2004;4:118–132.

110. Choi YS, Shim YM, Kim SH, et al. Prognostic significance of E-cadherin and β-catenin in resected stage I non-small cell lung cancer. Eur J Cardiothorac Surg 2003;24:441–449.

111. Liu D, Huang C, Kameyama K, et al. E-cadherin expression associated with differentiation and prognosis in

patients with non-small cell lung cancer. Ann Thorac Surg 2001;71:949–951; discussion 954–955.

112. Witta SE, Gemmill RM, Hirsch FR, et al. Restoring E-cadherin expression increases sensitivity to epidermal growth factor receptor inhibitors in lung cancer cell lines. Cancer Res 2006;66:944–950.

113. Fukuoka M, Yano S, Giaccone G, et al. Multi-institutional randomized phase II trial of gefitinib for previously treated patients with advanced non-small cell lung cancer (the IDEAL 1 Trial). J Clin Oncol 2003;21:2237–2246.

114. Kris MG, Natale RB, Herbst RS, et al. Efficacy of gefitinib, an inhibitor of the epidermal growth factor receptor tyrosine kinase, in symptomatic patients with non–small cell lung cancer: a randomized trial. JAMA 2003;290:2149–2158.

115. Shepherd FA, Rodrigues P, Jose C, et al. the National Cancer Institute of Canada Clinical Trials Group. Erlotinib in previously treated non-small-cell lung cancer. N Engl J Med 2005;353:123–132.

116. Paez JG, Janne PA, Lee JC, et al. EGFR mutations in lung cancer: correlation with clinical response to gefitinib therapy. Science 2004;304:1497–1500.

117. Tsao MS, Sakurada A, Cutz JC, et al. Erlotinib in lung cancer—molecular and clinical predictors of outcome. N Engl J Med 2005;353:133–144.

118. Cappuzzo F, Magrini E, Ceresoli GL, et al. Akt phosphorylation and gefitinib efficacy in patients with advanced non-small-cell lung cancer. J Natl Cancer Inst 2004;96:1133–1141.

119. Ohira T, Gemmill RM, Ferguson K, et al. WNT7a induces E-cadherin in lung cancer cells. Proc Natl Acad Sci USA 2003;100:10429–10434.

120. Verschuren K, Remacle JE, Collart C, et al. SIP1, a novel zinc finger/homeodomain repressor, interacts with Smad proteins and binds to 5′-CACCT sequences in candidate target genes. J Biol Chem 1999;27:20489–20498.

121. Chinnadurai G. CtBP, an unconventional transcriptional corepressor in development and oncogenesis. Mol Cell 2002;9:213–224.

122. Marks PA, Richon VM, Rifkind RA. Histone deacetylase inhibitors: inducers of differentiation or apoptosis of transformed cells. J Natl Cancer Inst 2000;92:1210–1216.

123. Gore L, Holden SN, Basche M, et al. Updated results from a phase I trial of the histone deacetylase (HCAC) inhibitor NS-275 in patients with refractory solid tumors. Proc Am Soc Clin Oncol 2004;22:3026(14S).

124. Deeb G, Want J, Ramnath N, et al. Altered E-cadherin and epidermal growth factor receptor expressions are associated with patient survival in lung cancer: a study utilizing high-density tissue microarray and immunohistochemistry. Mod Pathol 2004;17:430–439.

125. Al Moustafa AE, Yen L, Benlimame N, Alaoui-Jamali MA. Regulation of E-cadherin/catenin complex patterns by epidermal growth factor receptor modulation in human lung cancer cells. Lung Cancer 2002;37:49–56.

125. Al Moustafa AE, Yen L, Benlimame N, Alaoui-Jamali MA. Regulation of E-cadherin/catenin complex patterns by epidermal growth factor receptor modulation in human lung cancer cells. Lung Cancer 2002;37:49–56.

126. Zhong Y, Delgado Y, Gomez J, Lee SW, Perez-Soler R. Loss of H-cadherin protein expression in human non-small cell lung cancer is associated with tumorigenicity. Clin Cancer Res 2001;7:1683–1687.

127. Takeuchi T, Misaki A, Fujita J. T-cadherin (CDh13, H-cadherin) expression downregulated surfactant protein D in bronchioloalveolar cells. Virchows Arch 2001;438:370–375.

128. Toyooka KO, Toyooka S, Virmani AK, et al. Loss of expression and aberrant methylation of the CDH13 (H-cadherin) gene in breast and lung carcinomas. Cancer Res 2001;61:4556–4560.

129. Bremnes RM, Veve R, Gabrielson E, et al. High-throughput tissue microarray analysis used to evaluate biology and prognostic significance of the E-cadherin pathway in non–small-cell lung cancer. J Clin Oncol 2002;20:2417–2428.

130. Geng F, Shi BZ, Yuan YF, Wu XZ. The expression of core fucosylated E-cadherin in cancer cells and lung cancer patients: prognostic implications. Cell Res 2004;14:423–433.

131. Nakashima T, Huang C, Liu D, et al. Neural-cadherin expression associated with angiogenesis in non-small-cell lung cancer patients. Br J Cancer 2003;88:1227–1233.

132. Bremnes RM, Veve R, Hirsch FR, Franklin WA. The E-cadherin cell-cell adhesion complex and lung cancer invasion, metastasis, and prognosis. Lung Cancer 2002;36:115–124.

133. Chen XF, Zhang HT, Qi QY, Sung MM, Tao LY. Expression of E-cadherin and nm23 is associated with the clinico-pathological factors of human non-small cell lung cancer in China. Lung Cancer 2005;48:69–76.

134. Herbst RS, Yano S, Kuniyasu H, et al. Differential expression of E-cadherin and type IV collagenase genes predicts outcome in patients with stage I non–small cell lung carcinoma. Clin Cancer Res 2000;6:790–797.

135. Kimura K, Endo Y, Yonemura Y, et al. clinical significance of S100A4 and E-cadherin–related adhesion molecules in non-small cell lung cancer. Int J Oncol 2000;16:1125–1131.

136. Stefanou D, Goussia AC, Arkoumani E, Agnantis NJ. Expression of vascular endothelial growth factor and the adhesion molecule E-cadherin in non-small cell lung cancer. Anticancer Res 2003;23:4715–4720.

137. Shimamoto T, Ohyashiki HJ, Hirano T, Kato H, Ohyashiki K. Hypermethylation of E-cadherin gene is frequent and independent of p16INK4A methylation in non–small cell lung cancer: potential prognostic implications. Oncol Rep 2004;12:389–395.

138. Tang XJ, Zhou QH, Zhang SF, Liu LX. Expressions of nm23, E-cadherin, and beta-catenin in non–small cell lung cancer and their correlations with metastasis and prognosis. Al Zheng 2005;24:616–621.

139. Qiao GB, Wu YL, Ou W, et al. Expressions of E-cadherin in non–small cell lung cancer and its correlation and prognosis. Zhonghua Wai Ke Za Zhi 2005;43:913–917.

140. Charalabopoulos K, Gogali A, Dalavaga Y, et al. The clinical significance of soluble E-cadherin in nonsmall cell lung cancer. Exp Oncol 2006;28:83–85.

141. McEver RP. Properties of GMP-140, an inducible granule membrane protein of platelets and endothelium. Blood Cells 1990;16:73–80.

142. Carlos TM, Harlan JM. Leukocyte-endothelial adhesion molecules. Blood 1994;84:2068–2101.

143. Springer TA. Traffic signals for lymphocyte recirculation and leukocyte emigration: the multistep paradigm. Cell 1994;76:301–314.

144. Lowe JB, Ward PA. Therapeutic inhibition of carbohydrate-protein interactions in vivo. J Clin Invest 1997;100: S47–S51.

145. Li L, Short HJ, Qian KX, et al. Characterization of glycoprotein ligands for P-selectin on a human small cell lung cancer cell line NCI-H345. Biochem Biophys Res Commun 2001;288:637–644.

146. Tedder TF, Steeber DA, Chen A, Engle P. The selectins: vascular adhesion molecules. FASEB J 1995;9:866–873.

147. Stone JP, Wagner DD. P-selectin mediates adhesion of platelets to neuroblastoma and small cell lung cancer. J Clin Invest 1993;92:804–813.

148. Pottratz ST, hall TD, Scribner WM, Jayaram HN, Natarajan V. P-selectin–mediated attachment of small cell lung carcinoma to endothelial cells. Am J Physiol 1996;71: L918–L923.

149. Kaytes PS, Geng JG. P selectin mediates adhesion of the human melanoma cell line NKI-4: identification of glycoprotein ligands. Biochemistry 1998;37:10514–10521.

150. Yu CJ, Shih JY, Lee YC, et al. Sialyl Lewis antigens: association with MUC5AC protein and correlation with postoperative recurrence of non-small cell lung cancer. Lung Cancer 2005;47:59–67.

151. Rosen SD, Bertozzi CR. The selectins and their ligands. Curr Opin Cell Biol 1994;6:663–673.

152. Izumi Y, Taniuchi Y, Tsuji T, et al. characterization of human colon carcinoma variant cells selected for sialyl Le^x carbohydrate antigen: liver colonization and adhesion to vascular endothelial cells. Exp Cell Res 1995;216:215–221.

153. Laack E, Nikbakht H, Peters A, et al. Expression of CEA-CAM1 in adenocarcinoma of the lung: a factor of independent prognostic significance. J Clin Oncol 2002;20:4279–4284.

154. Yu CJ, shun CT, Yang PC, et al. Sialomucin expression is associated with erbB-2 oncoprotein overexpression, early recurrence and cancer death in non–small cell lung cancer. Am J Respir Crit Care Med 1997;155:1419–1427.

155. Yu CJ, Shew JY, Shun Ct, et al. Quantitative analysis of messenger ribonucleic acid encoding MUC1, MUC2, and MUC4AC genes: a correlation between specific mucin gene expression and sialomucin expression in non-small cell lung cancer. Am J Respir Cell Mol Biol 1998;18: 643–652.

156. Kristiansen G, Schluns K, Yongwei Y, et al. CD24 is an independent prognostic marker of survival in nonsmall cell lung cancer patients. Br J Cancer 2003;88:231–236.

157. D'Amico TA, Brooks KR, Joshi MBM, et al. Serum protein expression predicts recurrence in patients with early-stage lung cancer after resection. Ann Thorac Surg 2006;81: 1982–1987.

158. Rosselli M, Mineo TC, Martini F, et al. Soluble selectin levels in patients with lung cancer. Int J Biol Marker 2002;17:56–62.

159. Tsumatori G, Ozeki Y, Takagi K, Ogata T, Tanaka S. Relation between the serum E-selectin level and the survival rate of patients with resected non-small cell lung cancers. Jpn J Cancer Res 1999;90:301–307.

160. Gao Y, Wei M, Zheng S, Ba X. Chemically modified heparin inhibits the in vitro adhesion of nonsmall cell lung cancer cells to P-selectin. J Cancer Res Clin Oncol 2006;132:257–264.

161. Borsig L, Wong R, Hynes RQ, Varki NM, Varki A. synergistic effects of L- and P-selectin in facilitating tumor metastasis can involve non-mucin ligands and implicate leukocytes as enhancers of metastasis. Proc Natl Acad Sci USA 2002;99:2193–2198.

162. Borsig L, Wong R, Feramisco J, et al. Heparin and cancer revisited: mechanistic connections involving platelets, P-selectin, carcinoma mucins, and tumor metastasis. Proc Natl Acad Sci USA 2001;98:3352–3357.

163. Springer TA. Adhesion receptors of the immune system. Nature 1990;346:425–434.

164. Tessier-Lavigne M, Goodman CS. The molecular biology of axon guidance. Science 1996;274:1123–1133.

165. Pouniotis DS, Plebanski M, Apostolopoulos V, McDonald CF. Alveolar macrophage function is altered in patients with lung cancer. Clin Exp Immunol 2005;143:363–372.

166. Bingle L, Brown NJ, Lewis CE. The role of tumour-associated macrophages in tumour progression: implications for new anticancer therapies. J Pathol 2002;196:254–265.

167. Kim YG, Kim MJ, Lim JS, et al. ICAM-3–induced cancer cell proliferation through the PI3K/Akt pathway. Cancer Lett 2006;103–110.

168. van Buul JD, Mul FP, van der Schoot CE, Hordijk PL. ICAM-3 activation modulates cell–cell contacts of human bone marrow endothelial cells. J Vasc Res 2004;41:28–37.

169. Chung YM, Kim GB, Park CS, et al. Increased expression of ICAM3 is associated with radiation resistance in cervical cancer. Int J Cancer 2005;117:194–201.

170. Yasuda M, Tanaka Y, Tamura M, et al. Stimulation of β1 integrin down-regulates ICAM-1 expression and ICAM-1-dependent adhesion of lung cancer cells through focal adhesion kinase. Cancer Res 2001;61:2022–2030.

171. Schwartz RH. Models of T cell anergy: is there a common molecular mechanism? J Exp Med 1996;184:1–8.

172. Shen J, Devery JM, King NJ. Adherence status regulates the primary cellular activation responses to the *Flavivirus* West Nile. Immunology 1995;84:254–264.

173. Mukai S, Kagamu H, Shu S, Plautz GE. Critical role of CD11a (LFA-1) in therapeutic efficacy of systemically transferred antitumor effector T cells. Cell Immunol 1999;192:122–132.

174. Konishi J, Yamazaki K, Yokouchi H, et al. The characteristics of human NKT cells in lung cancer—CD1d independent cytotoxicity against lung cancer cells by NKT cells and decreased human NKT cell response in lung cancer patients. Hum Immunol 2004;65:1377–1388.

175. Zhang HW, Zhang L, Chen JH, Du JJ. The clinical significance of vascular endothelial growth factor and intercellular adhesion molecule-1 expression in non–small cell lung cancer. Zhonghua Wai Ke Za Zhi 2005;43: 354–357.

176. Shin HS, Jung CH, Park HD, Lee SS. The relationship between the serum intercellular adhesion molecule-1 level and the prognosis of the disease in lung cancer. Korean J Intern Med 2004;19:48.

177. Osaki T, Mitsudomi T, Yoshida Y, et al. Increased levels of serum intercellular adhesion molecule-1 (ICAM-1) in patients with non–small cell lung cancer. Surg Oncol 1996;5:107–113.

178. Dabrowska M, Grubek-Jaworska H, Hoser G, et al. Effect of IFN-gamma stimulation on expression of intercellular adhesion molecule-1 (ICAM-1) on alveolar macrophages in patients with non-small cell lung cancer. J Interferon Cytokine Res 2006;26:190–195.

179. Liu YJ, Yan PS, Li J, Jia JF. Expression and significance of CD44s, CD44v6, and nm23 mRNA in human cancer. World J Gastroenterol 2005;11:6601–6606.

180. Yasuda M, Nakano K, Yasumoto k, Tanaka Y. CD44: functional relevance to inflammation and malignancy. Histol Histopathol 2002;17:945–950.

181. Guo, YJ, Liu G, Wang X, et al. Potential use of soluble CD44 in serum as indicator of tumor burden and metastasis in patients with gastric or colon cancer. Cancer Res 1994;54:422–426.

182. Wielenga VJM, Heider KH, Offerhaus JA, et al. Expression of cD44 variant proteins in human colorectal cancer is related to tumor progression. Cancer Res 1993;53:4754–4756.

183. Backhus LM, Sievers E, Lin GY, et al. Perioperative cyclo-oxygenase 2 inhibition to reduce tumor cell adhesion and metastatic potential of circulating tumor cells in non–small cell lung cancer. J Thorac Cardiovasc Surg 2006;132:297–303.

184. Lee LN, Kuo SH, Lee YC, et al. CD44 splicing pattern is associated with disease progression in pulmonary adeno-carcinoma. J Formos Med Assoc 2005;104:541–548.

185. Yasuda M, Tanaka Y, Fujii k, Yasumoto K. CD44 stimulation down-regulates Fas expression and Fas-mediated apoptosis of lung cancer cells. Intern Immunol 2001;13:1309–1319.

186. Sneath RJ, Mangham DC. The normal structure and function of CD44 and its role in neoplasia. Mod Pathol 1998;51:191.

187. Suzuki H, Yamashiro K. Reduced expression of CD44 v3 and v6 is related to invasion in lung adenocarcinoma. Lung Cancer 2002;38:137–141.

188. Takahashi K, Takahashi F, Hirama M, Tanabe KK, Fukuchi Y. Restoration of CD44S in non–small cell lung cancer cells enhanced their susceptibility to the macrophage cyto-toxicity. Lung Cancer 2003;41:145–153.

189. Li M, Amizuka N, Takeuchi K, et al. Histochemical evidence of osteoclastic degradation of extracellular matrix in osteolytic metastasis originating from human lung small carcinoma (SBC-50) cells. Micro Res Tech 2006;69:73–83.

4
Apoptosis and Cell Death: Relevance to Lung

Pothana Saikumar and Rekha Kar

Introduction

In multicellular organisms, cell death plays an important role in development, morphogenesis, control of cell numbers, and removal of infected, mutated, or damaged cells. The term *apoptosis* was first coined in 1972 by Kerr et al.[1] to describe the morphologic features of a type of cell death that is distinct from necrosis and is today considered to represent programmed cell death. In fact, the evidence that a genetic program existed for physiologic cell death came from the developmental studies of the nematode *Caenorhabditis elegans*.[2] As time has progressed, however, apoptotic cell death has been shown to occur in many cell types under a variety of physiologic and pathologic conditions. Cells dying by apoptosis exhibit several characteristic morphologic features that include cell shrinkage, nuclear condensation, membrane blebbing, nuclear and cellular fragmentation into membrane-bound apoptotic bodies, and eventual phagocytosis of the fragmented cell (Figure 4.1).

Cell death is central to the normal development of multicellular organisms during embryogenesis and maintenance of tissue homeostasis in adults.[3] During development, sculpting of body parts is achieved through selective cell death, which imparts appropriate shape and creates required cavities in particular organs. In adults, cell death balances cell division as a homeostatic mechanism regulating constancy of tissue mass. Deletion of injured cells because of disease, genetic defects, aging, or exposure to toxins is also achieved by apoptosis. In essence, apoptotic cell death has important biologic roles not only in development and homeostasis but also in the pathogenesis of several disease processes.

Dysregulation of apoptosis is found in a wide spectrum of human diseases, including cancer, autoimmune diseases, neurodegenerative diseases, ischemic diseases, viral infections,[4] and lung diseases.[5] Our knowledge of cell death and the mechanisms of its regulation increased dramatically in the past two decades with the discovery of death genes in *C. elegans*[2] and their counterparts in mammals.

Apoptosis and Other Forms of Cell Death

Earlier, cell death was broadly classified into only two distinct types: apoptosis and necrosis. However, in recent years, it has become increasingly evident that such a classification is an oversimplification. Although 12 different types of cell death have been described in the literature, they can be grouped into five major types: apoptosis, necrosis, autophagy, paraptosis, and autoschizis. Some forms of death are classified under one of these other headings. For example, anoikis and oncosis are forms of apoptosis (triggered by cell detachment) and necrosis, respectively. Because of overlap and shared signaling pathways among different death programs, it is difficult to devise exclusive definitions for each of these cell death programs.

Necrosis

Necrosis results from a variety of accidental and lethal actions by toxins or physical stimuli or in association with pathologic conditions, such as ischemia. Necrosis is characterized by cellular edema, lysis of nuclear chromatin, disruption of the plasma membrane, and loss of cellular contents into the extracellular space, resulting in inflammation (see Figure 4.1). In contrast, in the setting of apoptosis, membrane damage occurs late in the process, and dead cells are engulfed by neighboring cells or phagocytes, leading to little or no inflammation (see Figure 4.1). Although necrosis has mostly been regarded as an accidental form of cell death, more recent data have suggested that necrosis can also occur as a programmed form of cell death. There is growing evidence that necrotic and apoptotic forms of cell death may have similarities.[6]

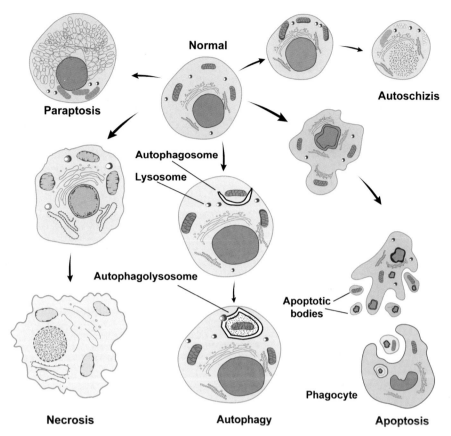

FIGURE 4.1. Morphologic features of cell death. *Necrosis*: Cells die by necrosis, and their organelles are characteristically swollen. There is early membrane damage with eventual loss of plasma membrane integrity and leakage of cytosol into extracellular space. Despite early clumping, the nuclear chromatin undergoes lysis (karyolysis). *Apoptosis*: Cells die by type I programmed cell death (also called apoptosis); they are shrunken and develop blebs containing dense cytoplasm. Membrane integrity is not lost until after cell death. Nuclear chromatin undergoes striking condensation and fragmentation. The cytoplasm becomes divided to form apoptotic bodies containing organelles and/or nuclear debris. Terminally, apoptotic cells and fragments are engulfed by phagocytes or surrounding cells. *Autophagy*: Cells die by type II programmed cell death, which is characterized by the accumulation of autophagic vesicles (autophagosomes and autophagolysosomes). One feature that distinguishes apoptosis from autophagic cell death is the source of the lysosomal enzymes used for most of the dying-cell degradation. Apoptotic cells use phagocytic cell lysosomes for this process, whereas cells with autophagic morphology use the endogenous lysosomal machinery of dying cells. *Paraptosis*: Cells die by type III programmed cell death, which is characterized by extensive cytoplasmic vacuolization and swelling and clumping of mitochondria, along with absence of nuclear fragmentation, membrane blebbing, or apoptotic body formation. *Autoschizis*: In this form of cell death, the cell membrane forms cuts or schisms that allow the cytoplasm to leak out. The cell shrinks to about one-third of its original size, and the nucleus and organelles remain surrounded by a tiny ribbon of cytoplasm. After further excisions of cytoplasm, the nuclei exhibit nucleolar segregation and chromatin decondensation followed by nuclear karyorrhexis and karyolysis.

Nevertheless, necrosis has been shown to occur in cells having defects in apoptotic machinery or upon inhibition of apoptosis,[7] and this form of cell death is emerging as an important therapeutic tool for cancer treatment.[8]

Autophagy

Autophagy, which is also referred to as *type II programmed cell death*, is characterized by sequestration of cytoplasm and organelles in double or multimembrane structures called *autophagic vesicles*, followed by degradation of the contents of these vesicles by the cell's own lysosomal system (see Figure 4.1). The precise role of autophagy in cell death or survival is not clearly understood. Autophagy has long been regarded as a cell survival mechanism whereby cells eliminate long-lived proteins and organelles. In this regard, it is argued that autophagy may help cancer cells survive under nutrient-limiting and low-oxygen conditions and against ionizing radiation.[9,10] However, recent observations that there is decreased autophagy during experimental carcinogenesis and heterologous disruption of an autophagy gene, *Beclin 1* (Bcn1), in cancer cells[11,12] suggest that breakdown of autophagic machinery may contribute to development of cancer. Other interesting studies have shed some light on the relationship between autophagy and apoptosis. These investigations have shown prevention of caspase inhibitor z-VAD–induced cell death in mouse L929 cells by RNA interference directed against autophagy genes *atg7* and Bcn1[13] and protection of *Bax*$^{-/-}$, *Bak*$^{-/-}$ murine embryonic fibroblasts against staurosporine- or etoposide-induced cell death by RNA interference against autophagy genes *atg5* and Bcn1.[14] However, both of these studies were done in cells whose apoptotic pathways had been compromised. Thus, it remains to be seen whether cells with intact apoptotic machinery can also die by autophagy and whether apoptotic-competent cells lacking autophagy genes will be resistant to different death stimuli.

Paraptosis

Paraptosis has recently been described as a form of cell death characterized by extensive cytoplasmic vacuolation (see Figure 4.1) caused by swelling of mitochondria and endoplasmic reticulum. This form of cell death does not involve caspase activation, is not inhibited by caspase inhibitors, but is inhibited by the inhibitors of transcription and translation, actinomycin D, and cycloheximide, respectively,[15] suggesting a requirement for new protein synthesis. The tumor necrosis factor receptor family TAJ/TROY and the insulin-like growth factor I receptor have been shown to trigger paraptosis.[16] Paraptosis appears to be mediated by mitogen-activated protein kinases and inhibited by AIP1/Alix, a protein interacting with the calcium-binding death-related protein ALG-2.[16]

Autoschizis

Autoschizis is a recently described type of cell death that differs from apoptosis and necrosis and is induced by oxidative stress.[17] In this type of death, cells lose cytoplasm by self-morsellation or self-excision (see Figure 4.1). Autoschizis usually affects contiguous groups of cells both in vitro and in vivo but can also occasionally affect scattered individual cells trapped in subcapsular sinuses of lymph nodes.[18] The nuclear envelope and pores remain intact while the cytoplasm is reduced to a narrow rim surrounding the nucleus. The chromatin marginates along the nuclear membrane, and mitochondria and other organelles around the nucleus aggregate as a result of cytoskeletal damage and condensation of the cytosol. Interestingly, the rough endoplasmic reticulum is preserved until the late stages of autoschizis, in which cells

fragment and the nucleolus becomes condensed and breaks into smaller fragments.[19] Eventually, the nuclear envelope and the remaining organelles dissipate with cell demise.

Apoptosis

Genetic studies in the nematode worm *C. elegans* led to the characterization of apoptosis. Activation of specific death genes during the development of this worm results in death of exactly 131 cells, leaving 959 cells intact.[2] Further studies revealed that apoptosis can be divided into three successive stages: (1) commitment phase, in which death is initiated by specific extracellular or intracellular signals; (2) execution phase; and (3) clean-up phase, in which dead cells are removed by other cells with eventual degradation of the dead cells in the lysosomes of phagocytic cells.[20] The apoptotic machinery is conserved through evolution from worm to human.[21] In *C. elegans*, execution of apoptosis is mediated by CED-3 and CED-4 proteins. Commitment to a death signal results in the activation of CED-3 by CED-4 binding. The CED-9 protein prevents activation of CED-3 by binding to CED-4.[22,23]

Mechanisms of Apoptosis

Caspases

Studies over the past decade have indicated that two distinct apoptotic pathways are followed in mammalian systems: the extrinsic or death receptor pathway and the intrinsic or mitochondrial pathway. The executioners in both intrinsic and extrinsic pathways of cell death are the caspases,[24] which are cysteine proteases with specificity to cleave their substrates after aspartic acid residues. The central role of caspases in apoptosis is underscored by the observation that apoptosis and all classic changes associated with apoptosis can be blocked by inhibition of caspase activity. To date, 12 mammalian caspases (caspase-1 to -10, caspase-14, and mouse caspase-12) have been identified.[25] Caspase-13 was later found to represent a bovine homolog and caspase-11 appears to be a murine homolog of human caspases-4 and -5, respectively.

Caspases are normally produced as inactive zymogens containing an N-terminal prodomain followed by a large and a small subunit that constitute the catalytic core of the protease. They have been categorized into two distinct classes: initiator and effector caspases. The upstream initiator caspases contain long N-terminal prodomains and one of the two characteristic protein–protein interaction motifs: the death effector domain (DED; caspase-8 and -10) and the caspase activation and recruitment domain (caspase-1, -2, -4, -5, -9, and -12). The downstream effector caspases (caspase-3, -6, and -7) are characterized by the presence of a short prodomain. Apart from the structural differences, a prominent difference between initiator and effector caspases is their basal state. Both the zymogen and the activated forms of effector caspases exist as constitutive homodimers, whereas initiator caspase-9 exists predominantly as a monomer both before and after proteolytic processing.[26] Initiator caspase-8 has been reported to exist in an equilibrium between monomers and homodimers.[27] Although the initiator caspases are capable of autocatalytic activation, the activation of effector caspases requires formation of oligomeric complexes with their adapter proteins and often intrachain cleavage within the initiator caspase.

Caspases have also been divided into three categories based on substrate specificity.[28] Group I members (caspase-1, -4, and -5) have a substrate specificity for the WEHD sequence with high promiscuity; group II members (caspase-2, -3, and -7 and CED-3) prefer the DEXD sequence and have an absolute requirement for aspartate (D) at P4; and members of group III (caspase-6, -8, and -9 and the "aspase" granzyme B) have a preference for (I/L/V)EXD sequences. Several reports have suggested a role for group I members in inflammation and that of group II and III members in apoptotic signaling events.

Extrinsic Death Pathway

The extrinsic pathway involves binding of death ligands such as tumor necrosis factor-α (TNF-α), CD95 ligand (Fas ligand), and TNF-related apoptosis-inducing ligand (TRAIL) to their cognate cell surface receptors TNFR1, CD95/Fas, TRAIL-R1, TRAIL-R2, and the DR series of receptors,[29] resulting in the activation of initiator caspase-8 (also known as FADD-homologous ICE/CED-3-like protease or FLICE) and subsequent activation of effector caspase-3 (Figure 4.2).[30] The cytoplasmic domains of death receptors contain the "death domain," which plays a crucial role in transmitting the signal from the cell's surface to intracellular signaling molecules. Binding of the ligands to their cognate receptors results in receptor trimerization and recruitment of adapter proteins to the cell membrane, which involves homophilic interactions between death domains of the receptors and the adapter proteins. The adapter protein for the receptors TNFR1 and DR3 is TNFR-associated death domain protein (TRADD)[31] and that for Fas, TRAIL-R1, TRAIL-R2, and DR4 is Fas-associated death domain protein (FADD).[32]

The receptor/ligand and FADD complex in turn recruits caspase-8 to the activated receptor, resulting in the formation of death-inducing signaling complex (DISC) and subsequent activation of caspase-8 through oligomerization and self-cleavage. Depending on the cell type and/or apoptotic stimulus, caspase-8 can also be activated by caspase-6.[33] Activated caspase-8 then activates effector caspase-3. In some cell types, cleavage of caspase-3 by caspase-8 also requires a mitochondrial amplification loop involving cleavage of proapoptotic protein Bid by caspase-8 and its translocation to the mitochondrial membrane, triggering the release of apoptogenic proteins from mitochondria into cytosol (see Figure 4.2). In these cell types, overexpression of *Bcl-2* and *Bcl-xL* can block CD95-induced apoptosis.[34]

Tumor necrosis factor-α is produced by T cells and activated macrophages in response to infection. Although TNF-α–mediated signaling can be propagated through either TNFR1 or TNFR2 receptors, the majority of biologic functions are initiated by TNFR1.[35] Binding of TNF-α to TNFR1 causes release of inhibitory protein silencer of death domain protein (SODD) from TNFR1, which enables recruitment of adapter protein TRADD. Signaling induced by activation of TNFR1 or DR3 diverges at the level of TRADD. In one pathway, nuclear translocation of the transcription factor nuclear factor-κB (NF-κB) and activation of c-Jun N-terminal kinase (JNK) are initiated, which results in the induction of a number of proinflammatory and immunomodulatory genes.[36] In another pathway, TNF-α signaling is coupled to Fas signaling events through interaction of TRADD with FADD.[37] The TNFR1–TRADD complex can alternatively engage TRAF2 protein, resulting in activation of transcription factor c-Jun, which is involved in survival signaling. Furthermore, binding of receptor interaction protein to TNFR1 through TRADD results in activation of transcription factor NF-κB, which suppresses apoptosis through transcriptional upregulation of antiapoptotic molecules such as TRAF1, TRAF2, cIAP1, cIAP2, and FLIP. The FLICE-associated huge protein was identified to be a CED-4 homolog interacting with the DED of caspase-8 and was shown to modulate Fas-mediated activation of caspase-8.[38] Another class of protein, FLIP (FLICE inhibitory protein), was shown to block Fas-induced and TNF-α–induced DISC formation and subsequent activation of caspase-8.[39]

Cytotoxic T cells play a major role in vertebrate defense against viral infection.[40] They induce cell death in infected cells to prevent viral multiplication and spread of infection.[41] Cytotoxic T cells can kill their targets either by activating the Fas ligand/Fas pathway or by injecting granzyme B, a serine protease, into target cells. Cytotoxic T cells carry Fas ligand on their surface but also carry granules containing the channel-forming protein perforin and granzyme B. Upon recognizing the infected cells, the lymphocytes bind and secrete granules onto the surface of infected cells. Perforin then assembles into transmembrane channels to allow the entry of granzyme B into the target cell. Upon entry, granzyme B, which cleaves after aspartate residues in proteins ("aspase"), activates one or

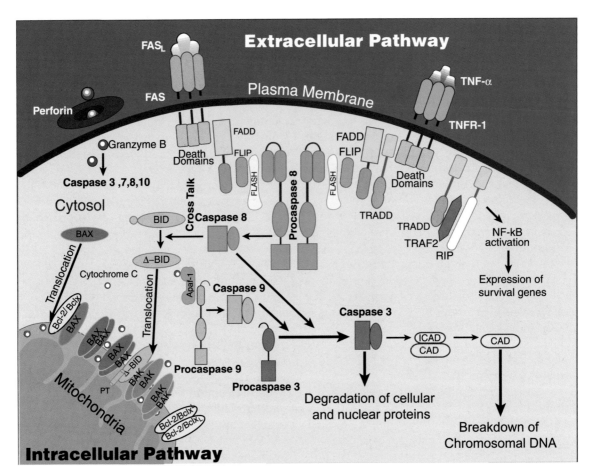

FIGURE 4.2. Schematic representation of apoptotic signaling pathways. *Extracellular Pathway:* Following the binding of peptides such as TNF-α or Fas ligand (FAS$_L$), the receptors oligomerize and recruit adapter proteins (Fas-associated death domain [FADD], tumor necrosis factor receptor [TNFR]–associated death domain [TRADD]) to form death-inducing signaling complexes, causing the activation of the initiator caspase-8, which sequentially activates effector caspases (e.g., caspase-3). Other adapter proteins (FLASH), inhibitory proteins (FLIP), or proteins involved in survival pathways as well as death mechanisms (receptor interaction protein [RIP]) may participate in complex mechanisms that determine life or death. The TNF-α TNFR1 complex can also elicit an antiapoptotic response by recruiting TRAF2, which results in NF-κB–mediated upregulation of antiapoptotic genes. In cytotoxic T lymphocyte–induced death, granzyme B, which enters the cell through membrane channels formed by the protein perforin, activates caspases by cleaving them directly or indirectly. *Intracellular Pathways:* Lack of survival stimuli (withdrawal of growth factor, hypoxia, genotoxic substances, etc.) is thought to generate apoptotic signals through ill-defined mechanisms, which

lead to translocation of proapoptotic proteins such as Bax to the outer mitochondrial membrane. In some cases, transcription mediated by p53 may be required to induce proteins such as Bax. Translocated Bax undergoes conformational changes in the outer membrane to form oligomeric structures (pores) that leak cytochrome c from mitochondria into the cytosol. Formation of a ternary complex of cytochrome c, the adapter protein Apaf-1, and the initiator caspase-9 results in the activation of caspase-9 followed by sequential activation of effector caspase(s) such as caspase-3 and others. The action of caspases, endonucleases, and possibly other enzymes leads to cellular disintegration. For example, the endonuclease CAD (caspase activated DNAse) becomes activated when it is released from its inhibitor ICAD upon cleavage of ICAD by an effector caspase. Antiapoptotic proteins such as Bcl-2 and Bcl-xL inhibit the membrane-permeabilizing effects of Bax and other proapoptotic proteins. Cross-talk between extra- and intracellular pathways occurs through caspase-8–mediated Bid cleavage, which yields a 15 kDa protein that migrates to mitochondria and releases cytochrome c, thereby setting in motion events that lead to apoptosis via caspase-9.

more of the apoptotic proteases (caspase-2, -3, -7, -8, and -10) to trigger the proteolytic death cascade (see Figure 4.2). Fas ligand/Fas and perforin/granzyme B systems are the main apoptotic machinery that regulates homeostasis in immune cell populations.

Intrinsic Death Pathway

Cells can respond to various stressful stimuli and metabolic disturbances by triggering apoptosis. Drugs, toxins, heat, radiation, hypoxia, and viral infections are some of the stimuli known to activate death pathways. Cell death, however, is not necessarily inevitable after exposure to these agents, and the mechanisms determining the outcome of the injury are a topic of active interest. The current consensus appears to be that it is the intensity and the duration of the stimulus that determine the outcome. The stimulus must go beyond a threshold to commit cells to apoptosis. Although the exact mechanism used by each stimulus may be unique and different, a few broad patterns can be identified. For example, agents that damage DNA, such as ionizing radiation and certain xenobiotics, lead to activation of p53-mediated mechanisms that commit cells to apoptosis, at least in part through transcriptional upregulation of proapoptotic proteins.[42] Other stresses induce increased activity of stress-activated protein kinases, which result ultimately in apoptotic commitment.[43] These different mechanisms converge in the activation of caspases.

A cascade of caspases plays the central executioner role by cleaving various mammalian cytosolic and nuclear proteins that play roles in cell division, maintenance of cytoskeletal structure, DNA replication and repair, RNA splicing, and other cellular processes. This proteolytic carnage produces the characteristic morphologic changes of apoptosis. Once the caspase cascade is initiated, the process of cell death has crossed the point of no return.

The roles of various caspases in apoptotic pathways and their relative importance for animal development have been examined in genetic studies involving knockout of different caspase genes. A caspase-1 (interleukin [IL]-1b converting enzyme [ICE]) knockout study suggested that ICE plays an important role in inflammation by activating cytokines such as IL-1b and IL-18. However, caspase-1 was not required to mediate apoptosis under normal circumstances and did not have a major role during development.[44] Surprisingly, ischemic brain injury was significantly reduced in caspase-1 knockout mice compared with wild-type mice,[45] suggesting that inflammation may contribute to ischemic injury. Caspase-3 deficiency leads to impaired brain development and premature death. Also, functional caspase-3 is required for some typical hallmarks of apoptosis such as formation of apoptotic bodies, chromatin condensation, and DNA fragmentation in many cell types.[46] Lack of caspase-8 results in the death of embryos at day 11 with abnormal formation of the heart,[47] suggesting that caspase-8 is required for cell death during mammalian development. In support of this finding, knockout of FADD, which is required for caspase-8 activation, resulted in fetal death with signs of abdominal hemorrhage and cardiac failure.[48] Moreover, caspase-8–deficient cells did not die in response to signals from members of the TNF receptor family.[47] However, cells lacking either FADD or caspase-8, which are resistant to TNF-α–mediated or CD95-mediated death, are susceptible to chemotherapeutic drugs, serum depriva-

tion, ceramide, γ-irradiation, and dexamethasone-induced killing.[48] In contrast, caspase-9 has a key role in apoptosis induced by intracellular activators, particularly those that cause DNA damage. Deletion of caspase-9 resulted in perinatal lethality, apoptotic failure in developing neurons, enlarged brains, and craniofacial abnormalities.[49] In caspase-9–deficient cells, caspase-3 was not activated, suggesting that caspase-9 is upstream of caspase-3 in the apoptotic cascade. As a consequence, caspase-9–deficient cells are resistant to dexamethasone or irradiation, whereas they retain their sensitivity to TNF-α–induced or CD95-induced death[49] because of the presence of caspase-8, the initiator caspase involved in death receptor signaling that can also activate caspase-3. Overall, these observations support the idea that different death signaling pathways converge on downstream effector caspases (see Figure 4.2). Indeed, caspase-3 is regarded as one of the key executioner molecules activated by apoptotic stimuli originating either at receptors for exogenous molecules or within cells through the action of drugs, toxins, or radiation.

Regulators of Caspases

In *C. elegans*, biochemical and genetic studies have indicated a role for CED-4 upstream of CED-3.[50] Upon receiving death commitment signals, CED-4 binds to pro-CED-3 and releases active CED-3.[50] However, when overexpressed, CED-9 can inhibit the activation of pro-CED-3 by binding to CED-4 and sequestering it away from pro-CED-3. Therefore, CED-3 and CED-4 are involved in activation of apoptosis, and CED-9 inhibits apoptosis. After the discovery of caspases as CED-3 homologs, a search for activators and inhibitors analogous to CED-4 and CED-9 led to the discovery of diverse mammalian regulators of apoptosis. The plethora of these molecules and their functional diversity allowed them to be classified into four broad categories: (1) adapter proteins, (2) the Bcl-2 family of regulators, (3) inhibitors of apoptosis (IAPs), and (4) other regulators.

Adapter Proteins

As stated earlier, two major pathways of apoptosis, involving either the initiator caspase-8 or the initiator caspase-9 (see Figure 4.2), have been recognized. Signaling by death receptors (CD95, TNFRI) occurs through a well-defined process of recruitment of caspase-8 to the death receptor by adapter proteins such as FADD. Recruitment occurs through interactions between the death domains that are present on both receptor and adapter proteins. Receptor-bound FADD then recruits caspase-8 through interactions between DEDs common to both caspase-8 and FADD forming a DISC. In the DISC, caspase-8 activation occurs through oligomerization and autocatalysis.

Activated caspase-8 then activates downstream caspase-3, culminating in apoptosis. The inhibitory protein, FLIP was shown to block Fas-induced and TNF-α–induced DISC formation and subsequent activation of caspase-8.[39] Of particular interest is cellular FLIP, which stimulates caspase-8 activation at physiologically relevant levels and inhibited apoptosis upon high ectopic expression.[51] Cellular FLIP contains two DEDs that can compete with caspase-8 for recruitment to the DISC. This limits the degree of association of caspase-8 with FADD and thus limits activation of the caspase cascade. It also forms a heterodimer with caspase-8 and caspase-10 through interactions between both the DEDs and the caspase-like domains of the proteins, thus activating both caspase-8 and caspase-10.[52]

Apoptotic protease activating factor-1 (Apaf-1), a CED-4 homolog in mammalian cells, affects the activation of initiator caspase-9.[53] This factor binds to procaspase-9 in the presence of cytochrome c and 2′-deoxyadenosine 5′-triphosphate (dATP) or adenosine triphosphate (ATP) and activates this protease, which in turn activates a downstream cascade of proteases (see Figure 4.2).[54] By and large, Apaf-1 deficiency is embryonically lethal and the embryos exhibit brain abnormalities similar to those seen in caspase-9 knockout mice.[55] These genetic findings support the idea that Apaf-1 is coupled to caspase-9 in the death pathway. Unlike CED-4 in nematodes, Apaf-1 requires the binding of ATP and cytochrome c to activate procaspase-9. The multiple WD40 repeats in the C-terminal end of Apaf-1 have a regulatory role in the activation of caspase-9.[56]

The Bcl-2 Family of Proteins

The CED-9 homolog in mammals is the Bcl-2 protein. Bcl-2 was first discovered in B-cell lymphoma as a proto-oncogene. Overexpression of Bcl-2 was shown to offer protection against a variety of death stimuli.[57] The Bcl-2 protein family includes both proapoptotic (Bcl-2, Bcl-xL, Bcl-w, Mcl-1, Nr13, and A1/Bfl-1) and antiapoptotic proteins (Bax, Bak, Bok, Diva, Bcl-Xs, Bik, Bim, Hrk, Nip3, Nix, Bad, and Bid).[58] These proteins are characterized by the presence of Bcl-2 homology (BH) domains: BH1, BH2, BH3, and BH4 (Figure 4.3). The proapoptotic members have two subfamilies: a multidomain and a BH3-only group (see Figure 4.3). The relative ratio of pro- and antiapoptotic proteins determines the sensitivity of cells to various apoptotic stimuli.

The best-studied proapoptotic members are Bax and Bid. Exposure to various apoptotic stimuli leads to translocation of cytosolic Bax from the cytosol to the mitochondrial membrane.[59] Bax oligomerizes on the mitochondrial membrane along with another proapoptotic protein, Bak, leading to the release of cytochrome c from the mitochondrial membrane into the cytosol.[60]

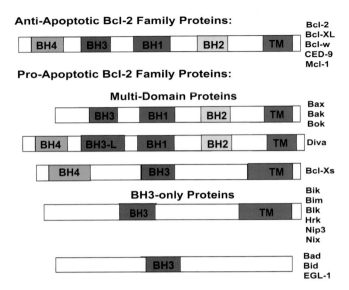

FIGURE 4.3. Structural homologies in anti- and proapoptotic proteins of the Bcl-2 family. Anti- and proapoptotic proteins of the Bcl-2 family proteins are depicted, indicating Bcl-2 homologous (BH) regions BH1, BH2, BH3, and BH4 and transmembrane (TM) domains.

Other proapoptotic proteins, mainly the BH3-only proteins, are thought to aid in Bax–Bak oligomerization on the mitochondrial membrane. The antiapoptotic Bcl-2 family members are known to block Bax–Bak oligomerization on the mitochondrial membrane and subsequent release of cytochrome c into the cytosol.[60,61] After release from the mitochondria, cytochrome c is known to interact with the WD40 repeats of the adaptor protein Apaf-1, resulting in the formation of the apoptosome complex.

Seven molecules of Apaf-1, interacting through their N-terminal caspase activation and recruitment domain, form the central hub region of the symmetric wheel-like structure, the apoptosome. Binding of ATP/dATP to Apaf-1 triggers the formation of the apoptosome, which subsequently recruits procaspase-9 into the apoptosome complex, resulting in its activation[62]. Activated caspase-9 then activates executioner caspases, such as caspase-3 and caspase-7, eventually leading to programmed cell death.

Inhibitors of Apoptosis Proteins

The IAPs, first discovered in baculoviruses and then in insects and *Drosophila*, inhibit activated caspases by directly binding to the active enzymes.[63] These proteins contain one or more baculovirus inhibitor of apoptosis repeat domains, which are responsible for the caspase inhibitory activity.[64] To date, eight mammalian IAPs have been identified. They include X-linked IAP (XIAP), c-IAP1, c-IAP2, Melanoma IAP (ML-IAP)/Livin, IAP-like protein-2 (ILP-2), neuronal apoptosis-inhibitory protein (NAIP), Bruce/Apollon, and Survivin. In mammals, caspase-3, -7, and -9 are inhibited by IAPs.[62] There are reports suggesting aberrant expression of IAPs in many cancer tissues. For example, cIAP1 is overexpressed in esophageal squamous cell sarcoma[65]; cIAP2 locus is translocated in mucosa-associate lymphoid lymphoma[66] and Survivin has been shown to be upregulated in many cancer cells.[67]

Other Regulators

The caspase inhibitory activity of IAPs is inhibited by proteins containing an IAP-binding tetrapeptide motif.[62] The founding member of this family is SMAC/DIABLO, which is released from the mitochondrial intermembrane space into the cytosol during apoptosis. In the cytosol, it interacts with several IAPs and inhibits their function. The other mitochondrial protein, Omi/HtrA2, is also known to antagonize XIAP-mediated inhibition of caspase-9 at high concentrations.[68] A serine protease, Omi/HtrA2 can proteolytically cleave and inactivate IAP proteins and thus is considered to be a more potent suppressor of IAPs than SMAC.[69]

It has been reported that the heat shock proteins Hsp90, Hsp70, and Hsp27 can inhibit caspase activation by cytochrome c either by interacting with Apaf-1 or other players in the pathway.[70–72] A high-throughput screen identified a compound called PETCM (α-[trichloromethyl]-4-pyridineethanol) as a caspase-3 activator. Further work with PETCM revealed its involvement in apoptosome regulation.[73] This pathway also includes oncoprotein prothymosin-α and tumor suppressor putative HLA-DR–associated proteins. These proteins were shown to promote caspase-9 activation after apoptosome formation, whereas prothymosin-α inhibited caspase-9 activation by inhibiting apoptosome formation.

Protein Targets of Caspases

In an apoptotic cell, the regulatory, structural, and housekeeping proteins are the main targets of the caspases. The regulatory proteins mitogen-activated protein/extracellular signal-regulated kinase kinase-1, p21-activated kinase-2, and Mst-1 are activated upon cleavage by caspases.[74] Caspase-mediated protein hydrolysis inactivates other proteins, including focal adhesion kinase, phosphatidylinositol-3 kinase, Akt, Raf-1, IAPs, and inhibitors of caspase-activated DNAse (ICAD). Caspases also convert the antiapoptotic protein Bcl-2 into a proapoptotic protein such as Bax upon cleavage. There are many structural protein targets of caspases, which include nuclear lamins, actin, and regulatory proteins such as spectrin, gelsolin, and fodrins.[75]

Degradation of nuclear DNA into internucleosomal chromatin fragments is one of the hallmarks of apoptotic cell death that occurs in response to various apoptotic stimuli in a wide variety of cells. A specific DNase, CAD (caspase-activated DNase), that cleaves chromosomal DNA in a caspase-dependent manner, is synthesized with the help of ICAD. In proliferating cells, CAD is always found to be associated with ICAD in the cytosol. When cells are undergoing apoptosis, caspases (particularly caspase-3) cleave ICAD to release CAD and allow its translocation to the nucleus to cleave chromosomal DNA. Thus, cells that are ICAD deficient or that express caspase-resistant ICAD mutant do not exhibit DNA fragmentation during apoptosis.

Apoptosis and the Pathogenesis of Lung Diseases

Apoptosis plays a critical role in the postnatal lung.[76] Regulated removal of inflammatory cells by apoptosis helps in the resolution of inflammation in the lung.[77] Recent evidence also supports a role for apoptosis in the remodeling of lung tissue after acute lung injury[78] and in the pathogenesis of chronic pulmonary hypertension,[79] idiopathic pulmonary fibrosis, and chronic obstructive pulmonary disease.[80,81]

Acute Lung Injury/Acute Respiratory Distress Syndrome

Acute lung injury, which clinically manifests itself as the acute respiratory distress syndrome (ARDS), involves disruption of the alveolar epithelium and endothelium, increased vascular permeability, and edema. Two main hypotheses link the pathogenesis of ARDS to apoptosis, namely, the "neutrophilic hypothesis" and the "epithelial hypothesis." These two hypotheses are not mutually exclusive, and both could play important roles in the pathogenesis of ARDS.

The neutrophilic hypothesis suggests that neutrophil apoptosis plays an important role in the resolution of inflammation and that the inhibition of neutrophil apoptosis or the inhibition of clearance of apoptotic neutrophils is deleterious in ARDS.[82,83] Studies in humans showed that bronchoalveolar lavage fluids from patients with early ARDS inhibit the rate at which neutrophils develop apoptosis in vitro.[84] The inhibitory effect of bronchoalveolar lavage fluids on neutrophil apoptosis is mediated by granulocyte/macrophage colony-stimulating factor, and possibly by IL-8 and IL-2.[85,86] A membrane surface molecule, CD44, has been shown to play an important role in the clearance of apoptotic cells in vivo and in vitro.[87] In a model of bleomycin-induced lung injury, CD44-deficient mice failed to clear apoptotic neutrophils, which was associated with worsened inflammation and increased mortality.[87] Activation of phagocytic cells inhibits production of proinflammatory cytokines, including IL-1β, IL-8, IL-10, granulocyte/ macrophage colony-stimulating factor, and TNF-α and increases release of anti-inflammatory mediators such as transforming growth factor-β, prostaglandin E_2, and platelet-activating factor.[88,89] The net effects of these changes could favor resolution of inflammation.

The epithelial hypothesis suggests that the apoptotic death of alveolar epithelial cells, in response to soluble mediators such as Fas ligand, contributes to the prominent alveolar epithelial injury characteristic of ARDS. Several lines of evidence suggest a role for the Fas/Fas ligand system in epithelial cell apoptosis.[90] Fas is expressed on alveolar and airway epithelial cells,[91,92] and its expression increases in response to inflammatory mediators such as lipopolysaccharide. Fas-mediated lung cell apoptosis is modulated by surfactant protein A, which inhibits apoptosis in vivo.[93]

Chronic Obstructive Pulmonary Disease

Chronic obstructive pulmonary disease, caused primarily by smoking, generally refers to chronic bronchitis and emphysema. Several factors, including protease/antiprotease imbalance, oxidative stress, cigarette smoke–derived toxins, and inflammation mediated by neutrophils, macrophages, and CD8+ T cells, have been shown to contribute to the disease process. Furthermore, matrix metalloproteinase[94] and vascular endothelial growth factor receptor inhibition,[95,96] but not Fas/Fas ligand, have been shown to play role in the development of emphysema.

Asthma

Allergic asthma is characterized by intermittent or persistent bronchoconstriction and has been linked to airway remodeling and chronic inflammation, with increased numbers of eosinophils, CD4+ T cells, and mast cells. Although at present a role for apoptosis in asthma is not confirmed, studies ex vivo have shown reduced apoptosis of circulating peripheral CD4+ T cells and eosinophils in asthma, which might contribute to inflammation. Corticosteroids used to reduce inflammation in asthma have been shown to induce eosinophil apoptosis.[97]

Pulmonary Fibrosis

Pulmonary fibrosis is characterized by epithelial damage, fibroblast proliferation, and deposition of collagen. Although the mechanism of alveolar epithelial cell apoptosis in pulmonary fibrosis is not known, several reports have suggested Fas pathway,[98] angiotensin pathway,[99] activated T cell-derived perforin,[100] IL-13 stimulation,[101]

and transforming growth factor-β1 activation[102] to play critical roles.

Lung Cancer

Because insufficient apoptosis is often associated with tumorigenesis, modulation of apoptotic and antiapoptotic targets seems to be an attractive approach to cancer therapy. Lung cancers can be divided into small cell lung cancers (SCLCs) and non–small cell lung cancers (NSCLCs).[103] The SCLCs are relatively more sensitive to anticancer drugs and irradiation than are the NSCLCs,[104] but the molecular basis for this difference is not clearly known. Evaluation of apoptosis-associated substances has shown that caspase-8, Fas, and Fas ligand are often downregulated in SCLCs but not in NSCLCs.[105] An investigation of the basis for these differences revealed that there were no differences in the levels of Bax and Bcl-xL, but the expression of Bcl-2 was found to be significantly higher in SCLC than in NSCLC cell lines. The observation that in some cases Bcl-2 can be converted into a proapoptotic Bax-like death molecule may offer an explanation for the paradoxic expression of Bcl-2 in SCLC.[106] The lack of expression of procaspase-1, -4, -8, and -10[107] reported in SCLC suggests that these caspases probably do not contribute to spontaneous apoptosis in these cells. Apoptosis regulators Apaf-1 and procaspase-3 are overexpressed and are functional in NSCLC cell lines. In both types of lung cancer, apoptotic stimuli result in cytochrome c release and activation of caspase-9 and caspase-3, but only SCLC cell lines showed a relocalization of caspase-3 into the nucleus[108]; this suggests that the resistance of NSCLC cell lines is probably due to defective relocalization of caspase-3. The expression of caspase-9 and caspase-7 in NSCLCs was found to be similar to normal lung tissue.[109] However, these cell lines express the apoptosis inhibitor and splice variant of caspase-9 CASP9b. In vitro, chemotherapy-resistant NSCLC cell lines exhibit decreased caspase-9 and caspase-3 expression,[110] which suggests an inhibition of apoptosis induction via apoptosome formation in NSCLC.

Additionally, both NSCLC and SCLC cells express high and almost equal levels of Survivin.[107] The resistant NSCLC cells showed higher expression of c-IAP2, and the radiosensitive SCLC cells exhibited increased expression of XIAP.[111] These results suggest no correlation between the level of expression of the IAPs and the difference in the radiosensitivity between NSCLC and SCLC cells.

Conclusion

Cell death has become an area of intense interest and investigation in science and medicine because of the recognition that cell death, in general, and apoptosis, in particular, are important features of many biologic processes. Involvement of many genes in the death process suggests that cell death is a complex phenomenon with many redundant mechanisms to ensure definitiveness. The realization that defective cell death plays a central role in the pathogenesis of diseases has stimulated work on therapies targeted to these processes, and this work will undoubtedly continue in the future.

References

1. Kerr JF, Wyllie AH, Currie AR. Apoptosis: a basic biological phenomenon with wide-ranging implications in tissue kinetics. Br J Cancer 1972;26(4):239–257.
2. Ellis HM, Horvitz HR. Genetic control of programmed cell death in the nematode *C. elegans*. Cell 1986;44(6):817–829.
3. Jacobson MD, Weil M, Raff MC. Programmed cell death in animal development. Cell 1997;88(3):347–354.
4. Saikumar P, Dong Z, Mikhailov V, et al. Apoptosis: definition, mechanisms, and relevance to disease. Am J Med 1999;107(5):489–506.
5. de Souza PM, Lindsay MA. Apoptosis as a therapeutic target for the treatment of lung disease. Curr Opin Pharmacol 2005;5(3):232–237.
6. Leist M, Jaattela M. Four deaths and a funeral: from caspases to alternative mechanisms. Nat Rev Mol Cell Biol 2001;2(8):589–598.
7. Vercammen D, Brouckaert G, Denecker G, et al. Dual signaling of the Fas receptor: initiation of both apoptotic and necrotic cell death pathways. J Exp Med 1998;188(5):919–930.
8. Zong WX, Ditsworth D, Bauer DE, et al. Alkylating DNA damage stimulates a regulated form of necrotic cell death. Genes Dev 2004;18(11):1272–1282.
9. Paglin S, Hollister T, Delohery T, et al. A novel response of cancer cells to radiation involves autophagy and formation of acidic vesicles. Cancer Res 2001;61(2):439–444.
10. Cuervo AM. Autophagy: in sickness and in health. Trends Cell Biol 2004;14(2):70–77.
11. Canuto RA, Tessitore L, Muzio G, et al. Tissue protein turnover during liver carcinogenesis. Carcinogenesis 1993;14(12):2581–2587.
12. Kisen GO, Tessitore L, Costelli P, et al. Reduced autophagic activity in primary rat hepatocellular carcinoma and ascites hepatoma cells. Carcinogenesis 1993;14(12):2501–2505.
13. Yu L, Alva A, Su H, et al. Regulation of an ATG7–beclin 1 program of autophagic cell death by caspase-8. Science 2004;304(5676):1500–1502.
14. Shimizu S, Kanaseki T, Mizushima N, et al. Role of Bcl-2 family proteins in a non-apoptotic programmed cell death dependent on autophagy genes. Nat Cell Biol 2004;6(12):1221–1228.
15. Sperandio S, de Belle I, Bredesen DE. An alternative, non-apoptotic form of programmed cell death. Proc Natl Acad Sci USA 2000;97(26):14376–14381.
16. Sperandio S, Poksay K, de Belle I, et al. Paraptosis: mediation by MAP kinases and inhibition by AIP-1/Alix. Cell Death Differ 2004;11(10):1066–1075.
17. Jamison JM, Gilloteaux J, Taper HS, et al. Autoschizis: a novel cell death. Biochem Pharmacol 2002;63(10):1773–1783.
18. Taper HS, Jamison JM, Gilloteaux J, et al. Inhibition of the development of metastases by dietary vitamin C:K3 combination. Life Sci 2004;75(8):955–967.
19. Gilloteaux J, Jamison JM, Lorimer HE, et al. Autoschizis: a new form of cell death for human ovarian carcinoma cells following ascorbate/menadione treatment. Nuclear and DNA degradation. Tissue Cell 2004;36(3):197–209.
20. Vaux DL, Strasser A. The molecular biology of apoptosis. Proc Natl Acad Sci USA 1996;93(6):2239–2244.
21. Yuan J. Evolutionary conservation of a genetic pathway of programmed cell death. J Cell Biochem 1996;60(1):4–11.
22. Spector MS, Desnoyers S, Hoeppner DJ, Hengartner MO. Interaction between the *C. elegans* cell-death regulators CED-9 and CED-4. Nature 1997;385(6617):653–656.
23. Wu D, Wallen HD, Inohara N, Nunez G. Interaction and regulation of the *Caenorhabditis elegans* death protease CED-3 by CED-4 and CED-9. J Biol Chem 1997;272(34):21449–21454.
24. Thornberry NA, Lazebnik Y. Caspases: enemies within. Science 1998;281(5381):1312–1316.
25. Launay S, Hermine O, Fontenay M, et al. Vital functions for lethal caspases. Oncogene 2005;24(33):5137–5148.
26. Shiozaki EN, Chai J, Rigotti DJ, et al. Mechanism of XIAP-mediated inhibition of caspase-9. Mol Cell 2003;11(2):519–527.
27. Donepudi M, Mac Sweeney A, Briand C, Grutter MG. Insights into the regulatory mechanism for caspase-8 activation. Mol Cell 2003;11(2):543–549.
28. Thornberry NA, Rano TA, Peterson EP, et al. A combinatorial approach defines specificities of members of the caspase family and granzyme B. Functional relationships established for key mediators of apoptosis. J Biol Chem 1997;272(29):17907–17911.
29. Magnusson C, Vaux DL. Signalling by CD95 and TNF receptors: not only life and death. Immunol Cell Biol 1999;77(1):41–46.
30. Ashkenazi A, Dixit VM. Apoptosis control by death and decoy receptors. Curr Opin Cell Biol 1999;11(2):255–260.
31. Hsu H, Xiong J, Goeddel DV. The TNF receptor 1–associated protein TRADD signals cell death and NF-kappa B activation. Cell 1995;81(4):495–504.
32. Chinnaiyan AM, O'Rourke K, Tewari M, Dixit VM. FADD, a novel death domain-containing protein, interacts with the death domain of Fas and initiates apoptosis. Cell 1995;81(4):505–512.
33. Cowling V, Downward J. Caspase-6 is the direct activator of caspase-8 in the cytochrome c–induced apoptosis pathway: absolute requirement for removal of caspase-6 prodomain. Cell Death Differ 2002;9(10):1046–1056.
34. Scaffidi C, Fulda S, Srinivasan A, et al. Two CD95 (APO-1/Fas) signaling pathways. EMBO J 1998;17(6):1675–1687.
35. Grell M, Zimmermann G, Gottfried E, et al. Induction of cell death by tumour necrosis factor (TNF) receptor 2, CD40 and CD30: a role for TNF-R1 activation by endogenous membrane-anchored TNF. EMBO J 1999;18(11):3034–3043.

36. Natoli G, Costanzo A, Moretti F, et al. Tumor necrosis factor (TNF) receptor 1 signaling downstream of TNF receptor-associated factor 2. Nuclear factor kappaB (NFkappaB)–inducing kinase requirement for activation of activating protein 1 and NFkappaB but not of c-Jun N-terminal kinase/stress-activated protein kinase. J Biol Chem 1997;272(42):26079–26082.

37. Boldin MP, Goncharov TM, Goltsev YV, Wallach D. Involvement of MACH, a novel MORT1/FADD-interacting protease, in Fas/APO-1- and TNF receptor-induced cell death. Cell 1996;85(6):803–815.

38. Imai Y, Kimura T, Murakami A, et al. The CED-4-homologous protein FLASH is involved in Fas-mediated activation of caspase-8 during apoptosis. Nature 1999;398(6730): 777–785.

39. Thome M, Schneider P, Hofmann K, et al. Viral FLICE-inhibitory proteins (FLIPs) prevent apoptosis induced by death receptors. Nature 1997;386(6624):517–521.

40. Offit PA, Cunningham SL, Dudzik KI. Memory and distribution of virus-specific cytotoxic T lymphocytes (CTLs) and CTL precursors after rotavirus infection. J Virol 1991;65(3):1318–1324.

41. Zajac AJ, Quinn DG, Cohen PL, Frelinger JA. Fas-dependent CD4+ cytotoxic T-cell–mediated pathogenesis during virus infection. Proc Natl Acad Sci USA 1996;93(25): 14730–14735.

42. Wu Q, Kirschmeier P, Hockenberry T, et al. Transcriptional regulation during p21WAF1/CIP1-induced apoptosis in human ovarian cancer cells. J Biol Chem 2002;277(39): 36329–36337.

43. Kunz M, Ibrahim S, Koczan D, et al. Activation of c-Jun NH2-terminal kinase/stress-activated protein kinase (JNK/SAPK) is critical for hypoxia-induced apoptosis of human malignant melanoma. Cell Growth Differ 2001;12(3): 137–145.

44. Li P, Allen H, Banerjee S, Seshadri T. Characterization of mice deficient in interleukin-1 beta converting enzyme. J Cell Biochem 1997;64(1):27–32.

45. Schielke GP, Yang GY, Shivers BD, Betz AL. Reduced ischemic brain injury in interleukin-1 beta converting enzyme-deficient mice. J Cereb Blood Flow Metab 1998; 18(2):180–185.

46. Janicke RU, Sprengart ML, Wati MR, Porter AG. Caspase-3 is required for DNA fragmentation and morphological changes associated with apoptosis. J Biol Chem 1998; 273(16):9357–9360.

47. Varfolomeev EE, Schuchmann M, Luria V, et al. Targeted disruption of the mouse caspase 8 gene ablates cell death induction by the TNF receptors, Fas/Apo1, and DR3 and is lethal prenatally. Immunity 1998;9(2):267–276.

48. Yeh WC, Pompa JL, McCurrach ME, et al. FADD: essential for embryo development and signaling from some, but not all, inducers of apoptosis. Science 1998;279(5358): 1954–1958.

49. Kuida K, Haydar TF, Kuan CY, et al. Reduced apoptosis and cytochrome c–mediated caspase activation in mice lacking caspase 9. Cell 1998;94(3):325–337.

50. Hengartner MO, Horvitz HR. The ins and outs of programmed cell death during C. elegans development. Philos Trans R Soc Lond B Biol Sci 1994;345(1313):243–246.

51. Chang DW, Xing Z, Pan Y, et al. c-FLIP(L) is a dual function regulator for caspase-8 activation and CD95-mediated apoptosis. EMBO J 2002;21(14):3704–3714.

52. Peter ME. The flip side of FLIP. Biochem J 2004;382(Pt 2): e1–e3.

53. Zou H, Henzel WJ, Liu X, et al. Apaf-1, a human protein homologous to C. elegans CED-4, participates in cytochrome c–dependent activation of caspase-3. Cell 1997; 90(3):405–413.

54. Zou H, Li Y, Liu X, Wang X. An APAF-1.cytochrome c multimeric complex is a functional apoptosome that activates procaspase-9. J Biol Chem 1999;274(17):11549–11556.

55. Cecconi F, Alvarez-Bolado G, Meyer BI, et al. Apaf1 (CED-4 homolog) regulates programmed cell death in mammalian development. Cell 1998;94(6):727–737.

56. Srinivasula SM, Ahmad M, Fernandes-Alnemri T, Alnemri ES. Autoactivation of procaspase-9 by Apaf-1–mediated oligomerization. Mol Cell 1998;1(7):949–957.

57. Zhong LT, Sarafian T, Kane DJ, et al. bcl-2 inhibits death of central neural cells induced by multiple agents. Proc Natl Acad Sci U S A 1993;90(10):4533–4537.

58. Reed JC. Bcl-2 family proteins. Oncogene 1998;17(25): 3225–3236.

59. Saikumar P, Dong Z, Patel Y, et al. Role of hypoxia-induced Bax translocation and cytochrome c release in reoxygenation injury. Oncogene 1998;17(26):3401–3415.

60. Mikhailov V, Mikhailova M, Degenhardt K, et al. Association of Bax and Bak homo-oligomers in mitochondria. Bax requirement for Bak reorganization and cytochrome c release. J Biol Chem 2003;278(7):5367–5376.

61. Mikhailov V, Mikhailova M, Pulkrabek DJ, et al. Bcl-2 prevents Bax oligomerization in the mitochondrial outer membrane. J Biol Chem 2001;276(21):18361–18374.

62. Shi Y. Mechanisms of caspase activation and inhibition during apoptosis. Mol Cell 2002;9(3):459–470.

63. Ekert PG, Silke J, Hawkins CJ, et al. DIABLO promotes apoptosis by removing MIHA/XIAP from processed caspase 9. J Cell Biol 2001;152(3):483–490.

64. Deveraux QL, Reed JC. IAP family proteins—suppressors of apoptosis. Genes Dev 1999;13(3):239–252.

65. Imoto I, Yang ZQ, Pimkhaokham A, et al. Identification of cIAP1 as a candidate target gene within an amplicon at 11q22 in esophageal squamous cell carcinomas. Cancer Res 2001;61(18):6629–6634.

66. Dierlamm J, Baens M, Wlodarska I, et al. The apoptosis inhibitor gene API2 and a novel 18q gene, MLT, are recurrently rearranged in the t(11;18)(q21;q21) associated with mucosa-associated lymphoid tissue lymphomas. Blood 1999;93(11):3601–3609.

67. Ambrosini G, Adida C, Altieri DC. A novel anti-apoptosis gene, survivin, expressed in cancer and lymphoma. Nat Med 1997;3(8):917–921.

68. Suzuki Y, Imai Y, Nakayama H, et al. A serine protease, HtrA2, is released from the mitochondria and interacts with XIAP, inducing cell death. Mol Cell 2001;8(3):613–621.

69. Yang QH, Church-Hajduk R, Ren J, et al. Omi/HtrA2 catalytic cleavage of inhibitor of apoptosis (IAP) irrevers-

ibly inactivates IAPs and facilitates caspase activity in apoptosis. Genes Dev 2003;17(12):1487–1496.

70. Pandey P, Farber R, Nakazawa A, et al. Hsp27 functions as a negative regulator of cytochrome c-dependent activation of procaspase-3. Oncogene 2000;19(16):1975–1981.

71. Beere HM, Wolf BB, Cain K, et al. Heat-shock protein 70 inhibits apoptosis by preventing recruitment of procaspase-9 to the Apaf-1 apoptosome. Nat Cell Biol 2000;2(8):469–475.

72. Pandey P, Saleh A, Nakazawa A, et al. Negative regulation of cytochrome c–mediated oligomerization of Apaf-1 and activation of procaspase-9 by heat shock protein 90. EMBO J 2000;19(16):4310–4322.

73. Jiang X, Kim HE, Shu H, et al. Distinctive roles of PHAP proteins and prothymosin-alpha in a death regulatory pathway. Science 2003;299(5604):223–226.

74. Widmann C, Gibson S, Johnson GL. Caspase-dependent cleavage of signaling proteins during apoptosis. A turn-off mechanism for anti-apoptotic signals. J Biol Chem 1998;273(12):7141–7147.

75. Sanghavi DM, Thelen M, Thornberry NA, et al. Caspase-mediated proteolysis during apoptosis: insights from apoptotic neutrophils. FEBS Lett 1998;422(2):179–184.

76. Schittny JC, Djonov V, Fine A, Burri PH. Programmed cell death contributes to postnatal lung development. Am J Respir Cell Mol Biol 1998;18(6):786–793.

77. Haslett C. Granulocyte apoptosis and its role in the resolution and control of lung inflammation. Am J Respir Crit Care Med 1999;160(5 Pt 2):S5–S11.

78. Bardales RH, Xie SS, Schaefer RF, Hsu SM. Apoptosis is a major pathway responsible for the resolution of type II pneumocytes in acute lung injury. Am J Pathol 1996;149(3):845–852.

79. Durmowicz AG, Stenmark KR. Mechanisms of structural remodeling in chronic pulmonary hypertension. Pediatr Rev 1999;20(11):e91–e102.

80. Hagimoto N, Kuwano K, Miyazaki H, et al. Induction of apoptosis and pulmonary fibrosis in mice in response to ligation of Fas antigen. Am J Respir Cell Mol Biol 1997;17(3):272–278.

81. Kuwano K, Hagimoto N, Kawasaki M, et al. Essential roles of the Fas–Fas ligand pathway in the development of pulmonary fibrosis. J Clin Invest 1999;104(1):13–19.

82. Haslett C, Savill JS, Whyte MK, et al. Granulocyte apoptosis and the control of inflammation. Philos Trans R Soc Lond B Biol Sci 1994;345(1313):327–333.

83. Cox G, Crossley J, Xing Z. Macrophage engulfment of apoptotic neutrophils contributes to the resolution of acute pulmonary inflammation in vivo. Am J Respir Cell Mol Biol 1995;12(2):232–237.

84. Matute-Bello G, Liles WC, Radella F 2nd, et al. Modulation of neutrophil apoptosis by granulocyte colony-stimulating factor and granulocyte/macrophage colony-stimulating factor during the course of acute respiratory distress syndrome. Crit Care Med 2000;28(1):1–7.

85. Aggarwal A, Baker CS, Evans TW, Haslam PL. G-CSF and IL-8 but not GM-CSF correlate with severity of pulmonary neutrophilia in acute respiratory distress syndrome. Eur Respir J 2000;15(5):895–901.

86. Lesur O, Kokis A, Hermans C, et al. Interleukin-2 involvement in early acute respiratory distress syndrome: relationship with polymorphonuclear neutrophil apoptosis and patient survival. Crit Care Med 2000;28(12):3814–3822.

87. Teder P, Vandivier RW, Jiang D, et al. Resolution of lung inflammation by CD44. Science 2002;296(5565):155–158.

88. Fadok VA, Bratton DL, Konowal A, et al. Macrophages that have ingested apoptotic cells in vitro inhibit proinflammatory cytokine production through autocrine/paracrine mechanisms involving TGF-beta, PGE2, and PAF. J Clin Invest 1998;101(4):890–898.

89. Huynh ML, Fadok VA, Henson PM. Phosphatidylserine-dependent ingestion of apoptotic cells promotes TGF-beta1 secretion and the resolution of inflammation. J Clin Invest 2002;109(1):41–50.

90. Matute-Bello G, Liles WC, Frevert CW, et al. Recombinant human Fas ligand induces alveolar epithelial cell apoptosis and lung injury in rabbits. Am J Physiol Lung Cell Mol Physiol 2001;281(2):L328–L335.

91. Fine A, Anderson NL, Rothstein TL, et al. Fas expression in pulmonary alveolar type II cells. Am J Physiol 1997;273(1 Pt 1):L64–L71.

92. Hamann KJ, Dorscheid DR, Ko FD, et al. Expression of Fas (CD95) and FasL (CD95L) in human airway epithelium. Am J Respir Cell Mol Biol 1998;19(4):537–542.

93. White MK, Baireddy V, Strayer DS. Natural protection from apoptosis by surfactant protein A in type II pneumocytes. Exp Cell Res 2001;263(2):183–192.

94. Segura-Valdez L, Pardo A, Gaxiola M, et al. Upregulation of gelatinases A and B, collagenases 1 and 2, and increased parenchymal cell death in COPD. Chest 2000;117(3):684–694.

95. Kasahara Y, Tuder RM, Taraseviciene-Stewart L, et al. Inhibition of VEGF receptors causes lung cell apoptosis and emphysema. J Clin Invest 2000;106(11):1311–1319.

96. Tuder RM, Zhen L, Cho CY, et al. Oxidative stress and apoptosis interact and cause emphysema due to vascular endothelial growth factor receptor blockade. Am J Respir Cell Mol Biol 2003;29(1):88–97.

97. Druilhe A, Letuve S, Pretolani M. Glucocorticoid-induced apoptosis in human eosinophils: mechanisms of action. Apoptosis 2003;8(5):481–495.

98. Kuwano K, Maeyama T, Inoshima I, et al. Increased circulating levels of soluble Fas ligand are correlated with disease activity in patients with fibrosing lung diseases. Respirology 2002;7(1):15–21.

99. Li X, Zhang H, Soledad-Conrad V, Zhuang J, Uhal BD. Bleomycin-induced apoptosis of alveolar epithelial cells requires angiotensin synthesis de novo. Am J Physiol Lung Cell Mol Physiol 2003;284(3):L501–L507.

100. Miyazaki H, Kuwano K, Yoshida K, et al. The perforin mediated apoptotic pathway in lung injury and fibrosis. J Clin Pathol 2004;57(12):1292–1298.

101. Lee CG, Homer RJ, Zhu Z, et al. Interleukin-13 induces tissue fibrosis by selectively stimulating and activating transforming growth factor beta(1). J Exp Med 2001;194(6):809–821.

102. Lee CG, Cho SJ, Kang MJ, et al. Early growth response gene 1-mediated apoptosis is essential for transforming growth factor beta1-induced pulmonary fibrosis. J Exp Med 2004;200(3):377–389.

103. Travis WD, Lubin J, Ries L, Devesa S. United States lung carcinoma incidence trends: declining for most histologic types among males, increasing among females. Cancer 1996;77(12):2464–2470.

104. Sekido Y, Fong KM, Minna JD. Progress in understanding the molecular pathogenesis of human lung cancer. Biochim Biophys Acta 1998;1378(1):F21–F59.

105. Shivapurkar N, Reddy J, Matta H, et al. Loss of expression of death-inducing signaling complex (DISC) components in lung cancer cell lines and the influence of MYC amplification. Oncogene 2002;21(55):8510–8514.

106. Cheng EH, Kirsch DG, Clem RJ, et al. Conversion of Bcl-2 to a Bax-like death effector by caspases. Science 1997; 278(5345):1966–1968.

107. Joseph B, Ekedahl J, Sirzen F, et al. Differences in expression of pro-caspases in small cell and non-small cell lung carcinoma. Biochem Biophys Res Commun 1999;262(2): 381–387.

108. Joseph B, Ekedahl J, Lewensohn R, et al. Defective caspase-3 relocalization in non-small cell lung carcinoma. Oncogene 2001;20(23):2877–2888.

109. Krepela E, Prochazka J, Liul X, et al. Increased expression of Apaf-1 and procaspase-3 and the functionality of intrinsic apoptosis apparatus in non–small cell lung carcinoma. Biol Chem 2004;385(2):153–168.

110. Okouoyo S, Herzer K, Ucur E, et al. Rescue of death receptor and mitochondrial apoptosis signaling in resistant human NSCLC in vivo. Int J Cancer 2004;108(4):580–587.

111. Ekedahl J, Joseph B, Grigoriev MY, et al. Expression of inhibitor of apoptosis proteins in small- and non-small-cell lung carcinoma cells. Exp Cell Res 2002;279(2):277–290.

5
Roles of Mutation and Epimutation in the Development of Lung Disease

William B. Coleman

Introduction

The diseases of the lung reflect a spectrum of pathologies and mechanisms of pathogenesis spanning genetic, infectious, inflammatory, obstructive, and neoplastic processes. Gene mutations and other genetic alterations play a significant role in many lung diseases. Likewise, nongenetic alterations affecting the expression of key genes (epimutations) may also contribute to the genesis of lung disease. In this chapter, the molecular bases of the major lung diseases are reviewed. This review is not intended to be comprehensive. Rather, the current state of understanding related to the genes and molecular mechanisms (genetic and epigenetic) that contribute to major forms of lung disease (such as lung cancer) is discussed. For the interested reader, more complete reviews of specific topics are cited in the text.

Pathogenesis of Lung Disease

Lung disease represents an important human health problem. Respiratory infections occur commonly among people of all ages and represent a major concern in clinical practice. Likewise, given the prevalence of cigarette smoking among the general population and the extent of air pollution (particularly in metropolitan areas), the development of lung diseases related to exposure to inhalants (including chronic bronchitis and emphysema) has significantly risen in recent decades.[1-3] Furthermore, the incidence of lung cancer has continued to increase at alarming rates, and lung cancer now represents the most common lethal neoplasm among men and women.[4] It is recognized that environmental exposures contribute in substantial ways to the development of various lung diseases. In addition, several genetic factors can predispose to or exacerbate environmentally induced lung diseases. This review focuses on (1) lung cancer, (2) emphysema, and (3) cystic fibrosis (CF) to illustrate the contributions of mutation and epimutation to the pathogenesis of lung disease.

Mutations and Epimutations

Mutation refers to a change in the genome that is characterized by an alteration in the nucleotide sequence of a specific gene and/or other alteration at the level of the primary structure of DNA. Point mutations, insertions, deletions, and chromosomal abnormalities are all classified as mutations. In contrast, *epimutation* refers to an alteration in the genome that does not involve a change in the primary sequence of the DNA. Aberrant DNA methylation and/or abnormal modifications of chromatin are considered epimutations. Despite the differences between mutation and epimutation, the consequences of these molecular processes on the normal expression and function of critical genes and proteins can be the same—reduction of normal gene expression and/or loss of normal protein function.

Genetic Alterations

Disease-related genetic alterations can be categorized into two major groups: (1) nucleotide sequence abnormalities and (2) chromosomal abnormalities. Examples of both of these forms of molecular lesions have been characterized in familial and acquired diseases of the lung.

Nucleotide sequence alterations include changes in individual genes involving single nucleotide changes (missense and nonsense) and small insertions or deletions (some of which result in frameshift mutations). Single nucleotide alterations that involve a change in the normal coding sequence of the gene (point mutations) can give rise to an alteration in the amino acid sequence of the encoded protein. Missense mutations alter the translation of the affected codon, whereas nonsense mutations alter codons that encode amino acids to produce stop codons. This results in premature termination of translation and the synthesis of a truncated protein product. Small deletions and insertions are typically classified as frameshift mutations, because deletion or insertion of a single nucleotide (for instance) will alter the reading frame of the gene on the 3′ side of the affected site. This alteration can result in the synthesis of a protein that bears very little resemblance to the normal gene product or production of an abnormal/truncated protein because of the presence of a stop codon in the altered reading frame. In addition, deletion or insertion of one or more groups of three nucleotides will not alter the reading frame of the gene but will alter the resulting polypeptide product, which will exhibit either loss of specific amino acids or the presence of additional amino acids within its primary structure.

Chromosomal alterations include the gain or loss of one or more chromosomes (aneuploidy), chromosomal rearrangements resulting from DNA strand breakage (translocations, inversions, and other rearrangements), and gain or loss of portions of chromosomes (amplification, large-scale deletion). The direct result of chromosomal translocation is the movement of some segment of DNA from its natural location into a new location within the genome, which can result in altered expression of the genes that are contained within the translocated region. If the chromosomal breakpoints utilized in a translocation are located within structural genes, then hybrid (chimeric) genes can be generated. The major consequence of chromosomal deletion (involving a whole chromosome or a large chromosomal region) is the loss of specific genes that are localized to the deleted chromosomal segment, resulting in changes in the copy number of the affected genes. Likewise, gain of chromosome number or amplification of chromosomal regions results in an increase in the copy numbers of genes found in these chromosomal locations.

Epigenetic Alterations

In contemporary terms, *epigenetics* refers to modifications of the genome that are heritable during cell division but do not involve a change in the DNA sequence.[5] Epigenetics describes heritable changes in gene expression that are not simply attributable to nucleotide sequence variation.[6] It is now recognized that epigenetic regulation of gene expression reflects contributions from both DNA methylation as well as complex modifications of histone proteins and chromatin structure.[7] Nonetheless, DNA methylation plays a central role in nongenomic inheritance and in the preservation of epigenetic states, and it remains the most accessible epigenomic feature because of its inherent stability. Thus, DNA methylation represents a target of fundamental importance for the charac-terization of the epigenome and for defining the role of epigenetics in disease pathogenesis.

Neoplastic Lung Diseases

Cancers of the lung and bronchus represent >90% of all respiratory system tumors.[8] The major forms of primary lung cancer include small cell lung carcinoma (SCLC) and non–small cell lung carcinoma (NSCLC). The SCLCs account for approximately 10% of lung cancers, and NSCLCs account for the balance.[9] Most NSCLCs can be classified as one of several major histologic subtypes: squamous cell carcinoma (approximately 35% of lung cancers), adenocarcinoma (approximately 35% of lung cancers), and large cell carcinoma (approximately 15% of lung cancers).[9]

Pathogenesis of Lung Cancer

Several risk factors for the development of lung cancer have been identified, and the majority of lung cancers can be linked to exposure to known carcinogenic agents, particularly cigarette smoke.[10,11] Numerous mutagenic and carcinogenic substances have been identified as constituents of the particulate or vapor phases of cigarette smoke, including benzo[a]pyrene, dibenza[a]anthracene, nickel, cadmium, polonium, urethane, formaldehyde, nitrogen oxides, and nitrosodiethylamine.[12–14] There is also evidence that smoking, combined with certain environmental (or occupational) exposures, results in potentiation of lung cancer risk. Urban smokers exhibit significantly higher incidences of lung cancer than smokers from rural areas, suggesting a possible role for air pollution in the development of lung cancer.[15] Occupational exposure to asbestos, bis(chloromethyl) ether, and chromium have been suggested to increase the risk of lung cancer development.[16,17] Likewise, high levels of exposure to the radioactive gas radon by miners working in uranium, iron, zinc, tin, and fluorspar mines may also contribute to increased lung cancer risk.[18,19] Common to all of these lung cancer risk factors are carcinogenic compounds with mutagenic properties, suggesting that a genotoxic event (resulting in mutation) contributes to disease pathogenesis.

Chromosomal Alterations in Lung Cancer

Chromosomal alterations have been widely documented in the various forms of lung cancer. In some cases, these alterations represent loss of individual chromosomes, chromosome arms, or specific chromosomal segments, consistent with deletion of a tumor suppressor locus. In other cases, these alterations represent gain of individual chromosomes or specific chromosomal segments, consistent with activation of a positive mediator of cell prolif-eration. In addition, some chromosomal rearrangements (such as translocation) have been characterized in lung cancer. In each of these cases, the result is alteration of gene dose (either as gene loss or gene amplification) and function (altered product or altered expression). The acti-vation and inactivation of specific genes that function as positive and negative mediators of cell proliferation cooperate in the neoplastic transformation of lung epi-thelial cells. A survey of chromosomal alterations found in lung cancer is provided below.

Amplification of the c-Myc Protooncogene in Lung Cancer

Several chromosomal regions have been characterized to be overrepresented in lung cancer,[20,21] suggestive of amplification of chromosomal regions. One such fre-quently overrepresented region is chromosome 8q, which harbors the c-*Myc* protooncogene.[22] The c-*Myc* protoon-cogene is a member of the basic helix-loop-helix super-family of nuclear transcription factors.[23] The Myc protein heterodimerizes with Max and the resulting Myc–Max protein complexes transcriptionally activate genes that contain a CAGCTG consensus binding sequence.[24-27] Increased expression of c-*Myc* has been reported for both SCLC and NSCLC.[28-32] Likewise, amplification of the c-*Myc* locus has been observed in both SCLC and NSCLC[33] but may be more prevalent in SCLC.[34] Thus, overexpression of c-*Myc* in lung cancer is the frequent consequence of gene amplification at 8q24.[35-37] Gene amplification and overexpression of c-*Myc* occurs more frequently in advanced neoplasms and metastatic lesions, suggesting a role for this event in tumor progression and partially explaining the significant correlation between c-*Myc* amplification and poor prognosis[36]. Unlike other cancers (such as lymphoma), point mutation of c-*Myc* and c-*Myc* gene translocation related to a specific chro-mosomal alteration have not been reported in lung cancer.

Common Chromosomal Deletions in Lung Cancer

Allelotype studies of lung cancer have identified several recurring chromosomal deletions. In SCLC, frequent loss of heterozygosity (LOH) occurs at 3p (91%), 5q (71%), 13q (96%), 17p (88%), and 22q (73%).[38] The NSCLCs display frequent LOH at 2q (68%), 3p (82%), 5q (60%), 9p (79%), 12q (63%), 13q (67%), 17p (89%), 18q (86%), and 22q (75%).[39] However, distinct differences in the patterns of chromosomal deletion have been noted for the histologic subtypes of NSCLC. Among squamous cell carcinomas, frequent LOH was noted for 3p (82%), 9q

(67%), 13q (60%), and 17p (88%).[40] In contrast, fewer chromosomal losses were noted among adenocarcino-mas, with 51% LOH at 17p representing the most fre-quent alteration.[40] In other studies, similar findings have been reported.[41-43]

Deletions affecting a specific chromosomal region (as measured by LOH) may be indicative of the presence of a tumor suppressor gene (or other negative mediator of cell proliferation) at that chromosomal location. Among lung cancers, frequent LOH affecting 3p, 5q, 13q, 17p, and 22q occurs in both SCLC and NSCLC. Several regions of chromosome 3p have been implicated in lung cancer, including 3p12–p14, 3p21, and 3p25.[44-46] These observa-tions suggest that there may be three (or more) tumor suppressor genes on human chromosome 3p[46]. Candidate tumor suppressor genes from chromosome 3p include *FHIT* at 3p12–p14[47] and *RASSF1* at 3p21.[48] Loss of het-erozygosity at chromosome 5q typically corresponds to loss at 5q13–q21.[49] A number of genes map to this chro-mosomal region, including *MCC* (for *mutated in colorec-tal cancer*) and *APC* (for *adenomatous polyposis coli*).[50-53] Although neither of these genes has been shown to be mutated in lung cancer,[54] frequent LOH at this chromo-somal region suggests the involvement of one of these or other candidate genes localized to this region in the molecular pathogenesis of lung cancer. The tumor sup-pressor gene *Rb1* localizes to chromosome 13q14.1.[55,56] The expression of *Rb1* is altered in a significant percent-age of primary lung cancer.[57,58] The *p53* tumor suppressor gene is located at 17p13.1[59] and is often lost because of chromosomal deletion of this region in all lung cancer types.[60] The precise nature of the putative lung cancer tumor suppressor locus at chromosome 22q is not yet defined. However, a candidate gene, termed *SEZ6L*, has been localized to 22q12.1 and shown to be mutated in a SCLC cell line.[61]

Complex Chromosomal Rearrangements in Lung Cancer

Progress toward characterization of complex chromo-somal rearrangements in lung cancer was hindered by technical limitations until recently when spectral karyo-typing became available. A number of studies using spec-tral karyotyping of lung cancer have now emerged.[42,62,63] These studies identified a number of unbalanced chromo-somal translocations, in many cases involving some of the same chromosomal regions that are frequently deleted in lung cancer. These complex chromosomal rearrange-ments may alter the structure or expression of genes localized to the affected chromosomal regions. However, additional investigation will be required to characterize the molecular consequences associated with specific chromosomal rearrangements in lung cancer.

Gene Mutations in Lung Cancer

Mutations affecting a variety of genes have been characterized in lung cancer. Some of these mutations represent activating mutations of protooncogenes (or other positive mediators of cell proliferation), and others represent inactivating mutations of tumor suppressor genes (or other negative mediators of cell proliferation). Mutations in these genes synergize with other genetic (chromosomal) and epigenetic abnormalities to drive neoplastic transformation and tumorigenesis in the lung. This review focuses on mutations affecting K-*ras*, *p53*, and *p16^{INK4A}*.

The ras *Gene Family*

Three genes constitute the *ras* gene family: H-*ras*, K-*ras*, and N-*ras*. The majority of *ras* mutations in human lung cancer occur in the K-*ras* gene.[64,65] K-*ras* is mutated in 15%–20% of all NSCLC and in 30%–50% of lung adenocarcinomas[34,64,66–70] but is infrequently mutated in other lung cancer types.[34,67] In lung adenocarcinomas, 85% of K-*ras* mutations affect codon 12.[65] Certain carcinogens found in cigarette smoke, such as benzo[a]pyrene, have been shown to preferentially adduct codon 12 of K-*ras*, and this adduct is not effectively repaired.[71,72] No K-*ras* mutations are found in adenocarcinomas of nonsmokers, supporting a specific role of tobacco carcinogens in the mutation of K-*ras*[73]. The majority of K-*ras* codon 12 mutations are G to T transversions,[74] resulting in either glycine to cysteine (GGT to TGT) or glycine to valine (GGT to GTT) amino acid substitutions in the mutant protein.

The ras protein functions in cell signaling like a heterotrimeric G protein, toggling between inactive and active forms. In response to a specific cell stimulus, inactive ras protein releases bound guanosine diphosphate (GDP) and binds a guanosine triphosphate (GTP) molecule.[75,76] In this GTP-bound active configuration, cell signaling occurs until the intrinsic GTPase activity of the ras protein itself cleaves the GTP to GDP, resulting in reacquisition of the inactive configuration.[75,76] Mutant K-ras proteins lack intrinsic GTPase activity and remain in a continuously active form.[77] The constitutive activation of K-*ras* through this mutational mechanism leads to the induction of multiple signaling pathways involved with cell proliferation and cell survival.[78]

Tumor Suppressor p53

The *p53* tumor suppressor gene is one of the most frequently mutated genes in cancer.[79,80] The *p53* gene may be involved in the molecular pathogenesis of lung cancer through chromosomal deletion of 17p13.1, as well as through gene mutation. Approximately 50% of NSCLCs and 90% of SCLCs harbor mutations in the *p53* gene.[81–83]

The *p53* mutational spectrum in lung cancer indicates that G to T transversions dominate and that specific hotspot codons are frequently mutated (including codons 157, 158, 175, 245, 248, 249, and 273).[84] The types of mutations detected may reflect the interaction of the DNA with specific carcinogens found in cigarette smoke.[85,86]

The p53 protein functions as a transcriptional regulator and mediator of cellular responses to DNA damage and stress.[87] Point mutation of *p53* leads to synthesis of mutant forms of the protein that do not fold properly,[88] resulting in a nonfunctional protein that will not bind DNA.[89,90] When this mutant protein oligomerizes with other p53 molecules (normal or mutant), the resultant tetramers (or higher order oligomers) are nonfunctional.[91] Thus, cells with mutant *p53* (or *p53* deficiency due to chromosomal deletion) become susceptible to progressive genomic instability and accumulation of additional genetic damage.[92,93]

Tumor Suppressor p16^{INK4A}

Inactivating mutations of the *p16^{INK4A}* tumor suppressor gene are common in lung cancer, particularly in NSCLCs[94]. *p16^{INK4A}* is also subject to inactivation through deletion of chromosome 9p21 or hypermethylation of its promoter CpG island[95]. Thus, three different molecular mechanisms can lead to the inactivation of the *p16^{INK4A}* gene in lung cancer.[96] The *p16^{INK4A}* tumor suppressor gene encodes a cyclin-dependent kinase (Cdk) inhibitor that plays a key role in *Rb1*-mediated cell cycle control pathway. The p16^{INK4A} protein inhibits the activities of Cdk4–cyclin D, Cdk6–cyclin D, and Cdk2–cyclin E, leading to a blockade of pRb phosphorylation (with persistence of E2F sequestration) and growth suppression.[97] When *p16^{INK4A}* is mutated, the function of the protein is lost, resulting in a loss of normal cell cycle control and a persistent progression of cells through the cell cycle.

Epimutations in Lung Cancer

Several genes are known to be hypermethylated in lung cancer, resulting in gene silencing.[98] Among these genes, *p16^{INK4A}* is found to be methylated in >40% of lung cancers examined.[95,96] Although it is recognized that hypermethylation of *p16^{INK4A}* occurs frequently in lung cancer, there is debate regarding the importance of this mechanism of inactivation among lung cancer patients who are smokers versus nonsmokers (or never smokers). In one study, deletion or mutation of the *p16^{INK4A}* gene was observed only in the lung cancers of smokers, whereas hypermethylation was found only among nonsmokers.[99] In contrast, other studies have found hypermethylation of *p16^{INK4A}* as the prevalent mechanism of inactivation among lung cancers from smokers.[100] Other epigenetically regulated genes in lung cancer include *CDH1*,[101]

CDKN1A,[102] DAPK1,[103] ESR1,[104] GJB2,[105] GSTP1,[106] HS3ST2,[107] PRDM2,[108] PRKCDBP,[109] RASSF1,[110] and SFN.[111] Like p16[INK4A], RASSF1 may be subject to inactivation through multiple molecular mechanisms, including hypermethylation[110] and deletion of chromosome 3p21.[48] Using recently developed array-based methods, a number of putative targets for promoter methylation in lung cancer (including some new gene targets) have been identified, including HIC1, IRF7, ASC, RIPK3, FABP3, and PAX3.[112]

Obstructive Lung Diseases

The major forms of obstructive lung disease include emphysema, chronic bronchitis, bronchiectasis, and asthma. Emphysema and chronic bronchitis are often grouped together and referred to as chronic obstructive pulmonary disease (COPD). Various factors contribute to the development of COPD, including cigarette smoking. The majority of patients with COPD are long-term heavy cigarette smokers, but only a minority of cigarette smokers develop COPD, suggesting a role for additional (possibly genetic) factors in the development of this condition. In addition, obstructive lung disease is a major clinical manifestation of CF, which is a multiorgan disease with a clear genetic component. In this section, genetic and epigenetic alterations in specific genes contributing to emphysema and CF are reviewed.

Pathogenesis of Emphysema

Emphysema is characterized by permanent enlargement of the airspaces distal to the terminal bronchiole, accompanied by bronchiolar wall damage, but without fibrosis. There are four major forms of emphysema, which are classified by their anatomic distribution within the lobule: (1) centriacinar, (2) panacinar, (3) paraseptal, and (4) irregular.[113] Centriacinar emphysema accounts for the majority (>95%) of cases. The clinical treatment of emphysema does not depend on the classification of the disease, however. The etiologic mechanisms for development of emphysema have not been firmly established, but the prevailing theory focuses on alterations in the balance between protease and antiprotease enzymes.[114] This theory holds that an imbalance between protease enzymes (particularly elastase) and antiproteases (such as α_1-antitrypsin) in the lung leads over time to alveolar wall destruction.[114] According to this idea, emphysema will develop when the elastase–antielastase balance is altered through a relative increase in elastase activity (perhaps in association with cigarette smoking or persistent lung infection) or a relative decrease in the antielastase defense mechanisms (as in the case of α_1-antitrypsin deficiency).[115]

Gene Mutations in Emphysema

The best-characterized genetic risk factor for emphysema is α_1-antitrypsin deficiency.[116] However, α_1-antitrypsin deficiency is a rare condition and accounts for only 1%–2% of patients with emphysema,[117] typically those with panacinar pathology.[115] α_1-Antitrypsin is a member of the serine protease inhibitor superfamily of proteins, which function to inactivate neutrophil elastase and other proteases to maintain the protease–antiprotease balance.[118] Normally, α_1-antitrypsin is synthesized in the liver and secreted into the blood, producing serum concentrations of 20–53 μmol/L.[115] In deficient individuals, α_1-antitrypsin levels in the serum fall below 20 μmol/L.[115] A number of different mutant alleles for α_1-antitrypsin have been identified and characterized.[119] Most clinically recognized cases of α_1-antitrypsin deficiency are due to the presence of the Z allele, which is characterized by the substitution of lysine for glutamic acid at position 342 (Glu342Lys).[115] The Glu342Lys mutation leads to polymerization of the Z form of α_1-antitrypsin within hepatocytes, resulting in impaired secretion and reduction of the plasma levels of α_1-antitrypsin to 15% of normal.[118,120] To compound the α_1-antitrypsin deficiency in these patients, the Z form of α_1-antitrypsin does not function properly.[121] Thus, deficiency in the antielastase activity of α_1-antitrypsin due to diminished serum levels and decreased activity of the defective protein (Z form) sets up a chronic condition in the patient characterized by a relative excess of elastase activity and destruction of lung tissue.

Pathogenesis of Cystic Fibrosis

Cystic fibrosis is a fairly common genetically based multiorgan disease caused by a disorder in epithelial transport function affecting fluid secretion in exocrine glands and the epithelial lining of the respiratory, gastrointestinal, and reproductive tracts.[122] Chronic lung disease is one of the major clinical manifestations of CF. Affected individuals have impaired lung clearance because of the production of thick mucus by the submucosal glands of the respiratory tree and develop secondary obstruction of the air passages. The inspissation of these mucus secretions leads to impaired air flow and creates a setting for frequent, persistent pulmonary infections culminating in bronchiectasis.[123]

Gene Mutations in Cystic Fibrosis

The molecular basis for the development of CF is mutation of the cystic fibrosis transmembrane conductance regulator (CFTR) gene.[124,125] The symptomatology of CF is highly variable from patient to patient, possibly owing to differences in CFTR function because of specific mutations.[126–128] Given that epithelia in CF patients behave as though they are impermeable to chloride ions,[129] it was expected that the *CFTR* gene would encode a chloride channel. However, it was found that the *CFTR* gene encodes an ABC transporter homolog that actually functions as a chloride channel that is directly activated by phosphorylation.[125] The most common mutation in the *CFTR* gene is designated ΔF508 and results in deletion of phenylalanine at position 508 within nucleotide binding domain 1 of the CFTR protein.[125] The ΔF508 mutation accounts for >65% of *CFTR* mutations, although >1,000 other *CFTR* mutations have been documented. The ΔF508–CFTR protein is not properly folded during post-translational processing and is rapidly degraded, resulting in deficiency of CFTR protein.[130]

Epimutations in Cystic Fibrosis

Evidence in the literature strongly suggests that loss of CFTR function causes CF, and a large number of mutations in the *CFTR* gene have been characterized.[125] However, there is some evidence that the *CFTR* gene may be subject to methylation-dependent epigenetic regulation. The promoter of the *CFTR* gene is remarkably GC rich.[131,132] Early studies found hypermethylation of the *CFTR* promoter in various cell lines analyzed, which correlated with low levels of expression.[133,134] However, a more detailed bisulfite sequencing analysis of the *CFTR* promoter has not been reported. Nevertheless, these results suggest that the *CFTR* gene may be subject to epigenetic regulation through promoter hypermethylation, possibly representing a nonmutational mechanism for inactivation of *CFTR* leading to CF.

References

1. Maziak W. The asthma epidemic and our artificial habitats. BMC Pulm Med 2005;5:5.
2. Walusiak J. Occupational upper airway disease. Curr Opin Allergy Clin Immunol 2006;6:1–6.
3. Wong GW, von Mutius E, Douwes J, Pearce N. Environmental determinants associated with the development of asthma in childhood. Int J Tuberc Lung Dis 2006;10:242–251.
4. Jemal A, Siegel R, Ward E, et al. Cancer statistics, 2006. CA Cancer J Clin 2006;56:106–130.
5. Coleman WB, Rivenbark AG. Quantitative DNA methylation analysis: the promise of high-throughput epigenomic diagnostic testing in human neoplastic disease. J Mol Diagn 2006;8:152–156.
6. Murrell A, Rakyan VK, Beck S. From genome to epigenome. Hum Mol Genet 2005;14 Spec No 1:R3–R10.
7. Fuks F. DNA methylation and histone modifications: teaming up to silence genes. Curr Opin Genet Dev 2005;15:490–495.
8. Landis SH, Murray T, Bolden S, Wingo PA. Cancer statistics, 1999. CA Cancer J Clin 1999;49:8–31.
9. Giaccone G, Smit E. Lung cancer. Cancer Chemother Biol Response Modif 2003;21:445–483.
10. Shopland DR, Eyre HJ, Pechacek TF. Smoking-attributable cancer mortality in 1991: is lung cancer now the leading cause of death among smokers in the United States? J Natl Cancer Inst 1991;83:1142–1148.
11. Garfinkel L, Silverberg E. Lung cancer and smoking trends in the United States over the past 25 years. CA Cancer J Clin 1991;41:137–145.
12. Smith CJ, Livingston SD, Doolittle DJ. An international literature survey of "IARC Group I carcinogens" reported in mainstream cigarette smoke. Food Chem Toxicol 1997;35:1107–1130.
13. Smith CJ, Perfetti TA, Mullens MA, et al. "IARC group 2B Carcinogens" reported in cigarette mainstream smoke. Food Chem Toxicol 2000;38:825–848.
14. Smith CJ, Perfetti TA, Rumple MA, et al. "IARC group 2A Carcinogens" reported in cigarette mainstream smoke. Food Chem Toxicol 2000;38:371–383.
15. Haenszel W, Loveland DB, Sirken MG. Lung-cancer mortality as related to residence and smoking histories. I. White males. J Natl Cancer Inst 1962;28:947–1001.
16. Hammond EC, Selikoff IJ, Seidman H. Asbestos exposure, cigarette smoking and death rates. Ann NY Acad Sci 1979;330:473–490.
17. Cancer IAfRo. An evaluation of chemicals and industrial processes associated with cancer in humans based on human and animal data: IARC Monographs Volumes 1 to 20. Report of an IARC Working Group. Cancer Res 1980;40:1–12.
18. Archer VE, Gillam JD, Wagoner JK. Respiratory disease mortality among uranium miners. Ann NY Acad Sci 1976;271:280–293.
19. Harley NH, Harley JH. Potential lung cancer risk from indoor radon exposure. CA Cancer J Clin 1990;40:265–275.
20. Berrieman HK, Ashman JN, Cowen ME, Greenman J, Lind MJ, Cawkwell L. Chromosomal analysis of non–small-cell lung cancer by multicolour fluorescent in situ hybridisation. Br J Cancer 2004;90:900–905.
21. Balsara BR, Sonoda G, du Manoir S, et al. Comparative genomic hybridization analysis detects frequent, often high-level, overrepresentation of DNA sequences at 3q, 5p, 7p, and 8q in human non–small cell lung carcinomas. Cancer Res 1997;57:2116–2120.
22. Nowell PC, Croce CM. Chromosomal approaches to the molecular basis of neoplasia. Symp Fundam Cancer Res 1986;39:17–29.
23. Grandori C, Eisenman RN. Myc target genes. Trends Biochem Sci 1997;22:177–181.
24. Hurlin PJ, Huang J. The MAX-interacting transcription factor network. Semin Cancer Biol 2006;16:265–274.
25. Blackwood EM, Eisenman RN. Max: a helix-loop-helix zipper protein that forms a sequence-specific DNA-binding complex with Myc. Science 1991;251:1211–1217.
26. Blackwood EM, Kretzner L, Eisenman RN. Myc and Max function as a nucleoprotein complex. Curr Opin Genet Dev 1992;2:227–235.
27. Blackwood EM, Luscher B, Kretzner L, Eisenman RN. The Myc:Max protein complex and cell growth regulation. Cold Spring Harb Symp Quant Biol 1991;56:109–117.

28. Gazzeri S, Brambilla E, Caron de Fromentel C, et al. p53 genetic abnormalities and myc activation in human lung carcinoma. Int J Cancer 1994;58:24–32.

29. Broers JL, Viallet J, Jensen SM, et al. Expression of c-myc in progenitor cells of the bronchopulmonary epithelium and in a large number of non–small cell lung cancers. Am J Respir Cell Mol Biol 1993;9:33–43.

30. Lorenz J, Friedberg T, Paulus R, et al. Oncogene overexpression in non–small-cell lung cancer tissue: prevalence and clinicopathological significance. Clin Invest 1994;72:156–163.

31. Volm M, Drings P, Wodrich W, van Kaick G. Expression of oncoproteins in primary human non–small cell lung cancer and incidence of metastases. Clin Exp Metastasis 1993;11:325–329.

32. Wodrich W, Volm M. Overexpression of oncoproteins in non–small cell lung carcinomas of smokers. Carcinogenesis 1993;14:1121–1124.

33. Mitani S, Kamata H, Fujiwara M, et al. Analysis of c-myc DNA amplification in non–small cell lung carcinoma in comparison with small cell lung carcinoma using polymerase chain reaction. Clin Exp Med 2001;1:105–111.

34. Richardson GE, Johnson BE. The biology of lung cancer. Semin Oncol 1993;20:105–127.

35. Krystal G, Birrer M, Way J, et al. Multiple mechanisms for transcriptional regulation of the myc gene family in small-cell lung cancer. Mol Cell Biol 1988;8:3373–3381.

36. Johnson BE, Russell E, Simmons AM, et al. MYC family DNA amplification in 126 tumor cell lines from patients with small cell lung cancer. J Cell Biochem Suppl 1996;24:210–217.

37. Levin NA, Brzoska P, Gupta N, et al. Identification of frequent novel genetic alterations in small cell lung carcinoma. Cancer Res 1994;54:5086–5091.

38. Kawanishi M, Kohno T, Otsuka T, et al. Allelotype and replication error phenotype of small cell lung carcinoma. Carcinogenesis 1997;18:2057–2062.

39. Shiseki M, Kohno T, Adachi J, et al. Comparative allelotype of early and advanced stage non–small cell lung carcinomas. Genes Chromosomes Cancer 1996;17:71–77.

40. Sato S, Nakamura Y, Tsuchiya E. Difference of allelotype between squamous cell carcinoma and adenocarcinoma of the lung. Cancer Res 1994;54:5652–5655.

41. Tsuchiya E, Nakamura Y, Weng SY, et al. Allelotype of non–small cell lung carcinoma—comparison between loss of heterozygosity in squamous cell carcinoma and adenocarcinoma. Cancer Res 1992;52:2478–2481.

42. Luk C, Tsao MS, Bayani J, et al. Molecular cytogenetic analysis of non–small cell lung carcinoma by spectral karyotyping and comparative genomic hybridization. Cancer Genet Cytogenet 2001;125:87–99.

43. Lui WO, Tanenbaum DM, Larsson C. High level amplification of 1p32–33 and 2p22–24 in small cell lung carcinomas. Int J Oncol 2001;19:451–457.

44. Hibi K, Takahashi T, Yamakawa K, et al. Three distinct regions involved in 3p deletion in human lung cancer. Oncogene 1992;7:445–449.

45. Brauch H, Tory K, Kotler F, et al. Molecular mapping of deletion sites in the short arm of chromosome 3 in human lung cancer. Genes Chromosomes Cancer 1990;1:240–246.

46. Wistuba II, Behrens C, Virmani AK, et al. High resolution chromosome 3p allelotyping of human lung cancer and preneoplastic/preinvasive bronchial epithelium reveals multiple, discontinuous sites of 3p allele loss and three regions of frequent breakpoints. Cancer Res 2000;60:1949–1960.

47. Zochbauer-Muller S, Wistuba II, Minna JD, Gazdar AF. Fragile histidine triad (FHIT) gene abnormalities in lung cancer. Clin Lung Cancer 2000;2:141–145.

48. Dammann R, Schagdarsurengin U, Seidel C, et al. The tumor suppressor RASSF1A in human carcinogenesis: an update. Histol Histopathol 2005;20:645–663.

49. Hosoe S, Ueno K, Shigedo Y, et al. A frequent deletion of chromosome 5q21 in advanced small cell and non–small cell carcinoma of the lung. Cancer Res 1994;54:1787–1790.

50. Kinzler KW, Nilbert MC, Su LK, et al. Identification of FAP locus genes from chromosome 5q21. Science 1991;253:661–665.

51. Kinzler KW, Nilbert MC, Vogelstein B, et al. Identification of a gene located at chromosome 5q21 that is mutated in colorectal cancers. Science 1991;251:1366–1370.

52. Groden J, Thliveris A, Samowitz W, et al. Identification and characterization of the familial adenomatous polyposis coli gene. Cell 1991;66:589–600.

53. Joslyn G, Carlson M, Thliveris A, et al. Identification of deletion mutations and three new genes at the familial polyposis locus. Cell 1991;66:601–613.

54. Horii A, Nakatsuru S, Miyoshi Y, et al. Frequent somatic mutations of the APC gene in human pancreatic cancer. Cancer Res 1992;52:6696–6698.

55. Fung YK, Murphree AL, T'Ang A, et al. Structural evidence for the authenticity of the human retinoblastoma gene. Science 1987;236:1657–1661.

56. Lee WH, Bookstein R, Hong F, et al. Human retinoblastoma susceptibility gene: cloning, identification, and sequence. Science 1987;235:1394–1399.

57. Hensel CH, Hsieh CL, Gazdar AF, et al. Altered structure and expression of the human retinoblastoma susceptibility gene in small cell lung cancer. Cancer Res 1990;50:3067–3072.

58. Xu HJ, Hu SX, Cagle PT, et al. Absence of retinoblastoma protein expression in primary non–small cell lung carcinomas. Cancer Res 1991;51:2735–2739.

59. McBride OW, Merry D, Givol D. The gene for human p53 cellular tumor antigen is located on chromosome 17 short arm (17p13). Proc Natl Acad Sci U S A 1986;83:130–134.

60. Yokota J, Wada M, Shimosato Y, et al. Loss of heterozygosity on chromosomes 3, 13, and 17 in small-cell carcinoma and on chromosome 3 in adenocarcinoma of the lung. Proc Natl Acad Sci USA 1987;84:9252–9256.

61. Nishioka M, Kohno T, Takahashi M, et al. Identification of a 428-kb homozygously deleted region disrupting the SEZ6L gene at 22q12.1 in a lung cancer cell line. Oncogene 2000;19:6251–6260.

62. Sy SM, Fan B, Lee TW, et al. Spectral karyotyping indicates complex rearrangements in lung adenocarcinoma of non-smokers. Cancer Genet Cytogenet 2004;153:57–59.

63. Sy SM, Wong N, Lee TW, et al. Distinct patterns of genetic alterations in adenocarcinoma and squamous cell carcinoma of the lung. Eur J Cancer 2004;40:1082–1094.

64. Mills NE, Fishman CL, Rom WN, et al. Increased prevalence of K-ras oncogene mutations in lung adenocarcinoma. Cancer Res 1995;55:1444–1447.

65. Slebos RJ, Kibbelaar RE, Dalesio O, et al. K-ras oncogene activation as a prognostic marker in adenocarcinoma of the lung. N Engl J Med 1990;323:561–565.

66. Rodenhuis S, Slebos RJ, Boot AJ, et al. Incidence and possible clinical significance of K-ras oncogene activation in adenocarcinoma of the human lung. Cancer Res 1988;48:5738–5741.

67. Rodenhuis S, Slebos RJ. Clinical significance of ras oncogene activation in human lung cancer. Cancer Res 1992;52:2665s–2669s.

68. Reynolds SH, Anna CK, Brown KC, et al. Activated protooncogenes in human lung tumors from smokers. Proc Natl Acad Sci USA 1991;88:1085–1089.

69. Suzuki Y, Orita M, Shiraishi M, et al. Detection of ras gene mutations in human lung cancers by single-strand conformation polymorphism analysis of polymerase chain reaction products. Oncogene 1990;5:1037–1043.

70. Li S, Rosell R, Urban A, et al. K-ras gene point mutation: a stable tumor marker in non–small cell lung carcinoma. Lung Cancer 1994;11:19–27.

71. Feng Z, Hu W, Chen JX, et al. Preferential DNA damage and poor repair determine ras gene mutational hotspot in human cancer. J Natl Cancer Inst 2002;94:1527–1536.

72. Hu W, Feng Z, Tang MS. Preferential carcinogen-DNA adduct formation at codons 12 and 14 in the human K-ras gene and their possible mechanisms. Biochemistry 2003;42:10012–10023.

73. Ahrendt SA, Decker PA, Alawi EA, et al. Cigarette smoking is strongly associated with mutation of the K-ras gene in patients with primary adenocarcinoma of the lung. Cancer 2001;92:1525–1530.

74. Slebos RJ, Hruban RH, Dalesio O, et al. Relationship between K-ras oncogene activation and smoking in adenocarcinoma of the human lung. J Natl Cancer Inst 1991;83:1024–1027.

75. Barbacid M. Ras genes. Annu Rev Biochem 1987;56:779–827.

76. Barbacid M. Ras oncogenes: their role in neoplasia. Eur J Clin Invest 1990;20:225–235.

77. Wittinghofer A, Scheffzek K, Ahmadian MR. The interaction of Ras with GTPase-activating proteins. FEBS Lett 1997;410:63–67.

78. Hancock JF. Ras proteins: different signals from different locations. Nat Rev Mol Cell Biol 2003;4:373–384.

79. Hollstein M, Sidransky D, Vogelstein B, Harris CC. p53 mutations in human cancers. Science 1991;253:49–53.

80. Hollstein M, Shomer B, Greenblatt M, et al. Somatic point mutations in the p53 gene of human tumors and cell lines: updated compilation. Nucleic Acids Res 1996;24:141–146.

81. Chiba I, Takahashi T, Nau MM, et al. Mutations in the p53 gene are frequent in primary, resected non–small cell lung cancer. Lung Cancer Study Group. Oncogene 1990;5:1603–1610.

82. Curiel DT, Buchhagen DL, Chiba I, D'Amico D. A chemical mismatch cleavage method useful for the detection of point mutations in the p53 gene in lung cancer. Am J Respir Cell Mol Biol 1990;3:405–411.

83. D'Amico D, Carbone D, Mitsudomi T, et al. High frequency of somatically acquired p53 mutations in small-cell lung cancer cell lines and tumors. Oncogene 1992;7:339–346.

84. Robles AI, Linke SP, Harris CC. The p53 network in lung carcinogenesis. Oncogene 2002;21:6898–6907.

85. Greenblatt MS, Bennett WP, Hollstein M, Harris CC. Mutations in the p53 tumor suppressor gene: clues to cancer etiology and molecular pathogenesis. Cancer Res 1994;54:4855–4878.

86. Denissenko MF, Pao A, Tang M, Pfeifer GP. Preferential formation of benzo[a]pyrene adducts at lung cancer mutational hotspots in P53. Science 1996;274:430–432.

87. Kastan MB, Onyekwere O, Sidransky D, et al. Participation of p53 protein in the cellular response to DNA damage. Cancer Res 1991;51:6304–6311.

88. Gannon JV, Greaves R, Iggo R, Lane DP. Activating mutations in p53 produce a common conformational effect. A monoclonal antibody specific for the mutant form. EMBO J 1990;9:1595–602.

89. Kern SE, Kinzler KW, Baker SJ, et al. Mutant p53 proteins bind DNA abnormally in vitro. Oncogene 1991;6:131–136.

90. Kern SE, Kinzler KW, Bruskin A, et al. Identification of p53 as a sequence-specific DNA-binding protein. Science 1991;252:1708–1711.

91. Kern SE, Pietenpol JA, Thiagalingam S, et al. Oncogenic forms of p53 inhibit p53-regulated gene expression. Science 1992;256:827–830.

92. Kramer A, Neben K, Ho AD. Centrosome replication, genomic instability and cancer. Leukemia 2002;16:767–775.

93. Wahl GM, Linke SP, Paulson TG, Huang LC. Maintaining genetic stability through TP53 mediated checkpoint control. Cancer Surv 1997;29:183–219.

94. Gazzeri S, Gouyer V, Vour'ch C, et al. Mechanisms of p16INK4A inactivation in non small-cell lung cancers. Oncogene 1998;16:497–504.

95. Tanaka R, Wang D, Morishita Y, et al. Loss of function of p16 gene and prognosis of pulmonary adenocarcinoma. Cancer 2005;103:608–615.

96. Shapiro GI, Park JE, Edwards CD, et al. Multiple mechanisms of p16INK4A inactivation in non–small cell lung cancer cell lines. Cancer Res 1995;55:6200–6209.

97. Chin L, Pomerantz J, DePinho RA. The INK4a/ARF tumor suppressor: one gene—two products—two pathways. Trends Biochem Sci 1998;23:291–296.

98. Toyooka S, Toyooka KO, Maruyama R, et al. DNA methylation profiles of lung tumors. Mol Cancer Ther 2001;1:61–67.

99. Sanchez-Cespedes M, Decker PA, Doffek KM, et al. Increased loss of chromosome 9p21 but not p16 inactivation in primary non–small cell lung cancer from smokers. Cancer Res 2001;61:2092–2096.

100. Liu Y, Lan Q, Siegfried JM, et al. Aberrant promoter methylation of p16 and MGMT genes in lung tumors from smoking and never-smoking lung cancer patients. Neoplasia 2006;8:46–51.

101. Tsou JA, Shen LY, Siegmund KD, et al. Distinct DNA methylation profiles in malignant mesothelioma, lung

adenocarcinoma, and non-tumor lung. Lung Cancer 2005; 47:193–204.

102. Zhu WG, Srinivasan K, Dai Z, et al. Methylation of adjacent CpG sites affects Sp1/Sp3 binding and activity in the p21(Cip1) promoter. Mol Cell Biol 2003;23:4056–4065.

103. Soria JC, Rodriguez M, Liu DD, et al. Aberrant promoter methylation of multiple genes in bronchial brush samples from former cigarette smokers. Cancer Res 2002;62: 351–355.

104. Lai JC, Cheng YW, Chiou HL, et al. Gender difference in estrogen receptor alpha promoter hypermethylation and its prognostic value in non–small cell lung cancer. Int J Cancer 2005;117:974–980.

105. Chen Y, Huhn D, Knosel T, et al. Downregulation of connexin 26 in human lung cancer is related to promoter methylation. Int J Cancer 2005;113:14–21.

106. Wistuba II, Gazdar AF, Minna JD. Molecular genetics of small cell lung carcinoma. Semin Oncol 2001;28:3–13.

107. Miyamoto K, Asada K, Fukutomi T, et al. Methylation-associated silencing of heparan sulfate D-glucosaminyl 3-O-sulfotransferase-2 (3-OST-2) in human breast, colon, lung and pancreatic cancers. Oncogene 2003;22:274–280.

108. Du Y, Carling T, Fang W, et al. Hypermethylation in human cancers of the RIZ1 tumor suppressor gene, a member of a histone/protein methyltransferase superfamily. Cancer Res 2001;61:8094–8099.

109. Xu XL, Wu LC, Du F, et al. Inactivation of human SRBC, located within the 11p15.5–p15.4 tumor suppressor region, in breast and lung cancers. Cancer Res 2001;61:7943–7949.

110. Dammann R, Takahashi T, Pfeifer GP. The CpG island of the novel tumor suppressor gene RASSF1A is intensely methylated in primary small cell lung carcinomas. Oncogene 2001;20:3563–3567.

111. Osada H, Tatematsu Y, Yatabe Y, et al. Frequent and histological type-specific inactivation of 14-3-3sigma in human lung cancers. Oncogene 2002;21:2418–2424.

112. Fukasawa M, Kimura M, Morita S, et al. Microarray analysis of promoter methylation in lung cancers. J Hum Genet 2006;51:368–374.

113. Wright JL, Churg A. Advances in the pathology of COPD. Histopathology 2006;49:1–9.

114. Janoff A. Elastases and emphysema. Current assessment of the protease–antiprotease hypothesis. Am Rev Respir Dis 1985;132:417–433.

115. Stoller JK, Aboussouan LS. Alpha1-antitrypsin deficiency. Lancet 2005;365:2225–2236.

116. Tomashefski JF Jr, Crystal RG, Wiedemann HP, et al. The bronchopulmonary pathology of alpha-1 antitrypsin (AAT) deficiency: findings of the Death Review Committee of the national registry for individuals with Severe Deficiency of Alpha-1 Antitrypsin. Hum Pathol 2004;35: 1452–1461.

117. Lieberman J, Winter B, Sastre A. Alpha 1-antitrypsin Pi-types in 965 COPD patients. Chest 1986;89:370–373.

118. Lomas DA, Mahadeva R. Alpha1-antitrypsin polymerization and the serpinopathies: pathobiology and prospects for therapy. J Clin Invest 2002;110:1585–1590.

119. DeMeo DL, Silverman EK. Alpha1-antitrypsin deficiency. 2: genetic aspects of alpha(1)-antitrypsin deficiency: phenotypes and genetic modifiers of emphysema risk. Thorax 2004;59:259–264.

120. Lomas DA, Evans DL, Finch JT, Carrell RW. The mechanism of Z alpha 1-antitrypsin accumulation in the liver. Nature 1992;357:605–607.

121. Ogushi F, Fells GA, Hubbard RC, et al. Z-type alpha 1-antitrypsin is less competent than M1-type alpha 1-antitrypsin as an inhibitor of neutrophil elastase. J Clin Invest 1987;80:1366–1374.

122. Lewis MJ, Lewis EH 3rd, Amos JA, Tsongalis GJ. Cystic fibrosis. Am J Clin Pathol 2003;120 Suppl:S3–S13.

123. Robinson P. Cystic fibrosis. Thorax 2001;56:237–241.

124. Riordan JR, Rommens JM, Kerem B, et al. Identification of the cystic fibrosis gene: cloning and characterization of complementary DNA. Science 1989;245:1066–1073.

125. Gadsby DC, Vergani P, Csanady L. The ABC protein turned chloride channel whose failure causes cystic fibrosis. Nature 2006;440:477–483.

126. Zielenski J, Tsui LC. Cystic fibrosis: genotypic and phenotypic variations. Annu Rev Genet 1995;29:777–807.

127. Mickle JE, Cutting GR. Genotype–phenotype relationships in cystic fibrosis. Med Clin North Am 2000;84: 597–607.

128. Zielenski J. Genotype and phenotype in cystic fibrosis. Respiration 2000;67:117–133.

129. Quinton PM. Chloride impermeability in cystic fibrosis. Nature 1983;301:421–422.

130. Du K, Sharma M, Lukacs GL. The DeltaF508 cystic fibrosis mutation impairs domain–domain interactions and arrests post-translational folding of CFTR. Nat Struct Mol Biol 2005;12:17–25.

131. Chou JL, Rozmahel R, Tsui LC. Characterization of the promoter region of the cystic fibrosis transmembrane conductance regulator gene. J Biol Chem 1991;266: 24471–2446.

132. Yoshimura K, Nakamura H, Trapnell BC, et al. The cystic fibrosis gene has a "housekeeping"-type promoter and is expressed at low levels in cells of epithelial origin. J Biol Chem 1991;266:9140–9144.

133. Denamur E, Chehab FF. Methylation status of CpG sites in the mouse and human CFTR promoters. DNA Cell Biol 1995;14:811–815.

134. Koh J, Sferra TJ, Collins FS. Characterization of the cystic fibrosis transmembrane conductance regulator promoter region. Chromatin context and tissue-specificity. J Biol Chem 1993;268:15912–15921.

Section 2
Techniques and Experimental Systems in Molecular Pathology

6
Bioinformatics and Omics

Timothy Craig Allen and Philip T. Cagle

Introduction

The term *genomics* originated in 1920 to describe the complete set of chromosomes and their associated genes; however, it has been in the past decade that the use of omics—genomics, transcriptomics, and proteomics—and bioinformatics has led to dramatic advances in the understanding of the molecular and genetic bases of disease.[1-29] This chapter briefly reviews the subject, with subsequent chapters providing more details on specific technologies.

Bioinformatics

Bioinformatics has become an essential part of omics research and requires unique practical and analytical skills for appropriate results interpretation. Bioinformatics uses computers and statistics to perform extensive omics-related research by searching biologic databases and comparing gene sequences and protein data on a vast scale to identify sequences or proteins that differ between diseased and healthy tissues or between different phenotypes of the same disease.[30-37] The techniques used in omics are called *high throughput* because they involve analysis of very large numbers of genes, gene expressions, or proteins in one procedure or combination of procedures. The vast amounts of data generated by these high-throughput studies typically require computers for analysis and comparison of differences between diseased and physiologic cells and tissues, a key feature of bioinformatics. Omics and bioinformatics are used not only for studying genes and signaling pathways involved in human diseases but also for identifying potential targets of therapy and the design of therapeutic drugs.

Omics

Omics—a suffix signifying the measurement of the entire complement of a given level of biologic molecules and information—today encompasses a variety of new technologies that can help explain normal and abnormal cell pathways, networks, and processes via the simultaneous monitoring of thousands of molecular components.[6,7]

Genomics

Genomics provides platforms for the study of genomes and their genes, including haplotyping and single nucleotide polymorphism detection by investigating single nucleotide polymorphisms (SNPs) and mutations using high-throughput genome sequencing techniques such as high-density DNA microarrays/DNA (oligonucleotide) chips.[7,38-44] The base sequence of the genes of the human mitochondrial genome was completed in 1981, and in 2003 the base sequence of the genes of the entire human genome was completed.[45-47] The human genomic sequence data from the International Human Genome Sequencing Consortium can be mined using tools that are now publicly available.[48] Public databases can also be mined for SNPs, human mitochondrial genomes, and other human DNA polymorphic markers.[49-54]

Transcriptomics

Also termed *functional genomics*, transcriptomics provides information about the expressions of individual genes at the messenger RNA (mRNA) level and correlates patterns of expression with biologic function.[7,55-64] A variety of techniques have been developed to investigate gene expression. These techniques include serial analysis of gene expression (SAGE), suppression subtractive hybridization (SSH), differential display (DD) analysis,

RNA arbitrarily primer–PCR (RAP-PCR), amplified restriction fragment-length polymorphism (AFLP), total gene expression analysis (TOGA), and use of internal standard competitive template primers in a quantitative multiplex RT-PCR method [StaRT-(PCR)], restriction endonucleolytic analysis of differentially expressed sequences (READS), differential screening (DS), high-density cDNA filter hybridization analysis (HDFCA), and gene expression microarrays.[65–67]

Proteomics

Proteomics is discussed in detail in Chapter 13. Proteomics investigates individual protein concentrations present in a biologic system and studies the structural, functional, and regulatory roles of proteins in the cell and in pathways, including how and where they are expressed.[7,68–86] Because gene function is ultimately performed by the proteins transcribed from the genes and mRNA, proteomics is essential to comprehend the actual definitive functioning of a gene or pathway.[3,4] Fortunately, proteomics can be performed on surgical specimens, including needle biopsy tissue, cytology specimens, serum, and other fluids.[3,4] Frequently, two-dimensional gel electrophoresis (two-dimensional polyacrylamide gel electrophoresis) and mass spectrometry are employed in proteomics to initially fractionate the groups of proteins in a specimen. Proteins in a given sample fraction may later be identified using fingerprinting or sequence tag techniques.[3,4]

Metabolomics

Metabolomics (also termed *metabonomics*) involves study of metabolic profiles by investigating the compounds in a process and the characterization and quantification of small organic molecules in either circulatory or cell tissue systems.[7,87–90] Nuclear magnetic resonance and mass spectrometry are techniques frequently used in metabolomics.[7,87–90]

DNA Microarrays

DNA microarrays are employed to simultaneously screen for the presence or expression of large numbers of genes.[91–98] Suppression subtractive hybridization selectively amplifies target cDNA fragments (differentially expressed genes) and suppresses nontarget DNA.[99,100] Serial analysis of gene expression is used for global analysis of gene expression and provides a comprehensive qualitative and quantitative expression profiles of virtually every gene in a cell population or tissue, and SAGE libraries from different cells and tissues have been created.[101–103]

Conclusion

Rapid medical advances in the laboratory have not necessarily translated into rapid treatment advances. However, continuing omics research to understand the conceptual framework of disease—including disease progression and treatment response—along with improved and more efficient bioinformatics tools to analyze the great amounts of data originating from omics investigations may permit future diagnostic, prognostic, and therapeutic benefit to arise from these technologies.[6]

References

1. Biron DG, Brun C, Lefevre T, et al. The pitfalls of proteomics experiments without the correct use of bioinformatics tools. Proteomics 2006; Sept 22; [Epub ahead of print].
2. McKusick VA. Genomics: structure and functional studies of genomes. Genomics 1997; 45:244–249.
3. Palagi PM, Hernandez P, Walther D, Appel RD. Proteome informatics I: bioinformatics tools for processing experimental data. Proteomics 2006; Sept. 22; [Epub ahead of print].
4. Lisacek F, Cohen-Boulakia S, Appel RD. Proteome informatics II: bioinformatics for comparative proteomics. Proteomics 2006; Sept. 22; [Epub ahead of print].
5. Maojo V, Martin-Sanchez F. Bioinformatics: towards new directions for public health. Methods Inf Med 2004; 43: 208–214.
6. Bilello JA. The agony and ecstasy of "OMIC" technologies in drug development. Curr Mol Med 2005; 5:39–52.
7. Morel NM, Holland JM, van der Greef P, et al. Primer on medial genomics part XIV: introduction to systems biology—a new approach to understanding disease and treatment. Mayo Clin Proc 2004; 79:651–658.
8. Provart NJ, McCourt P. Systems approaches to understanding cell signaling and gene regulation. Curr Opin Plant Biol 2004; 7:605–609.
9. Wheelock AM, Goto S. Effects of post-electrophoretic analysis on variance in gel-based proteomics. Expert Rev Proteomics 2006; 3:129–142.
10. Debouck C, Metcalf B. The impact of genomics on drug discovery. Annu Rev Pharmacol Toxicol 2000; 40:193–207.
11. Ghosh D. High throughput and global approaches to gene expression. Comb Chem High Throughput Screen 2000; 3:411–420.
12. Hanke J. Genomics and new technologies as catalysts for change in the drug discovery paradigm. J Law Med Ethics 2000; 28(4 Suppl):15–22.
13. Harris T. Genetics, genomics, and drug discovery. Med Res Rev 2000; 20:203–211.
14. Rudert F. Genomics and proteomics tools for the clinic. Curr Opin Mol Ther 2000; 2:633–642.
15. Merrick BA, Bruno ME. Genomic and proteomic profiling for biomarkers and signature profiles of toxicity. Curr Opin Mol Ther 2004; 6:600–607.

16. Chalkley RJ, Hansen KC, Baldwin MA. Bioinformatic methods to exploit mass spectrometric data for proteomic applications. Methods Enzymol 2005; 402:289–312.

17. Dennis JL, Oien KA. Hunting the primary: novel strategies for defining the origin of tumours. J Pathol 2005; 205:236–247.

18. Englbrecht CC, Facius A. Bioinformatics challenges in proteomics. Comb Chem High Throughput Screen 2005; 8:705–715.

19. Fung ET, Weinberger SR, Gavin E, Zhang F. Bioinformatics approaches in clinical proteomics. Expert Rev Proteomics 2005; 2:847–862.

20. Kremer A, Schneider R, Terstappen GC. A bioinformatics perspective on proteomics: data storage, analysis, and integration. Biosci Rep 2005; 25:95–106.

21. Mount DW, Pandey R. Using bioinformatics and genome analysis for new therapeutic interventions. Mol Cancer Ther 2005; 4:1636–1643.

22. Nishio K, Arao T, Shimoyama T, et al. Translational studies for target-based drugs. Cancer Chemother Pharmacol 2005; 56 Suppl 1:90–93.

23. Katoh M, Katoh M. Bioinformatics for cancer management in the post-genome era. Technol Cancer Res Treat 2006; 5:169–175.

24. Miles AK, Matharoo-Ball B, Li G, et al. The identification of human tumour antigens: current status and future developments. Cancer Immunol Immunother 2006; 55: 996–1003.

25. Quackenbush J. Microarray analysis and tumor classification. N Engl J Med 2006; 354:2463–2472.

26. Redfern O, Grant A, Maibaum M, Orengo C. Survey of current protein family databases and their application in comparative, structural and functional genomics. J Chromatogr B Analyt Technol Biomed Life Sci 2005; 815: 97–107.

27. Iqbal O, Fareed J. Clinical applications of bioinformatics, genomics, and pharmacogenomics. Methods Mol Biol 2006; 316:159–177.

28. Reeves GA, Thornton JM, BioSapiens Network of Excellence. Integrating biological data through the genome. Hum Mol Genet 2006; 15(Spec No 1):R81–R87.

29. Waggoner A. Fluorescent labels for proteomics and genomics. Curr Opin Chem Biol 2006; 10:62–66.

30. Ritchie MD. Bioinformatics approaches for detecting gene–gene and gene–environment interactions in studies of human disease. Neurosurg Focus 2005; 19:E2.

31. Hanai T, Hamada H, Okamoto M. Application of bioinformatics for DNA microarray data to bioscience, bioengineering and medical fields. J Biosci Bioeng 2006; 101:377–384.

32. Goodman N. Biological data becomes computer literate: new advances in bioinformatics. Curr Opin Biotechnol 2002; 13:68–71.

33. Ness SA. Basic microarray analysis: strategies for successful experiments. Methods Mol Biol 2006; 316:13–33.

34. Perco P, Rapberger R, Siehs C, et al. Transforming omics data into context: bioinformatics on genomics and proteomics raw data. Electrophoresis 2006; 27:2659–2675.

35. Haoudi A, Bensmail H. Bioinformatics and data mining in proteomics. Expert Rev Proteomics 2006; 3:333–343.

36. Ivanov AS, Veselovsky AV, Dubanov AV, Skvortsov VS. Bioinformatics platform development: from gene to lead compound. Methods Mol Biol 2006; 316:389–431.

37. Teufel A, Krupp M, Weinmann A, Galle PR. Current bioinformatics tools in genomic biomedical research [review]. Int J Mol Med 2006; 17:967–973.

38. Regnstrom K, Burgess DJ. Pharmacogenomics and its potential impact on drug and formulation development. Crit Rev Ther Drug Carrier Syst 2005; 22:465–492.

39. Willard HF, Angrist M, Ginsburg GS. Genomic medicine: genetic variation and its impact on the future of health care. Philos Trans R Soc Lond B Biol Sci 2005; 360:1543–1550.

40. Garraway LA, Seller WR. From integrated genomics to tumor lineage dependency. Cancer Res 2006; 66:2506–2508.

41. McDunn JE, Chung TP, Laramie JM, et al. Physiologic genomics. Surgery 2006; 139:133–139.

42. Tost J, Gut IG. Genotyping single nucleotide polymorphisms by mass spectrometry. Mass Spectrom Rev 2002; 21:388–418.

43. Thomas DC, Haile RW, Duggan D. Recent developments in genomewide association scans: a workshop summary and review. Am J Hum Genet 2005; 77:337–345.

44. Bernig T, Chanock SJ. Challenges of SNP genotyping and genetic variation: its future role in diagnosis and treatment of cancer. Expert Rev Mol Diagn 2006; 6:319–331.

45. Anderson S, Bankier AT, Barrell BG, et al. Sequence and organization of the human mitochondrial genome, Nature 1981; 290:457–465.

46. Mundy C. The human genome project: a historical perspective. Pharmacogenomics 2001; 2:37–49.

47. International Human Genome Sequencing Consortium. Finishing the euchromatic sequence of the human genome. Nature 2004; 431:931–945.

48. Baxevanis AD. Using genomic databases for sequence-based biological discovery. Mol Med 2003; 9:185–192.

49. The International HapMap Consortium. The International HapMap Project. Nature 2003; 426:789–796.

50. Thorisson GA, Stein LD. The SNP Consortium website: past, present and future, Nucleic Acids Res 2003; 31:124–127.

51. Liu T, Johnson JA, Casella G, Wu R. Sequencing complex diseases with HapMap. Genetics 2004; 168:503–511.

52. Riva A, Kohane IS. A SNP-centric database for the investigation of the human genome. BMC Bioinformatics 2004; 5:33.

53. Kong X, Matise TC. MAP-O-MAT: internet-based linkage mapping. Bioinformatics 2005; 21:557–559.

54. Brandon MC, Lott MT, Nguyen KC, et al. MITOMAP: a human mitochondrial genome database—2004 update. Nucleic Acids Res 2005; 33:D611–D613.

55. Carulli JP, Artinger M, Swain PM, et al. High throughput analysis of differential gene expression. J Cell Biochem Suppl 1998; 30–31:286–396.

56. Scheel J, Von Brevern MC, Horlein A, et al. Yellow pages to the transcriptome. Pharmacogenomics 2002; 3:791–807.

57. Hedge PS, White IR, Debouck C. Interplay of transcriptomics and proteomics. Curr Opin Biotechnol 2003; 14: 647–651.

58. Suzuki M, Hayashizaki Y. Mouse-centric comparative transcriptomics of protein coding and non-coding RNAs. Bioessays 2004; 26:833–843.

59. Breitling R, Herzyk P. Biological master games: using biologists' reasoning to guide algorithm development for integrated functional genomics. OMICS 2005; 9:225–232.

60. Storck T, von Brevern MC, Behrens CK, et al. Transcriptomics in predictive toxicology. Curr Opin Drug Discov Dev 2002; 5:90–97.

61. Hu YF, Kaplow J, He Y. From traditional biomarkers to transcriptome analysis in drug development. Curr Mol Med 2005; 5:29–38.

62. Kralj M, Kraljevic S, Sedic M, et al. Global approach to perinatal medicine: functional genomics and proteomics. J Perinat Med 2005; 33:5–16.

63. Morgan KT, Jayyosi Z, Hower MA, et al. The hepatic transcriptome as a window on whole-body physiology and pathophysiology. Toxicol Pathol 2005; 33:136–145.

64. Jansen BJ, Schalkwijk J. Transcriptomics and proteomics of human skin. Brief Funct Genomic Proteomic 2003; 1:326–341.

65. Liang P, Zhu W, Zhang X, et al. Differential display using one-base anchored oligo-dT primers. Nucleic Acids Res 1994; 22:5763–5764.

66. Ahmed FE. Molecular techniques for studying gene expression in carcinogenesis. J Environ Sci Health C Environ Carcinog Ecotoxicol Rev 2002; 20:77–116.

67. Muller-Hagen G, Beinert T, Sommer A. Aspects of lung cancer gene expression profiling. Curr Opin Drug Discov Dev 2004; 7:290–303.

68. Anderson JS, Mann M. Functional genomics by mass spectrometry. FEBS Lett 2000; 480:25–31.

69. Liotta LA, Petricoin EF 3rd. The promise of proteomics. Clin Adv Hematol Oncol 2003; 1:460–462.

70. Jain KK. Role of oncoproteomics in the personalized management of cancer. Expert Rev Proteomics 2004; 1:49–55.

71. Hanash S. Disease proteomics. Nature 2003; 422:226–32.

72. Baggerman G, Vierstraete E, De Loof A, Schoofs L. Gel-based versus gel-free proteomics: a review. Comb Chem High Throughput Screen 2005; 8:669–677.

73. Calvo KR, Liotta LA, Petricoin EF. Clinical proteomics: from biomarker discovery and cell signaling profiles to individualized personal therapy. Biosci Rep 2005; 25:107–125.

74. Brown RE. Morphoproteomics: exposing protein circuitries in tumors to identify potential therapeutic targets in cancer patients. Expert Rev Proteomics 2005; 2:337–348.

75. Kalia A, Gupta RP. Proteomics: a paradigm shift. Crit Rev Biotechnol 2005; 25:173–198.

76. Scaros O, Fisler R. Biomarker technology roundup: from discovery to clinical applications, a broad set of tools is required to translate from the lab to the clinic. Biotechniques 2005 April; (Suppl):30–32.

77. Clarke W, Chan DW. ProteinChips: the essential tools for proteomic biomarker discovery and future clinical diagnostics. Clin Chem Lab Med 2005; 43:1279–1280.

78. Kolch W, Mischak H, Pitt AR. The molecular make-up of a tumour: proteomics in cancer research. Clin Sci (Lond) 2005; 108:369–383.

79. Patel PS, Telang SD, Rawal RM, Shah MH. A review of proteomics in cancer research. Asian Pac J Cancer Prev 2005; 6:113–117.

80. Roboz J. Mass spectrometry in diagnostic oncoproteomics. Cancer Invest 2005; 23:465–478.

81. Waldburg N, Kahne T, Reisenauer A, et al. Clinical proteomics in lung diseases. Pathol Res Pract 2004; 200: 147–154.

82. Stroncek DF, Burns C, Martin BM, et al. Advancing cancer biotherapy with proteomics. J Immunother 2005; 28:183–192.

83. Fleming K, Kelley LA, Islam SA, et al. The proteome: structure, function and evolution. Philos Trans R Soc Lond B Biol Sci 2006; 361:441–451.

84. Domon B, Aebersold R. Mass spectrometry and protein analysis. Science 2006; 312:212–217.

85. Gulmann C, Sheehan KM, Kay EW, et al. Array-based proteomics: mapping of protein circuitries for diagnostics, prognostics, and therapy guidance in cancer. J Pathol 2006; 208:595–606.

86. Kingsmore SF. Multiplexed protein measurement: technologies and applications of protein and antibody arrays. Nat Rev Drug Discov 2006; 5:310–320.

87. Davis CD, Milner J. Frontiers in nutrigenomics, proteomics, metabolomics and cancer prevention. Mutat Res 2004; 551:51–64.

88. Griffin JL, Bollard ME. Metabonomics: its potential as a tool in toxicology for safety assessment and data integration. Curr Drug Metab 2004; 5:389–398.

89. Rochfort S. Metabolomics reviewed: a new "omics" platform technology for systems biology and implications for natural products research. J Nat Prod 2005; 68:1813–1820.

90. Griffin JL. The Cinderella story of metabolic profiling: does metabolomics get to go to the functional genomics ball? Philos Trans R Soc Lond B Biol Sci 2006; 361: 147–161.

91. Ramsay G. DNA chips: State-of-the art. Nature Biotechnol 1997; 16:40–44.

92. Duggan DJ, Bittner M, Chen Y, et al. Expression profiling using cDNA microarrays. Nat Genet 1999; 21(Suppl 1):10–14.

93. Chen l. Ren J. High-throughput DNA analysis by microchip electrophoresis. Comb Chem High Throughput Screen 2004; 7:29–43.

94. Heller MJ. DNA microarray technology: devices, systems, and applications. Annu Rev Biomed Eng 2002; 4:129–153.

95. Obeid PJ, Christopoulos TK. Microfabricated systems for nucleic acid analysis. Crit Rev Clin Lab Sci 2004; 41:429–465.

96. Shi L, Tong W, Goodsaid F, et al. QA/QC: challenges and pitfalls facing the microarray community and regulatory agencies. Expert Rev Mol Diagn 2004; 4:761–777.

97. Zhumabayeva B, Chenchik A, Siebert PD, Herrler M. Disease profiling arrays: reverse format cDNA arrays complimentary to microarrays. Adv Biochem Eng Biotechnol 2004; 86:191–213.

98. Brentani RR, Carraro DM, Verjovski-Almeida S, et al. Gene expression arrays in cancer research: methods

and applications. Crit Rev Oncol Hematol 2005; 54:95–105.

99. Diatchenko L, Lau YF, Campbell AP, et al. Suppression subtractive hybridization: a method for generating differentially regulated or tissue-specific cDNA probes and libraries. Proc Natl Acad Sci USA 1996; 93:6025–6030.

100. Wang X, Feuerstein GZ. Suppression subtractive hybridization: application in the discovery of novel pharmacological targets. Pharmacogenomics 2000; 1:101–108.

101. Velculescu VE, Vogelstein B, Kinzler KW. Analyzing uncharted transcriptomes with SAGE. Trends Genet 2000; 16:423–425.

102. Polyak K, Riggins GJ. Gene discovery using the serial analysis of gene expression technique: implications for cancer research. J Clin Oncol 2001; 19:2948–2958.

103. Riggins GJ. Using serial analysis of gene expression to identify tumor markers and antigens. Dis Markers 2001; 17:41–48.

7
General Approach to Molecular Pathology

Gregory L. Blakey and Daniel H. Farkas

Introduction

Once a highly specialized subdiscipline of laboratory medicine, molecular diagnostics now infiltrates all of anatomic and clinical pathology. The shift from dependence on a few, relatively cumbersome methods to a wider range of technologies has facilitated this expansion. In addition, the completion of the Human Genome Project and the growing amount of sequence data related to infection, cancer, and other disease states have yielded additional applications of molecular biology for the clinical laboratory (Figure 7.1). As the various phases of testing can be automated in many instances, molecular biologic experience is no longer a prerequisite. In fact, performance of nucleic acid extraction and amplification in a tabletop unit is possible.[1, 2] Increasingly, miniaturization will further move molecular testing to the point of care.[3]

Although varying from protocol to protocol, the workflow for many molecular pathologic tests follows a similar scheme (Figure 7.2). As with other laboratory tests, preanalytic variables can dramatically affect molecular assay results. Therefore, appropriate care should be paid to specimen collection, transport, processing, and storage. In particular, fresh samples submitted for analysis of RNA must be rapidly processed to prevent degradation.

Nucleic Acid Extraction

Although the traditional organic means of extracting nucleic acids, with phenol and chloroform, are useful in the clinical laboratory, less cumbersome methods now dominate. For instance, silica-based spin column technologies couple ease of use with adaptability. With these methods, a digested sample is loaded onto a column to which nucleic acids bind in the presence of chaotropic salts. Microcentrifugation of the column followed by washing removes proteins and other macromolecules. Finally, nucleic acids are eluted with buffer or water. As with more traditional techniques, conventional spin column–based nucleic acid isolation suffers from the need for manual labor, not an insignificant factor in the busy clinical laboratory.[4,5]

Automation of nucleic acid extraction techniques has increased laboratory efficiency and decreased turnaround time. Of particular importance for quantitative testing, reduced inter- and intraoperator variability also results. Commonly used automated nucleic acid extraction techniques often rely on magnetized glass beads. After cell lysis, nucleic acids bind the beads, which can be robotically manipulated with a magnet. The beads are washed, and then nucleic acids are eluted with water or an appropriate buffer. Throughput of automated extraction robots ranges from approximately 6 samples to 96 or more per run. Depending on the model, these machines are capable of processing various sample types, including plasma, whole blood, fresh tissue, and formalin-fixed tissue. Typical isolation choices include total nucleic acid, DNA, and RNA.

Although nucleic acids are most commonly purified for use in molecular protocols, crude cell lysates can be used in selected cases. Such an approach may be especially useful when only minute amounts of samples are available, as with macro- or microdissected cells. In these instances, the decrease in nucleic acid yield because of the extraction process might be unacceptable. Crude lysates have been successfully used as starting material for polymerase chain reaction (PCR)-based clinical diagnostics.[6]

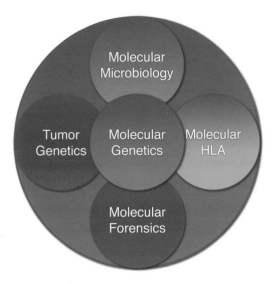

FIGURE 7.1. Molecular diagnostics encompasses the use of nucleic acids to diagnose infection, malignancy (hematologic and solid tumors), and genetic diseases. Other major foci include the investigation of human remains and crime scenes (forensics) and evaluation of transplant donors and recipients (human leukocyte antigen [HLA] testing).

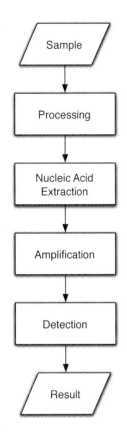

FIGURE 7.2. The general steps in many molecular diagnostic protocols are similar. For example, a blood sample received for genetic testing first may be processed to isolate white blood cells. Then, DNA is extracted from these cells and used to set up polymerase chain reaction. A multitude of detection methods are available (see text for further discussion).

Amplification Technologies

Target Amplification

Polymerase Chain Reaction

In combination with a variety of other methods (Figure 7.3), PCR remains the core molecular pathologic technique. It results in a many fold increase in target

FIGURE 7.3. Numerous techniques allow detection and analysis of polymerase chain reaction (PCR) products, amplicons. Amplicons can be sized by gel electrophoresis, detected in real-time with fluorescent probes, and sequenced with a variety of methods. Mass spectrometry approaches allow precise fragment sizing or base composition determination, and DNA "chips" permit parallel hybridization of amplicon and thousands of probes. (Sequencing diagram modified from Blakey and Farkas,[7] by permission of the Colorado Association for Continuing Medical Laboratory Education.)

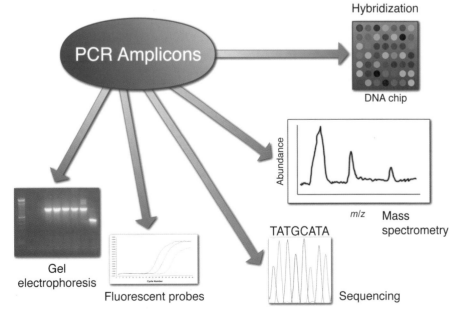

sequences by virtue of repeated cycles in which product becomes additional template. Despite the superior sensitivity and convenience of PCR versus Southern blotting and other venerable methods, the potential for contamination of the laboratory space and reagents with reaction products—amplicons—slowed entry of molecular diagnostics into traditional laboratory settings. The relatively recent availability of thermal cyclers that can continually monitor product formation has mitigated this problem. These instruments allow real-time PCR in which subsequent detection steps requiring opening of the reaction vessel are usually not needed. Besides lowering the risk of contamination, real-time PCR allows rapid turnaround time; the high-speed thermal cyclers used rapidly change the reaction temperature of metal blocks or air in which reaction vessels are suspended. Applications of real-time PCR include genotyping, pathogen identification, and target quantification.

Besides the standard reagents (primers flanking the target site, heat-resistant polymerase, deoxyribonucleotide triphosphates (dNTPs), and various buffer components), real-time PCR requires fluorescent molecules for ultimate product detection. Fluorescent dyes such as SYBR Green that nonspecifically bind double-stranded DNA can be used, but false-positive results may occur. More commonly, polymorphism and mutation detection are accomplished with fluorescently labeled oligonucleotide probes. Some of the most frequently used of the many such probe systems are hybridization probes, hydrolysis probes, and molecular beacons. Paired hybridization probes anneal to adjacent sites on the target sequence. One hybridization probe has an acceptor fluorophore, the other a donor fluorophore. When in close proximity, the energy from the donor excites the acceptor via fluorescence resonance energy transfer (FRET; Figure 7.4A). The real-time thermal cycler measures this signal. A hydrolysis probe consists of a single oligonucleotide labeled with reporter and quencher fluorophores; fluorescence is inhibited by FRET between the two. Upon dissociation of the two fluorophores by the exonuclease activity of the DNA polymerase during the extension phase of PCR, the reporter emits light (Figure 7.4B). Similarly, molecular beacons contain a stem-loop structure that brings together reporter and quencher fluorophores attached to the respective ends of the probe. When the probe binds to the target sequence, the reporter and quencher are physically separated (Figure 7.4C).

Melting curve analysis with hybridization probes can be used to distinguish different target sequences. Hybridized strands separate at the melting temperature (T_m). To determine T_m, after PCR is completed, the thermal cycler slowly increases the temperature while continuously monitoring fluorescence. As the temperature rises, probes that are less tightly bound to target, either by design or because of mismatches, dissociate first. Stronger, more stable, target–probe hybrids melt at higher temperatures. By plotting the change in fluorescence produced versus temperature, different target amplicon species, (e.g., normal vs. mutant or different pathogens) can be distinguished (Figure 7.5).

Real-time PCR permits relatively easy quantification of analytes such as microbial genomes or fusion transcripts. As the initial concentration of an analyte of interest increases, the reaction cycle number where fluorescence exceeds background decreases. Therefore, external calibrators can be used to construct a standard curve, permitting quantification.

Polymerase chain reaction systems with 96- and 384-well plates increase throughput. Multiplexing (more than one reaction per tube or well) enhances this. However, untoward interactions between the various components of a multiplexed reaction limit the number of analytes that can be interrogated simultaneously. High-throughput gene expression profiling may be accomplished by advances such as highly parallel picoliter-scale PCR.[8] With potentially superior dynamic range and reproducibility versus microarrays (see later), real-time PCR may allow gene expression profiling to enter more widespread clinical use.

Other Target Amplification Techniques

Besides PCR, target amplification techniques include the proprietary nucleic acid sequence based amplification and transcription-mediated amplification, both of which rely on the isothermal production of RNA intermediates.

Signal Amplification

Instead of increasing the number of targets to boost sensitivity, signal amplification techniques rely on multiplying the detection signal. Signal amplification techniques include Hybrid Capture, Invader, and branched chain DNA (bDNA), all proprietary.

With Hybrid Capture, in wide use for the identification of human papillomavirus, hybrids of viral DNA and probe RNA are bound by antibodies attached to a reaction well. Labeled antibodies complete the sandwich of the hybrids, allowing chemiluminescent detection.

Invader assays depend on recognition of the combination of the target, a probe, and a so-called Invader oligonucleotide by a proprietary enzyme (Cleavase); probe

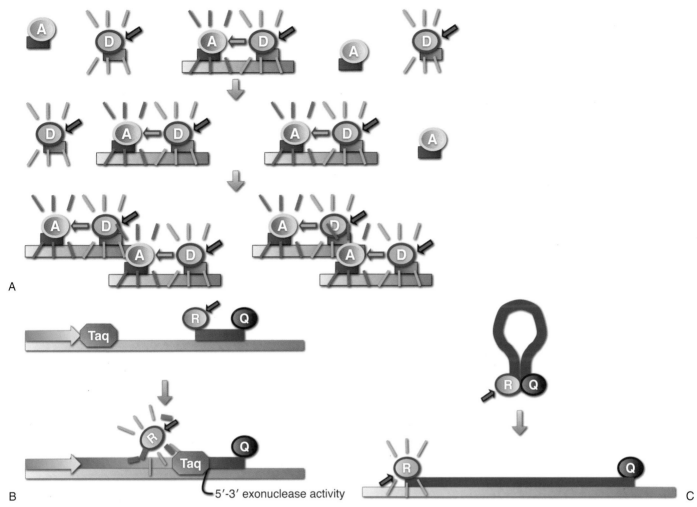

A

B

5'-3' exonuclease activity

C

FIGURE 7.4. Many different strategies allow detection of amplicons in real-time polymerase chain reaction (PCR). These three probe systems rely on fluorescence resonance energy transfer (FRET) between fluorophores. Blue arrows represent light emitted by the thermal cycler. **(A)** Dual hybridization probes bind the target sequence, whereupon the acceptor fluorophore (A) on one probe receives light from the adjacent donor fluorophore (D) on the other probe. As the PCR progresses, fluorescence increases. (Modified from Blakey and Farkas,[7] by permission of the Colorado Association for Continuing Medical Laboratory Education.) **(B)** A hydrolysis probe, an oligonucle-otide labeled with reporter (R) and quencher (Q) fluorophores, binds the target sequence during the extension phase of PCR. *Taq* polymerase hydrolyzes bound probe, freeing the reporter from the quencher. (Modified from Blakey and Farkas,[7] by permission of the Colorado Association for Continuing Medical Laboratory Education.) **(C)** A molecular beacon probe, composed of a stem-loop oligonucleotide structure with terminal reporter (R) and quencher (Q) fluorophores. Binding of the probe to the target sequence separates quencher from reporter, allowing fluorescence of the latter.

cleavage results. A probe fragment in turn interacts with a looped DNA structure labeled with reporter and quencher fluorophores (FRET cassette). Cleavage again results, releasing the reporter, which fluoresces. Invader chemistry is isothermal. Thus, a thermal cycler is not required. In addition, as amplicons are not produced, the risk of contamination is minimized. Genotyping is a common application.

bDNA technology uses a combination of capture molecules and labels to amplify the amount of signal. Applications include quantification of human immuno-deficiency, hepatitis B, and hepatitis C viruses.

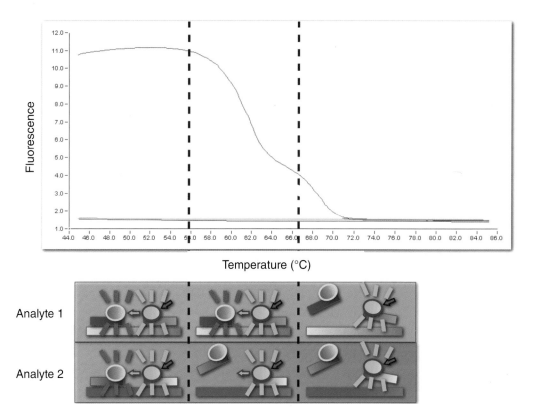

FIGURE 7.5. Amplicons can be distinguished by melting curve analysis. Two hybridization probe pairs differentiate between a mixture of analytes 1 and 2 in this illustration **(left)**. As the thermal cycler ramps up the temperature, one of the probes for analyte 2 dissociates first **(middle)**, resulting in drop in total fluorescence. The temperature at which this loss of fluorescence occurs is the melting temperature for analyte 2. A second drop indicates the dissociation of at least one of the analyte 1 probes **(right)**.

Restriction Fragment Analysis and Southern Blotting

Restriction Fragment-Length Polymorphism

Restriction fragment-length polymorphism (RFLP) analysis, previously a mainstay of genotyping, involves cutting target molecules (usually after amplification with PCR) with a restriction endonuclease, followed by gel electrophoresis. The resulting fragment patterns can be compared to those of controls to deduce the genotype. Many RLFP assays have been supplanted by those based on real-time PCR.

Southern Blotting

A particularly laborious and time-consuming (turnaround times of many days) technique, the Southern blot is still used in the clinical laboratory, particularly when target sequences are too long to safely amplify with PCR. In Southern blotting, relatively large quantities (microgram) of DNA are digested with a restriction endonuclease, fractionated via gel electrophoresis, and then transferred to a solid support, such as a nylon membrane. Labeled probes then hybridize to complementary target sequences, permitting detection.

Sequencing

Sequencing is used widely in genetics laboratories, particularly for the identification of heterogeneous mutations within a given gene or exon.

Sanger Sequencing

In Sanger sequencing, fluorescently labeled dideoxyribonucleotide triphosphates are incorporated into growing nucleotide strands, causing chain termination. The resulting fragments are resolved with slab gel or, more commonly, capillary electrophoresis, to yield the sequence. Sequence read lengths are in the hundreds of base pairs. Common sequencing primers and protocols, high-throughput 384-capillary sequencers, and sophisticated analysis software form the large-scale sequencing pipeline required for the timely detection of polymorphisms and mutations in the high-volume clinical molecular genetics laboratory.

Real-time Sequencing

Pyrosequencing, or real-time sequencing, depends on a proprietary chemical cascade that converts the pyrophosphate byproduct of nucleotide incorporation to light (Figure 7.6). With inkjet printer technology, the pyrosequencing instrument adds individual dNTPs in a specified order to reaction vessels. Only when a dNTP incorporates at a given position is light generated and detected by the instrument; therefore, the sequence of the target can be inferred.

Although Sanger sequencing remains the predominant sequencing technique, real-time sequencing offers several advantages. Sequence reads can begin immediately after the sequencing primers. In addition, detection occurs during the sequencing reaction, reducing turnaround time. Compared with real-time PCR, pyrosequencing has the advantage of quicker assay development in some instances, given that design and optimization of fluorescently labeled probes is not required. Limitations of pyrosequencing include difficulty reading homopolymeric repeats (several consecutive identical bases) and the relatively short sequence read lengths (less than approximately 100 base pairs).

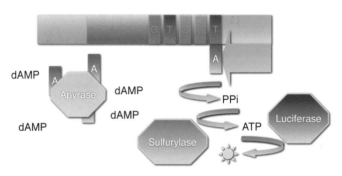

FIGURE 7.6. Pyrosequencing takes advantage of the pyrophosphate byproduct of nucleotide incorporation into a growing DNA strand. Pyrophosphate is converted to light by sulfurylase and luciferase. Apyrase degrades excess deoxyribonucleotide triphosphate. As nucleotides are added individually in a predetermined order, the target sequence can be deduced as the DNA strand grows. Hence, pyrosequencing is also known as *sequencing by synthesis*. The large arrow represents the sequencing primer. ATP, adenosine triphosphate; dAMP, deoxyadenosine monophosphate; PPi, inorganic phosphate. (Modified from Blakey and Farkas,[7] by permission of the Colorado Association for Continuing Medical Laboratory Education.)

Advanced Sequencing

Rapid progress in high-throughput sequencing technologies hastens the goal of quickly and inexpensively sequencing a human genome for clinical purposes. One recently introduced machine, based on pyrosequencing chemistry and the so-called shotgun sequencing approach, can sequence a bacterial genome in as little as a few hours.[9] An effort to more fully characterize genomic changes of malignancies, the National Institutes of Health's Cancer Genome Atlas project (http://cancergenome.nih.gov), could eventually generate new clinical assays based on new sequencing technologies.

Methylation Detection Methods

Epigenetic changes, modifications to the genome that do not alter the sequence itself, are involved in the regulation of gene expression. Means to identify one such class of epigenetic change, methylation of cytosines, include methylation-sensitive restriction enzymes that generate differential RFLP patterns and chemical conversion (bisulfite treatment) of methylated bases followed by sequencing.

Fluorescence In Situ Hybridization and Microarrays

Fluorescence In Situ Hybridization

Fluorescently labeled probes hybridized to histologic and cytologic preparations allow the detection of translocations, amplifications, and deletions. Fluorescence in situ hybridization (FISH) is used widely in the study of hematologic malignancies, solid tumors, and genetic disorders. Platforms with automated hybridization and analysis will increase the practicality of FISH in the clinical laboratory. Although generally less sensitive than PCR, FISH has the advantage of preserving histologic context.

Chromosomal Microarrays

Composed of hundreds or thousands of probes or clones representing every chromosome, chromosomal microarrays achieve a higher resolution than the staining techniques of classic cytogenetics. Thus, this technique, also known as array comparative genomic hybridization, may detect small deletions and duplications missed by traditional karyotyping. Prior to hybridization, samples may undergo whole genome amplification to increase sensitivity. Preliminary studies have shown that formalin-fixed cells and tissues may be successfully used with chromosomal microarrays,[10,11] raising the possibility of its routine use in anatomic pathology.

Oligonucleotide Microarrays

Oligonucleotide microarrays are constructed by spotting hundreds to thousands of oligonucleotide probes onto a glass slide or other substrate. Alternatively, probes can be incorporated in situ during construction of the array. By hybridizing cDNA, derived from cellular mRNA via reverse transcription, to these arrays, the expression levels of the various genes in a cell can be measured. Gene expression profiling has been repeatedly demonstrated to generate "signatures" that correlate with prognosis of different cancers, although variabilities in the means of assay performance and statistical analysis have sometimes rendered interlaboratory comparison difficult. Platform standardization and other efforts to improve reproducibility will likely pave the way for gene expression profiling to more fully enter routine clinical use. Selected example applications of microarray technologies are listed in Table 7.1.

Liquid Bead Microarrays

Liquid bead arrays consisting of sets of labeled polystyrene microbeads can be used to simultaneously interrogate numerous targets for genotyping, pathogen identification, and other purposes. As with traditional flow cytometry, beads are passed single file through a laser-based detector. One laser identifies the bead based on its unique color while another quantifies attached analyte. Besides nucleic acids, proteins, cytokines, and other biomolecules can be attached to the beads, enhancing the multiplexing power of this technology.

TABLE 7.1. Applications of microarray technologies.

Application	Format	Comment
Gene expression profiling	Solid phase, liquid bead	Can identify disease-specific signatures
Global chromosomal abnormality detection	Solid phase	Resolution depends on number of clones or probes; may not detect balanced translocations
Pathogen detection	Solid phase, liquid bead	Has potential to replace many conventional virologic and bacteriologic methods
Polymorphism and mutation detection	Solid phase, liquid bead	A pharmacogenetic test is the first Food and Drug Administration–approved microarray-based assay
Sequencing	Solid phase	Alternative to traditional sequencing techniques

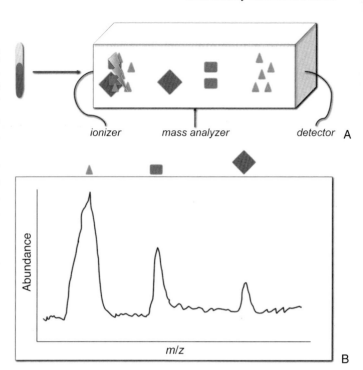

FIGURE 7.7. **(A)** Mass spectrometry can be used to separate serum proteins. Following ionization or other means of dissociation, proteins move through the mass analyzer based on the ratio of mass to charge. A detector measures this time of flight (TOF). **(B)** Mass spectrometry TOF yields quantitative "proteomic profiles," as shown in this simplified diagram. The species with the lowest mass/charge ratio (triangle) is more abundant than the two species with higher mass/charge ratios (rectangle and diamond). Serum proteomic signatures may be composed of the shed proteins and peptides of cancer and other diseases.

Mass Spectrometry

Although not "molecular pathology"—the diagnosis of disease using nucleic acids—in the strict sense, proteomic profiling with mass spectrometry is touted by some as a powerful tool for the screening and diagnosis of malignancies and the identification of pathogens. Numerous variants of mass spectrometry separate proteins by mass and charge (Figure 7.7A). The resultant protein mass fingerprints reveal the relative quantities of the protein and peptide species present (Figure 7.7B). Such patterns derived from blood may constitute proteomic disease signatures.[12] Confirmation of these sometimes controversial, nascent diagnostic approaches is needed before implementation in the clinical laboratory.

Systems Biology Approaches

The emerging field of systems biology seeks to more fully understand life in terms of its myriad molecular networks. This outlook contrasts with the reductionist bent of

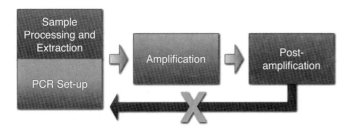

FIGURE 7.8. Unidirectional workflow in the molecular pathology laboratory prevents contamination of new samples and reagents with amplicons produced in previously performed polymerase chain reactions (PCRs).

molecular biology and the common clinical practice of employing one or a few biomarkers to diagnose a given disease. Much more predictive, less reactive medical care is promised by use of multiparameter, high-throughput molecular tools.[13] Although molecular diagnostic assays now serve primarily as adjuncts to other methods in surgical pathology, the use of global, systems-based approaches may challenge the dominance of histopathology.

Implementing Molecular Pathology

Laboratory Design Considerations

To prevent contamination, laboratories manipulating amplicons generated by PCR or other target amplification technologies must strictly observe a unidirectional workflow, from sample processing to detection (Figure 7.8). Reagent preparation should ideally be done in an area of the laboratory separate from sample processing and nucleic acid extraction. Both of these activities benefit from positive air pressure or "still boxes" and ultraviolet light to minimize airborne contaminants. Most importantly, the laboratory's postamplification room, where reaction vessels are opened post-PCR, must be kept separate from the rest of the laboratory. Dedicated gloves and gowns should be kept in this area. In addition, negative air flow can prevent escape of amplicons.

Laboratory Staffing

Early molecular pathology laboratories relied on staff trained in molecular biology to perform and troubleshoot assays. Now, those with more traditional medical technologist training increasingly perform these functions in part because of better educational opportunities. The

American Society for Clinical Pathology, the American Board of Bioanalysis, and the National Credentialing Agency for Laboratory Personnel offer certification in molecular diagnostics. In addition, there are several degree-granting programs. The Training and Education section of the Association for Molecular Pathology website provides an updated list of molecular training available for technologists (http://www.amp.org/T&E/training&edu.htm).

References

1. Hughes SJ, Xi L, Raja S, et al. A rapid, fully automated, molecular-based assay accurately analyzes sentinel lymph nodes for the presence of metastatic breast cancer. Ann Surg 2006; 243:389–398.
2. Ulrich MP, Christensen DR, Coyne SR, et al. Evaluation of the Cepheid GeneXpert system for detecting Bacillus anthracis. J Appl Microbiol 2006; 100:1011–1016.
3. Holland CA, Kiechle FL. Point-of-care molecular diagnostic systems—past, present and future. Curr Opin Microbiol 2005; 8:504–509.
4. Barkham T. BioRobot EZ1 workstation compares well with manual spin kits for extraction of viral RNA from sera and saves substantial staff time. J Clin Microbiol 2006; 44:1598.
5. Knepp JH, Geahr MA, Forman MS, et al. Comparison of automated and manual nucleic acid extraction methods for detection of enterovirus RNA. J Clin Microbiol 2003; 41:3532–3536.
6. Hatanpaa KJ, Burger PC, Eshleman JR, et al. Molecular diagnosis of oligodendroglioma in paraffin sections. Lab Invest 2003; 83:419–428.
7. Blakey GL, Farkas DH. Understanding Molecular Pathology: Methods and Applications. Denver: Colorado Association for Continuing Medical Laboratory Education; 2006.
8. Marcus JS, Anderson WF, Quake SR. Parallel picoliter RT-PCR assays using microfluidics. Anal Chem 2006; 78:956–958.
9. Margulies M, Egholm M, Altman WE, et al. Genome sequencing in microfabricated high-density picolitre reactors. Nature 2005; 437:367–380.
10. Ghazani AA, Arneson NC, Warren K, et al. Limited tissue fixation times and whole genomic amplification do not impact array CGH profiles. J Clin Pathol 2006; 59:311–315.
11. Johnson NA, Hamoudi RA, Ichimura K, et al. Application of array CGH on archival formalin-fixed paraffin-embedded tissues including small numbers of microdissected cells. Lab Invest 2006; 86:968–978.
12. Petricoin EF III, Ardekani AM, Hitt BA, et al. Use of proteomic patterns in serum to identify ovarian cancer. Lancet 2002; 359:572–577.
13. Hood L, Health JR, Phelps ME, et al. Systems biology and new technologies enable predictive and preventative medicine. Science 2004; 306:640–643.

8
Applications of Molecular Tests in Anatomic Pathology

Jennifer L. Hunt and Sanja Dacic

Introduction

Molecular testing in anatomic pathology is becoming increasingly important for most organ systems, including in the lung. Such tests are used both diagnostically and prognostically and are particularly important in the workup of neoplasia and for identification or subclassification for certain infectious processes. Fresh and frozen tissues are always considered to be the most optimal source of DNA and RNA that serves as the template for targeted molecular analysis. However, archival paraffin-embedded tissue is an attractive alternative source of tissue for clinical testing. Paraffin-embedded tissue can be a critical source of nucleic acid when unexpected diagnoses are rendered in the pathologic evaluation of tissue material. It also, however, provides the advantage of allowing for archival analysis with correlation to outcome.

Molecular analysis can be performed at different levels of resolution, from the whole chromosome down to the specific nucleotide sequence. At the chromosomal level, classic cytogenetics discerns chromosome structure and number and can detect most major translocations and deletions. This technique requires fresh cells that are capable of entering into cell division. The cells are arrested in metaphase in order for the chromosomes to be visualized individually for analysis. A newer technique that can be combined with classic cytogenetics is spectral karyotyping. For this specialized analysis, the metaphase chromosomes are subjected to fluorescent in situ hybridization (FISH) with specific probes that are labeled with combinations of five different fluorescent tags. The result involves the "painting" of each chromosome with a unique fluorescent signal that can be differentiated with the assistance of a computer detection system. This technique allows for resolution of complex karyotypes.

Chromogenic in situ hybridization (CISH) or FISH enables detection of known sequences of DNA and can be performed on whole cells or sections cut from paraffin or frozen tissue. The probes used in in situ hybridization can highlight amplifications, specific translocations, or genomic material from infectious organisms. In paraffin-embedded tissues, FISH is a particularly powerful tool for molecular analysis, given the known difficulties in DNA extraction from fixed material.

Comparative genomic hybridization (CGH) is another relatively new technique that can detect and map changes in copy number for specific DNA sequences. The DNA from a test genome (e.g., a tumor) and a reference genome (e.g., normal tissue) are differentially labeled and hybridized to normal metaphase chromosomes. In the past few years, microarray-based formats for CGH (array CGH) have been developed and are beginning to be widely used in preference to chromosome-based CGH. Overrepresentation (amplifications) or underrepresentation (deletions) of the test sample signal can be resolved with computer software. This technique is excellent for discovery of unique genetic alterations (deletions and amplifications) but is not commonly used as a diagnostic tool.

In anatomic pathology laboratories genetic material is often analyzed at the nucleic acid level, especially with the powerful tool of polymerase chain reaction (PCR). Currently many of the PCR-based diagnostic molecular tests yield positive or negative results to identify disease-specific genetic changes. As molecular testing becomes more focused on quantitation of molecular targets, the need for relatively pure cell populations will increase. Tissue microdissection is an excellent method to obtain relatively pure cellular samples of morphologically confirmed cell types.[1-3] This cellular purity will result in more accurate test results. Microdissection can be performed in a variety of ways, all of which have different advantages and disadvantages that have been reviewed elsewhere. Basically, these methods range from simple and inexpensive manual methods to laser-capture microdissection methods that require expensive and complex equipment. Microdissection of target tissue is followed by DNA or RNA extraction. The common sequence of tissue

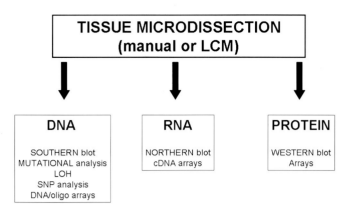

FIGURE 8.1. Tissue processing in anatomic, clinical, and developmental molecular pathology laboratories. Manual or laser capture microdissection (LCM) of frozen or paraffin-embedded target tissue is followed by DNA, RNA, or protein extraction and subsequently analyzed by the appropriate molecular techniques. LOH, loss of heterozygosity; SNP, single nucleotide polymorphism.

processing in anatomic clinical or developmental molecular pathology laboratories is illustrated in Figure 8.1.

Anatomic Pathology Testing to Detect or Characterize Neoplasia

Rapid advances in molecular technologies and expanding knowledge about lung tumor carcinogenesis has resulted in many studies of potential diagnostic and prognostic biomarkers. Based on current understanding, lung cancers have multiple genetic and epigenetic alterations, including inactivation of tumor suppressor genes and activation of oncogenes. These molecular changes can be correlated with the sequential morphologic changes of multistep carcinogenesis. The status of the many genes involved in tumorigenesis has been explored with multiple different molecular techniques, including loss of heterozygosity (LOH), array CGH, direct gene sequencing, gene expression profiling, FISH, and proteomics. Each of these assays is discussed in the relevant chapters on specific assays throughout this book. In the following discussion, a more general overview of molecular testing in lung carcinomas is presented.

Oncogenes

Protooncogenes are wild-type universally present genes that stimulate carcinogenesis when mutated. The mutant forms are designated as *oncogenes*. Oncogenes act as dominant genes, in which a mutation in only one copy of the gene leads to activation usually through overexpression of a protein product. A variety of mutational events can transform a protooncogene into an oncogene, including point mutations, translocations, amplifications, and deletions. Because most of these mutations are activating mutations and cause overexpression, the aberrant protein product may be detectable by immunohistochemistry. In some cases, an amplified gene will be detected by in situ hybridization. However, overexpression of an oncogene protein product by immunohistochemistry alone does not necessarily signify a mutation, because other nonmutational mechanisms can also be responsible for protein overexpression.

In surgical pathology, some of the most common oncogene assays detect translocations, particularly for sarcomas and hematologic malignancies. These tumorigenic translocations often reposition an oncogene partner next to a constitutively active gene. The oncogene is then aberrantly and constitutively activated in the cells harboring the translocation. Depending on the clustering of breakpoints, translocation assays can use reverse-transcription and polymerase chain reaction, PCR alone, or in situ hybridization. Most epithelial tumors do not have consistent useful translocations. The most common applications of translocation testing in lung pathology include FISH or PCR-based assays for t(11;22) in extraosseus Ewing's sarcoma/primitive neuroectodermal tumor and t(x;18) in synovial sarcoma of the pleura.

Most oncogenes that have been associated with epithelial tumors involve specific point mutations in notorious genes. One of the most important oncogenes in non–small cell carcinoma is KRAS. KRAS mutations usually involve one of three important codons (12, 13, or 61) and often consist of G to T transversions. These unique mutations have been associated with the genetic damage from tobacco.[4] KRAS mutations occur almost exclusively in adenocarcinoma and not usually squamous or small cell carcinomas. About 30% of adenocarcinomas harbor KRAS mutations.[5,6] Interestingly, KRAS mutations have been reported in 25%–40% of atypical adenomatous hyperplasia as well. This molecular alteration has been suggested to indicate a relationship between atypical adenomatous hyperplasia and carcinoma.[7] The clustering of mutations in KRAS mutations in lung adenocarcinoma makes it feasible to use a simple and rapid PCR-based sequencing assay for detection of these mutations. Even in small or low cellularity samples, such as sputum or bronchoalveolar lavage fluid samples, the assay can be applied.

In fact, mutational analysis has been proposed as an early indicator, because mutations at KRAS codon 12 can be detected up to 4 years before the clinical diagnosis of cancer. Unfortunately, KRAS mutations are not specific for carcinoma. They have also been detected in the sputum of patients whose tumors are negative for KRAS mutations and even in individuals with no clinically detectable carcinoma.[8–11] This highlights the fact that mutations in KRAS are a component of the carcinogenesis pathway but do not represent entirely specific correlation with malignant transformation. KRAS mutations are also associated with smoking tobacco. Therefore, their occurrence in individuals at high risk for lung cancer may also indicate widespread precancerous lesions that harbor these mutations. Although KRAS may be a good biomarker for early diagnosis of lung adenocarcinoma, the major limitation remains the relatively low frequency of KRAS mutations in primary lung cancers overall; only a small proportion of high-risk patients may potentially benefit from the test. In addition, this test does not entirely solve the problem of early detection of adenocarcinoma of the lung in nonsmokers, who do represent an important population of lung cancer patients in recent years.

Tumor Suppressor Genes

Tumor suppressor genes (TSGs) in the wild-type state have two active copies (alleles). These genes are thought to functionally suppress carcinogenesis in their routine cellular activity. Because both copies of the TSG must be mutated for tumorigenesis, TSGs are designated as recessive genes. This is in contrast to dominant protooncogenes, in which only one mutation is needed. We rarely test for both hits when assessing the status of TSGs. The most common assays for identifying TSGs include LOH, CGH, array CGH, and FISH. The LOH studies have provided clues to the localization of the many TSGs involved in lung carcinogenesis.

In general, alterations of chromosomes 3p, 9p21, 13q14, and 17p13 are frequently observed, even in the early precursor lesions.[12,13] These molecular alterations are thought to be cumulative and progressive. Advanced tumors frequently show widespread complete or partial loss of each chromosomal arm, whereas precursor lesions tend to show more focal and smaller chromosomal losses.[14] Most of these molecular alterations are thought to also correlate with smoking-related damage and may not necessarily indicate an increased risk for development of invasive carcinoma. Therefore, it is unlikely that any of these markers in isolation will be able to serve as a mechanism for diagnosis.

Molecular Anatomic Testing for Targeted Therapies in Lung Cancer

The development of small-molecule inhibitors of the epidermal growth factor receptor (EGFR) opened a new chapter for the treatment of patients with advanced lung cancer. It is clear from the experience with targeted therapy for breast cancer that standardized assays for assessing and predicting the effects of therapeutic agents are ideally developed in parallel with targeted therapies. The first assays used in the search for biomarkers for drug

therapy with EGFR inhibitors were tests for EGFR protein expression by immunohistochemistry and gene copy number by FISH.[15-17] There is a good correlation between immunohistochemistry and FISH results, meaning that amplification correlates with increased protein expression. Unfortunately, the assays were not able to predict patient response to EGFR inhibitors. In addition, impact of EGFR status on patient survival, as assessed by FISH and immunohistochemistry has also been controversial. In 2004, mutations in the EGFR gene were identified, and there appeared to be a strong relationship between clinical responsiveness to the tyrosine kinase inhibitor gefitinib and the presence of gene mutations.[18] Epidermal growth factor receptor mutations appear to be exclusive to lung cancer; only extremely rare mutations have been identified in other types of cancer, particularly in colorectal carcinoma.[19] The same deletion in exon 19 as is seen in lung cancer has also been rarely detected in squamous cell carcinoma of the head and neck.[20]

Epidermal growth factor receptor mutations have a unique pattern in terms of affected populations. They are usually seen in adenocarcinomas, most commonly in never smokers, and are more prevalent in East Asian women.[21] Although EGFR mutations correlate with the clinical response to tyrosine kinase inhibitors, recent clinical trials showed that survival benefit cannot be explained only by mutations. This led to renewed interest in the relationship between EGFR gene amplification or protein expression and survival after treatment with tyrosine kinase inhibitors. In addition, the genetic status of EGFR-related genes has also been explored. A recent study showed that gefitinib was most effective in non–small cell lung cancer patients with a high EGFR gene copy number, high protein expression, or EGFR mutations.[22] Because only high EGFR gene copy number determined by FISH correlated with prolonged survival, the authors proposed EGFR FISH analysis as an ideal clinical test for selecting patients for tyrosine kinase inhibitor therapy.

Anatomic Pathology Testing for Infectious Agents

As microbiology becomes more and more grounded in molecular technology, sophisticated assays can be readily applied to tissues in anatomic pathology. Molecular testing for infectious agents is increasingly useful as a diagnostic tool. Immunohistochemistry and in situ hybridization remain the popular ancillary techniques for surgical pathologists, because they can be applied to routine diagnostic material coupled with histologic evaluation. However, paraffin-embedded tissues can also serve as excellent source material for PCR-based organism identification assays. This is particularly useful when tissue was not sent directly for cultures or when suspicion is high but immunohistochemistry and in situ hybridization are negative or inconclusive. DNA and RNA extracted from formalin-fixed paraffin-embedded tissue are usually more fragmented than DNA from fresh or frozen tissue. Several laboratories are now equipped to do testing for *Mycobacterium* species and viruses, such as cytomegalovirus, in anatomic pathology material.

Despite the increase in isolates of *Mycobacterium tuberculosis* in the United States since 1985, there are now more isolates of nontuberculous mycobacteria (NTB) such as *Mycobacterium avium* complex. The diagnosis of tuberculosis for many years has been based on special stains of smears for acid-fast bacilli and mycobacterial cultures. The special stains for acid-fast bacilli are not sensitive and do not allow the identification of the different *Mycobacterium* species. Mycobacterial cultures are specific, but results are usually not available for 2 to 3 weeks or longer. Polymerase chain reaction using oligonucleotide primers specific for gene fragments in *M. tuberculosis* has been used to identify tuberculosis organisms from archival formalin-fixed paraffin-embedded tissue.[23] This method may detect organism with high specificity and sensitivity and is much faster than conventional cultures. The sensitivity of PCR is better than that of the special stains, in which a few mycobacteria might be missed on routine histologic sections. However, PCR results should always be interpreted in a clinical context. In diagnostic molecular pathology, sampling error is an important source of false-positive and false-negative results. The percentage of false-negative results after PCR amplification of *M. tuberculosis* from formalin-fixed, paraffin-embedded tissue varies among studies from 2% to 19% depending on the PCR technique employed.[24] The DNA extraction used for this method is performed from several whole thick sections, because the rate of PCR positivity seems to be at least partially related to the quantity of DNA used for amplification. Therefore, PCR techniques may have some disadvantages, such as possibly increased effect of tissue inhibitors or increased possibility of false-positive results due to contamination. Because of the relatively low amount of template DNA needed for amplification, PCR-based analysis is now increasingly performed on microdissected areas from tissue sections. For surgical pathologists, a molecular identification of mycobacteria can be the method of choice when the tissue obtained by biopsy is not sent for culture.

Several types of amplification assays are available for quantitation of cytomegalovirus and other viruses, most of which use a form of real-time or quantitative PCR. Currently, most assays are designed for peripheral blood, and therefore surgical pathologists are rarely involved in ordering these tests.

References

1. Hunt JL, Finkelstein SD. Microdissection techniques for molecular testing in surgical pathology. Arch Pathol Lab Med 2004;128:1372–1378.
2. Eltoum IA, Siegal GP, Frost AR. Microdissection of histologic sections: past, present, and future. Adv Anat Pathol 2002;9:316–322.
3. Simone NL, Paweletz CP, Charboneau L, et al. Laser capture microdissection: beyond functional genomics to proteomics. Mol Diagnosis 2000;5:301–307.
4. Rodenhuis S, Slebos RJ. The ras oncogenes in human lung cancer. Am Rev Respir Dis 1990;142: S27–S30.
5. Westra WH, Slebos RJ, Offerhaus GJ, et al. K-ras oncogene activation in lung adenocarcinomas from former smokers. Evidence that K-ras mutations are an early and irreversible event in the development of adenocarcinoma of the lung. Cancer 1993;72: 432–438.
6. Nelson HH, Christiani DC, Mark EJ, et al. Implications and prognostic value of K-ras mutation for early-stage lung cancer in women. J Natl Cancer Inst 1999;91:2032–2038.
7. Chapman AD, Kerr KM. The association between atypical adenomatous hyperplasia and primary lung cancer. Br J Cancer 2000;83:632–636.
8. Mao L, Hruban RH, Boyle JO, et al. Detection of oncogene mutations in sputum precedes diagnosis of lung cancer. Cancer Res 1994;54:1634–1637.
9. Ronai Z, Yabubovskaya MS, Zhang E, et al. K-ras mutation in sputum of patients with or without lung cancer. J Cell Biochem Suppl 1996;25:172–176.
10. Nakajima E, Hirano T, Konaka C, et al. K-ras mutation in sputum of primary lung cancer patients does not always reflect that of cancerous cells. Int J Oncol 2001;18:105–110.
11. Destro A, Bianchi P, Alloisio M, et al. K-ras and p16(INK4A)alterations in sputum of NSCLC patients and in heavy asymptomatic chronic smokers. Lung Cancer 2004; 44:23–32.
12. Wistuba II, Behrens C, Milchgrub S, et al. Sequential molecular abnormalities are involved in the multistage development of squamous cell lung carcinoma. Oncogene 1999;18:643–650.
13. Wistuba II, Lam S, Behrens C, et al. Molecular damage in the bronchial epithelium of current and former smokers. J Natl Cancer Inst 1997;89:1366–1373.
14. Wistuba II, Behrens C, Virmani AK, et al. High resolution chromosome 3p allelotyping of human lung cancer and preneoplastic/preinvasive bronchial epithelium reveals multiple, discontinuous sites of 3p allele loss and three regions of frequent breakpoints. Cancer Res 2000;60:1949–1960.
15. Nakamura H, Kawasaki N, Taguchi M, et al. Survival impact of epidermal growth factor receptor overexpression in patients with non–small cell lung cancer: a meta-analysis. Thorax 2006;61:140–145.
16. Suzuki S, Dobashi Y, Sakurai H, et al. Protein overexpression and gene amplification of epidermal growth factor receptor in nonsmall cell lung carcinomas. An immunohistochemical and fluorescence in situ hybridization study. Cancer 2005;103:1265–1273.

17. Hirsch FR, Varella-Garcia M, Bunn PA Jr, et al. Epidermal growth factor receptor in non–small-cell lung carcinomas: correlation between gene copy number and protein expression and impact on prognosis. J Clin Oncol 2003;21: 3798–3807.

18. Lynch TJ, Bell DW, Sordella R, et al. Activating mutations in the epidermal growth factor receptor underlying responsiveness of non–small-cell lung cancer to gefitinib. N Engl J Med 2004;350:2129–2139.

19. Nagahara H, Mimori K, Ohta M, et al. Somatic mutations of epidermal growth factor receptor in colorectal carcinoma. Clin Cancer Res 2005;11:1368–1371.

20. Lee JW, Soung YH, Kim SY, et al. Somatic mutations of EGFR gene in squamous cell carcinoma of the head and neck. Clin Cancer Res 2005;11:2879–2882.

21. Paez JG, Janne PA, Lee JC, et al. EGFR mutations in lung cancer: correlation with clinical response to gefitinib therapy. Science 2004;304:1497–1500.

22. Cappuzzo F, Hirsch FR, Rossi E, et al. Epidermal growth factor receptor gene and protein and gefitinib sensitivity in non–small-cell lung cancer. J Natl Cancer Inst 2005;97:643–655.

23. Johansen IS, Thomsen VO, Forsgren A, et al. Detection of Mycobacterium tuberculosis complex in formalin-fixed, paraffin-embedded tissue specimens with necrotizing granulomatous inflammation by strand displacement amplification. J Mol Diagn 2004;6:231–236.

24. Marchetti G, Gori A, Catozzi L, et al. Evaluation of PCR in detection of Mycobacterium tuberculosis from formalin-fixed, paraffin-embedded tissues: comparison of four amplification assays. J Clin Microbiol 1998;6:1512–1517.

9
Polymerase Chain Reaction and Reverse Transcription–Polymerase Chain Reaction

Dwight Oliver

Polymerase Chain Reaction

Polymerase chain reaction (PCR) enables one to determine if a specific needle is present in a haystack, and it can be used as a step toward the characterization of the needle. It is a quick, powerful, inexpensive DNA amplification technique that has become a fundamental tool in molecular pathology.

Theory

The PCR is one of the most significant technical innovations in molecular biology.[1] The PCR was devised by Kary Mullis and colleagues[2,3] at Cetus Corporation in California and was first described in a 1985 paper demonstrating its application in the prenatal diagnosis of sickle cell anemia[2] and then further described in an ensuing paper.[3] These works detailed how a DNA sequence could be enzymatically amplified in vitro using specific oligonucleotide primers and bacterial (Klenow) DNA polymerase. With refinement of PCR over the next 3 years, it was found that a robust PCR using a thermostable polymerase could amplify a DNA sequence by a factor of over 10^7, even when the target DNA made up only 1 of 100,000 DNA strands in a reaction.[4] Since then, additional improvements and variations to the original reaction have been made, affording even more efficiency, sensitivity, and utility to this tool. Its application specifically to diseases of the lungs has ranged from detection of infectious diseases[5-7] to study of inflammatory mechanisms,[8,9] to use in mutation analysis,[10-12] to detection of tumors and metastases.[13-15]

Principles

The principle of PCR is illustrated in Figure 9.11. The target DNA to be amplified in vitro can be human genomic, bacterial, viral, plasmid, or previously PCR-amplified DNA and is represented in the figure by the target's nucleotide base letters A, C, G, and T and the sugar phosphate backbone. Other components of PCR include a thermostable DNA polymerase such as *Taq* polymerase, two oligonucleotide primers, four deoxynucleotide triphosphates, magnesium, buffer, and a thermocycler. Polymerase chain reaction achieves amplification of the DNA by repeating a three-step cycle over and over. These three steps are denaturation, annealing, and extension.

In the denaturation step, target double-stranded DNA (dsDNA) is heated to a high temperature (94°–95°C) in order to break the hydrogen bonds between nucleotide bases on opposing strands. The dsDNA *denatures*, splitting into two intact single strands (ssDNA) that are *complementary* to each other. In the second (annealing) step, the reaction mix is cooled to typically 50°–65°C, allowing ssDNA oligonucleotide *primers* to bind (*anneal*) to the portion of the target ssDNA to which they have specifically been designed. The investigator must know the sequence of the target DNA (at least in the region of the primers) in order to design the primers. Two primers are required—one that is complementary to the $3' \rightarrow 5'$ oriented target strand in Figure 9.1 (the *forward* primer), and one primer that is complementary to the $5' \rightarrow 3'$ target strand in the figure (the *reverse* primer). Since these primers are in overwhelming abundance compared with the target DNA, they will anneal to the target DNA much more frequently than the full-length target DNA will anneal to its full-length complementary strand as the reaction is cooled. In the third (*extension*) step, as the temperature is raised to its working optimum (72°C), *Taq* polymerase recognizes these partially double-stranded DNAs and uses the forward and reverse primers as initiation points to begin extending the primers via polymerization in a $5' \rightarrow 3'$ direction along the two new (*nascent*) strands. DNA polymerase does this by selecting high-energy deoxynucleotide triphosphates (dNTPs) from solution and placing them in the nascent strands directly across from their complementary base in the template

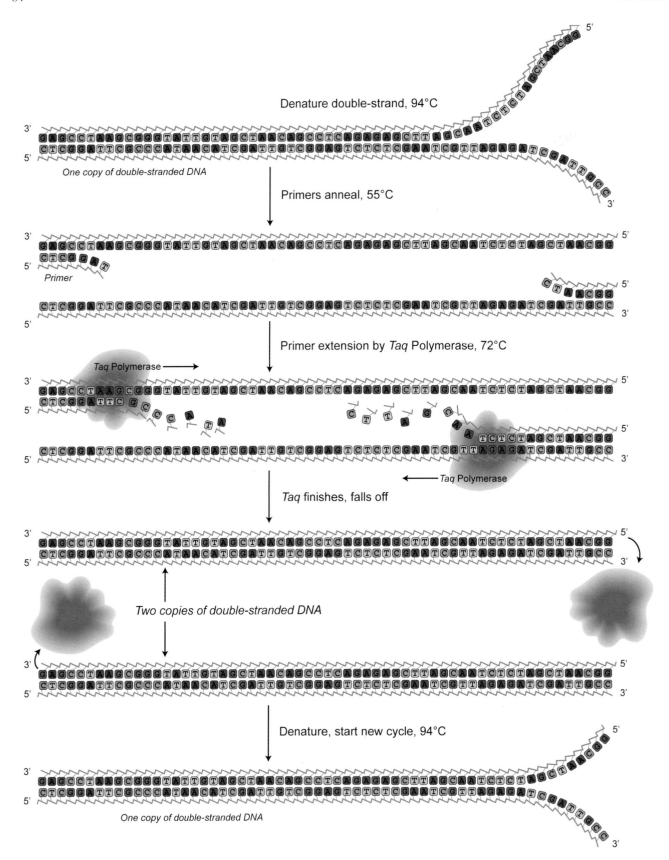

FIGURE 9.1. Polymerase chain reaction steps. A single double-stranded DNA fragment is denatured and cycled through three steps—denaturation, annealing, and extension—to create an exact copy of the original. *Taq* polymerase extends primers by selecting deoxyribonucleotide triphosphates from the reaction solution based on the nucleotide sequence of the target DNA.

(target) strand. During the first round (*cycle*) of PCR, the DNA polymerases extend the nascent strands for a relatively long distance before falling off. At the end of the first cycle, two double-stranded copies of a portion of the target DNA have been generated from one copy.

During the second cycle (Figure 9.2, where DNA strands are symbolized by lines) the same process happens, but now the polymerase can only proceed as far down the DNA as the point where the opposite primer started. At the end of the second cycle the PCR products (*amplicons*) include two relatively short fragments of ssDNA whose two ends now correspond exactly to the locations of the forward and reverse primers. Both the genomic DNA and new amplicons can serve as templates in successive PCR cycles.[16] With subsequent cycles, the longer dsDNA PCR products are diluted out by the more numerous shorter dsDNA PCR products.[17,18] In a perfect PCR the amount of dsDNA doubles with each cycle so that after 30 cycles there are more than 1 billion copies of the original dsDNA ($2^{30} = 1.1$ billion) and more than 1 trillion copies after 40 cycles ($2^{40} = 1.1$ trillion). Because the primers recognize only the target DNA they are designed for, only a specific segment of DNA is amplified, even if it makes up only a fraction of all the different DNA sequences in a reaction.[4] This preferential amplification greatly facilitates post-PCR analysis of the target sequence.

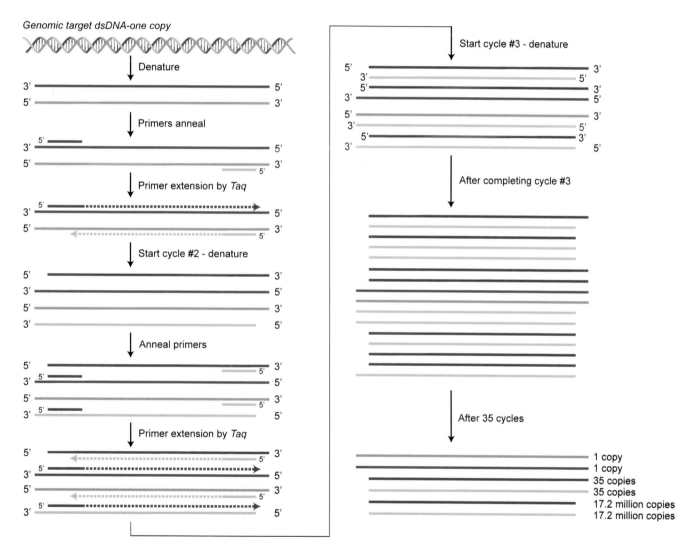

FIGURE 9.2. Thirty-five cycles of polymerase chain reaction (PCR). DNA strands are abbreviated as lines. In the first cycle, two long PCR products of variable length (red, green lines) are polymerized, but with ensuing cycles the overwhelming PCR product is short, as defined by the positions of the forward (red) and reverse (green) primers. In a perfect PCR, several million amplicons are present after 35 cycles and ready for post-PCR analysis.

TABLE 9.1. Typical polymerase chain reaction (PCR) thermocycler program.

	Temperature	Time
Initial denaturation	95°C	10 min
40 cycles of		
Denaturation step	95°C	30 sec
Annealing step	57°C	30 sec
Extension step	72°C	45 sec
Final polymerization	72°C	10 min
Post-PCR hold	4°C	Indefinite

Polymerase chain reaction cycling is done in a *thermocycler*, a small automated tabletop instrument programmed by the investigator. A typical program (Table 9.1) starts with a 5–10 min denaturation at 94°–95°C in order to ensure that the majority of the DNA (especially large chromosomal strands) is denatured. This is followed by 30–50 cycles of brief denaturation/annealing/extension. The PCR concludes with a 5–10-min final polymerization step at 72°C to ensure nearly all amplicons are extended to their full length.

Practical Polymerase Chain Reaction

Thermocyclers must be properly programmed in order to create an efficient PCR. Most programs are roughly similar (see Table 9.1), except for the annealing temperature and time intervals of each step. The annealing temperature is dependent on the melting temperature of the primers, and the time spent at the different steps is dictated by the size of the target DNA. The denaturation temperature is generally the same in all PCRs (94°–95°C), just as the extension temperature is usually 72°C, because most polymerases used in PCR work best at this temperature (but see later discussion of polymerases and real-time PCR).

Denaturation Step Programming

The initial denaturation, which occurs prior to any cycling, is typically 94°–95°C for 5–10 min. This gives human chromosomal DNA time to unravel and split into single strands. Smaller (e.g., viral) DNA targets may require only 3–5 min. Because ssDNA tends to reanneal while cooling, the dsDNA must be redenatured at 94°C for 10–60 sec at the beginning of each cycle. GC-rich targets may require hotter/longer denaturations, while formamide or dimethylsulfoxide (DMSO) can be added to promote denaturation.[19] Avoid temperatures above 95°C or excessive cycles, as *Taq* stability decreases under these conditions.[20]

Annealing Step Programming and Primer Design

The *annealing* temperature varies with every PCR and is a critical factor in the PCR program, as it helps dictate lower limit of detection, sensitivity, and specificity of the PCR. It must be calculated for each unique PCR reaction and is dependent on the melting temperature of the two oligonucleotide primers. The *melting* temperature (T_m) of a DNA fragment is the temperature at which half of it has denatured into the single-stranded form (e.g., the primer is *not* annealed to its complementary target) and half is still double-stranded (primer *is* annealed to its target), assuming the number of copies of the two complementary strands is equal. Melting temperature calculation of an oligonucleotide can be very complex, with formulas that employ thermodynamics and depend on nearest neighbor nucleotides[21,22] and the salt concentrations in the reaction. Numerous web sites, including those of companies that manufacture custom oligonucleotides, have free T_m calculators; after typing in a primer sequence the T_m is instantly calculated. Software is also available that will generate a list of potential primer pairs, with their T_ms, once the entire target sequence is entered.

Manual calculation of the approximate T_ms of short oligonucleotides can also be done using the abbreviated Wallace rule[23]:

$$T_m = 2(A + T) + 4(C + G)$$

Here T_m is in degrees Centigrade, and A, T, C, and G stand for the number of each of these bases in the single-stranded oligonucleotide sequence. Thus the approximate T_m of a 22 base pair (bp) (22mer) poly(A) oligonucleotide would be only 44°C, while the 21mer CGGCTG CACGCTGCGCCGTCC would have an approximate T_m of 76°C. Because Cs and Gs base pair with three hydrogen bonds, more heat is required to melt them apart in a dsDNA → ssDNA conversion compared with As and Ts, which base pair by sharing only two hydrogen bonds.

To design primers, one must first isolate the region of the gene of interest that will be amplified. The human genome and the genomes of many viruses and bacteria are available on the National Center of Biotechnology Information (NCBI) web site (www.ncbi.nlm.nih.gov/). Avoid placing primers in regions with known polymorphisms or splice variants or, in the case of viruses and bacteria, where any subtype/strain variations have been reported in the region of the proposed primers.

To ensure genomic DNA (and not reverse-transcribed mRNA) is being amplified, primers should be located at exon–intron junctions or within introns. To ensure reverse-transcribed RNA is being amplified (from the cDNA, see later), primers should span introns and be within exons.

In order to create a robust PCR, the size of the DNA region amplified (distance of the two primers from each other) should be less than 500 bp and preferably around 200–300 bp. Amplicons larger than 1 kb (kilobase or 1,000 bp) often require special polymerases (see later) with enhanced processivity. These forward and reverse primers should be only 18–25 bp long, have a 40%–60% G + C content, and T_ms in the 55°–65°C range. Melting temperatures outside this range may work, and in fact are sometimes necessary, but they have a greater likelihood of resulting in a less efficient or more nonspecific PCR. In addition, the primers should have T_ms that are within 2°C of each other: add or remove bases to meet this goal. Ideally, the last five bases in the primer should include three Cs or Gs, and the 3′ end of the primers should be a C or G to promote tight base pairing at the point of *Taq* recognition and initiation of polymerization.

Just as a primer will anneal to its complementary region in the target DNA, so a pair of primers might anneal to complementary regions within themselves or within each other. Thus, **TGGCCC**ATTACACTT**GGCC**ATTT is a poor primer choice because there will be some tendency for the boldface sequences to anneal to each other, forming a hairpin *stem-loop structure* within itself or to form *primer dimers* between two similar primers. Likewise, a 5′–TAGG–3′ sequence in the reverse primer could transiently anneal to a 5′–CCTA–3′ sequence in the forward primer. Many of the web sites that calculate T_ms also have a tool to check for these types of structures, as these aberrant forms can significantly reduce the yield of PCR product due to effective reduction of the available primer supply. Finally, avoid repetitive bases at the 3′ end of a primer, as this promotes slippage ("out of register") errors by *Taq* polymerase. Once all (or as many as feasible) of the above rules are met and two primer sequences have been found, the primers should be checked to be certain they are not complementary to DNA sequences unrelated to the target sequence by using the NCBI BLAST (basic local alignment search tool) database at www.ncbi.nlm.nih.gov/BLAST/. This web site will list all published DNA sequences that exactly or closely match the oligonucleotide sequences submitted. If one or both primers are close matches to nontarget DNA that may be present in the samples tested, new primer(s) may have to be designed.

The rules are empirical and do not guarantee a large PCR yield for reasons that are not always obvious or easily tested. It is often more expeditious to simply design more than one set of primers using the above rules and test all on a specimen to determine which pair gives the most robust PCR.

What annealing temperature should now be used in the PCR? This also requires trial and error. Initially the annealing temperature programmed into the thermocycler should be 5°–10°C below the lowest T_m of the forward and reverse primers. At such a low temperature there will be mispriming onto nontarget sequences, resulting in amplification of nonspecific products. To enhance the specificity and perhaps even the sensitivity of the PCR, the temperature should then be systematically raised until amplicon yield drops and hopefully nonspecific amplicons disappear. Alternatively, the annealing temperature can be lowered, potentially increasing sensitivity, at the risk of generating nonspecific amplicons in addition to the desired PCR product.

Polymerase Chain Reaction Components

Thermostable Polymerase

The first PCRs used an *Escherichia coli* DNA polymerase[2] that was thermolabile and had to be replaced at each cycle; extension at 37°C would allow the nonspecific priming of numerous genomic sites and thus formation of nonspecific amplicons. Because the cycling of PCR repeatedly raises the reaction to 95°C, a thermostable polymerase is required. *Taq* polymerase, the most frequently used, was first purified from the bacterium *Thermus aquaticus* in 1976,[24] years before PCR. The enzyme has optimal 5′ → 3′ polymerase activity at 80°C (but will inefficiently extend primers at much lower temperatures), requires a divalent cation (Mg^{2+}), extends at a rate of 60 nucleotides/sec,[25] and a polymerization per binding event (processivity) of 50–80 bases.[26] *Taq* has double-strand–specific 5′ → 3′ exonuclease activity (see later discussion of real-time PCR) but does not have 3′ → 5′ exonuclease (proofreading) ability; its estimated error rate is 2.1×10^{-4} errors per base per duplication.[27] *Taq* is inhibited in samples containing heparin, hemoglobin, phenol,[28] urine, urea,[29] ethanol and high formamide, DMSO, or ethylenediaminetetraacetic acid (EDTA) levels.

Polymerases with fidelity superior to *Taq* include *Pfu*, *Pwo*, *Tgo* (from *Pyrococcus furiosus, Pyrococcus woesei, Thermococcus gorgonarius*, respectively), and *Tli* (from *Thermococcus litoralis*) has superior thermostability.[30] *Thermus thermophilus* polymerase (*Tth*), unlike *Taq*, has reverse transcriptase activity (see later) as well as DNA polymerase activity. All of these polymerases are readily available from different distributors.

Deoxynucleotides

The four dNTPs needed to replicate DNA are deoxyadenosine triphosphate, deoxyguanosine triphosphate, deoxycytosine triphosphate, and deoxythymidine triphosphate (dATP, dGTP, dCTP, and dTTP). They are added in equal concentration to the PCR mix, typically with a final concentration of 50–250 μM each in the reaction (200–1,000 μM total for all four dNTPs).

To prevent contamination of a new PCR reaction by previously amplified DNA, deoxyuridine triphosphate (dUTP), instead of dTTP, is added to reactions and incorporated into the amplicons. When the bacterial enzyme uracil-N-glycosylase[31] is added and activated at the start of subsequent PCRs, it destroys any previously amplified PCR products that contain uracil, but it does not harm the natural TTP-containing DNA of the new sample. Uracil-N-glycosylase is deactivated at temperatures above 50°C and therefore does not destroy the newly polymerized DNA strands made during PCR.

Polymerase Chain Reaction Buffer

Taq requires the correct pH to function throughout the range of temperatures in PCR. The buffer Tris-HCl (10mM) provides a pH of 8.3 at 25°C but 7.2 at 72°C; *Taq* has improved fidelity at this pH or lower.[32] Potassium chloride (50mM) stabilizes the DNA and promotes primer annealing to its target. Nonionic detergents such as 0.01% Tween-20 or 0.1% Triton X-100 are often used, as well as gelatin. Fortunately, the above components (depending on manufacturer) are included in optimized 10× PCR buffer solutions provided by most *Taq* polymerase suppliers and do not have to be added individually to the reaction.

Magnesium

The magnesium concentration is important because it affects PCR specificity and efficiency through its interaction with *Taq,* whose function is dependent on the divalent cation.[33] A free $[Mg^{2+}]$ of 1.2–1.3mM is optimal for *Taq*, whereas much higher Mg^{2+} levels result in increased error rates due to base substitutions and frameshift errors.[32] Magnesium is often included in 10× PCR buffer solutions at a $[Mg^{2+}]$ of 1.5mM, which decreases to 1.3mM in the presence of 0.2mM dNTPs due to equimolar binding of dNTPs and Mg^{2+} by *Taq* polymerase.[33]

Polymerase Chain Reaction Set-Up

Prior to starting experiments using PCR, accommodations must be made in the laboratory. Because of the amplification power of PCR, contamination of even minute amounts of DNA from one sample to the next must be avoided. Master mixes, containing all components of the PCR except the DNA, should be set up in a separate, dedicated room or area (hood) away from specimens or post-PCR solutions. DNA or RNA should be isolated from samples in a second room or area. DNA of the samples can then be added to the master mix in a third area, ideally. The thermocycler should also be in a separate room or area of the lab. Keep a

TABLE 9.2. Typical polymerase chain reaction (PCR) reagent mix.

H₂O (nuclease-free) to final total volume of	25.0μL
dNTPs at 5–10mM each (20–40mM total)	0.5μL
Forward primer at 25μM	0.3μL
Reverse Primer at 25μM	0.3μL
10 × PCR buffer with Mg²⁺	2.5μL
Taq polymerase at 1 unit*/μL	1.0μL
Target DNA 100–500ng	1.0μL

*One unit of Taq is defined as the amount of enzyme that will incorporate 10nmol of deoxynucleotide triphosphates into acid-insoluble material in 30min at 75°C.

unidirectional flow of material from pre-PCR to post-PCR—do not allow PCR-amplified material into the master mix preparation or DNA isolation areas. Label dedicated pipettors and use only aerosol-resistant tips to prevent contamination of pipettor barrels. Wear protective disposable gloves at all times, and change them and laboratory coats when going from one room or area to the next. Use ultraviolet irradiation inside hoods or on benchtops to destroy possible contaminating DNA.

Use only autoclaved molecular biology–grade water in master mixes. Make certain that all plastic tubes and tips are DNAse and RNAse free, as these enzymes will digest the target nucleic acids in specimens.

There is no universal recipe for the PCR mix, but a typical mix, including the DNA, is shown in Table 9.2. However, this is just a start. All PCRs need some adjusting—annealing temperatures, cycle step times, reagents (concentration of each primer, Mg^{2+} concentration, etc.), primer sequences—to determine the optimal conditions to give the greatest yield, fastest time, or highest specificity.

Postprocedure Analysis

Polymerase chain reaction alone does not provide answers to an investigator's questions, but, because of the huge increase in a specific product, it makes the product's analysis much easier. To prove that a target sequence was present in a specimen, amplicons are run out on agarose or polyacrylamide electrophoresis gels to compare their lengths to DNA "ladder" markers; amplicons of the correct size are strong evidence that the target sequence was present. Southern blotting[34] with probe hybridization is an alternative. Bacterial restriction endonuclease digestion prior to electrophoresis or single-stranded conformation polymorphism studies can be done on PCR products to check for mutations.[33] DNA sequencing[35] of the amplicons or ligation into a plasmid for further analysis are other options, depending on the needs of the researcher.

Variations

Improvements and variations in PCR have been introduced over the past 20 years to meet the needs of researchers and clinical molecular diagnostics labs.

Hot start PCR[36–39] is a technique preventing *Taq* from extending primers until a temperature of 60°–80°C is reached, usually done by withholding *Taq* from the reaction until these temperatures have been reached. This prevents *Taq* extension of primer dimers or primers that have annealed to nonspecific regions of the specimen DNA at low temperatures, such as during the preparation of the reagent mix. The result is improved specificity and yield of the PCR and is especially helpful when the target DNA is a small percentage of the total DNA. There are two common hot start methods. The first uses a wax plug to separate key reagents (e.g., dNTPs from *Taq*) in the PCR tube; the wax melts at a temperature well above the primers' T_m and allows mixing of all reagents. The second uses a modified *Taq* that is activated only after the initial 95°C 10-min denaturation step.

Nested PCR[40,41] uses two pairs of primers to improve amplicon yield and specificity. The first pair ("outer primers") is designed to amplify a larger fragment of the target DNA. These amplicons are then used, usually in a second PCR, as the template DNA for the second set ("inner primers"), which necessarily makes a smaller PCR product. Even if two sequential PCRs are run there may still be four products in the final PCR, the smallest being defined by only the inner primers. If all four primers are added at once and only one PCR is run, the T_m of the inner primers should be lower than the outer primers' T_m.[33]

Methylation-specific PCR[42–44] is used on genomic DNA to determine if the CpG islands within the promoter of a gene are methylated on the cytosine residue (blocking the gene's expression in the cell[45]) or unmethylated (potentially allowing gene expression). For example, imprinted genes and silenced genes on X chromosomes are methylated,[46] as are the promoters of tumor suppressor genes in many cancers.[47–49] Methylation-specific PCR is based on the realization that a cytosine converts to a uracil after bisulfite treatment, whereas a methylated cytosine (5-methylcytosine) is refractory and remains as cytosine.[50] An unmethylated CpG will be converted to UpG after bisulfite, but a methylated one will remain as CpG. The change in DNA sequence of an unmethylated promoter compared with a methylated promoter after bisulfite treatment allows one to design primers that can discriminate between the two. Whichever of the two primers yields a PCR product indicates the methylation status of the promoter.

Multiplex PCR amplifies multiple different regions of DNA at one time by using multiple primer pairs in one reaction. Several targets can be analyzed in one specimen, including housekeeping genes and variably expressed genes, multiple microorganisms,[51] or multiple mutations in a genetic disorder[52] or malignancy.[53,54] Although ostensibly a timesaver, designing primers and optimizing reaction conditions so as to ensure equally robust amplification of all targets in multiplex PCR is a challenge. First, design individual primer pairs (but avoid primer dimers with every other primer), and program the thermocycler to allow optimal amplification of all targets on an individual basis. Then combine (equimolar) primers and run the same program to see which targets are weakly amplified. Adjust primer concentrations, annealing temperatures, $[Mg^{2+}]$, and so forth, to equalize yields of targets. Primer software is also available, but in all cases trial and error are necessary to arrive at the final set-up.

Other variations of PCR, each with its unique benefits, include the amplification refractory mutation system,[55] allele-specific oligonucleotide probes,[56] rapid amplification of cDNA ends,[57] and in situ PCR.[58] One variant that deserves special attention is real-time PCR.

Real-Time Polymerase Chain Reaction

Real-time PCR[59–62] is a recent innovation that has quickly become very popular in molecular biology research and molecular diagnostics. It circumvents the need for time-consuming post-PCR analysis, and it can detect DNA targets, quantify the original (before amplification) copy number of the target DNA present in a specimen, or detect specific mutations. Although very similar to conventional PCR, real-time PCR is based on two additional principles. First, *Taq* polymerase has a bonus 5′ *exonuclease* activity on partially double-stranded DNA[63]—it will digest it to a single-stranded target—just prior to polymerizing it into a double-stranded amplicon. Second, energy can be transferred between fluorescent molecules (fluorophores) attached to oligonucleotides when these small DNA fragments are used as probes against specific DNA targets. This second principle, first proposed in 1948 by Förster[64] and later supported by Stryer and Haugland,[65] indicates that electronic excitation energy can be transferred over short distances (≤ 50 Å) via dipole–dipole resonance between an energy donor and acceptor chromophore.[66] Transfer efficiency is proportional to the inverse sixth power of the distance separating the donor and acceptor.[65]

Fluorescence resonance energy transfer (FRET) in real-time PCR is demonstrated in the five frames in Figure 9.3. A single oligonucleotide (TaqMan® type) probe is designed so that it specifically anneals to its complementary region of a target DNA, somewhere between the forward and reverse primers (top frame of Figure 9.3). A donor/emitter fluorophore covalently attached to one end of this oligonucleotide is stimulated by monochromatic light from a laser, and the energy is

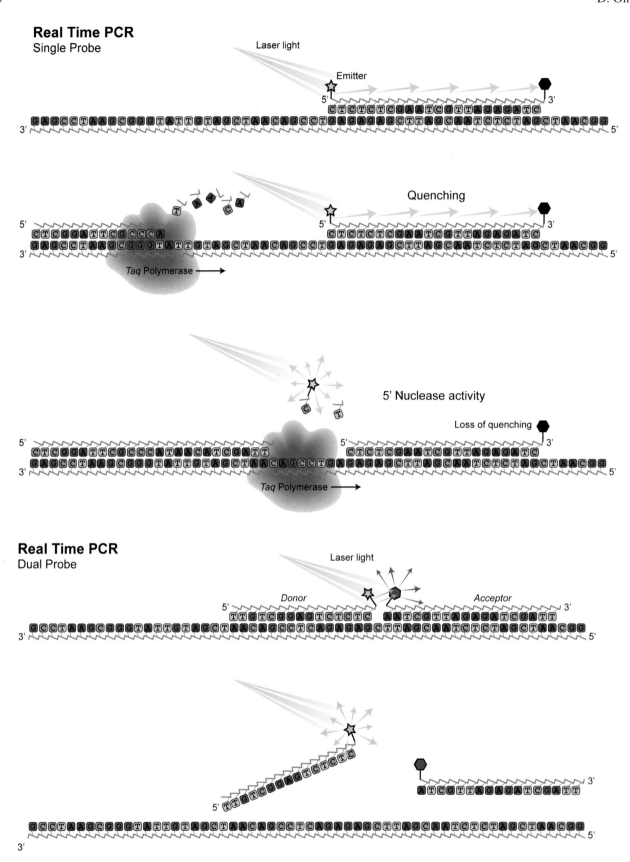

FIGURE 9.3. Real-time polymerase chain reaction (PCR). The top three frames demonstrate single-probe real-time PCR. Quenching ceases once the nucleotide bound to the emitter (yellow) is cleaved by *Taq*. In the third frame, the forward portion of *Taq* cleaves the probe (releasing nucleotides), while the back part of *Taq* extends the forward primer (consuming other nucleotides). The bottom two frames show a dual-probe assay in which probes attach to the target DNA and transfer energy from the yellow to the red fluorophore during the annealing step. They float away during the extension or denaturation step, terminating fluorescence energy transfer, and will not be cleaved by *Taq*.

transferred to a quencher fluorophore at the other end. In this kind of probe, light is either not reemitted by the quencher or is reemitted at a wavelength different from that of the donor fluorophore. During the primer *extension* step of PCR (see Figure 9.3, second frame) the probe remains intact—and the light remains quenched—until degraded into single nucleotides by the 5′ exonuclease activity of *Taq* as it passes through during polymerization of the target DNA (see Figure 9.3, third frame). Once cleaved, the emitter nucleotide drifts too far away for its emissions to be quenched, and its fluorescence is recorded in each PCR cycle by a sensitive photodetector and entered into the system's computer. With each PCR cycle the number of amplicons and the quantity of light double as more probes are cleaved.

Dual-probe real-time PCR (LightCycler® type or *hybridization probes;* see Figure 9.3, last two frames) uses donor/emitter and acceptor probes, designed to anneal side by side on the same target DNA. Fluorescent energy is transferred from the fluorophore of the 5′ donor probe (on the left) to the 3′ acceptor probe (on the right) during the *annealing* step of PCR. The acceptor immediately reemits at a wavelength unique to its fluorophore, and its signal strength doubles as the number of amplicons doubles with each PCR cycle. The probes separate, and FRET is terminated as the temperature is increased for the denaturation step.

Whether in single- or double-probe real-time PCR, the unique emission spectra of all fluorophores are captured and analyzed throughout each cycle by the real-time instrument software in order to generate curves such as those in Figure 9.4. Cycle number is plotted versus fluorescence, and each of the colored curves represents a different specimen. Flat lines indicate no target DNA was

in the specimen, and curves that begin rising at a low cycle number represent specimens that had more initial target DNA than those curves that rise later. Note that an exponential increase in fluorescence (and thus amplicon number) occurs only after numerous cycles, when PCR becomes its most efficient. To compare specimen target DNA copy number, a single horizontal *threshold* line can be drawn through all curves at this exponential phase and then a vertical line dropped from each intersection point to the X (cycle number) axis. This point on the X axis is the *cycle threshold* number of the specimen, and it *increases* as the original DNA copy number in a specimen *decreases*. Real-time PCR can be quantitative: a series of controls with a range of known DNA copy numbers are run to generate a standard curve of cycle threshold versus copy number. The cycle threshold values of specimens run simultaneously with the controls can then be converted into original DNA copy number by extrapolating from the standard curve.

Real-time instruments are able to detect fluorescence over a broad range of amplification—dynamic ranges of 7–8 logs can be obtained[61] (e.g., specimen DNA copy numbers from 10^1 to 10^8 or 10^2 to 10^9 can be detected on the same run). In addition, probes are able to detect even a single base pair change in target DNA, such as in allelic discrimination.[67,68]

In the design of real-time PCR reactions, the target should be short, preferably less than 150 bp, to maximize amplification efficiency. In some real-time instrument programs the annealing and extension steps are combined into one and run at a temperature of ~60°C. Probes should be designed before the primers and can bind the sense or antisense strand. They should be ≤35 bp long, have a GC content of 30%–80%, should not have runs

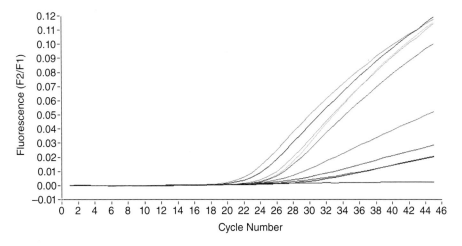

FIGURE 9.4. Amplification curves using a dual-probe real-time polymerase chain reaction (PCR). The PCR cycle number is plotted against fluorescence for seven samples of human genomic DNA being tested for a blood coagulation factor. Note that the specimen represented by the rising curve on the far left contains the most target DNA, as it shows exponential amplification at an earlier cycle. (Courtesy of Mai Le, M[ASCP].)

of four or more of the same nucleotide, should not partially anneal to each other or to either primer, and should have the 3′ end blocked by phosphorylation to prevent extension by *Taq*. TaqMan® probes should have a T_m of 68°–70°C (about 8°–10° higher than their associated primers, which should have T_ms of 58°–60°C), and the 5′ fluorophore should not be bound to a G. LightCycler® probes should optimally be 1–3bp apart, have a T_m between the extension and annealing step temperatures, and be 5°–10°C higher than the primers' T_m; the T_m of the two probes should be within 2°C of each other unless mutation detection is desired. Mutation detection is facilitated by looking for differential melting (denaturation and consequently loss of FRET) of probes from wild-type versus mutant target DNA sequences (*melting curve*).

Reverse Transcription

All normal cells in a human's body, with few exceptions, have the same chromosomal DNA sequence, that is, the same genetic code. Thus, genomic information obtained from the DNA of easily obtained normal white blood cells would be applicable to the genetic makeup of normal lung, brain, or colon cells. This does not apply to malignant cells, which can have a genetic composition that is profoundly different from that of normal cells.

Function and structure of various cell types differ because of the mRNA that they transcribe and ultimately the proteins that are translated. In other words, it is the protein expression profile of cells that differentiates them. Presently, the most practical way to study the specific genes expressed in a particular cell type is to analyze the mRNA the cells make. Because RNA is unstable and therefore difficult to work with in the laboratory, it can be converted into the complementary DNA (cDNA) by a process known as *reverse transcription*.[69–71] The resultant cDNA is much more stable than the mRNA. Reverse transcription is so named because RNA is used as the template to direct the production of DNA—the reverse of normal cellular transcription, where DNA is used by RNA polymerase to direct the production of mRNA.

Reverse transcriptase enzyme is an RNA-directed DNA polymerase made and used by some RNA viruses to complete their life cycle within a host. Viral reverse transcriptases have been characterized and/or cloned, and the enzymes are commercially available for use in research and clinical molecular laboratories.[72–76]

Reverse transcriptase, like DNA polymerase, requires a DNA primer (Figure 9.5) to initiate its function. Because mRNA has a poly(A) tail at its 3′ end, an ideal primer for reverse transcription of mRNA species would be a poly(T) oligonucleotide (oligo dT).[77,78] A replete collection of short DNA primers with random sequences can also be used; these primers are recommended if reverse transcription of ribosomal RNA (rRNA) is also desired along with mRNA. The enzyme starts transcription at the 3′ end of template RNA (the 5′ end of the nascent [new] cDNA strand) and proceeds in a 5′ → 3′ direction on the nascent strand ("first strand synthesis"). In this fashion, all of the mRNA (or total RNA) present in a cell can be transcribed into complementary DNA. Those mRNA sequences that are present at a high copy number in the cell will be reverse transcribed to a high cDNA copy number compared with those mRNA sequences that are rare in a cell.

A typical reverse transcription protocol is given in Table 9.3. The two most commonly used reverse transcriptases are from bird and mouse viruses: avian myeloblastosis virus (AMV) and Moloney murine leukemia virus (MMLV)[79]. Their recommended buffers should not be interchanged. RNAse inhibitors and diethylpyrocarbonate-treated water are needed to preserve the unstable RNA. The initial 70°C heating is to remove secondary structures from the RNA; the 42°C (AMV and some MMLV products) or 37°C (some MMLV products) incubations are the working temperature of the enzymes. The 90°–95°C is needed to inactivate the enzymes.

The cDNA made by reverse transcription of mRNA (and/or rRNA) can then be used as a template for PCR if the appropriate primers for the target DNA are present. During the first cycle of the PCR, only one (the forward) primer is needed because only one strand is polymerized, but this new strand will serve as the template for the opposite primer during the second PCR cycle, and polymerization of both strands will continue with each cycle. (Note that some bacteria such as *T. thermophilus* have an enzyme [*Tth*] that can both reverse transcribe RNA and polymerize DNA, allowing reverse transcription and PCR to proceed simultaneously in a single tube.)

Reverse transcription–PCR is thus an important tool that allows the investigator to study the genes expressed or not expressed in specific cells after isolation of the mRNA.[80–83] Additional (post-PCR) techniques such as gel electrophoresis, single-stranded conformation polymorphism gels, restriction fragment-length polymorphism analysis, DNA sequencing, microarrays, and so forth, can be applied to also determine if the genes expressed have mutations.

Under- or overexpression of a particular gene in neoplastic or reactive cells can be investigated by comparing their expression levels in normal cells. This could be done by comparing band strengths on Northern (RNA) blots. However, in these methods one must control for the number of tumor/reactive cells being the same as the number of normal cells. Analysis is much easier if done by real-time PCR, in which the ratio of the expression level of the gene of interest is compared with the expression level of a constitutively expressed housekeeping gene such as β-actin, 18S rRNA, cyclophilin, glyceralde-

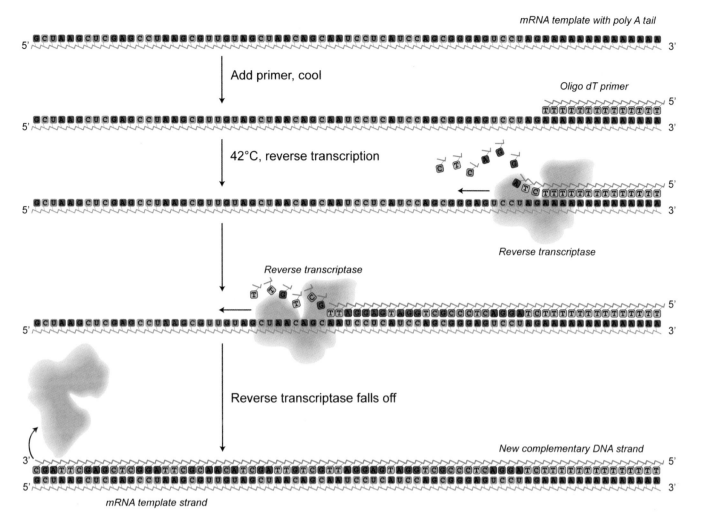

FIGURE 9.5. Reverse Transcription. Reverse transcriptase uses oligo dT as the primer on the target mRNA and polymerizes in the 5′ → 3′ direction on the new DNA strand. The original mRNA strand is then cleaved by an RNAse domain within the reverse transcriptase (not shown), thus allowing polymerization of the single-stranded DNA into double-stranded DNA during polymerase chain reaction.

TABLE 9.3. Typical reverse transcription reaction protocol.

RNA 1–2 µg	1.0 µL
DEPC-treated H₂O	8.5 µL
Oligo dT or random primers at 40 µM	2.0 µL
70°C ↓ 5 min	
4°C ↓ 5 min	
Quickly add 20.0 µL of prepared RT master mix:	
DEPC-treated H₂O add to total final volume	20.0 µL
MMLV (10×) or AMV (5×) buffer	2.0–4.0 µL
dNTP at 10 mmol	3.0 µL
RNAse inhibitor 10–40 units	1.0 µL
MMLV reverse transcriptase 200 units*	1.0 µL
AMV reverse transcriptase 30 units*	
37° or 42°C ↓ 60 min	
90°–95°C ↓ 5 min	
Use ~1–3 µL in the PCR reaction	

*One unit of reverse transcriptase is defined as the amount of enzyme that will incorporate 1 nmol of deoxythymidine triphosphate into acid-insoluble material in 10 min at 37°C using poly(rA). oligo(dT) as template primer.

Note: AMV, avian myeloblastosis virus; DEPC, diethylpyrocarbonate; dNTP, deoxynucleotide triphosphate; MMLV, Moloney murine leukemia virus; PCR, polymerase chain reaction; RT, reverse transcription.

hyde-3-phosphate dehydrogenase, and β_2-microglobulin. This ratio is calculated in both the normal and neoplastic/reactive cell, and then the ratios are compared to see if there is relative up- or downregulation of the gene of interest.

References

1. Bell J. The polymerase chain reaction. Immunol Today 1989;10:351–355.
2. Saiki RK, Scharf S, Faloona F, et al. Enzymatic amplification of beta-globin genomic sequences and restriction site analysis for diagnosis of sickle cell anemia. Science 1985;230:1350–1354.
3. Mullis K, Faloona F, Scharf S, et al. Specific enzymatic amplification of DNA in vitro: the polymerase chain reaction. Cold Spring Harb Symp Quant Biol 1986;51(Pt 1):263–273.
4. Saiki RK, Gelfand DH, Stoffel S, et al. Primer-directed enzymatic amplification of DNA with a thermostable DNA polymerase. Science 1988;239:487–491.
5. Saboor SA, Johnson NM, McFadden J. Detection of mycobacterial DNA in sarcoidosis and tuberculosis with polymerase chain reaction. Lancet 1992;339:1012–1015.
6. Myerson D, Lingenfelter PA, Gleaves CA, et al. Diagnosis of cytomegalovirus pneumonia by the polymerase chain reaction with archived frozen lung tissue and bronchoalveolar lavage fluid. Am J Clin Pathol 1993;100:407–413.
7. Raad I, Hanna H, Huaringa A, et al. Diagnosis of invasive pulmonary aspergillosis using polymerase chain reaction–based detection of aspergillus in BAL. Chest 2002;121:1171–1176.
8. Sundaresan S, Alevy YG, Steward N, et al. Cytokine gene transcripts for tumor necrosis factor-alpha, interleukin-2, and interferon-gamma in human pulmonary allografts. J Heart Lung Transplant 1995;14:512–518.
9. Lordan JL, Bucchieri F, Richter A, et al. Cooperative effects of Th2 cytokines and allergen on normal and asthmatic bronchial epithelial cells. J Immunol 2002;169:407–414.
10. Nogee LM, Dunbar AE 3rd, Wert SE, et al. A mutation in the surfactant protein C gene associated with familial interstitial lung disease. N Engl J Med 2001;344:573–579.
11. Pan Q, Pao W, Ladanyi M. Rapid polymerase chain reaction–based detection of epidermal growth factor receptor gene mutations in lung adenocarcinomas. J Mol Diagn 2005;7:396–403.
12. Westra WH, Baas IO, Hruban RH, et al. K-ras oncogene activation in atypical alveolar hyperplasias of the human lung. Cancer Res 1996;56:2224–2228.
13. Pulte D, Li E, Crawford BK, et al. Sentinel lymph node mapping and molecular staging in nonsmall cell lung carcinoma. Cancer 2005;104:1453–1461.
14. Bohlmeyer T, Le TN, Shroyer AL, et al. Detection of human papillomavirus in squamous cell carcinomas of the lung by polymerase chain reaction. Am J Respir Cell Mol Biol 1998;18:265–269.
15. Bremnes RM, Sirera R, Camps C. Circulating tumour-derived DNA and RNA markers in blood: a tool for early detection, diagnostics, and follow-up? Lung Cancer 2005;49:1–12.
16. Eisenstein BI. The polymerase chain reaction. A new method of using molecular genetics for medical diagnosis. N Engl J Med 1990;322:178–183.
17. Wenham PR. DNA-based techniques in clinical biochemistry: a beginner's guide to theory and practice. Ann Clin Biochem 1992;29 (Pt 6):598–624.
18. Remick DG, Kunkel SL, Holbrook EA, Hanson CA. Theory and applications of the polymerase chain reaction. Am J Clin Pathol 1990;93:S49–S54.
19. Chakrabarti R, Schutt CE. The enhancement of PCR amplification by low molecular-weight sulfones. Gene 2001;274:293–298.
20. Laksanalamai P, Pavlov AR, Slesarev AI, Robb FT. Stabilization of Taq DNA polymerase at high temperature by protein folding pathways from a hyperthermophilic archaeon, Pyrococcus furiosus. Biotechnol Bioeng 2006;93:1–5.
21. Breslauer KJ, Frank R, Blocker H, Marky LA. Predicting DNA duplex stability from the base sequence. Proc Natl Acad Sci USA 1986;83:3746–3750.
22. SantaLucia J Jr, Allawi HT, Seneviratne PA. Improved nearest-neighbor parameters for predicting DNA duplex stability. Biochemistry 1996;35:3555–3562.
23. Wallace RB, Shaffer J, Murphy RF, et al. Hybridization of synthetic oligodeoxyribonucleotides to phi chi 174 DNA: the effect of single base pair mismatch. Nucleic Acids Res 1979;6:3543–3557.
24. Chien A, Edgar DB, Trela JM. Deoxyribonucleic acid polymerase from the extreme thermophile Thermus aquaticus. J Bacteriol 1976;127:1550–1557.
25. Takagi M, Nishioka M, Kakihara H, et al. Characterization of DNA polymerase from Pyrococcus sp. strain KOD1 and its application to PCR. Appl Environ Microbiol 1997;63:4504–4510.
26. Davidson JF, Fox R, Harris DD, et al. Insertion of the T3 DNA polymerase thioredoxin binding domain enhances the processivity and fidelity of Taq DNA polymerase. Nucleic Acids Res 2003;31:4702–4709.
27. Keohavong P, Thilly WG. Fidelity of DNA polymerases in DNA amplification. Proc Natl Acad Sci USA 1989;86:9253–9257.
28. Wilson IG. Inhibition and facilitation of nucleic acid amplification. Appl Environ Microbiol 1997;63:3741–2751.
29. Khan G, Kangro HO, Coates PJ, Heath RB. Inhibitory effects of urine on the polymerase chain reaction for cytomegalovirus DNA. J Clin Pathol 1991;44:360–365.
30. Pavlov AR, Pavlova NV, Kozyavkin SA, Slesarev AI. Recent developments in the optimization of thermostable DNA polymerases for efficient applications. Trends Biotechnol 2004;22:253–260.
31. Longo MC, Berninger MS, Hartley JL. Use of uracil DNA glycosylase to control carry-over contamination in polymerase chain reactions. Gene 1990;93:125–128.
32. Eckert KA, Kunkel TA. High fidelity DNA synthesis by the Thermus aquaticus DNA polymerase. Nucleic Acids Res 1990;18:3739–3744.
33. McPherson MJ, Møller SG. PCR. Oxford, UK: BIOS Scientific Publications; 2000.
34. Southern EM. Detection of specific sequences among DNA fragments separated by gel electrophoresis. J Mol Biol 1975;98:503–517.

35. Bevan IS, Rapley R, Walker MR. Sequencing of PCR-amplified DNA. PCR Methods Appl 1992;1:222–228.

36. Moretti T, Koons B, Budowle B. Enhancement of PCR amplification yield and specificity using AmpliTaq Gold DNA polymerase. Biotechniques 1998;25:716–722.

37. Brandwein M, Zeitlin J, Nuovo GJ, et al. HPV detection using "hot start" polymerase chain reaction in patients with oral cancer: a clinicopathological study of 64 patients. Mod Pathol 1994;7:720–727.

38. Nuovo GJ, Gallery F, MacConnell P. Detection of amplified HPV 6 and 11 DNA in vulvar lesions by hot start PCR in situ hybridization. Mod Pathol 1992;5:444–448.

39. Chou Q, Russell M, Birch DE, et al. Prevention of pre-PCR mis-priming and primer dimerization improves low-copy-number amplifications. Nucleic Acids Res 1992;20:1717–1723.

40. Tilston P, Corbitt G. A single tube nested PCR for the detection of hepatitis C virus RNA. J Virol Methods 1995;53:121–129.

41. Smit VT, Boot AJ, Smits AM, et al. KRAS codon 12 mutations occur very frequently in pancreatic adenocarcinomas. Nucleic Acids Res 1988;16:7773–7782.

42. Herman JG, Graff JR, Myohanen S, et al. Methylation-specific PCR: a novel PCR assay for methylation status of CpG islands. Proc Natl Acad Sci USA 1996;93:9821–9826.

43. Curtis CD, Goggins M. DNA methylation analysis in human cancer. Methods Mol Med 2005;103:123–136.

44. Li LC, Dahiya R. MethPrimer: designing primers for methylation PCRs. Bioinformatics 2002;18:1427–1431.

45. Bird A. The essentials of DNA methylation. Cell 1992;70:5–8.

46. Robertson KD, Jones PA. DNA methylation: past, present and future directions. Carcinogenesis 2000;21:461–467.

47. Rhee I, Bachman KE, Park BH, et al. DNMT1 and DNMT3b cooperate to silence genes in human cancer cells. Nature 2002;416:552–556.

48. Dammann R, Takahashi T, Pfeifer GP. The CpG island of the novel tumor suppressor gene RASSF1A is intensely methylated in primary small cell lung carcinomas. Oncogene 2001;20:3563–3567.

49. Zochbauer-Muller S, Fong KM, Virmani AK, et al. Aberrant promoter methylation of multiple genes in non–small cell lung cancers. Cancer Res 2001;61:249–255.

50. Clark SJ, Harrison J, Paul CL, Frommer M. High sensitivity mapping of methylated cytosines. Nucleic Acids Res 1994;22:2990–2997.

51. Elnifro EM, Ashshi AM, Cooper RJ, Klapper PE. Multiplex PCR: optimization and application in diagnostic virology. Clin Microbiol Rev 2000;13:559–570.

52. Richards B, Skoletsky J, Shuber AP, et al. Multiplex PCR amplification from the CFTR gene using DNA prepared from buccal brushes/swabs. Hum Mol Genet 1993;2:159–163.

53. Scurto P, Hsu Rocha M, Kane JR, et al. A multiplex RT-PCR assay for the detection of chimeric transcripts encoded by the risk-stratifying translocations of pediatric acute lymphoblastic leukemia. Leukemia 1998;12:1994–2005.

54. Pallisgaard N, Hokland P, Riishoj DC, et al. Multiplex reverse transcription–polymerase chain reaction for simultaneous screening of 29 translocations and chromosomal aberrations in acute leukemia. Blood 1998;92:574–588.

55. Newton CR, Graham A, Heptinstall LE, et al. Analysis of any point mutation in DNA. The amplification refractory mutation system (ARMS). Nucleic Acids Res 1989;17:2503–2516.

56. Saiki RK, Bugawan TL, Horn GT, et al. Analysis of enzymatically amplified beta-globin and HLA-DQ alpha DNA with allele-specific oligonucleotide probes. Nature 1986;324:163–166.

57. Schaefer BC. Revolutions in rapid amplification of cDNA ends: new strategies for polymerase chain reaction cloning of full-length cDNA ends. Anal Biochem 1995;227:255–273.

58. Komminoth P, Long AA. In-situ polymerase chain reaction. An overview of methods, applications and limitations of a new molecular technique. Virchows Arch B Cell Pathol Incl Mol Pathol 1993;64:67–73.

59. Livak KJ, Flood SJ, Marmaro J, et al. Oligonucleotides with fluorescent dyes at opposite ends provide a quenched probe system useful for detecting PCR product and nucleic acid hybridization. PCR Methods Appl 1995;4:357–362.

60. Heid CA, Stevens J, Livak KJ, Williams PM. Real time quantitative PCR. Genome Res 1996;6:986–994.

61. Lie YS, Petropoulos CJ. Advances in quantitative PCR technology: 5′ nuclease assays. Curr Opin Biotechnol 1998;9:43–48.

62. Holland PM, Abramson RD, Watson R, Gelfand DH. Detection of specific polymerase chain reaction product by utilizing the 5′–3′ exonuclease activity of *Thermus aquaticus* DNA polymerase. Proc Natl Acad Sci USA 1991;88:7276–7280.

63. Longley MJ, Bennett SE, Mosbaugh DW. Characterization of the 5′ to 3′ exonuclease associated with *Thermus aquaticus* DNA polymerase. Nucleic Acids Res 1990;18:7317–7322.

64. Förster T. Zwischemolekulare energiewanderung und fluoreszenz. Ann Physik 1948;2:55–67.

65. Stryer L, Haugland RP. Energy transfer: a spectroscopic ruler. Proc Natl Acad Sci USA 1967;58:719–726.

66. Grinvald A, Haas E, Steinberg IZ. Evaluation of the distribution of distances between energy donors and acceptors by fluorescence decay. Proc Natl Acad Sci USA 1972;69:2273–2277.

67. Oliver DH, Thompson RE, Griffin CA, Eshleman JR. Use of single nucleotide polymorphisms (SNP) and real-time polymerase chain reaction for bone marrow engraftment analysis. J Mol Diagn 2000;2:202–208.

68. Lay MJ, Wittwer CT. Real-time fluorescence genotyping of factor V Leiden during rapid-cycle PCR. Clin Chem 1997;43:2262–2267.

69. Temin HM, Mizutani S. RNA-dependent DNA polymerase in virions of Rous sarcoma virus. Nature 1970;226:1211–1213.

70. Baltimore D. RNA-dependent DNA polymerase in virions of RNA tumour viruses. Nature 1970;226:1209–1211.

71. Spiegelman S, Burny A, Das MR, et al. Characterization of the products of DNA-directed DNA polymerases in oncogenic RNA viruses. Nature 1970;227:563–567.

72. Shinnick TM, Lerner RA, Sutcliffe JG. Nucleotide sequence of Moloney murine leukaemia virus. Nature 1981;293:543–548.

73. Reddy EP, Smith MJ, Aaronson SA. Complete nucleotide sequence and organization of the Moloney murine sarcoma virus genome. Science 1981;214:445–450.

74. Kotewicz ML, D'Alessio JM, Driftmier KM, et al. Cloning and overexpression of Moloney murine leukemia virus reverse transcriptase in *Escherichia coli*. Gene 1985;35: 249–258.

75. Verma IM, Baltimore D. Purification of the RNA-directed DNA polymerase from avian myeloblastosis virus and its assay with polynucleotide templates. Methods Enzymol 1974;29:125–130.

76. Houts GE, Miyagi M, Ellis C, et al. Reverse transcriptase from avian myeloblastosis virus. J Virol 1979;29:517–522.

77. Verma IM. Studies on reverse transcriptase of RNA tumor viruses III. Properties of purified Moloney murine leukemia virus DNA polymerase and associated RNase H. J Virol 1975;15:843–854.

78. Marcus SL, Modak MJ. Observations on template-specific conditions for DNA synthesis by avian myeloblastosis virus DNA polymerase. Nucleic Acids Res 1976;3: 1473–1486.

79. Sambrook J, Russell DW. Molecular Cloning, A Laboratory Manual, 3rd ed. Cold Spring Harbor, NY: Cold Spring Harbor Laboratory Press; 2001:A4.24.

80. Broackes-Carter FC, Mouchel N, Gill D, et al. Temporal regulation of CFTR expression during ovine lung development: implications for CF gene therapy. Hum Mol Genet 2002;11:125–131.

81. Dagnon K, Pacary E, Commo F, et al. Expression of erythropoietin and erythropoietin receptor in non–small cell lung carcinomas. Clin Cancer Res 2005;11:993–999.

82. Singhal S, Wiewrodt R, Malden LD, et al. Gene expression profiling of malignant mesothelioma. Clin Cancer Res 2003;9:3080–3097.

83. Lam KM, Oldenburg N, Khan MA, et al. Significance of reverse transcription polymerase chain reaction in the detection of human cytomegalovirus gene transcripts in thoracic organ transplant recipients. J Heart Lung Transplant 1998;17:555–565.

10
Array Comparative Genomic Hybridization in Pathology

Reinhard Ullmann

Principle of Comparative Genomic Hybridization

Comparative genomic hybridization (CGH) is a molecular cytogenetic method for the detection and mapping of chromosomal gains and losses.[1] It is based on the cohybridization of differentially labeled test and reference DNAs onto metaphase spreads, which usually have been prepared from peripheral blood lymphocytes of a healthy donor. The signal intensity ratios of the two labels along the chromosomes then reflect DNA copy number changes in the test genome relative to the reference genome. Although CGH has tremendously contributed to our knowledge of chromosomal aberrations, unfortunately its resolution is limited to about 3–10 Mb.[2] Resolution of CGH has significantly improved when samples were not hybridized to metaphase spreads but to DNA targets that have been arrayed on a glass substrate. This modification of the original technique has been named *array CGH*[3] or *matrix CGH*.[4] In theory, resolution of array CGH is only limited by number and quality of DNA targets arrayed on the slide. The principle of array CGH is illustrated in Figure 10.1.

Array Comparative Genomic Hybridization Platforms

Arrays Based on Clone Inserts

cDNA Arrays

The first genome wide application of array CGH was based on cDNA arrays, with each spot representing one reversely transcribed mRNA.[5] Apart from the fact that these arrays were readily available, the main advantage of cDNA arrays was that they facilitated a direct comparison of DNA copy number changes with gene expression data derived from the same tumor.[6,7] However, cDNA arrays are extremely gene focused, and thus only a small percentage of the genome is actually represented. DNA copy number changes concerning promoters, introns, or intergenic sequences are missed. Another problem arises from paralogous genes or shared sequence motifs. Together with the low signal to background ratio usually obtained with this kind of array, these disadvantages have limited the use of cDNAs for the detection of DNA copy number changes.

Large-Insert Clone Arrays

Until now the most widely used array CGH platforms are based on large-insert clones, mainly bacterial artificial chromosome (BAC) and P1 artificial chromosome (PAC) clones and to a lesser extent cosmids (Figure 10.2). The first large-insert clone sets for whole-genome analysis provided a resolution of about 1 Mb.[8,9] Subsequently, a more comprehensive clone set has been assembled,[10,11] and, in 2004, the first submegabase resolution whole-genome tiling path array CGH study was published, which was based on an array comprising 32,433 large-insert clones covering the whole genome in an overlapping fashion[12] (further information can be found at http://bacpac.chori.org/). Because of the overlap of clones, tiling path arrays can provide a theoretical resolution that is below the average insert size of a BAC (150 kb). In a recent study, Garnis et al. used this platform to study DNA copy number changes in 28 non–small cell lung carcinomas.[13] Figure 10.3 shows the array CGH analysis of a squamous cell lung carcinoma using a submegabase resolution whole-genome tiling path with more than 36,000 clones.

Despite its robustness and widespread application, the BAC array has some limitations. The low copy number of BACs and PACs within the propagating bacteria requires special isolation methods that preserve the integrity of the clone insert while at the same time eliminate as much bacterial genomic DNA as possible. Most laboratories

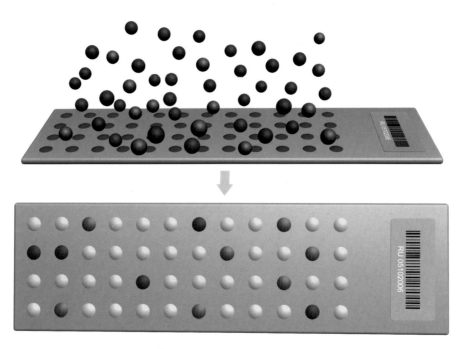

FIGURE 10.1. Principle of array comparative genomic hybridization. Differentially labeled test and reference DNA (green and red spheres, respectively) are cohybridized onto an array of DNA spots printed on a glass slide. In the case of a deletion in the test DNA, fewer test DNA will bind to the corresponding spots and the red label of the reference DNA will prevail. Gains in the test genome can be identified by a dominance of the green label of the test DNA. Spots, representing sequences with the same copy number in the test genome relative to the reference genome, appear yellow. For bacterial artificial chromosome arrays, an excess of repetitive Cot DNA (blue spheres) has to be added in order to suppress otherwise nonspecifically binding repetitive sequences.

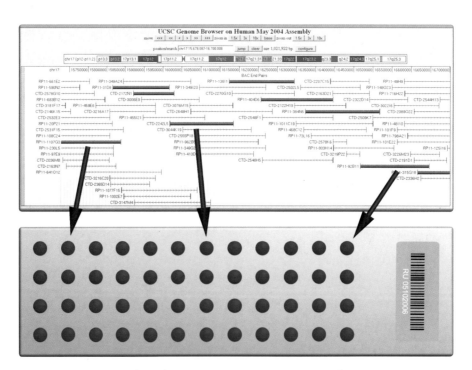

FIGURE 10.2. Bacterial artificial chromosome (BAC) array. Each spot on a BAC array represents the very specific part of the genome that is contained in the BAC. A whole-genome tiling path BAC array comprises as many BAC clones as necessary to cover the whole genome in an overlapping manner (~32,400 for the human genome). The upper part of the image is based on a screenshot of the UCSC Human Genome Browser. The red lines illustrate the selection of overlapping clones out of a comprehensive BAC library.

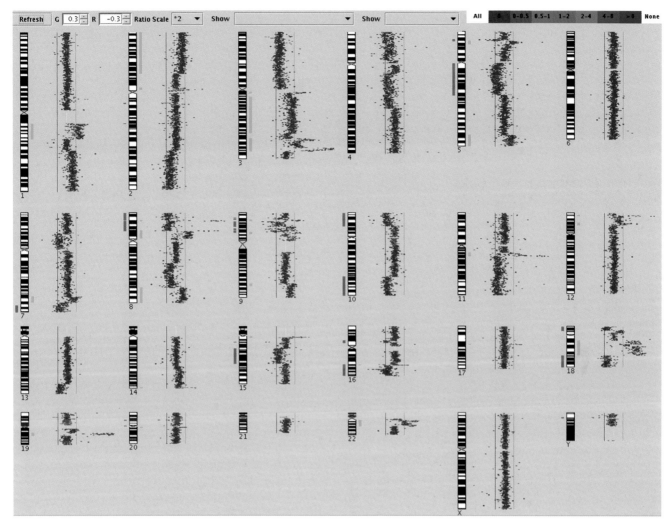

FIGURE 10.3. Array comparative genomic hybridization analysis of a squamous cell lung carcinoma using a submegabase resolution whole-genome tiling path bacterial artificial chromosome array comprising more than 36,000 spots. The Cy3/Cy5 intensity ratios of each clone are plotted in a size-dependent manner along the chromosome ideograms. The red and green lines indicate the log2 ratio thresholds −0.3 (loss) and 0.3 (gain), respectively. Note the very small high-copy amplicons that would have been missed by low-resolution methods.

are not spotting this isolated DNA directly but instead amplify the material to generate a renewable stock of amplicons that can be printed several times (amplification methods are discussed later). A protocol for the high-throughput isolation and amplification of BAC/ PAC clone inserts can be downloaded from our website (http://www.molgen.mpg.de/~abt_rop/molecular_cyto-genetics/Protocols.html). Whatever protocol is followed, the set up of a comprehensive BAC array platform remains time consuming and costly. Other shortcomings of BAC arrays are directly related to specific features of the respective genomic sequence. Otherwise unspecific binding repetitive sequences must be blocked using a considerable excess of (expensive) Cot-DNA. Low-copy repeats (i.e., stretches of DNA, which are longer than 1 kb and have a sequence similarity of more than 90% to other locations in the genome) can lead to ambiguous results. This especially applies to tiling path arrays, because low-resolution arrays usually avoid low-copy repeats. Finally, with the coming of tiling path arrays, BAC arrays have met the limits of resolution, which are simply given by clone insert size.

Repeat-Free and Nonredundant Sequence Arrays

In light of the problems connected to the presence of repetitive sequences in the genome, researches have set out to generate genomic arrays that are depleted for repetitive and redundant sequences. This depletion, for example, has been accomplished by means of selective amplification using sequence-specific primers.

Mantripragada et al. used this approach to create arrays focusing on the DiGeorge region (22q11 deletion syndrome).[14] Another array, based on sequence-specific polymerase chain reaction (PCR) products of 162 exons of five genes, has been generated to test a spectrum of inherited human disorders.[15] However, workload and high costs associated with this approach, as well as the coming of commercial oligonucleotide arrays, have hampered the widespread use of this approach.

Oligonucleotide Arrays Using Presynthesized Oligonucleotides

In contrast to the oligonucleotide platforms described later, arrays using presynthesized oligonucleotides are generated by either printing prefabricated, commercially available sets of oligonucleotides on glass slides or by coupling oligonucleotides to beads, which are assembled on the slide afterward. One example of the use of printed arrays is reported by Carvalho et al., who used a set of 18,861 oligos to identify DNA copy number changes in several tumor cell lines.[16] Presynthesized oligos coupled to beads are used for a platform developed by Illumina (see http://www.illumina.com). The company provides several designs that are dedicated to gene expression, linkage, or DNA copy number analysis. Some of their array designs allow the simultaneous detection of DNA copy number changes and loss of heterozygosity.[17]

Although prefabrication of oligonucleotides enables highly efficient synthesis, at the same time it also reduces flexibility in terms of sequences on the array. Custom design gets considerably expensive and requires a minimal batch size to pay off.

Oligonucleotide Arrays Based on In Situ Synthesis

Meanwhile there are numerous ways to synthesize an oligonucleotide directly on the slide. Despite this diversity, the common principle is shared and is already known from PCR primer synthesis: the growing oligonucleotide is alternatively exposed to As, Gs, Cs, and Ts, but only when the last oligonucleotide of the growing chain is activated by splitting off a protective group can a new nucleotide be attached. The main difference between the platforms comes from how this protective group is inactivated. Some companies use light, selectively distributed through fixed photolithographic masks (www.affymetrix.com) or micromirrors (http://www.nimblegen.com/ or http://www.febit.de). Others deprotect by means of a current-induced change of pH value (http://www.combimatrix.com/) or control synthesis by specifically addressing each spot separately with high-resolution printers (http://www.home.agilent.com). Usually, oligonucleotides on such arrays are designed to be both isothermal (i.e.,

share the same melting temperature) and single-copy sequences. This sometimes results in an uneven distribution of oligonucleotides leading to considerable variability in terms of resolution across the genome. Nevertheless, given the current developments, it can be expected that oligonucleotide arrays will replace all other platforms in the near future. Shortcomings with respect to hybridization kinetics (see later discussion) and coverage will be compensated by the incredible increase in features on the array. Oligonucleotide arrays with more than 500,000 features are readily available. Especially those platforms that are not dependent on fixed photolithographic masks can offer extreme flexibility, which is only limited by the setup fees charged by some companies. Single nucleotide polymorphism arrays, consisting of short oligonucleotides in the range of 16–20 mers and originally dedicated to linkage analysis, have been successfully used for the simultaneous detection of loss of heterozygosity and DNA copy number changes.[18]

General Platform Considerations

Before setting up an array CGH facility, several decisions have to be made. The first one is to determine the expected number of array CGH experiments. In many cases, it will be much cheaper to cooperate with other groups that already have established the technique or to send the samples to a company that provides a hybridization service. The next decision concerns the type of array to be used. Certainly, this decision depends on the scientific problem that will be addressed with the analysis, but often the consequences of this decision are far ranging. Frequently it necessitates the purchase of expensive machines that can be used only with arrays sold by the same company. This is especially true for the most expensive devices necessary for array CGH analysis, namely, the hybridization machine and the scanner.

A hybridization machine is designed to provide controlled temperature and even circulation of the hybridization mix to promote hybridization efficiency (see later discussion). Some of these machines also accomplish the posthybridization washing of slides. Important criteria to consider when choosing a machine are slide formats, handling, maintenance/follow-up costs, and, most important, performance in their own laboratory.

High-quality scanners are essential for the errorless readout of hybridization results. Reliability, flexibility, and resolution, the latter especially in light of the continuing minimization of feature sizes on the array, are important issues. Other arguments can be the availability of auto loaders to support high-throughput analysis or the need for more than two-color channels. Note that there are devices that are scanning from the back of the slide and need transparent substrates.

DNA Preparation and Hybridization

DNA Isolation and Quality

DNA quality has a great influence on the outcome of an array CGH experiment. In general, oligonucleotide platforms, especially when used for one-color experiments, are more sensitive to compromised DNA quality than are BAC arrays. One source of trouble can be the DNA isolation procedure, for example, contaminants that could hamper the subsequent labeling process and introduce noise in the data. Although such problems can be avoided quite easily by improving or changing the isolation protocol, the situation is much more difficult when it comes to retrospective studies using formalin-fixed, paraffin-embedded material. This kind of fixation very frequently results in damage of DNA.[19] To cope with such damage, several adaptations of the DNA isolation and labeling protocols are required. Modifications can include prolonging the tissue digestion time, with addition of fresh proteinase each day, or switching from enzymatic to chemical labeling systems. For other applications, some laboratories have even tried to repair fixation-induced DNA strand breaks by protocols following the principle of nick translation assay or employed sodium thiocyanate to revert DNA–protein cross-linking. Unfortunately, it is not always possible to reliably predict the performance of formalin-fixed, paraffin-embedded DNA in an array CGH experiment, but verifying the average fragment size of the single-stranded DNA by gel electrophoresis and testing DNA performance in PCR reactions with different sized amplicons can give a good estimate.

In light of the increasing impact of molecular (cytogenetic) techniques on research and routine diagnostics, optimization of fixation protocols gains increasing importance. Short-term measures, including correct buffering of formalin regular control of the pH value and reducing fixation time to the minimum necessary to ensure proper histologic evaluation and storage, should be considered. In the long run it may be beneficial to abandon old traditions and switch to alternative fixation protocols.[19] In this context, it is also worth note that many institutes have started to establish tissue banks in which, in addition to usual formalin fixation, tissues are especially preserved for various applications.

Microdissection and DNA Amplification

In many instances, for example, when trying to avoid normal cell contamination in compact growing tumors, it is sufficient to manually scratch out regions of interest from the section using a needle. Unfortunately, this low-budget solution may not be applicable to other problems in pathology. For single cells or small cell clusters interspersed in the tissue (e.g., suspected tumor stem cells, micrometastasis, or preneoplasias), laser microdissection has to be employed.[20] Figure 10.4 demonstrates the microdissection of a bronchiolar columnar cell dysplasia.[21]

The amount of DNA isolated from laser-microdissected samples usually is not sufficient for array CGH analysis. Thus uniform amplification of the whole genome is required to make such samples amenable to array CGH. Fortunately, in the meantime, numerous protocols for whole-genome amplification exist, and many

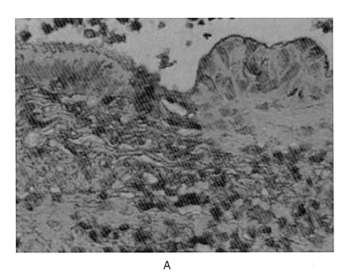
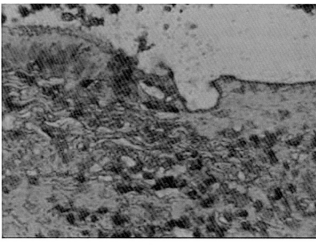

A   B

FIGURE 10.4. Laser microdissection. The selective isolation of bronchiolar columnar cell dysplasia is shown before (A) and after (B) laser microdissection.

companies are providing advanced whole-genome amplification kits. Roughly, whole-genome amplification methods can be divided into PCR-based and non–PCR-based approaches. Probably the best-known PCR-based technique is degenerate oligonucleotide primer–PCR.[22] The name of this technique refers to the specific primer that contains a central cassette of six degenerated bases (at each of these six positions one out of the four bases can be present).

In the first cycles of PCR with very low annealing temperature, this primer promotes the priming of DNA synthesis from multiple evenly dispersed sites within the genome, resulting in amplicons that are flanked by the primer sequence, which then can serve as the annealing site in the subsequent amplification step using high stringency conditions (Figure 10-5A). The initial priming is supposed to occur at approximately 10^6 sites in the human genome,[22] resulting in a genomic representation sufficient for chromosomal CGH. However, with the coming of high-resolution, array-based CGH techniques, many laboratories have shifted to alternative methods that promise better coverage of the genomic complexity. Among the PCR-based methods, this capability is mainly ascribed to ligation-mediated PCR techniques, which have already been successfully used for the analysis of single cells by CGH.[23] The principle of ligation-mediated PCR is based on enzymatic,[23–25] hydrodynamic,[26] or chemical fragmentation (http://www.rubicongenomics.com) of DNA followed by the ligation of an adaptor complex, which serves as a universal priming site for uniform amplification (Figure 10.5B). Certainly, PCR-based approaches imply the risk of amplification bias and experimental errors, and therefore some researchers prefer non–PCR-based approaches, including strand displacement amplification using enzymes such as phi29 DNA polymerase. Hughes et al. provide a more comprehensive review and discussion of the pros and cons of the diverse whole-genome amplification WGA.[27]

Unfortunately, whole-genome amplification usually cannot distinguish DNA that should be amplified from DNA that has been introduced without purpose. There-fore, precautions have to be taken to avoid any contamination with DNAs from other sources. This includes cleaning the carving board before sectioning the resected tumor, regular cleaning or replacement of microtome blades, exchanging water used to stretch paraffin sections, and so forth. Especially when dealing with formalin-fixed, paraffin-embedded material, one has to be aware that nondegraded, contaminating DNA is preferentially amplified. Amplicons generated in previous PCR reactions, distributed through aerosols, are an extremely good template. Therefore, strict compliance to the general rules of PCR setup is mandatory to produce reliable results.

Reference DNA

In a typical array CGH experiment, test DNA is compared with DNA from a healthy donor or with a DNA pool of healthy individuals. Many laboratories hybridize in a sex-matched manner (i.e., test and reference DNA have the same sex), whereas others prefer sex-mismatched hybridizations in which the ratio changes at the sex chromosomes can serve as an internal control of hybridization quality but eventually render the interpretation of DNA copy number changes at the sex chromosomes complicated. Using DNA from the same individual as the test DNA, but isolated from normal-looking tissue far away from the tumor, may be advantageous in terms of hybridization quality, but it contains the risk of missing DNA copy number changes present in both DNAs,[28] for example, constitutional changes that may predispose to tumor formation or chromosomal imbalances also present in the tumor microenvironment.[29]

For chromosomal CGH, it has already been shown that matching the quality of the test and reference DNAs can significantly improve the results of an experiment. Thus it has been realized that combining amplified test DNA with nonamplified reference DNA can introduce hybridization artifacts that can be avoided when a PCR-amplified reference DNA is used.[30] A related observation has been made in our laboratory when working with formalin-fixed, paraffin-embedded DNA, where the use of

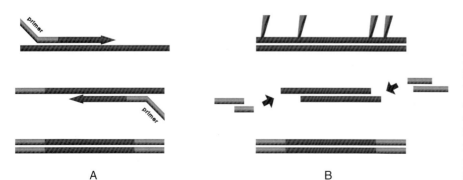

A   B

FIGURE 10.5. Two examples of polymerase chain reaction (PCR)–based whole-genome amplification techniques are shown: **(A)** Degenerate oligonucleotide primer–PCR. **(B)** Linker-mediated PCR. Primer and oligo complexes, respectively, are depicted in gray; template DNA is drawn in black. See text for further discussion.

reference DNA also isolated from formalin-fixed, paraffin-embedded tissue has significantly improved results. In one-color array CGH experiments using short oligonucleotides arrays, the reference DNA is not tested within the same experiment, but data are compared with a reference dataset either generated in the same laboratory by analyzing a cohort of several normal individuals or provided by the array selling company. This in silico comparison can hardly compensate for intraexperimental variation and thus is more prone to noise.

DNA Labeling

Problems in labeling DNA can result in artifacts and failure of the array CGH experiment. Despite a great variety of direct and indirect labeling protocols, at the moment the prevailing method for DNA labeling is direct incorporation of fluorochromes into the DNA by means of a random priming assay, which, as a nice side effect, also results in a net gain of DNA. However, in some instances, for example, when dealing with highly degraded DNA isolated from formalin-fixed, paraffin-embedded tissue, chemical labeling may be superior, because this method does not depend on long DNA fragments and DNA synthesis.[31] As it is true for DNA quality, in our experience it is essential that test and reference DNA do also match in the way they have been labeled so that a possible bias introduced by problems in labeling of specific sequences can be compensated. Commercial arrays frequently require different labeling protocols and the use of specialized kits, usually sold by the same company.

Hybridization

Disadvantageous hybridization kinetics is the greatest problem of array CGH based on oligonucleotide arrays. Even long oligonucleotides represent an extremely low complex target—a diversity of 3 billion bases in the hybridization mix versus ~60 bases represented by each specific spot (Figure 10.6). Circulation of the hybridization mix can only partially compensate for this discrepancy. Representational oligonucleotide microarray analysis (ROMA) is one technical approach to address the problem of complexity.[32] Representational oligonucleotide microarray analysis is based on a linker-mediated PCR (see Figure 10.4B) using the restriction enzyme *Bgl*II. The following PCR is optimized to result in the preferential amplification of fragments smaller than 1.2 kb and thus reduce the complexity down to about 2.5%. Given the known recognition sequence of the restriction enzyme and the maximum spacing between two sites, the authors expected the amplification of about 200,000 sites across the genome and designed a corresponding array specific for the expected sites. It is clear

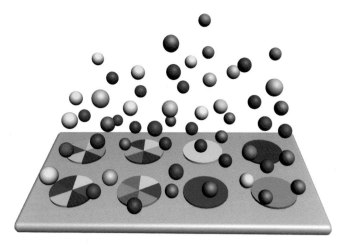

FIGURE 10.6. Comparison of hybridization efficiency of oligonucleotide and BAC arrays. With more than 3 billion different bases, the human genome is very complex (indicated by the differentially colored spheres). Therefore, the relative concentration for a given oligonucleotide that is complementary to the oligonucleotides on the array (shown as four single-color disks) is extremely low. In contrast, an average bacterial artificial chromosome clone represents 150 kb (illustrated by the colored disks). This increases the chance of binding and thus signal intensity.

that this approach is technical and computationally demanding and requires optimal settings and standardization to avoid introducing artifacts.

Data Analysis

A typical array CGH experiment yields several thousand data points that have to be displayed in a comprehensive and illustrative way. Hardly ever are raw data presented in a manuscript. Instead, data have already passed several steps of manipulation. For many readers the computational analysis appears like a "black box," and the brief descriptions of the procedures in many manuscripts are not always able to shed light into this box. However, availability and understanding of information concerning data analysis are essential not only for appreciating the quality of a microarray experiment, the functional (real) resolution of an experiment, and so forth, but also for judging whether or not a comparison of two different studies is feasible. It is beyond the scope of this chapter to provide in depth insights into data analysis; instead, the following is meant as a rough overview that should enable a basic understanding of the data analysis workflow and highlight key points of data interpretation of an array CGH experiment. Chari et al. provide a more comprehensive review of computational aspects of array CGH.[33]

Image Processing

The wet lab part of a typical two-color array CGH experiment ends with putting the hybridized array into the scanner, where the signal intensities of the two different fluorochromes are recorded as two gray scale images either simultaneously or one by one. Usually the scanner output is two 16-bit TIFF images, which provide 2^{16} (65,536) different gray scales. These images are then imported into specialized image processing software, frequently sold as a package together with the laser scanner. There, DNA spots are defined by superimposition of a grid, which reflects the architecture of the array in terms of rows and columns and links each spot with information on clone/sequence identity and chromosomal location.

Background Subtraction

Global background subtraction is based on the averaged signal intensities of all pixels outside those areas that have been identified as DNA spots. This method does not take into account the possible uneven distribution of background signal intensities across the array. Therefore, most people favor local subtraction methods based on background intensity values determined in the vicinity of each spot in order to cope with spatial bias. In our laboratory we do not subtract background at all. At this stage data can be exported to array CGH–specific analysis tools.

Normalization

The absolute signal intensities measured in each channel can be subject to systematic, spatial, or intensity-dependent bias, which can influence array CGH results[34] and has to be removed before calculating the signal intensity ratios. Systematic bias of signal intensities can arise because of differences in input of test and reference DNA, fluorochromes and labeling efficiency, laser settings (laser power as well as amplification through photomultiplier tubes), and so forth. The simplest way to eliminate systematic bias is to normalize by equalizing the median intensities of the two channels.

Unfortunately, calculating the global median intensity does not take into account spatial effects, that is, areas on the array that appear to show trends of higher and lower intensity, respectively. For this reason, many researches apply this normalization method to small subgrids separately. Meanwhile, more sophisticated programs are also available that can detect and remove spatial bias.[35] Sometimes, evaluation of intensity scatterplots reveals an intensity dependent trend, for example, the ratios of low intensity spots show always the same tendency. Normalization algorithms like LOWESS or subgrid LOWESS, which are based on regression models, can be employed to tackle this problem.

Whatever algorithm is applied to normalize the data, it relies on the assumption that for many, if not most, of the data points DNA copy number is the same in test and reference DNA. This may be a problem with tumors with complex aberrations or customized arrays focusing on very small regions of interest. Therefore, for some projects it may be advisable to skip normalization altogether to avoid loss of dynamic range.

Identifying an Aberration

In the beginning of array CGH, most researchers have analyzed and plotted their data using Excel, Access, and/or similar programs, but meanwhile, luckily, more sophisticated tools are available that ease the analysis and visualization of data.[36] Ratios are frequently plotted as log2 values, because this transformation displays deletions and gains within the same scale. If replicas are present on the array, usually the averaged ratios are displayed.

Defining the presence or absence of an aberration is not as trivial at it may appear in the beginning. The simplest way to identify an aberration would be to determine fixed thresholds with every clone that is beyond these thresholds counted as a change of DNA copy number at the respective chromosomal site. Alternatively to the use of fixed thresholds, which do not take into account variable data quality, thresholds can be defined based on standard deviation.

However, given the considerable number of outliers that can occur in one experiment, false-positive results will pose a problem. Smoothing data by means of sliding windows (moving average) has been frequently applied in order to be less sensitive to outliers (Figure 10.7). Although this method dramatically reduces the false-positive rate, it also entails loss of resolution, which depends on the size of the window (i.e., the number of clones/oligos that are averaged).

Examples of more sophisticated algorithms dedicated to the objective determination of DNA copy number changes are Hidden Markow Models (HMM),[37] BioHMM,[38] circular binary segmentation,[39] and wavelet-based approaches.[40]

There are other issues to consider as well when it comes to identifying disease-associated aberrations. Because of the high resolution of array CGH, several DNA copy number variants have been found to occur in the normal population (a comprehensive database can be found at http://projects.tcag.ca/variation/). Although these variants can be several hundred kilobases in size, many of them are supposed to be phenotypically neutral; but they also may predispose to disease.

Especially in tumor cytogenetics, biology introduces another layer of complexity that renders data interpretation difficult. Imagine the following scenario: a tetraploid cell loses one chromosome. In a tetraploid cell with four

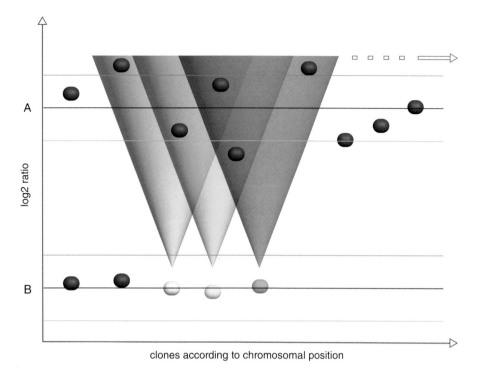

FIGURE 10.7. Data smoothening by sliding window. In this illustration, a sliding window of three clones/oligonucleotides is shown. Instead of the original ratio (row a, upper part of the triangle), the averaged ratio of three adjacent clones/oligonucleotides is plotted (row b, tip of each triangle). The differentially colored triangles symbolize the moving of the windows (red triangle is the latest window). Note that the size of the window determines both the quality of data smoothening and the functional resolution of the array.

copies of each chromosome, this means a relative loss of 25%. There may also be some polyclonality in the tumor specimen, with some cells having this aberration and others not. Some cells may even be euploid, especially those normal cells that are contaminating the tumor sample. In short, DNA copy number changes are not necessarily changing as integers, and it is up to the scientist to determine those thresholds that reflect the best compromise between sensitivity and specificity. This decision can dramatically influence the outcome of an array CGH study and can hamper the comparability of different array CGH studies. In this context it is of great interest that authors of array CGH papers are increasingly following the so-called MIAME criteria, Minimal Information About a Microarray Experiment,[41] which also include the deposition of primary data to a public database such as Gene Expression Omnibus (http://www.ncbi.nlm.nih.gov/geo/) or Array Express (http://www.ebi.ac.uk/arrayexpress/). Every scientist interested in a specific published dataset can download the respective files and perform in silico reanalysis of the datasets with different analysis parameters or a different focus. Meanwhile, a number of array CGH analysis and visualization tools are available for free[36,42] to assist in the exploitation of this valuable data source.

Conclusion

The accumulation of chromosomal imbalances is a typical feature of lung tumors. The specific composition of chromosomal changes creates a unique genomic setting that influences the biologic behavior of the tumor. Currently, array CGH using high-resolution platforms is the most advanced technique to detect DNA copy number changes. Because of the introduction of commercial platforms, the technique is no longer restricted to highly specialized laboratories, and therefore molecular cytogenetics profiling by means of array CGH will gain increasing importance in routine pathology. Array CGH data can be employed to identify chromosomal signatures useful for differential diagnosis and therapeutic decisions. Some aberrations may serve as discriminators in differential diagnosis, especially for tumors, which are hardly distinguishable by classic pathologic approaches, while the finding of other chromosomal changes may be useful to anticipate the risk of metastasis or the likelihood of recurrence. The detection of genes frequently amplified in tumors will help identify new therapy targets, and customized therapy arrays help predict responses to such therapies.

References

1. Kallioniemi A, Kallioniemi OP, Sudar D, et al. Comparative genomic hybridization for molecular cytogenetic analysis of solid tumors. Science 1992;258:818–821.
2. Kirchhoff M, Gerdes T, Maahr J, et al. Deletions below 10 megabasepairs are detected in comparative genomic hybridization by standard reference intervals. Genes Chromosomes Cancer 1999;25:410–413.
3. Pinkel D, Segraves R, Sudar D, et al. High resolution analysis of DNA copy number variation using comparative genomic hybridization to microarrays. Nat Genet 1998;20:207–211.
4. Solinas-Toldo S, Lampel S, Stilgenbauer S, et al. Matrix-based comparative genomic hybridization: biochips to screen for genomic imbalances. Genes Chromosomes Cancer 1997;20:399–407.
5. Pollack JR, Perou CM, Alizadeh AA, et al. Genome-wide analysis of DNA copy-number changes using cDNA microarrays. Nat Genet 1999;23:41–46.
6. Pollack JR, Sorlie T, Perou CM, et al. Microarray analysis reveals a major direct role of DNA copy number alteration in the transcriptional program of human breast tumors. Proc Natl Acad Sci USA 2002;99:12963–12968.
7. Monni O, Barlund M, Mousses S, et al. Comprehensive copy number and gene expression profiling of the 17q23 amplicon in human breast cancer. Proc Natl Acad Sci USA 2001;98:5711–5716.
8. Fiegler H, Carr P, Douglas EJ, et al. DNA microarrays for comparative genomic hybridization based on DOP-PCR amplification of BAC and PAC clones. Genes Chromosomes Cancer 2003;36:361–374.
9. Snijders AM, Nowak N, Segraves R, et al. Assembly of microarrays for genome-wide measurement of DNA copy number. Nat Genet 2001;29:263–264.
10. Krzywinski M, Bosdet I, Smailus D, et al. A set of BAC clones spanning the human genome. Nucleic Acids Res 2004;32:3651–3660.
11. Osoegawa K, Mammoser AG, Wu C, et al. A bacterial artificial chromosome library for sequencing the complete human genome. Genome Res 2001;11:483–496.
12. Ishkanian AS, Malloff CA, Watson SK, et al. A tiling resolution DNA microarray with complete coverage of the human genome. Methods for high throughput validation of amplified fragment pools of BAC DNA for constructing high resolution CGH arrays. Nat Genet 2004;36:299–303.
13. Garnis C, Lockwood WW, Vucic E, et al. High resolution analysis of non–small cell lung cancer cell lines by whole genome tiling path array CGH. Int J Cancer 2006;118:1556–1564.
14. Mantripragada KK, Tapia-Paez I, Blennow E, et al. DNA copy-number analysis of the 22q11 deletion-syndrome region using array-CGH with genomic and PCR-based targets. Int J Mol Med 2004;13:273–279.
15. Dhami P, Coffey AJ, Abbs S, et al. Exon array CGH: detection of copy-number changes at the resolution of individual exons in the human genome. Am J Hum Genet 2005;76:750–762.
16. Carvalho B, Ouwerkerk E, Meijer GA, Ylstra B. High resolution microarray comparative genomic hybridisation analysis using spotted oligonucleotides. J Clin Pathol 2004;57:644–646.
17. Peiffer DA, Le JM, Steemers FJ, et al. High-resolution genomic profiling of chromosomal aberrations using Infinium whole-genome genotyping. Genome Res 2006;16:1136–1148.
18. Bignell GR, Huang J, Greshock J, et al. High-resolution analysis of DNA copy number using oligonucleotide microarrays. Genome Res 2004;14:287–295.
19. Srinivasan M, Sedmak D, Jewell S. Effect of fixatives and tissue processing on the content and integrity of nucleic acids. Am J Pathol 2002;161:1961–1971.
20. Hernandez S, Lloreta J. Manual versus laser microdissection in molecular biology. Ultrastruct Pathol 2006;30:221–228.
21. Ullmann R, Bongiovanni M, Halbwedl I, et al. Bronchiolar columnar cell dysplasia—genetic analysis of a novel preneoplastic lesion of peripheral lung. Virchows Arch 2003;442:429–436.
22. Telenius H, Pelmear AH, Tunnacliffe A, et al. Cytogenetic analysis by chromosome painting using DOP-PCR amplified flow-sorted chromosomes. Genes Chromosomes Cancer 1992;4:257–263.
23. Klein CA, Schmidt-Kittler O, Schardt JA, et al. Comparative genomic hybridization, loss of heterozygosity, and DNA sequence analysis of single cells. Proc Natl Acad Sci USA 1999;96:4494–4499.
24. Ludecke HJ, Senger G, Claussen U, Horsthemke B. Cloning defined regions of the human genome by microdissection of banded chromosomes and enzymatic amplification. Nature 1989;338:348–350.
25. Saunders RD, Glover DM, Ashburner M, et al. PCR amplification of DNA microdissected from a single polytene chromosome band: a comparison with conventional microcloning. Nucleic Acids Res 1989;17:9027–9037.
26. Tanabe C, Aoyagi K, Sakiyama T, et al. Evaluation of a whole-genome amplification method based on adaptor-ligation PCR of randomly sheared genomic DNA. Genes Chromosomes Cancer 2003;38:168–176.
27. Hughes S, Arneson N, Done S, Squire J. The use of whole genome amplification in the study of human disease. Prog Biophys Mol Biol 2005;88:173–189.
28. Petzmann S, Ullmann R, Halbwedl I, Popper HH. Analysis of chromosome-11 aberrations in pulmonary and gastrointestinal carcinoids: an array comparative genomic hybridization-based study. Virchows Arch 2004;445:151–159.
29. Moinfar F, Man YG, Arnould L, et al. Concurrent and independent genetic alterations in the stromal and epithelial cells of mammary carcinoma: implications for tumorigenesis. Cancer Res 2000;60:2562–2566.
30. Huang Q, Schantz SP, Rao PH, et al. Improving degenerate oligonucleotide primed PCR-comparative genomic hybridization for analysis of DNA copy number changes in tumors. Genes Chromosomes Cancer 2000;28:395–403.
31. van Gijlswijk RP, Talman EG, Janssen PJ, et al. Universal Linkage System: versatile nucleic acid labeling technique. Expert Rev Mol Diagn 200;11:81–91.
32. Lucito R, Healy J, Alexander J, et al. Representational oligonucleotide microarray analysis: a high-resolution method

to detect genome copy number variation. Genome Res 2003;13:2291–2305.

33. Chari R, Lockwood WW, Lam WL. Computational methods in array CGH. Cancer Informatics 2006;2:48–58.

34. Khojasteh M, Lam WL, Ward RK, MacAulay C. A stepwise framework for the normalization of array CGH data. BMC Bioinformatics 2005;6:274.

35. Neuvial P, Hupe P, Brito I, et al. Spatial normalization of array-CGH data. BMC Bioinformatics 2006;7:264.

36. Chari R, Lockwood WW, Lam1 WL. Computational methods for the analysis of array comparative genomic hybridization. Cancer Informatics 2006;2:48–58.

37. Fridlyand J, Pinkel D, Albertson DG, et al. Application of Hidden Markov Models to the analysis of the array CGH data. J Multivariate Analysis [Spec Issue] 2004;90:132–153.

38. Marioni JC, Thorne NP, Tavare S. BioHMM: a heterogeneous hidden Markov model for segmenting array CGH data. Bioinformatics 2006;22:1144–1146.

39. Olshen AB, Venkatraman ES, Lucito R, Wigler M. Circular binary segmentation for the analysis of array-based DNA copy number data. Biostatistics 2004;5:557–572.

40. Hsu L, Self SG, Grove D, et al. Denoising array-based comparative genomic hybridization data using wavelets. Biostatistics 2005;6:211–226.

41. Brazma A, Hingamp P, Quackenbush J, et al. Minimum information about a microarray experiment (MIAME)—toward standards for microarray data. Nat Genet 2001;29:365–371.

42. Chen W, Erdogan F, Ropers HH, et al. CGHPRO—a comprehensive data analysis tool for array CGH. BMC Bioinformatics 2005;6:85.

11
Loss of Heterozygosity in Lung Diseases

Sharon C. Presnell

Introduction

Lung cancer remains the leading cause of cancer-related death, accounting for over 1 million deaths per year worldwide.[1-3] Exposure to insult, primarily tobacco smoke, is the indisputable root cause of most lung cancers,[4] but it is the consequential epigenetic and genetic changes (promoter methylation, mutations, deletions, and amplifications) that drive tumor formation, progression, and metastasis. Loss of heterozygosity (LOH) is an extremely common genetic feature of lung cancer and is a significant mechanism by which critical genes involved in growth regulation and homeostasis become inactivated, or silenced, during disease evolution. This chapter reviews LOH and its implications in the major classes of lung cancer as well as in nonmalignant lung diseases.

What Is Loss of Heterozygosity?

Within the entire human genome (3 billion base pairs), only 0.08% of the sites vary within any two humans, and only 0.02% of these variations actually result in a different amino acid being specified as a result of the change.[5] Even more remarkable, 90% of these variations are changes that are common in the population and lead to normal variation in traits among individuals—eye color, for example. In a normal individual's DNA, every genetic locus is composed of two alleles, one inherited from each parent. Most genetic loci are composed of two homozygous alleles, meaning that both copies of the gene are exactly the same such that the loss of one allele leaves another in its place and results in no pathology. A limited number of genetic loci are heterozygous, meaning that the two copies of that gene are different, usually the result of single nucleotide polymorphisms in one copy, making it one nucleotide different from the "wild-type" copy.[5] Most (90%) of this variance is normal within the population, but ~10% of the heterozygous sites in any

individual's DNA are the result of deleterious genetic variations that have the potential to cause disease. Loss or silencing of one allele can occur, usually through mitotic recombination, at any locus, homozygous or heterozygous. Allelic loss of the wild-type allele at a heterozygous site results in "loss of heterozygosity" in a single step, leaving the cell with a single copy of a gene that is aberrant and has the potential to disrupt cellular homeostasis. More commonly, allelic loss occurs at a homozygous site followed by point mutation or gene silencing (via promoter methylation in the remaining allele). The latter is a well-documented mechanism by which tumor suppressor genes are lost during the formation and progression of many types of cancer, including lung cancer.[6,7]

Detecting Loss of Heterozygosity

Methods to detect LOH rely on the ability to assess copy number and determine that one copy is missing or reduced compared with the other copy. Technical methods such as comparative genomic hybridization allow detection of regions of chromosomal gain or loss but generally do not have the resolution to detect LOH at specific loci.[8] Classic methods for detection of LOH involved tedious, low-throughput methods of restriction fragment-length polymorphism analysis and Southern blotting. In the past decade, researchers have taken advantage of simple sequence length polymorphisms (or microsatellites) as genetic markers for studying LOH,[9,10] which has led to more comprehensive PCR-based "allelotyping" studies of LOH in larger sample sets and has enabled studies aimed at identifying clusters or linkages of loci altered by LOH in specific disease states.[9] More recently, the use of single nucleotide polymorphism arrays has facilitated reasonably high-throughput studies aimed at assessing LOH across the genome rather than targeting studies to a defined set of suspected loci.[11] Regardless of the methods used, studies of LOH typically provide several key measurements helpful in understanding the potential role of LOH in the sample set being studied. The areas of the genome that are commonly targeted for allelic loss throughout the sample set are defined as the *minimally deleted regions,* and these hotspots are likely to contain key genes that when altered play a role in the development and/or progression of the cancer. The extent of allelic loss in a given sample is expressed as *fractional allelic loss* and is defined as the number of LOH events in a sample divided by the total number of informative heterozygous markers in the corresponding normal DNA.[12] Breakpoints can also be determined and are defined as the junction between a specific marker displaying LOH and an adjacent marker that retains heterozygosity (LOH:HET).[12]

Conducting LOH analysis requires gaining access to tumor cells. In the case of surgical resection or postmortem analysis of specimens, cells can be obtained directly from lung tissue via macro- or microdissection. Cells have also been harvested successfully from biopsy specimens and bronchial brushings.[13] Caution must be exercised with respect to purity of the cells or tissue obtained, as contaminating stroma, blood vessels, lymphocytes, and other normal cells are inevitably present and can confound results substantially.[11,14] Another caveat of LOH analysis is the phenomenon by which one allele becomes genetically amplified, leading to experimental evidence that the other allele has been deleted when it is intact.[14]

Tobacco Smoke and Loss of Heterozygosity

The evidence linking exposure to tobacco smoke and lung cancer is overwhelming, with smoking named as the greatest etiologic factor contributing to an individual's risk of developing the disease.[3,15–17] The mechanisms by which tobacco carcinogens contribute to the development and progression of lung cancer are multivariate and are only partially understood. Tobacco smoke produces reactive chemical species, including benzo(a)pyrenes and polycyclic aromatic hydrocarbons, that can form physical complexes at sites within the DNA.[18] These so-called "DNA adducts" have been associated with *p53* mutations as well as LOH events at fragile sites on chromosome 3, both of which occur at the very early stages of tobacco-induced carcinogenesis.[18,19] The linkage between tobacco carcinogen exposure and LOH on chromosome 3p is particularly strong in individuals who initiated smoking at an early age.[16,18]

In two studies, LOH at a locus near the *hMLH1* gene on chromosome 3p21 was correlated strongly with early age of smoking initiation, level of hydrophobic DNA adducts, and level of polycyclic aromatic hydrocarbon–

DNA adducts.[17,20] When adolescents smoke, it is believed that normal lung epithelium is "preconditioned" by exposure to tobacco carcinogens at a time of critical lung development, resulting in somatic mutations in an entire "field" of epithelium rather than in a single cell or cluster of cells.[16] These genetically altered cells are replicated during normal adolescent lung growth, leading to the presence of a large number of cells that are "primed" for subsequent events (such as allelic loss), thus rendering the individual highly susceptible to the development of lung cancer. Smoking during adolescence may increase the risk that if lung cancer develops it will develop as many clonal cancers that progress concomitantly and aggressively, a concept first described as "field cancerization."[16,21]

Other Factors Influencing Loss of Heterozygosity

Asbestos

Asbestos is an important pulmonary carcinogen, linked in particular to the formation of mesotheliomas—lung tumors that usually develop in individuals with a history of asbestos exposure, typically with a long period of latency between exposure and clinical presentation.[22] Studies have linked exposure to asbestos to allelic deletion of the *FHIT* gene on chromosome 3p14 and a significant reduction in Fhit protein expression,[23] although the specific mechanisms by which asbestos contributes to LOH are not known. Mutagenicity studies carried out using a lymphocyte model demonstrated that the LOH rate upon exposure to asbestos fibers was greater than the spontaneous LOH rate of the assay,[24] suggesting a direct connection between the fibers and LOH. A recent study of asbestos-exposed individuals in Turkey found LOH on regions of chromosome 6q in >50% of the cases analyzed.[25]

Pathogens

Inflammation associated with chronic infection can be a contributing risk factor for carcinogenesis. One well-known example is infection of the gastric wall with *Helicobacter pylori* as a predisposing factor for gastric cancer.[26] Similarly, lung cancer has been linked with chronic *Chlamydia pneumoniae* infections as well as *Mycobacterium tuberculosis* (M-TB) infections[27,28] Infection with M-TB is, like asbestos, associated with LOH in the *FHIT* gene on chromosome 3p14.[27,28] Studies indicate that the mechanism of DNA damage in relation to infections is indirect and comes from the host's activated inflammatory cells sent to fight the infection. Cumulative evidence suggests that free radicals, such as nitric oxide, produced by activated inflammatory cells can contribute to cancer, as they are known to be able to cause direct damage to DNA.[29]

Patterns of Loss of Heterozygosity in Lung Cancer

Lung cancers are divided into two major categories: small cell lung cancers (SCLCs) and non–small cell lung cancers (NSCLCs), the latter of which can be further classified based on the cell type(s) of which they are comprised. The two most common classifications of NSCLC are adenocarcinomas and squamous cell carcinomas, but mesotheliomas, large cell carcinomas, and adenosquamous varieties exist as well. The SCLCs account for around 20%–25% of all cases of lung cancer and carries with it a relatively poor prognosis.[30] The remaining 75%–80% of diagnosed lung cancers are NSCLCs, with adenocarcinomas and squamous cell carcinomas equally prevalent and jointly representing ~80% of all NSCLCs.[30]

While all types of lung cancer share pathologic and genetic features, there are some clear type-specific differences with regard to incidence and pattern of LOH. Table 11.1 summarizes the chromosomal regions most frequently targeted for LOH in lung cancer, including their relative frequencies in SCLC and NSCLC and the tumor suppressor genes (if known) that are targeted by LOH events. Association of each LOH-targeted area with insult (tobacco smoke, asbestos, and pathogens) is also reported in Table 11.1. Allelic losses occur most fre-

quently, in both SCLC (~90%) and NSCLC (~70%), on chromosomes 3p, 13q, and 17p—likely representing the inactivation of key tumor suppressor genes, which include fragile histidine triad (*FHIT*), *p53*, and Retinoblastoma (*RB*).[9,31,32] In SCLC, LOH occurs at a relatively high frequency on chromosomes 3p (>90%), 5q (>50%), 4q (>40%), 10q (>80%), 13q (>90%), 15q (>40%), and 17p (>90%),[13] and concordance between some of these sites has been suggested by cluster analysis.[9] The pattern of LOH is distinct in NCSLC and frequently involves the targeting of genes on chromosomes 1p (>60%), 3p (>50%), 8p (>70%), 9p (>70%), 13q (>60%), 17p (>80%), 19p (>70%), Xp (>60%), and Xq (>60%).[9,32,33] In general, more alterations are detected in NSCLCs than in SCLCs, but this may be due to variability incurred when histologically and pathologically distinct tumors (adenocarcinomas, squamous cell carcinomas, and so forth) are grouped together as "NSCLC" and treated as a single sample set, as is common in many studies. When adenocarcinomas and squamous cell carcinomas are considered as separate sample sets, it is clear that LOH is a more common feature of squamous cell carcinomas, with >90% of them exhibiting LOH (compared with ~70% of adenocarcinomas) as well as a greater number of LOH events per sample.[33] Furthermore, the occurrence and degree of LOH in adenocarcinomas is correlated positively with exposure to tobacco smoke.[34,35] Patterns of allelic loss have been identified in studies of tobacco smoke–exposed bronchial epithelial cells and NSCLCs, leading to the hypothesis that LOHs at 8p, 9p, 11q, and 13q are early lesions that occur upon exposure to tobacco smoke.[34,35] Transition to the cancerous stage is associated temporally

TABLE 11.1. Major loss of heterozygosity (LOS)–targeted regions in small cell lung cancer (SCLC) and non–small cell lung cancer (NSCLC).

Chromosome	Candidate target gene(s)	SCLC	NSCLC	Smoking	Asbestos	Pathogens
				Insult		
1p	*p73, TNFR2*	>40%	>60%	X		
3p	***FHIT***, *MLH1, VHL, TGFBR2, DLC1, RASSF1A, BAP1, RARβ*	>90%	>50%	X	X	X
4q		>40%	>40%			
5q	*SPARC, MCC, APC, IRF1*	>50%	>70%	X		
8p		>50%	>70%	X		
9p	***p16***^{INK4A}, *p15*^{INK4B}, *p*^{14ARF}	>30%	>70%	X		
10q	*PTEN/MMAC1*	>80%	>30%			
13q	***RB1***, *BRCA2*	>90%	>60%	X		
15q		>40%	>40%			
17p	***TP53***	>90%	>80%	X	X	
19p		NR	>70%			
Xp		NR	>60%			
Xq		NR	>60%			

Note: Candidate LOH-targeted genes are listed. Well-characterized and defined tumor suppressor genes associated with lung cancer are in bold-face. Relative frequencies of detection (compiled from studies cited in this chapter) are shown for both SCLC and NSCLC. Regions associated with LOH-targeting in response to exposure to smoking, asbestos, or pathogens are marked (X). NR, not reported.

with LOH at 1p, followed by additional LOH events at 3p and 17p in the progression of squamous cell carcinomas or at 5q and 18q in the progression of adenocarcinomas.[33-35]

Broader "genome-wide" allelotyping studies that employ higher throughput methods for detecting LOH (see earlier discussion) have enabled the detection of novel "hotspots" for allelic loss, making these areas of the genome likely to contain tumor suppressor genes that have yet to be described. Many laboratories are focused on mapping and identifying candidate tumor suppressor genes in these areas of the genome. To date, there is not strong experimental evidence suggesting that specific patterns of LOH in lung cancer have prognostic value by correlating with clinical parameters such as disease stage, tumor size, mitotic rate, degree of angiogenesis, or tumor recurrence.[10,36,37] However, the mechanistic role(s) of some specific genes lost via LOH have been studied, and a summary of each major LOH target is provided below.

Loss of Heterozygosity at 1p

Loss of heterozygosity at 1p36 occurs in SCLC (~40%) but is more common in NSCLC (>60%) and encompasses several candidate tumor suppressor genes, including *p73* and tumor necrosis factor receptor 2 (*TNFR2*).[9,38-40] Additional targets of LOH have been identified in NSCLC samples at 1p21 and 1p22, although no tumor suppressor gene candidates have been described in these regions. *p73* is a member of the *p53* family and is capable of mimicking some of the effector functions of *p53*, including induction of permanent growth arrest and promotion of apoptosis.[41] *TNFR2* binds and mediates signals from lymphotoxin-α, lymphotoxin-β, and tumor necrosis factor, three cytokines associated with receptor-mediated induction of cell death.[42]

Loss of Heterozygosity at 3p

The best-described and best-documented gene targeted for LOH in nearly all lung cancers is *FHIT* on 3p14. Loss of heterozygosity at 3p14 is strongly correlated with exposure to tobacco smoke and occurs early in carcinogen-exposed lung epithelium.[14,43-48] The *FHIT* gene encodes a small protein with diadenosine triphosphate hydrolase activity, but its tumor suppressor activity is presumed to be independent from this enzymatic activity.[47] FRA3B, the most fragile site in the human genome, maps to the *FHIT* gene region and is believed to play a role in cancer susceptibility.[49] Evidence for *FHIT* as a tumor suppressor gene includes the observations that *FHIT*-deficient mice are more susceptible to carcinogen-induced tumor formation[49] and that expression of *FHIT* suppresses the growth of cancer cells through promotion of apoptosis and growth inhibition.[50] Although the *FHIT* gene is considered a candidate tumor suppressor gene, some studies have failed to support this hypothesis[51,52] such that the precise mechanisms by which *FHIT* contributes to lung cancer development remain undetermined.

Additional regions of 3p are targeted for LOH in both SCLC and NSCLC, as extensively reviewed in several publications.[9,14,43,44,53,54] Tumor suppressor gene candidates targeted by LOH in the same region (3p12-3p22) as the *FHIT* gene include transforming growth factor receptor-β2 (*TGFRβ2*), *MLH/HNPCC2*, deleted in lung Cancer-1 (*DLC1*), *RASSF1A*, retinoic acid receptor-β (*RARβ*), and *BRCA1*-associated protein 1 (*BAP1*).[9,14,43,44,53,54] Loss of heterozygosity at 3p25, which includes the von Hippel-Lindau (*VHL*) locus, has also been reported as a frequent event in both SCLC and NSCLC.[14,55]

Loss of Heterozygosity at 4q

Two regions on chromosome 4q (4q21-28 and 4q34-ter) are frequently targeted by LOH in both SCLC and NSCLC.[9,11,32,34,35] Despite consistent observations of LOH in these areas, to date clear tumor suppressor gene candidates have not been identified.

Loss of Heterozygosity at 5q

Small cell carcinoma is characterized by a high frequency of LOH at 5q32-ter, and, although no candidate tumor suppressor genes have been identified, the *SPARC* (secreted protein acidic and rich in cysteine) gene maps to 5q32 and has been associated with LOH in idiopathic pulmonary fibrosis.[56] The SPARC protein, which is involved in the regulation of cell adhesion and growth, is methylated aberrantly in lung cancers.[57] Although NSCLC has not been associated with LOH at 5q32, there is often LOH at 5q21.3-31, a region that contains several key tumor suppressor genes, including *MCC* (mutated in colorectal cancer), *APC* (adenomatous polyposis coli), and *IRF*.[9]

Loss of heterozygosity at 5q21 has been documented in preneoplastic cells, suggesting that it may be an early genetic change, and it is more prevalent in squamous cell carcinomas than in adenocarcinomas.[33,58] However, as for other LOH events, studies have failed to provide a strong correlation between these events and patient prognosis. In lung cancer, it appears that LOH at the *APC* locus is relatively frequent but that the mechanism by which the remaining allele is silenced is usually promoter methylation rather than mutation.[59]

Loss of Heterozygosity at 8p

Loss of heterozygosity on chromosome 8p21-23 is a frequent and early occurrence in NSCLC, believed to occur after LOH events at 3p and 9p.[60,61] Despite consistent observations of LOH in this region in lung cancer, specific tumor suppressor genes have not been mapped to 8p21–23 and implicated in the development and progression of lung cancer. LOH at 8p21–23 is also a frequent event in hepatocellular carcinoma, and a gene encoding a growth-inhibitory protein, *HCRP1* (hepatocellular carcinoma related protein-1), has been mapped to that area and implicated in hepatocellular carcinoma.[62] Additional work will be needed to define the tumor suppressor genes, perhaps including *HCRP1*, involved in lung cancer.

Loss of Heterozygosity at 9p

Chromosome 9p is frequently altered in NSCLC not only by LOH but also by homozygous deletion and gene silencing via promoter hypermethylation.[9,10,63] The redundancy in mechanisms aimed at silencing genes in this region and the prevalence of these alterations in smoke-exposed preneoplastic epithelium point to the importance of 9p in the development of lung cancer. The gene most frequently identified in LOH studies of 9p (9p21) in NSCLC is *p16^{INK4A}*, a gene that encodes a cell cycle protein that inhibits Cdk4, Cdk6, and cyclin-dependent phosphorylation of the *Rb* gene product.[64–66] Loss of the *p16^{INK4A}* gene effectively removes key negative regulation of the cell cycle at the G1 → S phase transition.[67] Interestingly, experimental evidence suggests that the silencing of the remaining p16^{INK4A} allele after allelic loss is predominantly due to epigenetic methylation rather than mutation.[68]

Loss of Heterozygosity at 10q

Loss of heterozygosity at 10q22–23 is a frequent observation in SCLC. Although no tumor suppressor genes in this region have been definitively associated with lung cancer, multiple studies have identified LOH targeted to the *PTEN/MMAC* locus at 10q23.[69–71] The encoded PTEN protein is a lipid phosphatase that negatively regulates the phosphatidylinositol 3-kinase/Akt pathway. Loss of *PTEN* function results in reduced apoptosis and stimulation of cellular proliferation and migration.[69]

Loss of Heterozygosity at 13q

Chromosome 13q12–14 is a prevalent hotspot for LOH in both SCLC and NSCLC. The retinoblastoma (*RB1*) gene is a well-characterized tumor suppressor gene at 13q12, the product of which is a key regulator of entry into S phase of the cell cycle.[72] The critical pathway regulated by *RB*, *p16^{INK4A}*, cyclin D1, and cyclin-dependent kinases (Cdks) is disturbed, usually via multiple components, in nearly every case of lung cancer, thus rendering cells insensitive to the signaling involved in regulating mitosis.[72] Loss of heterozygosity on 13q12.1–13.1 can be

identified in cells obtained from bronchial washing specimens from SCLC and NSCLC patients and is proposed as one of a set of markers that could be used for early detection of lung cancer.[73] Another gene targeted to 13q12–14 is *BRCA2*, a gene associated with cancer susceptibility and with possible linkages to *p53* in the context of DNA damage repair.[74]

Loss of Heterozygosity at 15q

Broader studies of LOH have consistently identified LOH at 15q as a common occurrence in SCLC.[9,75–77] Several microsatellite markers targeted to the long arm of chromosome 15 demonstrate LOH in these studies, but the region between D15S1012 and D15S1016 was the most frequently altered.[75] As for chromosomes 1, 4, and 8, much work is needed to identify the LOH-targeted tumor suppressor genes on chromosome 15q.

Loss of Heterozygosity at 17p

The *TP53* gene at 17p13 is the most frequently altered tumor suppressor gene in human cancers, including lung cancers. *TP53* is targeted by mutation, methylation, and homozygous deletion, in addition to LOH. The redundancy by which *TP53* is inactivated in lung cancer and the prevalence of its inactivation point to its critical role in the development of the disease. *TP53* modulates a broad network of cellular responses, including cell cycle arrest, apoptosis, DNA repair, cellular senescence, and inflammation, and therefore plays a central role in homeostasis.[78] *TP53* mutations can be found in precancerous lesions, but to date studies of LOH at 17p indicate that allelic loss of *TP53* occurs during disease progression, after LOH events on chromosome 3p.[34]

Loss of Heterozygosity at 19p

Loss of heterozygosity at 19p13.3 is a very frequent event in NSCLC but is not targeted in SCLC.[9] One tumor suppressor gene candidate residing at this locus is *STK11/LKB1*, a gene implicated in Peutz-Jeghers syndrome.[79,80] Loss of heterozygosity at this locus has been documented in breast cancer and in brain metastases from a variety of human cancers.[79,81] Although mutations and LOH of *STK11/LKB1* have been reported in isolated cases of lung cancer, additional work is needed to define the role of this gene in lung carcinogenesis.

Loss of Heterozygosity on the X Chromosome

The X chromosome is targeted for LOH at Xp–q21 and Xq22.1 in NSCLC.[9] Specific tumor suppressor genes have not been mapped to these regions or implicated in lung cancer.

Loss of Heterozygosity in Benign Lung Diseases

There is evidence to suggest that many common lung diseases, such as chronic obstructive pulmonary disease (COPD) and asthma, have a genetic predisposition and probably arise via the interaction between multiple gene products.[82] Studies of microsatellite instability and LOH have been employed to study these diseases with the goals of identifying causative genes and/or developing genetic screening tools for use in epidemiology. Loss of heterozygosity in several prevalent lung diseases is discussed.

Idiopathic Pulmonary Fibrosis

Idiopathic pulmonary fibrosis is a serious disease believed to be the result of immune response to tissue damage in the lung.[83] Although idiopathic pulmonary fibrosis is a benign disease, it progresses to bronchogenic carcinoma in ~10% of idiopathic pulmonary fibrosis patients.[82] The observation that the incidence of lung cancer in idiopathic pulmonary fibrosis patients is much higher than the incidence in the general population lends support to the hypothesis that idiopathic pulmonary fibrosis contains precancerous lesions that may progress to peripheral-type lung tumors through the inactivation of critical tumor suppressor genes.[84] Indeed, LOH at several common loci (3p21, 5q32, 9p21, and 17p13) has been documented in idiopathic pulmonary fibrosis.[56]

Sarcoidosis

Sarcoidosis is a multisystem disease characterized by the formation of noncaseating granulomatous lesions in affected organs, especially the lungs. These lesions can progress to cause fibrosis and, like idiopathic pulmonary fibrosis, lead to a higher incidence of lung cancer.[82] Studies of LOH have identified targeted loci on 9p, 9q, and 17q.[85,86] The genes targeted by LOH were within or proximal to DNA mismatch repair genes and genes associated with lymphocyte activation. This pattern is somewhat distinct from lung cancer or idiopathic pulmonary fibrosis and may reflect the absence of linkage with exposure to tobacco smoke.[86]

Chronic Obstructive Pulmonary Disease and Asthma

Loss of heterozygosity has been detected in COPD and asthma, although the number of studies is limited and have focused on analysis of chromosomal regions that contain genes suspected in the diseases.[82] There are genes implicated in the development and progression of asthma throughout the genome, although the hotspot for altera-

tions via LOH is chromosome 14q, which contains several target genes that have been implicated in asthma, including prostaglandin E receptor 2 (PTGER2), arginase II (ARG2), and α_1-antichymotrypsin precursor (AACT).[87-88] Within asthmatic patients, those with the greater number of genetic alterations have higher mean immunoglobulin E and blood eosinophils,[89] both of which are indicators of inflammation and bronchial hyperresponsiveness. Analyses of COPD samples demonstrate that LOH occurs most frequently at the thyroid hormone receptor-$\alpha 1$ (THRA1) locus on chromosome 17q21.[90] It is believed that exposure to tobacco smoke is a risk factor for the genetic changes associated with COPD, and individuals with COPD (like those with idiopathic pulmonary fibrosis) carry a greater risk for the development of lung cancer.[91]

Conclusion

Clearly, LOH is a well-documented occurrence in benign, premalignant, and malignant lung diseases. Although some genes targeted by LOH represent key early events in pathogenesis, many occur at later stages of disease progression, thus making their specific contributions difficult to discern. Continued comprehensive genome-wide studies of LOH in lung diseases, in large sample sets, may ultimately provide the researcher and clinician with tools for diagnosis and prognosis based on patterns of LOH.

References

1. Coleman MP, Gatta G, Verdecchia A, et al. EUROCARE-3 summary: cancer survival in Europe at the end of the 20th century. Ann Oncol 2003;14(Suppl 5):v128–v149.
2. Edwards BK, Brown ML, Wingo PA, et al. Annual report to the nation on the status of cancer, 1975–2002, featuring population-based trends in cancer treatment. J Natl Cancer Inst 2005;97(19):1407–1427.
3. Knoke JD, Shanks TG, Vaughn JW, Thun MJ, Burns DM. Lung cancer mortality is related to age in addition to duration and intensity of cigarette smoking: an analysis of CPS-I data. Cancer Epidemiol Biomarkers Prev 2004;13(6):949–957.
4. Jemal A, Murray T, Ward E, et al. Cancer statistics, 2005. CA Cancer J Clin 2005;55(1):10–30.
5. Cecil RL, Goldman L, Ausiello DA. Cecil Textbook of Medicine. 23rd ed. Philadelphia: Saunders Elsevier; 2007.
6. Fong KM, Sekido Y, Minna JD. Molecular pathogenesis of lung cancer. J Thorac Cardiovasc Surg 1999;118(6):1136–1152.
7. Sekido Y, Fong KM, Minna JD. Progress in understanding the molecular pathogenesis of human lung cancer. Biochim Biophys Acta 1998;1378(1):F21–F59.
8. Pinkel D, Segraves R, Sudar D, et al. High resolution analysis of DNA copy number variation using comparative genomic hybridization to microarrays. Nat Genet 1998; 20(2):207–211.

9. Girard L, Zochbauer-Muller S, Virmani AK, Gazdar AF, Minna JD. Genome-wide allelotyping of lung cancer identifies new regions of allelic loss, differences between small cell lung cancer and non–small cell lung cancer, and loci clustering. Cancer Res 2000;60(17):4894–4906.

10. Virmani AK, Fong KM, Kodagoda D, et al. Allelotyping demonstrates common and distinct patterns of chromosomal loss in human lung cancer types. Genes Chromosomes Cancer 1998;21(4):308–319.

11. Lindblad-Toh K, Tanenbaum DM, Daly MJ, et al. Loss-of-heterozygosity analysis of small-cell lung carcinomas using single-nucleotide polymorphism arrays. Nat Biotechnol 2000;18(9):1001–1005.

12. Vogelstein B, Fearon ER, Kern SE, et al. Allelotype of colorectal carcinomas. Science 1989;244(4901):207–211.

13. Powell CA, Klares S, O'Connor G, Brody JS. Loss of heterozygosity in epithelial cells obtained by bronchial brushing: clinical utility in lung cancer. Clin Cancer Res 1999;5(8): 2025–2034.

14. Zabarovsky ER, Lerman MI, Minna JD. Tumor suppressor genes on chromosome 3p involved in the pathogenesis of lung and other cancers. Oncogene 2002;21(45):6915–6935.

15. Halpern MT, Gillespie BW, Warner KE. Patterns of absolute risk of lung cancer mortality in former smokers. J Natl Cancer Inst 1993;85(6):457–464.

16. Wiencke JK, Kelsey KT. Teen smoking, field cancerization, and a "critical period" hypothesis for lung cancer susceptibility. Environ Health Perspect 2002;110(6):555–558.

17. Hirao T, Nelson HH, Ashok TD, et al. Tobacco smoke–induced DNA damage and an early age of smoking initiation induce chromosome loss at 3p21 in lung cancer. Cancer Res 2001;61(2):612–615.

18. Wiencke JK. DNA adduct burden and tobacco carcinogenesis. Oncogene 2002;21(48):7376–7391.

19. Wiencke JK, Nelson HH, Wain JC, Mark EJ, Christiani DC, Kelsey KT. Association of increased PAH-DNA adducts and p53 mutations in lung cancer. Proc Natl Acad Sci USA 1998;39:562.

20. Zienolddiny S, Ryberg D, Arab MO, Skaug V, Haugen A. Loss of heterozygosity is related to p53 mutations and smoking in lung cancer. Br J Cancer 2001;84(2):226–231.

21. Slaughter DP, Southwick HW, Smejkal W. Field cancerization in oral stratified squamous epithelium ;clinical implications of multicentric origin. Cancer 1953;6(5):963–968.

22. Craighead J, Mossman B. The pathogenesis of asbestos-associated diseases. N Engl J Med 1982;306:1446–1455.

23. Pylkkanen L, Wolff H, Stjernvall T, et al. Reduced Fhit protein expression and loss of heterozygosity at FHIT gene in tumours from smoking and asbestos-exposed lung cancer patients. Int J Oncol 2002;20(2):285–290.

24. Both K, Henderson DW, Tumer DR. Asbestos and erionite fibres can induce mutations in human lymphocytes that result in loss of heterozygosity. Int J Cancer 1994;59(4): 538–542.

25. Tug E, Tug T, Elyas H, et al. Tumor suppressor gene alterations in patients with malignant mesothelioma due to environmental asbestos exposure in Turkey. J Carcinog 2006;5:23–25.

26. Wu MS, Shun CT, Wang HP, et al. Genetic alterations in gastric cancer: relation to histological subtypes, tumor stage, and *Helicobacter pylori* infection. Gastroenterology 1997; 112(5):1457–1465.

27. Song L, Yan W, Deng M, Song S, Zhang J, Zhao T. Aberrations in the fragile histidine triad (FHIT) gene may be involved in lung carcinogenesis in patients with chronic pulmonary tuberculosis. Tumour Biol 2004;25(5–6):270–275.

28. Song L, Yan W, Zhao T, et al. *Mycobacterium tuberculosis* infection and FHIT gene alterations in lung cancer. Cancer Lett 2005;219(2):155–162.

29. Brenner C, Bieganowski P, Pace HC, Huebner K. The histidine triad superfamily of nucleotide-binding proteins. J Cell Physiol 1999;181(2):179–187.

30. Minna JD, ed. Neoplasms of the Lung. New York: McGraw-Hill; 1994.

31. Shiseki MT, Kohno J, Adachi J, et al. Comparative allelotype of early and advanced stage non–small cell lung carcinomas. Genes Chromosomes Cancer 1996;17:71–77.

32. Tseng RC, Chang JW, Hsien FJ, et al. Genomewide loss of heterozygosity and its clinical associations in non small cell lung cancer. Int J Cancer 2005;117(2):241–247.

33. Yoshino I, Osoegawa A, Yohena T, et al. Loss of heterozygosity (LOH) in non–small cell lung cancer: difference between adenocarcinoma and squamous cell carcinoma. Respir Med 2005;99(3):308–312.

34. Pan H, Califano J, Ponte JF, et al. Loss of heterozygosity patterns provide fingerprints for genetic heterogeneity in multistep cancer progression of tobacco smoke–induced non–small cell lung cancer. Cancer Res 2005;65(5):1664–1669.

35. Powell CA, Bueno R, Borczuk AC, et al. Patterns of allelic loss differ in lung adenocarcinomas of smokers and non-smokers. Lung Cancer 2003;39(1):23–29.

36. Baksh FK, Dacic S, Finkelstein SD, et al. Widespread molecular alterations present in stage I non–small cell lung carcinoma fail to predict tumor recurrence. Mod Pathol 2003;16(1):28–34.

37. Zhou X, Kemp BL, Khuri FR, et al. Prognostic implication of microsatellite alteration profiles in early-stage non–small cell lung cancer. Clin Cancer Res 2000;6(2):559–565.

38. Dacic S, Ionescu DN, Finkelstein S, Yousem SA. Patterns of allelic loss of synchronous adenocarcinomas of the lung. Am J Surg Pathol 2005;29(7):897–902.

39. Sasatomi E, Johnson LR, Aldeeb DN, et al. Genetic profile of cumulative mutational damage associated with early pulmonary adenocarcinoma: bronchioloalveolar carcinoma vs. stage I invasive adenocarcinoma. Am J Surg Pathol 2004; 28(10):1280–1288.

40. Ragnarsson G, Eiriksdottir G, Johannsdottir JT, Jonasson JG, Egilsson V, Ingvarsson S. Loss of heterozygosity at chromosome 1p in different solid human tumours: association with survival. Br J Cancer 1999;79(9–10):1468–1474.

41. Fang L, Lee SW, Aaronson SA. Comparative analysis of p73 and p53 regulation and effector functions. J Cell Biol 1999;147(4):823–830.

42. Gupta S. Molecular steps of tumor necrosis factor receptor–mediated apoptosis. Curr Mol Med 2001;1(3):317–324.

43. Wistuba, II, Behrens C, Virmani AK, et al. High resolution chromosome 3p allelotyping of human lung cancer and preneoplastic/preinvasive bronchial epithelium reveals multiple, discontinuous sites of 3p allele loss and three

regions of frequent breakpoints. Cancer Res 2000;60(7): 1949–1960.

44. Yokota J, Wada M, Shimosato Y, Terada M, Sugimura T. Loss of heterozygosity on chromosomes 3, 13, and 17 in small-cell carcinoma and on chromosome 3 in adenocarcinoma of the lung. Proc Natl Acad Sci USA 1987;84(24):9252–9256.

45. Toledo G, Sola JJ, Lozano MD, Soria E, Pardo J. Loss of FHIT protein expression is related to high proliferation, low apoptosis and worse prognosis in non–small-cell lung cancer. Mod Pathol 2004;17(4):440–448.

46. Ohta M, Inoue H, Cotticelli MG, et al. The FHIT gene, spanning the chromosome 3p14.2 fragile site and renal carcinoma–associated t(3;8) breakpoint, is abnormal in digestive tract cancers. Cell 1996;84(4):587–597.

47. Fong KM, Biesterveld EJ, Virmani A, et al. FHIT and FRA3B 3p14.2 allele loss are common in lung cancer and preneoplastic bronchial lesions and are associated with cancer-related FHIT cDNA splicing aberrations. Cancer Res 1997;57(11):2256–2267.

48. Woenckhaus M, Grepmeier U, Wild PJ, et al. Multitarget FISH and LOH analyses at chromosome 3p in non–small cell lung cancer and adjacent bronchial epithelium. Am J Clin Pathol 2005;123(5):752–761.

49. Zanesi N, Fidanza V, Fong LY, et al. The tumor spectrum in FHIT-deficient mice. Proc Natl Acad Sci USA 2001;98(18): 10250–10255.

50. Ji L, Fang B, Yen N, Fong K, Minna JD, Roth JA. Induction of apoptosis and inhibition of tumorigenicity and tumor growth by adenovirus vector–mediated fragile histidine triad (FHIT) gene overexpression. Cancer Res 1999;59(14): 3333–3339.

51. Otterson GA, Xiao GH, Geradts J, et al. Protein expression and functional analysis of the FHIT gene in human tumor cells. J Natl Cancer Inst 1998;90(6):426–432.

52. Werner NS, Siprashvili Z, Fong LY, et al. Differential susceptibility of renal carcinoma cell lines to tumor suppression by exogenous Fhit expression. Cancer Res 2000;60(11): 2780–2785.

53. Marsit CJ, Hasegawa M, Hirao T, et al. Loss of heterozygosity of chromosome 3p21 is associated with mutant TP53 and better patient survival in non–small-cell lung cancer. Cancer Res 2004;64(23):8702–8707.

54. Chmara M, Wozniak A, Ochman K, et al. Loss of heterozygosity at chromosomes 3p and 17p in primary non–small cell lung cancer. Anticancer Res 2004;24(6):4259–4263.

55. Ho WL, Chang JW, Tseng RC, et al. Loss of heterozygosity at loci of candidate tumor suppressor genes in microdissected primary non–small cell lung cancer. Cancer Detect Prev 2002;26(5):343–349.

56. Demopoulos K, Arvanitis DA, Vassilakis DA, Siafakas NM, Spandidos DA. MYCL1, FHIT, SPARC, p16(INK4) and TP53 genes associated to lung cancer in idiopathic pulmonary fibrosis. J Cell Mol Med 2002;6(2):215–222.

57. Suzuki M, Hao C, Takahashi T, et al. Aberrant methylation of SPARC in human lung cancers. Br J Cancer 2005;92(5): 942–948.

58. Sanz-Ortega J, Bryant B, Sanz-Esponera J, et al. LOH at the APC/MCC gene (5Q21) is frequent in early stages of non–small cell lung cancer. Pathol Res Pract 1999;195(10): 677–680.

59. Brabender J, Usadel H, Danenberg KD, et al. Adenomatous polyposis coli gene promoter hypermethylation in non–small cell lung cancer is associated with survival. Oncogene 2001;20(27):3528–3532.

60. Kurimoto F, Gemma A, Hosoya Y, et al. Unchanged frequency of loss of heterozygosity and size of the deleted region at 8p21–23 during metastasis of lung cancer. Int J Mol Med 2001;8(1):89–93.

61. Wistuba, II, Behrens C, Virmani AK, et al. Allelic losses at chromosome 8p21–23 are early and frequent events in the pathogenesis of lung cancer. Cancer Res 1999;59(8):1973–1979.

62. Xu Z, Liang L, Wang H, Li T, Zhao M. HCRP1, a novel gene that is downregulated in hepatocellular carcinoma, encodes a growth-inhibitory protein. Biochem Biophys Res Commun 2003;311(4):1057–1066.

63. Marsit CJ, Wiencke JK, Nelson HH, et al. Alterations of 9p in squamous cell carcinoma and adenocarcinoma of the lung: association with smoking, TP53, and survival. Cancer Genet Cytogenet 2005;162(2):115–121.

64. Ohtani N, Yamakoshi K, Takahashi A, Hara E. The p16INK4a–RB pathway: molecular link between cellular senescence and tumor suppression. J Med Invest 2004; 51(3–4):146–153.

65. Sumitomo K, Shimizu E, Shinohara A, Yokota J, Sone S. Activation of RB tumor suppressor protein and growth suppression of small cell lung carcinoma cells by reintroduction of p16INK4A gene. Int J Oncol 1999;14(6): 1075–1080.

66. Kratzke RA, Greatens TM, Rubins JB, et al. Rb and p16INK4a expression in resected non–small cell lung tumors. Cancer Res 1996;56(15):3415–2340.

67. Quesnel B, Preudhomme C, Fenaux P. p16ink4a gene and hematological malignancies. Leuk Lymphoma 1996; 22(1–2):11–24.

68. Awaya H, Takeshima Y, Amatya VJ, et al. Inactivation of the p16 gene by hypermethylation and loss of heterozygosity in adenocarcinoma of the lung. Pathol Int 2004;54(7):486–489.

69. Marsit CJ, Zheng S, Aldape K, et al. PTEN expression in non–small-cell lung cancer: evaluating its relation to tumor characteristics, allelic loss, and epigenetic alteration. Hum Pathol 2005;36(7):768–776.

70. Kim SK, Su LK, Oh Y, et al.. Alterations of PTEN/MMAC1, a candidate tumor suppressor gene, and its homologue, PTH2, in small cell lung cancer cell lines. Oncogene 1998; 16(1):89–93.

71. Hosoya Y, Gemma A, Seike M, et al. Alteration of the PTEN/MMAC1 gene locus in primary lung cancer with distant metastasis. Lung Cancer 1999;25(2):87–93.

72. Wikman H, Kettunen E. Regulation of the G1/S phase of the cell cycle and alterations in the RB pathway in human lung cancer. Expert Rev Anticancer Ther 2006;6(4):515–350.

73. Arvanitis DA, Papadakis E, Zafiropoulos A, Spandidos DA. Fractional allele loss is a valuable marker for human lung cancer detection in sputum. Lung Cancer 2003;40(1):55–66.

74. Gorgoulis VG, Zacharatos P, Kotsinas A, et al. Alterations of the p16–pRb pathway and the chromosome locus

9p21–22 in non–small-cell lung carcinomas: relationship with p53 and MDM2 protein expression. Am J Pathol 1998;153(6):1749–1765.

75. Kee HJ, Shin JH, Chang J, et al. Identification of tumor suppressor loci on the long arm of chromosome 15 in primary small cell lung cancer. Yonsei Med J 2003;44(1):65–74.

76. Stanton SE, Shin SW, Johnson BE, Meyerson M. Recurrent allelic deletions of chromosome arms 15q and 16q in human small cell lung carcinomas. Genes Chromosomes Cancer 2000;27(3):323–331.

77. Petersen I, Langreck H, Wolf G, et al. Small-cell lung cancer is characterized by a high incidence of deletions on chromosomes 3p, 4q, 5q, 10q, 13q and 17p. Br J Cancer 1997; 75(1):79–86.

78. Hussain SP, Harris CC. p53 biological network: at the crossroads of the cellular-stress response pathway and molecular carcinogenesis. J Nippon Med Sch 2006;73(2):54–64.

79. Yang TL, Su YR, Huang CS, et al. High-resolution 19p13.2–13.3 allelotyping of breast carcinomas demonstrates frequent loss of heterozygosity. Genes Chromosomes Cancer 2004;41(3):250–256.

80. von Herbay A, Arens N, Friedl W, et al. Bronchioloalveolar carcinoma: a new cancer in Peutz-Jeghers syndrome. Lung Cancer 2005;47(2):283–288.

81. Sobottka SB, Haase M, Fitze G, Hahn M, Schackert HK, Schackert G. Frequent loss of heterozygosity at the 19p13.3 locus without LKB1/STK11 mutations in human carcinoma metastases to the brain. J Neurooncol 2000;49(3): 187–195.

82. Samara K, Zervou M, Siafakas NM, Tzortzaki EG. Microsatellite DNA instability in benign lung diseases. Respir Med 2006;100(2):202–211.

83. King T. Idiopathic pulmonary fibrosis. In: Schwartz M, King T, eds. Interstitial Lung Disease. Ontario, Canada: Decker BC, Inc.; 1998:597–644.

84. Uematsu K, Yoshimura A, Gemma A, et al. Aberrations in the fragile histidine triad (FHIT) gene in idiopathic pulmonary fibrosis. Cancer Res 2001;61(23):8527–8533.

85. Vassilakis DA, Sourvinos G, Pantelidis P, Spandidos DA, Siafakas NM, Bouros D. Extended genetic alterations in a patient with pulmonary sarcoidosis, a benign disease. Sarcoidosis Vasc Diffuse Lung Dis 2001;18(3):307–310.

86. Demopoulos K, Arvanitis DA, Vassilakis DA, Siafakas NM, Spandidos DA. Genomic instability on hMSH2, hMLH1, CD48 and IRF4 loci in pulmonary sarcoidosis. Int J Biol Markers 2002;17(4):224–230.

87. Xu J, Meyers DA, Ober C, et al. Genomewide screen and identification of gene–gene interactions for asthma-susceptibility loci in three U.S. populations: collaborative study on the genetics of asthma. Am J Hum Genet 2001;68(6): 1437–1446.

88. Sandford AJ, Pare PD. The genetics of asthma. The important questions. Am J Respir Crit Care Med 2000;161(3 Pt 2):S202–S206.

89. Paraskakis E, Sourvinos G, Passam F, et al. Microsatellite DNA instability and loss of heterozygosity in bronchial asthma. Eur Respir J 2003;22(6):951–955.

90. Siafakas NM, Tzortzaki EG, Sourvinos G, et al. Microsatellite DNA instability in COPD. Chest 1999;116(1):47–51.

91. Anderson GP, Bozinovski S. Acquired somatic mutations in the molecular pathogenesis of COPD. Trends Pharmacol Sci 2003;24(2):71–76.

12
In Situ Hybridization: Principles and Applications for Pulmonary Medicine

Kevin C. Halling and Amy J. Wendel

Introduction

In situ hybridization is a technique that utilizes nucleic acid (DNA or RNA) probes to assess intact cells for various types of genetic alterations. In situ hybridization has become an extremely useful tool for the clinical pathology laboratory to aid oncologists, geneticists, and infectious disease specialists in the diagnosis and treatment of their patients. Common applications of in situ hybridization include its use to detect cancer cells in cytologic specimens, chromosomal alterations in resected tumor specimens that predict prognosis, and response to therapy of certain cancer types and microorganisms in various specimen types.

In situ hybridization is typically performed either with fluorescently labeled probes or with probes that are subsequently visualized with a chromogen such as diaminobenzidine. If performed with fluorescently labeled probes, the technique is referred to as fluorescence in situ hybridization (FISH). Alternatively, if the technique is performed with a probe that requires subsequent visualization with a chemical reaction that produces a colored chemical at the site of the probe (a chromogen), the technique is referred to as chromogenic in situ hybridization (CISH).

An advantage that in situ hybridization has over other techniques, such as polymerase chain reaction (PCR), which is also used to assess cells for genetic alterations, is that with in situ hybridization the cells remain intact. This allows one to determine which specific cells have the abnormality. An additional advantage that in situ hybridization has over some genetic techniques is that it can sensitively detect alterations that occur in only a small subset of cells analyzed. This is quite important, for example, in oncology, because tumors tend to be quite heterogeneous, and the alteration that is being assessed for may be present in only a small percentage of the cells. Other molecular techniques in which the tissue is homogenized prior to analysis often cannot detect these altera-

tions because of dilution by cells not carrying the alteration (e.g., by benign stromal or inflammatory cells that are invariably present in tumors).

In Situ Hybridization: General Principles

To understand how in situ hybridization works, one should be familiar with (1) DNA and RNA composition and structure, (2) principles of base pairing, (3) denaturation and hybridization, and (4) factors that influence denaturation and hybridization. It is not possible to cover these topics extensively; however, the following paragraphs briefly touch on the most important aspects of these topics.

DNA Composition and Structure

DNA and RNA are each composed of four nucleotides that form long chains. The nucleotides that comprise DNA contain one of four bases, adenine, cytosine, guanine, or thymine (Figure 12.1). RNA is composed of nucleotides that also contain the same nucleotides except that uracil substitutes for thymine. Another important difference between DNA and RNA is that DNA is double stranded and RNA is single stranded.

Principles of Base Pairing

To comprehend hybridization, it is essential to understand how base pairing occurs in double stranded DNA or DNA/RNA hybrids. In double stranded DNA, nucleotides with an adenine (A) or thymine (T) pair with one another (referred to as *base pairing*) through two hydrogen bonds while guanine (G) and cytosine (C) pair with one another through three hydrogen bonds (see Figure 12.1). The only difference with DNA/RNA hybrids is that

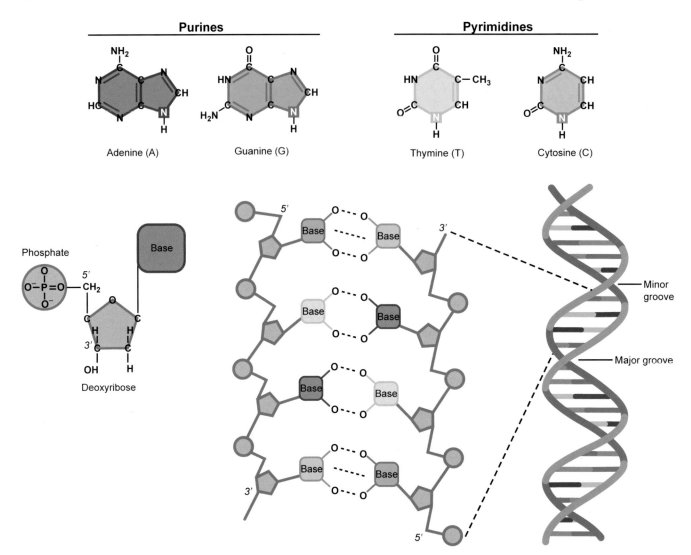

FIGURE 12.1. DNA structure. Nucleotides are the building blocks of both DNA and RNA. Nucleotides are composed of the sugar deoxyribose (DNA) or ribose (RNA), a phosphate group, and a base. The four bases found in DNA are the purines, guanine and adenine, and the pyrimidines, cytosine and thymine. Uracil substitutes for thymine in RNA. Single-stranded DNA is a polymer of nucleotides. The 5′ end of a single-stranded DNA molecule is the end that has a free phosphate group, and the 3′ end is the end that has a free 3′-OH group. Double-stranded DNA is composed of two single-stranded DNA molecules that run in opposite directions. In double-stranded DNA, guanine pairs with cytosine through three hydrogen bonds, and adenine pairs with thymine through two hydrogen bonds.

uracil (U) rather than thymine base pairs with adenine. It is the pairing of As to Ts (or Us in the case of RNA) and of Cs to Gs that keeps the two strands of DNA or the two strands of a DNA/RNA hybrid paired to one another. Because GC base pairs have three hydrogen bonds, they are stronger and require more energy to break than AT base pairs. If two strands of DNA have bases that pair perfectly, that is, every A, C, G, or T on one strand is matched with a T, G, C, or A, respectively, on the opposite strand, then the two strands are said to be 100% complementary.

Denaturation, Renaturation, and Influencing Factors

Denaturation refers to the process of making double-stranded DNA (or DNA/RNA hybrids) single stranded. Denaturation is also sometimes referred to as *melting* the DNA. Denaturation is brought about by breaking the hydrogen bonds that hold the two strands of DNA together. This is most commonly achieved by applying heat (i.e., raising the temperature of the sample). In addition, certain chemicals such as formamide can be used to promote denaturation. Because G/C base pairs are stronger than A/T or A/U base pairs, double-stranded DNA fragments (or DNA/RNA hybrids) with a higher percentage of Gs and Cs will require more heat (i.e., higher temperatures) to denature than will dsDNA fragments (or DNA/RNA hybrids) with a higher percentage of As and Ts. *Renaturation* refers to the process of bringing two complementary strands of DNA (or complementary DNA and RNA) back together.

Hybridization occurs when two strands of complementary single-stranded DNA or RNA molecules "stick to" one another. The greater the complementarity of the two single-stranded molecules, the more likely two strands will hybridize to one another. In addition, because of stronger base pairing, DNA/DNA or DNA/RNA hybrids that are 100% complementary will be more stable and require more energy to break apart than those that are less complementary. Two strands that are less complementary (e.g., only 95% complementary) can hybridize to one another under certain conditions that are referred to as *less stringent* conditions. The tendency for a DNA or RNA probe to stick to sequences that are not complementary is referred to as *nonspecific hybridization*. Nonspecific hybridization can be prevented by maintaining conditions, referred to as *stringent conditions*, that favor hybridization of the most complementary sequences but prevent the hybridization of less complementary sequences. Stringent conditions are generally achieved by keeping the temperature at the highest possible temperature that allows the most complementary single-stranded DNA or RNA probe to anneal to its completely complementary target without allowing it to anneal to targets that are less complementary. Depending on how similar the noncomplementary sequence is to the complementary sequence, the difference between stringent and nonstringent conditions may be just a degree or two. For example, 37°C may favor the annealing of a probe that is 100% complementary to its target sequence but prevent a probe that is only 95% complementary to bind to its target sequence. However, dropping the hybridization temperature just a couple of degrees to 35°C may favor the binding of both probes to the target sequence.

The melting temperature (T_m) of double-stranded DNA in solution is approximated by the following formula:

$$T_m = 81.5 + 16.6 \log (Na^+) + 0.41 \,(\% \text{ GC})$$
$$-0.63 \,(\% \text{ formamide}) - (300 + 2{,}000) \,(Na^+)/N$$

where T_m is the melting temperature in degrees centigrade, Na^+ is the molar concentration of sodium ions, % GC is the percentage of GC base pairs in the hybridized molecules, % formamide is the percentage of formamide (volume/volume), and N is the length in bases of the hybrid.[1] This formula may appear somewhat daunting to those of us who are less mathematically inclined, but,

conceptually, the important points to note are that increasing the salt concentration inhibits melting and increasing the formamide promotes melting. This is because high salt concentrations favor hydrogen bonding of the two strands of a DNA/DNA or DNA/RNA hybrid, whereas formamide helps break those hydrogen bonds. Likewise, it is important to note that, under identical conditions, shorter fragments of DNA melt at lower temperatures than longer fragments of DNA. A familiarity with this formula can be helpful when trying to troubleshoot problems with nonspecific or incomplete hybridization.

Probes

Types of Probes

All in situ hybridization techniques utilize DNA or RNA probes. These probes are designed to hybridize to specific target sequences of interest such as genes that have been implicated in inherited diseases or cancer as well as to microorganisms of various types. DNA probes that are commonly used for genetic and/or oncologic applications have been categorized as chromosome enumeration (CEP) probes, locus-specific indicator probes, telomeric probes, and chromosome paints.

Chromosome Enumeration Probes

Chromosome enumeration probes hybridize to repetitive DNA sequences found near the centromeres of chromosomes, which are referred to as α-satellite DNA. These regions are composed of ~171 base pair (bp) sequences that are tandemly repeated thousands of times and span approximately 250,000 to 5,000,000 bases.[2] The repeat regions of the different chromosomal centromeres exhibit substantial sequence divergence of approximately 20%–40%.[2] Because of this, probes specific for each of the centromeres are available for most but not all chromosomes. A few chromosomes, for example, chromosomes 13 and 21, 14 and 22, as well as 5 and 19, have α-satellite repeat sequences that are too similar to allow one to distinguish these chromosomes from each another due to cross-hybridization.

Chromosome enumeration probes are used to enumerate the number of copies of a given chromosome in a cell. They are able to enumerate chromosome copy number because the centromere of a chromosome is lost the whole chromosome will generally be lost. One advantage of CEP probes is that because they hybridize to sequences that have a high copy number, they provide strong (i.e., bright) signals. In addition, because these regions are tightly compacted in the heterochromatic regions of the chromosome, the signals provided with CEP probes are generally tight ("crisp") rather than diffuse.

Locus-Specific Probes

Locus-specific probes hybridize to unique sequences (i.e., nonrepetitive DNA sequences) and are generally used to determine if specific genes are amplified (e.g., *HER2*), deleted (e.g., *P53* or *P16*), or translocated (e.g., *BCR/ABL* translocation). These probes typically hybridize to a region that ranges from 40 to 500 kilobases (kb). Probes that hybridize to regions smaller than 40 kb often produce weak signals that can be difficult to see. Probes larger than this can produce diffuse signals that are difficult to distinguish as single spots.

Telomeric Probes

Telomeric probes are not actually probes to telomeric sequences but to unique DNA sequences found very near the telomeres (so-called subtelomeric probes).[3,4] Unique telomeric probes are available for 41 of the 46 chromosomal telomeres. The only telomeres for which there are not probes are those for the p arms of the acrocentric chromosomes 13, 14, 15, 21, and 22. However, these regions are composed primarily of ribosomal DNA, and deletions or duplications of these regions are not generally thought to have clinical significance.[4]

Chromosomal Paints

Chromosomal paints are mixtures of probes that hybridize to the entire length of one or more chromosomes. The probes that comprise chromosomal paints are generally prepared by isolating individual chromosomes by flow cytometry and then performing PCR amplification with degenerate oligonucleotide primers. The fluorescently labeled probes generated from this can then be used as a "paint" that highlights the entire chromosome homogeneously along its length. Chromosomal paints can be used to identify specific chromosomes in a metaphase spread. This can be particularly helpful when standard karyotyping is unable to identify a chromosome (e.g., marker chromosomes).

Probe Preparation

Probes are generally prepared from fragments of DNA that have been cloned into bacterial (BAC), P1 (PAC), or yeast (YAC) artificial chromosomes. Probes that are used for FISH can either be directly or indirectly labeled with a fluorophore.[5] A fluorophore is a molecule that fluoresces when excited by light of a specific wavelength. There are a wide variety of fluorophores that can be used for FISH.[5] Two of the more commonly used fluorophores are fluorescein isothiocyanate (FITC) and Texas Red, which fluoresce green and red, respectively.

Directly Labeled Probes

Directly labeled probes are prepared by incorporating a fluorophore-labeled nucleotide into the probe usually by nick translation or random priming. Because the fluorescently labeled probe is bound to its cellular target in a single hybridization step, no further processing is required to visualize the probe. Directly labeled CEP and locus-specific probes are commercially available singly or as probe mixtures of up to four different probes and are generally labeled with red, green, aqua, or yellow fluorophores.

Indirectly Labeled Probes

Indirectly labeled probes contain nucleotides that have covalently attached reporter molecules such as biotin or digoxigenin. These probes require an additional step after hybridization in which the probe is generally visualized by applying fluorophore-labeled avidin or fluorophore labeled antidigoxigenin in a second step. A significant disadvantage of using indirectly labeled probes is that it adds extra steps to the procedure. However, potential advantages of indirectly labeled probes include the possibility obtaining stronger signals due to an ability to achieve greater signal amplification. In addition, indirect labeling allows for greater versatility in probe use because one can visualize any probe that has been labeled with biotinylated 2′-deoxyuridine 5′-triphosphate (dUTP) or digoxigenin.

In-House Developed Probes

Most diagnostic laboratories utilize commercially available probes. However, a laboratory may want to prepare its own in-house probe if one is not commercially available. If a laboratory prepares its own probes for diagnostic use, it is important to extensively validate the probe prior to clinical implementation to ensure that it hybridizes to the intended target and provides the expected results on normal and abnormal specimens. Wiktor et al. have recently provided recommendations for the validation of probes for clinical use.[6]

Fluorescence In Situ Hybridization

Procedure

The steps involved in performing FISH are as follows: (1) obtain specimen for FISH, (2) prepare specimen for hybridization ("prehybridization"), (3) hybridize probes to target DNA in specimen, (4) remove nonspecifically bound probe by washing, and (5) assess signals in specimen using fluorescence microscopy (Figure 12.2). Each of these steps is described in more detail.

1. Protease treatment to ease accessibility of double-stranded cellular DNA to probe DNA

2. Denature double-stranded DNA, 73°C

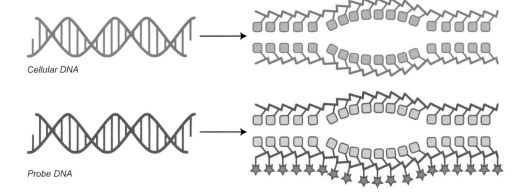

Cellular DNA

Probe DNA

3. Hybridize probe to cellular DNA, 37°C

4. Removal of non-specifically bound probe DNA

5. Microscopic assessment of fluorescent signals in cells

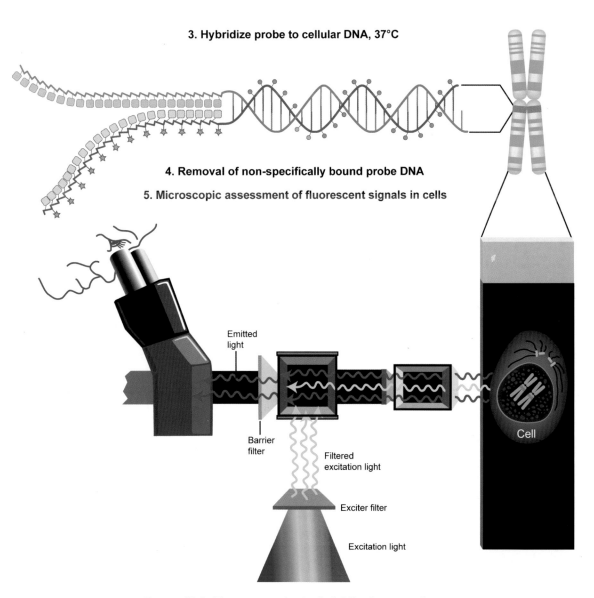

FIGURE 12.2. Fluorescence in situ hybridization procedure.

Specimens

Fluorescence in situ hybridization can be performed on a wide range of specimens, including peripheral blood, paraffin-embedded tissue, and cytology specimens (e.g., urine, sputum, or endoscopic brushings). Frozen tissue will not work well because freezing results in intracellular ice crystals that disrupt the morphology of the cells. The fixative that gives the best FISH results for paraffin-embedded tissue is neutral buffered formalin. However, tissue that has been left in formalin too long (>48hr) prior to paraffin embedding will not provide good FISH results.[7] Specimens that have been fixed in B5 fixative, which is often used for hematologic specimens, may require isolation of nuclei prior to FISH to obtain good results.[8] Some fixatives such as Prefer work poorly if at all for FISH.[9]

Prehybridization

The goal of prehybridization is to prepare the cells in the specimen so that the probe can efficiently hybridize to its cellular DNA target but do so without significantly disrupting the morphology of the cells. Detailed protocols for prehybridization and hybridization can be found elsewhere.[10,11] The pretreatment required for different specimen types (e.g., fresh cells versus paraffin-embedded tissue) is similar but frequently has some important differences. For example, certain specimens such as paraffin-embedded tissue generally need to be treated with a protease such as pepsin to increase the accessibility of the probe DNA to its nuclear DNA target. It is important to not over- or underdigest the tissue with pepsin. Overdigestion can lead to a decrease in signal intensity and destroy nuclear morphology. Underdigestion can lead to autofluorescence, and an underestimation of signal copy number may result. Other methods that have been used to facilitate entry of the probe into the cell include treatment with dilute acid or nonionic detergents.[12]

Denaturation and Hybridization

Denaturation and hybridization involve denaturing the probe and cellular DNA and then allowing the probe to hybridize to its cellular DNA target. The probe hybridization solution contains not only the probe DNA but a type of DNA that is referred to as Cot DNA. Cot DNA is DNA that hybridizes to highly repetitive DNA sequences that are present throughout the genome. Without Cot DNA, the probe DNA would nonspecifically bind to these repetitive DNA sequences, resulting in many nonspecific signals rather than the specific signals that are desired. In one of the more widely utilized FISH hybrid-

ization protocols, the probe and target DNA are codenatured at about 73°C for about 3 min in 50% formamide. Formamide is added to lower the temperature at which the probe and cellular DNA melt. This is important because high temperatures can destroy the cellular morphology that needs to be maintained. The temperature is then lowered to about 37°C to allow the probe DNA to hybridize to its specific target.

The hybridization temperature is less fastidious for FISH assays than for PCR assays because FISH probes are much longer than PCR probes. Hybridization is generally allowed to occur over about 4 to 12hr. Factors that can influence the efficiency and specificity of the hybridization include the probe sequence and hybridization temperature. If the probe sequence is not unique, additional signals may present that represent crosshybridizing sequences. If the hybridization temperature is too high, the signals may be weak, and if the hybridization temperature is too low, there may be an abundance of nonspecific background signal.

Removing Nonspecifically Bound Probe

Following hybridization, the slide is washed with a specific washing solution. The goal of this step is to remove any probe that is not specifically bound to the desired target without removing the probe that has bound to the desired target. This is generally done by washing the slide in a solution that is heated to 73°C and contains 0.4× SSC/0.3% NP40 (nonformalin-fixed samples) or 2.0× SSC/0.3% NP40 (formalin-fixed samples). A higher salt concentration (less stringent wash) is used for paraffin-embedded specimens because the probe/target hybrids are less strong for paraffin-embedded specimens than for nonformalin-fixed samples. This may be due to shorter length of target DNA sequences in paraffin-embedded tissue or to persistence of protein in the hybridized region that causes hybrid destabilization.[10] If the posthybridization wash is too stringent, all or most of the probe may be washed off, and there may be either no signals or weak signals when viewed under the microscope. On the other hand, if the wash is not stringent enough, there may be an excessive amount of nonspecific hybridization background when viewed under the microscope. If indirectly labeled probes are used, an additional step is required at this point to attach the fluorophore to the probe. The procedure used will depend on the type of reporter molecule (biotin, digoxigenin, other) that has been previously chosen.

Finally, approximately 10μL of a solution that contains 4'-6-diamidino-2-phenylindole (DAPI) and "antifade" is placed on the slide, and the slide is coverslipped. 4'-6-diamidino-2-phenylindole is a nuclear counterstain that fluoresces blue-gray when viewed with a fluorescent microscope. It allows one to see the nuclei. Without

DAPI, the FISH signals would appear to be free-floating in a dark background. Antifade is used to inhibit photobleaching, which is the tendency of fluorophores to fade with exposure to light and heat.[13] Because fluorophores are susceptible to photobleaching, it is best to store hybridized slides and probe in a refrigerator and in the dark. In addition, when viewing the slide on the microscope, it is important to remove the slide from the path of light by closing the condenser when not viewing. If a slide has lost its fluorescence, it can generally be rehybridized with good results if the target DNA is still intact. We have successfully rehybridized slides that are several years old.

Fluorescence Microscopy

Following hybridization, FISH signals are assessed with a fluorescence microscope (usually an epifluorescence microscope) equipped with the appropriate filters necessary to see the probe signals. A detailed discussion of fluorescence microscopy is beyond the scope of this chapter, but there are several excellent reviews of the subject.[14] Nonetheless, it is important to understand at least a few basic aspects of how fluorescence microscopy works.

As noted earlier, a fluorophore is a molecule that absorbs light of a certain wavelength (actually a certain range of wavelengths) and then reemits that energy as light of longer wavelengths. For example, as shown in Figure 12.3, the fluorophore that is referred to as Spectrum Green™ absorbs light that ranges from about 470 to 510 nm and then reemits it (i.e., fluoresces) as light of higher wavelengths that range from about 500 to 550 nm. The goal of FISH is to cause the fluorophore-labeled DNA or RNA probe to fluoresce and highlight the target of interest in the specimen. To do this, the fluorescence

microscope must have a light source that is capable of exciting the fluorophore. Mercury or xenon arc lamps are typically relied-upon light sources for fluorescence microscopes. These lamps emit light of wavelengths that can be absorbed by the fluorophores. A combination of filters (excitation, beam splitting interference, and barrier) select an appropriate wavelength of light to excite the fluorophore and ensure that the main light that reaches the observer's eye is the desired fluorescence wavelength. These filters are generally incorporated into a single housing device that is referred to as a *filter cube*. The appropriate combination of filters depends on the fluorophore(s) that are being utilized. Cubes are available for most fluorophores. Most cubes contain filters that allow one to look at only one probe at a time. However, dual-pass and triple-pass filters that allow one to see red and green signals or the red signal, green signal, and DAPI counterstain simultaneously are available and very useful.

It is frequently necessary to take a picture of the cells and their fluorescent signals. This requires the use of imaging systems and software that enable one to capture the different colored probe signals in a single composite image. When a multicolor probe set has been used, it may be particularly difficult to take a picture that shows all the signals when using a normal camera. This is because the signals are often present in different planes. This can be overcome with a device known as a Z-stack camera, which allows one to easily capture all the signals in a cell as a single image.

Chromogenic In Situ Hybridization

Chromogenic in situ hybridization is another type of in situ hybridization that is very similar to FISH except that the probe is visualized by a chromogenic reaction after it has hybridized to its target rather than being visualized as a fluorescent signal. There are several ways to perform CISH. One method incorporates biotinylated dUTP into the probe. After hybridization of the probe to its target, horseradish peroxidase–labeled streptavidin is added to the slide. The streptavidin attaches to the biotin. Diaminobenzidine (DAB) is then added, and the horseradish peroxidase converts the DAB to a brown chromogen at the site of the probe. Another CISH method utilizes digoxigenin-labeled probes instead of biotin-labeled probes but also utilizes peroxidase and DAB to visualize the probe.

Chromogenic in situ hybridization has several advantages over FISH. One major advantage is that CISH slides can be viewed with a light microscope, and the tissue architecture is much easier to discern. This makes it easier to correlate molecular alterations with histologic or cytologic features with CISH than with FISH. In

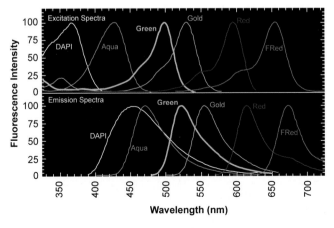

FIGURE 12.3. Excitation (absorption) and emission spectra for commonly used fluorophores.

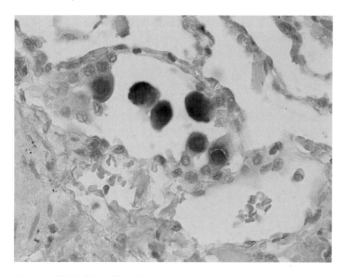

FIGURE 12.4. Identification of cytomegalovirus in lung tissue section utilizing chromogenic in situ hybridization. The purple stained nuclei contain cytomegalovirus.

addition, CISH can be performed in conjunction with immunohistochemistry to assess for correlations between chromosomal alterations and protein expression.[15] A final important advantage of CISH is that the permanent slides obtained after CISH analysis do not fade and thus are suitable for long-term archiving.

Disadvantages of CISH (relative to FISH) include that it can easily identify only a single target at a time, and the signals produced with CISH are less discrete than those produced by FISH, which makes signal enumeration less precise than what is possible by FISH. The inability of CISH to identify more than one target may or may not be important depending on the application. For example, CISH is frequently used to identify viruses such as Epstein-Barr virus and cytomegalovirus in lung tissue sections (Figure 12.4). For this particular application, the inability of CISH to identify more than a single target is not a limitation.

However, the inability to detect more than one target at a time could be a limitation for some applications. For example, one commercially available FISH assay for *HER2* amplification utilizes two probes, a green probe to the chromosome 17 centromere and a red probe to the *HER2* gene. With this FISH assay, a *HER2*/CEP17 signal ratio of >2.0 is considered evidence of *HER2* amplification and justification for Herceptin therapy. The rationale for including the CEP17 probe in this probe set was that some tumors may exhibit gains (i.e., more than two copies) of the *HER2* gene because of polysomy (i.e., extra copies) of chromosome 17 in the tumor but not because of true amplification of the *HER2* gene. It is not fully known at this time whether the absolute *HER2* copy number by itself is predictive of response to Herceptin or whether knowing the ratio of *HER2*/CEP17 is important. However, if knowing the ratio is important, this informa-

tion would not be available with the CISH assay. Other probe sets, for example, a FISH probe set for bladder cancer detection, utilize as many as four different probes in a single cocktail to achieve high sensitivities for bladder tumor detection.[16] Studies have shown that the use of a multiprobe FISH cocktail provides higher sensitivity than is achievable with probe sets that contain only one or two probe sets.

Other Techniques That Utilize In Situ Hybridization

Comparative Genomic Hybridization

Comparative genomic hybridization (CGH) is a powerful technique that can, similar to conventional karyotyping, be used to analyze the entire genome of cells for chromosomal abnormalities.[17] The CGH technique is particularly useful for assessing solid tumors for chromosomal abnormalities. As first described, CGH is preformed by isolating DNA from tumor tissue and labeling it with a green fluorophore and isolating DNA from normal tissue and labeling it with a red fluorophore.[18] Equal amounts of the green-labeled tumor DNA and red-labeled normal DNA are then cohybridized to a normal metaphase spread (i.e., a karyotype without any abnormalities). If there are no chromosomal abnormalities in the tumor tissue, then equal amounts of green and red probe will hybridize to the chromosomes in the normal metaphase spread, and the color of all the chromosomes in the metaphase spread will be yellow (because equal amounts of red and green make yellow). However, if there are, for example, three copies of chromosome 1 in the tumor, then there will be more green-labeled than red-labeled chromosome 1 DNA, and chromosome 1 in the metaphase spread will appear green. Thus, areas in the metaphase spread that appear green represent chromosomal areas that have been gained in the tumor while areas that appear red represent chromosomal areas that have been deleted in the tumor. In this fashion, CGH can be used to identify many of the chromosomal abnormalities present in a tumor.

Comparative genomic hybridization is generally not performed with metaphase spreads anymore but instead with microarrays of DNA clones that are largely representative of all the loci along the length of the 24 chromosomes.[19] This technique, which is referred to as *array CGH*, has the potential for higher resolution and greater reproducibility than can be obtained with metaphase spreads. A representative example of an array CGH is shown in Figure 12.5.

Comparative genomic hybridization has several advantages over conventional karyotyping, including the following: (1) the tumor can be grown in culture prior to analysis; (2) the cells do not have to be in

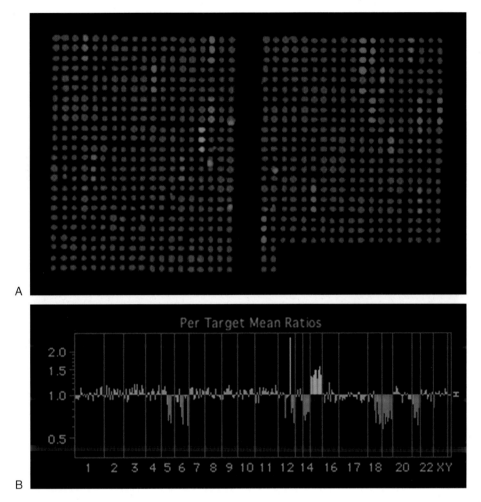

FIGURE 12.5. Array comparative genomic hybridization. **(A)** Genomic array spotted with DNA from 287 targets in the genome. The targets include subtelomeric regions, oncogenes, tumor suppressor genes, and microdeletion loci. Each target is spotted in triplicate. Green-labeled tumor DNA from a single tumor (a bile duct tumor) and red-labeled normal DNA were cohybridized to the DNA spots on the array. Gene amplifica- tions within the tumor appear as green spots (in triplicate), and deletions within the tumor appear as red spots (in triplicate). **(B)** Illustration of the chromosomal locations of the gene ampli- fications and deletions shown in A. The tumor shows deletions of 5q, 6q, 12q, 14q, 18q, 19, and 21, a gain of 15, and amplification of the *MDM2* gene at 12q14.3–q15.

metaphase to determine the types of chromosomal abnormalities present; and (3) it has higher resolution, typically down to about 1 megabase, whereas karyo- typing has a resolution down to about 5 megabases. The main disadvantage of CGH relative to conven- tional karyotyping is that it cannot detect balanced chromosomal alterations (e.g., reciprocal transloca- tions). Although CGH is generally not used clinically, it has been a powerful research tool for identifying the most common chromosomal abnormalities that are present in various tumor types, including both non– small cell and small cell lung cancer.[20–36] Comparative genomic hybridization studies have, for instance, shown that gains of 1q31, 3q26, 5p13, and 8q24 and deletions at 3p21, 8p22, 9p21, 13q22, and 17p13 are common in lung cancer and likely important in the pathogenesis of these tumors.[30,31–33]

Multicolor Whole-Chromosome Painting

Spectral karyotyping and multicolor FISH are highly sophisticated techniques that allow one to generate a color-coded karyotype.[37,38] In other words, these tech- niques produce a karyotype in which each chromosome has its own unique color. The generation of chromosomal paints for each chromosome is accomplished with com- binatorial labeling of the chromosome-specific probes with just five fluorophores. Spectral karyotyping and mul- ticolor FISH can be helpful in identifying chromosomes that are difficult to identify such as marker chromosomes or chromosomes that are involved in complex rearrange- ments. This can be particularly helpful for solid tumor genetics because solid tumors often have very complex karyotypes that are difficult to elucidate (Figure 12.6).

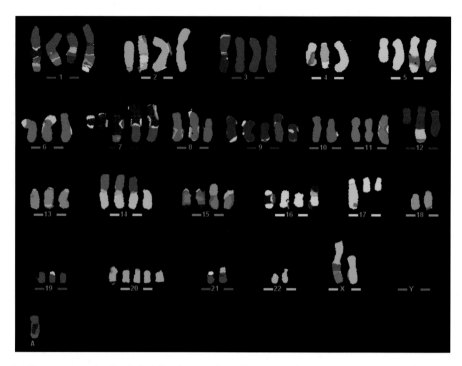

FIGURE 12.6. Multicolor fluorescence in situ hybridization analysis of a karyotype from a pediatric osteosarcoma. The technique reveals numerous complex rearrangements in this tumor. For example, there is a complex rearrangement involving the X chromosome (light aqua), chromosomes 1 (red), 11 (dark aqua), and 6 (dark pink).

Clinical Applications

Oncology

Fluorescence and chromogenic in situ hybridization have been used in oncology to help detect and type tumors, to prognosticate, and to guide therapy.

Tumor Detection

Fluorescence in situ hybridization is being increasingly utilized by cytotechnologists and cytopathologists to identify malignant cells in various types of cytologic specimens. The technique works well for this purpose because most solid tumors have chromosomal alterations that are readily detectable by FISH. Examples of how FISH has been used to identify tumor cells in cytologic specimens include its use to identify bladder cancer in urine specimens,[39,40] biliary tract malignancy in biliary tract brushing specimens,[41] and lung cancer in bronchoscopic brushing and sputum specimens.[42–45]

The FISH assay that has been used for lung cancer detection contains probes to 5p15.2, 7p21, 8q24 and to the pericentromeric region of chromosome 6, which are labeled with green, red, gold, and aqua fluorophores, respectively. The 7p21 and 8q24 probes hybridize to the *EGFR* and *C-MYC* genes, which are both implicated in lung cancer tumorigenesis. The 5p15 probe hybridizes to a region near the gene for the reverse transcriptase subunit of the telomerase enzyme, which is also implicated in lung cancer tumorigenesis. The finding of as few as five (or more) cells with gains of two or more of the four probes in this probe set on a cytologic slide prepared from a bronchial brushing is consistent with a diagnosis of lung cancer (Figure 12.7). Several studies suggest that FISH with this probe set is significantly more sensitive but slightly less specific than conventional cytology at detecting lung cancer.[42–45]

Tumor Typing

Fluorescence in situ hybridization has been extensively used to help type hematologic tumors such as chronic myelogenous leukemia, promyelocytic leukemia, Burkitt's lymphoma,[46,47] and soft tissue sarcomas such as synovial and Ewing's sarcomas,[48] because these malignancies often have characteristic chromosomal translocations. For example, virtually all patients with chronic myelogenous leukemia have a reciprocal translocation involving chromosomes 9 and 22, and this particular translocation is generally found only in chronic myelogenous leukemia. Consequently, the identification of this translocation by FISH can be used to type this tumor. Solid tumors have much more complicated chromosomal abnormalities

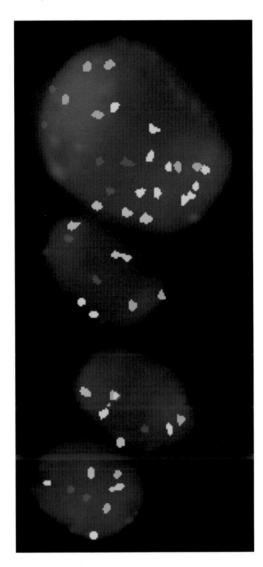

FIGURE 12.7. Fluorescence in situ hybridization detection of lung cancer in bronchoscopic brushing specimen using the LAVysion™ probe set: 5p15 (green), CEP6 (aqua), 7p12 (red), 8q24 (gold). Note that the three normal cells on the bottom show only two copies for each of the four probes, while the malignant cell (top) shows extra copies for all four of the probes.

than are found in hematologic malignancies and soft tissue sarcomas, and chromosomal abnormalities that are specific for one solid tumor versus another have not been identified. Consequently, in situ hybridization has not as yet been helpful for distinguishing different types of lung cancer or other solid tumor types.

Prognostication and Guiding Treatment

The best example of how in situ hybridization has been used to assess prognosis and guide therapy in oncology is its use to detect *HER2* gene amplification in breast cancer. Studies have shown that women whose breast cancer demonstrates *HER2* amplification (~25% of the cases) have a worse survival than those whose breast cancer does not.[49] In addition, women whose tumor shows *HER2* amplification respond more favorably to Herceptin, a humanized monoclonal antibody that is directed to the *HER2* receptor, than women whose tumor does not show *HER2* amplification.[50,51] Recent studies suggest that *EGFR* amplification detected by FISH in lung cancer may predict worse survival but a more favorable response to Iressa (gefitinib), an immunotherapeutic drug to the *EGFR* receptor.[52–56]

Infectious Disease

In situ hybridization has been used to detect viruses, bacteria, and fungi in various specimen types. The probes used for the detection of bacteria, mycobacteria, or fungi are generally directed to either the 16S or 23S rRNA of the organism. The rRNA sequences make ideal targets because they are well characterized among different organisms and are known to be relatively specific for given microorganisms. In addition, there are often as many as 10,000 to 100,000 ribosomes, and thus 10,000 to 100,000 rRNA copies in growing bacterial cells, providing many targets for these probes. This produces strong signals without the need for further signal amplification.

In situ hybridization can be used not only to identify the presence of an organism in tissue but also to provide important additional information about the position and abundance of the organism in the specimen. The ability to identify a microorganism without prior culture can be a definite advantage for microorganisms such as *Mycobacterium* that are not easily cultured or that take a long time to culture.

Inherited Diseases

Fluorescence in situ hybridization is frequently used to detect chromosomal alterations that are associated with certain inherited disorders. For example, FISH is used to identify chromosomal alterations associated with congenital disorders, such as Down, Edwards, and Patau syndromes, neurofibromatosis.[57,58] DiGeorge syndrome, mental retardation (using subtelomeric probes),[59] and Charcot-Marie-Tooth syndrome.

Conclusion

In situ hybridization is a technique that utilizes nucleic acid (DNA or RNA) probes to assess intact cells for various types of alterations. To understand how in situ hybridization works, one should be familiar with DNA and RNA composition and structure, principles of base pairing, and factors which influence denaturation and hybridization. Techniques that utilize ISH include FISH, CISH, comparative genomic hybridization, spectral karyotyping, and multicolor FISH. These techniques have found many important applications in oncology, genetics, and infectious disease.

Acknowledgments. We thank Lisa Peterson (Figure 12.5), Renan Mota and Reid Meyer (Figure 12.6), and Jesse Voss (Figure 12.7) for their technical assistance in preparing these figures for publication.

References

1. Beltz GA, Jacobs KA, Eickbush TH, et al. Isolation of multigene families and determination of homologies by filter hybridization methods. Methods Enzymol 1983;100:266–285.
2. Lee C, Wevrick R, Fisher RB, et al. Human Centromeric DNA's. Hum Genet 1997;100:291–304.
3. Knight SJ, Flint J. Perfect endings: a review of subtelomeric probes and their use in clinical diagnosis. J Med Genet 2000;37:401–409.
4. Moog U, Arens YH, van Lent-Albrechts JC, et al. Subtelomeric chromosome aberrations: still a lot to learn. Clin Genet 2005;68:397–407.
5. Morrison LE, Ramakrishnan R, Ruffalo TM, et al. Labeling fluorescence in situ hybridization probes for genomic targets. In Fan Y-S, ed. Molecular Cytogenetics: Protocols and Applications, vol 204. Totowa, NJ: Humana Press; 2002:21–40.
6. Wiktor AE, Van Dyke DL, Stupca PJ, et al. Preclinical validation of fluorescence in situ hybridization assays for clinical practice. Genet Med 2006;8:16–23.
7. Petersen BL, Sorensen MC, Pedersen S, et al. Fluorescence in situ hybridization on formalin-fixed and paraffin-embedded tissue: optimizing the method. Applied Immunohistochemistry Mol Morphol 2004;12:259–265.
8. Schurter MJ, LeBrun DP, Harrison KJ. Improved technique for fluorescence in situ hybridisation analysis of isolated nuclei from archival, B5 or formalin fixed, paraffin wax embedded tissue. Mol Pathol 2002;55:121–124.
9. Tubbs RR, Hsi ED, Hicks D, et al. Molecular pathology testing of tissues fixed in prefer solution. Am J Surg Pathol 2004;28:417–419.
10. Van Stedum S, King W. Basic FISH techniques and troubleshooting. In Fan Y-S, ed. Molecular Cytogenetics: Protocols and Applications, vol 204. Totowa, NJ: Humana Press; 2002:51–63.
11. Solovei I, Walter J, Cremer C, et al. FISH on three-dimensionally preserved nuclei. In Beatty B, Mai S, Squire J, eds. FISH: A Practical Approach. Oxford: Oxford University Press; 2002:119–158.
12. McNicol AM, Farquharson MA. In situ hybridization and its diagnostic applications in pathology. J Pathol 1997;182:250–261.
13. Florijn RJ, Bonnet J, Vrolijk H, et al. Effect of chromatic errors in microscopy on the visualization of multi-color fluorescence in situ hybridization. Cytometry 1996;23:8–14.
14. Tanke HJ. Fluorescence microscopy for quantitative fluorescence in situ hybridization analysis. In: Andreeff M, Pinkel D, eds. Introduction to Fluorescence In Situ Hybridization: Principles and Clinical Applications. New York: Wiley-Liss, 1999:33–52.
15. Downs-Kelly E, Pettay J, Hicks D, et al. Analytical validation and interobserver reproducibility of EnzMet GenePro: a second-generation bright-field metallography assay for concomitant detection of HER2 gene status and protein expression in invasive carcinoma of the breast. Am J Surg Pathol 2005;29:1505–1511.
16. Sokolova IA, Halling KC, Jenkins RB, et al. The development of a multitarget, multicolor fluorescence in situ hybridization assay for the detection of urothelial carcinoma in urine. J Mol Diagn 2000;2:116–123.
17. Lapierre JM, Tachdjian G. Detection of chromosomal abnormalities by comparative genomic hybridization. Curr Opin Obstet Gynecol 2005;17:171–177.
18. Kallioniemi OP, Kallioniemi A, Sudar D, et al. Comparative genomic hybridization: a rapid new method for detecting and mapping DNA amplification in tumors. Semin Cancer Biol 1993;4:41–46.
19. Vissers LE, Veltman JA, van Kessel AG, et al. Identification of disease genes by whole genome CGH arrays. Hum Mol Genet 2005;14(Spec Issue 2):R215–R223.
20. Kim TM, Yim SH, Lee JS, et al. Genome-wide screening of genomic alterations and their clinicopathologic implications in non–small cell lung cancers. Clin Cancer Res 2005;11: 8235–8242.
21. Peng WX, Shibata T, Katoh H, et al. Array-based comparative genomic hybridization analysis of high-grade neuroendocrine tumors of the lung. Cancer Sci 2005;96:661–667.
22. Shibata T, Uryu S, Kokubu A, et al. Genetic classification of lung adenocarcinoma based on array-based comparative genomic hybridization analysis: its association with clinicopathologic features. Clin Cancer Res 2005;11:6177–6185.
23. Tonon G, Wong KK, Maulik G, et al. High-resolution genomic profiles of human lung cancer. Proc Natl Acad Sci USA 2005;102 9625–9630.
24. Petersen I. Comparative genomic hybridization of human lung cancer. Methods Mol Med 2003;75:209–237.
25. Ashman JN, Brigham J, Cowen ME, et al. Chromosomal alterations in small cell lung cancer revealed by multicolour fluorescence in situ hybridization. Int J Cancer 2002;102: 230–236.
26. Chujo M, Noguchi T, Miura T, et al. Comparative genomic hybridization analysis detected frequent overrepresentation of chromosome 3q in squamous cell carcinoma of the lung. Lung Cancer 2002;38:23–29.
27. Massion PP, Kuo WL, Stokoe D, et al. Genomic copy number analysis of non–small cell lung cancer using array comparative genomic hybridization: implications of the phosphatidylinositol 3-kinase pathway. Cancer Res 2002;62:3636–3640.
28. Lindstrom I, Nordling S, Nissen AM, et al. DNA copy number changes in lung adenocarcinoma in younger patients. Mod Pathol 2002;15:372–378.
29. Goeze A, Schluns K, Wolf G, et al. Chromosomal imbalances of primary and metastatic lung adenocarcinomas. J Pathol 2002;196:8–16.

30. Pei J, Balsara BR, Li W, et al. Genomic imbalances in human lung adenocarcinomas and squamous cell carcinomas. Genes Chromosomes Cancer 2001;31:282–287.
31. Petersen I, Bujard M, Petersen S, et al. Patterns of chromosomal imbalances in adenocarcinoma and squamous cell carcinoma of the lung. Cancer Res 1997;57:2331–2335.
32. Balsara BR, Sonoda G, du Manoir S, et al. Comparative genomic hybridization analysis detects frequent, often high-level, overrepresentation of DNA sequences at 3q, 5p, 7p, and 8q in human non–small cell lung carcinomas. Cancer Res 1997;57:2116–2120.
33. Petersen I, Langreck H, Wolf G, et al. Small-cell lung cancer is characterized by a high incidence of deletions on chromosomes 3p, 4q, 5q, 10q, 13q and 17p. Br J Cancer 1997;75:79–86.
34. Levin NA, Brzoska PM, Warnock ML, et al. Identification of novel regions of altered DNA copy number in small cell lung tumors. Genes Chromosomes Cancer 1995;13:175–185.
35. Levin NA, Brzoska P, Gupta N, et al. Identification of frequent novel genetic alterations in small cell lung carcinoma. Cancer Res 1994;54:5086–5091.
36. Ried T, Petersen I, Holtgreve-Grez H, et al. Mapping of multiple DNA gains and losses in primary small cell lung carcinomas by comparative genomic hybridization. Cancer Res 1994;54:1801–1806.
37. Schrock E, du Manoir S, Veldman T, et al. Multicolor spectral karyotyping of human chromosomes. Science 1996;273:494–497.
38. Speicher MR, Gwyn Ballard S, Ward DC. Karyotyping human chromosomes by combinatorial multi-fluor FISH. Nat Genet 1996;12:368–375.
39. Skacel M, Fahmy M, Brainard JA, et al. Multitarget fluorescence in situ hybridization assay detects transitional cell carcinoma in the majority of patients with bladder cancer and atypical or negative urine cytology. J Urol 2003;169:2101–2105.
40. Halling KC, King W, Sokolova IA, et al. A comparison of cytology and fluorescence in situ hybridization for the detection of urothelial carcinoma. J Urol 2000;164:1768–1775.
41. Kipp BR, Stadheim LM, Halling SA, et al. A comparison of routine cytology and fluorescence in situ hybridization for the detection of malignant bile duct strictures. Am J Gastroenterol 2004;99:1675–1681.
42. Bubendorf L, Muller P, Joos L, et al. Multitarget FISH analysis in the diagnosis of lung cancer. Am J Clin Pathol 2005;123:516–523.
43. Varella-Garcia M, Kittelson J, Schulte AP, et al. Multitarget interphase fluorescence in situ hybridization assay increases sensitivity of sputum cytology as a predictor of lung cancer. Cancer Detect Prev 2004;28:244–251.
44. Romeo MS, Sokolova IA, Morrison LE, et al. Chromosomal abnormalities in non–small cell lung carcinomas and in bronchial epithelia of high-risk smokers detected by multi-target interphase fluorescence in situ hybridization. J Mol Diagn 2003;5:103–112.
45. Halling KC, Rickman OB, Kipp BR, et al. A comparison of cytology and fluorescence in situ hybridization for the detection of lung cancer in bronchoscopic specimens. Chest 2006;130:694–701.
46. Kearney L, Horsley SW. Molecular cytogenetics in haematological malignancy: current technology and future prospects. Chromosoma 2005;114:286–294.
47. Frohling S, Scholl C, Gilliland DG, et al. Genetics of myeloid malignancies: pathogenetic and clinical implications. J Clin Oncol 2005;23:6285–6295.
48. Bennicelli JL, Barr FG. Chromosomal translocations and sarcomas. Curr Opin Oncol 2002;14:412–419.
49. Press MF, Bernstein L, Thomas PA, et al. HER-2/neu gene amplification characterized by fluorescence in situ hybridization: poor prognosis in node-negative breast carcinomas. J Clin Oncol 1997;115:2894–2904.
50. Vogel CL, Cobleigh MA, Tripathy D, et al. Efficacy and safety of trastuzumab as a single agent in first-line treatment of HER2-overexpressing metastatic breast cancer. J Clin Oncol 2002;20:719–726.
51. Hicks DG, Tubbs RR. Assessment of the HER2 status in breast cancer by fluorescence in situ hybridization: a technical review with interpretive guidelines. Hum Pathol 2005;36:250–261.
52. Cappuzzo F, Toschi L, Domenichini I, et al. HER3 genomic gain and sensitivity to gefitinib in advanced non–small-cell lung cancer patients. Br J Cancer 2005;93:1334–1340.
53. Hirsch FR, Varella-Garcia M, McCoy J, et al. Increased epidermal growth factor receptor gene copy number detected by fluorescence in situ hybridization associates with increased sensitivity to gefitinib in patients with bronchioloalveolar carcinoma subtypes: a Southwest Oncology Group Study [see comment]. J Clin Oncol 2005;23:6838–6845.
54. Cappuzzo F, Varella-Garcia M, Shigematsu H, et al. Increased HER2 gene copy number is associated with response to gefitinib therapy in epidermal growth factor receptor-positive non–small-cell lung cancer patients. J Clin Oncol 2005;23:5007–5018.
55. Suzuki S, Dobashi Y, Sakurai H, et al. Protein overexpression and gene amplification of epidermal growth factor receptor in nonsmall cell lung carcinomas. An immunohistochemical and fluorescence in situ hybridization study. Cancer 2005;103:1265–1273.
56. Cappuzzo F, Hirsch FR, Rossi E, et al. Epidermal growth factor receptor gene and protein and gefitinib sensitivity in non–small-cell lung cancer. J Natl Cancer Inst 2005;97:643–655.
57. Kluwe L, Siebert R, Gesk S, et al. Screening 500 unselected neurofibromatosis 1 patients for deletions of the NF1 gene. Hum Mutat 2004;123:111–116.
58. Riva P, Corrado L, Natacci F, et al. NF1 microdeletion syndrome: refined FISH characterization of sporadic and familial deletions with locus-specific probes. Am J Hum Genet 2000;66:100–109.
59. Xu J, Chen Z. Advances in molecular cytogenetics for the evaluation of mental retardation. Am J Med Genet Part C Semin Med Genet 2003;117:15–24.

13
Proteomics

Larry Fowler and Wieslaw Furmaga

Omics

The establishment of a complete human genome sequence has opened a new era in biology referred to as *omics*. The term designates a complete analysis of biologic systems in which entire metabolic pathways are studied. This new methodologic approach becomes possible because of the dynamic development of advanced instrumentation unique for each of the omics subdisciplines. By increasing analytical sensitivity and through transformation into high-throughput analysis, such technologies as DNA and protein microarray or mass spectrometry have become a driving force for omics research. The amount of information derived from omics disciplines has in turn stimulated the development of bioinformatics. By improving the methods of storage and analysis of large amounts of data, an improved system of bioinformatics allows efficient exchange of information among researchers and contributes significantly to the development of omics disciplines. Despite its short history, this new methodology has proved its effectiveness by advancing our understanding of biologic processes, which brings hope for more accurate diagnosis and treatment of diseases.

Genomics and Transcriptomics

In light of omics as a "method of thinking large," *genomics* can be defined as a comprehensive study of DNA structure and function. Genomics studies single nucleotide polymorphisms and DNA mutations and investigates gene expression in cells. The analysis of gene expression has evolved into transcriptomics, an independent field with specific methodology and instrumentation. The main shortcoming of both genomics and transcriptomics is their inability to predict phenotypic and functional consequences of mutations or single nucleotide polymor-

phisms. To gather that information, analysis at the effector protein level is necessary.

Proteomics

The ambition of proteomics is to perform a systematic study of proteins and to present a complete explanation of the structural, functional, and regulatory roles of these proteins in a particular biologic system. The technologic and methodologic evolutions have made it possible to go beyond a simple biochemical analysis of a single protein and to progress into investigation of the complex protein mixtures. In conjunction with highly advanced bioinformatics, proteomics is able to explain physiologic and pathologic processes in both normal and diseased cells, and therefore it has a chance to become an essential component in laboratory diagnostics.

The first tool that helped evolve protein biochemistry into proteomics was two-dimensional gel electrophoresis. Despite its imperfections, two-dimensional gel electrophoresis is still used for protein profiling and/or quantitation of protein expression. The main limitation of this method is its low sensitivity, making it unfeasible for analysis of posttranslational modifications and protein–protein interactions. However, rapid progression in mass spectrometry and protein microarray technology has offered solutions to the two-dimensional electrophoresis limitations. The new generation of user-friendly mass spectrometers is able to analyze a protein mixture with high sensitivity and specificity as well as perform in a high-throughput mode on different types of specimens (serum, bronchoalveolar lavage [BAL], tissue and cell extracts). The improvements in protein microarray technology and in affinity chromatography permit efficient isolation of protein complexes and study of protein—protein interactions. All of these bring proteomics closer to being a useful diagnostic tool for lung disease.

Proteomics: A New Diagnostic Tool for Lung Diseases

Genomics and transcriptomics measure gene expression and transcriptional activities of the cells. It has been widely recognized that the changes in protein expression cannot be predicted at the level of gene amplification or at the level of mRNA production.[1] For this reason, as well as the fact that proteins are the true effectors that change a functional state of cells, it is the proteins that should be examined as the most pertinent markers for cellular function.[2] Performed on cytologic or surgical specimens, proteomics shows a complete picture of cellular activity and, along with other omics, provides new information about physiology, pathology, and cellular reaction to treatment. If cytologic or histologic diagnostic material is not accessible, or when the main goal is the discovery of a new marker, protein profiling in biologic fluids such as blood, urine, BAL, and pleural fluid may be performed.[3] The primary objective for protein profiling is the discovery of a protein that is different in the pathologic than in the physiologic state. It is accomplished by a comparison of an entire collection of proteins present in the specimen derived from healthy and diseased organisms.

The Ideal Proteomics

The ideal proteomics can be described as a method, or a series of methods, that can analyze an unmodified specimen in its entirety in both the control and the testing groups and is able to detect 100% of the proteins present in these sets. The results of proteomics experiments are submitted for evaluation, which analyzes the entire data and recognizes the proteins that differ between the control and the testing groups (proteins of difference). These selected proteins are subsequently used as a characteristic signature for a particular state of a cell or an organism and can be used for both an explanation of the biochemical pathways and for diagnosis.

This simple model of proteomics becomes complicated by what is referred to as *abundance*. There are approximately 35,000 human genes encoding proteins. Most of the proteins undergo posttranslational modifications so that the actual number of functionally active proteins exceeds 1 million.[4] Therefore, if a particular metabolic process involves 0.1% of the total protein composition (proteome) in order to fulfill the proteomics requirement that the entire spectrum of proteins must be detected, the protein collection characteristic for this state exceeds 1,000 individual particles.[4]

The problem of abundance affects both the laboratory (separation and identification) and the analytical (data analysis) portions of the proteomics process. For separation and identification, the problem is not only to detect the low-abundance proteins but also to avoid recording artificial peptides that are not naturally produced. Similarly, abundance makes it more difficult to obtain sufficient statistical power for data analysis and to prove that the detected protein of difference is systematic and not incidental.[4]

Shotgun and Protein Profiling

For diagnostic purposes, proteomics methods are not restricted to surgically removed lung tissue but can also be used to analyze fine-needle aspirates, BAL, pleural effusions and serum. For all of these specimens, proteomics provides a unique opportunity to evaluate the entire protein content.

Because the amount of analyzed proteins is large, to improve the identification process and to alleviate overload, the original specimen is fractionated and divided into portions containing the proteins with similar physicochemical properties. The process of fractionation is performed on gel electrophoresis or by mass spectrometry. The information received during the fractionation process can be used in two different ways. The first one is the shotgun protocol, in which the identification process of proteins present in a chosen fraction is performed. The proteins are identified by using fingerprinting and/or a sequence tag methodology and subsequently they are evaluated as a potential diagnostic marker. The second approach is protein profiling, in which the electrophoretic spots or mass spectrometric peaks obtained from control and test groups are compared and the pattern of difference (discriminatory pattern) is detected. In this methodology, the pattern by itself consists of characteristics of a particular cellular state or state of the organism. The electrophoretic pattern is defined as the presence or absence of protein spots at particular locations, as well as the intensity of their staining. The mass spectrometry pattern is described as either the presence or absence of spectral peaks and their amplitudes. The discriminatory pattern that separates the control from the testing group is usually related to the small subset of proteins or peptides present in the barely visible electrophoretic spots or that shows up as small spectrometric peaks hiding in the background of the spectra.

To differentiate between the groups, the amount of data to be analyzed is so large that for most instances it exceeds the capacity of the human brain. For this reason, to evaluate data from two-dimensional gel electrophoresis or from mass spectrometry, the advanced pattern recognition software are used as integrative tools of proteomics protocols. Despite difficulties, the protein profiling approach has noted some successes. The pattern of mass spectrometry peaks has been successfully used as a marker for differentiation between ovarian carcinoma and noncancer cases with a sensitivity of 100% (95% CI, 93–100), a specificity of 95% (87%–99%), and a positive predictive value of 94% (84%–99%) [5].

Protein Identification

For protein identification, a chosen fraction received by two-dimensional electrophoresis separation is enzymatically digested and submitted for mass spectrometry analysis. There are two general methods for protein identification used by proteomics: protein mass fingerprinting[6] and protein sequence tagging. In fingerprinting methods, the molecular mass of the chosen peptide from the specimen is compared with the database that contains a collection of proteins and peptides derived from these proteins after enzymatic digestion. Based on the similarity of masses, a cluster of protein candidates is selected that can potentially be present in the mixture. For each of these protein candidates, a matching score is calculated that reflects the probability that this candidate is a factual protein present in the specimen. The higher the score, the higher the probability that a given protein is truly present in the specimen.

The protocol of protein identification based on a sequence tag is similar to fingerprinting, with the only difference being that rather than the molecular mass, the sequence of amino acids is compared between peptides from the specimen and from the database. The calculation and interpretation of the matching scores are similar for both methods. The most efficient way for high-throughput protein identification is to combine the tagging and fingerprinting methods.

Data Validation

Because the amount of data collected with each proteomics run is oversized, a separate field of bioinformatics has been developed to support researchers and to increase the efficiency of data analysis. For this purpose, a new proteomics-specialized software operating with modern statistical methods has been developed. The example is software packet for biomarker discovery that comprises hierarchical clustering, principal component etc. and which is sold by Bio-Rad along with the SELDI mass spectrometer.

Proteomics Instrumentation

Two-Dimensional Gel Electrophoresis

The first protein separation method that met omics criteria was two-dimensional polyacrylamide gel electrophoresis (PAGE). This technique is able to accept minimally prepared specimens and to separate all proteins present in the mixture. Because of its contribution to proteomics and its popularity among researchers, the name *two-dimensional electrophoresis* has become almost synonymous with the term *proteomics*. Two-dimensional PAGE can be divided into two procedural steps. The first is isoelectric focusing (IEF), which separates proteins based on differences in isoelectric (pI) points. During IFE separation, proteins migrate along a pH gradient until they reach a point where the pH is equal to the pI. At that point, the net charge of the protein becomes zero and migration stops. At the end of this step, the original mixture of proteins is divided into fractions with the same pI. The second step of two-dimensional PAGE separates proteins based on their molecular mass and is performed on sodium dodecylsulfate (SDS)–polyacrylamide gel. To visualize separated proteins located in the spots that share the same pI and molecular weight, staining with silver or Coomassie Blue G-250 is performed. In an ideal situation, in which the sensitivity of separation is 100%, each spot would contain one protein. Unfortunately, the sensitivity of two-dimensional PAGE is not perfect, which contributes to several serious methodologic problems.

Methodologic Obstacles of PAGE

Two-dimensional PAGE requires considerable manual operation. For both shotgun and protein profiling approaches, precise and reproducible placement of spots on the gel is critical. Even minute changes in protocol and/or environment may lead to misplacement of identical spots, which could be mistakenly evaluated as spots of difference. During IEF, even minimal changes in the pH gradient from one experiment to the other deposit the same proteins in different locations on the strip and change their placement on the final gel. This problem was significantly reduced when an immobilized pH gradient was introduced. Despite improvement in the procedure, large hydrophobic proteins failed to be separated by IFE because of their tendency to aggregate and precipitate around their pI. The problem of precipitation also plagues separation of strong acidic or basic proteins, which occurs on the extreme points of the IEF strip.

The second step of the two-dimensional PAGE separation requires a precise placement of IFE strips on the SDS-polyacrylamide gel slab because any inconsistency changes the final location of the same protein from run to run. To secure precise and reproducible placement of the IFE strip on the gel slab, new hardware that is capable of consistent transfers of immobilized pH gradient strips onto the SDS-PAGE has been introduced. If performed on polyacrylamide gel the second dimension of separation is limited to the proteins with sizes larger than 10kDa. The smaller proteins, as well as low-abundance proteins with the number of copies fewer than 1,000 per cell, do not separate. This system is also unable to separate hydrophobic proteins such as the membrane proteins, which consist of low-abundance proteins with large hydrophobic domains. Two-dimensional PAGE also does not support separation of posttranslationally modified proteins, because these proteins are present in low concentrations, far below the sensitivity of this system.

Protein Staining

The next step in the two-dimensional PAGE separation is protein visualization. The staining not only reveals individual proteins but also, by its intensity, provides information about protein concentration. Unfortunately, most of the dyes also stain the background and quantitation of the protein is not simple. It requires statistical calculation that separates the intensity of background from spot staining.

There are a number of stains used, each with its own strengths and weaknesses. Silver (without glutaraldehyde) and Coomassie Blue G-250 stains are the most commonly used, with a preference for the former because of its significantly higher sensitivity. Silver staining is not specific for peptides but also stains the background, which drastically decreases its sensitivity. To minimize background stain and to increase the sensitivity for protein detection, glutaraldehyde is used. There is no end-point for the silver staining reaction, which means that the intensity of the color is directly proportional to time of staining.[7] The silver stain procedure is also not compatible with mass spectrometry and with fingerprinting protein identification. This incompatibility is due to protein oxidation and covalent modification during contact with silver and formaldehyde as well as to peptide—peptide binding occurring during background discoloration with glutaraldehyde.

The Coomassie Brilliant Blue stains proteins by chemical interaction with arginine residues. The staining process is not time dependent but relates to amino acid composition and stops when all arginine amino acids are saturated. For this reason, the relationship between staining intensity and protein concentration is not linear.[8] To establish this relationship, several gels with different protein concentrations must be run simultaneously. This solves the problem but slows down the process of identification.[7] The sensitivity for protein detection by Coomassie Brilliant Blue is much lower than that of the silver stain, but it possesses a higher compatibility with mass spectrometry. To take advantage of the high sensitivity of the silver stain and the mass spectrometry compatibility of the Coomassie Brilliant Blue, both techniques should be used in tandem.[9]

The sensitivity of protein visualization has been significantly improved through the use of fluorescent labeling agents such as ruthenium II tris, SYPRO dyes, and cyanine dyes to the extent that posttranslationally modified proteins can be revealed as a distinct spot. Another advantage of using fluorescent dyes is that the intensity of the staining is not time dependent, and it produces minimal background staining. Although special protocols and equipment are required, a fluorescent stain can be used for detection of low-abundance proteins. This method cannot, however, be used for protein quantitation, because the intensity is proportional to the amino acid composition rather than to the protein concentration.

To improve quantification of proteins, a special staining technique using stable isotopes was developed. In this procedure, both light and heavy isotopes of hydrogen, nitrogen, and carbon are used for in vitro or in vivo protein labeling. In vitro labeling is used mostly for relative quantification of the differences in protein concentrations between two states of a cellular culture or an organism.[7] The protein concentrations present at different cellular states can be calculated from the difference of signal intensities detected by mass spectrometry between the heavy and the light forms of protein. Thus far, in vitro labeling has generally been tested on samples of low complexity, such as commercially available proteins or simple systems such as viruses. Despite its promise, this method requires significant improvement before utilization with more complex systems.

Enzymatic and Nonenzymatic Digestion

The spots present on two-dimensional PAGE contain groups of similarly sized and charged proteins. To perform protein identification, the spots are excised and digested using enzymatic or nonenzymatic methods. During this process the proteins present in the spots are cleaved into smaller peptides suitable for mass spectrometry. The most common enzyme used for this process is trypsin. Its popularity is related to its low cost and to its generation of peptides of a size that is ideal for mass spectrometry analysis. The other proteases such as Glu-C endoprotease are used sparingly because of its production of large amounts of autoproteolytic peptides.[9] Cyanogen bromide is the most commonly used nonenzymatic agent. It produces peptides that are too large for mass spectrometry, and it must thus undergo additional cleavage with trypsin.

All of the enzymes used in preparatory digestion cleave proteins at well-defined sites. If the sequences of the protein and the digesting enzyme are known, it is possible to deduce the number, sequence, and molecular weight of all peptides produced by digestion. This information has been collected in databases that are readily accessible through the Internet. Database information such as peptide molecular mass and peptide sequence is used during the process of protein identification by fingerprinting and by protein sequence tag methods.

Like any other PAGE stages, enzymatic preparatory digestion carries several methodologic problems that need to be solved. For example, proteins with small lysine and arginine residues are not good targets for trypsinization, because they produce large fragments not suitable for mass spectrometric analysis. In addition, tryptic fragmentation of proteins is a very imprecise process that not only skips certain cleavage sites but also targets amino acids other than lysine and arginine, which complicates the fingerprinting method of protein identification.[10]

Mass Spectrometry

Mass spectrometry became a potential diagnostic technology at the time when electrospray ionization (ESI) and matrix-assisted laser desorption/ionization (MALDI) instruments were developed. These tools combine both high sensitivity and easy utility, which makes them ideal for commercialization. The new mass spectrometry technology coupled with automated and semiautomated specimen delivery systems provides the ability to perform high-throughput operations, an important aspect of diagnostic tools. Analyzing proteins in their original complex forms and performing this operation in high-throughput mode fulfills the omics criteria and makes modern mass spectrometry useful for proteomics procedures.

Matrix-Assisted Laser Desorption/Ionization

Originally described in 1987,[11] MALDI is a mass spectrometer in which the specimen is imbedded into matrix in a 1:1,000 ratio. Matrix is composed of small molecules that absorb ultraviolet waves. In the MALDI instrument, ultraviolet laser is pointed at the matrix, which induces solvent vaporization and matrix crystallization. During crystallization, the specimen is incorporated into matrix crystals and vaporized. The vaporized clouds of ionized crystals are directed into a detector, most commonly the time of flight (TOF) mass analyzer. The MALDI-TOF technique is used to analyze thousands of different components, but its role in proteomics seems to be the most significant. Because of its ability for precise measurement of the peptides' molecular masses, MALDI has become the most important instrument in the fingerprinting method of protein identification. With current technology, in which samples are automatically processed and deposited on the MALDI target plate, the procedure is rapid and requires no more than 2 min for processing one sample.[12]

The most common mass detector coupled with MALDI is the TOF analyzer. The analytical sensitivity of modern TOF is high enough to allow for fingerprinting identification of proteins present in a mixture even at very low concentration.

Protein identification based on amino acid sequence is performed on two variants of the MALDI mass spectrometer, MALDI-Oq-TOF (Oq indicating quadrupole-quadrupole time of flight) and MALDI-TOF/TOF.[13] These instruments operate with a collision chamber located between the first and second mass analyzer. The first analyzer measures molecular masses of peptides present in the specimen. One peptide is chosen from the mixture and is directed to the collision chamber for fragmentation. The second analyzer measures the molecular masses of the fragments produced in the collision chamber, which is the basis for sequencing of the chosen peptide.

Imaging Mass Spectrometry

A technologic improvement of MALDI mass spectrometry evolved into a new method called *imaging mass spectrometry* in which the mass spectrometer produces a two-dimensional ion image of the sample with labeled localizations of target molecules.[14] There are two techniques used for imaging mass spectrometry. The blotting technique requires fresh tissue to be placed on a methanol-wetted organic membrane, which allows for protein to be bound. After the tissue is removed, the blotted area is submitted for MALDI-TOF mass spectrometry analysis. The second technique calls for frozen tissue to be placed on a flat metal MALDI target plate and to be covered by the matrix. The image is constructed by mapping the m/z value over the target area. Imaging mass spectrometry allows gathering of information about protein distribution directly from the tissue and measuring their relative concentration and local composition. This technique has been successfully used for protein visualization in glioblastoma of the brain and in non–small cell carcinoma of the lung. In clinical practice, it can be used to identify different populations of cells based on their molecular differentiation, which can be used to clear surgical margins at the molecular level.[14]

Although this technology seems extremely attractive, several serious limitations must be overcome before its implementation in diagnosis. The size of the analyzing spats is limited by the laser spat, which is 30 μm in diameter. The polar solvent used cannot dissolve membrane proteins, leaving them unanalyzed. The use of this technique in anatomic pathology is limited by the overshadowing effect. In the overshadowing effect, a low signal is suppressed by a higher one, which most often comes from hemoglobin on the cut surface. In addition, every limitation of the MALDI is also pertinent in this system.

Surface-Enhanced Laser Desorption/ Ionization Mass Spectrometry

The other spectrometric system that has gained interest is surface-enhanced laser desorption/ionization (SELDI) mass spectrometry. This system uses microchip technology and is promoted predominantly by Bio-Rad. A minimally prepared or nonprepared specimen containing a mixture of proteins is applied to an aluminium or steel microchip support platform measuring 1–2 mm in diameter. The surface of the miniplate is coated with chemical matrices ("bites") similar to chromatographic columns and composed of hydrophobic, cationic or anionic phases. With these types of bites, proteins are separated based on their physicochemical properties such as pI point. The mixture of proteins and peptides present in the specimen is applied to the chip, and groups of proteins with similar physicochemical properties bind to the surface. The unbound proteins are removed during the washing process. The chips can also be coated with more specific matrices such as antibodies, enzymes, ligands, proteins, receptors, or DNA oligonucleotides. These specifically reacting chips are designed to interact with a single target protein and are used to study specific molecular interactions such as protein–protein, protein–antibody, as well as protein–receptor or protein–DNA interactions.[16] The bound "bite" proteins of interest are subsequently analyzed by MALDI-TOF or MALDI-TOF/TOF mass spectrometry. Microchips are suitable for analyzing all possible specimens, including cellular lysate, BAL, pleural fluid, sputum, and serum.

To enhance the analyzing efficiency of the results, the instrument is equipped with pattern recognition software. This program analyzes configuration of spectrometric peaks and recognizes a difference in the patterns between healthy and diseased cells, as well as between different stages of disease or different states of normal organisms. This approach provides a basis for discovering biomarkers, a strategy called *proteomics pattern diagnostics*.[17] This strategy has been successfully applied to the development of diagnostic patterns for ovarian cancer,[18] prostate cancer,[19] and breast cancer.[20] To validate biomarker correlation with progression of various cancers, an artificial neuronal network logarithm has been integrated with the SELDI mass spectrometry instrument. Artificial neural network is a statistical tool that imitates the learning ability of the human brain. PRoPeak software provided by Bio-Rad is based on an artificial neural network and is able to "learn" to recognize universal elements based on repeat analysis of the complex data from at lest two experimental groups. Based on the "experience" gained during the training set, the instrument develops criteria and rules that are validated during subsequent test runs. Each run is used to validate and modify the rules, similar to the typical learning process.

The usage of the pattern of mass spectrometric peaks as a marker for disease is a completely new approach in laboratory diagnostics and carries several methodologic and technical issues. The most serious ones are related to the low sensitivity of SELDI instrumentation, its limited reproducibility, and difficulties in protein identification.[21] In addition, several questions not specifically related to the SELDI instrumentation such as the validation of results among different laboratories, influence of different sample handling on results and different experimental designs have been raised.[21]

Other Types of Spectrometry

The other type of mass spectrometry used in proteomics is electrospray ionization (ESI) mass spectrometry. This operates on soft ionization, which allows the generation of ions from large (>100 kDa) nonvolatile analytes, such as proteins, with no fragmentation. The main difference between MALDI and ESI is that the latter produces multicharged ions and consequently more complex spectra. It collects more information, but at the same time its results seem to be more difficult to interpret than the less complex spectra from MALDI.[22] At the same time, MALDI possesses lower resolution and limited sequence information, which makes it less useful for identification of protein isoforms, posttranslational modifications, and protein complexes. In the recent years ESI has become a more user-friendly instrument and is more widely used than MALDI.

A "Dream Team" Mass Spectrometry System

The technologic challenge for today's proteomics is to develop a system that will allow rapid fractionation of the sample and efficient identification of proteins in the mixture in high-throughput mode. In 2004, Schrader and Klein published a paper describing the ideal proteomics system.[23] This scheme consists of a high-performance liquid chromatography–based separation system coupled with Fourier Transform Ion Cyclotron Resonance (LC-FTICR) mass spectrometry. The Schrader system helps to overcome the limited sensitivity of gel-based separation and limited accuracy of mass spectrometry. High-performance liquid chromatography is able to fractionate an entire specimen in a liquid environment into fractions containing proteins with precisely defined m/z. The FTICR detects ions in the mixture by measuring their frequency of resonance. Because frequency of resonance changes with mass, precise measurement of frequency allows for mass measurement with high resolution and accuracy. It seems to be the solution for problems related to the currently used, less accurate mass spectrometers. The FTICR is also able to analyze unfractionated samples. It can provide fast fractionation of a complex protein mixture, and it is able to perform mass measurement with precision, allowing for library-based protein identification using very narrow mass tolerances.

At the same time, Infrared Multiphoton Dissociation (IRMPD), a fragmentation method used for FTICR, produces peptide fragments similar to those obtained in the collision chamber in a tandem mass spectrometry system. The analysis of fragments is similar to that obtained by a tandem mass spectrometry system but with significantly higher mass accuracy and efficiency. This technique has been successfully employed for protein and oligonucleotide sequencing.

Proteomics Protocols

Protein Identification

Mass Fingerprinting Identification

There are two basic methods for high-throughput protein identification used by proteomics. They are mass fingerprinting identification and sequence base identification methods such as protein sequence tag.[24]

Mass fingerprinting identification was the first and is the most often utilized method by proteomics investigators. It is based on the fact that proteolytic enzymes cleave proteins at precisely defined points, and the numbers of peptides and their sequences and molecular masses can be predicted based on protein amino acid composition and on the characteristics of enzymatic action. The information about proteins and theoretical sets of peptides derived from them after enzymatic digestions are stored in a database. To identify proteins present in the specimen, molecular masses of experimental peptides are compared against molecular masses present in the database. If the molecular masses match, the peptide and its "mother" protein are identified. This perfect picture of protein identification is complicated in real life by several factors. The main obstacles are the mass spectrometer's instrumental sensitivity or degree of precision for molecular mass measurement and the database completeness for particular proteins.

The general rule for peptides matching is that the shorter fragments have a higher chance to be present in the experimental mixture and to be found in the database. On the other hand, the longer peptides are more specific for the "mother" protein. To obtain a search result with higher specificity, longer peptides are more desirable. Unfortunately, during the spectrometric procedure large peptides do not ionize as well as small ones do. For this reason, to increase the efficiency of mass measurement during an experiment, a larger number of small peptides is more desirable than a smaller number of large ones. The peptides with an average length of 8–10 amino

acid pairs are optimal for spectrometric analysis. The peptides with these characteristics are produced by trypsin, the proteolytic enzyme most widely used for preparatory digestion. Also, small proteins have a lower chance of being identified by the fingerprinting method than the large ones. This is because they produce a much lower number of digested fragments that are evaluated against the database. On the other hand, if two-dimensional PAGE is used for sample prefractionation, most of the large proteins with a molecular mass higher than 100 kDa are not identified because they are missed due to their incompatibility with IEF.

To increase the chance of correct protein identification, it is crucial to measure the mass of the ions with the highest possible accuracy. The number of peptides that differ from each other in the mass range of 0.5 Da is four times higher than the number of different peptides in the mass range higher than 0.5 Da. For the mass spectrometer with a mass resolution higher than 0.5 Da, the probability that dissimilar peptides are differentiated is higher than if the resolution is lower than 0.5 Da. The instrumental sensitivity is even more important for the detection of posttranslational modification or for the uncovering of a single element from a complex eukaryotic proteome.

A general rule for successful protein identification is that the most intense peaks should be submitted for this process. However, peak intensity is not always related to peptide abundance. An example is MALDI-TOF, which creates peaks with intensity depending more on arginine content than on peptide concentration. It indicates that arginine-rich proteins have a greater chance of being identified by MALDI-TOF spectrometry than proteins with low arginine contents.

Sequence-Based Identification

It is possible that in a digested protein mixture, especially one derived from eukaryotic organisms, there are a number of peptides with the same molecular mass but with different amino acid compositions. It is also possible that the same mixture contains peptides with slightly different masses that are not discriminated by the mass spectrometer. For these cases, molecular mass alone cannot be the basis for protein identification, and to increase scoring and certainty for protein identification, amino acid sequencing is added to the protocol. Peptide sequencing is performed with tandem mass spectrometry, in which the spectrometers are separated by a collision chamber. When the mixture of ions reaches the first mass spectrometer, the molecular masses are measured and one of the ions is chosen for future sequencing. This ion is directed to the collision chamber, where the peptide is fragmented into a unique spectrum of derived ions. The molecular masses of the derived ions are measured in the second mass spectrometer. As a result, a series of increasing m/z is received, progressing from a single C amino acid to the entire peptide, where every subsequent ion differs from the previous by the mass of one amino acid.[25] Detailed analysis of the molecular masses of these fragments allows for the construction of amino acid sequences. For protein identification, the collision-induced spectra are compared with a comprehensive protein sequence in the database by using one of the identification algorithms. The simplest one starts with a match of the experimental ion mass with the masses of peptides present in the database. Usually, a wide window of mass tolerance is chosen, and a broad range of peptides is selected. In the next step, a theoretical sequence for each peptide candidate is created, which is then compared with the sequence of the experimental one. The identification process by collision-induced spectra is very efficient, because a sequence analysis brings supportive information to the identification process performed by the fingerprinting method.

Database Searching

There are several available databases that allow for comprehensive searches for molecular mass and for sequence matching. No matter which database is used, the peaks produced by internal standards and the peaks of autolytic peptides must be excluded from the search. For comprehensive fingerprint and sequence tag protein identification, the MASCOT, NCBI and Swiss-Prot databases are most widely used. The Swiss-Prot is not as complete as the other two, but it contains several tools for sequence analysis.

The NCBI can be searched entirely during each entry, but it requires more specific information, such as keratin contamination, the proteolytic enzyme used, the number of allowed missed cleavages, the usage of iodo-acetamide for cysteine modification, and the fixative modification in cysteine residues. This information narrows the spectrum of the search and reduces searching time.[26]

The MASCOT provides a complex search report expressed in numbers. The score of 100 identifies a protein, but any score between 70 and 100 indicates that a chosen protein is a good candidate for identification. The MASCOT also provides a list of unassigned masses. The most common reasons for unmatched peaks are tryptophan oxidation, methylation of aspartic and glutamic acids, and (not as often, but most excitingly) a new protein.

A very advanced tool for fingerprint identification is "iterative analysis," which analyzes in depth the two-dimensional PAGE protein distribution and protein composition within a single two-dimension spot. The software for the database search can be obtained from the Internet. Similar to the NCBI method, before the search is performed, masses of contaminants such as keratins, products of trypsin autolysis, and dye, must be removed from the spectra. The second step of interactive analysis consists of removing the peaks caused by neighboring spats and is done by MASCOT software. The final results of protein identification are reevaluated for the major components and contaminants. Unassigned peaks created by posttranslational modification can be detected and subsequently validated by tandem mass spectrometry.[27]

Validation of Protein Match

To validate matching accuracy for each candidate protein, various scoring methods are available. In the simplest one, the peak intensities of the experimental peptides are compared with those of the theoretical group. The most serious bias for this method is that the intensity of peaks depends on the collision energy. Any inconsistency in collision energy significantly changes the matching results. The most popular scoring systems using signal intensity produced by tandem mass spectrometry is MASCOT. The second generation of scoring methods is a series of more advanced validation systems that calculate the matching score based on intensity of collision energy and internal properties of the peptides.[28] The popularity of more advanced analytical methods is very low, and simpler MASCOT and SEQUEST systems still dominate the market.[29]

The sequence-based identification process may be obscured if the reference database for a particular organism is not available, if the identified protein underwent posttranslational modification not listed in the database, or if spectrometric peak intensity is doubtful because of low signal-to-noise ratio. These situations can be overcome by using a de novo sequencing method. There are three basic approaches to the de novo sequencing method: the exhaustive listing method, the subsequencing method, and the "graph theoretical" approach. Detailed descriptions of these methods are available elsewhere.[29]

A simpler version of de novo sequencing identification is the partial sequence method. It is based on the mass-sequence-mass protocol, which matches a molecular mass and established sequence for an experimental peptide with a theoretical partial sequence and the masses of peptide candidates.[29] The other group of methods is based on calculating the theoretical mass from peptide sequences in the database and comparing the results with observed peaks.

Although a large number of methods used for validation of sequence-based matching are used, it is difficult to assess which one is the best because there is no consistent evaluation protocol that can be used for method comparison.[30] No matter what kind of validation method is used, it seems obvious that the comprehensive identification method, which includes the fingerprinting and sequencing approach, increases the chance of correct identification not only of common proteins but also of proteins with extremely low and extremely high molecular masses.

Protein Quantification

For higher organisms, in which a large number of isoforms are produced from a single gene and proteins undergo extensive posttranslational modifications, the old concept of "one gene, one protein" does not hold anymore. The different isoforms of the same protein play important regulatory roles and may have the opposite effect on cellular function. The idea that a solitary protein participates in cellular metabolism as a single factor has been revised and changed to the theory that a protein network governs cellular functions. The function of these complexes is regulated not only by the actions of different isoforms but also by different concentrations of the participating proteins. Although the importance of different protein concentrations for cellular metabolism is well known, to this day there is no good method which measures absolute concentrations of the proteins or their isoforms. The only well-established method uses a stable isotope and measures a relative concentration of a protein in prokaryotic cells. This strategy is based on the ability of mass spectrometry to separate chemically identical proteins that differ by the stable isotope. The other method that brings hope of obtaining a solution to this problem is a new technology based on the multiphoton detection methodology. The sensitivity of this method is as high as 600 molecules per 1 L, and protein isoforms can be detected.[31]

There is no single method that can be used for simultaneous protein identification and quantification. The most widely used tactic is to identify and quantify individual components separately and to subsequently integrate these results using analytical tools. If two-dimensional PAGE is used for separation, protein spots are stained and the concentration of the protein is assessed by measuring stain intensity. The selected spot is subsequently excised, digested, and submitted for protein identification. The gel base approach carries several obstacles described earlier, of which the most important is the inability to detect low-abundance proteins, posttranslational modification, and protein complexes.[30]

The second approach for protein identification and quantification is a mass spectrometry–based protocol in which an entire protein mixture is submitted for analysis. Although more efficient than the gel-based approach, mass spectrometry protocols are still imperfect. One of the problems is related to low analytical sensitivity of single-dimension mass spectrometry and its insufficiency in detecting low-abundance proteins. The other shortcoming for this method is the poor relationship between peak intensity and analyte concentration. To surmount this problem, the known concentration of the substance, serving as an internal standard, must be added to the specimen. The obstacle to low instrumental sensitivity can be overcome by using a "dream team" mass spectrometry system comprised of high-performance liquid chromatography for prefractionation coupled with LC-FTICR.

Detection of Posttranslational Modification

Posttranslational modification is a reversible event serving as a regulatory process that modifies protein activity. During this process, proteins become mature and ready for their physiologic function. There is no single and efficient method to determine posttranslational modification in purified proteins or in any protein mixture. The most popular method of posttranslational modification detection is the use of different enzymes interacting with post-translationally modified proteins/peptides and subsequent analysis of the differences in molecular masses.

The most commonly observed modifications are phosphorylation, splicing, and disulfide bridges. Phosphorylation is an important regulatory mechanism and occurs at the serine, threonine, and tyrosine residues. During this modification, 80 Da is added to the molecular mass of the peptide, which can be detected by comparative mass measurement before and after treatment with alkaline phosphatase. However, this method is complicated by a low consistency in peptide ionization and by unpredictable protein fragmentation.[32] The nonenzymatic approach for detection of phosphorylation and other posttranslational modifications is based on a specific database search aimed at evaluation of modified and nonmodified peptides.[33]

Splicing is a regulatory mechanism for gene expression present in higher organisms that leads to the production of multiple proteins from a single transcript. Splicing can be detected by adding amino acid sequencing as a complementary identification method to the fingerprinting protocol. Disulfide bridging is formed between cysteine residues and can be produced in vivo or during sample preparation. It can occur within the same protein, producing a change in the tertiary structure, or between molecules with the formation of multimers. This modification changes the molecular mass and subsequently behavior during electrophoretic separation. The formation of multimers is suspected if the same amino acid sequence is detected in several bands or spats on the electrophoretic gel and can be confirmed by the presence of a molecular mass two or more times higher than the mass of a basic peptide.

The modification of proteins not only occurs in vivo as a regulatory process of protein activity but also can be artificially produced during laboratory procedures. For example, during electrophoresis, proteins react with non-polymerized acrylamide monomers and produce unusually modified amino acids such as alkalysated cysteine or propionamide. Similarly, during the staining procedure in the presence of acetic acid and methanol, asparic and glutamic acids are methylated.[34] For practical reasons it is important to be aware of these artificial modifications and not misinterpret them as naturally occurring.

Protein Complexes and Protein Interactions

In a physiologic environment, proteins do not exist as single entities but rather as a complex system responsible for cellular function and regulation. The methods of studying protein complexes must be able to evaluate not one but multiple elements, as one-on-one interaction between proteins is more an exception than a rule. Proteins interact not only with other proteins but also with nucleic acids, small molecules, and other components, such as drugs.

The classic system for studying the interaction between proteins or between a protein and other molecules is a design in which one component is used as bait for the isolation of its binding partner. The most serious obstacle to this system is its low reproducibility, even if the same bait is used for protein binding.[35]

The protein–protein interaction depends on changes in protein affinity, which is regulated by changes in the cytoplasmic environment. Because the environment of mass spectrometry is completely different from that in the cytoplasm, mass spectrometry is not a good method for studying protein–protein interaction. In recent years, new and more advanced methods for protein complex study have been developed. One is the "complex walking" strategy in which the complex is studied sequentially. The other method uses stable isotopes for labeling the different components of the protein complexes. This method allows for the identification of dynamic changes in protein composition in relation to different cellular states.

Applications to Pulmonary Pathology

All pathologic diseases of the lung have proteomics fluctuations, upregulated or downregulated, compared with the normal physiologic state. However, we remain on the cusp of proving whether these can be reliably detected by protein profile changes that will assist with the screening for specific disease states, differential diagnosis, prognosis, and/or therapeutic choices. Protein markers detected by monoclonal antibody techniques have been utilized clinically since the 1970s with variable success

but mainly for pulmonary neoplasm differentiation. The newer proteomics methodologies, as previously discussed, should allow comparison of pathologic changes from the "normal" physiologic state with the discovery of new differentiating proteins for all pathologic conditions. Early reports using more recent proteomics methodologies have tended to concentrate on screening for lung cancer[36,37] via serologic testing or bronchoalveolar washes,[38] but the potential exists for proteomic profile comparisons to be useful for the differential diagnosis of infection versus neoplasia and infections versus transplant rejection, diagnosis of chronic lung disorders, assessment of disease activity,[39] as well as the categorization and management of neoplastic pulmonary disease.

Advantages of this methodology include that it can also be utilized on "cell-poor" samples that by microscopic examination are not sufficient for diagnosis; and product expression can be more easily detected without "amplification," thus diminishing risks for confusion with contaminants as well as improving turn-around time. Proteomics assessment also fits within the current classifications of diseases by histology, cytology, and immunohistochemistry. Disadvantages currently include lack of standardization of methodologies as discussed earlier, thus affecting reproducibility, and a lack of knowledge of proteomics patterns from a host of potential "contaminants" as noted in serologic samples previously (medications, nonpulmonary disease states, etc.). With pulmonary specimens there is an even greater potential for respiratory specimen contamination (by talc, lidocaine gel, pollen, tobacco products, etc., located throughout the oral and respiratory tree other than the lung specifically)[40] as has been seen in cytologic examinations of respiratory specimens. In the following sections we discuss the potential of proteomics profiling for general pathologic conditions of the lungs as per particular clinical scenarios/differential diagnoses and provide currently published supportive references.

Noninfectious Inflammatory Diseases of the Lung

Tissue injury is mediated by a host of pathways that involve both the epithelial and stromal components of the lung as well as inflammatory cells. The building blocks to further define the dynamics of lung inflammatory processes and especially the understanding of chronic lung diseases are being established to connect to the clinical disease processes. Extensive study of the pulmonary fibroblast proteome has been reported by Malmström and colleagues.[41] They reported close to 2,000 protein identities from the pulmonary fibroblast alone.

Sepper and Prikk have also shown how proteomics can help us to understand and monitor some of the proteins that may serve as markers of ongoing inflammation, such as serine and the matrix metalloproteinases (MMPs).[42] They found elevated levels of MMP-8, -13, -14, and -2 mainly in active forms within BAL fluids by proteomics methodology. The MMP-8 levels in BAL fluid appeared to correlate inversely with the degree of airflow obstruction in bronchial asthma. They proposed that enhanced levels of different MMPs could reflect continuing tissue injury. Thus proteomics can potentially monitor beyond what cytologic features of the BAL fluid presently do without the potential variability of the pathologist's description of cellular features by microscopy. Many have voiced the hope that through the better and quicker detection of expressed protein products via modern methods with conditions such as asthma that further therapeutic targets will also be discovered.[39]

There have been suggestions that proteomics may be able to predict which smokers are developing or are at risk to develop chronic obstructive pulmonary disease.[43] Although sufficient screening tests may be currently available for some pulmonary diseases such as cystic fibrosis (CF), recent evaluations of protein differentials may also lead to newer specific therapies. Pollard et al.[44] showed, via mass spectrometry studies of cultured CF cells, a high abundance of proteins associated with inflammation, including the classic NF-κB, p65 (RelA) and NF-κB, p65 (RelB), and suggested that this high-abundance CF lung epithelial proteome could serve as a reference database for future studies of candidate CF drugs. Kriegova et al.[45] have recently reported 40 differentially expressed protein entities (2.75–185.62 kD) that were detected in patients with pulmonary sarcoidosis versus control subjects ($p < 0.05$) by SELDI-TOF performed on BAL samples. Differences also existed between stages of the disease.

Infectious Diseases of the Lung

Department of Defense grants[46] have been awarded to utilize proteomics profiling for rapid detection of a host of bacterial, viral, fungal, parasitic, and prion infectious agents not only for natural disease states but also for the detection of biologic agents that could be utilized as part of terrorist activities. The protein antigens of these agents also remain the target of vaccine and other therapies. Whether the complicated proteomics profile of respiratory specimens, including the inhaled "artifact" superimposed on preexisting or concomitant lung diseases, may be deciphered is yet to be determined. At least one report[47] indicated that utilizing the proteomics profile in the acute respiratory distress syndrome was helpful in the diagnosis and management of a severe acute respiratory syndrome outbreak. Infectious agents associated with neoplastic processes are also a target for proteomics research. Proteomics should be helpful in determining not only the presence of infectious agents in cancer

patients but also the progression of a neoplastic process associated with the infections and hopefully in identifying proteins that can be targets for therapy as well as screening (see later discussion).[48]

Transplant Rejection Versus Infection

A National Heart, Lung, and Blood Institute workshop in 2004 reviewed current difficulties with lung transplantation with suggestions on future pathways for exploration, including improved diagnosis and monitoring of acute and chronic rejection. Bronchoalveolar lavage samples at the time of endobronchial biopsy have been a target for evaluating acute and chronic rejection of lung transplants as well as for attempts at serologic testing.

Although gene expression has had limited success at detecting acute rejection,[49] hope remains that protein expression will be more useful. Whether detection of chemokines or other proteins in respiratory or serologic sampling by newer proteomics methodology will be helpful for detection and management of acute rejection remains to be determined.

Nelsestuen et al.[50] have reported three unusually intense peaks at m/z = 3,373, 3,444, and 3,488 that were identified as human neutrophil peptides 1–3. These were detected in archived BAL samples from lung transplant recipients using mass spectrometry. Eighty-nine percent of patients who developed bronchiolitis obliterans syndrome had sustained elevation of human neutrophil peptide levels on repetitive BAL samples, reaching as high as 6% of the total BAL protein. Some control patients demonstrated a slightly elevated human neutrophil peptide level that later declined in subsequent BAL samples. Human neutrophil peptide levels did not appear to correlate with episodes of acute rejection, cytomegalovirus, or fungal infections in their study. They found that the elevated human neutrophil peptide levels associated with the onset of bronchiolitis obliterans syndrome could predate the clinical onset of disease by up to 15 months.

Neoplastic Diseases of the Lung

The 5-year survival rate for lung cancer is <15% from the time of diagnosis[36] in large part because of the late stage of the disease at diagnosis. Great hope has been expressed that newer proteomics methods can bring about clinically useful screening for early stage lung cancer or identification of premalignant lesions.

Many researchers have already moved from investigations to definitively identify unique proteins within actual tumor samples to protein peak signatures or profiles of serologic samples for screening of lung cancer. Sensitivities of up to 93.3% and specificities of 96.7% have been reported for lung cancer,[51] results similar to those for screening of ovarian, prostate, and other primary malig-

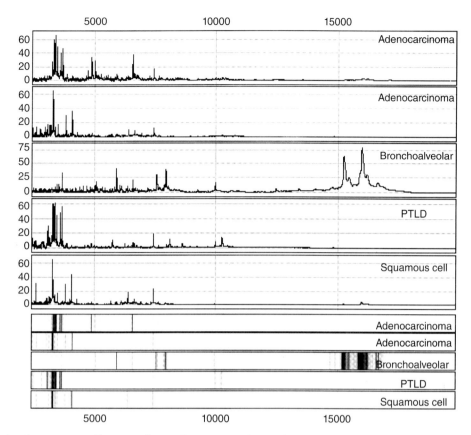

FIGURE 13.1. Protein signature profiles revealing unique patterns from fine-needle aspiration samples placed in Preserv-Cyt® and then processed by surface-enhanced laser desorption/ionization—time of flight mass spectrometry. PTLD, posttransplantation lymphoproliferative disease.

nancies by serologic sampling utilizing SELDI-TOF along with computational software. The benefit of such screening is potential detection of cancer at an earlier tumor stage when therapy may be more beneficial. Commercial laboratories and technical companies have already begun jumping on the bandwagon, promising to offer serologic testing for risk assessment of pulmonary malignancies, including mesothelioma.[52]

However, despite these headline-inducing reports, in-depth identification and characterization of lung malignancies remains ongoing. Zhukov at al., utilizing SELDI-TOF on laser-captured cells from frozen sections, were able to identify distinct protein profiles (signatures) specific for both lung tumors and the premalignant lesion of atypical adenomatous hyperplasia.[53] They found that three protein peaks between 17 and 23 kDa were markedly increased in malignant compared with normal cells, and the peak at 17,250 Da was not detected in any of the normal respiratory epithelial cells. Two peaks at the 17–18 kDa mass range were also increased in the "premalignant" cells of atypical adenomatous hyperplasia.

Yanagisawa et al., utilizing MALDI-TOF on laser-captured cells from tumor specimens as well as cultured cells, also revealed protein peak differences between normal and malignant cells.[54] Campa et al., using MALDI-TOF, not only revealed unique patterns in non–small cell malignancies but also identified overexpression of macrophage migration inhibitory factor and cyclophilin A.[55] We have noted similar protein signature (profile) differences in our own laboratory from fine-needle aspiration samples of fresh tumor specimens placed in PreservCyt® and processed as previously published[56] and evaluated by SELDI-TOF (Figure 13.1). Tyan et al. have shown that proteomics evaluation of pleural effusions can be helpful for staging and further evaluating patients with adenocarcinoma of the lung.[57]

Once unique profiles are determined that differentiate between normal tissue, premalignant conditions, and varying types of malignancies in a standardized, reproducible manner, then these proteins or portions of these proteins can be identified in sputum, BAL, pleural fluid, and serologic samples for screening, diagnosis, prognosis, and evaluation for tumor recurrence. Further identification of unique proteins may also lead to additional protein targets for future therapy, while the profile will allow the selection of therapies to which a given tumor is most likely sensitive. Table 13.1 lists some proteins identified as important in pulmonary disease.

TABLE 13.1. Some proteins identified as important in pulmonary disease.

Pulmonary protein	Expression	Disease process	Reference
Bax	Decreased	Dysplasia and cancer	37
Bcl-2	Increased	Dysplasia and cancer	37
Cyclin D1	Increased	Dysplasia and cancer	37
Cyclin E	Increased	Dysplasia and cancer	37
Cyclophylin A	Present	Cancer	56
Fibronectin	Increased	Lung remodeling	41
Alternatively spliced fibronectin (EDA fibronectin)	Increased	Lung remodeling	41
Human neutrophil peptides 1–3	Increased	Chronic transplant rejection	50
Migration inhibitory factor	Present	Cancer	55
Matrix metalloproteinase-8, -13, -14, and -2	Increased	Acute inflammation and asthma	42
Neuropilin-1 and -2	Increased	Dysplasia and cancer	37
NF-κB, p65 (RelA) and (RelB)	Increased	Cystic fibrosis	44
p16	Decreased	Dysplasia and cancer	37
p53	Increased	Dysplasia and cancer	37
p-Akt	Present	Dysplasia and cancer	37
SUMO-2	Present	Cancer	37
Thymosin-β4	Present	Cancer	37
Tob	Increased	Dysplasia and cancer	37
VEGF	Increased	Dysplasia and cancer	37

References

1. Gygi SP, Rochon Y, Franza BR, Aebersold R. Correlation between protein and mRNA abundance in yeast. Mol Cell Biol 1999;19:1720–1730.
2. Karin DR. Proteomics and cancer diagnosis: the potential of mass spectrometry. Clin Biochem 2004;37:579–583.
3. Patterson DS. Proteomics: beginning to realize its promise? Arthritis Rheum 2004;12:3741–3744.
4. Check E. Proteomics and cancer: running before we can walk? Nature 1004;429(6991):496–497.
5. Petricoin III FE, Ardekani MA, Hitt AB, et al. Use of proteomics patterns in serum to identify ovarian cancer. Lancet 2002;359:572–577
6. Henzel WJ, Stults JT, Wong SC, et al. Identifying proteins from two-dimensional gels by molecular mass searching of peptide fragments in protein sequence databases. Proc Natl Acad Sci USA 1993;90:5011–5015.
7. Moritz B, Meyer HE. Approaches for the quantification of protein concentration ratios. Proteomics 2003;3:2208–2220.
8. Consoli L, Damerval C. Quantification of individual zein isoforms resolved by two-dimensional electrophoresis: genetic variability in 45 maize inbred lines. Electrophoresis 2001;22:2983–2989.
9. Thiedea B, Höhenwarterb W, Kraha A, et al. Peptide mass fingerprinting. Methods 2005;35:237–247.
10. Godovac-Zimmermann J, Kleiner O, Brown RL, Drukier KA. Perspectives in spicing up proteomics with splicing. Proteomics 2005;5:699–709.
11. Karas M, Bachnann D, Bahr U, Hillenkamp F, Matrix. Assisted ultraviolet laser desorption of non-volatile compounds. Int J Mass Spectrom Ion Process 1987;78:53–68.
12. Burtis AC, Ashwood RE, Burns D. Tietz Textbook of Clinical Chemistry and Molecular Diagnosis, 4th ed. Philadelphia: Elsevier; 2006:170.

13. Loboda AV, Krutchinsky AN, Bromirski M, et al. A tandem quadrupole/time-of-flight mass spectrometer with a matrix-assisted laser desorption/ionization source: design and performance. Rapid Commun Mass Spectrom 2000;14:1047–1057.
14. Chaurand P, Caprioli MR. Direct profiling and imaging of peptides and proteins from mammalian cells and tissue sections by mass spectrometry. Electrophoresis 2002;23:3125–3135.
15. Stoeckli M, Farmer TB, Caprioli RM. Automated mass spectrometry imaging with a matrix-assisted laser desorption ionization time-of-flight instrument. J Am Soc Mass Spectrom 1999;10(1):67–71.
16. Poetz O, Schwenk MJ, Kramer S, et al. Protein microarrays: catching the proteome. Mech Ageing Dev 2005;126:161–170.
17. Petricoin E, Paweletz C, Liotta L. Clinical applications of proteomics: proteomic pattern diagnostics. J Mammary Gland Biol Neoplasia 2002;7:433–440.
18. Petricoin EF, Ardekani AM, Hitt BA, et al. Use of proteomic patterns in serum to identify ovarian cancer. Lancet 2002;359:572–577.
19. Petricoin EI, Ornstein D, Paweletz C, et al. Serum proteomic patterns for detection of prostate cancer. J Natl Cancer Inst 2002;94:1576–1578.
20. Zhang L, Rosenzweig J, Wang Y, Chan D. Proteomics and bioinformatics approaches for identification of serum biomarkers to detect breast cancer. Clin Chem 2002;48:1296–1304.
21. Rodland DK. Proteomics and cancer diagnosis: the potential of mass spectrometry. Clin Bioch 2004;37:579–583.
22. Reinders J, Lewandrowski U, Moebius J, et al. Challenges in mass spectrometry–based proteomics. Proteomics 2004;4:3686–3703.

23. Schrader W, Klein WH. Liquid chromatography/Fourier transform ion cyclotron resonance mass spectrometry (LC-FTICR MS): an early overview. Anal Bioanal Chem 2004;379:1013–1024.

24. Johnsona RS, Davisa MT, Taylorb JA, Pattersona SD. Informatics for protein identification by mass spectrometry. Methods 2005;35:223–236.

25. Papayannopoulos IA. The analysis of progressive spectra yields information about the amino acid sequence for the chosen peptide. Mass Spectrom Rev 1995;14:49–73.

26. Thiedea B, Höhenwarterb W, Kraha A, et al. Peptide mass fingerprinting. Methods 2005;35:237–247.

27. Schmidt F, Schmid M, Jungblut PR, et al. Iterative data analysis is the key for exhaustive analysis of peptide mass fingerprints from proteins separated by two-dimensional electrophoresis J Am Soc Mass Spectrom 2004;14:943–956.

28. Tabb LD, Smith LL, Breci AL, et al. Statistical characterization of ion trap tandem mass spectra from doubly charged tryptic peptides. Anal Chem 2003;75:1155–1163.

29. Shadforth I, Crowther D, Bessant C. Protein and peptide identification algorithms using MS for use in high-throughput, automated pipelines. Proteomics 2005;5:4082–4095.

30. Gygi SP, Corthals GL, Zhang Y, et al. Evaluation of two-dimensional gel electrophoresis-based proteome analysis technology. Proc Natl Acad Sci USA 2000;97:9390–9395.

31. Kleiner O, Price DA, Ossetrova N, et al. Ultra-high sensitivity multi-photon detection imaging in proteomics analyses. Proteomics 2005;5(9):2322–2330.

32. Mann M. Analysis of protein phosphorylation using mass spectrometry: deciphering the phosphoproteome. Trends Biotechnol 2002;20:261–268.

33. MacCoss M J. Shotgun identification of protein modifications from protein complexes and lens tissue. Proc Natl Acad Sci USA 2002;99:7900–7905.

34. Galvani M, Hamdan M, Herbert B, Righetti GP. Alkylation kinetics of proteins in preparation for two-dimensional maps: a matrix assisted laser desorption/ionization—mass spectrometry investigation. Electrophoresis 2001;22:2058–2065.

35. Rotheneder H, Geymayer S, Haidweger E. Transcription factors of the Sp1 family: interaction with E2F and regulation of the murine thymidine kinase promoter. J Mol Biol 1999;293:1005–1015.

36. Granville CA, Dennis PA. An overview of lung cancer genomics and proteomics. Am J Respir Cell Mol Biol 2005;32:169–176.

37. Chanin TD, Merrick DT, Franklin WA, Hirsch FR. Recent developments in biomarkers for the early detection of lung cancer: perspectives based on publications 2003 to present. Curr Opin Pulm Med 2004;10(4):242–247.

38. Noël-Georis I, Bernard A, Falmagne P, Wattiez R. Proteomics as the tool to search for lung disease markers in bronchoalveolar lavage. Dis Markers 2001;17(4):271–284.

39. Houtman R, van den Worm E. Asthma, the ugly duckling of lung disease proteomics? J Chromatograph B 2005; 815(1–2):285–294.

40. Hirsch J, Hansen KC, Burlingame AL, Matthay MA. Proteomics: current techniques and potential applications to lung disease. Am J Physiol Lung Cell Mol Physiol 2004;287: 1–23.

41. Malmström J, Larsen K, Malmström L, et al. Proteome annotations and identifications of the human pulmonary fibroblast. J Proteome Res 2004;3(3):525–537.

42. Sepper R, Prikk K. Proteomics: is it an approach to understand the progression of chronic lung disorders? J Proteome Res 2004;3(2):277–281.

43. Merkel D, Rist W, Seither P, et al. Proteomic study of human bronchoalveolar lavage fluids from smokers with chronic obstructive pulmonary disease by combining surface-enhanced laser desorption/ionization—mass spectrometry profiling with mass spectrometric protein identification. Proteomics 2005;5(11):2972–2980.

44. Pollard HB, Ji X-D, Jozwik C, Jacobowitz DM. High abundance protein profiling of cystic fibrosis lung epithelial cells. Proteomics 2005;8:2210–2226.

45. Kriegova E, Melle C, Kolek V, et al. Protein profiles of bronchoalveolar lavage fluid from patients with pulmonary sarcoidosis. Am J Respir Crit Care Med 2006;173:1145–1154.

46. Drake RR, Deng Y, Schwegler EE, Gravenstein S. Proteomics for biodefense applications: progress and opportunities. Expert Rev Proteomics 2005;2(2):203–213.

47. Kang X, Xu Y, Wu X. Proteomic fingerprints for potential application to early diagnosis of severe acute respiratory syndrome. Clin Chem 2005;51(1):56–64.

48. Srivastava S, Verma M, Gopal-Srivastava R. Proteomic maps of the cancer-associated infectious agents. J Proteome Res 2005;4:1171–1180.

49. Gimino VJ, Lande JD, Berryman TR, et al. Gene expression profiling of bronchoalveolar lavage cells in acute lung rejection. Am J Respir Crit Care Med 2003;168:1237–1242.

50. Nelsestuen GL, Michael B, Martinez MB, et al. Proteomic identification of human neutrophil alpha-defensins in chronic lung allograft rejection. Proteomics 2005;5(6): 1705–1713.

51. Xiao X, Liu D, Tang Y, Guo et al. Development of proteomic patterns for detecting lung cancer. Dis Markers 2003–2004;19(1):33–39.

52. Robinson BWS, Creaney J, Lake R, et al. Mesothelin-family proteins and diagnosis of mesothelioma. Lancet 2003; 362(9396):1612–1616.

53. Zhukov TA, Johanson RA, Cantor AB. Discovery of distinct protein profiles specific for lung tumors and pre-malignant lung lesions by SELDI mass spectrometry. Lung Cancer 2003;40:267–279.

54. Yanagisawa K, Shyr Y, Xu BJ. Proteomic patterns of tumour subsets in non–small-cell lung cancer. Lancet 2003;362: 433–439.

55. Campa MJ, Wang MZ, Howard B, et al, Protein expression profiling identifies macrophage migration inhibitory factor and cyclophilin as potential molecular targets in non—small cell lung cancer. Cancer Res 2003, 63:1652–1656.

56. Fowler LJ, Lovell MO, Izbicka E. Fine-needle aspiration in PreservCyt®: a novel and reproducible method for ancillary proteomic pattern evaluation of breast neoplasms by SELDI-TOF. Mod Pathol 2004;17:1012–1020.

57. Tyan YC, Wu HY, Su WC, et al. Proteomic analysis of human pleural effusion. Proteomics 2001;5(4):1062–1074.

14
Animal Models of Lung Disease

Roberto Barrios

Introduction

The lung is a complex organ composed of many different cell types. Its architecture is difficult to dissect so that a researcher can analyze specific pathways and early lesions. Animal models afford the opportunity for investigators to experimentally manipulate a number of controlled variables such as strain of animal, environment, and the genome in order to investigate the molecular interactions involved in the pathogenesis of many lung diseases.[1] They also provide a unique opportunity to test potential therapeutic interventions. Transgenic mouse technology has provided a powerful tool for both neoplastic and noneoplastic disease investigation. Although the basic molecular biology terminology is covered in the first two chapters of this book, it is convenient to briefly review it here regarding the development of transgenic mice.

Transgenic Mouse Models

Injection of exogenous DNA into fertilized eggs (zygotes) is known as transgenesis and is the most common method to modify the germline of mice. The offspring of transgenic founders are usually examined for a specific phenotype and are used to characterize genes and gene regulatory elements. The procedure involves a construct made of a segment of DNA that contains the sequence of interest and that has been cut with restriction enzymes. This segment may be ligated to a promoter, which will induce expression of the transgene. Injection of the construct into mouse embryos results in a random integration of variable copy numbers into the mouse genome. The result will be expression of the transgene contained in the construct. Random integration and the copy number of the transgene are factors that cannot be controlled in the classic transgenic mouse technology.

The procedure necessitates the generation and characterization of several founders to ensure that the phenotype is dependent on the transgene and not a result of alterations in the function of an endogenous gene. The standard protocol involves injection of the DNA construct into the pronucleus of fertilized eggs (0.5-day post-coital embryos). These injected eggs are then implanted into the oviduct of a pseudopregnant foster mother. The injected DNA integrates randomly into the genome in a fraction of the implanted embryos. Founders are mated to demonstrate germline transmission and to establish a transgenic line.[2]

Nonneoplastic Diseases

Chronic Bronchitis and Emphysema

Chronic obstructive pulmonary disease (COPD) is one of the most common pulmonary diseases seen in clinical practice. Smoking is by far the most important risk factor for COPD. Because it is produced by a combination of environmental and genetic factors, animal models are ideal to study the pathogenesis of these conditions. A number of species have been proposed in the literature.[3] In recent years, mice have been shown to be excellent for these studies because mouse and human genomes are very similar[4] and because of the ability to modify the genetic constitution of the mouse by inducing a protein, knocking out genes, or creating new mutations. In addition, the physiology and general aspects of mouse biology are well known and a large number of inbred strains are commercially available.[5,6]

There are several experimental models of COPD and emphysema.[7–9] Some depend on endobronchial perfusion of proteolytic enzymes in guinea pigs, hamsters, and mice.[10] Others depend on tobacco smoke.[11,12] There are also mouse strains that develop emphysema spontaneously.[8]

An imbalance between collagen synthesis and degradation and between proteases and their inhibitors has been proposed for many years as a possible pathogenetic mechanism for the development of emphysema. It is not surprising that this hypothesis has been studied in experimental models. In theory, this imbalance may be due to an excessive production of proteases by inflammatory cells or by reduced synthesis or increased breakdown of antiproteases. This hypothesis generated a number of experimental models that included intratracheal instillation of papain, trypsin, porcine elastase, and human neutrophil elastase as well as a large number of other proteases.[13,14]

More recently, transgenic mice have allowed expression or overexpression of proteases, such as human interstitial collagenase (matrix metalloproteinase-1).[15,16] These mice develop emphysema that is very similar to that seen in human α_1-antitrypsin deficiency. The emphysematous changes are induced by degradation of type III collagen. Overexpression of interleukin-13 or interferon-γ increase the expression of matrix metalloproteinases that are most likely responsible for the emphysematous changes. Knockout of TIMP-3 and, in other models, knockout of surfactant protein D, induce "spontaneous," age-related emphysema.[17,18] A number of the previously mentioned models support the hypothesis of an imbalance between protein formation and degradation, a hypothesis that has also been proposed for the development of interstitial fibrosis.[19]

Asthma

A large number of animal models have been proposed to study asthma under experimental conditions.[20–23] These models have aided in the study of mechanisms and pathways leading to the development of airway hyperreactivity and inflammation. The majority of described models depend on previous sensitization and challenge with the offending antigen. Most of these models are reminiscent of the changes seen in individuals with airway hyperreactivity; however, the morphologic changes seen in these animals do not show the changes that the pathologist sees in patients with asthma. Sensitization and challenge with interleukins, such as interleukin-13 have provided new knowledge related to the roles of leukotrienes and the glutathione pathway in this disease.[24]

Cystic Fibrosis

With the discovery of the cystic fibrosis (CF) gene in 1989,[25–28] a number of models have been attempted. Three years later, the first CF mouse model was described.[29] Approximately 11 CF mouse models have been described.[30,31] Cystic fibrosis, the most common genetic disease among Caucasians, is caused by mutations in the gene encoding the cystic fibrosis transmembrane conductance regulator (CFTR). However, CFTR null mice did not develop pathology resembling human CF lesions.[32] A more promising model was that of Mall et al. in which they enhanced sodium absorption in mouse airways manipulating the epithelial sodium channel. This model has provided new insight into the pathogenesis of CF and the study of ion transport defects.[33]

Interstitial Lung Diseases

To understand the pathogenesis and possible therapeutic interventions in interstitial diseases that progress to fibrosis, animal models are of valuable help. Pathologists have known for decades that the pathogenesis of fibrosis is associated with a number of conditions, such as infections, collagen vascular disease, allergic alveolitis, and trauma. However, the origin and mechanisms of development of idiopathic interstitial pulmonary fibrosis remain uncertain, probably in part because of a lack of a good experimental model analog to human interstitial fibrosis. Despite the number of experimental models, we still lack a model that re-creates all the characteristics of human disease.

Similar to the approach for emphysema, researchers have attempted to instill fibrogenic agents intratracheally into various experimental models. Although these approaches attempt to elucidate some mechanisms of fibrogenesis, it is uncertain whether they really can be extrapolated to human disease. Nevertheless, our understanding of the basic pathology of the development of fibrosis has increased dramatically because of many of these models. A number of pioneer studies demonstrated that mice and other species were susceptible to the development of fibrosis after bleomycin (a profibrotic drug) instillation.[34–37] These models have been well studied; however, they do not resemble human idiopathic pulmonary fibrosis.[38] Paraquat-induced fibrosis has also been well described in experimental models,[39] but the lesions tend to be heterogeneous. With the development of transgenic technology, induced abnormal expression of extracellular matrix proteins, cytokines, and proteases have provided additional information.[40]

Although some of these models mimic pulmonary fibrosis, interpretation of the results requires critical analysis. At present, it is impossible to reproduce the natural history of human pulmonary fibrosis in an experimental model. Recent advances, however, such as microarray analysis, are providing better scrutiny of the initial mechanisms of disease. For example, it has been shown that bleomycin alters the gene transcription pattern in the mouse lung by increasing genes associated with inflammation, which reached maximum levels at 5 days after bleomycin administration, while genes involved in the development of fibrosis increased gradually up to 14 days after bleomycin treatment. These changes in gene expression signature were well correlated with observed histopathologic changes.[41] This approach will provide a sensitive method to assess gene expression and may help identify genes involved in clinical pulmonary fibrosis.

Animal Models of Lung Cancer

A large number of animal models of neoplastic diseases have been developed. Urethane-induced lung tumors in some strains of mice is a well known model that has been studied for many years,[42–47] and the mechanisms for the increased susceptibility of some mouse strains have been studied[48–50] with and without transgenic manipulation.[51] There are, however, many complications in establishing animal models of lung cancer, among them a good correlation between histologic patterns of human and animal malignancies, natural strain susceptibility, and time frames.

The first oncogene targeted specifically to the lung was the Simian virus (SV) large T antigen.[52] A model of pulmonary adenocarcinomas has been produced in transgenic mice harboring a chimeric gene comprising the SV40 large T antigen under the control of a transcriptional region derived from the human surfactant protein C gene.[53] In these studies, transgenic mice succumbed with pulmonary tumors within 4–5 months of age. By histology, the tumors were adenocarcinomas with lepidic, papillary, and solid growth patterns that were indistinguishable from adenocarcinomas occurring in humans. This model has been useful in our understanding of regulatory pathways disrupted during tumor progression.[54]

Surfactant protein C promoter has also been used to express c-Myc, epidermal growth factor, the recepteur d'origine nantais (RON), receptor tyrosine kinase (a member of the MET protooncogene family), and Raf-1. These models have been very useful for specifically targeting certain cell types such that other lung cell types are not directly affected.[55,56] Animal models for squamous cell carcinomas and small cell carcinomas are needed. Failure to develop specific tumor types is probably due to variability of the transgene expression early in lung development. Another limiting factor in the study of these models is that once transcription of the transgene is initiated, it is irreversible.

Apparently, conditional transgenic models have overcome these limitations. The ligand-inducible binary transgenic systems provide effective regulatory models. They consist of at least two transgene constructions, a regulatory transgene and a target transgene, to provide regulated expression of a specific gene. The regulator transgene encodes a transcription factor whose activity is determined by the administration of an exogenous compound. The regulator is placed under the control of a tissue-specific promoter in order to express the transcription factor in the tissue of interest. This regulator does not activate transcription of the target transgene until the animal receives an exogenous compound. When this compound is administered, the regulator activates only the target transgene. The other construct that contains the target gene also contains the sequence of a protein of interest under the transcriptional control of cis-actin DNA elements that are responsive to the DNA-binding domain of the regulator transgene. The currently used ligand-inducible binary transgenic systems are the tetracycline transactivator inducible system, the mifepristone gene switch, and the ecdysone regulatory system.[57]

Knockout Mouse Models

Knockout mouse production implies mutation or ablation of an endogenous gene by homologous recombination in embryonic stem cells. Basically, the embryonic stem cells with the appropriate target are injected into the blastocyst of a mouse embryo; mice born contain cells from both the host embryo and the targeted embryonic stem cells. If these embryonic stem cells incorporate themselves into the germline, the mutation can be transmitted to future generations.[2] There are limitations for the use of these models in lung cancer because the mutated or knockout gene will provide either a silent phenotype or will not allow the study of new neoplastic transformation in the adult mouse.

Ligand-dependent Cre recombinase provides a clever mechanism to produce controlled lesions. The technique depends on the Cre protein, which is encoded by the coliphage P1. It is a 38-kDa protein that efficiently promotes both intra- and intermolecular synapses and recombination of DNA both in *Escherichia coli* and in vitro. Recombination occurs at a specific site, called *lox*, and does not require any other protein factors. The Cre protein causes synapsis of DNA and site-specific recombination in a mammalian cell line. Cre protein activity is directly regulated by a ligand, which binds to the Cre recombinase and causes changes in conformation that allow the recombinase to edit floxed genes. Cre, the product of the *Cre* (cyclization recombination) gene of bacteriophage P1, catalyzes the reciprocal recombination of genomic segments that are flanked by *loxP* sequences. The recombinase Cre acts on the DNA site *loxP*. If there are two *loxP* sites in the same orientation near each other, Cre can act to loop out the sequence between the two sites, leaving a single *loxP* site in the original DNA and a second *loxP* in a circular piece of DNA containing the intervening sequence. Therefore, a properly designed targeting construct containing *loxP* sites can be used for introducing subtle mutations or for a temporally or spatially controlled knockout (see also Chapter 1).[2] Although this technology appears promising, it has not been applied successfully to the study of lung malignancies.[58,59]

Animal Models of Mesothelioma

Malignant mesothelioma has been linked to asbestos exposure and generally has a poor prognosis, because it is often diagnosed in advanced stages and is refractory to conventional therapy. Mouse models of pleural and peritoneal mesotheliomas have been produced by exposure to asbestos fibers, radionuclides, particulate nickel compounds, and chemicals such as 3-methylcholanthrene. The role of SV40 virus as a cofactor with asbestos fibers in the development of diffuse malignant mesotheliomas in humans has also been explored in animal models. Some models have shown that SV40 virus alone induces mesotheliomas in hamsters. Because human malignant mesotheliomas frequently show hypermethylation or deletions at the *CDKN2A/ARF* and *CDKN2B* gene loci and deletions or mutations at the *NF2* gene locus, heterozygous *NF2*(+/−) experiments with mice exposed to crocidolite asbestos fibers have been published. These mice exhibited accelerated development of malignant mesotheliomas compared with wild-type littermates.

An interesting study by Altomare et al.[60,61] in a mouse model of mesothelioma, demonstrated that mesotheliomas from asbestos-treated *Nf2*(+/−) mice show somatic genetic changes, including homozygous deletion of the tumor suppressor genes $p16^{INK4A}$, $p14^{ARF}/p19^{ARF}$, and/or $p15^{INK4B}$ that are very similar to events found in human malignant mesotheliomas. Moreover, they show that in both mouse and human malignant mesotheliomas, a similar reciprocal pattern of *ARF* loss versus *p53* alteration are present. Taken together, these data implicate a common set of cellular perturbations in both human and mouse malignant mesotheliomas. Thus, from these studies it seems that alterations of the p53/ARF and $p16^{INK4A}$ cell cycle regulatory pathways and the Akt and p21-activated kinase–merlin signal transduction pathways seem to be critical events that cooperate to drive malignant mesothelioma tumorigenesis in both human and murine malignant mesotheliomas. These findings are consistent with the view that cancer is a multistep process involving the accumulation of somatic genetic changes that enable tumor cells to override failsafe mechanisms regulating normal cell proliferation.[60,61]

Conclusion

Animal models of lung disease have provided extraordinary information to understand human disease. They are powerful tools that enable the study of the mechanisms and natural history of human diseases. Several species have provided good models for certain diseases; however, murine models have several intrinsic advantages compared with other animal models, including lower cost, less maintenance, and rapid reproduction rate. Transgenic or knockout mice can be generated in the laboratory in a relatively short time compared with other species. Nevertheless, anatomic and immunologic differences between mice and humans mean that murine models have limitations that must be considered when interpreting the results obtained from experimental models and applying these to the pathogenesis of human diseases. The methodology is limited by a number of factors, including species differences, lack of models that truly resemble human disease, and strain variations.

Although transgenic and knock out mice have been used in research for many years, the sequencing of the mouse and human genomes and high-density DNA expression analysis have recently added powerful tools to researchers using animal models. Furthermore, new knowledge of certain pathways altered in some diseases, obtained from animal models, may provide an opportunity for pharmacologic intervention.

References

1. Kumar RK. Experimental models in pulmonary pathology. Pathology 1995;27(2):130–132.
2. Argmann C, Dierich A, Auwrex J. Current Protocols in Molecular Biology. John Wiley & Sons; 2006.
3. Brusselle GG, Bracke KR, Maes AI, et al. Murine models of COPD. Pulm Pharmacol Ther 2006;19:155–165.
4. Paigen K. A miracle enough: the power of mice. Nat Med 1995;1(3):215–220.
5. Glasser SW, Korfhagen TR, Wert SE, Whitsett JA. Transgenic models for study of pulmonary development and disease. Am J Physiol 1994;267(5 Pt 1):L489–L497.
6. Ho YS. Transgenic models for the study of lung biology and disease. Am J Physiol 1994;266(4 Pt 1):L319–L353.
7. Shapiro SD. Animal models for COPD. Chest 2000;117 (5 Suppl 1):223S–227S.
8. Shapiro SD. Animal models for chronic obstructive pulmonary disease: age of klotho and Marlboro mice. Am J Respir Cell Mol Biol 2000;22(1):4–7.
9. Lucey EC. Experimental emphysema. Clin Chest Med 1983; 4(3):389–403.
10. Snider GL, Lucey EC, Stone PJ. Animal models of emphysema. Am Rev Respir Dis 1986;133(1):149–169.
11. Guerassimov A, Hoshino Y, Takubo Y, et al. The development of emphysema in cigarette smoke–exposed mice is strain dependent. Am J Respir Crit Care Med 2004;170(9): 974–980.
12. Bartalesi B, Cavarra E, Fineschi S, et al. Different lung responses to cigarette smoke in two strains of mice sensitive to oxidants. Eur Respir J 2005;25(1):15–22.
13. Valentine R, Rucker RB, Chrisp CE, Fisher GL. Morphological and biochemical features of elastase-induced emphysema in strain A/J mice. Toxicol Appl Pharmacol 1983;68(3): 451–461.
14. Gross P, Pfitzer EA, Tolker E, Babyak MA, Kaschak M. Experimental emphysema: its production with papain in normal and silicotic rats. Arch Environ Health 1965;11: 50–58.

15. Shiomi T, Okada Y, Foronjy R, et al. Emphysematous changes are caused by degradation of type III collagen in transgenic mice expressing MMP-1. Exp Lung Res 2003; 29(1):1–15.

16. Foronjy RF, Okada Y, Cole R, D'Armiento J. Progressive adult-onset emphysema in transgenic mice expressing human MMP-1 in the lung. Am J Physiol Lung Cell Mol Physiol 2003;284(5):L727–L737.

17. Zheng T, Zhu Z, Wang Z, et al. Inducible targeting of IL-13 to the adult lung causes matrix metalloproteinase- and cathepsin-dependent emphysema. J Clin Invest 2000;106(9): 1081–93.

18. Wang Z, Zheng T, Zhu Z, et al. Interferon gamma induction of pulmonary emphysema in the adult murine lung. J Exp Med 2000;192(11):1587–1600.

19. Elkington PT, Friedland JS. Matrix metalloproteinases in destructive pulmonary pathology. Thorax 2006;61(3):259–266.

20. Elwood W, Lotvall JO, Barnes PJ, Chung KF. Characterization of allergen-induced bronchial hyperresponsiveness and airway inflammation in actively sensitized brown-Norway rats. J Allergy Clin Immunol 1991;88(6):951–960.

21. Nagai H, Yamaguchi S, Inagaki N, et al. Effect of anti-IL-5 monoclonal antibody on allergic bronchial eosinophilia and airway hyperresponsiveness in mice. Life Sci 1993;53(15): PL243–PL247.

22. Renz H, Saloga J, Bradley KL, et al. Specific V beta T cell subsets mediate the immediate hypersensitivity response to ragweed allergen. J Immunol 1993;151(4):1907–1917.

23. Kung TT, Jones H, Adams GK 3rd, et al. Characterization of a murine model of allergic pulmonary inflammation. Int Arch Allergy Immunol 1994;105(1):83–90.

24. Chavez J, Young HW, Corry DB, Lieberman MW. Interactions between leukotriene C4 and interleukin 13 signaling pathways in a mouse model of airway disease. Arch Pathol Lab Med 2006;130(4):440–446.

25. Kerem B, Rommens JM, Buchanan JA, et al. Identification of the cystic fibrosis gene: genetic analysis. Science 1989; 245(4922):1073–1080.

26. Buchwald M, Tsui LC, Riordan JR. The search for the cystic fibrosis gene. Am J Physiol 1989;257(2 Pt 1):L47–L52.

27. Riordan JR, Rommens JM, Kerem B, et al. Identification of the cystic fibrosis gene: cloning and characterization of complementary DNA. Science 1989;245(4922):1066–1073.

28. Rommens JM, Iannuzzi MC, Kerem B, et al. Identification of the cystic fibrosis gene: chromosome walking and jumping. Science 1989;245(4922):1059–1065.

29. Snouwaert JN, Brigman KK, Latour AM, et al. An animal model for cystic fibrosis made by gene targeting. Science 1992;257(5073):1083–1088.

30. Davidson DJ, Rolfe M. Mouse models of cystic fibrosis. Trends Genet 2001;17(10):S29–S37.

31. Guilbault C, Saeed Z, Downey GP, Radzioch D. Cystic fibrosis mouse models. Am J Respir Cell Mol Biol 2007; 36(1):1–7.

32. Frizzell RA, Pilewski JM. Finally, mice with CF lung disease. Nat Med 2004;10(5):452–454.

33. Mall M, Grubb BR, Harkema JR, et al. Increased airway epithelial Na+ absorption produces cystic fibrosis-like lung disease in mice. Nat Med 2004;10(5):487–493.

34. Fleischman RW, Baker JR, Thompson GR, et al. Bleomycin-induced interstitial pneumonia in dogs. Thorax 1971;26(6): 675–682.

35. Adamson IY, Bowden DH. The pathogenesis of bleomycin-induced pulmonary fibrosis in mice. Am J Pathol 1974;77(2): 185–197.

36. Adamson IY, Bowden DH. Bleomycin-induced injury and metaplasia of alveolar type 2 cells. Relationship of cellular responses to drug presence in the lung. Am J Pathol 1979; 96(2):531–544.

37. Snider GL, Hayes JA, Korthy AL. Chronic interstitial pulmonary fibrosis produced in hamsters by endotracheal bleomycin: pathology and stereology. Am Rev Respir Dis 1978;117(6):1099–1108.

38. Borzone G, Moreno R, Urrea R, et al. Bleomycin-induced chronic lung damage does not resemble human idiopathic pulmonary fibrosis. Am J Respir Crit Care Med 2001;163(7): 1648–1653.

39. Popenoe D. Effects of paraquat aerosol on mouse lung. Arch Pathol Lab Med 1979;103(7):331–334.

40. Yoshida M, Sakuma J, Hayashi S, et al. A histologically distinctive interstitial pneumonia induced by overexpression of the interleukin 6, transforming growth factor beta 1, or platelet-derived growth factor B gene. Proc Natl Acad Sci USA 1995;92(21):9570–9574.

41. Katsuma S, Nishi K, Tanigawara K, et al. Molecular monitoring of bleomycin-induced pulmonary fibrosis by cDNA microarray-based gene expression profiling. Biochem Biophys Res Commun 2001;288(4):747–751.

42. Driessens J, Clay A, Vanlerenberghe J, Adenis L. [The urethane-induced experimental pulmonary adenoma in the mouse. I. Histological study.] CR Seances Soc Biol Fil 1962; 156:655–657.

43. Mirvish SS. The carcinogenic action and metabolism of urethane and N hydroxyurethane. Adv Cancer Res 1968;11: 1–42.

44. Brooks RE. Pulmonary adenoma of strain A mice: an electron microscopic study. J Natl Cancer Inst 1968;41(3):719–742.

45. Gargus JL, Paynter OE, Reese WH, Jr. Utilization of newborn mice in the bioassay of chemical carcinogens. Toxicol Appl Pharmacol 1969;15(3):552–559.

46. Shabad LM. Dose–response studies in experimentally induced lung tumours. Environ Res 1971;4(4):305–315.

47. Snyder C, Malone B, Nettesheim P, Snyder F. Urethane-induced pulmonary adenoma as a tool for the study of surfactant biosynthesis. Cancer Res 1973;33(10):2437–2443.

48. Cazorla M, Hernandez L, Fernandez PL, et al. Ki-ras gene mutations and absence of p53 gene mutations in spontaneous and urethane-induced early lung lesions in CBA/J mice. Mol Carcinog 1998;21(4):251–260.

49. Lin L, Festing MF, Devereux TR, et al. Additional evidence that the K-ras protooncogene is a candidate for the major mouse pulmonary adenoma susceptibility (Pas-1) gene. Exp Lung Res 1998;24(4):481–497.

50. Avanzo JL, Mesnil M, Hernandez-Blazquez FJ, et al. Altered expression of connexins in urethane-induced mouse lung adenomas. Life Sci 2006;79(23):2202–8.

51. Umemura T, Kodama Y, Hioki K, et al. Susceptibility to urethane carcinogenesis of transgenic mice carrying a

human prototype c-Ha-ras gene (rasH2 mice) and its modification by butylhydroxytoluene. Cancer Lett 1999;145(1–2): 101–106.

52. Furth PA. SV40 rodent tumour models as paradigms of human disease: transgenic mouse models. Dev Biol Stand 1998;94:281–287.

53. Wikenheiser KA, Clark JC, Linnoila RI, et al. Simian virus 40 large T antigen directed by transcriptional elements of the human surfactant protein C gene produces pulmonary adenocarcinomas in transgenic mice. Cancer Res 1992; 52(19):5342–5352.

54. Wikenheiser KA, Whitsett JA. Tumor progression and cellular differentiation of pulmonary adenocarcinomas in SV40 large T antigen transgenic mice. Am J Respir Cell Mol Biol 1997;16(6):713–723.

55. Kwak I, Tsai SY, DeMayo FJ. Genetically engineered mouse models for lung cancer. Annu Rev Physiol 2004;66:647–663.

56. Zhao B, Magdaleno S, Chua S, et al. Transgenic mouse models for lung cancer. Exp Lung Res 2000;26(8):567–579.

57. Albanese C, Hulit J, Sakamaki T, Pestell RG. Recent advances in inducible expression in transgenic mice. Semin Cell Dev Biol 2002;13(2):129–141.

58. Matsuda I, Aiba A. Receptor knock-out and knock-in strategies. Methods Mol Biol 2004;259:379–390.

59. Sato Y, Endo H, Ajiki T, et al. Establishment of Cre/LoxP recombination system in transgenic rats. Biochem Biophys Res Commun 2004;319(4):1197–1202.

60. Altomare DA, Vaslet CA, Skele KL, et al. A mouse model recapitulating molecular features of human mesothelioma. Cancer Res 2005;65(18):8090–8095.

61. Altomare DA, You H, Xiao GH, et al. Human and mouse mesotheliomas exhibit elevated AKT/PKB activity, which can be targeted pharmacologically to inhibit tumor cell growth. Oncogene 2005;24(40):6080–6089.

15
Tissue Culture Models

Roger A. Vertrees, Thomas Goodwin, Jeffrey M. Jordan, and Joseph B. Zwischenberger

Introduction

The use of tissue cultures as a research tool to investigate the pathophysiologic bases of diseases has become essential in the current age of molecular biomedical research. Although it will always be necessary to translate and validate the observations seen in vitro to the patient or animal, the ability to investigate the role(s) of individual variables free from confounders is paramount toward increasing our understanding of the physiology of the lung and the role of its cellular components in disease. Additionally, it is not feasible to conduct certain research in humans because of ethical constraints, yet investigators may still be interested in the physiologic response in human tissues; in vitro characterization of human tissue is an acceptable choice.

Tissue culture techniques have been utilized extensively to investigate questions pertaining to lung physiology and disease. The isolation and propagation of human bronchial epithelial cells has allowed investigators to begin to characterize the interactions and reactions that occur in response to various stimuli. Moreover, the culture of human airway smooth muscle has allowed researchers to investigate a pathologic cascade that occurs in asthma as well as other physiologic responses in the smooth muscle of the lung. Numerous lung cancer cell lines have been established to investigate their responses to chemotherapy and determine their biologic properties. Overall, the use of cultured human lung tissue has provided a windfall of information on the pathogenesis of diseases that affect the lung and on the basic physiology and development of the lung in general. Despite this wealth of information in the literature, this chapter is the first to discuss the use of tissue culture models to examine the physiology and pathologic basis of lung diseases. In light of this, we briefly discuss the history and principles behind the utilization of tissue culture. We then discuss the current use of tissue culture to examine many of the unanswered questions involved in pulmonary physiology and pathology.

History of Tissue Culture

The technique of tissue culture is generally accepted to have arisen following the experiment of Ross Harrison, around the turn of the twentieth century. In 1907, Harrison began by adapting a previously established bacteriology technique, the "hanging-drop" method, to culture a frog neuron.[1] In 1912, Alexis Carrel built upon this work by successfully culturing small tissue samples from an 18-day-old chick embryo heart, thereby becoming the first scientist to propagate mammalian cells in vitro.[2] Carrel's demonstration that cells could be passaged 18 times, remain viable over 3 months, and continue to maintain cardiac rhythm was the first to show that cardiac tissues in vitro could retain normal characteristics for a prolonged period of time. These elegant studies, conceived by Carrel, initiated the modern day art of *histoculture* as it is now known.[3,4]

Although only a small "sect" of researchers embraced early tissue culture as a methodology to investigate the pathogenesis of disease, it is appropriate to describe Carrel as the father of mammalian tissue culture. In fact, Sven Gard, in his presentation speech for the Nobel Prize in Physiology or Medicine in 1954 referred to tissue culture as a "tissue cult . . . with Carrel as their high priest." In that year, Drs. Weller, Enders, and Robbins shared the prize for their work in propagating poliovirus in tissue culture. This work was the first Nobel Prize awarded in medicine and physiology for work accomplished primarily utilizing tissue culture as a methodology.

An additional important milestone in the use of tissue culture in biomedical research was the establishment of the first human cell line. In 1951, cervical cancer cells from Henrietta Lacks were cultivated into the first immortal cell line—"HeLa."[5] HeLa cells are still one of the most widely used cell lines today. Since the 1950s, tissue culture has become firmly established as a mechanism to answer many questions in biomedical research. Today, tissue culture is widely used to investigate diseases that affect the lung, and through this work we have been able to increase our understanding of the pathologic cascades that occur in lung diseases, as well as the normal physiologies of the lung.

Types of Tissue Culture

Tissue culture is a commonly used generic term for the in vitro cultivation of cells, attributed to the early cultures that generally consisted of heterogeneous cultures of crudely disaggregated tissues. Currently, many terms are used that can be encompassed by the term: organ culture, cell culture, primary explants, and ex vivo propagation all deal with the in vitro cultivation of cells or tissues. *Cell culture* in general can be applied either to primary cells (e.g., those with a finite life span) or to cell lines (e.g., HeLa cells). Additionally, these cultures can be either a homogenous or a heterogenous group of cells.

Primary cell culture involves the isolation of cells from a tissue by disaggregation. Single cell suspensions from tissues can be completed through either enzymatic digestion of extracellular matrix surrounding the cells—such as with ethylenediaminetetraacetic acid, trypsin, or collagenase—or mechanical disaggregation. These disaggregation procedures have the disadvantage of possibly injuring cells. If the cells of interest are adherent viable cells, they will be separated from nonviable cells when the medium is changed. Alternatively, viable cells can be separated from nonviable cells prior to culture by subjecting the single cell suspension to density gradient centrifugation (e.g., Hypaque). Primary cells have an advantage of possessing many of the biologic properties that they possessed in vivo because they are not transformed. Primary cells, unlike cell lines, are not immortal and have only a finite survival time in culture before becoming senescent. Variant cells, however, as well as those obtained from neoplastic tissue, may proliferate infinitely, thus becoming immortal in vitro. This will eventually allow the immortal cell to take over the culture and can be thought of as a cell line. In general, primary human cultures will survive for 30–80 passages in vitro, although this number is dependent on cell type, conditions, and possibly other unknown factors. Primary cells are widely used to examine the effects of toxins, infectious agents, or other cellular interactions that would not be feasible in vivo. Primary cells have a disadvantage of being a heterogeneous mixture of cells upon primary isolation, with the type of cell obtained generally a component of the disag-

gregation method used. The most common contaminant seen following isolation of primary cells is cells of mesenchymal origin (e.g., fibroblasts). However, advances have been made that allow the culture of homogenous populations of cells. For instance, cell surface molecules specific for the cells of interest may be tagged with monoclonal antibodies. Techniques such as fluorescence-activated cell sorting or the use of magnetic beads can be utilized to enrich the single cell suspension for the cell type of interest. Additionally, some investigators have recently exploited unique characteristics of certain cells, such as the presence of P-glycoprotein or multidrug resistance-associated proteins expressed on endothelial cells, to poison other contaminating cells in culture.[6]

Another type of primary cell culture is "primary explants." This type of culture is not subjected to a disaggregation procedure like the primary cell technique described earlier. Therefore, single cell suspensions do not occur. Briefly, tissue samples are dissected and finely minced. These tissue pieces are then placed onto the surface of a tissue culture plate. Following plating of tissue pieces, cells have been shown to migrate out of the tissue and onto the tissue culture surface.[7] This technique is useful when cells of interest may become damaged or lost in the disaggregation technique described earlier and is often used to culture human bronchial epithelial cells.[8]

Cell lines are another useful source of cells to investigate questions in biomedical research. These cells have the advantage of being immortal as opposed to the finite life spans that primary cells possess. Additionally, they are generally well studied and characterized, leaving few experimental variables to worry about. These cells however, are prone to dedifferentiation—a process by which they lose the phenotypic characteristics of the cell from which they began. Many of the early cell lines were established from tumor tissue and as such possess abnormal growth characteristics. Newer cell lines have been established by molecular techniques such as inserting a telomerase gene into a cell to allow it to replicate infinitely.[9] Because of the phenotypic changes that allow cell lines to replicate infinitely in culture, they are often a first choice for experiments; however, they are also highly criticized in light of their nonnatural phenotype.

Organ culture, as the name implies, involves ex vivo culture of the whole or significant portion of the organ. The main advantage to this type of culture is the retention and preservation of the original cell–cell interaction and extracellular architecture. This type of culture may be particularly important when experimental design necessitates the use of an ex vivo system, but researchers still need to retain the original organ architecture to answer questions posed. These types of cultures do not grow rapidly, however, and are therefore not suitable for experiments needing large numbers of a particular cell type.[10]

Advantages and Limitations of Tissue Culture

Tissue culture has become the penultimate tool of the reductionist biologist. The utilization of tissue culture as a research methodology has allowed investigators to study isolated interactions in its near-normal environment. These experiments by their very nature introduce artifacts; however, they do minimize the number of confounding variables that may affect a particular experiment. For instance, tissue culture allows investigators to determine the effects of one particular treatment on a particular cell type, which would not be feasible in vivo. Additionally, tissue culture models of disease allow investigators to obtain samples and make observations more readily than those done in vivo. However, it is the relative simplicity of experiments done in vitro that allows models of disease or physiology to come under frequent and warranted criticism. These models do not take into consideration the complexity of biologic systems. Diminishing possible confounding variables by culturing cells in vitro brings up the constant criticism of how applicable results are because of alterations of the normal cellular environment in vivo. For example, cell–cell interactions in vitro are reduced and unnatural. Moreover, the culture does not contain the normal heterogeneity and three-dimensional architecture that is seen in vivo. This said, however, tissue culture biology has proved to be successful in many ways.

Cell Culture and the Study of Disease Processes

We have briefly discussed the advantages that experimental systems using tissue culture affords researchers studying physiology and pathogenesis. Because of its ability to isolate individual variables and determine their role(s) in physiology, cell culture has become an integral tool in deciphering the pathologic cascades that occur in human disease. Diseases that affect lung are no exception.

Many diseases that affect the lung, and humans in general, are multifactorial. This begs the question how can cell culture, because of its reductionist nature only dealing with a minimal number of variables, help to solve the unknown questions and decipher the components involved in disease? Often, clinical observations, and the questions arising therein, have been the launching pad for investigation.

For instance, observations of massive inflammation in the bronchoalveolar lavage samples of patients with acute respiratory disease syndrome (ARDS), consistent with damage seen in histologic samples, prompted investigators to determine the role(s) of inflammation in the etiology of ARDS. Through the use of cell culture, investigators were able to determine individual interactions that occurred in the disease process. Investigators have utilized culture models employing microcapillary endothelial cells under flow conditions to understand the role of proinflammatory cytokines in the cytokinesis and emigration of neutrophils in disease. Using a model of pulmonary endothelium under flow conditions allowed investigators to demonstrate the importance of certain proinflammatory cytokines in ARDS.[11]

The role of inhaled toxicants in lung injury, and the mechanism(s) by which they cause disease, is another area of investigation that has utilized cell culture. Scientists have developed diverse and unique tissue culture systems that contain air–liquid barriers of lung epithelium and subjected these cells to various gaseous toxicants to determine what occurs following inhalation of various chemicals. Utilizing these types of systems, investigators are able to control the exposure time and other variables that may be difficult when determining inhaled toxicant effects in vivo. Moreover, the use of tissue culture, as opposed to an animal model, allows investigators to observe effects kinetically, without undue changes (e.g., sacrifice) and expense in the experimental model.[11]

A tissue culture model also permits an investigator to observe multiple changes in real time, such as cellular integrity, cell signaling and intracellular trafficking, protein expression changes, oxidant-induced cellular damage, and more. Deciphering each of these changes in an animal model would be extremely difficult; through employing a tissue culture model, researchers are able to tightly control the experimental system while isolating the events of interest. Further examples of how tissue culture models are currently being used to elucidate questions in lung physiology and disease are discussed later in the section on lung tissue cell lines.

Biology of the Cultured Cell

Culture Environment

Maintaining cells in vitro was initially a very difficult task. Many characteristics need to be fulfilled before a successful cell culture occurs. Some of these characteristics are dependent on the type of tissue being studied; others may depend on specific requirements of the individual cells. Various chemically defined media are now available commercially to support the growth and differentiation of numerous cell types. The creation of defined media has allowed investigators to culture a multitude of cell types while controlling the local environment to answer pertinent questions. For example, glucose can be removed from a culture medium in order to study its effects on cellular metabolism, relative position in the cell cycle, and many other effects. Each chemical component is known in these media. Additionally, investigators can add growth factors to nourish their cell cultures.

The medium chosen when culturing cells in tissue culture must fit two main requirements: (1) it must allow cells to continue to proliferate in vitro, and (2) it must allow the preservation of the certain specialized functions of interest.[7] The most common medium formulations used currently in lung research are Dulbecco's modified Eagle's medium, minimum essential medium, RPMI 1640, and Ham's F-12. Occasionally, investigators develop new medium types to attain a formulation that optimizes their own experimental conditions. Fetal bovine serum is a common additive to most tissue culture media, although some investigators choose to forgo this additive for more defined supplementation. Additionally, others may choose sera from other sources such as human serum when culturing cells of human origin. Inactivation of complement by heat treating serum for 1 hr at 56°C was initially very popular in tissue culture. However, it has become clear that this treatment may in fact damage some of the proteinaceous growth factors present in the medium, rendering it less effective. Currently, many experts recommend heat inactivation only if the cell type of interest is particularly sensitive to complement.[12] More specific examples of medium utilized in lung tissue culture models are given later in the section on lung tissue cell lines.

When deciphering if the current culture conditions are sufficient for the experimental design, the investigator must determine which cellular characteristics are important. Not only are the general characteristics, such as adhesion, multiplication, and immortalization of cell types important, but so are tissue-specific characteristics. Of importance to pulmonary research, the lung is a unique environment to simulate in vitro because of the air–liquid interface. Recently, investigators have made use of culture insert wells (e.g., Transwells, Corning) in order to study this interaction.[6]

Cell Adhesion

Nearly all normal or neoplastic human epithelial cells will attach with relative ease to tissue culture surfaces. Most tissue culture models utilizing tissue of lung origin fit this description, with the notable exception of small cell lung carcinoma cell lines. However, for culture cells that may loosely adhere, or may not adhere at all, scientists coat tissue culture surfaces with extracellular matrix proteins. Incubating tissue culture surfaces with serum, as well as laminin, fibronectin, or collagen, prior to culture has been shown to improve attachment of finicky cells.[8] These treatments also help in replicating the normal attachment of cells to extracellular matrix proteins in vivo.

Development of Continuous Cell Lines

The development of continuous cell lines may be serendipitous, as was the development of early cell lines. In brief, many investigators would continue splitting primary cell cultures until one or more cell clones became immortal. Unfortunately, the changes that generally occurred in culture led to cells with abnormal phenotypes that had undergone dedifferentiation. Today, many investigators choose to use molecular biology techniques, exploiting our current knowledge of oncogenic viruses and enzymatic processes of cellular aging to transform primary cells in vitro to an immortal phenotype. It is known that the large T antigen present in the SV (Simian virus) 40 virus is capable of transforming cells to an abnormal phenotype.[11,13,14] Moreover, transfection of primary cells with a transposase enzyme has also been shown to induce an immortal phenotypic change while preserving most normal cellular functions and phenotypes.[11]

Dedifferentiation

A commonly encountered problem in tissue culture is dedifferentiation. This loss of phenotype may be insignificant to the research at hand or it may be critical, and it must be dealt with on a case by case basis. When a cell culture undergoes dedifferentiation it is often unclear whether undifferentiated cells took over the culture of terminally differentiated cells or whether a primary cell of interest became immortal under the culture conditions.

Functional Environment

The functional environment in which cells are cultured is critical when correlating experimental results to those seen in vivo. We previously alluded to the importance of the environment in which cells are cultured when discussing the advantages and limitations of tissue culture. Investigators have frequently strived to replicate integral in vivo environments in vitro in order to increase the significance of their experimental results.

The development of cell culture insert wells (e.g., Transwells, Corning) has allowed investigators to culture bronchial or alveolar epithelial cells at an air–liquid interface. This ability allows investigators to begin to replicate a significant aspect of these cells' functional environment in vitro, thereby increasing their understanding of the effects of gaseous particles on pulmonary epithelial cells. Alternatively, scientists have also cultured epithelial cells on a roller bottle apparatus. This method allows investigators to determine the amount of time the apical epithelial cell surface is in contact with the air.

Capillary cell cultures have also come under frequent criticism when cultured in a monolayer in a tissue culture plate. Investigators have been able to utilize gel matrices in which capillary cells form tubule-like structures, more closely replicating the architecture these cells maintain in vivo. Additionally, endothelial cells are constantly under flow conditions in vivo. Addressing this condition in vitro has allowed investigators to look at the role of endothelial cells during inflammation—helping to increase the understanding of the role endothelium plays in acute lung injury.

At times, researchers may also choose to determine the effects of soluble factors (e.g., cytokines, hormones, neurotransmitters) from acute patients or animal models in a cell culture model. The milieu of soluble factors present in the serum that may play a role in a disease state is considerable. Moreover, these factors may have actions alone that are different when combined with other soluble factors. Reconstituting every factor presents a difficulty in vitro and leaves the possibility that an unknown factor may be missing. To address this, investigators have harvested sera from patients or animal models and used these samples as additives in their media formulations. For instance, through the use of serum samples from an animal model of smoke/burn injury–induced acute lung injury, investigators have demonstrated that use of arteriovenous CO_2 removal in acute lung injury significantly reduces apoptotic cell death in epithelial cells.[15]

Lung Tissue Cell Lines: Establishment and Significance

The diversity of research fields utilizing tissue culture models of lung diseases is extensive. In this section, we will give a brief overview of the main lung cell types that are being utilized in research today to answer pressing questions about lung physiology and the pathophysiology of pulmonary disease. Included in this discussion is also an overview of cell isolation and culture.

Normal Human Bronchial Epithelial Cells

The use of normal human bronchial epithelial (HBE) cells is extensively reported in the literature. Based on a method pioneered by Lechner et al.,[16] bronchial fragments obtained from surgery, autopsy, or biopsy specimens may be used as explants. The outgrowth of bronchial epithelial cells occurs readily from these explants when grown in medium supplemented with bovine pituitary extract and epidermal growth factor. Alternatively, these cells have also been demonstrated to grow in basal keratinocyte serum-free medium without supplementation; however, they demonstrate a slower growth rate and earlier senescence.[8]

Cultures of HBE cells are valuable for determining the responses to toxic inhaled pollutants. In vitro exposure systems based on these methods have several advantages. First, in vitro exposure systems can be stringently controlled and reproduced much better than in animal systems; second, individual determination of the cell types' responses to pollutants allows for a better characterization of the individual involvement of the cell type to a biologic response. Finally, in vitro determination of the responses to toxic agents allows investigators to observe the reactions of human cells when testing in humans is not feasible because of ethical restraints.

In vitro study of the responses of bronchial cells to gaseous pollutants is not without its difficulties. Wallaert et al.[17] have described these constraints well. Briefly, because of the gaseous nature of the pollutants, culture systems should be designed that allow significant exposure times to pollutants while also taking care to inhibit cells from drying out when exposed to air. To facilitate these experiments, roller bottle cultures have been developed that allow cells direct contact with the ambient air. Alternatively, cells have been grown on a membrane filter and cultured at an air–liquid interface, which allows constant exposure to the experimental treatment. The same type of experiments that are used to determine the responses of cells to inhaled toxicants have also been used to characterize responses to inhaled pharmaceuticals.

In addition to the characterization of responses to inhaled agents, epithelial cell cultures, notably alveolar epithelium obtained from fetal lung tissue, have allowed investigators to characterize the liquid transport phenotype that occurs in the developing lung. Characterization of the Cl^- ion secretion system, which occurs in the distal lung epithelium throughout gestation, has been shown to be integral in the stimulation of growth of the developing lung by regulating liquid secretion. Likewise, a phenotypic switch of Na^+ absorptive capacity has been described toward the end of gestation, which is important for preparation of the lung to function postpartum and beyond. These culture systems have elucidated important physiologic changes that occur in the developing lung. Similar experiments have demonstrated that while ion transport plays a crucial role in this process other hormones and neurotransmitters are also important.

Pulmonary Endothelial Cells

Pulmonary endothelial cells represent a unique type of endothelium because of their paradoxical responses to hypoxia. This uniqueness highlights the need to utilize cell culture models of pulmonary endothelium as opposed to other endothelia when interested in investigating their role(s) in pulmonary physiology. Several investigators have described the isolation and culture of pulmonary endothelial cells. Persistent pulmonary hypertension of the newborn, also known as neonatal pulmonary hypertension, is caused by a disorder of the pulmonary vasculature from fetal to neonatal circulation, culminating in hypoxemic respiratory failure and death. The inciting events that culminate in neonatal pulmonary hypertension are multifactorial. Despite this, decreased production of vasodilator molecules such as nitric oxide and prostaglandin I_2 in the pulmonary endothelium has been shown to be a critical component of disease progression.[18]

Airway Smooth Muscle and Asthma

Primary cell cultures of human airway smooth muscle tissue can be obtained utilizing a method described by Halayko et al.[19] in which they isolated and characterized airway smooth muscle cells obtained from canine tracheal tissue. Briefly, airway smooth muscle cells were obtained by finely mincing tissue and subjecting it to an enzymatic disaggregation solution containing collagenase, type IV elastase, and type XXVII Nagarse protease. Following generation of a single cell suspension, cells may be grown in Dulbecco's modified Eagle's medium supplemented with 10% fetal bovine serum. Halayko et al.[20] obtained approximately 1.3×10^6 smooth muscle cells per gram of tissue using this method. Although Halayko et al.[21] pioneered this technique using trachealis tissue, many other investigators have obtained airway smooth muscle cells from a variety of biopsy specimens.

Airway smooth muscle hyperreactivity and hypertrophy has been known for nearly 100 years[2] to be an important end response of asthma. The use of airway smooth muscle in vitro has been vital toward delineating the pathologic steps that occur in asthma, as well as testing of potential therapeutics that may help to decrease the morbidity and mortality of asthma. Additionally, the relative paucity of in vivo models of asthma further illustrates the value of isolation and characterization of smooth muscle cells from asthmatic patients in vitro.

Using airway smooth muscle cell culture, investigators have characterized both the hypertrophic and hyperplastic growth of smooth muscle in individuals. Investigation of the potential stimuli that lead to airway smooth muscle proliferation and hypertrophy have led researchers to implicate the mitogen-activated protein kinase family members, extracellular signal-regulated kinase-1 and -2, and the phosphoinositol-3 kinase pathways in pathogenesis.[22] Additionally, mediators directing smooth muscle migration have also been observed in vitro and may play a role in the progression of asthma. Platelet-derived growth factor, fibroblast growth factor-2, and transforming growth factor-β (TGF-β) have all been shown to play a role in the migratory response of smooth muscle cells seen in asthma.[22] Additionally, contractile agonists such as leukotriene E_4 have been shown to potentiate the migratory responses seen with platelet-derived growth factor treatment.[22]

Human airway smooth muscle cell culture has also been utilized to investigate possible pharmacologic interventions for the treatment of asthma. $β_2$-Agonists have been shown to decrease the rate of DNA synthesis and likewise decrease the hyperplasia seen in airway smooth muscle cells in response to mitogenic stimuli through an increase in cyclic adenosine monophosphate. Like $β_2$-agonists, glucocorticoids have similar antiproliferative activities.

Lung Cancer Tissue and the Development of Novel Therapeutics

Culture of neoplastic cells from human tumors has allowed investigators to harvest a wealth of knowledge into the biology of lung cancers; moreover, these cultures have provided potential models to test potential therapeutics. The propagation of lung cancer cells in vitro has been covered in great depth previously.[8] In contrast to primary cell cultures, cultures of neoplastic cells are immortal, allowing their easy growth in culture with less chance of being overgrown by mesenchymal cells such as fibroblasts. The relative ease of growth in culture has led to many cell lines of lung cancer tissue. The National Cancer Institute, recognizing the need for a variety of lung cancer cell lines (both small cell and non–small cell), helped establish over 300 cell lines.[23] These lines are a wonderful resource for investigators given that they are extensively characterized, and many have full clinical data available. Moreover, many of these cell lines are now easily available through the American Type Culture Collection for a modest handling fee. Additionally, if investigators do not wish to use currently established lung cancer cell lines, obtaining clinical samples for use in tissue culture models is relatively easy. The same methods used to obtain biopsy specimens for clinical staging can also be used to begin cell cultures. Following culture and initial characterization of lung cancer cell lines, many investigators have demonstrated that lung cancer cell lines maintain a similar phenotype after establishment. Specifically, it has been verified that injection of lung cancer cell lines into nude mice exhibit similar histopathology to the original tumor, indicating minimal change occurred following establishment of the cell lines.

Small cell lung carcinoma (SCLC) cell lines have been established from a multitude of biopsy specimens, including bone marrow, lymph nodes, and pleural effusions.[8,24] Once viable cells have been obtained from clinical samples, cells are easily maintained in a basal cell culture medium such as RPMI 1640 in a humidified incubator at 37°C and 5% CO_2, although the initial isolations of SCLC lines utilized HITES and ACL-4 media.[25] Most established SCLC cell lines maintain a neuroendocrine phenotype in culture; however, Baillie-Johnson et al.[24] noticed considerable heterogeneity in the cell lines they established, highlighting the significance that establishing a cell line from the clinical sample of interest may provide investigators with a line that possesses the exact phenotypic properties of interest.

Small cell carcinoma poses many difficulties to surgical treatment, owing to its early and widespread metastasis. Therefore, combination chemotherapy is generally utilized in treatment. Unfortunately, despite initial sensitivities, SCLC tumors become resistant to further treatment. Utilizing in vitro cultures of SCLC cell lines, Sethi et al.[26] began to describe how extracellular matrix proteins can protect SCLC against apoptosis-inducing chemotherapeutics through β_1-integrin–mediated survival signals. These data indicate that extracellular matrix proteins surrounding SCLC may play a role in the local recurrence seen in patients following chemotherapy in vivo and suggest novel therapeutics aimed at blocking these survival signals.

Non–small cell lung carcinoma (NSCLC) cell lines including squamous cell carcinoma, adenocarcinoma, and large cell carcinoma have all been established. Despite the fact that NSCLC cells comprise three distinct histologic cell types, all cell types can be established relatively easily. The primary treatment protocol for patients afflicted by NSCLC is generally surgical resection of the tumor; therefore, tumor cells for culture are readily available. These cell types can be grown under conditions similar to those described for SCLC.

Infectious Diseases

Infectious diseases play a unique role in lung pathology in light of their roles as either important contributors or consequences of many lung diseases. For instance, certain lung diseases may predispose patients to infection: patients afflicted with obstructive lung diseases, as well as cystic fibrosis patients, commonly suffer from severe and recurrent bacterial infections. Additionally, patients may become superinfected following a viral respiratory infection. Systemic infections, such as gram-negative bacterial sepsis, may lead to lung diseases such as ARDS.

Human Type II Alveolar Pneumocytes and Acute Lung Injury/Acute Respiratory Distress Syndrome

Pulmonary alveolar type II cells are a unique cell subset that carries out highly specialized functions that include synthesis and secretion of surfactant, a unique composition of lipoproteins that act to reduce surface tension at the alveolar air–liquid interface.[27] Defining the molecular mechanisms leading to production of surfactant by type II pneumocytes is important in many disease processes.

The pathogenic sequence that results in ARDS, the most severe manifestation of alveolar lung injury, is generally thought to be initiated by a systemic inflammatory response.[28] Despite this knowledge, there still exist many questions about the initial triggers and pathologic steps that occur in ARDS. Greater understanding of these steps may help to develop new treatment regimes. Currently, treatment of ARDS consists of mechanical ventilation, which helps to stabilize blood gases. However, mechanical ventilation itself may provoke further inflammation in the alveoli, thereby decreasing compliance and gas exchange in the alveoli.[29]

The cell type of particular interest in ARDS and diffuse alveolar damage is the type II pneumocytes.[30–34] Until recently, studies trying to decipher the pathologic sequence in acute lung injury have had to rely on standard lung epithelial cell lines. Recently, however, human type II alveolar epithelial cells (pneumocytes) have been successfully isolated from fetal human lung tissue by collagenase digestion.[35] Briefly, fetal lung tissues were minced and incubated in a serum-free medium containing dibutyryl cyclic adenosine monophosphate for 5 days. The tissue explants were then treated with collagenase and incubated with DEAE-dextran to eliminate contaminating fibroblasts. Cells were then plated onto tissue culture dishes treated with extracellular matrix derived from MDCK cells and cultured overnight in Waymouth's medium containing 10% serum. These steps resulted in relatively pure populations of human type II pneumocytes that were then cultured at an air–liquid interface. Using these methods, Alcorn et al.[35] were able to maintain a primary culture that retained the morphologic and biochemical characteristics of type II pneumocytes for up to 2 weeks.

Three-Dimensional Biology

Conventional Bioreactors and Three-Dimensionality: The Origins of Three-Dimensional Culture

Carrel postulated that tissue development was linked to access to nutrient supply, noting that peripheral cells grew readily, and internal cells became necrotic presumably based on their distance from the nutrient source. To circumvent this issue, Carrel implemented cultures on silk veils, preventing the plasma clots of the growth media from deforming or becoming spherical, thus facilitating the internal cell's ability to obtain nutrient replenishment. Many attempts were made in standard culture systems (bioreactors) and other culture apparatuses to escape the constraints of two-dimensional cell culture, with the intent of yielding high-fidelity human and mammalian tissues, and thus emphasizing the need for development of three-dimensional biology.

Another famous researcher, Leighton, improved on Carrel's techniques in the 1950s and 1960s. Leighton's major contribution to three-dimensional culture technology was the introduction of the idea of a sponge matrix as a substrate on which to culture tissues.[36,37] Leighton first experimented on cellulose sponges surrounded by plasma clots resident within glass tubes. He devised a system to grow 1- to 5-mm^3 tissue explants on sponges, using small amounts of chick plasma and embryo extract. After the mixture solidified on the sponge Leighton added the nutrient media and inserted the "histoculture" in a roller apparatus to facilitate nutrient mass transfer. He experimented with many sponge combinations, discovering that collagen-impregnated cellulose sponges were optimal for sustaining the growth of native tissue architecture.[3,38]

Leighton was successful in growing many different tissue types on the sponge-matrix cultures.[3,38] Leighton also found that C3HBA mouse mammary adenocarcinoma cells, when grown on sponge-matrix histoculture, aggregated "much like the original tumor, forming distinct structures within the tumors such as lumina and stromal elements, and glandular structures." An extremely important difference of this three-dimensional histoculture from the standard two-dimensional culture is the apparent quiescence of the stromal component and the balanced growth of these cells with regard to the overall culture. Leighton further advanced the concept of three-dimensional histoculture to histophysiologic gradient cultures.[39] These cultures are conducted in chambers that allow metabolic exchange between "the pool of medium and the culture chamber by diffusion across a membrane." Histophysiologic gradient cultures mimic, to some degree, diffusion in tissues.[38]

From the pioneering work of Carrel and Leighton, other methods of emulating three-dimensional cultures have been developed, such as embedding cells and tissues in collagenous gels of rat tail as per the techniques of Nandi and colleagues. Many of the advantages of three-dimensional cultures seen by Leighton, Nandi, and others may be attributed to permitting the cells to retain their normal shape and special associations.[3] This global concept will be important as we begin to understand and recall the physical and environmental characteristics of the rotating-wall vessel systems.

Other methods of three-dimensional culture encompass a technique known as *organ culture* or *culture on a filter*, a strategy developed by Strangeways[40] and Fell and Robinson.[41] Tissue explants were grown on lens paper in a watch glass containing liquid culture medium. Browning and Trier[42] found "that for some tissues, it is critical to keep the cultures at the air–liquid interface," thus allowing the tissues to experience conditions similar to the in vivo environment.

Another strategy is the use of three-dimensional cultures known as *proto-tissues*, or aggregates of cells, used to form spheroids. This technique was popularized by Sutherland and colleagues more than 20 years ago when they manipulated aggregates of cells into a spherical configuration by spinning agitation of the cells in spinner flasks.[43] This technique produced pseudo-tissue-like organoids useful for research evaluations. Each of these methodologies will be of benefit as we continue to examine strategies for achieving three-dimensional lung tissue constructs.[3,38]

Finally, membrane bioreactors are capable of retaining enzymes, organelles, and microbial, animal, and plant cells behind a membrane barrier, trapped in a matrix or adherent to the membrane surface. In 1963, Gallup and Gerhardt[44] first used the membrane bioreactor for dialysis culture of *Serratia marcescens*. Immobilized enzyme microencapsulation was pioneered by Chang,[45] but Butterworth et al.[46] first developed the enzyme membrane reactor to successfully accomplish starch hydrolysis with α-amylase. Likewise, for animal cell culturing, Knazek et al.[47] first cultured human choriocarcinoma cells on compacted bundles of Amicon fibers. Many reviews on the particular applications of hollow fiber and immobilized bioreactant bioreactors for enzyme catalysts, microbial cells, and animal cell culture are available.[48–53]

As presented previously, tissue-engineering applications of three-dimensional function and structure are well known in medical science research.[54] In microgravity three-dimensional aggregates form, facilitating the expression of differentiated organotypic assemblies. Investigations to determine the effect of composite matrices, spiked with esterified hyaluronic acid and gelatin, to augment osteochondral differentiation of cultured, bone marrow–derived mesenchymal progenitor cells and the effects of the matrix on cellular differentiation have been examined in vitro and in vivo.[54]

Briefly, empty and populated matrices cultured for 28 days, with and without TGF-β_1 demonstrated the following results. Cells implanted in the matrix produced a robust type II collagen extracellular matrix in vitro. Matrices placed in immunodeficient mice yielded no differentiation in empty constructs, osteochondral differentiation in loaded implants, and an enhanced level of differentiation in preimplantation in vitro–cultured matrices containing TGF-β_1. These results demonstrate the utility of three-dimensional matrix for presentation of bone mesenchymal progenitor cells in vivo for repair of cartilage and bone defects as well as indicate the efficacy for in vitro tissue engineering regimes.[54] These techniques lend themselves to microgravity and ground-based research tissue cultures alike.

Many earth-based laboratories are researching and developing hemopoietic bone marrow cultures of stem cell origin, and three-dimensional configurations are providing promising results as illustrated by Schoeters and coworkers.[55] They report that murine bone marrow cells, cultured under long-term hemopoietic conditions, produce mineralized tissue and bone matrix proteins in vitro but only when precipitated by the presence of adherent bone stroma cells in three-dimensional collagen matrices. At a concentration of 8×10^6 stromal cells, mineralization occurs in 6 days. In contrast, two-dimensionally oriented marrow fragments at 1×10^7 cells require requires more than 10 days before mineralization can similarly be detected.[55]

Two-dimensional long-term marrow culture facilitates and enhances expansion of the stromal component and rudimentary differentiation of osteogenic-like cells in the adherent stromal layer as verified by type I collagen or cells positive for alkaline phosphatase. Production of osteonectin and osteocalcin, a bone-specific protein, combined with calcification is observed only in three-dimensional cultures. These studies demonstrate the need for and benefit of three-dimensionality and the application to the microgravity environment.[55] As we can see, this further reinforces the quest for three-dimensionality and the potential of modeling the microgravity environment.

Three-Dimensional Models for Physiological Study

Investigations clearly show the need for the application of three-dimensional study techniques in lung pathophysiologic studies. Interestingly, three-dimensional biology has facilitated full-scale investigations into most areas of tissue engineering, cell biology and physiology, immunology, and cancer research.

Anchorage-dependent cells are widely cultured on microcarriers.[56] Studies show that for the purposes of improved surface-to-volume ratio and scale up, the microcarrier suspension culture provides excellent potential for high-density cell growth.[57] In addition, microcarriers serve well as structural supports for three-dimensional assembly, the composite of which is the basis for three-dimensional tissue growth.[58]

Conventional culture systems for microcarrier cultures (i.e., bioreactors) use mechanical agitation to suspend microcarriers and thus induce impeller strikes as well as fluid shear and turbulence at the boundary layer between the wall and the fluid. Investigators have attempted to make a complete study of the most efficient bioreactor designs and agitation regimens.[59] They concluded that virtually all stirred-tank bioreactors operate in the turbulent regimen. It has been demonstrated that bead-to-bead bridging of cells is enhanced significantly at lower agitation rates in a stirred reactor.[60] Excessive agitation from either stirring or gas bubble sparging has been documented as a cause of cell damage in microcarrier cell cultures.[61,62] To overcome the problems induced by these mechanisms, investigators developed alternative culture techniques such as porous microcarriers to entrap cells,[63] increased viscosity of culture medium,[64] bubble-free oxygenation,[65] and improved methods for quiescent inoculation.[66,67] These steps decreased the damage attributed to turbulence and shear forces but failed to significantly rectify the problems. Reactor systems of substantially increased volume exhibit less agitation-related cell damage. This is presumably because of the decreased frequency of cell–microcarrier contact with the agitation devices in the systems. Research-scale investigations do not afford the luxury of experimenting with large-scale production systems. Therefore, if a large-volume system is indeed more quiescent, an improved bioreactor system should emulate the fluid dynamics present in the upper regions of large-scale reactors in which cells and microcarriers reside with minimal agitation. The problem, then, is to suspend microcarriers and cells without inducing turbulence or shear while providing adequate oxygenation and nutritional replenishment.

The term *rotating-wall vessel* comprises a family of vessels, batch fed and perfused, that embody the same fluid dynamic operating principles. These principles are (1) solid body rotation about a horizontal axis that is characterized by (a) colocation of particles of different sedimentation rates, (b) extremely low fluid shear stress and turbulence, and (c) three dimensional spatial freedom; and (2) oxygenation by active or passive diffusion to the exclusion of all but dissolved gasses from the reactor chamber, yielding a vessel devoid of gas bubbles and gas–fluid interface (zero head space).[68,69]

Three-Dimensional Models of Lung Disease

Lung Cancer

Current cell culture models have shortcomings resulting in unreliable tumor growth, uncharacteristic tumor development, nonhuman tumors, and inadequate methods of detection. Cells propagated under traditional culture conditions differ widely in their expression of differentiated markers, adhesion receptors, and growth factor receptors compared with cells in situ or those grown as tissue-like structures.[70,71] This is of concern because the phenotypic changes leading to malignant transformation often stem from alterations in the balanced and multifaceted roles of growth factors, receptors, and cytokines (reviewed by Herlyn et al.[71]). With increasing evidence of the importance of adhesive contacts, paracrine cross-talk between different cell types, and signaling cascades that link the cell with a complex substratum, there is now recognition that models must be developed that better simulate these complexities. There is still much to learn about the dynamic relationships among the different phenotypes found in the normal lung and in lung cancers. Until a cell culture system is developed that allows differentiation to occur,[72] it is difficult to make any firm statement about relating effects in cell culture to clinical practice. Tissue engineering is very embryonic in development and currently nearly universally focused on building replacement tissues. A new technology developed at the NASA Johnson Space Center used to study colon cancer has been adapted to three-dimensional in vitro lung tissue culture models but has not been reported on to date.

Rotating-wall vessels are horizontally rotating cylindrical tissue culture vessels that provide controlled supplies of oxygen and nutrients with minimal turbulence and extremely low shear.[69] These vessels suspend cells and microcarriers homogeneously in a nutrient-rich environment, which allows the three-dimensional assembly of cells to tissue. Prior to seeding rotating-wall vessels (Synthecon, Inc, Houston, TX), cells were cultured in standard T flasks (Corning, Corning, NY) in GTSF-2 medium (1993 PSEBM) in a humidified 37°C, 5% CO_2 incubator. The rotating-wall vessels were seeded with 1–2 mg/mL Cultispher-GL microcarriers (Hyclone Laboratories, Inc., Logan, UT) followed by BEAS2-B or BZR-T33 cells (ATCC, Baltimore, MD) at a density of 2×10^5 cells/mL. Cultures were grown in the rotating-wall vessels for 14–21 days for formation of 3- to 5-mm diameter tumor masses. Rotating-wall vessel rotation was initiated at 25 rpm and increased as aggregate size became larger. Stationary control cultures were initiated under the same conditions using FEP Teflon bags (American Fluoroseal, Columbia, MD). At 24-hour intervals pH, dissolved CO_2, and dissolved O_2 were determined using a Corning 238 model clinical blood gas analyzer. Glucose concentration was determined using a Beckman 2 model clinical glucose analyzer (Beckman, Fullerton, CA). Cell samples were harvested every 48 hr and fixed with Omnifix (Xenetics, Tustin, CA) for immunohistochemistry or fixed with 3% glutaraldehyde/2% paraformaldehyde in 0.1 M cacodylic buffer (Electron Microscopy Sciences, Fort Washington, PA) for scanning electron microscopy.

Cancer models already developed by NASA investigators include growth and differentiation of an ovarian tumor cell line,[72–74] growth of colon carcinoma lines,[72] and three-dimensional aggregate and microvillus formation in a human bladder carcinoma cell line.[74] In support as an appropriate model for cancer, even the most rudimentary three-dimensional cellular structures exhibit different phenotypes than cell lines cultured under two-dimensional conditions. Properties such as responses to TGF-β, drug resistance to cisplatin or cyclophosphamide, and resistance to apoptosis are all altered in various types of cell aggregates.[75]

Many investigations sustain consistent evidence that cells growing in three-dimensional arrays appear more resistant to cytotoxic chemoagents than cells in monolayer culture.[38] Li et al. found that spheroids were more resistant to cytosine arabinoside by 11-fold and methotrexate by 125-fold when compared with single cell suspensions.[76] Further monolayer cultures of colon carcinoma cells were sensitive to piericidin C in contrast to responses within in vivo colon tumors or three-dimensional slices of tumors grown in vitro.[77] Numerous other investigations have revealed increased levels of drug resistance of spheroids compared with single cell monolayers.[3,38]

Questions of poor diffusion and insufficient drug absorption within spheroids and a relatively frequent high proportion of resting cells have clouded differences in drug resistance, which could be the result of nutrient deprivation and hypoxia. Heppner and colleagues executed precise experiments that confirmed three-dimensional structure and function as the causative agent and was responsible for drug resistance rather than simple inaccessibility to nutrients or the drug concentration. Heppner embedded tumor specimens or cell aggregates in collagen gels, exposed the culture to various cytotoxic drugs, and compared the drug responses of the same cells in monolayers. These experiments revealed an increased resistance in the three-dimensional tumor arrays of a remarkable 1,000-fold greater than in monolayer cultures, and a similar result was seen in three-dimensional histocultures in collagen. The tumor cells grew in the presence of drug concentrations that rendered monolayers to a viability less than 0.1% of control cultures. Amazingly, Heppner observed that the cells became sensitive again when replated as monolayers and finally showed that even when exposed to melphalan and 5-fluorouracil in monolayer cells transferred to collagen gels were again resistant based on three-dimensional architecture. Thus, the cells were exposed to the drugs as monolayers, facilitating access to the drugs, and, once the cells were transferred after drug exposure to a three-dimensional structure, high resistance to the drugs was sustained.[38,78–81]

Based on the caliber of data referenced above, Teicher et al.[82] serially passaged through multiple (10) transfers EMT-6 tumors in mice that were treated with thiotepa, cisplatin, and cyclophosphamide over a prolonged 6-month period, thus producing extremely drug-resistant tumors in vivo. When these tumors were grown as monolayer cultures, they were as drug sensitive as the parental cells. Kobayashi and colleagues[83] grew the same in vivo drug-resistant tumor cell lines as spheroids in three-dimensional arrays, and resistance was almost 5,000 times that of the parent line with selected drugs, an example being the active form of cyclophosphamide used in vitro. Similarly extreme resistance was also observed to cisplatin and thiotepa. This resistance was not seen in monolayer cultures, even when the monolayers were cultured on traditional extracellular matrix substrates. These experiments reconfirmed that cells in a three-dimensional array are more drug resistant than monolayer cells in vitro and demonstrated that three-dimensional cellular configurations can and do become resistant to super pharmacologic doses of drugs by forming compact structures.[38]

Rotating-Wall Vessel Tumor Models

Several important human tumor models have been created in rotating-wall vessel cultures, specifically, lung, prostate, colon, and ovarian.[14,58,73,84] Many of these models involve cancers that are leading killers in our society. We present two such examples in this section, colon and prostate carcinoma. As previously reviewed, the literature indicates the remarkable difference between chemotherapeutic cytotoxicity in two-dimensional and three-dimensional cellular constructs, which may be predicated on a number of criteria. Therefore, a three-dimensional tumor model that emulates differentiated in vivo–like characteristics would provide unique insights into tumor biology.

Goodwin et al.[58] detail the first construction of a complex three-dimensional ex vivo tumor in rotating-wall vessel culture composed of a normal mesenchymal base layer (as would be seen in vivo) and either of two established human colon adenocarcinoma cell lines, HT-29, an undifferentiated line, and HT-29KM a stable, moderately differentiated subline of HT-29. Each of these engineered tumor tissues produced tissue-like aggregates (TLAs) with glandular structures, apical and internal glandular microvilli, tight intercellular junctions, desmosomes, cellular polarity, sinusoid development, internalized mucin, and structural organization akin to normal colon crypt development. Necrosis was minimal throughout the tissue masses up to 60 days of culture while achieving >1.0 cm in diameter. Other notable results included enhanced growth of neoplastic colonic epithelium in the presence of mixed normal human colonic mesenchyme. These results mimic the cellular differentiation seen in vivo and are similar to results obtained with other tumor types.

Prostate carcinoma has also been modeled in the rotating-wall vessel system by several investigators.[85–87] One of the most comprehensive descriptions of these engineered tissues is detailed by Wang et al.[88] In that review, the authors describe the ability of the rotating-wall vessel system to recapitulate human prostate carcinoma (LNCaP) and bone stroma (MG63) to illuminate the evolution of prostate tumorigenesis to the metastatic condition. In particular, the LNCaP and ARCaP models represented in the review are known to be lethal in the human, being androgen independent and metastatic. Rotating-wall vessel TLA engineering also allowed in-depth study of epithelial and stromal interactions, which

are the facilitating elements of the continuance of LNCaP prostate-specific antigen production in vitro. When LNCaP was cultured in three dimensions without stroma, production of prostate-specific antigen ceased and metastatic markers were not observed. The authors outline the process of malignant transformation, demonstrating that these metastatic models are only possible in three-dimensional TLAs and are achieved by specific geometric relationships in three-dimensional configuration. Furthermore, they show through direct comparison with other culture systems the advantages of the rotating-wall vessel system to allow synergistic relationships to study this disease state.[88]

Unlike two-dimensional models, these rotating-wall vessel tumor tissues were devoid of metabolic and nutrient deficiencies and demonstrated in vivo–like architecture. These data suggest that the rotating-wall vessel affords a new model for investigation and isolation of growth, regulatory, and structural processes within neoplastic and normal tissues.

Rotating-Wall Vessel Normal Human Tissue Models as Disease Targets

In this section, we explore the utility of rotating-wall vessel TLAs as targets for microbial infection and disease. Several studies have been conducted recently that indicate that three-dimensional tissues respond to infective agents with greater fidelity and with a more in vivo–like response than traditional two-dimensional cultures. Nickerson et al.[89] describe the development of a three-dimensional TLA engineered from INT-407 cells of the human small intestine, which were used as targets for the study of Salmonella typhimurium. In this study, three-dimensional TLAs were used to study the attachment, invasion, and infectivity of Salmonella into human intestinal epithelium. Immunocytochemical characterization and scanning and transmission electron microscopic analyses of the three-dimensional TLAs revealed that the TLAs more accurately modeled human in vivo differentiated tissues than did two-dimensional cultures. The level of differentiation in the INT-407 TLAs was analogous to that found in previously discussed small intestine TLAs[72] and from other organ tissues reconstructed in rotating-wall vessels. Analysis of the infectivity studies revealed Salmonella attached and infected in a manner significantly different from that in control two-dimensional cultures. During an identical exposure period of infection with Salmonella, the three-dimensional TLAs displayed a minor loss of structural integrity when compared with the two-dimensional INT-407 cultures. Furthermore, Salmonella demonstrated a greatly reduced ability to adhere, invade, and induce the apoptotic event in these INT-407 three-dimensional TLAs than in two-dimensional cultures. This result is not unlike the in vivo human response. Two-dimensional cultures were significantly damaged within several hours of contact with the bacteria; conversely, although "pot marks" could be seen on the surfaces of the three-dimensional TLAs, they remained structurally sound.

Cytokine analysis and expression postinfection of three-dimensional TLAs and two-dimensional cultures with *Salmonella* exhibited remarkable differences in expressed levels of interleukin (IL)-1α, IL-1β, IL-6, IL-1Ra, and tumor necrosis factor-α mRNAs. Additionally, noninfected three-dimensional TLAs constitutively demonstrated elevated levels of TGF-β$_1$ mRNA and prostaglandin E$_2$ compared with noninfected two-dimensional cultures of INT-407.[89]

As previously stated, traditional two-dimensional cell monolayers lack adequate fidelity to emulate the infection dynamics of in vivo microbial adhesion and invasion. The respiratory epithelium is of critical importance in protecting humans from disease. Exposed to the environment, the respiratory epithelium acts as a barrier to invading microbes present in the air, defending the host through a multilayered complex system.[90] The three major layers of the human respiratory epithelium are pseudostratified epithelial cells, a basement membrane, and underlying mesenchymal cells. Ciliated, secretory, and basal epithelial cells are connected by intercellular junctions and anchored to the basement membrane through desmosomal interactions. Together with tight junctions and the mucociliary layer, the basement membrane maintains the polarity of the epithelium and provides a physical barrier between the mesenchymal layer and the airway.[91,92] Infiltrating inflammatory and immune cells move freely between the epithelial and subepithelial compartments.

Airway epithelial cells play a vital role in host defense[90] by blocking paracellular permeability and modulating airway function through cellular interactions. Ciliated epithelial cells block invasion of countless inhaled microorganisms by transporting them away from the airways.[93] As regulators of the innate immune response, epithelial cells induce potent immunomodulatory and inflammatory mediators such as cytokines and chemokines that recruit phagocytic and inflammatory cells that remove microbes and enhance protection.[90,91,94,95]

Ideally, cell-based models should reproduce the structural organization, multicellular complexity, differentiation state, and function of the human respiratory epithelium. Immortalized human epithelial cell lines, such as BEAS-2B,[96] primary normal human bronchial epithelial cells,[97] and air–liquid interface cultures,[98] are used to study respiratory virus infections in vitro. Traditional monolayer cultures (two-dimensional) of immortalized human bronchoepithelial cells represent homogenous lineages. Although growing cells in monolayers is convenient and proliferation rates are high, such models lack

the morphology and cell–cell and cell–matrix interactions characteristic of human respiratory epithelia. Thus, their state of differentiation and intracellular signaling pathways most likely differ from those of epithelial cells in vivo. Primary cell lines of human bronchoepithelial cells provide a differentiated model similar to the structure and function of epithelial cells in vivo; however, this state is short lived in vitro.[97,99] Air–liquid interface cultures of primary human bronchoepithelial cells (or submerged cultures of human adenoid epithelial cells) are grown on collagen-coated filters in wells on top of a permeable filter. These cells receive nutrients basolaterally, and their apical side is exposed to humidified air. The result is a culture of well-differentiated heterogeneous (ciliated, secretory, basal) epithelial cells essentially identical to airway epithelium in situ.[98,100] Although this model shows fidelity to the human respiratory epithelium in structure and function, maintenance of consistent cultures is not only difficult and time consuming but also limited to small-scale production and thus limits industrial research capability.

True cellular differentiation involves sustained complex cellular interactions[101–103] in which cell membrane junctions, extracellular matrices (e.g., basement membrane and ground substances), and soluble signals (endocrine, autocrine, and paracrine) play important roles.[104–107] This process is also influenced by the spatial relationships of cells to each other. Each epithelial cell has three membrane surfaces: a free apical surface, a lateral surface that connects neighboring cells, and a basal surface that interacts with mesenchymal cells.[108]

Recently viral studies by Goodwin et al.[109] and Suderman et al.[110] were conducted with rotating-well vessel–engineered TLA models of normal human lung. This model is composed of a coculture of in vitro three-dimensional human bronchoepithelial TLAs engineered using a rotating-wall vessel to mimic the characteristics of in vivo tissue and to provide a tool to study human respiratory viruses and host–pathogen cell interactions. The TLAs were bioengineered onto collagen-coated cyclodextran beads using primary human mesenchymal bronchial-tracheal cells as the foundation matrix and an adult human bronchial epithelial immortalized cell line (BEAS-2B) as the overlying component. The resulting TLAs share significant characteristics with in vivo human respiratory epithelium, including polarization, tight junctions, desmosomes, and microvilli. The presence of tissue-like differentiation markers, including villin, keratins, and specific lung epithelium markers, as well as the production of tissue mucin, further confirm these TLAs differentiated into tissues functionally similar to in vivo tissues. Increasing virus titers for human respiratory syncytial virus (*wt*RSVA2) and parainfluenza virus type 3 (*wt*PIV3 JS) and the detection of membrane-bound glycoproteins (F and G) over time confirm productive infections with both viruses. Viral growth kinetics up to day 21 pi with *wt*RSVA2 and *wt*PIV3 JS were as follows: *wt*PIV3 JS replicated more efficiently than *wt*RSVA2 in TLAs. Peak replication was on day 7 for *wt*PIV3 JS (approximately $7\log_{10}$ particle forming units [pfu] per milliliter) and on day 10 for *wt*RSVA2 (approximately $6\log_{10}$ pfu/mL). Viral proliferation remained high through day 21 when the experiments were terminated. Viral titers for severe acute respiratory syndrome–coronavirus were approximately $2\log_{10}$ pfu/mL at 2 day pi.

Conclusion

Human lung TLAs mimic aspects of the human respiratory epithelium well and provide a unique opportunity to study the host–pathogen interaction of respiratory viruses and their primary human target tissue independent of the host's immune system, as there can be no secondary response without the necessary immune cells. These rotating-wall vessel–engineered tissues represent a valuable tool in the quest to develop models that allow analysis and investigation of cancers and infectious disease in models engineered with human cells alone.

We have explored the creation of three-dimensional TLAs for normal and neoplastic studies and finally as targets for microbial infections. Perhaps Carrel and Leighton would be fascinated to know that from their early experiments in three-dimensional modeling and the contributions they made has sprung the inventive spirit to discover a truly space age method for cellular recapitulation.

References

1. Clements JA, King RJ. Composition of surface active material. In: Crystal RG, ed. The Biochemical Basis of Pulmonary Function. New York: Marcel Dekker; 1976: 363–387.
2. Huber HL, Koessler KK. The pathology of bronchial asthma. Arch Int Med 1922;30:689–760.
3. Hoffman RM. Three-dimensional histoculture: origins and applications in cancer research. Cancer Cells 1991;3:86–92.
4. Sherwin RP, Richters A, Yellin AE, et al. Histoculture of human breast cancers. J Surg Oncol 1980;13:9–20.
5. Scherer WF, Syverton JT, Gey GO. Studies on the propagation in vitro of poliomyelitis viruses. IV. Viral multiplication in a stable strain of human malignant epithelial cells (strain HeLa) derived from an epidermoid carcinoma of the cervix. J Exp Med 1953;97:695–710.
6. Look DC, Walter MJ, Williamson MR, et al. Effects of paramyxoviral infection on airway epithelial cell Foxj1 expression, ciliogenesis, and mucociliary function. Am J Pathol 2001;159:2055–2069.
7. Freshney RI. Culture of Animal Cells: A Manual of Basic Technique, 3rd ed. New York: Wiley-Liss; 1994.
8. Tsao M, Viallet J. Preclinical models of lung cancer: cultured cells and organ culture. In: Lenfant C, ed. Biology of Lung Cancer. New York: Marcel Dekker; 1998:215–246.
9. Walboomers JM, Meijer CJ, Steenbergen RD, et al. [Human papillomavirus and the development of cervical cancer: concept of carcinogenesis.] Ned Tijdschr Geneeskd 2000; 144:1671–1674.
10. Adamson IY, Young L, Bowden DH. Relationship of alveolar epithelial injury and repair to the induction of pulmonary fibrosis. Am J Pathol 1988;130:377–383.
11. Krump-Konvalinkova V, Bittinger F, Unger RE, et al. Generation of human pulmonary microvascular endothelial cell lines. Lab Invest 2001;81:1717–1727.
12. Rep M, van Dijl JM, Suda K, et al. Promotion of mitochondrial membrane complex assembly by a proteolytically inactive yeast Lon. Science 1996;274:103–106.
13. Gruenert DC, Finkbeiner WE, Widdicombe JH. Culture and transformation of human airway epithelial cells. Am J Physiol 1995;268:L347–L360.
14. Vertrees RA, Das GC, Coscio AM, et al. A mechanism of hyperthermia-induced apoptosis in ras-transformed lung cells. Mol Carcinog 2005;44:111–121.
15. Vertrees RA, Nason R, Hold MD, et al. Smoke/burn injury–induced respiratory failure elicits apoptosis in ovine lungs and cultured lung cells, ameliorated with arteriovenous CO_2 removal. Chest 2004;125:1472–1482.
16. Lechner JF, Haugen A, Autrup H, et al. Clonal growth of epithelial cells from normal adult human bronchus. Cancer Res 1981;41:2294–2304.
17. Wallaert B, Fahy O, Tsicopoulos A, et al. Experimental systems for mechanistic studies of toxicant induced lung inflammation. Toxicol Lett 2000;112–113:157–163.
18. Shaul PW. Regulation of vasodilator synthesis during lung development. Early Hum Dev 1999;54:271–294.
19. Halayko AJ, Salari H, Ma X, et al. Markers of airway smooth muscle cell phenotype. Am J Physiol 1996;270: L1040–L1051.
20. Halayko AJ, Rector E, Stephens NL. Airway smooth muscle cell proliferation: characterization of subpopulations by sensitivity to heparin inhibition. Am J Physiol 1998;274:L17–L25.
21. Halayko AJ, Camoretti-Mercado B, Forsythe SM, et al. Divergent differentiation paths in airway smooth muscle culture: induction of functionally contractile myocytes. Am J Physiol 1999;276:L197–L206.
22. Stewart AG. Airway wall remodelling and hyperresponsiveness: modelling remodelling in vitro and in vivo. Pulm Pharmacol Ther 2001;14:255–265.
23. Gazdar AF, Minna JD. NCI series of cell lines: an historical perspective. J Cell Biochem Suppl 1996;24:1–11.
24. Baillie-Johnson H, Twentyman PR, Fox NE, et al. Establishment and characterisation of cell lines from patients with lung cancer (predominantly small cell carcinoma). Br J Cancer 1985;52:495–504.
25. Oie HK, Russell EK, Carney DN, et al. Cell culture methods for the establishment of the NCI series of lung cancer cell lines. J Cell Biochem Suppl 1996;24:24–31.
26. Sethi T, Rintoul RC, Moore SM, et al. Extracellular matrix proteins protect small cell lung cancer cells against apop-

tosis: a mechanism for small cell lung cancer growth and drug resistance in vivo. Nat Med 1999;5:662–668.

27. Gikas EG, King RJ, Mescher EJ, et al. Radioimmunoassay of pulmonary surface-active material in the tracheal fluid of the fetal lamb. Am Rev Respir Dis 1977;115:587–593.

28. Goodwin MN Jr. Selected anatomic burn pathology review for clinicians and pathologists. Aviat Space Environ Med 1989;60:B39–B43.

29. Lionetti V, Recchia FA, Ranieri VM. Overview of ventilator-induced lung injury mechanisms. Curr Opin Crit Care 2005;11:82–86.

30. Balamugesh T, Kaur S, Majumdar S, et al. Surfactant protein-A levels in patients with acute respiratory distress syndrome. Indian J Med Res 2003;117:129–133.

31. Herrera MT, Toledo C, Valladares F, et al. Positive end-expiratory pressure modulates local and systemic inflammatory responses in a sepsis-induced lung injury model. Intensive Care Med 2003;29:1345–1353.

32. Imai Y, Parodo J, Kajikawa O, et al. Injurious mechanical ventilation and end-organ epithelial cell apoptosis and organ dysfunction in an experimental model of acute respiratory distress syndrome. JAMA 2003;289:2104–2112.

33. Schiller HJ, Steinberg J, Halter J, et al. Alveolar inflation during generation of a quasi-static pressure/volume curve in the acutely injured lung. Crit Care Med 2003;31:1126–1133.

34. Song ZF, Yu KL, Shan HW, et al. [Evaluation of mechanical ventilation for patients with acute respiratory distress syndrome as a result of interstitial pneumonia after renal transplantation.] Zhongguo Wei Zhong Bing Ji Jiu Yi Xue 2003;15:358–361.

35. Alcorn JL, Smith ME, Smith JF, et al. Primary cell culture of human type II pneumonocytes: maintenance of a differentiated phenotype and transfection with recombinant adenoviruses. Am J Respir Cell Mol Biol 1997;17:672–682.

36. Leighton J, Justh G, Esper M, et al. Collagen-coated cellulose sponge: three dimensional matrix for tissue culture of Walker tumor 256. Science 1967;155:1259–1261.

37. Leighton J, Tchao R, Stein R, et al. Histophysiologic gradient culture of stratified epithelium. Methods Cell Biol 1980;21B:287–307.

38. Hoffman RM. The three-dimensional question: can clinically relevant tumor drug resistance be measured in vitro? Cancer Metastasis Rev 1994;13:169–173.

39. Leighton J. Structural biology of epithelial tissue in histophysiologic gradient culture. In Vitro Cell Dev Biol 1992;28A:482–492.

40. Strangeways T. Tissue culture in relation to growth and differentiation. Cambridge, England: W Heffer and Sons; 1924.

41. Fell HB, Robinson R. The growth, development and phosphatase activity of embryonic avian femora and end-buds cultivated in vitro. Biochem J 1929;23:767–784.

42. Browning TH, Trier JS. Organ culture of mucosal biopsies of human small intestine. J Clin Invest 1969;48:1423–1432.

43. Inch WR, McCredie JA, Sutherland RM. Growth of nodular carcinomas in rodents compared with multi-

cell spheroids in tissue culture. Growth 1970;34:271–282.

44. Gallup DM, Gerhardt P. Dialysis fermentor systems for concentrated culture of microorganisms. Appl Microbiol 1963;11:506–512.

45. Chang TM. Semipermeable microcapsules. Science 1964;146:524–525.

46. Butterworth TA, Wang DI, Sinskey AJ. Application of ultrafiltration for enzyme retention during continuous enzymatic reaction. Biotechnol Bioeng 1970;12:615–631.

47. Knazek RA, Gullino PM, Kohler PO, et al. Cell culture on artificial capillaries: an approach to tissue growth in vitro. Science 1972;178:65–67.

48. Belfort G. Membranes and bioreactors: a technical challenge in biotechnology. Biotechnol Bioeng 1989;33:1047–1066.

49. Chang HN. Membrane bioreactors: engineering aspects. Biotechnol Adv 1987;5:129–145.

50. Chang HN, Furusaki S. Membrane bioreactors: present and prospects. Adv Biochem Eng Biotechnol 1991;44:27–64.

51. Gekas VC. Artificial membrane as carrier for the immobilization of biocatalysts. Enz Microb Technol 1986;8:450–460.

52. Hopkinson J. Hollow fiber cell culture in industry. In: Mattiasson B, ed. Immobilized Cells and Organelles. Boca Raton, FL: CRC Press; 1983.

53. Kitano H, Ise N. Hollow fiber enzyme reactors. Trends Biotechnol 1984;2:5–7.

54. Angele P, Kujat R, Nerlich M, et al. Engineering of osteochondral tissue with bone marrow mesenchymal progenitor cells in a derivatized hyaluronan-gelatin composite sponge. Tissue Eng 1999;5:545–554.

55. Schoeters G, Leppens H, Van Gorp U, et al. Haemopoietic long-term bone marrow cultures from adult mice show osteogenic capacity in vitro on 3-dimensional collagen sponges. Cell Prolif 1992;25:587–603.

56. Van Wezel AL. Microcarrier/cultures of animal cells. In: Paterson MK, ed. Tissue Culture: Methods and Applications. New York: Academic Press; 1973.

57. Glacken MW, Fleishaker RJ, Sinskey AJ. Mammalian cell culture: engineering principles and scale-up. Trends in Biotech 1983;1:102–108.

58. Goodwin TJ, Jessup JM, Wolf DA. Morphologic differentiation of colon carcinoma cell lines HT-29 and HT-29KM in rotating-wall vessels. In Vitro Cell Dev Biol 1992;28A:47–60.

59. Croughan MS, Hammel JF, Wang DIC. Hydrodynamic effects on animal cells in microcarrier cultures. Biotechnol Bioeng 1987;29:130–141.

60. Cherry RS, Papoutsakis ET. Physical mechanisms of cell damage in microcarrier cell culture bioreactors. Biotechnol Bioeng 1988;32:1001–1004.

61. Croughan MS, Wang DI. Growth and death in over agitated microcarrier cell cultures. Biotechnol Bioeng 1989;33:731–744.

62. Cherry RS, Hulle CT. Cell death in the thin films of bursting bubbles. Biotechnol Prog 1992;8:11–18.

63. Nilsson K, Buzsaky F, Mosbach K. Growth of anchorage-dependent cells on macroporous microcarriers. Biotechnology 1986;4:989–990.

64. Croughan MS, Sayre SS, Wang DI. Viscous reduction of turbulent damage in animal cell culture. Biotechnol Bioeng 1989;33:862–872.

65. Thalmann E. Biological experiences in bubble-free aeration system. Acta Biotechnol 1989;39:511–516.

66. Clark J, Hirstenstein H, Gebb C. Critical parameters in the microcarrier culture of animal cells. Dev Biol Stand 1980; 46:117–124.

67. Feder J, Tolbert WR. The large-scale cultivation of mammalian cells. Sci Am 1983;248:36–43.

68. Wolf DA, Schwarz RP. Analysis of gravity-induced particle motion and fluid perfusion flow in the NASA-designed rotating zero-head-space tissue culture vessel. NASA Tech Paper 1991:3143.

69. Schwarz RP, Goodwin TJ, Wolf DA. Cell culture for three-dimensional modeling in rotating-wall vessels: an application of simulated microgravity. J Tissue Cult Methods 1992;14:51–57.

70. Shih IM, Herlyn M. Autocrine and paracrine roles for growth factors in melanoma. In Vivo 1994;8:113–123.

71. Herlyn M, Kath R, Williams N, et al. Growth-regulatory factors for normal, premalignant, and malignant human cells in vitro. Adv Cancer Res 1990;54:213–234.

72. Goodwin TJ, Prewett TL, Wolf DA, et al. Reduced shear stress: a major component in the ability of mammalian tissues to form three-dimensional assemblies in simulated microgravity. J Cell Biochem 1993;51:301–311.

73. Goodwin TJ, Prewett TL, Spaulding GF, et al. Three-dimensional culture of a mixed mullerian tumor of the ovary: expression of in vivo characteristics. In Vitro Cell Dev Biol Anim 1997;33:366–374.

74. Prewett TL, Goodwin TJ, Spaulding GF. Three-dimensional modeling of T-24 human bladder carcinoma cell line: a new simulated microgravity vessel. J Tissue Cult Methods 1993;15:29–36.

75. Kerbel RS, Rak J, Kobayashi H, et al. Multicellular resistance: a new paradigm to explain aspects of acquired drug resistance of solid tumors. Cold Spring Harb Symp Quant Biol 1994;59:661–672.

76. Li LH, Bhuyan BK, Wallace TL. Comparison of cytotoxicity of agents on monolayer and spheroid systems. Proc Am Assoc Cancer Res 1989;30:2435A.

77. Smith KS, Badiner GJ, Adams FG, et al. Modified 2-tumour (L1210, colon 38) assay to screen for solid tumor selective agents. Proc Symp Anticancer Drug Discovery Dev 2006 (in press).

78. Lawler EM, Miller FR, Heppner GH. Significance of three-dimensional growth patterns of mammary tissues in collagen gels. In Vitro 1983;19:600–610.

79. Miller BE, Miller FR, Heppner GH. Assessing tumor drug sensitivity by a new in vitro assay which preserves tumor heterogeneity and subpopulation interactions. J Cell Physiol Suppl 1984;3:105–116.

80. Miller BE, Miller FR, Heppner GH. Factors affecting growth and drug sensitivity of mouse mammary tumor lines in collagen gel cultures. Cancer Res 1985;45:4200–4205.

81. Simon-Assmann P, Bouziges F, Vigny M, et al. Origin and deposition of basement membrane heparan sulfate proteoglycan in the developing intestine. J Cell Biol 1989; 109:1837–1848.

82. Teicher BA, Herman TS, Holden SA, et al. Tumor resistance to alkylating agents conferred by mechanisms operative only in vivo. Science 1990;247:1457–1461.

83. Kobayashi H, Man S, Graham CH, et al. Acquired multicellular-mediated resistance to alkylating agents in cancer. Proc Natl Acad Sci USA 1993;90:3294–3298.

84. Margolis J, Li ZP. Heat sterilisation to inactivate AIDS virus in lyophilised factor VIII [lett]. Aust NZ J Med 1986;16:413.

85. Ingram M, Techy GB, Saroufeem R, et al. Three-dimensional growth patterns of various human tumor cell lines in simulated microgravity of a NASA bioreactor. In Vitro Cell Dev Biol Anim 1997;33:459–466.

86. Margolis L, Hatfill S, Chuaqui R, et al. Long term organ culture of human prostate tissue in a NASA-designed rotating wall bioreactor. J Urol 1999;161:290–297.

87. Zhau HE, Goodwin TJ, Chang SM, et al. Establishment of a three-dimensional human prostate organoid coculture under microgravity-simulated conditions: evaluation of androgen-induced growth and PSA expression. In Vitro Cell Dev Biol Anim 1997;33:375–380.

88. Wang R, Xu J, Juliette L, et al. Three-dimensional coculture models to study prostate cancer growth, progression, and metastasis to bone. Semin Cancer Biol 2005;15: 353–364.

89. Nickerson CA, Goodwin TJ, Terlonge J, et al. Three-dimensional tissue assemblies: novel models for the study of Salmonella enterica serovar typhimurium pathogenesis. Infect Immun 2001;69:7106–7120.

90. Hiemstra PS, Bals R. Series introduction: Innate host defense of the respiratory epithelium. J Leuk Biol 2004;75: 3–4.

91. Knight DA, Holgate ST. The airway epithelium: structural and functional properties in health and disease. Respirology 2003;8:432–446.

92. Gibson MC, Perrimon N. Apicobasal polarization: epithelial form and function. Curr Opin Cell Biol 2003;15:747–752.

93. Cotran R, Kumar V, Collins T. Robbins Infectious Diseases, 6th ed. Philadelphia: WB Saunders; 1999.

94. Garofalo RP, Haeberle H. Epithelial regulation of innate immunity to respiratory syncytial virus. Am J Respir Cell Mol Biol 2000;23:581–585.

95. Polito AJ, Proud D. Epithelia cells as regulators of airway inflammation. J Allergy Clin Immunol 1998;102:714–718.

96. Ke Y, Reddel RR, Gerwin BI, et al. Human bronchial epithelial cells with integrated SV40 virus T antigen genes retain the ability to undergo squamous differentiation. Differentiation 1988;38:60–66.

97. Stoner GD, Katoh Y, Foidart JM, et al. Identification and culture of human bronchial epithelial cells. Methods Cell Biol 1980;21A:15–35.

98. Wu R, Sato GH, Whitcutt MJ. Developing differentiated epithelial cell cultures: airway epithelial cells. Fundam Appl Toxicol 1986;6:580–590.

99. Gray GD, Wickstrom E. Evaluation of anchorage-independent proliferation in tumorigenic cells using the redox dye alamar Blue. Biotechniques 1996;21:780–782.

100. Adler KB, Li Y. Airway epithelium and mucus: intracellular signaling pathways for gene expression and secretion. Am J Respir Cell Mol Biol 2001;25:397–400.

101. Fukamachi H. Disorganization of stroma alters epithelial differentiation of the glandular stomach in adult mice. Cell Tissue Res 1986;243:65–68.

102. Sutherland AE, Calarco PG, Damsky CH. Expression and function of cell surface extracellular matrix receptors in mouse blastocyst attachment and outgrowth. J Cell Biol 1988;106:1331–1348.

103. Wiens D, Park CS, Stockdale FE. Milk protein expression and ductal morphogenesis in the mammary gland in vitro: hormone-dependent and -independent phases of adipocyte-mammary epithelial cell interaction. Dev Biol 1987; 120:245–258.

104. Kaye GI, Siegel LF, Pascal RR. Cell replication of mesenchymal elements in adult tissues. I. The replication and migration of mesenchymal cells in the adult rabbit dermis. Anat Rec 1971;169:593–611.

105. Buset M, Winawer S, Friedman E. Defining conditions to promote the attachment of adult human colonic epithelial cells. In Vitro Cell Dev Biol 1987;23:403–412.

106. Daneker GW Jr., Mercurio AM, Guerra L, et al. Laminin expression in colorectal carcinomas varying in degree of differentiation. Arch Surg 1987;122:1470–1474.

107. Durban EM, Knepper JE, Medina D, et al. Influence of mammary cell differentiation on the expression of proteins encoded by endogenous BALB/c mouse mammary tumor virus genes. Virus Res 1990;16:307–323.

108. O'Brien LE, Zegers MM, Mostov KE. Opinion: Building epithelial architecture: insights from three-dimensional culture models. Nat Rev Mol Cell Biol 2002;3:531–537.

109. Goodwin TJ, Deatly AM, Suderman MT, et al. Three-dimensional engineered high fidelity normal human lung tissue-like assemblies (TLA) as targets for human respiratory virus infection. In: American Society for Virology 22nd Annual Meeting, 2003 (abstr).

110. Suderman MT, Mossel E, Watts DM, et al. Severe acute respiratory syndrome (SARS)-CoV infection in a three-dimensional human bronchial-tracheal (HBTE) tissue-like assembly. In: American Society for Virology 23rd Annual Meeting, 2004 (abstr).

Section 3
Molecular Pathology of Pulmonary and Pleural Neoplasms: General Principles

16
Molecular Oncogenesis of Lung Cancer

Arwen A. Stelter and Jingwu Xie

Introduction

In 2005, cancer surpassed heart disease as the leading cause for death in Americans under the age of 80 years. Among all types of human cancer, lung cancer is the leading cause of cancer-related death, claiming more than 150,000 lives every year in the United States alone (which exceeds the combined mortality from breast, prostate, colorectal, and pancreatic cancers). Patients with advanced stages of lung cancer, representing 75% of all new cases, have a median survival time of only 10 months.[1] In contrast to the significant medical burden associated with lung cancer, research on lung cancer is underfunded. According to National Institutes of Health data (http://planning.cancer.gov/disease), the U.S. government spent approximately $1,200 per lung cancer death in 2002 on research compared with $11,425 for breast cancer, $8,190 for prostate cancer, and $3,350 for colorectal cancer. Approximately $31,000 was spent on research per HIV/AIDS death in 2002. Understanding the molecular basis of lung cancer progression and tumor metastasis is an essential step to reducing the mortality from lung cancer.

Lung cancer can broadly be divided into two categories: small cell lung cancer (SCLC) (~20%) and non–small cell lung cancer (NSCLC) (80%).[2] Small cell lung cancer is typically composed of cells that have scanty cytoplasm, a neuroendocrine phenotype, inconspicuous nucleoli, and frequent metastases.[3,4] Non–small cell lung cancer can be further subdivided into adenocarcinomas, squamous cell carcinomas, large cell carcinomas, and several infrequent subtypes.[3–5]

The TNM staging method is the currently accepted system for staging NSCLC in which T indicates the size and location of the primary tumor, N indicates the location of involved lymph nodes, and M indicates the presence of metastatic lesions.[3] Lung cancer with stages I, II, and IIIA, but not stages IIIB and IV, can be treated with surgery; the latter can be treated by chemotherapy and radiation therapy.[3,4] Five-year survival rates decline sharply as the stage increases: 61% for stage IA, 38% for stage IB, 22%–34% for stage II, 9%–13% for stage III, and less than 5% for stage IV.[3,6] The staging of SCLC is less complex, with a distinction made only between limited stage and extensive stage disease.[3] Most SCLC cases are diagnosed when metastasis has already occurred, and the 5-year survival rates for all SCLC cases are 3% or less.[3]

Lung cancer is a primarily environmental disease with risk factors that include radon exposure and asbestos exposure, but the risk factor with the highest correlation by far is cigarette smoking. From 80% to 90% of lung cancer patients have a history of cigarette smoking, and the relative risk for lung cancer for current smokers is 20 times greater than the risk to those who have never smoked.[3,7] The contribution of cigarette smoking to lung cancer is believed to be related to a "field cancerization" effect where simultaneous mutations accumulate throughout the bronchial epithelium, increasing the chances of mutations leading to cancer.[7,8] Because studies suggest that this accumulation must reach at least 10 significant mutations to proceed to apparent oncogenic transformation, the broad effects of field cancerization significantly decrease the barriers to lung cancer development.[9]

In this chapter, we summarize recent advances in our understanding of the molecular oncogenesis of lung cancer, particularly with regard to alterations of oncogenes, tumor suppressor genes, and growth factors and their receptors. Recent insights into novel genetic changes, such as MiRNA silencing, are also be discussed.

Oncogene Activation

Figure 16.1 shows the major genetic changes associated with lung cancer. Activation of protooncogenes and growth factor signaling play a critical role in the oncogenesis of lung cancer. Common oncogenes in lung cancer

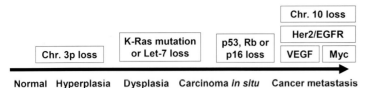

FIGURE 16.1. A proposed model for major genetic alterations in lung cancer development from normal tissue to metastatic tumor.

include K-*ras* and c-*Myc*. In addition, mutations of *EGFR* (epidermal growth factor receptor) are associated with aggressive metastasis of lung cancer. Elevated expression of growth factor receptors is quite common in lung cancer.

K-*ras* Activation

In normal cells, Ras protein functions as a signal transducer between growth factor signaling at the cell membrane and the mitogen-activated protein kinase (MAPK) pathways. Growth factors bind to receptor tyrosine kinases that indirectly stimulate guanosine triphosphate for guanosine diphosphate exchange on Ras. Guanosine triphosphate–bound Ras (the active form) then serves to propagate the signal through its downstream effectors, which results in many cellular changes, many of which promote cell growth and proliferation (see Figure 16.2 for details). Ras is actually a superfamily of proteins, and of these the isoform K-Ras is mutated in 17%–25% of human tumors and in 20%–50% of NSCLCs.[2,10,11] Studies in mouse models of lung cancer indicate that mutation of K-*ras* is an early essential event during lung cancer oncogenesis, further emphasizing the essential role of K-Ras in lung cancer.[12]

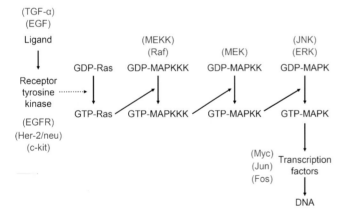

FIGURE 16.2. Growth factor signaling and the Ras/MAP kinase pathway. The basic pathway components are given in black with examples in gray parentheses. EGF, epidermal growth factor; GDP, guanosine diphosphate; GTP, guanosine triphosphate; MAPK, mitogen-activated protein kinase; MAPKK, MAPK kinase; MAPKKK, MAPKK kinase; TGF-α, transforming growth factor-α.

Erb Family Activation: ErbB1 (*EGFR*) and ErbB2 (*HER2/neu*)

Epidermal growth factor receptor (EGFR), which is also known as ErbB1, is a receptor tyrosine kinase. Receptor tyrosine kinases are transmembrane spanning proteins whose activation by ligand binding, such as epidermal growth factor and transforming growth factor α (TGF-α), to their extracellular binding domain causes dimerization followed by autophosphorylation of intracellular tyrosine residues. This phosphorylation leads to binding of kinase substrates and adapter proteins that stimulate downstream activation of cell signaling pathways (see Figure 16.2), such as Ras/MAPK, and phosphatidylinositol-3 kinase, that then propagate signals for proliferation, differentiation, motility, invasion, adhesion, and blocking of apoptosis,[13,14] through signal transduction and activation of transcription proteins.

EGFR mutations have been found in approximately 20% of NSCLC, and all of these are located in the tyrosine kinase domain of the protein.[15] Additionally, the overexpression of EGFR ligands and amplification of *EGFR* contribute to EGFR-dependent phenotypes. Because of the availability of tyrosine kinase inhibitors and because of the low survival rates for lung cancer chemotherapy, the application of these inhibitors in the treatment of lung cancer has been explored (see Chapter 17).

HER2/neu, which is also known as ErbB2, is another member of the same family of receptor tyrosine kinases as EGFR, and it has also been implicated in NSCLC. HER2/neu has been shown to be upregulated in a subset of NSCLC.[3] The anti-HER2/neu monoclonal antibody trastuzumab, which has shown success in HER2/neu-positive breast cancer when used in combination with chemotherapy, has not shown the same level of success in NSCLC (see Chapter 17).[16]

Myc Activation

The Myc proteins can be regulated by the Ras/MAPK pathway and are transcription factors that regulate the expression of genes important in cell cycle regulation, proliferation, and DNA synthesis. There are three members: c-Myc, N-Myc, and L-Myc. Through a mechanism that is unclear, Myc proteins also induce p14[ARF], which serves as a negative feedback loop triggering apoptosis through p53 if cellular conditions are not appropriate for proliferation. Because of this, Myc upregulation in cancer cells is usually accompanied by mutations in p53 pathway components.

Overexpression of Myc proteins by either gene amplification or transcriptional dysregulation has been observed in 10%–40% of SCLCs the majority of which are the N-Myc and L-Myc subtypes.[3,5] Myc overexpression has been observed in only 8%–20% of NSCLCs.[5]

Other Alterations: Vascular Endothelial Growth Factor, *Bcl-2, Myb, Fms, Rlf, Kit/SCR, GRP/GRPR, Raf*

Expression of vascular endothelial growth factor (VEGF), an important molecule in the regulation of tumor angiogenesis, is associated with poor outcomes of chemotherapy of metastatic NSCLC and SCLC. Recent clinical trials indicate that the angiogenesis inhibitor bevacizumab in combination with chemotherapy can significantly extend survival in patients with advanced lung cancer. The list of additional oncogenes in lung cancer includes *Raf, Fes, Fur, Sis, Bcl-2*, and *IGF-1* for NSCLC and *Raf, Myb, Fms, Kit/SCF, Rlf* and *GRP/GRP*R SCLC.[7] *Raf* is another member of the MAPK pathway (see Figure 16.2) acting as a kinase downstream of *Ras. Raf* mutations are rare in lung cancer with detection in less than 3% of case.[15] c-Kit is a receptor tyrosine kinase that upon ligand binding activates signaling pathways such as the MAPK pathway.[17] Its ligands include stem cell factor (SCF), which has been shown to be aberrantly expressed with the c-Kit receptor in SCLC, thereby producing autocrine proliferation signals.[17,18] Activating mutations of c-*Kit* have been discovered in SCLC but are not common.[17]

Gastrin-releasing peptide (GRP) is a peptide hormone that binds to the GRP receptor (GRPR), a G protein–coupled receptor (GPCR) that activates the phosphatidylinositol-3 kinase pathway.[19] Gastrinreleasing peptide and its receptor have been detected in many cases of SCLC, indicating that they may act in an autocrine manner to stimulate proliferation of SCLC cells.[18,19]

Bcl-2 promotes cell survival by acting as a negative regulator of mitochondrial-stimulated apoptosis. It has been shown to be overexpressed in 10%–27% of NSCLC.[2,8] Recent studies indicate that hedgehog signaling is activated in subsets of lung cancer.[20–22] Loss of the tumor suppressor *PTCH* in the hedgehog signaling pathway by chromosomal deletion of 9q is just one of several ways that this pathway may be activated in SCLC.[9,23] These and many other potential oncogenes have been proposed, but the clinical significance of their actions has not been determined.

Alterations of Tumor Suppressor Genes in Lung Cancers

The p53 Pathway

The transcription factor p53 protein is well known as a key regulator of cell cycle progression that is frequently targeted for inactivation in neoplastic cells. Functional inactivation of p53 and its pathway components occurs with high frequency in lung cancer. p53 responds to a variety of signals such as DNA damage and oncoprotein expression, and it responds by initiating cell cycle arrest, senescence, apoptosis, differentiation, DNA repair, or other p53-dependent pathways depending on the cell conditions (see Figure 16.3).[24–26] The p53 protein

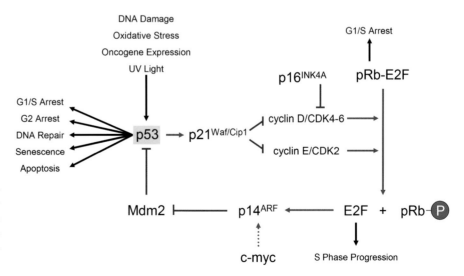

FIGURE 16.3. The p53 and retinoblastoma (Rb) pathways. The main pathway connections between components of the p53 pathway and the Rb pathway are shown. The purple P indicates a phosphate residue. UV, ultraviolet.

promotes the transcription of several target genes, including $p21^{WAF/Cip1}$, which contribute to G1 cell cycle arrest. Cell cycle arrest gives the cell time to initiate and complete DNA repair before replication. If repair is unsuccessful, p53 can initiate apoptosis by initiating transcription of *Bim1, Bax, PERP*, and others.[27] The primary mechanism for regulation of p53 is through its concentration in the cell where the negative regulator MDM2 (HDM2) plays a crucial role as an E3 ubiquitin ligase specific for p53. The *p53* gene is located on chromosome 17p13.

Because of the crucial role that p53 plays as a monitor of DNA damage, it is a logical target in cancer progression. The *p53* mutations are found in 70% of SCLC and 50% of NSCLC, and loss of the second wild-type allele via chromosomal deletion of the 17p13 region is common.[27-29] For additional information on specific *p53* mutations, one can review the database of published mutations for *p53* at http://www-p53.iarc.fr, maintained by the International Agency for Research on Cancer.[30] Several studies have proposed that the G to T transversion mutations in *p53* are directly caused by the carcinogenic components of smoke or the reactive oxygen species that they promote.[28,31] Contributing to the mutagenic selection of *p53* is the fact that cigarette smoke may also inhibit repair.[28,32] Unfortunately, there is controversy regarding the use of *p53* status as an indicator for prognosis (see Chapter 15).[29] It is likely that alterations to other p53 pathway components such as $p21^{WAF/Cip1}$ and MDM2 contribute to treatment outcome as well (see Chapter 17).[29] In fact, accumulation of MDM2 has been shown to occur in more than 24% of NSCLC and in more than 40% of SCLC.[33] Also, $p14^{ARF}$, an inhibitor for MDM2 (see Figure 16.3), has shown to be inactivated in 19%–37% of NSCLC, adding to the proliferative controls inactivated in lung cancers.[34]

The Retinoblastoma Pathway: Rb and P16^{INK4}

The retinoblastoma (Rb) pathway is another important regulator of the cell cycle. It has cross-talk with the p53 pathway through p14^{ARF} and p21$^{Waf/Cip1}$ (see Figure 16.3). Active Rb exists in a hypophosphorylated state and therefore is inactivated by phosphorylation. Cell cycle promoting complexes such as cyclin D–Cdk4–6 and cyclin E–Cdk2 promote this phosphorylation, thus relieving the inhibition of Rb on cell cycle progression. Active p53 promotes the transcription of $p21^{WAF/Cip1}$, which inhibits these two cyclin complexes, thereby promoting Rb-dependent inhibition of cell cycle progression. In turn, active Rb binds to E2F proteins, preventing them from acting as transcription factors for the transcription of genes necessary for entry into and progression through S phase of the cell cycle.[35] E2F proteins also increase the transcription of $p14^{ARF}$, which inhibits MDM2. This serves as a negative feedback loop to increase p53 concentration

in the cell and to prevent dysfunctional Rb from allowing cell cycle progression. As such, Rb pathway inactivation is commonly associated with p53 pathway inactivation. Expression of $p14^{ARF}$ is also induced by other oncoproteins such as *Myc* and *Ras*, increasing its ability to control hyperproliferation.[36] Protein p16^{INK4A} functions in the Rb pathway by binding to CDK4 and CDK6 and inhibiting the cyclin D–CDK4–6 complex.[37] By inhibiting the inactivation of Rb, p16^{INK4A} also inhibits G1/S phase progression. The *Rb* gene is located on chromosome 13q14.[9]

It has been postulated that components of the Rb pathway are inactivated in most human lung cancers. There appears to be a selection preference for Rb pathway components that differs between SCLC and NSCLC. Rb inactivation occurs in approximately 90% of SCLC but substantially less frequently in NSCLC, whereas the upstream regulator p16^{INK4A} seems to have the opposite pattern, with 70% inactivation in NSCLC and little in SCLC.[38] This interesting dichotomy has yet to be explained but is likely related to inherent differences in protein expression patterns between NSCLC and SCLC. Approximately 40% of NSCLC show overexpression of cyclin D1, which would contribute to phosphorylation and thus inactivation of Rb.[39]

Taken together, the high frequency of alterations in the Rb and p53 pathways indicates that these pathways are crucial obstacles to lung cancer oncogenesis. The inactivation of individual components leads to slightly different phenotypes even when inactivated components are within the same pathway. This is because the above pathway descriptions have been simplified and do not include information on the different isoforms of each pathway member and the heterogeneity of pathway cross-talk. Because of the complexity of these different phenotypes, it has been difficult to definitively determine the prognostic implications of each mutation (see Chapter 15).

Other Chromosomal Deletions

While the p53 and Rb pathways represent two of the best-studied tumor suppressor pathways, other chromosomal deletions have been shown to occur in lung cancer specimens with a frequency that suggests that important but as of yet unconfirmed tumor suppressors are encoded in these regions. Using allelotyping studies of lung cancer cell lines, it has been demonstrated that the following regions are frequently lost: in SCLC, 4p, 5p, and 10q; in NSCLC, 6p, 6q, 10q, 11q, 12p, 16q, 19p, 19q, 21q, 22p, Xp, and Xq; and in both, 1p, 1q, 3p, 4q, 5q, 8p, 9p, 9q, 10p, 11p, 15q, 16q, 18q, and 20p.[9]

Additionally, the locus for p53 (17p) and Rb (13q) are frequently lost in both SCLC and NSCLC. The 9p site encodes both $p16^{INK4A}$ and $p14^{ARF}$ genes whose genes partially overlap in the same coding sequence.[9,36] The 9q site for SCLC is known to contain the *PTCH* locus, which is a known tumor suppressor functioning in the hedgehog signaling pathway.[9,23] The 3p region has several candidate tumor suppressor genes whose functional significance has yet to be determined. These include *FHIT, VHL, TGFBR2, DLC1, MLH1/HNPCC2, PTPG, BAP1, RARβ, RASSF1A, SEMA3B, FUS1,* and *ROBO1.*[9,40–43] Tumor suppressor gene(s) in the 3p locus are likely to be important to lung cancer development, as loss of the region appears to be an early event in lung cancer formation.[8] Recent work indicates that alteration of microRNA may be responsible for some of these changes.

Gene Silencing by MicroRNA

Micro (mi) RNAs were initially discovered through studies of embryonic development of *Caenorhabditis elegans.*[44] They are 22 nucleotide (nt) noncoding RNAs that control essential processes during normal development, such as cell differentiation, proliferation, apoptosis, and metabolism. It is estimated that the human genome contains about 1,000 MiRNAs, which are generated from large RNA precursors (pre-miRNAs) in the nucleus by RNase III enzyme. The pre-miRNAs form hairpin structures and are transported into cytoplasm.[45] Maturation of miRNAs requires Dicer, another RNase III enzyme. The exact mechanism for miRNA-mediated gene expression regulation is not entirely clear at present, but the function of miRNA requires its binding to the complimentary sequences of the target mRNA transcripts, leading to either degradation or translational block of the target genes.

Mounting evidence indicates that miRNA expression patterns are altered in human cancer, including lung cancer. MicroRNA genes are frequently located at fragile sites, as well as in minimal regions of loss of heterozygosity, minimal regions of amplification, and common breakpoint regions, suggesting that miRNAs might be a new class of genes involved in human tumorigenesis. Cancer patients with a low level of *let-7* expression in the tumor have significantly shorter survival.[45] Further studies show that *let-7* can inhibit K-*ras* expression.[46] In support of this, microarray analysis of miRNAs revealed specific downregulation of *let-7* expression in samples of lung but not of breast or colon cancer compared with normal adjacent tissue. Direct comparison of squamous cell carcinoma of the lung and adjacent normal tissue reveals reduced expression of *let-7* miRNA and concomitant overexpression of *ras* in the lung carcinomas. A comprehensive study of miRNA expression in 104 paired specimens of lung cancer has recently been performed. It shows that human lung cancer has extensive alterations of miRNA expression that may deregulate cancer-related genes. The miRNA molecular profiles of lung adenocarcinoma, particularly *mir-155* and *let-7,* also correlate with patient survival.[47] However, much work remains to identify the targets of these miRNA.

More work is needed in order to understand the genetic alterations involved in lung cancer progression. More knowledge about these alterations in tumor suppressor genes, oncogenes, and miRNA in the tumor will provide a better understanding of molecular oncogenesis of lung.

Perspectives

Significant progress has been made in understanding lung oncogenesis. The challenges for us are to translate this knowledge into clinically relevant strategies to diagnose cancer early, to prevent formation of the tumors, and to treat lung cancers with novel and specific compounds, which will require tremendous synergy and collaboration between basic scientists and clinical researchers. On the one hand, basic information about lung cancer biology, such as early diagnosis and therapeutic interventions, needs to be applied in cancer patient care. The results of these applications, in return, will feed back basic research. Clinical findings of lung cancer drive the research to a higher level.

With new technologies now available for large-scale testing of clinical specimens, such as tissue microarray, gene chip analysis, and large-scale screening of small molecule chemicals with biologic activities, we are very hopeful that the next decade will be a golden age for researchers in lung cancer biology. In particular, we believe the following two areas of research will advance significantly. First, early diagnosis of lung cancer utilizing multiple biomarkers and ultrasound-guided fine aspiration will significantly improve lung cancer detection. Second, novel small molecule compounds with specific biologic activities will be discovered and applied to clinical trials or even clinical use, particularly small interference RNA. Again, these advances will require high synergy and collaboration between basic researchers and clinical scientists.

References

1. Medley LT, Cullen MT. Best supportive care versus palliative chemotherapy in nonsmall-cell lung cancer. Curr Opin Oncol 2002;14(4):384–388.
2. American Cancer Society. Cancer Facts and Figures 2006. Atlanta: American Cancer Society; 2006.
3. Tuveson DA, Jacks T. Modeling human lung cancer in mice: similarities and shortcomings. Oncogene 1999;18:5318–5324.
4. Xie J. Identifying biomarkers of lung cancer in the postgenomic era. Curr Pharmacogenomics 2005;3(4):319–331.
5. Sekido Y, Fong KM, Minna JD. Molecular genetics of lung cancer. Annu Rev Med 2003;54:73–87.

6. Mountain CF. Revisions in the international system for staging lung cancer. Chest 1997;111:1710–1717.

7. Toloza EM, Roth JA, Swisher SG. Molecular events in bronchogenic carcinoma and their implications for therapy. Semin Surg Oncol 2000;18:91–99.

8. Hilbe W, Dirnhofer S, Greil R, et al. Biomarkers in non–small cell lung cancer prevention. Eur J Cancer Prev 2004; 13:425–436.

9. Girard L, Zochbauer-Muller S, Virmani AK, et al. Genome-wide allelotyping of lung cancer identifies new regions of allelic loss, differences between small cell lung cancer and non–small cell lung cancer, and loci clustering. Cancer Res 2000;60:4894–4906.

10. Kranenburg O. The KRAS oncogene: past, present, and future. Biochim Biophys Acta 2005;1756(2):81–82.

11. Mascaux C, Iannino N, Martin B, et al. The role of RAS oncogene in survival of patients with lung cancer: a systemic review of the literature with meta-analysis. Br J Cancer 2005;92:131–139.

12. Johnson L, Mercer K, Greenbaum D, et al. Somatic activation of the K-ras oncogene causes early onset lung cancer in mice. Nature 2001;410:1111–1116.

13. Janne PA, Engelman JA, Johnson BE. Epidermal growth factor receptor mutations in non–small-cell lung cancer: implications for treatment and tumor biology. J Clin Oncol 2005;23(14):3227–3234.

14. Martin P, Kelly CM, Carney D. Epidermal growth factor receptor-targeted agents for lung cancer. Cancer Control 2006;13(2):129–140.

15. Shigematsu H, Gazdar AF. Somatic mutation of epidermal growth factor receptor signaling pathway in lung cancers. Int J Cancer 2006;118(2):257–262.

16. Spicer J, Harper P. Targeted therapies for non–small cell lung cancer. Int J Clin Pract 2005;59(9):1055–1062.

17. Miettinen M, Lasota J. KIT (CD117): a review on expression in normal and neoplastic tissues, and mutations and their clinicopathologic correlation. Appl Immunohistochem Mol Morphol 2005;13:205–220.

18. Jackman DM, Johnson BE. Small-cell lung cancer. Lancet 2005;366:1385–1396.

19. Patel O, Shulkes A, Baldwin GS. Gastrin-releasing peptide and cancer. Biochim Biophys Acta 2006; [Epub ahead of print].

20. Watkins DN, Berman DM, Burkholder SG, et al. Hedgehog signalling within airway epithelial progenitors and in small-cell lung cancer. Nature 2003;422(6929):313–317.

21. Chi S, Huang S, Li C, et al. Activation of the hedgehog pathway in a subset of lung cancers. Cancer Lett 2006; [Epub ahead of print].

22. He N, Li C, Zhang X, et al. Regulation of lung cancer cell growth and invasiveness by beta-TRCP. Mol Carcinog 2005; 42(1):18–28.

23. Haque AK, Au W, Cajas-Salazar N, et al. Association of patient smoking history, cyp2E1 polymorphism and p53 expression with patient survival in non–small cell lung cancer. Appl Immunohistochem Mol Morphol 2004;12(4): 315–322.

24. Prives C, Hall PA. The p53 pathway. J Pathol 1999;187:112–126.

25. Pietsch EC, Humbey O, Murphy ME. Polymorphisms in the p53 pathway. Oncogene 2006;25:1602–1611.

26. Liu G, Chen X. Regulation of p53 transcriptional activity. J Cell Biochem 2006;97:448–458.

27. Robles AI, Linke SP, Harris CC. The p53 network in lung carcinogenesis. Oncogene 2002;21:6898–6907.

28. Rodin SN, Rodin AS. Origins and selection of p53 mutations in lung carcinogenesis. Semin Cancer Biol 2005;15:103–112.

29. Viktorsson K, De Petris L, Lewensohn R. The role of p53 in treatment responses of lung cancer. Biochem Biophys Res Commun 2005;331:868–880.

30. Olivier M, Eeles R, Hollstein M, et al. The IARC TP53 database: new online mutation analysis and recommendations to users. Hum Mutat 2002;19:607–614.

31. Yu D, Berlin JA, Penning TM, et al. Reactive oxygen species generated by PAH o-quinones cause change-in-function mutations in p53. Chem Res Toxicol 2002;15:832–842.

32. Wani MA, Zhu Q, El-Mahdy M, et al. Enhanced sensitivity to anti-benzo(a)pyrene-diol-epoxide DNA damage correlates with decreased global genomic repair attributable to abrogated p53 function in human cells. Cancer Res 2000; 60:2273–2280.

33. Eymin B, Gazzeri S, Brambilla C, et al. Mdm2 overexpression and p14(ARF) inactivation are two mutually exclusive events in primary human lung tumors. Oncogene 2002; 21:2750–2761.

34. Nicholson SA, Okby NT, Khan MA, et al. Alterations in p14(ARF), p53 and p73 genes involved in the e2f-1–mediated apoptotic pathways in non–small cell lung carcinoma. Cancer Res 2001;61:5636–5643.

35. Dimova DK, Dyson NJ. The E2F transcriptional network: old acquaintances with new faces. Oncogene 2005;24:2810–2826.

36. Sherr CJ. The INK4a/ARF network in tumour suppression. Nat Rev Mol Cell Biol 2001;2:731–737.

37. Rocco JW, Sidransky D. p16(MTS-1/CDKN2/INK4a) in cancer progression. Exp Cell Res 2001;264:42–55.

38. Yokota J, Kohno T. Molecular footprints of human lung cancer progression. Cancer Sci 2004;95(3):197–204.

39. Brambilla E, Moro D, Gazzeri S, et al. Alterations of expression of Rb, p16(INK4A) and cyclin D1 in non–small cell lung carcinoma and their clinical significance. J Pathol 1999;188:351–360.

40. Zou CP, Youssef EM, Zou CC, et al. Differential effects of chromosome 3p deletion on the expression of the putative tumor suppressor RARbeta and on retinoid resistance in human squamous carcinoma cells. Oncogene 2001;20:6820–6827.

41. Minna JD, Fong K, Zochbauer-Muller S, et al. Molecular pathogenesis of lung cancer and potential translational applications. Cancer J 2002;8(Suppl1):S41–S54.

42. Ito I, Ji L, Tanaka F, et al. Liposomal vector mediated delivery of the 3p FUS1 gene demonstrates potent antitumor activity against human lung cancer in vivo. Cancer Gene Ther 2004;11:733–739.

43. Xian J, Clark KJ, Fordham R, et al. Inadequate lung development and bronchial hyperplasia in mice with a targeted deletion in the Dutt1/Robo1 gene. Proc Natl Acad Sci USA 2001;98(26):15062–15066.

44. Ambros V. MicroRNA pathways in flies and worms: growth, death, fat, stress, and timing. Cell 2003;113:673–676.

45. Takamizawa J, Konishi H, Yanagisawa K, et al. Reduced expression of the let-7 microRNAs in human lung cancers in association with shortened postoperative survival. Cancer Res 2004;64:3753–3756.

46. Johnson SM, Grosshans H, Shingara J, et al. RAS is regulated by the let-7 microRNA family. Cell 2005;120:635–647.

47. Yanaihara N, Caplen N, Bowman E, et al. Unique microRNA molecular profiles in lung cancer diagnosis and prognosis. Cancer Cell 2006;9(3):189–198.

17
Genetic Susceptibility

Philip T. Cagle and Timothy Craig Allen

Lung Cancer Risk

Tobacco smoke, with its many associated carcinogens, procarcinogens, and suspected carcinogens such as nitrosamines, aromatic amines, polycyclic aromatic hydrocarbons (PAHs), and free radical species, is strongly linked to lung cancer risk. Compared with tobacco smoke, other environmental exposures implicated in lung cancer have little impact on lung cancer risk. However, not every one with the same or similar tobacco exposure develops lung cancer. Why do only 10%–20% of smokers develop lung cancer, even with similar smoking histories, while up to 15% of lung cancers occur in individuals who have never smoked? Although never-smokers may have been exposed to environmental carcinogens or procarcinogens, their lung cancers are often considered to be idiopathic. Still, many people have similar environmental exposures without developing lung cancer. What factors can be used to distinguish between never-smokers with similar environmental exposures who develop lung cancer and those who do not?

People are generally thought to have different susceptibilities to cancer risk factors, including lung cancer risk factors.[1–19] These different susceptibilities might explain why some people exposed to a certain risk factor develop cancer while others similarly exposed do not and why some people with minimal exposure, or younger than average for that group of exposed individuals, develop cancer. A genetic basis for different susceptibilities to cancer risk factors has been proposed based on the observation that different susceptibilities seem to be inherited based on aggregation of cancers within families.[20–47] Inherited susceptibilities would help explain why some people develop lung cancer, such as individuals with minimal or no tobacco smoke exposure,[48–54] frequently in association with family histories positive for cancer,[55–59] or those who develop lung cancer from exposure at a significantly earlier-than-average age.[60–63] This genetic susceptibility to cancer may arise from inherited polymorphisms of genes the products of which affect an individual's ability to repair DNA damage from carcinogen exposures, to metabolize carcinogens to more potent forms, or to detoxify carcinogens. Although these inherited polymorphisms are not themselves cancer causing, they affect a certain exposure's effect or affect an individual's response to that exposure.

Familial Lung Cancer Risk

Many authors have reported increased incidences of lung and other cancers in lung cancer patients' family members.[20–47] As family members have common genetics, but also typically live in common environments, a familial increase in cancer risk could possibly be caused by exposures common to the family members sharing the same environment or common lifestyles. Potentially confounding factors such as secondhand smoke, similar smoking habits, and common occupational exposures must be taken into account before a familial cluster of cancer can legitimately be considered to be from a genetic cause. Studies examining these confounding factors have identified a statistically significant increased lung cancer risk in relatives of lung cancer patients.[22,26–36,40–47] Specifically, studies of families of lung cancer patients who were nonsmokers or significantly younger than average showed an increased familial lung cancer risk—further evidence that genetic susceptibility is a factor in lung cancer development.[29,31,41,48–63]

Most likely, some degree of familial lung cancer risk is caused by inherited polymorphisms in the DNA repair genes, as noted earlier, and xenobiotic-metabolizing enzyme genes, discussed later. Potential chromosomal loci for lung cancer susceptibility in families can be investigated with current techniques. In a study of multigenerational families with lung, throat, and laryngeal cancer, for example, a lung cancer susceptibility locus was mapped to chromosome 6q23–25.[38]

Lung Cancer Risk in Women and Men

Multiple studies have investigated possible gender differences in lung cancer susceptibility.[64-71] Some suggest that women smokers have an increased risk of developing lung cancer relative to men smokers with the same smoking histories,[72-74] whereas others have not identified any differences.[75,76] The International Early Lung Cancer Action Program Investigators, studying 7,498 women and 9,427 men, found an increased susceptibility to tobacco carcinogens in women.[71] Conversely, neither the Nurses' Health Study, studying smoking and lung cancers in more than 60,000 women, nor the Health Professionals Follow-Up Study, examining more than 25,000 men, identified an increased lung cancer risk in women.[76] Hormonal influences and environmental factors have been proposed as reasons for reported differences in gender-associated lung cancer susceptibility, as have differences in xenobiotic-metabolizing enzymes, between men and women.[77,78]

Xenobiotic-Metabolizing Enzymes

Xenobiotics, chemicals within the body such as drugs, toxins, solvents, and poisons, are altered by xenobiotic-metabolizing enzymes. Xenobiotics may induce xenobiotic-metabolizing enzymes by various methods, such as by acting as substrate ligands that bind receptors, by activating the xenobiotic enzymes by transcription, or by stabilizing the protein product. Phase I xenobiotic-metabolizing enzymes can metabolize the xenobiotic chemicals into other compounds but paradoxically may cause metabolic bioactivation of xenobiotic substrates and transform them into active or more potent toxins or carcinogens, so-called reactive intermediates. The cytochrome P450s, or CYPs, are an important group of phase I xenobiotic-metabolizing enzymes. Phase II enzymes can detoxify reactive intermediates and transform them into compounds that can be removed from the body. The glutathione-S-transferases (GSTs) are an important class of phase II enzymes. Phase III transporters, including P-glycoprotein, multidrug resistance–associated proteins, and organic anion transporting polypeptide 2, are important for xenobiotic transport and excretion.[79-89]

The primary activity of the phase I enzymes P450s or CYPs is to catalyze xenobiotic oxidation; however, they also may catalyze reduction reactions. These enzymes are also involved in other processes, such as biosynthesis of steroid hormones and prostaglandins.[90-101] These reactions primarily occur in the liver but can take place in other tissues, including lung tissue.[102-106] Cytochrome P450–dependent metabolism frequently produces intermediate compounds—reactive intermediates—that may be more potent carcinogens than their parent compounds and that could covalently bind to DNA and form adducts.

DNA adduct formation is thought to be an important step in carcinogenesis. These intermediate compounds are also converted to more soluble, inactive products that can be excreted or compartmentalized by phase II enzyme-dependent conjugation reactions. As such, CYP metabolism may be a double-edged sword, leading to production of reactive intermediates that are more carcinogenic than the original compounds—but also more readily detoxified and removed than the original compounds. Nearly 60 active human P450 genes have been identified, and most are polymorphic. The *CYP* allele homepage address is http://www.imm.ki.se/cypalleles/. The CYP enzymes and genes are designated by family number (an Arabic number), subfamily letter (A, B, C, etc.), and individual members of a subfamily (also an Arabic number). Class I polymorphic CYP enzymes, which include CYP1A1, CYP1A2, CYP1B1, CYP2A6, CYP2E1, and CYP3A4, metabolize procarcinogens. In particular, CYP1A1 and CYP1B1 are important for the metabolism of PAHs from tobacco smoke, and CYP2A6 and CYP2E1 are involved in the metabolism of nitrosamines from tobacco smoke.[90-101]

A number of CYPs are induced by the aryl hydrocarbon receptor (AhR), which dimerizes with the AhR nuclear translocator (Arnt) and induces expression of *CYP1A1* and *CYP1B1*. *CYP1A1* and *CYP1B1* encode aryl hydrocarbon hydroxylases as well as *CYP1A2*. Ligands for AhR include PAHs and other xenobiotics that are also substrates for the activated CYP enzymes. Aryl hydrocarbon receptor may exhibit either low affinity or high affinity for its ligands, producing low or high inducibility of CYP1 enzymes. After binding its ligand, AhR translocates into the nucleus and dimerizes with Arnt protein. The AhR–Arnt dimer binds to xenobiotic responsive elements (XREs) of the *CYP1A1* gene, thereby activating its transcription.[107-110]

Benzo(a)pyrene, a PAH in tobacco smoke, has been extensively studied. Benzo(a)pyrene binds to AhR upon entering the lungs, resulting in the induction of *CYP1A1* and *CYP1B1*. The CYP enzymes metabolically activate benzo(a)pyrene to benzo[*a*]pyrene-7,8-diol-9,10-epoxide (BPDE); BPDE is a carcinogen that damages DNA by covalently bonding to the DNA, forming bulky chemical adducts, for example by binding to guanine nucleobases in codons 157, 248, and 273 of *p53*—mutational "hotspots" in smoking-related lung cancers.[111-118] Besides PAHs, tobacco smoke contains *N*-nitrosamines, including 4-(methylnitrosamino)-1-(3-pyridyl)-1-butanone, *N*-dimethylnitrosamine, *N*-diethylnitrosamine, *N*-nitrosophenylmethyl-amine, and *N*-nitrosonornicotine. These inhaled *N*-nitrosamines are metabolically activated by CYP2A6 and CYP2E1 to compounds that form chemical adducts with DNA.[119-124]

The phase II enzyme GSTs primarily act to catalyze the conjugation of glutathione to xenobiotics containing an electrophilic center, forming more soluble, nontoxic peptides that can be excreted or compartmentalized by other enzymes—phase III enzymes. The GST superfamily consists of enzymes that catalyze the conjunction of glutathione to xenobiotics. It is divided into three subfamilies, each composed of multigene families—soluble or cytosolic (canonical) GSTs, microsomal or MAPEG (membrane-associated proteins involved in eicosanoid and glutathione metabolism) GST, and the plasmid-encoded bacterial fosfomycin-resistance GSTs. The cytosolic GSTs are polymorphic and are divided into seven classes—alpha, mu, and pi are regarded as specific and sigma, omega, theta, and zeta as common. Of particular interest among the cytosolic GSTs in the metabolism of tobacco-derived carcinogens are GSTM1, GSTM3, and GSTP1, which detoxify reactive intermediates of PAHs such as benzo(a)pyrene, and GSTT1, which detoxifies reactive oxidants such as ethylene oxide.[125–129] Other phase II enzymes include N-acetyltransferases (NATs), sulfotransferases, UDP-glucuronosyltransferases, and NAD(P)H:quinone oxidoreductase (NQO1). Microsomal epoxide hydrolase (mEH) is a phase II enzyme that also acts as a phase I enzyme. Microsomal epoxide hydrolase catalyzes the trans-addition of water to xenobiotics such as PAHs, including benzo(a)pyrene, producing dihydro-diol reactive intermediates involved in PAH-initiated carcinogenesis.[130–134]

DNA Adducts and Lung Cancer

DNA adducts from metabolically activated intermediates of compounds found in tobacco smoke are mutagenic and carcinogenic.[135–138] Bulky DNA adducts can be identified with ^{32}P-postlabeling of tumor tissues, peripheral blood lymphocytes, and other tissues; immunoassays and immunohistochemistry; mass spectrometry; fluorescence; high performance liquid chromatography electrochemical detection; and phosphorescence spectroscopy.[139] Polycyclic aromatic hydrocarbon–DNA adducts can be identified by BPDE-DNA immunoassays such as the BPDE-DNA chemiluminescence immunoassay.[140]

Elevated DNA adduct levels have been found in smokers' lung and other tissues. More DNA adducts are found in patients with smoking-related cancers such as lung cancer than in patients without cancer.[141–147] Veglia et al., in a metaanalysis that included data on 691 cancer patients and 632 controls from six studies (five studies involved lung cancer, one study oral cancer, and one study bladder cancer) found that current smokers with smoking-related cancers had a statistically significant (83% higher) level of DNA adducts than controls.[145] Gyorffy et al., studying 85 lung cancer patients—47 smokers, 23 long-term former smokers, 15 never-smokers—identified increased levels of DNA adducts in smokers' lungs relative to non-smokers' and never-smokers' lungs.[146]

These studies, along with studies demonstrating the carcinogenicity of DNA adducts from tobacco smoke, suggest a link between the number of DNA adducts and the development of lung cancer. However, in retrospective case–control studies, the possibility that the levels of DNA adducts are the result of, rather than the cause of, the disease cannot be completely excluded. Nonetheless, that DNA adducts are a cause of, rather than an effect of, cancer is strongly supported by prospective studies in which DNA adducts were measured in blood samples collected years before cancer onset. Tang et al., comparing blood samples from 89 subjects enrolled in the prospective Physicians' Health Study who developed primary lung cancers with 173 controls, found that disease-free current smokers with elevated levels of DNA adducts in blood leukocytes were three times more likely to be diagnosed with lung cancer 1–13 years later than current smokers with lower DNA adduct levels.[142]

In a case–control study of patients enrolled in the European Prospective Investigation into Cancer and Nutrition investigation, Peluso et al. measured the levels of DNA adducts in blood samples collected several years before the onset of cancer and noted that levels of leukocyte DNA adducts were associated with the subsequent risk of lung cancer.[147] The lung cancer association was stronger in never-smokers—whose sources would be environmental, such as second-hand tobacco smoke and air pollution—and in younger patients. These prospective studies strongly suggest a relationship between DNA adduct levels and lung cancer risk and further suggest that individual patients have differing susceptibilities to carcinogen exposures, highlighted by the risks observed in those with fewer years of exposure—younger patients—and those with lesser levels of exposure—never-smokers.

Polymorphisms and DNA Adduct Levels

Differences in levels of DNA adduct are related not only to exposure levels but also to the activity levels of xenobiotic enzymes.[148–154] Some alleles of specific xenobiotic enzymes are more active than other alleles. A variant of a phase I enzyme that is highly active (extensive metabolizer) may produce a greater number of reactive intermediates and, as a result, more DNA adducts than a less active variant of the same phase I enzyme (poor metabolizer). A less active variant of a phase II enzyme might detoxify reactive intermediates more slowly than a more active variant, resulting in a greater accumulation of reactive intermediates and therefore potentially creating more DNA adducts. Consequently, polymorphisms of xenobiotic enzymes could possibly contribute to differing DNA adduct levels in patients, which might cause patients to exhibit different susceptibilities to lung cancer. The same is true when less active variants of DNA repair genes repair damage from DNA adducts, or other sources, at a reduced rate.

Studies have found that differing levels of DNA adducts may occur in association with different variants of xenobiotic enzymes.[148–154] Patients lacking the GSTM1 enzyme have higher DNA adduct levels compared with GSTM1-positive patients. GPX1 is a phase II enzyme that conjugates PAH-diols to glutathione. In GPX1, the Pro198Leu allelic variant has lower enzyme activity, which results in less detoxification and therefore higher levels of DNA adduct compared with wild-type patients. Microsomal epoxide hydrolase is a phase II enzyme, and the slow allelic variant mEH*2 results in increased epoxide intermediates and therefore higher DNA adduct levels.[154]

Investigations of Specific Polymorphisms and Susceptibility to Lung Cancer

As described later, studies of polymorphisms of xenobiotic-metabolizing genes and DNA repair genes have identified potential allelic variants associated with greater or lesser risk of lung cancer.[155–158] Although the concept of polymorphisms of xenobiotic-metabolizing enzymes and DNA repair enzymes is appealing, studies correlating single-locus alleles with lung cancer risk have generally produced conflicting results. These conflicting results probably arise from a variety of factors. The number of cases might be too few in some studies to reliably gauge any moderate effects on lung cancer risk. The polymorphisms studied might vary. Different ethnic groups have widely differing frequencies of some polymorphisms that affect results according to the ethnic group studied. As the metabolism, detoxification, and repair processes involved in DNA adducts are complex, one single polymorphism most likely does not account for differences in DNA adduct levels. Studies analyzing several or many polymorphisms simultaneously in a single population are more likely to yield more comprehensive and consistent results. Newer technologies, permitting study of single nucleotide polymorphisms and haplotypes, increase statistical sensitivity.[158] Linkage disequilibrium–based strategies are likely to improve detection of the DNA alleles that contribute to common diseases, such as lung cancer.[155–158]

Xenobiotic-Metabolizing Genes

Cytochrome P450 Polymorphisms and Lung Cancer Susceptibility

Ayesh et al. proposed in 1984 that there was a relationship between risk of lung cancer and a polymorphism of CYP (debrisoquine 4-hydroxylase or CYP2D6).[159] In 1990, Kawajiri et al. suggested that CYP1A1 polymorphisms may impact on lung cancer risk.[160] Ensuing studies of CYP2D6 polymorphisms have produced mixed results.[161–166] Several CYP1A1 alleles have been extensively studied.

The CYP1A1 m1 allele, also known as MspI, has a T to C transition in the 3′ noncoding flanking region. It has increased enzyme activity. Hayashi et al. in 1991 first described a transition of adenine to guanine at position 2455 in exon 7 of CYP1A1, causing an isoleucine to valine amino acid substitution at codon 462 (Ile462Val).[167] Similar to the MspI allele, the valine allele, or CYP1A1 m2 allele—also termed CYP1A1*2C—has increased enzymatic activity (extensive metabolizer), believed to cause greater carcinogenic DNA adduct production and higher risk of tobacco smoke–related lung cancer. The CYP1A1 m3 allele, with a mutation in intron 7, is thought to be specific to African Americans, whereas the CYP1A1 m4 allele has a transition in exon 7 that causes a Thr for Asn substitution.[167–179]

Many studies have investigated the possible association between CYP1A1 polymorphisms and lung cancer risk in various ethnic populations.[180–220] CYP1A1 m1 and m2 polymorphisms correlated strongly with lung cancer risk in several Japanese studies, especially with respect to tobacco smokers and squamous cell carcinoma of the lung.[180,183,185,186,191,193,201] Song et al., examining 217 Chinese lung cancer cases and 404 controls, identified an increased risk for pulmonary squamous cell carcinoma in patients with at least one CYP1A1 m1 allele or at least one CYP1A1 m2 allele.[211] Lin et al. has reported similar findings.[207] Persson et al. did not identify any association of lung cancer and CYP1A1 polymorphisms in Chinese patients who were predominantly women with adenocarcinomas.[203]

Because the prevalence of the CYP1A1 m1 and m2 alleles is very low in Caucasians, studies have generally exhibited mixed results regarding these polymorphisms and Caucasian patient lung cancer risk.[184,187,188,197,199,200] Le Marchand et al., examining pooled data from Caucasians from 11 studies with a total of 1,153 lung cancer cases and 1,449 control patients, identified an increased risk of lung cancer, predominantly squamous cell carcinoma, related to the presence of the CYP1A1 m2 allele.[212] In a study of 1,050 lung cancer patients and 581 controls, Larsen et al. identified an association between the CYP1A1 m2 allele and the risk of lung cancer, especially among women patients, younger patients, and patients with lesser smoking histories.[217] Studies of populations of Americans with mixed ethnicity have also identified an increased risk of lung cancer associated with the CYP1A1 m1 allele,[197,199,200] and Brazilian studies have identified an increased lung cancer risk associated with the CYP1A1 m2 allele.[190,194] An increased risk for pulmonary adenocarcinoma, but not other types of lung cancer, associated with the CYP1A1 m3 allele has been reported in African Americans.[189,192,195,202]

CYP2A6

CYP2A6 metabolically bioactivates N-nitrosamines in tobacco smoke. Several alleles of *CYP2A6* have been identified, including *CYP2A6*4C*, *CYP2A6*7*, *CYP2A6*9*, and *CYP2A6*10*, and the alleles have decreased the enzyme activity or decreased expression of *CYP2A6*. These variant alleles of *CYP2A6* are associated with a decreased lung cancer risk, especially for squamous cell carcinoma and small cell carcinoma, and a decreased risk in heavy smokers compared with light smokers and never smokers, a finding compatible with the decreased metabolic bioactivation of N-nitorsamines.[221–224]

Other *CYP* Alleles

Several other *CYP* gene alleles have been studied as potential markers of lung cancer susceptibility, including *CYP2A13*,[235,236] *CYP2E*,[237,238] and *CYP3A*.[239] Data regarding their use as lung cancer susceptibility markers is limited, however.

Aryl Hydrocarbon Receptor

The AhR alleles have received some scrutiny for their use as possible markers of lung cancer susceptibility. However, no association with increased lung cancer risk has yet been found.[240,241]

Microsomal Epoxide Hydrolase

A number of authors have noted that mEH alleles with high activity show an association with a higher risk of smoking-related lung cancers relative to alleles with low activity.[242–247]

Glutathione-S-Transferase and Lung Cancer Susceptibility

Glutathione-S-transferase variants have been studied with respect to risk of lung cancer, but the studies have produced mixed results.[248–276] Glutathione-S-transferase polymorphisms could also affect lung cancer cell type.[277–279] These alleles occur in the *GSTM1*, *GSTT1*, *GSTP1*, and *GSTM3* genes and are associated with the reduced activity or deletion, with loss of all activity, of these phase II enzymes. These alleles include the *GSTM1*0* (*GSTM1* null) allele, a deletion of the *GSTM1* gene; the *GSTT1*0* (*GSTT1* null) allele, a deletion of the *GSTT1* gene; the *GSTP1* Ile105Val variant (I105V), caused by an A to G transition; the *GSTP1* Ala114Val variant (A114V), caused by a C to T transition; and the *GSTM3* intron 6 polymorphism, a three-base pair deletion in intron 6. Perera et al., in a nested case–control study that included 89 lung cancer cases and 173 controls (within the prospective

Physicians' Health Study), found, after controlling for smoking level, that adducts significant predicted lung cancer risk; that the combined *GSTM1* null/*GSTP1* Val genotype was associated with lung cancer generally, especially in patients who were former smokers; and that adducts were significantly higher in patients who were current or former smokers with lung cancer who exhibited the *GSTM1* non-null/*GSTP1* Ile genotype.[266] Ye et al., in a metaanalysis of data from 130 studies containing 23,452 lung cancer cases and 30,397 controls, found a weak association of the *GSTM1* null and *GSTT1* null polymorphisms with lung cancer risk and possibly weaker associations in studies of patients of European descent, whereas the *GSTP1*105V, *GSTP1*114V, and *GSTM3* intron 6 polymorphisms showed no significant overall associations with lung cancer.[276]

Other Phase II Xenobiotic Enzymes

Studies of *NQO1* alleles and possible lung cancer risk have shown mixed results.[280–284] Saldiver et al. noted that the *NQO1* variant allele associated with reduced activity was associated with increased lung cancer risk in younger patients, in women, and in never-smokers.[284] Other authors studying *NAT1* alleles and lung cancer risk have reached conflicting conclusions.[285–289] Habalova et al. found a slow acetylation variant—**5B/*6*—to be associated with squamous cell carcinoma risk in younger patients, in nonsmokers, and in women;[289] whereas Wang et al. noted an increased risk of lung cancer in association with the *SULT1A1*2 allele* (*variant A-allele*) which codes for a SULT1A1 sulfotransferase enzyme with decreased activity.[290]

Multiple Xenobiotic-Metabolizing Enzymes

Because xenobiotic metabolism is a complex process involving many enzymes, an accurate understanding of lung cancer susceptibility requires an understanding of the interactions among multiple genes and the effects of multiple enzymes. Several studies have examined the combined effects of two or more xenobiotic enzymes.[291–299] In a pooled analysis of data from 14 case–control studies that included 302 lung cancer cases and 1,631 controls in Caucasian nonsmokers from the International Collaborative Study on Genetic Susceptibility to Environmental Carcinogens, Hung et al. identified an increased lung cancer risk with the combined *CYP1A1 Ile462Val* variant and *GSTM1* null genotype relative to the *CYP1A1* wild type and *GSTM1* non-null genotype.[294] Raimondi et al. performed a metaanalysis of data from 21 case–control studies from the International Collaborative Study on Genetic Susceptibility to Environmental Carcinogens that included 2,764 Caucasians—555 lung cancer cases and 2,209 controls—and 383 Asians—113 lung cancer cases and 270 controls—who had never smoked on a regular basis.[299] In their analysis of multiple xenobiotic metabolizing enzymes, the investigators found (1) a significant association between lung cancer and *CYP1A1-Ile462Val* polymorphism in Caucasians; (2) *GSTT1* deletion was a risk factor for lung cancer in Caucasian nonsmokers only in studies including healthy controls; and (3) the combination of *CYP1A1* wild type, *GSTM1* null, and *GSTT1* non-null genotypes was associated with a lower lung cancer risk. None of the polymorphisms studied by Raimondi et al. were associated with lung cancer in Asian nonsmokers.[299]

DNA Repair Gene Polymorphisms and Lung Cancer Susceptibility

The genes and their products involved in DNA damage repair have been discussed elsewhere. In cultured lymphocytes, DNA repair capacity (DRC) can be measured using the host–cell reactivation assay and a reporter gene damaged by the activated tobacco carcinogen BPDE. A fivefold variation in DRC has been found in the general population. Also, decreased DRC has been associated with increased lung cancer risk.[300–304] Polymorphisms in DNA repair genes may be related to differences in efficiency of DNA repair. Decreased or increased ability to repair DNA damage is thought to impact the accumulation of significant genetic abnormalities required for cancer development. This has led to research regarding inherited polymorphisms of the DNA repair genes as factors in lung cancer susceptibility.

Nucleotide Excision Repair Pathway Polymorphisms

As discussed elsewhere, the nucleotide excision repair pathway removes bulky PAH–DNA adducts and as such has been an important focus of research investigating lung cancer susceptibility. After the recognition of DNA damage, such as bulky adducts, by the XPC–hHR23B complex, the helicase activities of XPD (also termed ERCC2) and XPB permit opening of the DNA double helix, which allows the damaged DNA segment to be excised and removed. The XPD protein is a required for the nucleotide excision repair pathway. Point mutations in *XPD* cause DNA repair-deficiency diseases, such as trichothiodystrophy, Cockayne syndrome, and xeroderma pigmentosum. Xeroderma pigmentosum patients have a very high predilection for cancers, which stresses the importance of the association between DNA repair efficiency and the risk of cancer.

The prevalence of *XPD* alleles and genotypes varies greatly by ethnicity. Polymorphisms in codons 156, 312, 711, and 751 of the *XPD* gene are noted commonly, with an allele frequency greater than 20%. Polymorphisms of codon G23592A (Asp312Asn) of exon 10 and codon A35931C (Lys751Gln) of exon 23 cause amino acid changes in the XPD protein and have been studied with respect to lung cancer susceptibility.[305–325] Studies have examined the levels of DNA adducts associated with these polymorphisms as an indication of the efficiency of the different alleles at DNA repair. Most likely a higher level of adducts suggests that the allele has less efficiency at excising DNA adducts. With respect to codon 312 polymorphisms, the majority of studies have found a higher level of DNA adducts in association with the *Asn* allele than with the *Asp* allele. With regard to the 751 polymorphism, the majority of studies have identified a higher level of DNA adducts in association with the *Gln* allele. As such, most studies indicate a difference in DNA repair efficiency between these specific *XPD* alleles.[305–325] Hu et al., in a metaanalysis of data from nine case–control studies including 3,725 lung cancer cases and 4,152 controls, found that patients with the *XPD751CC* genotype had a 21% higher risk of lung cancer compared with patients with the *XPD751AA* genotype and that patients with the *XPD312AA* genotype had a 27% higher risk of lung cancer than those with the *XPD312GG* genotype.[320]

Performing a meta-analysis derived from the same studies as Hu et al.,[320] including 2,886 lung cancer cases and 3,085 controls for the *XPD312* polymorphism from six studies and 3,374 lung cancer cases and 3,880 controls for the *XPD751* polymorphism from seven studies, Benhamou and Sarasin[322] were unable to conclude that one or the other of these polymorphisms was associated with an increased risk of lung cancer. After the conflicting metaanalyses, Hu et al. performed a case–control study that included 1,010 lung cancer cases and 1,011 age- and sex-matched cancer-free controls in a Chinese population.[324] They studied eight single nucleotide polymorphisms–deletion/insertion polymorphisms of *XPD/ERCC2* and *XPB/ERCC3* and found that none of the eight polymorphisms was individually associated with lung cancer risk; however, the combination of genetic variants in *ERCC2* and *ERCC3* contributed to the risk of lung cancer in a dose–response manner.

Other studies have shown an increased lung cancer risk with combinations of *XPD* polymorphisms and polymorphisms of other DNA repair genes. Zhou et al. identified a significantly increased lung cancer risk in patients with five or six variant alleles of *XPD* Asp312Asn, *XPD* Lys751Gln, and *XRCC1* Arg399Gln polymorphisms compared with patients with no variant alleles.[319] Chen et al. found that patients with variant alleles for both *XPD* Lys751Gln and *XRCC1* Arg194Trp polymorphisms had a higher lung cancer risk than patients with only one variant allele in a Chinese population.[310]

Other DNA Repair Genes

Other DNA repair gene polymorphisms, including *XPA*,[326-328] *XPC*,[329,330] *XPG*,[331] *XRCC1*,[332-338] *XRCC3*,[339] *MMH/OGG1*, the base excision repair pathway,[340-345] and *MGMT*,[346-348] have been examined with respect to lung cancer susceptibility, generally yielding conflicting or unconfirmed results, Kim et al., examining *ATM* genotypes in 616 lung cancer patients and 616 cancer-free controls, noted that the A allele at the site (IVS62+60G > A) was associated with a higher lung cancer risk than the G allele.[349] Patients with the ATTA haplotype showed significantly increased lung cancer risk versus patients with the common GCCA haplotype; and patients with the (NN)TA haplotype showed an increased lung cancer risk versus patients without the (NN)TA haplotype.

Multiple DNA Repair Genes

Zienolddiny et al., studying 44 single nucleotide polymorphisms in 20 DNA repair genes in 343 non–small cell carcinoma patients and 413 controls from the general population of Norway, found that (1) for the nucleotide excision repair pathway, *ERCC1* (Asn118Asn, C > T), *ERCC1* (C15310G), and *ERCC2* (Lys751Gln) variants were related to increased lung cancer risk, and *XPA*, *G23A*, and *ERCC5/XPG* (His46His) variants were related to decreased lung cancer risk; (2) for the base excision repair pathway, *OGG1* (Ser326Cys) and *PCNA* (A1876G) variants were associated with increased lung cancer risk, the *APE1/APEX* (Ile64Val) variant was associated with decreased lung cancer risk, and the variant T allele of PCNA2352 single nucleotide polymorphism had a marginal effect on cancer risk; (3) for the double-strand break repair pathway, the *XRCC2* (Arg188His) variant was related to increased lung cancer risk, and the *XRCC9* (Thr297Ile) and *ATR* (Thr211Met) variants were associated with decreased lung cancer risk; and (4) for the death receptor pathway, the *MGMT/AGT* (Leu-84Phe) variant in exon 3 exhibited a slight tendency toward a higher lung cancer risk.[350]

References

1. Caporaso NE, Landi MT. Molecular epidemiology: a new perspective for the study of toxic exposures in man. A consideration of the influence of genetic susceptibility factors on risk in different lung cancer histologies. Med Lav 1994;85:68–77.
2. Ikawa S, Uematsu F, Watanabe K, et al. Assessment of cancer susceptibility in humans by use of genetic polymorphisms in carcinogen metabolism. Pharmacogenetics 1995; 5(Spec. No.):S154–S160.
3. el-Zein R, Conforti-Froes N, Au WW. Interactions between genetic predisposition and environmental toxicants for development of lung cancer. Environ Mol Mutagen 1997; 30:196–204.
4. Mooney LA, Bell DA, Santella RM, et al. Contribution of genetic and nutritional factors to DNA damage in heavy smokers. Carcinogenesis 1997;18:503–509.
5. Amos CI, Xu W, Spitz MR. Is there a genetic basis for lung cancer susceptibility? Recent Results Cancer Res 1999;151:3–12.
6. Fryer AA, Jones PW. Interactions between detoxifying enzyme polymorphisms and susceptibility to cancer. IARC Sci Publ 1999;(148):303–322.
7. Kaminsky LS, Spivack SD. Cytochromes P450 and cancer. Mol Aspects Med 1999;20:70–84, 137.
8. Hirvonen A. Polymorphic NATs and cancer predisposition. IARC Sci Publ 1999;148:251–270.
9. Spitz MR, Wei Q, Li G, Wu X. Genetic susceptibility to tobacco carcinogenesis. Cancer Invest 1999;17:645–659.
10. Bartsch H, Nair U, Risch A, et al. Genetic polymorphism of CYP genes, alone or in combination, as a risk modifier of tobacco-related cancers. Cancer Epidemiol Biomarkers Prev 2000;9:3–28.
11. Houlston RS. CYP1A1 polymorphisms and lung cancer risk: a meta-analysis. Pharmacogenetics 2000;10:105–114.
12. Bouchardy C, Benhamou S, Jourenkova N, Dayer P, Hirvonen A. Metabolic genetic polymorphisms and susceptibility to lung cancer. Lung Cancer 2001;32:109–112.
13. Goode EL, Ulrich CM, Potter JD. Polymorphisms in DNA repair genes and associations with cancer risk. Cancer Epidemiol Biomarkers Prev 2002;11:1513–1530.
14. Kiyohara C, Otsu A, Shirakawa T, Fukuda S, Hopkin JM. Genetic polymorphisms and lung cancer susceptibility: a review. Lung Cancer 2002;37:241–256.
15. Gorlova OY, Amos C, Henschke C, et al. Genetic susceptibility for lung cancer: interactions with gender and smoking history and impact on early detection policies. Hum Hered 2003;56:139–145.
16. Schwartz AG. Genetic predisposition to lung cancer. Chest 2004;125(5 Suppl):86S–89S.
17. Kiyohara C, Yoshimasu K, Shirakawa T, Hopkin JM. Genetic polymorphisms and environmental risk of lung cancer: a review. Rev Environ Health 2004;19:15–38.
18. Miller YE, Fain P. Genetic susceptibility to lung cancer. Semin Respir Crit Care Med 2003;24:197–204.
19. Christiani DC. Genetic susceptibility to lung cancer. J Clin Oncol 2006;24:1651–1652.
20. Anderson D. Familial susceptibility to cancer. CA Cancer J Clin 1976;26:143–149.
21. Ooi WL, Elston RC, Chen VW, et al. Increased familial risk for lung cancer. J Natl Cancer Inst 1986;76:217–222.
22. Ooi WL, Elston RC, Chen VW, et al. Familial lung cancer—correcting an error in calculation. J Natl Cancer Inst 1986; 77:990.
23. Sellers TA, Ooi WL, Elston RC, et al. Increased familial risk for non-lung cancer among relatives of lung cancer patients. Am J Epidemiol 1987;126:237–246.
24. McDuffie HH. Clustering of cancer in families of patients with primary lung cancer. J Clin Epidemiol 1991;44:69–76.
25. Ambrosone CB, Rao U, Michalek AM, et al. Lung cancer histologic types and family history of cancer. Analysis of histologic subtypes of 872 patients with primary lung cancer. Cancer 1993;72:1192–1198.

26. Sellers TA, Chen PL, Potter JD, et al. Segregation analysis of smoking-associated malignancies: evidence for Mendelian inheritance. Am J Med Genet 1994;52:308–314.

27. Dragani TA, Manenti G, Pierotti MA. Polygenic inheritance of predisposition to lung cancer. Ann Ist Super Sanita 1996;32:145–150.

28. Ahlbom A, Lichtenstein P, Malmstrom H, et al. Cancer in twins: genetic and nongenetic familial risk factors. J Natl Cancer Inst 1997;89:287–293.

29. Li H, Yang P, Schwartz AG. Analysis of age of onset data from case–control family studies. Biometrics 1998;54:1030–1039.

30. Suzuki K, Ogura T, Yokose T, et al. Microsatellite instability in female non–small-cell lung cancer patients with familial clustering of malignancy. Br J Cancer 1998;77:1003–1008.

31. Hemminki K, Vaittinen P. Familial cancers in a nationwide family cancer database: age distribution and prevalence. Eur J Cancer 1999;35:1109–1117.

32. Bromen K, Pohlabeln H, Jahn I, et al. Aggregation of lung cancer in families: results from a population-based case–control study in Germany. Am J Epidemiol 2000;152:497–505.

33. Gupta D, Aggarwal AN, Vikrant S, Jindal SK. Familial aggregation of cancer in patients with bronchogenic carcinoma. Indian J Cancer 2000;37:43–49.

34. Wunsch-Filho V, Boffetta P, Colin D, Moncau JE. Familial cancer aggregation and the risk of lung cancer. Sao Paulo Med J 2002;120:38–44.

35. Etzel CJ, Amos CI, Spitz MR. Risk for smoking-related cancer among relatives of lung cancer patients. Cancer Res 2003;63:8531–8535.

36. Li X, Hemminki K. Familial and second lung cancers: a nation-wide epidemiologic study from Sweden. Lung Cancer 2003;39:255–263.

37. Rooney A. Family history reveals lung-cancer risk. Lancet Oncol 2003;4:267.

38. Bailey-Wilson JE, Amos CI, Pinney SM, et al. A major lung cancer susceptibility locus maps to chromosome 6q23–25. Am J Hum Genet 2004;75:460–474.

39. Hemminki K, Li X, Czene K. Familial risk of cancer: data for clinical counseling and cancer genetics. Int J Cancer 2004;108:109–114.

40. Jonsson S, Thorsteinsdottir U, Gudbjartsson DF, et al. Familial risk of lung carcinoma in the Icelandic population. JAMA 2004;292:2977–2983.

41. Hemminki K, Li X. Familial risk for lung cancer by histology and age of onset: evidence for recessive inheritance. Exp Lung Res 2005;31:205–215.

42. Jin YT, Xu YC, Yang RD, et al. Familial aggregation of lung cancer in a high incidence area in China. Br J Cancer 2005;92:1321–1325.

43. Jin Y, Xu Y, Xu M, Xue S. Increased risk of cancer among relatives of patients with lung cancer in China. BMC Cancer 2005;5:146.

44. Keith RL, Miller YE. Lung cancer: genetics of risk and advances in chemoprevention. Curr Opin Pulm Med 2005;11:265–271.

45. Li X, Hemminki K. Familial multiple primary lung cancers: a population-based analysis from Sweden. Lung Cancer 2005;47:301–307.

46. Matakidou A, Eisen T, Houlston RS. Systematic review of the relationship between family history and lung cancer risk. Br J Cancer 2005;93:825–833.

47. Schwartz AG, Ruckdeschel JC. Familial lung cancer: genetic susceptibility and relationship to chronic obstructive pulmonary disease. Am J Respir Crit Care Med 2006;173:16–22.

48. Bennett WP, Alavanja MC, Blomeke B, et al. Environmental tobacco smoke, genetic susceptibility, and risk of lung cancer in never-smoking women. J Natl Cancer Inst 1999;91:2009–2014.

49. Yang P, Yokomizo A, Tazelaar HD, et al. Genetic determinants of lung cancer short-term survival: the role of glutathione-related genes. Lung Cancer 2002;35:221–229.

50. Kiyohara C, Wakai K, Mikami H, et al. Risk modification by CYP1A1 and GSTM1 polymorphisms in the association of environmental tobacco smoke and lung cancer: a case–control study in Japanese nonsmoking women. Int J Cancer 2003;107:139–144.

51. Cohet C, Borel S, Nyberg F, et al. Exon 5 polymorphisms in the O6-alkylguanine DNA alkyltransferase gene and lung cancer risk in non-smokers exposed to second-hand smoke. Cancer Epidemiol Biomarkers Prev 2004;13:320–323.

52. Wenzlaff AS, Cote ML, Bock CH, et al. CYP1A1 and CYP1B1 polymorphisms and risk of lung cancer among never smokers: a population-based study. Carcinogenesis 2005;26:2207–2212.

53. Wenzlaff AS, Cote ML, Bock CH, et al. GSTM1, GSTT1 and GSTP1 polymorphisms, environmental tobacco smoke exposure and risk of lung cancer among never smokers: a population-based study. Carcinogenesis 2005;26:395–401.

54. Gorlova OY, Zhang Y, Schabath MB, et al. Never smokers and lung cancer risk: a case-control study of epidemiological factors. Int J Cancer 2006;118:1798–1804.

55. Schwartz AG, Yang P, Swanson GM. Familial risk of lung cancer among nonsmokers and their relatives. Am J Epidemiol 1996;144:554–562.

56. Yang P, Schwartz AG, McAllister AE, et al. Genetic analysis of families with nonsmoking lung cancer probands. Genet Epidemiol 1997;14:181–197.

57. Mayne ST, Buenconsejo J, Janerich DT. Familial cancer history and lung cancer risk in United States nonsmoking men and women. Cancer Epidemiol Biomarkers Prev 1999;8:1065–1069.

58. Schwartz AG, Rothrock M, Yang P, Swanson GM. Increased cancer risk among relatives of nonsmoking lung cancer cases. Genet Epidemiol 1999;17:1–15.

59. Yang P, Schwartz AG, McAllister AE, et al. Lung cancer risk in families of nonsmoking probands: heterogeneity by age at diagnosis. Genet Epidemiol 1999;17:253–273.

60. Kreuzer M, Kreienbrock L, Gerken M, et al. Risk factors for lung cancer in young adults. Am J Epidemiol 1998;147:1028–1037.

61. Gauderman WJ, Morrison JL. Evidence for age-specific genetic relative risks in lung cancer. Am J Epidemiol 2000;151:41–49.

62. Li X, Hemminki K. Inherited predisposition to early onset lung cancer according to histological type. Int J Cancer 2004;112:451–457.

63. Cote ML, Kardia SL, Wenzlaff AS, et al. Combinations of glutathione S-transferase genotypes and risk of early-onset lung cancer in Caucasians and African Americans: a population-based study. Carcinogenesis 2005;26:811–819.

64. Dresler CM, Fratelli C, Babb J, et al. Gender differences in genetic susceptibility for lung cancer. Lung Cancer 2000;30:153–160.

65. Kreuzer M, Wichmann HE. Lung cancer in young females. Eur Respir J 2001;17:1333–1334.

66. Haugen A. Women who smoke: are women more susceptible to tobacco-induced lung cancer? Carcinogenesis 2002;23:227–229.

67. Stabile LP, Siegfried JM. Sex and gender differences in lung cancer. J Gend Specif Med 2003;6:37–48.

68. Pauk N, Kubik A, Zatloukal P, Krepela E. Lung cancer in women. Lung Cancer 2005;48:1–9.

69. Matakidou A, Eisen T, Bridle H, et al. Case–control study of familial lung cancer risks in UK women. Int J Cancer 2005;116:445–450.

70. Patel JD. Lung cancer in women. J Clin Oncol 2005;23:3212–3218.

71. International Early Lung Cancer Action Program Investigators, Henschke CI, Yip R, Miettinen OS. Women's susceptibility to tobacco carcinogens and survival after diagnosis of lung cancer. JAMA 2006;296:180–184.

72. Risch HA, Howe GR, Jain M, et al. Are female smokers at higher risk for lung cancer than male smokers? A case–control analysis by histologic type. Am J Epidemiol 1993;138:281–293.

73. Zang EA, Wynder EL. Differences in lung cancer risk between men and women: examination of the evidence. J Natl Cancer Inst 1996;88:183–192.

74. Henschke CI, Miettinen O. Women's susceptibility to tobacco carcinogens. Lung Cancer 2004;43:1–5.

75. Bach PB, Kattan MW, Thornquist MD, et al. Variations in lung cancer risk among smokers. J Natl Cancer Inst 2003;95:470–478.

76. Bain C, Feskanich D, Speizer FE, et al. Lung cancer rates in men and women with comparable histories of smoking. J Natl Cancer Inst 2004;96:826–834.

77. Ng DP, Tan KW, Zhao B, Seow A. CYP1A1 polymorphisms and risk of lung cancer in non-smoking Chinese women: influence of environmental tobacco smoke exposure and GSTM1/T1 genetic variation. Cancer Causes Control 2005;16:399–405.

78. Mollerup S, Berge G, Baera R, et al. Sex differences in risk of lung cancer: expression of genes in the PAH bioactivation pathway in relation to smoking and bulky DNA adducts. Int J Cancer 2006;119:741–744.

79. Bond JA. Metabolism and elimination of inhaled drugs and airborne chemicals from the lungs. Pharmacol Toxicol 1993;72 Suppl 3:36–47.

80. Raunio H, Husgafvel-Pursiainen K, Anttila S, et al. Diagnosis of polymorphisms in carcinogen-activating and inactivating enzymes and cancer susceptibility—a review. Gene 1995;159:113–121.

81. Wormhoudt LW, Commandeur JN, Vermeulen NP. Genetic polymorphisms of human N-acetyltransferase, cytochrome P450, glutathione-S-transferase, and epoxide hydrolase

enzymes: relevance to xenobiotic metabolism and toxicity. Crit Rev Toxicol 1999;29:59–124.

82. Nakajima T, Aoyama T. Polymorphism of drug-metabolizing enzymes in relation to individual susceptibility to industrial chemicals. Ind Health 2000;38:143–152.

83. Miller MC 3rd, Mohrenweiser HW, Bell DA. Genetic variability in susceptibility and response to toxicants. Toxicol Lett 2001;120:269–280.

84. Rushmore TH, Kong AN. Pharmacogenomics, regulation and signaling pathways of phase I and II drug metabolizing enzymes. Curr Drug Metab 2002;3:481–490.

85. Daly AK. Pharmacogenetics of the major polymorphic metabolizing enzymes. Fundam Clin Pharmacol 2003;17:27–41.

86. Sheweita SA, Tilmisany AK. Cancer and phase II drug-metabolizing enzymes. Curr Drug Metab 2003;4:45–58.

87. Xu C, Li CY, Kong AN. Induction of phase I, II and III drug metabolism/transport by xenobiotics. Arch Pharm Res 2005;28:249–268.

88. Nishikawa A, Mori Y, Lee IS, et al. Cigarette smoking, metabolic activation and carcinogenesis. Curr Drug Metab 2004;5:363–373.

89. Cascorbi I. Genetic basis of toxic reactions to drugs and chemicals. Toxicol Lett 2006;162:16–28.

90. Raunio H, Husgafvel-Pursiainen K, Anttila S, et al. Diagnosis of polymorphisms in carcinogen-activating and inactivating enzymes and cancer susceptibility—a review. Gene 1995;159:113–121.

91. Kerremans AL. Cytochrome P450 isoenzymes—importance for the internist. Neth J Med 1996;48:237–243.

92. Dogra SC, Whitelaw ML, May BK. Transcriptional activation of cytochrome P450 genes by different classes of chemical inducers. Clin Exp Pharmacol Physiol 1998;25:1–9.

93. Lewis DF, Watson E, Lake BG. Evolution of the cytochrome P450 superfamily: sequence alignments and pharmacogenetics. Mutat Res 1998;410:245–270.

94. McKinnon RA, Nebert DW. Cytochrome P450 knockout mice: new toxicological models. Clin Exp Pharmacol Physiol 1998;25:783–787.

95. Ingelman-Sundberg M. Genetic susceptibility to adverse effects of drugs and environmental toxicants. The role of the CYP family of enzymes. Mutat Res 2001;482:11–19.

96. Ingelman-Sundberg M. Polymorphism of cytochrome P450 and xenobiotic toxicity. Toxicology 2002;181–182:447–452.

97. Lewis DF. Human cytochromes P450 associated with the phase 1 metabolism of drugs and other xenobiotics: a compilation of substrates and inhibitors of the CYP1, CYP2 and CYP3 families. Curr Med Chem 2003;10:1955–1972.

98. Shimada T, Fujii-Kuriyama Y. Metabolic activation of polycyclic aromatic hydrocarbons to carcinogens by cytochromes P450 1A1 and 1B1. Cancer Sci 2004;95:1–6.

99. Lewis DF. 57 varieties: the human cytochromes P450. Pharmacogenomics 2004;5:305–318.

100. Rodriguez-Antona C, Ingelman-Sundberg M. Cytochrome P450 pharmacogenetics and cancer. Oncogene 2006;25:1679–1691.

101. Sim SC, Ingelman-Sundberg M. The human cytochrome P450 Allele Nomenclature Committee Web site: submis-

sion criteria, procedures, and objectives. Methods Mol Biol 2006;320:183–191.

102. Raunio H, Hakkola J, Hukkanen J, et al. Expression of xenobiotic-metabolizing CYPs in human pulmonary tissue. Exp Toxicol Pathol 1999;51:412–417.

103. Hukkanen J, Pelkonen O, Raunio H. Expression of xeno-biotic-metabolizing enzymes in human pulmonary tissue: possible role in susceptibility for ILD. Eur Respir J Suppl 2001;32:122s–126s.

104. Hukkanen J, Pelkonen O, Hakkola J, Raunio H. Expres-sion and regulation of xenobiotic-metabolizing cytochrome P450 (CYP) enzymes in human lung. Crit Rev Toxicol 2002;32:391–411.

105. Ding X, Kaminsky LS. Human extrahepatic cytochromes P450: function in xenobiotic metabolism and tissue-selective chemical toxicity in the respiratory and gastroin-testinal tracts. Annu Rev Pharmacol Toxicol 2003;43:149–173.

106. Castell JV, Donato MT, Gomez-Lechon MJ. Metabolism and bioactivation of toxicants in the lung. The in vitro cellular approach. Exp Toxicol Pathol 2005;57(Suppl 1): 189–204.

107. Fujii-Kuriyama Y, Ema M, Mimura J, et al. Polymorphic forms of the Ah receptor and induction of the CYP1A1 gene. Pharmacogenetics 1995;5(Spec No):S149–S153.

108. Denison MS, Nagy SR. Activation of the aryl hydrocarbon receptor by structurally diverse exogenous and endo-genous chemicals. Annu Rev Pharmacol Toxicol 2003;43: 309–334.

109. Fujii-Kuriyama Y, Mimura J. Molecular mechanisms of AhR functions in the regulation of cytochrome P450 genes. Biochem Biophys Res Commun 2005;338:311–317.

110. Hankinson O. Role of coactivators in transcriptional acti-vation by the aryl hydrocarbon receptor. Arch Biochem Biophys 2005;433:379–386.

111. Gelboin HV. Benzo(a)pyrene metabolism, activation, and carcinogenesis. role and regulation of mixed function oxi-dases and related enzymes. Physiol Rev 1980;60:1107–1166.

112. Phillips DH. Fifty years of benzo(a)pyrene. Nature (Lond) 1983;303:468–472.

113. Jeffrey AM. DNA modification by chemical carcinogens. Pharmacol Ther 1985;28:237–272.

114. Graslund A, Jernstrom B. DNA-carcinogen interaction: covalent DNA-adducts of benzo(a)pyrene 7,8-dihydrodiol 9,10-epoxides studied by biochemical and biophysical techniques. Q Rev Biophys 1989;22:1–37.

115. Denissenko MF, Pao A, Tang M-S, Pfeifer GP. Preferential formation of benzo[a]pyrene adducts at lung cancer muta-tional hotspots in p53. Science 1996;274:430–432.

116. Kozack R, Seo KY, Jelinsky SA, Loechler EL. Toward an understanding of the role of DNA adduct conformation in defining mutagenic mechanism based on studies of the major adduct (formed at N(2)-dG) of the potent environ-mental carcinogen, benzo[a]pyrene. Mutat Res 2000;450: 41–59.

117. Pfeifer GP, Denissenko MF, Olivier M, et al. Tobacco smoke carcinogens, DNA damage and p53 mutations in smoking-associated cancers. Oncogene 2002;21:7435–7451.

118. Baird WM, Hooven LA, Mahadevan B. Carcinogenic polycyclic aromatic hydrocarbon–DNA adducts and mechanism of action. Environ Mol Mutagen 2005;45: 106–114.

119. Hoffmann D, Brunnemann KD, Adams JD, Hecht SS. For-mation and analysis of N-nitrosamines in tobacco products and their endogenous formation in consumers. IARC Sci Publ 1984;57:743–762.

120. Brunnemann KD, Hoffmann D. Analytical studies on tobacco-specific N-nitrosamines in tobacco and tobacco smoke. Crit Rev Toxicol 1991;21:235–240.

121. Amin S, Desai D, Hecht SS, Hoffmann D. Synthesis of tobacco-specific N-nitrosamines and their metabolites and results of related bioassays. Crit Rev Toxicol 1996;26: 139–147.

122. Brunnemann KD, Prokopczyk B, Djordjevic MV, Hoffmann D. Formation and analysis of tobacco-specific N-nitrosamines. Crit Rev Toxicol 1996;26:121–137.

123. Hecht SS, Biochemistry, biology, and carcinogenicity of tobacco-specific N-nitrosamines. Chem Res Toxicol 1998; 11:559–603.

124. Hecht SS. DNA adduct formation from tobacco-specific N-nitrosamines. Mutat Res 1999;424:127–142.

125. Vos RM, Van Bladeren PJ. Glutathione S-transferases in relation to their role in the biotransformation of xenobiot-ics. Chem Biol Interact 1990;75:241–265.

126. Daniel V. Glutathione S-transferases: gene structure and regulation of expression. Crit Rev Biochem Mol Biol 1993;28:173–207.

127. Hayes JD, Pulford DJ. The glutathione S-transferase supergene family: regulation of GST and the contribu-tion of the isoenzymes to cancer chemoprotection and drug resistance. Crit Rev Biochem Mol Biol 1995;30:445–600.

128. Rahman Q, Abidi P, Afaq F, et al. Glutathione redox system in oxidative lung injury. Crit Rev Toxicol 1999;29:543–568.

129. Salinas AE, Wong MG. Glutathione S-transferases—a review. Curr Med Chem 1999;6:279–309.

130. Baron J, Voigt JM. Localization, distribution, and induction of xenobiotic-metabolizing enzymes and aryl hydrocarbon hydroxylase activity within lung. Pharmacol Ther 1990;47: 419–445.

131. Seidegard J, Ekstrom G. The role of human glutathione transferases and epoxide hydrolases in the metabolism of xenobiotics. Environ Health Perspect 1997;105(Suppl 4): 791–799.

132. Omiecinski CJ, Hassett C, Hosagrahara V. Epoxide hydro-lase—polymorphism and role in toxicology. Toxicol Lett 2000;112–113:365–370.

133. Fretland AJ, Omiecinski CJ. Epoxide hydrolases: bio-chemistry and molecular biology. Chem Biol Interact 2000; 129:41–59.

134. Arand M, Cronin A, Adamska M, Oesch F. Epoxide hydro-lases: structure, function, mechanism, and assay. Methods Enzymol 2005;400:569–588.

135. Miller EC, Miller JA. Searches for ultimate chemical car-cinogens and their reaction with cellular macromolecules. Cancer 1981;47:2327–2345.

136. Pelkonen O, Nebert DW. Metabolism of polycyclic aromatic hydrocarbons: etiologic role in carcinogenesis. Pharmacol Rev 1982;34:189–222.

137. Poirier MC, Beland FA. DNA adduct measurement and tumor incidence during chronic carcinogen exposure in animal models: implications for DNA adduct-based human cancer risk assessment. Chem Res Toxicol 1992;5:749–755.

138. Bartsch H, Rojas M, Nair U, et al. Genetic cancer susceptibility and DNA adducts: studies in smokers, tobacco chewers, and coke oven workers. Cancer Detect Prev 1999;23:445–453.

139. Poirier MC, Santella RM, Weston A. Carcinogen macromolecular adducts and their measurement. Carcinogenesis 2000;21:353–359.

140. Weston A, Manchester DK, Poirier MC, et al. Derivative fluorescence spectral analysis of polycyclic aromatic hydrocarbon-DNA adducts in human placenta. Chem Res Toxicol 1989;2:104–108.

141. Vulimiri SV, Wu X, Baer-Dubowska W, et al. Analysis of aromatic DNA adducts and 7,8-dihydro-8-oxo-2′-deoxyguanosine in lymphocyte DNA from a case–control study of lung cancer involving minority populations. Mol Carcinog 2000;27:34–46.

142. Tang D, Phillips DH, Stampfer M, et al. Association between carcinogen DNA adducts in white blood cells and lung cancer risk in the Physicians Health Study. Cancer Res 2001;61:6708–6712.

143. Phillips DH. Smoking-related DNA and protein adducts in human tissues. Carcinogenesis 2002;23:1979–2004.

144. Wiencke JD. DNA adduct burden and tobacco carcinogenesis. Oncogene 2002;21:7376–7391.

145. Veglia F, Matullo G, Vineis P. Bulky DNA adducts and risk of cancer: a meta-analysis. Cancer Epidemiol Biomarkers Prev 2003;12:157–160.

146. Gyorffy E, Anna L, Gyori Z, et al. DNA adducts in tumour, normal peripheral lung and bronchus, and peripheral blood lymphocytes from smoking and non-smoking lung cancer patients: correlations between tissues and detection by 32P-postlabelling and immunoassay. Carcinogenesis 2004;25:1201–1209.

147. Peluso M, Munnia A, Hoek G, et al. DNA adducts and lung cancer risk: a prospective study. Cancer Res 2005;65:8042–8048.

148. Hassett C, Robinson KB, Beck NB, Omiecinski CJ. The human microsomal epoxide hydrolase gene (EPHX1): complete nucleotide sequence and structural characterization. Genomics 1994;23:433–442.

149. Kato S, Bowman ED, Harrington AM, et al. Human lung carcinogen–DNA adduct levels mediated by genetic polymorphisms in vivo. J Natl Cancer Inst 1995;87:902–907.

150. Butkiewicz D, Grzybowska E, Hemminki K, et al. Modulation of DNA adduct levels in human mononuclear white blood cells and granulocytes by CYP1A1 CYP2D6 and GSTM1 genetic polymorphisms. Mutat Res 1998;415:97–108.

151. Rojas M, Alexandrov K, Cascorbi I, et al. High benzo[a]pyrene diol-epoxide DNA adduct levels in lung and blood cells from individuals with combined CYP1A1 MspI/Msp-GSTM1*0/*0 genotypes. Pharmacogenetics 1998;8:109–118.

152. Ratnasinghe D, Tangrea JA, Andersen MR, et al. Glutathione peroxidase codon 198 polymorphism variant increases lung cancer risk. Cancer Res 2000;60:6381–6383.

153. Godschalk RW, Dallinga JW, Wikman H, et al. Modulation of DNA and protein adducts in smokers by genetic polymorphisms in GSTM1, GSTT1, NAT1 and NAT2. Pharmacogenetics 2001;11:389–398.

154. Ketelslegers HB, Gottschalk RW, Godschalk RW, et al. Interindividual variations in DNA adduct levels assessed by analysis of multiple genetic polymorphisms in smokers. Cancer Epidemiol Biomarkers Prev 2006;15:624–629.

155. Kawajiri K, Watanabe J, Eguchi H, Hayashi S. Genetic polymorphisms of drug-metabolizing enzymes and lung cancer susceptibility. Pharmacogenetics 1995;5(Spec No.): S70–S73.

156. Watanabe M. Polymorphic CYP genes and disease predisposition—what have the studies shown so far? Toxicol Lett 1998;102–103:167–171.

157. Smith GB, Harper PA, Wong JM, et al. Human lung microsomal cytochrome P4501A1 (CYP1A1) activities: impact of smoking status and CYP1A1, aryl hydrocarbon receptor, and glutathione S-transferase M1 genetic polymorphisms. Cancer Epidemiol Biomarkers Prev 2001;10: 839–853.

158. Liang G, Pu Y, Yin L. Rapid detection of single nucleotide polymorphisms related with lung cancer susceptibility of Chinese population. Cancer Lett 2005;223:265–274.

159. Ayesh R, Idle JR, Ritchie JC, et al. Metabolic oxidation phenotypes as markers for susceptibility to lung cancer. Nature 1984;312:169–170.

160. Kawajiri K, Nakachi K, Imai K, et al. Identification of genetically high risk individuals to lung cancer by DNA polymorphisms of the cytochrome P450IA1 gene. FEBS Lett 1990;263:131–133.

161. Caporaso N, Pickle LW, Bale S, et al. The distribution of debrisoquine metabolic phenotypes and implications for the suggested association with lung cancer risk. Genet Epidemiol 1989;6:517–524.

162. Nebert DW. Polymorphism of human CYP2D genes involved in drug metabolism: possible relationship to individual cancer risk. Cancer Cells 1991;3:93–96.

163. Puchetti V, Faccini GB, Micciolo R, et al. Dextromethorphan test for evaluation of congenital predisposition to lung cancer. Chest 1994;105:449–453.

164. Caporaso N, DeBaun MR, Rothman N. Lung cancer and CYP2D6 (the debrisoquine polymorphism): sources of heterogeneity in the proposed association. Pharmacogenetics 1995;5:S129–S134.

165. Gao Y, Zhang Q. Polymorphisms of the GSTM1 and CYP2D6 genes associated with susceptibility to lung cancer in Chinese. Mutat Res 1999;444:441–449.

166. Laforest L, Wikman H, Benhamou S, et al. CYP2D6 gene polymorphism in Caucasian smokers: lung cancer susceptibility and phenotype–genotype relationships. Eur J Cancer 2000;36:1825–1832.

167. Hayashi S, Watanabe J, Nakachi K, Kawajiri K. Genetic linkage of lung cancer-associated MspI polymorphisms with amino acid replacement in the heme binding region of the human cytochrome P450IA1 gene. J Biochem (Tokyo) 1991;110:407–411.

168. Petersen DD, Mckinney CE, Ikeya K, et al. Human CYP1A1 gene: cosegregation of the enzyme inducibility phenotype and an RFLP. Am J Hum Genet 1991;48:720–725.

169. Ingelman-Sundberg M, Johansson I, Persson I, et al. Genetic polymorphism of cytochromes P450: interethnic differences and relationship to incidence of lung cancer. Pharmacogenetics 1992;2:264–271.

170. Cosma G, Crofts F, Taioli E, et al. Relationship between genotype and function of the human CYP1A1 gene. J Toxicol Environ Health 1993;40:309–316.

171. Crofts F, Cosma GN, Taioli E, et al. A novel CYP1A1 gene polymorphism in African-Americans. Carcinogenesis 1993;14:1729–1731.

172. Kawajiri K, Nakachi K, Imai K, et al. The CYP1A1 gene and cancer susceptibility. Crit Rev Oncol Hematol 1993;14:77–87.

173. Crofts F, Taioli E, Trachman J, et al. Functional significance of different human CYP1A1 genotypes. Carcinogenesis 1994;15:2961–2963.

174. Drakoulis N, Cascorbi I, Brockmoller J, et al. Polymorphisms in the human CYP1A1 gene as susceptibility factors for lung cancer: exon-7 mutation (4889 A to G), and a T to C mutation in the 3′-flanking region. Clin Invest 1994;72:240–248.

175. Landi MT, Bertazzi PA, Shields PG, et al. Association between CYP1A1 genotype, mRNA expression and enzymatic activity in humans. Pharmacogenetics 1994;4:242–246.

176. Nakachi K, Hayashi S, Kawajiri K, Imai K. Association of cigarette smoking and CYP1A1 polymorphisms with adenocarcinoma of the lung by grades of differentiation. Carcinogenesis 1995;16:2209–2213.

177. Kawajiri K, Eguchi H, Nakachi K, et al. Association of CYP1A1 germ line polymorphisms with mutations of the p53 gene in lung cancer. Cancer Res 1996;56:72–76.

178. Kiyohara C, Hirohata T, Inutsuka S. The relationship between aryl hydrocarbon hydroxylase and polymorphisms of the CYP1A1 gene. Jpn J Cancer Res 1996;87:18–24.

179. Kiyohara C, Nakanishi Y, Inutsuka S, et al. The relationship between CYP1A1 aryl hydrocarbon hydroxylase activity and lung cancer in a Japanese population. Pharmacogenetics 1998;8:315–323.

180. Kawajiri K, Nakachi K, Imai K, et al. Individual differences in lung cancer susceptibility in relation to polymorphisms of P-450IA1 gene and cigarette dose. Princess Takamatsu Symp 1990;21:55–61.

181. Nakachi K, Imai K, Hayashi S, et al. Genetic susceptibility to squamous cell carcinoma of the lung in relation to cigarette smoking dose. Cancer Res 1991;51:5177–5180.

182. Uematsu F, Kikuchi H, Motomiya M, et al. Association between restriction fragment length polymorphism of the human cytochrome P450IIE1 gene and susceptibility to lung cancer. Jpn J Cancer Res 1991;82:254–256.

183. Hayashi S, Watanabe J, Kawajiri K. High susceptibility to lung cancer analyzed in term of combined genotypes of CYP1A1 and Mu-class glutathione S-transferase genes. Jpn J Cancer Res 1992;83:866–870.

184. Hirvonen A, Husgafvel-Pursiainen K, Karjalainen A, et al. Point-mutational MspI and Ile-Val polymorphisms closely linked in the CYP1A1 gene: lack of association with susceptibility to lung cancer in a Finnish study population. Cancer Epidemiol Biomarkers Prev 1992;1:485–489.

185. Kawajiri K, Nakachi K, Imai K, et al. The CYP1A1 gene and cancer susceptibility. Crit Rev Oncol Hematol 1993;14:77–87.

186. Nakachi K, Imai K, Hayashi S, Kawajiri K. Polymorphisms of the CYP1A1 and glutathione S-transferase genes associated with susceptibility to lung cancer in relation to cigarette dose in a Japanese population. Cancer Res 1993;53:2994–2999.

187. Shields PG, Caporaso NE, Falk RT, et al. Lung cancer, race, and a CYP1A1 genetic polymorphism. Cancer Epidemiol Biomarkers Prev 1993;2:481–485.

188. Alexandrie AK, Sundberg MI, Seidegard J, et al. Genetic susceptibility to lung cancer with special emphasis to CYP1A1 and GSTM1: a study on host factors in relation to age at onset, gender and histological cancer types. Carcinogenesis 1994;15:1785–1790.

189. Kelsey KT, Wiencke JK, Spitz MR. A race-specific genetic polymorphism in the CYP1A1 gene is not associated with lung cancer in African-Americans. Carcinogenesis 1994;15:1121–1124.

190. Hamada GS, Sugimura H, Suzuki I, et al. The heme-binding region polymorphism of cytochrome P450IA1 (CypIA1), rather than the RsaI polymorphism of IIE1 (CypIIE1), is associated with lung cancer in Rio de Janeiro. Cancer Epidemiol Biomarkers Prev 1995;4:63–67.

191. Kihara M, Kihara M, Noda K. Risk of smoking for squamous and small cell carcinomas of the lung modulated by combinations of CYP1A1 and GSTM1 gene polymorphisms in a Japanese population. Carcinogenesis 1995;16:2331–2336.

192. London SJ, Daly AK, Fairbrother KS, et al. Lung cancer risk in African-Americans in relation to a race-specific polymorphism. Cancer Res 1995;55:6035–6037.

193. Nakachi K, Hayashi S, Kawajiri K, Imai K. Association of cigarette smoking and CYP1A1 polymorphisms with adenocarcinoma of the lung by grades of differentiation. Carcinogenesis 1995;16:2209–2213.

194. Sugimura H, Hamada GS, Suzuki I, et al. CYP1A1 and CYP2E1 polymorphism and lung cancer, case-control study in Rio de Janeiro, Brazil. Pharmacogenetics 1995;5(Spec. Issue):145–148.

195. Taioli E, Crofts F, Demopoulos R, et al. An African American specific CYP1A1 polymorphism is associated with adenocarcinoma of the lung. Cancer Res 1995;55:472–473.

196. Cascorbi I, Brockmoller J, Roots I. A C4887A polymorphism in exon 7 of human CYP1A1: population frequency, mutation linkages, and impact on lung cancer susceptibility. Cancer Res 1996;56:4965–4969.

197. Xu X, Kelsey KT, Wiencke JK, et al. Cytochrome P450 CYP1A1 MspI polymorphism and lung cancer susceptibility. Cancer Epidemiol Biomarkers Prev 1996;5:687–692.

198. Bouchardy C, Wikman H, Benhamou S, et al. CYP1A1 genetic polymorphisms, tobacco smoking and lung cancer

risk in a French Caucasian population. Biomarkers 1997;2:131–134.

199. Garcia Closas M, Kelsey KT, Wiencke JK, et al. A case–control study of cytochrome P450 1A1, glutathione S-transferase M1, cigarette smoking and lung cancer susceptibility (Massachusetts, United States). Cancer Causes Control 1997;8:544–553.

200. Le Marchand L, Sivaraman L, Pierce L, et al. Association of CYP1A1, GSTM1, and CYP2E1 polymorphisms with lung cancer suggest cell type specificities to tobacco carcinogens. Cancer Res 1998;58:4858–4863.

201. Sugimura H, Wakai K, Genka K, et al. Association of Ile462Val (exon 7) polymorphism of cytochrome P450 IA1 with lung cancer in the Asian population: further evidence from a case–control study in Okinawa. Cancer Epidemiol Biomarkers Prev 1998;7:413–417.

202. Taioli E, Fordd J, Li Y, et al. Lung cancer risk and CYP1A1 genotype in African Americans. Carcinogenesis 1998;19:813–817.

203. Persson I, Johansson I, Lou Y-C, et al. Genetic polymorphism of xenobiotic metabolizing enzymes among Chinese lung cancer patients. Int J Cancer 1999;81:325–329.

204. Quinones L, Berthou F, Varela N, et al. Ethnic susceptibility to lung cancer: differences in CYP2E1, CYP1A1 and GSTM1 genetic polymorphisms between French Caucasian and Chilean populations. Cancer Lett 1999;141:167–171.

205. Dolzan V, Rudolf Z, Breskvar K. Genetic polymorphism of xenobiotic metabolising enzymes in Slovenian lung cancer patients. Pflugers Arch 2000;439(3 Suppl):R29–R30.

206. Han XM, Zhou HH. Polymorphism of CYP450 and cancer susceptibility. Acta Pharmacol Sin 2000;21:673–679.

207. Lin P, Wang S-L, Wang H-J, et al. Association of CYP1A1 and microsomal epoxide hydrolase polymorphisms with lung squamous cell carcinoma. Br J Cancer 2000;82:852–857.

208. Chen S, Xue K, Xu L, et al. Polymorphisms of the CYP1A1 and GSTM1 genes in relation to individual susceptibility to lung carcinoma in Chinese population. Mutat Res 2001;458:41–47.

209. Gsur A, Haidinger G, Hollaus P, et al. Genetic polymorphisms of CYP1A1 and GSTM1 and lung cancer risk. Anticancer Res 2001;21:2237–2242.

210. Quinones L, Lucas D, Godoy J, et al. CYP1A1, CYP2E1 and GSTM1 genetic polymorphisms. The effect of single and combined genotypes on lung cancer susceptibility in Chilean people. Cancer Lett 2001;174:35–44.

211. Song N, Tan W, Xing D, Lin D. CYP 1A1 polymorphism and risk of lung cancer in relation to tobacco smoking: a case-control study in China. Carcinogenesis 2001;22:11–16.

212. Le Marchand L, Guo C, Benhamou S, et al. Pooled analysis of the CYP1A1 exon 7 polymorphism and lung cancer (United States). Cancer Causes Control 2003;14:339–346.

213. Vineis P, Veglia F, Benhamou S, et al. CYP1A1 T3801 C polymorphism and lung cancer: a pooled analysis of 2451 cases and 3358 controls. Int J Cancer 2003;104:650–657.

214. Wang J, Deng Y, Li L, et al. Association of GSTM1, CYP1A1 and CYP2E1 genetic polymorphisms with susceptibility

to lung adenocarcinoma: a case–control study in Chinese population. Cancer Sci 2003;94:448–452.

215. Sobti RC, Sharma S, Joshi A, et al. Genetic polymorphism of the CYP1A1, CYP2E1, GSTM1 and GSTT1 genes and lung cancer susceptibility in a north Indian population. Mol Cell Biochem 2004;266:1–9.

216. Demir A, Altin S, Demir I, et al. The role of CYP1A1 Msp1 gene polymorphisms on lung cancer development in Turkey. Tuberk Toraks 2005;53:5–9.

217. Larsen JE, Colosimo ML, Yang IA, et al. Risk of non-small cell lung cancer and the cytochrome P4501A1 Ile462Val polymorphism. Cancer Causes Control 2005;16:579–585.

218. Sreeja L, Syamala V, Hariharan S, et al. Possible risk modification by CYP1A1, GSTM1 and GSTT1 gene polymorphisms in lung cancer susceptibility in a South Indian population. J Hum Genet 2005;50:618–627.

219. Larsen JE, Colosimo ML, Yang IA, et al. CYP1A1 Ile462Val and MPO G-463A interact to increase risk of adenocarcinoma but not squamous cell carcinoma of the lung. Carcinogenesis 2006;27:525–532.

220. Pisani P, Srivatanakul P, Randerson-Moor J, et al. GSTM1 and CYP1A1 polymorphisms, tobacco, air pollution, and lung cancer: a study in rural Thailand. Cancer Epidemiol Biomarkers Prev 2006;15:667–674.

221. Kamataki T, Nunoya K, Sakai Y, et al. Genetic polymorphism of CYP2A6 in relation to cancer. Mutat Res 1999;428:125–130.

222. Miyamoto M, Umetsu Y, Dosaka-Akita H, et al. CYP2A6 gene deletion reduces susceptibility to lung cancer. Biochem Biophys Res Commun 1999;261:658–660.

223. Nunoya KI, Yokoi T, Kimura K, et al. A new CYP2A6 gene deletion responsible for the in vivo polymorphic metabolism of (+)-cis-3,5-dimethyl-2-(3-pyridyl)thiazolidin-4-one hydrochloride in humans. J Pharmacol Exp Ther 1999;289:437–442.

224. Nunoya K, Yokoi T, Takahashi Y, et al. Homologous unequal cross-over within the human CYP2A gene cluster as a mechanism for the deletion of the entire CYP2A6 gene associated with the poor metabolizer phenotype. J Biochem (Tokyo) 1999;126:402–407.

225. Ariyoshi N, Takahashi Y, Miyamoto M, et al. Structural characterization of a new variant of the CYP2A6 gene (CYP2A6*1B) apparently diagnosed as heterozygotes of CYP2A6*1A and CYP2A6*4C. Pharmacogenetics 2000;10:687–693.

226. Kushida H, Fujita K, Suzuki A, et al. Development of a *Salmonella* tester strain sensitive to promutagenic N-nitrosamines: expression of recombinant CYP2A6 and human NADPH-cytochrome P450 reductase in S. typhimurium YG7108. Mutat Res 2000;471:135–143.

227. Ariyoshi N, Sawamura Y, Kamataki T. A novel single nucleotide polymorphism altering stability and activity of CYP2A6. Biochem Biophys Res Commun 2001;281:810–84.

228. Loriot MA, Rebuissou S, Oscarson M, et al. Genetic polymorphisms of cytochrome P450 2A6 in a case-control study on lung cancer in a French population. Pharmacogenetics 2001;11:39–44.

229. Pitarque M, von Richter O, Oke B, et al. Identification of a single nucleotide polymorphism in the TATA box of

the CYP2A6 gene: impairment of its promoter activity. Biochem Biophys Res Commun 2001;284:455–460.

230. Tan W, Chen GF, Xing DY, et al. Frequency of CYP2A6 gene deletion and its relation to risk of lung and esophageal cancer in the Chinese population. Int J Cancer 2001;95:96–101.

231. Xu C, Rao YS, Xu B, et al. An in vivo pilot study characterizing the new CYP2A6*7, *, and *10 alleles. Biochem Biophys Res Commun 2002;290:318–324.

232. Kiyotani K, Yamazaki H, Fujieda M, et al. Decreased coumarin 7-hydroxylase activities and CYP2A6 expression levels in humans caused by genetic polymorphism in CYP2A6 promoter region (CYP2A6*9). Pharmacogenetics 2003;13:689–695.

233. Fujieda M, Yamazaki H, Saito T, et al. Evaluation of CYP2A6 genetic polymorphisms as determinants of smoking behavior and tobacco-related lung cancer risk in male Japanese smokers. Carcinogenesis 2004;25:2451–2458.

234. Kamataki T, Fujieda M, Kiyotani K, et al. Genetic polymorphism of CYP2A6 as one of the potential determinants of tobacco-related cancer risk. Biochem Biophys Res Commun 2005;338:306–610.

235. Wang H, Tan W, Hao B, et al. Substantial reduction in risk of lung adenocarcinoma associated with genetic polymorphism in CYP2A13, the most active cytochrome P450 for the metabolic activation of tobacco-specific carcinogen NNK. Cancer Res 2003;63:8057–8061.

236. Cauffiez C, Lo-Guidice JM, Quaranta S, et al. Genetic polymorphism of the human cytochrome CYP2A13 in a French population: implication in lung cancer susceptibility. Biochem Biophys Res Commun 2004;317:662–669.

237. Itoga S, Nomura F, Makino Y, et al. Tandem repeat polymorphism of the CYP2E1 gene: an association study with esophageal cancer and lung cancer. Alcohol Clin Exp Res 2002;26(8 Suppl):15S–19S.

238. Iizasa T, Baba M, Saitoh Y, et al. A polymorphism in the 5′-flanking region of the CYP2E1 gene and elevated lung adenocarcinoma risk in a Japanese population. Oncol Rep 2005;14:919–23.

239. Dally H, Edler L, Jager B, et al. The CYP3A4*1B allele increases risk for small cell lung cancer: effect of gender and smoking dose. Pharmacogenetics 2003;13:607–618.

240. Cauchi S, Stucker I, Solas C, et al. Polymorphisms of human aryl hydrocarbon receptor (AhR) gene in a French population: relationship with CYP1A1 inducibility and lung cancer. Carcinogenesis 2001;22:1819–1824.

241. Cauchi S, Stucker I, Cenee S, et al. Structure and polymorphisms of human aryl hydrocarbon receptor repressor (AhRR) gene in a French population: relationship with CYP1A1 inducibility and lung cancer. Pharmacogenetics 2003;13:339–347.

242. Persson I, Johansson I, Lou YC, et al. Genetic polymorphism of xenobiotic metabolizing enzymes among Chinese lung cancer patients. Int J Cancer 1999;81:325–329.

243. London SJ, Smart J, Daly AK. Lung cancer risk in relation to genetic polymorphisms of microsomal epoxide hydrolase among African-Americans and Caucasians in Los Angeles County. Lung Cancer 2000;28:147–155.

244. Wu X, Gwyn K, Amos CI, et al. The association of microsomal epoxide hydrolase polymorphisms and lung cancer risk in African-Americans and Mexican-Americans. Carcinogenesis 2001;22:923–928.

245. To-Figueras J, Gene M, Gomez-Catalan J, et al. Lung cancer susceptibility in relation to combined polymorphisms of microsomal epoxide hydrolase and glutathione S-transferase P1. Cancer Lett 2001;173:155–162.

246. Cajas-Salazar N, Au WW, Zwischenberger JB, et al. Effect of epoxide hydrolase polymorphisms on chromosome aberrations and risk for lung cancer. Cancer Genet Cytogenet 2003;145:97–102.

247. Park JY, Chen L, Elahi A, et al. Genetic analysis of microsomal epoxide hydrolase gene and its association with lung cancer risk. Eur J Cancer Prev 2005;14:223–230.

248. Seidegard J, Pero RW, Markowitz MM, et al. Isoenzyme(s) of glutathione transferase (class Mu) as a marker for the susceptibility to lung cancer: a follow up study. Carcinogenesis 1990;11:33–36.

249. Zhong S, Howie AF, Ketterer B, et al. Glutathione S-transferase mu locus: use of genotyping and phenotyping assays to assess association with lung cancer susceptibility. Carcinogenesis 1991;12:1533–1537.

250. Hirvonen A, Husgafvel-Pursiainen K, Anttila S, Vainio H. The GSTM1 null genotype as a potential risk modifier for squamous cell carcinoma of the lung. Carcinogenesis 1993;14:1479–1481.

251. Kihara M, Kihara M, Noda K, Okamoto N. Increased risk of lung cancer in Japanese smokers with class mu glutathione S-transferase gene deficiency. Cancer Lett 1993;71:151–155.

252. Nazar-Stewart V, Motulsky AG, Eaton DL, et al. The glutathione S-transferase mu polymorphism as a marker for susceptibility to lung carcinoma. Cancer Res 1993;5 3(10 Suppl):2313–2318.

253. Deakin M, Elder J, Hendrickse C, et al. Glutathione S-transferase GSTT1 genotypes and susceptibility to cancer: studies of interactions with GSTM1 in lung, oral, gastric and colorectal cancers. Carcinogenesis 1996;17:881–884.

254. To-Figueras J, Gene M, Gomez-Catalan J, et al. Glutathione-S-Transferase M1 and codon 72 p53 polymorphisms in a northwestern Mediterranean population and their relation to lung cancer susceptibility. Cancer Epidemiol Biomarkers Prev 1996;5:337–342.

255. Kelsey KT, Spitz MR, Zuo ZF, Wiencke JK. Polymorphisms in the glutathione S-transferase class mu and theta genes interact and increase susceptibility to lung cancer in minority populations (Texas, United States). Cancer Causes Control 1997;8:554–559.

256. Sun GF, Shimojo N, Pi JB, Lee S, Kumagai Y. Gene deficiency of glutathione S-transferase mu isoform associated with susceptibility to lung cancer in a Chinese population. Cancer Lett 1997;113:169–172.

257. Jourenkova-Mironova N, Wikman H, Bouchardy C, et al. A. Role of glutathione S-transferase GSTM1, GSTM3, GSTP1 and GSTT1 genotypes in modulating susceptibility to smoking-related lung cancer. Pharmacogenetics 1998;8:495–502.

258. Stucker I, de Waziers I, Cenee S, et al. GSTM1, smoking and lung cancer: a case–control study. Int J Epidemiol 1999;28:829–835.

259. To-Figueras J, Gene M, Gomez-Catalan J, et al. Genetic polymorphism of glutathione S-transferase P1 gene and lung cancer risk. Cancer Causes Control 1999;10:65–70.

260. Belogubova EV, Togo AV, Kondratieva TV, et al. GSTM1 genotypes in elderly tumour-free smokers and non-smokers. Lung Cancer 2000;29:189–195.

261. Reszka E, Wasowicz W. Significance of genetic polymorphisms in glutathione S-transferase multigene family and lung cancer risk. Int J Occup Med Environ Health 2001;14: 99–113.

262. Benhamou S, Lee WJ, Alexandrie AK, et al. Meta- and pooled analyses of the effects of glutathione S-transferase M1 polymorphisms and smoking on lung cancer risk. Carcinogenesis 2002;23:1343–1350.

263. Cerrahoglu K, Kunter E, Isitmangil T, et al. Can't lung cancer patients detoxify procarcinogens? Allerg Immunol (Paris) 2002 Feb;34:51–55.

264. Lewis SJ, Cherry NM, Niven RM, et al. GSTM1, GSTT1 and GSTP1 polymorphisms and lung cancer risk. Cancer Lett 2002;180:165–171.

265. Liloglou T, Walters M, Maloney P, et al. A T2517C polymorphism in the GSTM4 gene is associated with risk of developing lung cancer. Lung Cancer 2002;37:143–146.

266. Perera FP, Mooney LA, Stampfer M, et al. Physicians' Health Cohort Study. Associations between carcinogen-DNA damage, glutathione S-transferase genotypes, and risk of lung cancer in the prospective Physicians' Health Cohort Study. Carcinogenesis 2002;23:1641–1646.

267. Stucker I, Hirvonen A, de Waziers I, et al. Genetic polymorphisms of glutathione S-transferases as modulators of lung cancer susceptibility. Carcinogenesis 2002;23:1475–1481.

268. Nazar-Stewart V, Vaughan TL, Stapleton P, et al. A population-based study of glutathione S-transferase M1, T1 and P1 genotypes and risk for lung cancer. Lung Cancer 2003;40:247–258.

269. Mohr LC, Rodgers JK, Silvestri GA. Glutathione S-transferase M1 polymorphism and the risk of lung cancer. Anticancer Res 2003;23:2111–2124.

270. Pinarbasi H, Silig Y, Cetinkaya O, et al. Strong association between the GSTM1-null genotype and lung cancer in a Turkish population. Cancer Genet Cytogenet 2003;146: 125–129.

271. Wang J, Deng Y, Cheng J, et al. GST genetic polymorphisms and lung adenocarcinoma susceptibility in a Chinese population. Cancer Lett 2003;201:185–193.

272. Reszka E, Wasowicz W, Rydzynski K, et al. Glutathione S-transferase M1 and P1 metabolic polymorphism and lung cancer predisposition. Neoplasma 2003;50:357–362.

273. Schneider J, Bernges U, Philipp M, Woitowitz HJ. GSTM1, GSTT1, and GSTP1 polymorphism and lung cancer risk in relation to tobacco smoking. Cancer Lett 2004;208:65–74.

274. Yang P, Bamlet WR, Ebbert JO, et al. Glutathione pathway genes and lung cancer risk in young and old populations. Carcinogenesis 2004;25:1935–1944.

275. Chan-Yeung M, Tan-Un KC, Ip MS, et al. Lung cancer susceptibility and polymorphisms of glutathione-S-transferase genes in Hong Kong. Lung Cancer 2004;45:155–160.

276. Ye Z, Song H, Higgins JP, et al. Five glutathione s-transferase gene variants in 23,452 cases of lung cancer and 30,397 controls: meta-analysis of 130 studies. PLoS Med 2006;3: e91.

277. Le Marchand L, Sivaraman L, Pierce L, et al. Associations of CYP1A1, GSTM1, and CYP2E1 polymorphisms with lung cancer suggest cell type specificities to tobacco carcinogens. Cancer Res 1998;58:4858–4863.

278. Liu G, Miller DP, Zhou W, et al. Differential association of the codon 72 p53 and GSTM1 polymorphisms on histological subtype of non-small cell lung carcinoma. Cancer Res 2001;61:8718–8722.

279. Risch A, Wikman H, Thiel S, et al. Glutathione-S-transferase M1, M3, T1 and P1 polymorphisms and susceptibility to non–small-cell lung cancer subtypes and hamartomas. Pharmacogenetics 2001;11:757–764.

280. Rosvold EA, McGlynn KA, Lustbader ED, Buetow KH. Identification of an NAD(P)H:quinone oxidoreductase polymorphism and its association with lung cancer and smoking. Pharmacogenetics 1995;5:199–206.

281. Wiencke JK, Spitz MR, McMillan A, Kelsey KT. Lung cancer in Mexican-Americans and African-Americans is associated with the wild-type genotype of the NAD(P)H: quinone oxidoreductase polymorphism. Cancer Epidemiol Biomarkers Prev 1997;6:87–92.

282. Xu LL, Wain JC, Miller DP, et al. The NAD(P)H: quinone oxidoreductase 1 gene polymorphism and lung cancer: differential susceptibility based on smoking behavior. Cancer Epidemiol Biomarkers Prev 2001;10: 303–309.

283. Lawson KA, Woodson K, Virtamo J, Albanes D. Association of the NAD(P)H:quinone oxidoreductase (NQO1) 609C->T polymorphism with lung cancer risk among male smokers. Cancer Epidemiol Biomarkers Prev 2005; 14:2275–2276.

284. Saldivar SJ, Wang Y, Zhao H, et al. An association between a NQO1 genetic polymorphism and risk of lung cancer. Mutat Res 2005;582:71–78.

285. Abdel-Rahman SZ, El-Zein RA, Zwischenberger JB, Au WW. Association of the NAT1*10 genotype with increased chromosome aberrations and higher lung cancer risk in cigarette smokers. Mutat Res 1998;398:43–54.

286. Seow A, Zhao B, Poh WT, et al. NAT2 slow acetylator genotype is associated with increased risk of lung cancer among non-smoking Chinese women in Singapore. Carcinogenesis 1999;20:1877–1881.

287. Wikman H, Thiel S, Jager B, et al. Relevance of N-acetyltransferase 1 and 2 (NAT1, NAT2) genetic polymorphisms in non-small cell lung cancer susceptibility. Pharmacogenetics 2001;11:157–168.

288. Belogubova EV, Kuligina ESh, Togo AV, et al. "Comparison of extremes" approach provides evidence against the modifying role of NAT2 polymorphism in lung cancer susceptibility. Cancer Lett 2005;221:177–183.

289. Habalova V, Salagovic J, Kalina I, Stubna J. A pilot study testing the genetic polymorphism of N-acetyltransferase 2 as a risk factor in lung cancer. Neoplasma 2005;52:364–368.

290. Wang Y, Spitz MR, Tsou AM, et al. Sulfotransferase (SULT) 1A1 polymorphism as a predisposition factor for lung cancer: a case-control analysis. Lung Cancer 2002;35: 137–142.

291. Roots I, Brockmoller J, Drakoulis N, Loddenkemper R. Mutant genes of cytochrome P-450IID6, glutathione S-transferase class Mu, and arylamine N-acetyltransferase in lung cancer patients. Clin Invest 1992;70:307–319.

292. Miller DP, Liu G, De Vivo I, et al. Combinations of the variant genotypes of GSTP1, GSTM1, and p53 are associated with an increased lung cancer risk. Cancer Res 2002;62:2819–2823.

293. Sunaga N, Kohno T, Yanagitani N, et al. Contribution of the NQO1 and GSTT1 polymorphisms to lung adenocarcinoma susceptibility. Cancer Epidemiol Biomarkers Prev 2002;11:730–738.

294. Hung RJ, Boffetta P, Brockmoller J, et al. CYP1A1 and GSTM1 genetic polymorphisms and lung cancer risk in Caucasian non-smokers: a pooled analysis. Carcinogenesis 2003;24:875–882.

295. Cajas-Salazar N, Sierra-Torres CH, Salama SA, et al. Combined effect of MPO, GSTM1 and GSTT1 polymorphisms on chromosome aberrations and lung cancer risk. Int J Hyg Environ Health 2003;206:473–483.

296. Lin P, Hsueh YM, Ko JL, et al. Analysis of NQO1, GSTP1, and MnSOD genetic polymorphisms on lung cancer risk in Taiwan. Lung Cancer 2003;40:123–129.

297. Alexandrie AK, Nyberg F, Warholm M, Rannug A. Influence of CYP1A1, GSTM1, GSTT1, and NQO1 genotypes and cumulative smoking dose on lung cancer risk in a Swedish population. Cancer Epidemiol Biomarkers Prev 2004;13:908–914.

298. Liu G, Zhou W, Park S, et al. The SOD2 Val/Val genotype enhances the risk of nonsmall cell lung carcinoma by p53 and XRCC1 polymorphisms. Cancer 2004;101:2802–2808.

299. Raimondi S, Boffetta P, Anttila S, et al. Metabolic gene polymorphisms and lung cancer risk in non-smokers: An update of the GSEC study. Mutat Res 2005;592:45–57.

300. Wei Q, Cheng L, Hong WK, Spitz MR. Reduced DNA repair capacity in lung cancer patients. Cancer Res 1996;56: 4103–4107.

301. Wei Q, Spitz MR. The role of DNA repair capacity in susceptibility to lung cancer: a review. Cancer Metastasis Rev 1997;16:295–307.

302. Wei Q, Cheng L, Amos CI, et al. Repair of tobacco carcinogen-induced DNA adducts and lung cancer risk: a molecular epidemiologic study. J Natl Cancer Inst 2000;92: 1764–1772.

303. Shen H, Spitz MR, Qiao Y, et al. Smoking, DNA repair capacity and risk of nonsmall cell lung cancer. Int J Cancer 2003;107:84–88.

304. Spitz MR, Wei Q, Dong Q, et al. Genetic susceptibility to lung cancer: the role of DNA damage and repair. Cancer Epidemiol Biomarkers Prev 2003;12:689–698.

305. Duell EJ, Wiencke JK, Cheng TJ, et al. Polymorphisms in the DNA repair genes XRCC1 and ERCC2 and biomarkers of DNA damage in human blood mononuclear cells. Carcinogenesis 2000;21:965–971.

306. Butkiewicz D, Rusin M, Enewold L, et al. Genetic polymorphisms in DNA repair genes and risk of lung cancer. Carcinogenesis 2001;22:593–597.

307. David-Beabes GL, Lunn RM, London SJ. No association between the XPD (Lys751Gln) polymorphism or the XRCC3 (Thr241Met) polymorphism and lung cancer risk. Cancer Epidemiol Biomarkers Prev 2001;10:911–912.

308. Palli D, Russo A, Masala G, et al. DNA adduct levels and DNA repair polymorphisms in traffic-exposed workers and a general population sample. Int J Cancer 2001;94: 121–127.

309. Spitz MR, Wu X, Wang Y, et al. Modulation of nucleotide excision repair capacity by XPD polymorphisms in lung cancer patients. Cancer Res 2001;61:1354–1357.

310. Chen S, Tang D, Xue K, et al. DNA repair gene XRCC1 and XPD polymorphisms and risk of lung cancer in a Chinese population. Carcinogenesis 2002;23:1321–1325.

311. Hou SM, Falt S, Angelini S, et al. The XPD variant alleles are associated with increased aromatic DNA adduct level and lung cancer risk. Carcinogenesis 2002;23:599–603.

312. Qiao Y, Spitz MR, Guo Z, et al. Rapid assessment of repair of ultraviolet DNA damage with a modified host-cell reactivation assay using a luciferase reporter gene and correlation with polymorphisms of DNA repair genes in normal human lymphocytes. Mutat Res 2002;509:165–174.

313. Park JY, Lee SY, Jeon HS, et al. Lys751Gln polymorphism in the DNA repair gene XPD and risk of primary lung cancer. (Letter). Lung Cancer 2002;36:15–16.

314. Tang D, Cho S, Rundle A, et al. Polymorphisms in the DNA repair enzyme XPD are associated with increased levels of PAH–DNA adducts in a case–control study of breast cancer. Breast Cancer Res Treat 2002;75:159–166.

315. Xing D, Tan W, Wei Q, Lin D. Polymorphisms of the DNA repair gene XPD and risk of lung cancer in a Chinese population. Lung Cancer 2002;38:123–129.

316. Liang G, Xing D, Miao X, et al. Sequence variations in the DNA repair gene XPD and risk of lung cancer in a Chinese population. Int J Cancer 2003;105:669–673.

317. Matullo G, Peluso M, Polidoro S, et al. Combination of DNA repair gene single nucleotide polymorphisms and increased levels of DNA adducts in a population-based study. Cancer Epidemiol Biomarkers Prev 2003;12:674–677.

318. Misra RR, Ratnasinghe D, Tangrea JA, et al. Polymorphisms in the DNA repair genes XPD, XRCC1, XRCC3, and APE/ref-1, and the risk of lung cancer among male smokers in Finland. Cancer Lett 2003;191:171–178.

319. Zhou W, Liu G, Miller DP, et al. Polymorphisms in the DNA repair genes XRCC1 and ERCC2, smoking, and lung cancer risk. Cancer Epidemiol Biomarkers Prev 2003;12:359–365.

320. Hu Z, Wei Q, Wang X, Shen H. DNA repair gene XPD polymorphism and lung cancer risk: a meta-analysis. Lung Cancer 2004;46:1–10.

321. Vogel U, Laros I, Jacobsen NR, et al. Two regions in chromosome 19q13.2–3 are associated with risk of lung cancer. Mutat Res 2004;546:65–74.

322. Benhamou S, Sarasin A. ERCC2 /XPD gene polymorphisms and lung cancer: a HuGE review. Am J Epidemiol. 2005;161:1–14.

323. Yin J, Li J, Ma Y, et al. The DNA repair gene ERCC2/ XPD polymorphism Arg156Arg (A22541C) and risk of lung cancer in a Chinese population. Cancer Lett 2005;223: 219–226.

324. Hu Z, Xu L, Shao M, et al. Polymorphisms in the two helicases ERCC2/XPD and ERCC3/XPB of the transcription factor IIH complex and risk of lung cancer: a case–control analysis in a Chinese population. Cancer Epidemiol Biomarkers Prev 2006;15:1336–1340.

325. Yin J, Vogel U, Ma Y, et al. Polymorphism of the DNA repair gene ERCC2 Lys751Gln and risk of lung cancer in a northeastern Chinese population. Cancer Genet Cytogenet 2006;169:27–32.

326. Park JY, Park SH, Choi JE, et al. Polymorphisms of the DNA repair gene xeroderma pigmentosum group A and risk of primary lung cancer. Cancer Epidemiol Biomarkers Prev 2002;11:993–997.

327. Butkiewicz D, Popanda O, Risch A, et al. Association between the risk for lung adenocarcinoma and a (-4) G-to-A polymorphism in the XPA gene. Cancer Epidemiol Biomarkers Prev 2004;13:2242–2246.

328. Vogel U, Overvad K, Wallin H, et al. Combinations of polymorphisms in XPD, XPC and XPA in relation to risk of lung cancer. Cancer Lett 2005;222:67–74.

329. Hu Z, Wang Y, Wang X, et al. DNA repair gene XPC genotypes/haplotypes and risk of lung cancer in a Chinese population. Int J Cancer 2005;115:478–483.

330. Lee GY, Jang JS, Lee SY, et al. XPC polymorphisms and lung cancer risk. Int J Cancer 2005;115:807–813.

331. Jeon HS, Kim KM, Park SH, et al. Relationship between XPG codon 1104 polymorphism and risk of primary lung cancer. Carcinogenesis 2003;24:1677–1681.

332. David-Beabes GL, London SJ. Genetic polymorphism of XRCC1 and lung cancer risk among African-Americans and Caucasians. Lung Cancer 2001;34:333–339.

333. Divine KK, Gilliland FD, Crowell RE, et al. The XRCC1 399 glutamine allele is a risk factor for adenocarcinoma of the lung. Mutat Res 2001;461:273–278.

334. Ito H, Matsuo K, Hamajima N, et al. Gene–environment interactions between the smoking habit and polymorphisms in the DNA repair genes, APE1 Asp148Glu and XRCC1 Arg399Gln, in Japanese lung cancer risk. Carcinogenesis 2004;25:1395–1401.

335. Vogel U, Nexo BA, Wallin H, et al. No association between base excision repair gene polymorphisms and risk of lung cancer. Biochem Genet 2004;42:453–460.

336. Schneider J, Classen V, Bernges U, Philipp M. XRCC1 polymorphism and lung cancer risk in relation to tobacco smoking. Int J Mol Med 2005;16:709–716.

337. Zhang X, Miao X, Liang G, et al. Polymorphisms in DNA base excision repair genes ADPRT and XRCC1 and risk of lung cancer. Cancer Res 2005;65:722–726.

338. Yin J, Vogel U, Guo L, et al. Lack of association between DNA repair gene ERCC1 polymorphism and risk of lung cancer in a Chinese population. Cancer Genet Cytogenet 2006;164:66–70.

339. Jacobsen NR, Raaschou-Nielsen O, Nexo B, et al. XRCC3 polymorphisms and risk of lung cancer. Cancer Lett 2004; 213:67–72.

340. Ishida T, Takashima R, Fukayama M, et al. New DNA polymorphisms of human MMH/OGG1 gene: prevalence of one polymorphism among lung-adenocarcinoma patients in Japanese. Int J Cancer 1999;80:18–21.

341. Sugimura H, Kohno T, Wakai K, et al. hOGG1 Ser326Cys polymorphism and lung cancer susceptibility. Cancer Epidemiol Biomarkers Prev 1999;8:669–674.

342. Wikman H, Risch A, Klimek F, et al. hOGG1 polymorphism and loss of heterozygosity (LOH): significance for lung cancer susceptibility in a Caucasian population. Int J Cancer 2000;88:932–937.

343. Ito H, Hamajima N, Takezaki T, et al. A limited association of OGG1 Ser326Cys polymorphism for adenocarcinoma of the lung. J Epidemiol 2002;12:258–265.

344. Hu YC, Ahrendt SA. hOGG1 Ser326Cys polymorphism and G:C-to-T:A mutations: no evidence for a role in tobacco-related non small cell lung cancer. Int J Cancer 2005;114:387–393.

345. Kohno T, Kunitoh H, Toyama K, et al. Association of the OGG1-Ser326Cys polymorphism with lung adenocarcinoma risk. Cancer Sci 2006 Jun 23; [Epub ahead of print].

346. Gackowski D, Speina E, Zielinska M, et al. Products of oxidative DNA damage and repair as possible biomarkers of susceptibility to lung cancer. Cancer Res 2003;63:4899–4902.

347. Yang M, Coles BF, Caporaso NE, et al. Lack of association between Caucasian lung cancer risk and O6-methylguanine-DNA methyltransferase-codon 178 genetic polymorphism. Lung Cancer 2004;44:281–286.

348. Chae MH, Jang JS, Kang HG, et al. O6-alkylguanine-DNA alkyltransferase gene polymorphisms and the risk of primary lung cancer. Mol Carcinog 2006;45:239–249.

349. Kim JH, Kim H, Lee KY, et al. Genetic polymorphisms of ataxia telangiectasia mutated affect lung cancer risk. Hum Mol Genet 2006 Apr 1;15(7):1181–1186.

350. Zienolddiny S, Campa D, Lind H, et al. Polymorphisms of DNA repair genes and risk of non-small cell lung cancer. Carcinogenesis 2006;27:560–567.

18
Prognostic Markers

Anna Sienko, Timothy Craig Allen, and Philip T. Cagle

Prognostic Markers

DNA damage in lung cancers results in molecular genetic abnormalities that contribute to their pathogenesis and progression.[1] Many studies have examined the predictive value of specific molecular genetic abnormalities involving cell cycle regulation, apoptosis, and so forth, in individual tumors on the clinical outcomes of lung cancer patients.[2-4] Both loss of specific tumor-suppressor gene function and the activation of specific oncogenes have been studied as potential prognostic indicators, as have other molecular abnormalities, for example, epigenetic phenomena such as hypermethylation.[3-22] Ultimately, no one molecular marker is expected to predict prognosis by itself because development and progression of cancer involves the accumulation of multiple genetic abnormalities with complex pathways, feedback loops, and redundancies such that abnormalities of any of several proteins in a pathway can produce similar effects on the cells. Therefore, molecular profiles of multiple markers are likely to be more useful than examination of one or two markers alone in predicting prognosis.[19] The markers presented here are those that have undergone the most investigation to date.

Non–Small Cell Lung Cancers

The presence of resectable tumor is the best established indicator of non–small cell lung carcinoma (NSCLC) prognosis because, while the 5-year survival rate for all NSCLC is 13%, early stage tumors treated surgically attain a 5-year survival rate of 47%.[23] Nonetheless, about half of the patients with early stage resected cancers relapse, suggesting differing degrees of aggressiveness, recurrence, and occult metastasis in similarly staged NSCLC.[23] Considerable clinical and basic science research has been performed examining the prognostic potential of molecular biologic markers that might help stratify lung cancer

patients in therapeutic trials and identify those patients who may be more likely to benefit from adjuvant therapies.[24] Table 18.1 lists a number of studies examining or reviewing potential prognostic implications from various molecular genetic abnormalities in NSCLC.[25-68]

c-erbB2

The c-erbB2 protooncogene (p185, HER2/neu), located on chromosome 17 q21, a well-established prognostic marker for breast cancer, codes for a transmembrane protein with tyrosine kinase activity.[23,69] It shares a large part of sequence homology with, and is structurally similar to, the epidermal growth factor receptor gene.[23,69] c-erbB2 is normally found in low levels in ciliated lung cells, type II pneumocytes, and bronchial submucosal glands.[23] ErbB2 receptor helps regulate DNA repair, cell cycle checkpoints, and apoptosis in NSCLC.[25] Kern et al. examined 44 NSCLC, all adenocarcinomas, and found overexpression of c-erbB2, especially in association with Ki-Ras mutations, to be associated with poorer prognosis for NSCLC patients.[25] Giatromanolaki et al. identified a worse prognosis with c-erbB2 immunopositivity in 107 NSCLC patients.[26] Other studies contradict this finding. Moldvay et al.,[23] examining 227 NSCLC patients, Pfeiffer et al.,[27] examining 186 NSCLC patients, and Pollan et al.,[28] examining 465 NSCLC patients, found no prognostic significance with c-erbB2 tumor cell immunopositivity. Tateishi et al., examining 203 NSCLC patients who showed improved survival with c-erbB2 overexpression, reported a 5-year survival rate of 52% for patients with c-erbB2 immunopositive tumors and 30% for patients with immunonegative tumors.[29] The contradictory results may be due to differing interpretations of immunostaining and cut-off values and to technique heterogeneity.[23,25] Some studies evaluate cytoplasmic staining, and others evaluate membranous staining.[23] Additional studies may clarify the role of c-erbB2 as a prognostic marker with NSCLC.

TABLE 18.1. Commonly studied prognostic markers.

Marker	Authors	Year
c-erbB2	Kern et al.[25]	1994
	Giatromanolaki et al.[26]	1996
	Pfeiffer et al.[27]	1996
	Moldvay et al.[23]	2000
	Pollan et al.[28]	2003
	Tateishi et al.[29]	1991
Bcl-2	Pezzella et al.[30]	1996
	Cox et al.[31]	2001
	Anton et al.[18]	1997
	Silvestrini et al.[32]	1998
	Poleri et al.[33]	2003
p53	Pastorino et al.[34]	1997
	Xu et al.[16]	1996
	Greatens et al.[35]	1998
	Lee et al.[36]	1999
	Quinlan et al.[15]	1992
	D'Amico et al.[37]	1999
	Kwaitkowski et al.[38]	1998
	Dalquen et al.[39]	1996
	Huang et al.[40]	1998
	Ahrendt et al.[41]	2003
	Fukuyama et al.[42]	1997
	Schiller et al.[43]	2001
p63	Au et al.[44]	2004
	Massion et al.[45]	2003
	Iwata et al.[46]	2005
Retinoblastoma protein	Dworakowska et al.[47]	2004
	Reissmann et al.[48]	1993
	Haga et al.[49]	2003
	D'Amico et al.[37]	1999
Other cell cycle proteins	Esposito et al.[50]	1999
	Anton et al.[22]	2000
Epidermal growth factor receptor	Sonnweber et al.[51]	2006
	Nakamura et al.[52]	2006
	Shepherd et al.[53]	2005
Murine double minute 2	Dworakowska et al.[54]	2004
	Higashiyama et al.[55]	1997
	Ko et al.[56]	2000
ras	Mascaux et al.[57]	2005
	Grossi et al.[58]	2003
	Keohavong et al.[59]	1996
L-Myc	Shih et al.[60]	2002
	Ge et al.[61]	1996
	Tefre et al.[62]	1990
	Spinola et al.[63]	2001
Neuroendocrine tumors	Johnson et al.[64]	1996
	Rodriguez-Salas et al.[65]	2001
	Micke et al.[66]	2001
	Beasley et al.[67]	2003
	Casali et al.[68]	2004

Bcl-2

The Bcl-2 (B-cell lymphoma/leukemia-2 gene mapping on chromosome 18 q21) protooncogene family is located on the inner mitochondrial membranes and makes up important control points in the intrinsic apoptotic pathway.[70] The family possesses two groups of control proteins: one group (Bcl-2, Bcl-xL, Bcl-w, Mcl-1) preserves mitochondrial membrane potential and prevents cell apoptosis by suppression of the release of apoptotic factors such as cytochrome c and apoptosis-inducing factor; and a second group (Bax, Bak, Bid, Bad, Bok, Bim) acts as proapoptotic factors, inducing via mitochondrial dysfunction the release of proapoptotic mediators, which then activate caspase-9.[70] Bcl-2 is abnormally expressed in over half of small cell lung cancers, but there is no prognostic benefit.[71]

Researchers, including Pezzella et al.,[30] examining 122 NSCLC patients, Cox et al.,[31] examining 167 NSCLC patients, Ohsaki et al.,[72] examining 99 NSCLC patients, and Silvestrini et al.,[32] examining 229 NSCLC patients, have found Bcl-2 overexpression to be associated with improved prognosis in lung adenocarcinomas, possibly from the loss of its antiapoptotic activity from Bcl-2 phosphorylation or from its association with other Bcl-2 family members, such as Bax and Bcl-x.[23,30–32,72] Other possible explanations include altered Bcl-2:Bax ratio and Bcl-2-induced inhibition of tumor angiogenesis.[23,31,32,72] However, one study by Poleri et al, examining 53 NSCLC patients, showed a poorer prognosis with increased Bcl-2 expression.[33] Bcl-2 acts by inhibiting programmed cell death and has a suppressive function over vascular endothelial growth factor and thymidine phosphorylase, involved in angiogenesis, and over c-erbB2, involved in cell migration.[73–75]

p53

p53 is a tumor suppressor gene associated with G1 arrest and apoptosis caused by cytotoxic stress, including DNA damage and various genetic abnormalities in the gene sequence. The cytotoxic stress stabilizes p53 and allows for its detection by immunohistochemistry. Its immunopositivity correlates with p53 missense mutation, but other types of p53 mutations, making up about 20% of mutations, cause an absence of functional p53 protein. These mutations, called null phenotype mutations, are not immunohistochemically identifiable. Also physiologically stabilized p53 accumulates and is detectable by immunohistochemistry in reactive processes. Therefore, presence or absence of p53 immunostaining is not an absolute indicator of p53 mutation.

Overexpression of p53 protein, and sometimes p53 mutations, may be found prior to invasive disease. Squamous cell dysplasia and in situ carcinoma demonstrate p53 accumulation, identifiable immunohistochemically, increasingly in the continuum of mild dysplasia to in situ carcinoma, from approximately 20% to approximately 60%. p53 alterations are the most common genetic changes found in lung cancer.[25] Between 40% and 60% NSCLC patients have p53 alterations detected by immunohistochemistry.[1,25,76] Reports have shown unique p53 changes in NSCLC patients who smoked, specifically an excess of G:C to T:A transversions.[1] Non–small cell lung cancer in never-smokers had a reciprocal increase in G: C to A:T transitions.[1] Squamous cell NSCLC patients have the greatest frequency of p53 mutations, approximately 70%.[1]

Studies regarding the prognostic role of *p53* have yielded conflicting results.[33] This may be caused by differing methods, immunohistochemistry techniques, or gene analysis used in identifying *p53* alterations.[77] Although some researchers examine specific *p53* gene mutations, others examine p53 protein expression by immunohistochemistry. The short half-life of wild-type *p53* allows little or no immunopositivity in normal cells, whereas the longer half-life of *p53* mutations generally results in visible immunopositivity.[77] Studies of the prognostic impact in NSCLC of p53 expression are numerous. Pastorino et al.[34] examined 515 NSCLC patients and Pappot et al.[78] examined 228 NSCLC patients, and neither group identified any prognostic effect with p53 expression by immunohistochemistry. Several other large studies have yielded similar results.[23,35,36,78,79]

Other studies including large numbers of NSCLC patients have found a worse prognosis with p53 tumor cell immunopositivity.[37–39,80] Several researchers using *p53* mutation analysis rather than immunohistochemistry, including Huang et al.,[40] who examined 204 tumors, Ahrendt et al.,[41] who examined 188 tumors, and Fukuyama et al.,[42] who examined 159 NSCLC patients, found a poorer prognosis for NSCLC patients with tumor cells containing mutated *p53*. Schiller et al. examined 183 stages II and III NSCLC patients with both techniques and found no prognostic effect by either mutational analysis or immunohistochemistry.[43] These conflicting studies suggest further research is necessary before p53 status can be used as a clinical prognostic marker.

p63

p63 is a member of the *p53* family with similar structural and functional features; however, unlike *p53*, *p63* has several isoforms.[81] *p63* is important in epithelial development, craniofacial development, and the development of limbs and may induce growth suppression and cell death in tumor cell lines.[81] Au et al.,[44] evaluating 284 NSCLC patients, and Massion et al.,[45] examining 217 NSCLC patients, found that p63 tumor cell immunopositivity was associated with a better prognosis in squamous cell NSCLC patients. Pelosi et al. examined 221 NSCLC patients and identified a high prevalence of p63 immunopositivity in squamous cell NSCLC, as well as in squamous metaplasia and dysplasia; however, tumor cell immunostaining did not correlate with prognosis of the NSCLC patients.[81] Iwata et al., studying 161 squamous cell NSCLC patients, did not identify any prognostic significance of p63 immunostaining.[46] Additional large prospective studies may establish the role of *p63* as a clinically useful prognostic marker.

Retinoblastoma Protein

Retinoblastoma protein (pRb) is a nuclear phosphoprotein that helps control G1 phase and cell proliferation. It is in turn regulated by phosphorylation by the cyclin D1 complex. Dworakowska et al.,[47] examining 195 NSCLC patients, Reissmann et al.,[48] examining 219 NSCLC patients, and Haga et al.,[49] evaluating 187 NSCLC patients, found no effect on prognosis with pRb tumor cell immunostaining. D'Amico et al. studied 408 NSCLC patients and identified a trend for better prognosis in patients with pRb tumor cell immunopositivity, but the results were not statistically significant.[37] By itself, pRb is not presently clinically useful as a prognostic marker.

Cell Cycle Proteins

Noting the key role performed by cell cycle kinase–cyclin complexes, their inhibitors, and p53 in regulating the cell cycle, and the role performed by proliferating cell nuclear antigen (PCNA) in DNA repair and replication, Esposito et al. examined cell cycle–related proteins p21, p16, p53, and PCNA as a group in 68 NSCLC patients for any prognostic implications and found that tumor cell immunopositivity with p53, p21, and p16, but not PCNA was significantly correlated with survival.[50] Those NSCLC patients having tumor cell immunonegativity with both p21 and p16 had significantly shorter overall survival.[50] Esposito et al. suggests that with cell cycle protein mutations occurring frequently in NSCLC, functional cooperation between the various cell cycle inhibitor proteins may helps regulate tumor cell growth and suppression.[50] Esposito et al. then examined 105 NSCLC patients for the simultaneous loss of cell cycle–related proteins and found that the simultaneous loss of cyclin D1, p16, and pRb correlated with survival.[82] Esposito et al. concludes that the cyclin D1–p16–retinoblastoma tumor suppressor pathway is inactivated in most NSCLC, supporting the authors' premise regarding cell cycle inhibitor protein cooperation.[82]

Epidermal Growth Factor Receptor

Epidermal growth factor receptor (EGFR), a receptor tyrosine kinase, is a glycoprotein involved with cell proliferation, differentiation, migration, and cell survival that is frequently overexpressed in NSCLC.[83] Epidermal growth factor receptor is most commonly expressed in squamous cell NSCLC but is also frequently found in adenocarcinoma and large cell NSCLC.[83] Research results regarding the relationship between EGFR protein overexpression and prognosis are inconsistent. Sonnweber et al. examined 78 NSCLC patients and found that phosphorylated EGFR is correlated with poor prognosis.[51] Nakamura et al.[52] performed a metaanalysis of 18 studies, including 15 immunohistochemical studies and containing 2,972 NSCLC patients, and found that EGFR was overexpressed in 58% of squamous cell NSCLC, 39% of adenocarcinomas, and 38% of large cell NSCLC. Nakamura et al. found that EGFR overexpression was not associated with poorer prognosis.[52] The results were the same whether or not the nonimmunohistochemical studies were excluded.[52]

With two EGFR inhibitors, gefitinib and erlotinib, approved in the United States for use as second or third line treatment for advanced NSCLC, the relationship between EGFR and prognosis after EGFR inhibitor therapy has been studied.[51] Shepherd et al. has shown improved survival of patients with advanced NSCLC who received erlotinib; however, the improved survival was not related to the status of the patients' EGFR overexpression.[53] Further studies might elucidate whether there is a clinically important role for examination of EGFR overexpression not only in the context of treatment of advanced NSCLC patients but also in the context of potential therapy for less advanced NSCLC patients.

Murine Double Minute 2

Murine double minute 2 (MDM2), an oncoprotein physically associated with p53, forms an autoregulatory feedback loop with p53, with p53 positively regulating MDM2 levels and MDM2 inhibiting p53 expression and activity.[54] Murine double minute 2 may have a p53-independent role in tumor development.[54] The prognostic implications of MDM2 overexpression are controversial. Higashiyama et al. identified MDM2 overexpression in 24% of 201 NSCLC patients and found MDM2 overexpression indicate an improved prognosis.[55] Murine double minute 2 immunopositive NSCLC patients who were also immunonegative for p53had an even better prognosis.[55] While 24% of patients had MDM2 protein overexpression, MDM2 gene amplification was identified in only 7% of 30 NSCLC patients in that study.[55] Ko et al., examining 81 NSCLC patients of whom 51.5% showed MDM2 protein overexpression, did not find the status of MDM2 protein overexpression to be prognostically helpful; however, MDM2 mRNA expression was found to be a favorable prognostic factor.[56] Dworakowska et al., studying 116 NSCLC patients of whom 21% were found to have MDM2 amplification by real-time polymerase chain reaction, noted a poorer prognosis for NSCLC patients with MDM2 gene amplification.[54] Further research is necessary to resolve these conflicting studies regarding the prognostic benefit of MDM2 gene amplification, mRNA expression, and MDM2 protein overexpression.

ras

The ras oncogene, involved in lung cancer development, is made up of three ras genes, the H-ras gene, the K-ras-2 gene, and the N-ras gene.[57] These genes code for four highly homologous p21 proteins.[58] ras is mutated in 15%–20% of NSCLC cases and in 30%–50% of adenocarcinomas.[57] The literature is unsettled as to whether ras mutations affect prognosis. Grossi et al. examined 269 NSCLC patients and found that K-ras mutations were associated with poorer prognosis.[58] Keohavong et al. examined 173 NSCLC patients with a combination of polymerase chain reaction and denaturing gradient gel electrophoresis and identified 43 NSCLCs with K-ras mutations, 41 within adenocarcinomas, 1 in an adenosquamous NSCLC, and 1 in a squamous cell NSCLC.[59] The authors found no prognostic difference between adenocarcinomas with K-ras mutations and K-ras–negative adenocarcinomas.[59] In an attempt to clarify whether ras is of any prognostic value, Mascaux et al. performed a metaanalysis of 28 studies and found that NSCLC patients with K-ras-2 mutations or with p21 overexpression, especially in adenocarcinomas, had a poorer prognosis.[57]

L-Myc

L-Myc, a member of the Myc gene family, including c-Myc and N-Myc, encodes for transcription factors affecting cell proliferation, apoptosis, and tumor development.[84] Some authors have identified an association between L-Myc polymorphism and NSCLC prognosis; however, other studies have not found any prognostic association.[84] Shih et al., examining 169 NSCLC patients, found poorer prognosis correlating with patients with an S allele of the L-Myc gene, along with a Pro/Pro variant genotype of p53.[60] Ge et al. evaluated 98 NSCLC patients and found a poorer prognosis for patients with the LL L-Myc genotype than for patients with the SS L-Myc genotype.[61] In contrast, Tefre et al. studied 83 NSCLC patients and found no prognostic value based on the presence or absence of an L-Myc polymorphism.[62] Spinola et al. examined 199 Italian patients with NSCLC and found no significant association between NSCLC prognosis and an L-Myc polymorphism.[63] Additional large studies are necessary to determine whether L-Myc polymorphism is a clinically significant prognostic factor in NSCLC patients.

Neuroendocrine Lung Cancers

The prognostic features of molecular markers for patients with neuroendocrine lung cancers have not been extensively examined. Johnson et al.[64] noted that over-expressions of c-*Myc*, N-*Myc*, and L-*Myc* have been identified in small cell lung carcinoma (SCLC) cell lines, and *Myc* dysregulation has been correlated with poor prognosis.[85] Rodriguez-Salas et al. examined 50 SCLC biopsies for β-catenin expression and found that β-catenin cytoplasmic overexpression correlated with shorter time to progression and shorter overall survival in the patients.[65] Micke et al., studying 107 SCLC patients, found that c-*erbB2* was identified in 13% and correlated with shorter survival.[66] Beasley et al., examining 25 atypical carcinoids, 42 large cell neuroendocrine carcinomas, and 79 SCLCs, found that p16 loss, cyclin D1 overexpression, and Rb loss were not prognostically significant.[67] Casali et al. examined 33 large cell neuroendocrine carcinomas and reported that c-kit expression correlated with a poorer prognosis in the patients.[68]

Conclusion

As a group, both NSCLC and neuroendocrine carcinomas have shown predictable prognosis with profiles of specific molecular genetic abnormalities in individual tumors that include common markers for tumor proliferation, cellular growth, apoptosis, and metastatic potential. The factors discussed in this chapter have been shown to be the more common molecular genetic abnormalities with implications for potential therapeutic trials and adjuvant therapies.

References

1. Brambilla E. Histopathological classification and phenotype of lung tumors. In Hayat MA, ed. Handbook of Immunohistochemistry and In Situ Hybridization of Human Carcinomas: Molecular Genetics; Lung and Breast Carcinomas. Boston: Elsevier; 2004:105–114.
2. Cagle PT. The cytogenetics and molecular genetics of lung cancer: implications for pathologists. In Rosen PP, Fechner RE, eds. Pathology Annual. East Norwalk, CT: Appleton & Lange; 1990:317–329.
3. Cagle PT. Carcinoma of the lung. In Churg AM, Myers JL, Taxelaar HD, Wright JL, eds. Thurlbeck's Pathology of the Lung, 3rd ed. New York: Thieme; 2005:413–480.
4. Fong KM, Sekido Y, Mina J. The molecular basis of lung carcinogenesis. In Coleman WB, Tsongalis GJ, eds. The Molecular Basis of Human Cancer. Totowa, NJ: Humana Press; 2002:379–405.
5. Fong KM, Sekido Y, Gazdar AF, Minna JD. Lung cancer. 9: Molecular biology of lung cancer: clinical implications. Thorax 2003;58:892–900.
6. Sekido Y, Fong KM, Minna JD. Molecular genetics of lung cancer. Annu Rev Med 2003;54:73–87.
7. Johnson BE, Ihde DC, Makuch RW, et al. myc family oncogene amplification in tumor cell lines established from small cell lung cancer patients and its relationship to clinical status and course. J Clin Invest 1987;79:1629–1634.
8. Harada M, Dosaka-Akita H, Miyamoto H, et al. Prognostic significance of the expression of ras oncogene product in non–small cell lung cancer. Cancer 1991;69:72–77.
9. Miyamoto H, Harada M, Isobe H, et al. Prognostic value of nuclear DNA content and expression of the ras oncogene product in lung cancer. Cancer Res 1991;51:6346–6350.
10. Slebos RJC, Kibbelaar RE, Dalesio O, et al. K-ras oncogene activation as a prognostic marker in adenocarcinoma of the lung. N Engl J Med 1990;323:561–565.
11. Kern JA, Schwartz DA, Nordberg JE, et al. p185[neu] expression in human lung adenocarcinomas predicts shortened survival. Cancer Res 1990;50:5184–191.
12. Volm M, Efferth T, Mattern J. Oncoprotein (c-myc, c-erbB1, c-erbB2, c-fos) and suppressor gene product (p53) expression in squamous cell carcinomas of the lung. Anticancer Res 1992;12:11–20.
13. Funa K, Steinholtz L, Nou E, Bergh J. Increased expression of N-myc in human small cell lung cancer biopsies predicts lack of response to chemotherapy and poor prognosis. Am J Clin Pathol 1987;88:216–220.
14. Xu H-J, Hu S-X, Cagle PT, Moore GE, Benedict WF. Absence of retinoblastoma protein expression in primary non–small cell lung carcinomas. Cancer Res 1991;51:2735–2739.
15. Quinlan D, Davidson A, Summers C, Doshi H. Production of mutant p53 protein correlates with a poor prognosis in human lung cancer. Proc Am Assoc Cancer Res 1992;33:379.
16. Xu H-J, Cagle PT, Hu S-X, Li J, Benedict WF. Altered retinoblastoma and p53 protein status in non–small cell carcinoma of the lung: potential synergistic effects on prognosis. Clin Cancer Res 1996;2:1169–1176.
17. Younes M, Brown RW, Stephenson M, Gondo M, Cagle PT. Overexpression of Glut1 and Glut3 in stage I non–small cell carcinoma is associated with poor survival. Cancer 1997;80:1046–1051.
18. Anton RC, Brown RW, Younes M, Gondo MM, Stephenson MA, Cagle PT. Absence of prognostic significance of bcl-2 immunopositivity in non–small cell lung cancer: Analysis of 427 cases. Hum Pathol 1997;28:1079–1082.
19. Marchevsky AM, Patel S, Wiley KJ, Stephenson MA, Gondo M, Brown R, Yi ES, Benedict WF, Anton RC, Cagle PT. Artificial neural networks and logistic regression as tools for prediction of survival in patients with stages I and II non–small cell lung cancer. Mod Pathol 1998;11:618–625.
20. Yi ES, Harclerode D, Gondo M, Stephenson M, Brown RW, Younes M, Cagle PT. High c-erbB-3 protein expression is associated with shorter survival in advanced non–small cell lung carcinomas. Mod Pathol 1997;10:142–148.
21. Castro CY, Stephenson M, Gondo MM, Medeiros LJ, Cagle PT. Prognostic implications of calbindin-D28K expression in lung cancer: analysis of 452 cases. Mod Pathol 2000;13:808–813.
22. Anton RC, Coffey DM, Gondo MM, Stephenson MA, Brown RW, Cagle PT. The expression of cyclins D1 and E in predicting short-term survival in squamous cell carcinoma of the lung. Mod Pathol 2000;13:1167–1172.
23. Moldvay J, Scheid P, Wild P, et al. Predictive survival markers in patients with surgically resected non–small cell lung carcinoma. Clin Cancer Res 2000;6:1125–1134.

24. Brundage MD, Davies D, Backillop WJ. Prognostic factors in non–small cell lung cancer: a decade of progress. Chest 2002;122:1037–1057.

25. Kern JA, Slebos RJC, Top B, et al. C-erB-2 expression and codon 12 k-ras mutations both predict shortened survival for patients with pulmonary adenocarcinomas. J Clin Invest 1994;93:516–520.

26. Giatromanolaki A, Gorgoulis V, Chetty R, et al. C-erbB-2 oncoprotein expression in operable non–small cell lung cancer. Anticancer Res 1996;16:987–994.

27. Pfeiffer P, Clausen PP, Anderson K, Rose C. Lack of prognostic significance of epidermal growth factor receptor and the oncoprotein p185^{her-2} in patients with systemically untreated non–small cell lung cancer: an immunohistochemical study on cryosections. Br J Cancer 1996;74:86–91.

28. Pollan M, Varela G, Torres A, et al. Clinical value of p53, c-erbB-2, CEA and CA125 regarding relapse metastasis and death in resectable non–small cell lung cancer. Int J Cancer 2003;107:781–790.

29. Tateishi M, Ishida T, Mitsudomi T, et al. Prognostic value of c-erbB-2 protein expression in human lung adenocarcinoma and squamous cell lung carcinoma. Eur J Cancer 1991;27:1372–1375.

30. Pezzella F, Turley H, Kuzu I, et al. Bcl-2 protein expression in non–small cell lung cancers: correlation with survival time. Clin Cancer Res 1996;2:690–694.

31. Cox G, Louise-Jones J, Andi A, et al. Bcl-2 is an independent prognostic factor and adds to a biological model for predicting outcome in operable non–small cell lung cancer. Lung Cancer 2001;34:417–426.

32. Silvestrini R. Costa A, Lequaglie C, et al. Bcl-2 protein and prognosis in patients with potentially curable non–small-cell lung cancer. Virchows Arch 1998;432:441–444.

33. Poleri C, Morero JL, Nieva B, et al. Risk of recurrence in patients with surgically resected stage I non–small cell lung carcinoma: histopathologic and immunohistochemical analysis. Chest 2003;123:1858–1867.

34. Pastorino U, Andreola S, Tagliabue E, et al. Immunocytochemical markers in stage I lung cancer: relevance to prognosis. J Clin Oncol 1997;15:2858–2865.

35. Greatens TM, Niehans GA, Rubins JB, et al. Do molecular markers predict survival in non–small-cell lung cancer? Am J Respir Crit Care Med 1998;157:1093–1097.

36. Lee YC, Chang YL, Luh SP, et al. Significance of p53 and Rb protein expression in surgically treated non–small cell lung cancers. Ann Thorac Surg 1999;68:343–347.

37. D'Amico TA, Massey M, Herndon JE, et al. A biologic risk model for stage I lung cancer: immunohistochemical analysis of 408 patients with the use of ten molecular markers. J Thorac Cardiovasc Surg 1999;117:736–743.

38. Kwiatkowski DJ, Harpole DH, Godleski J, et al. Molecular pathologic substaging in 244 stage I non–small-cell lung cancer patients: clinical implications. J Clin Oncol 1998;16:2468–2477.

39. Dalquen P, Sauter G, Torhorst J, et al. Nuclear p53 overexpression is an independent prognostic parameter in node-negative non–small cell lung carcinoma. J Pathol 1996;178:53–58.

40. Huang C, Taki T, Adachi M, et al. Mutations in exon 7 and 8 of p53 as poor prognostic factors in patients with non–small cell lung cancer. Oncogene 1998;16:2469–2477.

41. Ahrendt SA, Hu Y, Buta M, et al. p53 mutations and survival in stage I non–small-cell lung cancer: results of a prospective study. J Natl Cancer Inst 2003;95:961–970.

42. Fukuyama Y, Mitsudomi T, Sugio K, et al. K-ras and p53 mutations are an independent unfavourable prognostic indicator in patients with non–small-cell lung cancer. Br J Cancer 1997;75:1125–1130.

43. Schiller JH, Adak S, Reins RH, et al. Lack of prognostic significance of p53 and K-ras mutations in primary resected non–small-cell lung cancer on E4592: a laboratory ancillary study on an Eastern Cooperative Oncology Group Prospective Randomized Trial of Postoperative Adjuvant Therapy. J Clin Oncol 2001;19:448–457.

44. Au NCH, Cheang M, Huntsman DG, et al. Evaluation of immunohistochemical markers in non–small cell lung cancer by unsupervised hierarchical clustering analysis: a tissue microarray study of 284 cases and 18 markers. J Pathol 2004;204:101–109.

45. Massion PP, Taflan PM, Jamshedur Rahman SM, et al. Significance of p63 amplification and overexpression in lung cancer development and prognosis. Cancer Res 2003;63:7113–7121.

46. Iwata T, Uramoto H, Sugio K, et al. A lack of prognostic significance regarding ΔNp63 immunoreactivity in lung cancer. Lung Cancer 2005;50:67–73.

47. Dworakowska D, Jassem E, Jassem J, et al. Prognostic relevance of altered pRb and p53 protein expression in surgically treated non–small cell lung cancer patients. Oncology 2004;67:60–66.

48. Reissmann PT, Koga H, Takahashi R, et al. Inactivation of the retinoblastoma susceptibility gene in non–small-cell lung cancer. The Lung Cancer Study Group. Oncogene 1993;8:1913–1919.

49. Haga Y, Hiroshima K, Iyoda A, et al. Ki-67 expression and prognosis for smokers with resected stage I non–small cell lung cancer. Ann Thorac Surg 2003;75:1727–32; discussion 1732.

50. Esposito V, Baldi A, Tonini G, et al. Analysis of cell cycle regulator proteins in non–small cell lung cancer. J Clin Pathol 2004;57:58–63.

51. Sonnweber B, Dlaska M, Skvortsov S, et al. High predictive value of epidermal growth factor receptor phosphorylation but not of EGFRvIII mutation in resected stage I non–small cell lung cancer. J Clin Pathol 2006;59:255–259.

52. Nakamura H, Kawasaki N, Taguchi M, Kabasawa K. Survival impact of epidermal growth factor receptor in patients with non–small cell lung cancer: a meta-analysis. Thorax 2006;61:140–145.

53. Shepherd FA, Pereira J, Ciuleanu TE, et al. Erlotinib in previously treated non–small-cell lung cancer. N Engl J Med 2005;353:123–132.

54. Dworakowska D, Jassem E, Jassem J, et al. MDM2 gene amplification: a new independent factor of adverse prognosis in non–small cell lung cancer. Lung Cancer 2004;43:285–295.

55. Higashiyama M, Doi O, Kodama K, et al. MDM2 gene amplification and expression in non–small-cell lung cancer: immunohistochemical expression of its protein is a favourable prognostic marker in patients without p53 protein accumulation. Br J Cancer 1997;75:1302-1308.

56. Ko JL, Cheng YW, Change SL, et al. MDM2 mRNA expression is a favorable prognostic factor in non–small-cell lung cancer. Int J Cancer 2000;89:265–270.

57. Mascaux C, Iannino N, Martin B, et al. The role of RAS oncogene in survival of patients with lung cancer: a systemic review of the literature with meta-analysis. Br J Cancer 2005;92:131–139.

58. Grossi F, Loprevite M, Chiaramondia M, et al. Prognostic significance of K-ras, p53, bcl-2, PCNA, CD34 in radically resected non–small cell lung cancers. Eur J Cancer 2003;39: 1242–1250.

59. Keohavong P, De Michele MMA, Melacrinos AC, et al. Detection of K-ras mutations in lung carcinomas: relationship to prognosis. Clin Cancer Res 1996;2:411–418.

60. Shih CM, Kuo YY, Want YC, et al. Association of L-myc polymorphism with lung cancer susceptibility and prognosis in relation to age-selected controls and stratified cases. Lung Cancer 2002;32:125–132.

61. Ge H, Lam WK, Lee J, et al. Analysis of L-myc and GSTM1 genotypes in Chinese non–small cell lung carcinoma patients. Lung Cancer 1996;15:355–366.

62. Tefre T, Borresen AL, Aamdal S, Brogger A. Studies of the L-myc DNA polymorphism and relation to metastasis in Norwegian lung cancer patients. Br J Cancer 1990;61:809–812.

63. Spinola M, Nomoto T, Manenti G, et al. Linkage disequilibrium pattern in the L-myc gene in Italian and Japanese non–small-cell lung-cancer patients. Int J Cancer 2001;95: 329–331.

64. Johnson BE, Russell E, Simmons AM, et al. Myc family DNA amplification in 126 tumor cell lines from patients with small cell lung cancer. J Cell Biochem 1996;24:210–217.

65. Rodriguez-Salas N, Palacios J, de Castro J, et al. Beta-catenin expression pattern in small cell lung cancer: correlation with clinical and evolutive features. Histol Histopathol 2001;16: 353–358.

66. Micke P, Hengstler JG, Ros R, et al. c-erbB-2 expression in small-cell lung cancer is associated with poor prognosis. Int J Cancer 2001;92:474–479.

67. Beasley MB, Lantuejoul S, Abbondanzo S, et al. The p16/ cyclin D1/Rb pathway in neuroendocrine tumors of the lung. Hum Pathol 2003;34:136–140.

68. Casali C, Stefani A, Rossi G, et al. The prognostic role of c-kit protein expression in resected large cell neuroendocrine carcinoma of the lung. Ann Thorac Surg 2004;77:247–253.

69. Bakir K, Ucak R, Tuncozgur B, Elbeyli L. Prognostic factors and c-erbB-2 expression in non–small-cell lung carcinoma (c-erB-2 in non–small cell lung carcinoma). Thorac Cardiovasc Surg 2002;50:55–8.

70. Choi S, Kim M, Kang C, et al. Activation of Bak and Bax through c-Abl-protein kinase Cδ-p38 MAPK signaling in response to ionizing radiation in human non–small cell lung cancer cells. J Biol Chem 2006;281:7049–7059.

71. Jiang SX, Sato Y, Kuwao S, Kameya T. Expression of bcl-2 oncogene protein is prevalent in small cell lung carcinomas. J Pathol 1995;177:135–138.

72. Ohsaki Y, Toyoshima E, Fujiuchi S, et al. Bcl-2 and p53 protein expression in non–small cell lung cancers: correlation with survival time. Clin Cancer Res 1996;2:915–920.

73. Reed JC. Double identity for proteins of the bcl-2 family. Nature (Lond) 1997;387:773–776.

74. Koukourakis MI, Giatromanolaki A, O'Byrne KJ, et al. Potential role of Bcl-2 as a supressor of tumor angiogenesis in non–small cell lung cancer. Intl J Cancer 1997;74:565–570.

75. Yilmaz A, Savas I, Dizbay-Sak S, et al. Distribution of Bcl-2 gene expression and its prognostic value in non–small cell lung cancer. Tuberkuloz ve Toraks Dergisi 2005;53:323–329.

76. Maddau C, Confortini M, Bisanzi S, et al. Prognostic significance of p53 and Ki-67 antigen expression in surgically treated non–small cell lung cancer. Am J Clin Pathol 2006;125:425–431.

77. Singhal S, Vachani A, Antin-Ozerkis D, et al. Prognostic implications of cell cycle, apoptosis, and angiogenesis biomarkers in non–small cell lung cancer: a review. Clin Cancer Res 2005;11:3974–3986.

78. Pappot H, Francis D, Brunner N, et al. p53 protein in non–small cell lung cancers as quantitated by enzyme-linked immunosorbent assay: relation to prognosis. Clin Cancer Res 1996;2:155–160.

79. Nishio M, Koshikawa T, Kuroishi T, et al. Prognostic significance of abnormal p53 accumulation in primary, resected non–small-cell lung cancers. J Clin Oncol 1996;14: 497–502.

80. Harpole DH, Herndon JE, Wolfe WG, et al. A prognostic model of recurrence and death in stage I non–small cell lung cancer utilizing presentation, histopathology, and oncoprotein expression. Cancer Res 1995;55:51–56.

81. Pelosi, G, Pasini F, Stehnolm CO, et al. p63 immunoreactivity in lung cancer: yet another player in the development of squamous cell carcinomas? J Pathol 2002;198:100–109.

82. Esposito V, Baldi A, De Luca A, et al. Cell cycle related proteins as prognostic parameters in radically resected non–small cell lung cancer. J Clin Pathol 2005;58: 734–739.

83. Lee SM. Is EGFR expression important in non–small cell lung cancer? Thorax 2006;66:98–99.

84. Spinola M, Pedotti P, Dragani TA, Taioli E. Meta-analysis suggests association of L-myc EcoR1 polymorphism with cancer prognosis. Clin Cancer Res 2004;10:4769–4775.

85. Campbell AM, Camling BG, Algazy KM, El-Deiry WS. Clinical and molecular features of small cell lung cancer. Cancer Biol Ther 2002;1:105–112.

19
Pulmonary Angiogenesis in Neoplastic and Nonneoplastic Disorders

Michael P. Keane and Robert M. Strieter

Introduction

Angiogenesis is the process of new blood vessel growth and is a critical biologic process in both physiologic and pathologic conditions. Angiogenesis can occur in physiologic conditions, including normal wound repair and embryogenesis. In contrast, pathologic angiogenesis is associated with chronic inflammatory and fibroproliferative disorders, as well as growth of tumors. A variety of factors have been described that either promote or inhibit angiogenesis, including the CXC chemokines, endothelin-1 (ET-1), vascular endothelial growth factor (VEGF), and basic fibroblast growth factor (bFGF). In the local microenvironment, net angiogenesis is determined by the balance between angiogenic and angiostatic factors.

The CXC chemokines are heparin-binding proteins that display unique disparate roles in the regulation of angiogenesis. The family has four highly conserved cysteine amino acid residues, with the first two cysteines separated by a nonconserved amino acid residue.[1,2] A second structural domain dictates their functional activity. The NH2-terminus of several CXC chemokines contains three amino acid residues (Glu-Leu-Arg, the "ELR" motif), which immediately precede the first cysteine amino acid residue.[1,2] The CXC chemokines with the ELR motif (ELR$^+$) promote angiogenesis (Tables 19.1 and 19.2).[1] In contrast, the CXC chemokines that are, in general, interferon inducible and lack the ELR motif (ELR$^-$) inhibit angiogenesis (Tables 19.1 and 19.3).[1] The dissimilarity in structure dictates interaction with different CXC chemokine receptors on endothelial cells, which ultimately leads to signal coupling and either promotion or inhibition of angiogenesis. CXCR2 mediates the angiogenic signals of the ELR$^+$ CXC chemokines, whereas the ELR$^-$ CXC chemokines mediate their angiostatic actions through CXCR3. Furthermore, it has recently been suggested that angiostatic signals are specifically mediated through CXCR3B, whereas CXCR3A may mediate angiogenic signals.[3,4]

Endothelin-1 mediates it effects through two receptors, ETA and ETB. Endothelin A appears to be more important in angiogenesis. The dual ET-1 receptor antagonist bosentan has been shown to have beneficial effects in the treatment of pulmonary hypertension, but the precise mechanism underlying the beneficial effect is unclear.

The VEGF family of proteins is perhaps the best known of all angiogenic agents. There are six growth factors, VEGF-A, B, C, D, and E, and three receptors, VEGFR-1 (Flt-1), VEGFR-2 (KDR/flk-1), and VEGFR-3 (Flt-4). Vascular endothelial growth factor A, the best characterized of the family, is a 36–46 kDa glycoprotein that is induced by hypoxia and oncogenic mutation.[5] It mediates its effects through VEGFR-1 and -2 and has been implicated in the growth of several tumors. Much interest has been generated for understanding the mechanism of VEGF-mediated angiogenesis, and this has lead to the development of inhibitors of VEGF. The recombinant humanized monoclonal antibody to VEGF, bevacizumab, has been studied in clinical trials of various cancers, particularly colon cancer, with variable results.[6,7] Although use of bevacizumab alone has failed to show a survival benefit, when this agent is used in combination with other agents it has had positive effects on survival in colon and lung cancers.[6] Possible explanations for the variable results with bevacizumab are discussed later.

The CXC Chemokines

The CXC chemokines can be divided into two groups on the basis of a structure/function domain consisting of the presence or absence of three amino acid residues (Glu-Leu-Arg, the ELR motif) that precedes the first cysteine amino acid residue in the primary structure of these cytokines. The ELR$^+$ CXC chemokines are chemoattractants for neutrophils and act as potent angiogenic factors.[8] In contrast, the ELR$^-$ CXC chemokines are chemoattrac-

TABLE 19.1. The CXC chemokines that display disparate angiogenic activities.

Angiogenic CXC chemokines containing the ELR motif	
CXCL1	Growth-related oncogene-α (GRO-α)
CXCL2	Growth-related oncogene-β (GRO-β)
CXCL3	Growth-related oncogene-γ (GRO-γ)
CXCL5	Epithelial neutrophil activating protein-78 (ENA-78)
CXCL6	Granulocyte chemotactic protein-2 (GCP-2)
CXCL7	Neutrophil activating protein-2 (NAP-2)
CXCL8	Interleukin-8 (IL-8)
Angiostatic CXC chemokines lacking the ELR motif	
CXCL4	Platelet factor-4 (PF4)
CXCL9	Monokine induced by interferon-γ (MIG)
CXCL10	Interferon-γ–inducible protein (IP-10)
CXCL11	Interferon-inducible T cell α–chemoattractant (ITAC)
CXCL12	Stromal cell–derived factor-1 (SDF-1)
CXCL14	Breast and kidney–expressed chemokine (BRAK)

TABLE 19.3. CXC chemokine ligands and receptors that have been implicated in angiostasis.

Receptor	Ligand
CXCR3B	CXCL4,* CXCL9, CXCL10, CXCL11
Unknown/nonreceptor mediated	CXCL4,* CXCL14

*CXCL4 may act through CXCR3B or nonreceptor-mediated mechanisms.

tants for mononuclear cells and are potent inhibitors of angiogenesis (see Table 19.1).[8]

Based on structural/functional differences, the members of the CXC chemokine family are unique cytokines in their ability to behave in a disparate manner in the regulation of angiogenesis. The angiogenic members include CXCLs 1, 2, 3, 5, 6, 7, and 8. CXCL1, CXCL2, and CXCL3 are closely related CXC chemokines, with CXCL1 originally described for its melanoma growth stimulatory activity (see Table 19.1). CXCL5, CXCL6, and CXCL8 were all initially identified on the basis of neutrophil activation and chemotaxis. The angiostatic (ELR⁻) members of the CXC chemokine family include CXCL4, which was originally described for its ability to bind heparin and inactivate heparin's anticoagulation function. Other angiostatic ELR⁻ CXC chemokines are listed in Table 19.1.

CXCR2 Is the Receptor for Angiogenic ELR⁺ CXC Chemokine-Mediated Angiogenesis

The fact that all ELR⁺ CXC chemokines mediate angiogenesis highlights the importance of identifying a common receptor that mediates their biologic function in promoting angiogenesis. While the candidate CXC chemokine receptors are CXCR1 and/or CXCR2, only CXCL8 and CXCL6 specifically bind to CXCR1, whereas all ELR⁺

TABLE 19.2. CXC chemokine ligands and receptors that have been implicated in angiogenesis.

Receptor	Ligand
CXCR2	CXCL1, CXCL2, CXCL3, CXCL5, CXCL6, CXCL7, CXCL8
CXCR4	CXCL12

CXC chemokines bind to CXCR2.[9] The ability of all ELR⁺ CXC chemokine ligands to bind to CXCR2 supports the idea that this receptor mediates the angiogenic activity of ELR⁺ CXC chemokines.

Although CXCR1 and CXCR2 are both detected in endothelial cells,[9–11] it is CXCR2, and not CXCR1, that has been found to be the primary functional chemokine receptor in mediating endothelial cell chemotaxis.[9,10] Endothelial cells respond to CXCL8 with rapid stress fiber assembly, chemotaxis, enhanced proliferation, and phosphorylation of extracellular signal-regulated protein kinase 1/2 (ERK1/2) related to activation of CXCR2.[12] Blocking the function of CXCR2 by either specific neutralizing antibodies or inhibiting downstream signaling using specific inhibitors of ERK1/2 and phosphatidylinositol-3 kinase (PI3K) impaired CXCL8-induced stress fiber assembly, chemotaxis, and endothelial tube formation in endothelial cells.[12]

Activation of CXCR2 leads to receptor internalization and recycling of the receptor back to the cell membrane or targets CXCR2 for degradation. ELR⁺ CXC chemokine activation of CXCR2 under conditions in which the receptor is transiently exposed or stimulated with less than saturable concentrations results in movement of CXCR2 into clathrin-coated pits, movement into the early (sorting) endosome, and then to the recycling endosome, with trafficking back to the plasma membrane compartment and reexpression on the cell surface.[13] However, if CXCR2 is exposed to prolonged saturating concentrations of ELR⁺ CXC chemokines, a significant proportion of CXCR2 will move into the late endosome and on to the lysosome for degradation.[13] Interestingly, CXCR2 internalization is necessary for generating a chemotactic response. Mutation of CXCR2, which impairs receptor internalization by altering the binding of adaptor proteins AP-2 or β-arrestin to the receptor, results in a marked reduction in the chemotactic response.[13]

The importance of CXCR2 in mediating ELR⁺ CXC chemokine-induced angiogenesis has been shown in vivo using the corneal micropocket assay of angiogenesis in *CXCR2⁺/⁺* and *CXCR2⁻/⁻* animals. ELR⁺ CXC chemokine-mediated angiogenesis was inhibited in the corneas of *CXCR2⁻/⁻* mice and in the presence of neutralizing antibodies to CXCR2 in the rat corneal micropocket assay.[9] These studies have been further substantiated using *CXCR2*[-/-] mice in a wound repair model system in which significant delays in wound healing parameters, including decreased neovascularization, were found in *CXCR2*[-/-] mice.[14]

Virally Encoded Chemokine Receptors and Angiogenesis

Given the finding that CXCR2 is the receptor that mediates the angiogenic activity of ELR[+] CXC chemokines, it is logical to hypothesize that a relationship exists between aberrant expression of this receptor, or a homolog of this receptor, and the process of neoplastic transformation. The pathogenesis of lung cancer is a multistep process that involves sequential morphologic and molecular changes that precede invasive lung cancer, and similar events occur in the genesis of other neoplasms. For example, the human Kaposi's sarcoma herpes virus (KSHV) that mediates the pathogenesis of Kaposi's sarcoma (KS) encodes a seven-transmembrane G protein–coupled receptor (7TM-GPCR) (KSHV-GPCR) that is homologous to CXCR2.[15,16] Activation of 7TM-GPCR leads to dissociation of the heterotrimeric protein complex ($G_{\alpha\beta\gamma}$) to α- and βγ-subunits that mediate downstream regulation of several intracellular signaling pathways (i.e., cyclic adenosine monophosphate/AMP/protein kinase A, protein kinase C, phospholipase C, PI3K/Akt/mTOR, Ras/Raf/MEK/JNK/p38/ERK1/ERK2) and activate NF-κB pathways.[17–20] Some of these signaling pathways are identical to signal transduction by receptor protein tyrosine kinases that are important for cellular proliferation, migration, and regulation of apoptosis.[17–19] These findings support the idea that 7TM-GPCRs, like CXCR2, may be involved in preneoplastic to neoplastic transformation.

The KSHV-GPCR has been determined to constitutively signal couple, and signal coupling of this receptor can be further augmented with CXC chemokine ligand binding, (i.e., CXCL8 and/or CXCL1).[21–23] To ascertain the relevance of KSHV-GPCR in promoting the pathogenesis of KS, transgenic mice overexpressing expressing KSHV-GPCR have been found to constitutively produce tumors similar to KS.[24,25] The mice develop angioproliferative lesions in multiple organs that morphologically resemble KS lesions.[24,25] These findings suggest that the expression of only one viral chemokine receptor-like gene can lead to the histopathologic recapitulation of KS with cellular transformation and the development of a lesion that resembles an angiosarcoma. This supports the idea that a CXCR2-like receptor facilitates preneoplastic to neoplastic cellular transformation. The KSHV-GPCR has been found to signal couple a number of signaling pathways relevant to cellular transformation. In further support of this contention is the finding that a point muta-

tion of CXCR2, but not of CXCR1, results in constitutive signaling of the receptor and cellular transformation of transfected cells in a similar manner as KSHV-GPCR.[15] Furthermore, the persistent activation of CXCR2 by specific CXC chemokine ligands can lead to a similar cellular transformation as seen with either the point mutation of CXCR2 or KSHV-GPCR.[15] CXCR2 has been further identified in the cellular transformation of melanocytes into melanoma.[26] Therefore, the expression of CXCR2 on certain cells, in the presence of persistent autocrine and paracrine stimulation with specific CXC chemokine ligands, has important implications in promoting cellular transformation that may be relevant to the process of preneoplastic to neoplastic transformation.

Similar to KSHV-GPCR, another virally encoded chemokine receptor, US28, has been shown to signal and induce a proangiogenic phenotype and activate various pathways linked to proliferation.[27] Cells expressing US28 promote tumorigenesis and angiogenesis in mice.[27] This is mediated through the expression of VEGF, indicating important interactions between chemokines/chemokine receptors and VEGF in promoting tumor growth. Furthermore, these findings indicate potential mechanisms for viral involvement in tumorigenesis and angiogenesis.

CXCR3 Is the Major Receptor for CXC Chemokines That Inhibit Angiogenesis

The major receptor that has been identified for angiostatic CXC chemokines is CXCR3, which is involved in mediating recruitment of type 1 helper T cells and acts as the receptor for inhibition of angiogenesis.[28–32] Endothelial expression of CXCR3 was originally identified on murine endothelial cells;[33] subsequent studies demonstrated that CXCR3 ligands could block both human microvascular endothelial cell migration and proliferation in response to a variety of angiogenic factors.[11,34] Further clarification of the role of CXCR3 in mediating angiostatic activity has come from the discovery that CXCR3 exists as two alternative splice forms.[3] These variants have been termed CXCR3A and CXCR3B.[3] CXCR3A mediates the CXCR3 ligand-dependent chemotactic activity of mononuclear cells.[3] CXCR3B mediates the angiostatic activity of CXCL4, CXCL9, CXCL10, and CXCL11 on human microvascular endothelial cells.[3] Moreover, specific antibodies to CXCR3B immunolocalize to endothelial cells within neoplastic tissues.[3] This supports the idea that if CXCR3 ligands can be spatially expressed within the tumor, then CXCR3B activation can inhibit tumor-associated angiogenesis.[3] To add to the complexity of CXCR3 biology, a variant of human CXCR3 has been recently identified that is generated by posttranscriptional exon skipping, referred to as CXCR3-alt.[32] This receptor is expressed and responds to CXCL11 and, to a lesser extent, to CXCL9 and CXCL10.[32] These findings support the idea that augmenting CXCR3/CXCR3-ligand biology will be a therapeutic strategy to enhance angiostasis within the tumor.

Although the above studies support the idea that CXCR3 is the receptor for CXCL4, CXCL9, CXCL10, and CXCL11, it remains unclear whether, in vivo, these CXCR3 ligands use CXCR3 on endothelium to mediate their angiostatic effect. Yang and Richmond[35] have recently demonstrated that CXCL10 mediates its angiostatic activity in vivo by binding to CXCR3 and not via binding to glycosaminoglycans. To clarify this issue, they created expression constructs for mutants of CXCL10 that exhibit partial or total loss of binding to CXCR3 or loss of binding to glycosaminoglycans. They transfected a human melanoma cell line with these expression vectors, and stable clones were selected and inoculated into immunodeficient mice.[35] Tumor cells expressing wild-type CXCL10 showed remarkable reduction in tumor growth compared with control vector–transfected tumor cells. Surprisingly, mutation of CXCL10 resulting in partial loss of receptor binding (IP-10C) or loss of glycosaminoglycan binding (IP-10H) did not significantly alter the ability to inhibit tumor growth. The reduction in tumor growth was associated with a reduction in tumor-associated angiogenesis, leading to an observed increase in both tumor cell apoptosis and necrosis.[35] In contrast, expression of the CXCL10 mutant that fails to bind to CXCR3 failed to inhibit tumor growth.[35] These data suggest that CXCR3 receptor binding, but not glycosaminoglycan binding, is essential for the tumor angiostatic activity of CXCR3 ligands.

Endothelin-1 and Angiogenesis

Endothelin-1 is a potent mitogen for vascular endothelial cells in vitro and stimulates angiogenesis in vivo.[36–40] Endothelin-1 stimulates release of the angiogenic cytokines VEGF and interleukin (IL)-8 and directly stimulates neovascularization in the corneal micropocket model with an efficacy similar to that of either VEGF or CXCL8.[41] This corneal neovascular response could be inhibited by either ETA antagonism or mixed ETA and ETB antagonism using bosentan.[41] Interestingly, inhibition of ETB alone had no effect on the response to ET-1.[41] Chinese hamster ovary cells stably transfected with ET-1 stimulated angiogenesis in both the chick chorioallantoic membrane and gelatin sponge assays.[40] In addition, there was an increase in endothelial cell proliferation.[40] The angiogenic response could be inhibited by combined ETA/ETB antagonism with bosentan, selective ETA receptor antagonism, and inhibition of endothelin-converting enzyme-1.[40] Some of the effects appeared to be mediated through VEGF, as the angiogenic response

could be inhibited by inhibition of VEGF tyrosine kinase receptor activity.[40] Similarly, ischemia-mediated angiogenesis has been shown to be associated with upregulation of ETA and ET-1 but not ETB.[42,43] Endothelin receptor A is expressed during the healing and scar tissue phase of gastric ulcers, suggesting a role for endothelin in late angiogenesis, as opposed to the earlier expression of VEGF that is observed.[43] The hypoxia-induced factor HIF-1α, which is induced by the interaction of ET-1 with ETA, further promotes angiogenesis by inducing VEGF.[42]

Angiogenesis has probably received the most attention as it relates to tumor growth and invasion. Phaeochromocytomas are usually highly vascular tumors but demonstrate variable vascularity between tumors.[44] Recently, Favier et al. studied the vascularity of malignant and benign phaeochromocytomas to try and identify a vascular pattern characteristic of malignant lesions.[44] In situ hybridization demonstrated increased expression of ETA and ETB in pericytes and tumor cells in malignant as opposed to benign tumors, suggesting an important role for endothelin in the angiogenesis associated with the malignant phenotype.[44] Furthermore, there was a distinct vascular pattern that was associated with malignant tumors.[44] Similarly, ETA is overexpressed in ovarian cancer, and the selective ETA inhibitor atrasentan significantly inhibited tumor growth.[45] There was a significant reduction in microvessel density and levels of VEGF and matrix metalloproteinase-2 and an increase in the numbers of apoptotic cells.[45] This adds further support for the role of ET-1 in the regulation of angiogenesis associated with tumor growth.

Angiogenesis and Pulmonary Hypertension

Pulmonary hypertension is a rare and progressive disease that is characterized by vascular remodeling. Endothelin-1 has been implicated in the pathogenesis of pulmonary hypertension, and indeed antagonism of ET-1 effects with bosentan has been shown to have significant therapeutic efficacy.[46,47] The histopathologic hallmark of idiopathic pulmonary hypertension is the plexiform lesion, which has been shown to arise from monoclonal proliferation of endothelial cells.[48] These plexiform lesions show similarities to the renal glomerulus and the vascular hyperplasia that is seen around glioblastoma multiforme.[49] They demonstrate disorganized growth with areas of solid core and vascular channels and express markers of angiogenesis indicating that they are areas of vascular remodeling.[49] This suggests that the beneficial effects of endothelin antagonism in idiopathic pulmonary hypertension may be related to both antiproliferative and antiangiogenic effects. Tuder et al. have demonstrated the presence of markers of angiogenesis in the plexiform lesions of idiopathic pulmonary hypertension.[50] There were increased levels of VEGF, VEGFR2, and both HIF-1α and HIF-1β, all of which are involved in angiogenesis. Interestingly, the same group developed a rat model of severe pulmonary hypertension and vascular remodeling with the use of a VEGFR2 antagonist in combination with hypoxia.[51]

Angiogenesis and Fibroproliferation in the Lung

The existence of neovascularization in idiopathic pulmonary fibrosis was originally identified in 1963 by Turner-Warwick, who demonstrated that within areas of pulmonary fibrosis there was extensive neovascularization with anastomoses between the systemic and pulmonary microvasculature.[52] Further evidence of neovascularization as a component of the pathogenesis of pulmonary fibrosis has been demonstrated in bleomycin-induced pulmonary fibrosis, following the perfusion of the vascular tree of rat lungs with methacrylate resin at a time of maximal bleomycin-induced pulmonary fibrosis.[53] Angiogenesis has been shown to develop in the mouse lung within 6 days in response to ischemia, with the new vessels arising between the parietal and visceral pleura, supplied by intercostal arteries.[54] In a mouse model of pulmonary artery ligation it has been demonstrated that the angiogenic chemokines CXCL1 and CXCL2 are highly expressed in ischemic lung and associated with angiogenesis.[55] Recently, an imbalance in the levels of angiogenic chemokines compared with angiostatic chemokines, which favors net angiogenesis, has been demonstrated in both animal models and tissue specimens from patients with idiopathic pulmonary fibrosis.[56–59] Renzoni et al. have demonstrated vascular remodeling in both idiopathic pulmonary fibrosis and fibrosing alveolitis associated with systemic sclerosis.[60] Cosgrove et al. provided further support for the concept of vascular remodeling in idiopathic pulmonary fibrosis when they studied the expression of pigment epithelium-derived factor and VEGF in lung specimens of patients with idiopathic pulmonary fibrosis.[61] Immunolocalization demonstrated a relative absence of vessels in the fibroblastic foci of idiopathic pulmonary fibrosis. This appeared to correlate with increased expression of pigment epithelium-derived factor in the fibroblastic foci. Interestingly, they also noted significant vascularity in the areas of fibrosis around the fibroblastic foci, with numerous abnormal vessels in the regions of severe architectural distortion. These findings are similar to those of Renzoni et al.[61] and support the concept of regional heterogeneity of vascularity in idiopathic pulmonary fibrosis. This heterogeneity is not surprising, since usual interstitial pneumonia, which

is the pathologic manifestation of idiopathic pulmonary fibrosis, is defined by its regional and temporal heterogeneity.

Although studies have suggested an important role for CXCL8 in mediating neutrophil recruitment, CXC chemokines have been found to exert disparate effects in regulating angiogenesis.[8] This latter issue is relevant to idiopathic pulmonary fibrosis, as the pathology of idiopathic pulmonary fibrosis demonstrates features of dysregulated and abnormal repair with exaggerated angiogenesis, fibroproliferation, and deposition of extracellular matrix, leading to progressive fibrosis and loss of lung function. In idiopathic pulmonary fibrosis lung tissue, there is an imbalance in the presence of CXC chemokines that behave as either promoters of angiogenesis (CXCL8) or inhibitors of angiogenesis (CXCL10).[56] This imbalance favors augmented net angiogenic activity.[56] Immunolocalization of CXCL8 demonstrated that the pulmonary fibroblast was the predominant interstitial cellular source of this chemokine, and areas of CXCL8 expression were essentially devoid of neutrophil infiltration.[56] This supports an alternative biologic role for CXCL8 or other ELR+ CXC chemokines in the interstitium of idiopathic pulmonary fibrosis lung tissue.

CXCL5 is an additional important regulator of angiogenic activity in idiopathic pulmonary fibrosis.[59] Lung tissue from patients with idiopathic pulmonary fibrosis expressed greater levels of CXCL5 than did normal control lung tissue. The predominant cellular sources of CXCL5 were hyperplastic type II cells and macrophages. These hyperplastic type II cells are associated with areas of active inflammation and are often found in proximity to fibroblastic foci. This provides further support for the role of nonimmune cells in the pathogenesis of idiopathic pulmonary fibrosis and may help to explain the failure of conventional immunosuppressive agents in this disease. As both CXCL8 and CXCL5 bind to CXCR2, this may represent an attractive therapeutic target with respect to the inhibition of angiogenesis, which may lead to a slowing of the progression of idiopathic pulmonary fibrosis.

In contrast to the increased angiogenic activity attributable to CXCL5 and CXCL8, there is a deficiency of the production of the angiostatic factor CXCL10 in idiopathic pulmonary fibrosis compared with controls (56). Interestingly, interferon (IFN)-γ, a major inducer of CXCL10 from a number of cells, is a known inhibitor of wound repair in part because of its angiostatic properties, and it has been shown to attenuate fibrosis in bleomycin-induced pulmonary fibrosis.[62] This suggests that CXCL10 is a distal mediator of the effects of IFN-γ, and an imbalance in the expression of angiostatic CXCL10 is found in idiopathic pulmonary fibrosis. Attenuation of the angiogenic (CXCL8) or augmentation of the angiostatic (CXCL10) CXC chemokines may represent a viable therapeutic approach to the treatment of idiopathic pulmonary fibrosis. Indeed, IFN-γ treatment of patients with either systemic sclerosis or idiopathic pulmonary fibrosis has received increasing attention.[63]

In the murine model of bleomycin-induced pulmonary fibrosis, CXCL2 and CXCL10 were found to be directly and inversely correlated, respectively, with fibrosis.[57,58] Moreover, if either endogenous CXCL2 was depleted by passive immunization or exogenous CXCL10 was administered to the animals during bleomycin exposure, there resulted marked attenuation of pulmonary fibrosis that was entirely attributable to a reduction in angiogenesis in the lung.[57,58] Furthermore, a phase II study of the administration of IFN-γ to patients with idiopathic pulmonary fibrosis demonstrated a significant upregulation of lung CXCL11 gene expression and bronchoalveolar lavage (BAL) and plasma protein levels of CXCL11.[64] The administration of CXCL11 to bleomycin-treated mice attenuated the development of pulmonary fibrosis via inhibition of vascular remodeling.[65] These findings support the idea that vascular remodeling is a critical biologic event that supports fibroplasia and deposition of extracellular matrix in the lung during pulmonary fibrosis.

Further support for a role of vascular remodeling in pulmonary fibrosis was found in the study by Hamada et al.[66] They transfected the gene for the soluble VEGF receptor (*sFlt-1*) into the skeletal muscle of mice that received intratracheal bleomycin.[66] This expression of the soluble receptor and the subsequent inhibition of VEGF activity were associated with a decrease in vascular remodeling as assessed by the expression of von Willebrand factor.[66] Furthermore, there was an associated reduction in fibrosis.[66]

Chemokines and Angiogenesis in Lung Cancer

CXC chemokine-mediated angiogenesis has been shown to play an important role in tumor growth in a variety of tumors, including melanoma, lung cancer, pancreatic cancer, ovarian cancer, brain tumors, gastric carcinoma, breast cancer, and head and neck cancer.[67–72]

CXCL8 is markedly elevated and contributes to the overall angiogenic activity of non–small cell lung cancer (NSCLC).[73] Extending these studies to an in vivo model system of human tumorigenesis (i.e., human NSCLC/SCID mouse chimera),[74] tumor-derived CXCL8 was found to be directly correlated with tumorigenesis.[74] Tumor-bearing animals depleted of IL-8/CXCL8 demonstrated a >40% reduction in tumor growth and a reduction in spontaneous metastases, which correlated with reduced angiogenesis.[74] These findings have been further corroborated with several human NSCLC cell lines grown in immunoincompetent mice. Non–small cell lung cancer

cell lines that constitutively express CXCL8 display greater tumorigenicity that is directly correlated with angiogenesis.[75]

Although CXCL8 was the first angiogenic ELR⁺ CXC chemokine to be discovered in NSCLC, CXCL5 has now been determined to have a higher degree of correlation with NSCLC-derived angiogenesis.[76] Surgical specimens of NSCLC tumors demonstrate a direct correlation between CXCL5 expression and tumor angiogenesis. These studies were extended to a SCID mouse model of human NSCLC tumorigenesis. CXCL5 expression was directly correlated with tumor growth.[76] Moreover, when NSCLC-bearing animals were depleted of CXCL5, both tumor growth and spontaneous metastases were markedly attenuated.[76] The reduction of angiogenesis was also accompanied by an increase in tumor cell apoptosis, consistent with the previous observation that inhibition of tumor-derived angiogenesis is associated with increased tumor cell apoptosis.[76] Although CXCL5 expression correlates significantly with tumor-derived angiogenesis, tumor growth, and metastases, CXCL5 depletion does not completely inhibit tumor growth.[76] This reflects the fact that the angiogenic activity of NSCLC tumors is related to many overlapping and potentially redundant factors acting in a parallel or serial manner. Furthermore, when all ELR⁺ CXC chemokines are evaluated in human NSCLC, it appears that they correlate with patient mortality.[77,78]

These studies have been further extended to a lung cancer syngeneic tumor model system in $CXCR2^{-/-}$ compared with $CXCR2^{+/+}$ mice. Lung cancer in $CXCR2^{-/-}$ mice demonstrate reduced growth, increased tumor-associated necrosis, and inhibited tumor-associated angiogenesis and metastatic potential.[79] These in vitro and in vivo studies establish that CXCR2 is an important receptor that mediates ELR⁺ CXC chemokine-dependent angiogenic activity.

Non-ELR⁺ CXC Chemokines Attenuate Angiogenesis Associated with Tumorigenesis

Non-ELR⁺ CXC chemokines have been shown to inhibit angiogenesis in several model systems, for example, in Burkitt's lymphoma cell lines in immunoincompetent mice.[80] Angiogenesis is essential for tumorigenesis of these lymphomas, analogous to carcinomas. The expressions of CXCL9 and CXCL10 were found to be higher in tumors that demonstrated spontaneous regression and were directly related to impaired angiogenesis.[81] To determine whether this effect was attributable to CXCL9 or to CXCL10, more virulent Burkitt's lymphoma cell lines were grown in immunodeficient mice and subjected to intratumor inoculation with either CXCL9 or CXCL10. Both conditions resulted in marked reduction in tumor-associated angiogenesis. Although these CXCR3 ligands have been shown to bind to CXCR3 on mononuclear cells, the ability of these non-ELR[+] CXC chemokines to inhibit angiogenesis and induce lymphoma regression in immunodeficient mice supports the idea that these chemokines can mediate their effects in a T-cell–independent manner.

To examine the role of CXCL10 in the regulation of angiogenesis in lung carcinoma, the level of CXCL10 from human surgical NSCLC tumor specimens was examined and found to be significantly higher in the tumor specimens than in normal adjacent lung tissue.[82] The increase in CXCL10 from human NSCLC tissue was entirely attributable to the higher levels of CXCL10 present in squamous cell carcinomas compared with adenocarcinomas.[82] Moreover, depletion of CXCL10 from squamous cell carcinoma surgical specimens resulted in augmented angiogenic activity.[82] The marked differences in the levels and bioactivities of CXCL10 in squamous cell carcinomas and adenocarcinomas are clinically and pathophysiologically relevant and represent a possible explanation for the biologic differences between these two types of NSCLC. Patient survival is lower, metastatic potential is higher, and evidence of angiogenesis is greater for adenocarcinomas than for squamous cell carcinomas of the lung.

These studies were extended to a SCID mouse system to examine the effect of CXCL10 on human NSCLC cell line tumor growth in a T- and B-cell–independent manner. The SCID mice were inoculated with either an adenocarcinoma or a squamous cell carcinoma cell line.[82] The production of CXCL10 from adenocarcinoma and squamous cell carcinoma tumors was inversely correlated with tumor growth.[82] However, CXCL10 levels were significantly higher in squamous cell carcinomas than in adenocarcinomas.[82] The appearance of spontaneous lung metastases in SCID mice bearing adenocarcinomas occurred after CXCL10 levels from either the primary tumor or plasma had reached a nadir.[82] In subsequent experiments, SCID mice bearing squamous cell carcinomas were depleted of CXCL10, whereas animals bearing adenocarcinomas were treated with intratumor CXCL10.[82] Depletion of CXCL10 in squamous cell carcinoma tumors resulted in an increase in their size.[82] In contrast, intratumor supplementation with CXCL10 in adenocarcinomas reduced both tumor size and metastatic potential and was directly associated with a reduction in tumor-associated angiogenesis.[82] Similar results have been found for CXCL10 in melanoma involving a gene therapeutic strategy.[83]

Similar to CXCL10, CXCL9 also plays a significant role in regulating angiogenesis associated with NSCLC. Levels of CXCL9 in human specimens of NSCLC were not significantly different from those found in normal lung tissue.[84] However, these results suggested that the increased expression of ELR[+] CXC chemokines and other angiogenic factors found in these tumors was not counterregulated by a concomitant increase in the expression of the angiostatic CXC chemokine CXCL9. Thus, this imbalance could promote a microenvironment that fosters angiogenesis. To alter this imbalance, studies were performed to overexpress CXCL9 by three different strategies, including gene transfer.[84] These experiments resulted in the inhibition of NSCLC tumor growth and metastasis via a decrease in tumor-associated angiogenesis.[84] These findings support the importance of the IFN-inducible non-ELR[+] CXC chemokines in inhibiting NSCLC tumor growth by attenuation of tumor-associated angiogenesis. In addition, the above study demonstrates the potential efficacy of gene therapy as an alternative means to deliver and overexpress a potent angiostatic CXC chemokine.

Molecular Mechanisms of Angiogenesis

The tumor vascular system must rapidly respond to increased metabolic demands with generation of increased tumor microvasculature. In contrast to the normally tightly controlled angiogenic process that is characteristic of the menstrual cycle or wound repair, tumor-associated angiogenesis shows evidence of multiple adaptive strategies to perpetuate aberrant angiogenesis. The complexity and redundancy of these processes explain why therapeutic target of only one factor that promotes angiogenesis within a tumor may not lead to a dramatic outcome. To better understand aberrant angiogenesis within a tumor, it will be necessary to appreciate the temporal and spatial master switches that control specific gene products that promote and perpetuate aberrant tumor-associated angiogenesis, even when the microenvironmental cues change over time or in response to therapeutic intervention.

Two major transcription factors that respond to microenvironmental cues relevant to changes in metabolic needs and redox potential of tumor cells, and are activated in several tumors, are HIF-1α and the nuclear factor-κB (NF-κB). Hypoxia-induced factor-1α acts as a master transcription switch for regulation of oxygen homeostasis.[85] Hypoxia-induced factor-1 consists of a heterodimer of HIF-1α and HIF-1β subunits.[85] Normally, HIF-1α expression is under strict regulation. The von Hippel-Lindau tumor suppressor protein targets HIF-1α for rapid ubiquitination under nonhypoxic conditions,[85,86] whereas activation of PI3K/Akt and mitogen-activated protein kinase/extracellular signal-regulated kinase pathways are involved in activating HIF-1α under both normoxic and hypoxic conditions.[85,87,88] In contrast, HIF-1β is constitutively expressed.[85,86] The HIF-1 heterodimer recognizes and binds to specific cis-elements in the promoters of specific genes that are necessary for glycolysis and angiogenesis (i.e., VEGF).[85,86,89]

Nuclear factor-κB is a member of a heterodimeric family of transcription factors. Classic NF-κB is a heterodimer protein that is formed by p50/p65 proteins.[90,91] Normally NF-κB is under strict regulation by its sequestration in the cytoplasm in association with a heterotrimeric complex of NF-κB with the inhibitor of κB (IκB). Activation of NF-κB is related to phosphorylation of IκB by IκB kinases, followed by IκB ubiquitination and degradation by the proteasome and release of NF-κB for intranuclear localization and transactivation of a specific cis-element.[90,91] Change in the redox potential of the cell due to generation of reactive oxygen species and to activation of the PI3K/Akt and mitogen-activated protein kinase/extracellular signal-regulated kinase pathways is involved in activation of NF-κB. Nuclear factor-κB activates a number of genes that are relevant to innate and adaptive immunity, cellular proliferation, cell survival, and angiogenesis (i.e., ELR+ CXC chemokines).[2,91]

To link these two master switches of angiogenesis to aberrant angiogenesis in colon cancer, Mizukami and colleagues[92] used a strategy to target human colon cancer cells for stable knockdown of HIF-1α. They inoculated nude mice with wild-type and HIF-1α knockdown colon cancer cells and found that both cell types generated tumor growth in vivo. However, the HIF-1α knockdown colon cancer cells formed smaller tumors. When the histopathologies of the two types of tumors were examined, large differences were found in the areas of tumor necrosis, with larger areas of tumor necrosis in the wild-type colon cancer cells. In addition, the investigators found greater tumor cell proliferation, yet greater apoptotic rate, in the wild-type colon cancer cell tumors. These histopathologic changes were linked to changes in the expected levels of VEGF in these two tumor types. In vivo, VEGF mRNA and protein levels were reduced 51% and 52%, respectively, in HIF-1α knockdown colon cancer cell tumors. However, when the microdensity of vessels was assessed in the two tumor types, no difference was found in the magnitude of angiogenesis in the two tumor types to account for the difference in the sizes of areas of necrosis.[92] With regard to VEGF, this was an unexpected result, and this finding supported the conclusion that either high levels of VEGF were not required to stimulate angiogenesis or that other angiogenic factors may be expressed in a compensatory manner to maintain tumor-associated angiogenesis in the HIF-1α knockdown colon cancer cell tumors.

Interestingly, there was a twofold increase in the expression of the proangiogenic ELR+ CXC chemokine (i.e.,

IL-8; CXCL8) under hypoxic conditions in the HIF-1α knockdown colon cancer cells[92] These findings were confirmed by a 2.5-fold increase by quantitative polymerase chain reaction and measured levels of CXCL8 protein from cellular conditioned media. While CXCL8 protein levels were basally present in the wild-type colon cancer cells, there was no change in the magnitude of CXCL8 expression under conditions of hypoxia. This observation was confirmed in vivo in the tumor xenografts. These data support the idea that in the absence of HIF-1α within the tumor microenvironment there is a molecular switch that preserves tumor-associated angiogenesis in an HIF-1α–independent manner. Because NF-κB is the major regulator of proangiogenic ELR+ CXC chemokines,[2,93] including CXCL8, the investigators found that NF-κB was activated in the HIF-1α knockdown but not in the wild-type colon cancer cells. Pharmaceutical attenuation of NF-κB activation had a negative impact on CXCL8 expression by the HIF-1α knockdown colon cancer cells. The investigators further determined that the mechanism for NF-κB activation under conditions of hypoxia and in the absence of HIF-1α was related to increased generation of reactive oxygen species and signaling of the mutant K-ras oncogene.

To determine whether these molecular changes were specific to CXCL8-mediated aberrant tumor-associated angiogenesis of HIF-1α knockdown colon cancer cells in vivo, Mizukami and colleagues passively immunized tumor-bearing animals with specific neutralizing CXCL8 antibodies.[92] Depletion of CXCL8 in these tumors resulted in marked attenuation of tumor growth, decrease in tumor cell proliferation, increase in apoptotic index of the tumors, and reduction in tumor-associated angiogenesis. These studies confirmed the importance of two master angiogenesis switches in the preservation of tumor-associated angiogenesis and tumor growth of colon cancer cells. These findings may not be unique to colon cancer and imply that one should be cognizant of additional angiogenic factors within the tumor microenvironment prior to embarking on therapeutic strategies that treat only one angiogenic factor in cancer.

Although tremendous effort has been made to target VEGF in cancer, findings from studies using a monoclonal antibody against VEGF in patients with renal cell carcinoma or colon cancer have not produced overwhelming results.[94] Does this mean that tumor-associated angiogenesis is not important? Does this mean that VEGF is not as important as we have previously thought, or do these studies, together with the findings of Mizukami and colleagues,[92] highlight the importance of finding other angiogenic pathways? Nuclear factor-κB activation and induction of proangiogenic ELR+ CXC chemokines cannot be discounted for their important role in preserving aberrant angiogenesis in cancer. Future clinical studies designed to impair tumor-associated angiogenesis will benefit from the work of Mizukami and colleagues,[92] which emphasizes the need to develop strategies that will target both master switches of angiogenesis.[95]

Further insights into the mechanisms of angiogenesis associated with tumors have been gained from studies of glioblastoma. A hallmark of glioblastomas is the marked presence of angiogenesis,[96] which suggests that it may be necessary for malignant progression of this tumor. Garkavtsev and associates have recently identified a candidate tumor suppressor gene, *ING4*, which is involved in regulating glioblastoma tumor growth and angiogenesis.[96] In this study, the expression of *ING4* was found to be significantly reduced in glioblastomas compared to normal human brain tissue, and the extent of reduction correlated with the progression from lower to higher tumor grade.[96] Human glioblastomas that exhibited decreased expression of *ING4* when engrafted into immunoincompetent mice grew markedly faster and displayed greater angiogenesis than control tumors.[96] The mechanism for increased tumorigenicity in glioblastomas that expressed lower levels of *ING4* was related to *ING4*'s physical ability to bind the p65 (RelA) subunit of NF-κB, impair its nuclear translocation, and subsequently inhibit transactivation of NF-κB–dependent genes.[96] In fact, the mechanism for the angiogenic activity of glioblastomas that expressed low levels of *ING4* was CXCL8 dependent, as inhibition of CXCL8 in vivo markedly reduced tumor growth and tumor-associated angiogenesis.[96] These findings link a tumor suppressor gene to function and control of the expression of angiogenic ELR$^+$ CXC chemokines in human tumors and provide a unique opportunity to consider targeting ELR$^+$ CXC chemokine-mediated angiogenesis.

The Duffy Antigen Receptor for Chemokines and Tumor Angiogenesis

The Duffy antigen receptor for chemokines (DARC) is known to be a promiscuous chemokine receptor that binds chemokines in the absence of any detectable signal transduction events.[97] Within the group of ELR$^+$ CXC chemokines, DARC binds the angiogenic CXC chemokines including CXCL1, CXCL5, and CXCL8, all of which have previously been shown to be important for promoting tumor growth in a variety of tumors, including NSCLCs.[76,98,99] Addison and colleagues demonstrated that stable transfection and overexpression of DARC in an NSCLC tumor cell line resulted in the binding of the angiogenic ELR$^+$ CXC chemokines by the tumor cells.[97] The binding of tumor cell–derived ELR$^+$ CXC chemokines to the tumor cells themselves interfered with the local tumor paracrine microenvironment of tumor cell interaction with host responding endothelial cells by preventing the stimulation of endothelial cells by these angiogenic factors.[97] The NSCLC tumor cells that constitutively expressed DARC in vitro were similar in their growth characteristics to control-transfected cells. However, tumors derived from DARC-expressing cells were significantly larger than tumors derived from control-transfected cells. Interestingly, upon histologic examination, DARC-expressing tumors had significantly more necrosis and decreased tumor cellularity than control tumors.

Expression of DARC by NSCLC cells was also associated with a marked decrease in tumor-associated vasculature and a reduction in metastatic potential. Similarly, in a murine model of prostate cancer, $DARC^{-/-}$ mice had increased tumor growth, intratumoral levels of CXC chemokines, and increased intratumoral vessel density, indicating an important role for DARC in inhibiting the biologic effects of CXC chemokines in tumor growth.[100] The findings of this study suggested that competitive binding of ELR$^+$ CXC chemokines by tumor cells expressing a decoy receptor could prevent paracrine activation of endothelial cells in the tumor microenvironment and reduce tumor-associated angiogenesis.

Possible Nonreceptor-Mediated Inhibition of Angiogenesis

Platelet factor 4 (PF4)/CXCL4 was the first chemokine described to inhibit neovascularization.[101] Although this angiostatic chemokine was the subject of extensive research as a candidate anticancer drug,[102] its nonallelic gene variant PF4$_{alt}$/PF4$_{var1}$/SCYB4V1 has not been previously investigated.[103,104] The product of the nonallelic variant gene of CXCL4, PF4$_{var1}$/PF4$_{alt}$, designated CXCL4L1, was recently isolated from thrombin-stimulated human platelets and purified to homogeneity.[105] Although secreted CXCL4 and CXCL4L1 differ in only three amino acid residues, CXCL4L1 is more potent for inhibiting angiogenesis in response to angiogenic factors in both in vitro and in vivo models of angiogenesis.[105]

The molecular mechanism for the angiostatic function of CXCL4 is still a matter of debate. Brandt et al. suggested that CXCL4 is a unique chemokine that does not bind to a G protein–coupled receptor; rather, it activates cells (i.e., neutrophils) through binding to cell surface glycosaminoglycans.[106] However, it is not clear whether CXCL4 binding to glycosaminoglycan sites alone is both necessary and sufficient to trigger endothelial cell signaling. For instance, CXCL4 is reported to prevent activation of the extracellular signal-regulated kinase by bFGF and to inhibit downregulation of the cyclin-dependent kinase inhibitor p21.[108] Furthermore, CXCL4 function is not abrogated in heparan sulfate–deficient cells, and CXCL4 mutants or peptides lacking heparin affinity are capable of inhibiting angiogenesis.[102,109] Recently, Lasagni et al. identified a splice variant of CXCR3, designated CXCR3B, and found that this G protein–coupled receptor binds CXCL4 and mediates its angiostatic activity.[3] Finally, other studies have reported that the inhibitory effect of CXCL4 is mediated through complex formation with bFGF or CXCL8.[109,110] These findings suggest that the mechanisms involved in CXCL4L1-mediated attenuation of angiogenesis are complex. Furthermore, the important discovery of a variant of CXCL4 that is more efficacious for inhibiting angiogenesis than authentic CXCL4 has significant implications for the use of this angiostatic factor as a therapeutic tool to inhibit aberrant angiogenesis in a variety of diseases.

Breast and kidney-expressed chemokine/CXCL14 is another non-ELR⁺ CXC chemokine that has been recently identified to inhibit angiogenesis.[111] CXCL14 appears to be downregulated in tumor specimens as compared with normal adjacent tissue.[112] The biologic significance of the absence of CXCL14 in these tumors remained to be elucidated until Shellenberger and associates discovered that CXCL14 inhibited microvascular endothelial cell chemotaxis in vitro in response to CXCL8, bFGF, and VEGF and inhibited neovascularization in vivo in response to the same angiogenic agonists.[111] Schwarze and associates observed that CXCL14 is expressed in normal and neoplastic prostatic epithelium and focally in stromal cells adjacent to prostate cancer.[113] Interestingly, CXCL14 was found to be significantly upregulated in localized prostate cancer and positively correlated with Gleason score.[113] In contrast, CXCL14 levels were unchanged in benign prostate hypertrophy specimens.[113] In a model of human prostate cancer in immunodeficient mice, prostate cancer cells transfected with CXCL14 were found to have a 43% reduction in tumor growth compared with controls.[113] These studies support the idea that the loss or inadequate expression of CXCL14 is associated with the transformation of normal epithelial cells to cancer and may be due to the promotion of a proangiogenic microenvironment suitable for tumor growth. The receptor that mediates the actions of CXCL14 remains to be determined.

Conclusion

Angiogenesis is a pivotal process in a number of pathologic processes in the lung, including lung cancer, pulmonary hypertension, and pulmonary fibrosis. Studies performed on extrapulmonary neoplasms have also yielded results that contribute to our understanding of the mechanisms of angiogenesis in neoplasia. The mechanisms that are responsible for angiogenesis are diverse

and complex. Targeting a single distal mediator may not have significant effects. In contrast, targeting a proximal mediator or a "master switch" such as NF-κB has the potential to have profound effects on angiogenesis and therefore impact several disease processes. Similarly, the different profiles of angiogenic mediators produced by different tumors may aid in targeting therapies toward specific tumors.

References

1. Strieter RM, Polverini PJ, Kunkel SL, et al. The functional role of the ELR motif in CXC chemokine-mediated angiogenesis. J Biol Chem 1995;270(45):27348–27357.
2. Belperio JA, Keane MP, Arenberg DA, et al. CXC chemokines in angiogenesis. J Leuk Biol 2000;68(1):1–8.
3. Lasagni L, Francalanci M, Annunziato F, et al. An alternatively spliced variant of CXCR3 mediates the inhibition of endothelial cell growth induced by IP-10, Mig, and I-TAC, and acts as functional receptor for platelet factor 4. J Exp Med 2003;197(11):1537–1549.
4. Boulday G, Haskova Z, Reinders ME, Pal S, Briscoe DM. Vascular endothelial growth factor–induced signaling pathways in endothelial cells that mediate overexpression of the chemokine IFN-{gamma}-inducible protein of 10kDa in vitro and in vivo. J Immunol 2006;176(5): 3098–3107.
5. Ranieri G, Patruno R, Ruggieri E, et al. Vascular endothelial growth factor (VEGF) as a target of bevacizumab in cancer: from the biology to the clinic. Curr Med Chem 2006;13(16):1845–1857.
6. Jain RK, Duda DG, Clark JW, Loeffler JS. Lessons from phase III clinical trials on anti-VEGF therapy for cancer. Nat Clin Pract Oncol 2006;3(1):24–40.
7. Giatromanolaki A, Sivridis E, Koukourakis MI. Angiogenesis in colorectal cancer: prognostic and therapeutic implications. Am J Clin Oncol 2006;29(4):408–417.
8. Strieter RM, Polverini PJ, Kunkel SL, et al. The functional role of the "ELR" motif in CXC chemokine-mediated angiogenesis. J Biol Chem 1995;270(45):27348–27357.
9. Addison CL, Daniel TO, Burdick MD, et al. The CXC chemokine receptor 2, CXCR2, is the putative receptor for ELR(+) CXC chemokine-induced angiogenic activity. J Immunol 2000;165(9):5269–5277.
10. Murdoch C, Monk PN, Finn A. CXC chemokine receptor expression on human endothelial cells. Cytokine 1999; 11(9):704–712.
11. Salcedo R, Resau JH, Halverson D, et al. Differential expression and responsiveness of chemokine receptors (CXCR1–3) by human microvascular endothelial cells and umbilical vein endothelial cells. FASEB J 2000;14(13): 2055–2064.
12. Heidemann J, Ogawa H, Dwinell MB, et al. Angiogenic effects of interleukin 8 (CXCL8) in human intestinal microvascular endothelial cells are mediated by CXCR2. J Biol Chem 2003;278(10):8508–8515.
13. Richmond A, Fan GH, Dhawan P, Yang J. How do chemokine/chemokine receptor activations affect tumorigenesis?

Novartis Found Symp 2004;256:74–89, 91, 106–111, 266–269.

14. Devalaraja RM, Nanney LB, Du J, et al. Delayed wound healing in CXCR2 knockout mice. J Invest Dermatol 2000;115(2):234–244.

15. Burger M, Burger JA, Hoch RC, et al. Point mutation causing constitutive signaling of CXCR2 leads to transforming activity similar to Kaposi's sarcoma herpesvirus–G protein–coupled receptor. J Immunol 1999;163(4):2017–2022.

16. Gershengorn MC, Geras-Raaka E, Varma A, Clark-Lewis I. Chemokines activate Kaposi's sarcoma–associated herpesvirus G protein–coupled receptor in mammalian cells in culture. J Clin Invest 1998;102(8):1469–1472.

17. Sugden PH, Clerk A. Regulation of the ERK subgroup of MAP kinase cascades through G protein–coupled receptors. Cell Signal 1997;9(5):337–351.

18. Pawson T, Scott JD. Signaling through scaffold, anchoring, and adaptor proteins. Science 1997;278(5346):2075–2080.

19. Shyamala V, Khoja H. Interleukin-8 receptors R1 and R2 activate mitogen-activated protein kinases and induce c-fos, independent of Ras and Raf-1 in Chinese hamster ovary cells. Biochemistry 1998;37(45):15918–15924.

20. Couty JP, Gershengorn MC. Insights into the viral G protein–coupled receptor encoded by human herpesvirus type 8 (HHV-8). Biol Cell 2004;96(5):349–354.

21. Arvanitakis L, Geras-Raaka E, Varma A, et al. Human herpesvirus KSHV encodes a constitutively active G-protein–coupled receptor linked to cell proliferation. Nature 1997;385(6614):347–350.

22. Bais C, Santomasso B, Coso O, et al. G-protein–coupled receptor of Kaposi's sarcoma–associated herpesvirus is a viral oncogene and angiogenesis activator. Nature 1998;391(6662):86–89.

23. Geras-Raaka E, Arvanitakis L, Bais C, et al. Inhibition of constitutive signaling of Kaposi's sarcoma–associated herpesvirus G protein–coupled receptor by protein kinases in mammalian cells in culture. J Exp Med 1998;187(5):801–806.

24. Yang TY, Chen SC, Leach MW, et al. Transgenic expression of the chemokine receptor encoded by human herpesvirus 8 induces an angioproliferative disease resembling Kaposi's sarcoma. J Exp Med 2000;191(3):445–454.

25. Guo HG, Sadowska M, Reid W, et al. Kaposi's sarcoma–like tumors in a human herpesvirus 8 ORF74 transgenic mouse. J Virol 2003;77(4):2631–2639.

26. Luan J, Shattuck-Brandt R, Haghnegahdar H, et al. Mechanism and biological significance of constitutive expression of MGSA/GRO chemokines in malignant melanoma tumor progression. J Leuk Biol 1997;62(5):588–597.

27. Maussang D, Verzijl D, van Walsum M, et al. Human cytomegalovirus-encoded chemokine receptor US28 promotes tumorigenesis. Proc Natl Acad Sci USA 2006;103:13068–13073.

28. Luster AD, Cardiff RD, MacLean JA, et al. Delayed wound healing and disorganized neovascularization in transgenic mice expressing the IP-10 chemokine. Proc Assoc Am Physicians 1998;110(3):183–196.

29. Rollins BJ. Chemokines. Blood 1997;90(3):909–928.

30. Balkwill F. The molecular and cellular biology of the chemokines. J Viral Hepat 1998;5(1):1–14.

31. Loetscher M, Loetscher P, Brass N, Meese E, Moser B. Lymphocyte-specific chemokine receptor CXCR3: regulation, chemokine binding and gene localization. Eur J Immunol 1998;28(11):3696–705.

32. Ehlert JE, Addison CA, Burdick MD, et al. Identification and partial characterization of a variant of human CXCR3 generated by posttranscriptional exon skipping. J Immunol 2004;173(10):6234–6240.

33. Soto H, Wang W, Strieter RM, et al. The CC chemokine 6Ckine binds the CXC chemokine receptor CXCR3. Proc Natl Acad Sci U S A 1998;95(14):8205–8210.

34. Romagnani P, Annunziato F, Lasagni L, et al. Cell cycle–dependent expression of CXC chemokine receptor 3 by endothelial cells mediates angiostatic activity. J Clin Invest 2001;107(1):53–63.

35. Yang J, Richmond A. The angiostatic activity of interferon-inducible protein-10/CXCL10 in human melanoma depends on binding to CXCR3 but not to glycosaminoglycan. Mol Ther 2004;9(6):846–855.

36. Salani D, Di Castro V, Nicotra MR, et al. Role of endothelin-1 in neovascularization of ovarian carcinoma. Am J Pathol 2000;157(5):1537–1547.

37. Salani D, Taraboletti G, Rosano L, et al. Endothelin-1 induces an angiogenic phenotype in cultured endothelial cells and stimulates neovascularization in vivo. Am J Pathol 2000;157(5):1703–1711.

38. Pedram A, Razandi M, Hu RM, Levin ER. Vasoactive peptides modulate vascular endothelial cell growth factor production and endothelial cell proliferation and invasion. J Biol Chem 1997;272(27):17097–17103.

39. Venuti A, Salani D, Manni V, et al. Expression of endothelin 1 and endothelin A receptor in HPV-associated cervical carcinoma: new potential targets for anticancer therapy. FASEB J 2000;14(14):2277–2283.

40. Cruz A, Parnot C, Ribatti D, et al. Endothelin-1, a regulator of angiogenesis in the chick chorioallantoic membrane. J Vasc Res 2001;38(6):536–545.

41. Bek EL, McMillen MA. Endothelins are angiogenic. J Cardiovasc Pharmacol 2000;36(5 Suppl 1):S135–S139.

42. Akimoto M, Hashimoto H, Maeda A, et al. Roles of angiogenic factors and endothelin-1 in gastric ulcer healing. Clin Sci (Lond) 2002;103(Suppl 48):450S–454S.

43. Tsui JC, Baker DM, Biecker E, et al. Potential role of endothelin 1 in ischaemia-induced angiogenesis in critical leg ischaemia. Br J Surg 2002;89(6):741–747.

44. Favier J, Plouin P-F, Corvol P, Gasc J-M. Angiogenesis and vascular architecture in pheochromocytomas: distinctive traits in malignant tumors. Am J Pathol 2002;161(4):1235–1246.

45. Rosano L, Spinella F, Salani D, et al. Therapeutic targeting of the endothelin a receptor in human ovarian carcinoma. Cancer Res 2003;63(10):2447–2453.

46. Fagan KA, McMurtry IF, Rodman DM. Role of endothelin-1 in lung disease. Respir Res 2001;2(2):90–101.

47. Hoeper MM, Galie N, Simonneau G, Rubin LJ. New treatments for pulmonary arterial hypertension. Am J Respir Crit Care Med 2002;165(9):1209–1216.

48. Lee SD, Shroyer KR, Markham NE, et al. Monoclonal endothelial cell proliferation is present in primary but not secondary pulmonary hypertension. J Clin Invest 1998; 101(5):927–934.

49. Tuder RM, Voelkel NF. Angiogenesis and pulmonary hypertension: a unique process in a unique disease. Antioxid Redox Signal 2002;4(5):833–843.

50. Tuder RM, Chacon M, Alger L, et al. Expression of angiogenesis-related molecules in plexiform lesions in severe pulmonary hypertension: evidence for a process of disordered angiogenesis. J Pathol 2001;195(3):367–374.

51. Taraseviciene-Stewart L, Kasahara Y, Alger L, et al. Inhibition of the VEGF receptor 2 combined with chronic hypoxia causes cell death–dependent pulmonary endothelial cell proliferation and severe pulmonary hypertension. FASEB J 2001;15(2):427–438.

52. Turner-Warwick M. Precapillary systemic–pulmonary anastomoses. Thorax 1963;18:225–237.

53. Peao MND, Aguas AP, DeSa CM, Grande NR. Neoformation of blood vessels in association with rat lung fibrosis induced by bleomycin. Anat Rec 1994;238:57–67.

54. Mitzner W, Lee W, Georgakopoulos D, Wagner E. Angiogenesis in the mouse lung. Am J Pathol 2000;157(1): 93–101.

55. Srisuma S, Biswal SS, Mitzner WA, et al. Identification of genes promoting angiogenesis in mouse lung by transcriptional profiling. Am J Respir Cell Mol Biol 2003;29(2): 172–179.

56. Keane MP, Arenberg DA, Lynch JPr, et al. The CXC chemokines, IL-8 and IP-10, regulate angiogenic activity in idiopathic pulmonary fibrosis. J Immunol 1997;159(3): 1437–1443.

57. Keane MP, Belperio JA, Arenberg DA, et al. IFN-gamma–inducible protein-10 attenuates bleomycin-induced pulmonary fibrosis via inhibition of angiogenesis. J Immunol 1999;163(10):5686–5692.

58. Keane MP, Belperio JA, Moore TA, et al. Neutralization of the CXC chemokine, macrophage inflammatory protein-2, attenuates bleomycin-induced pulmonary fibrosis [In Process Citation]. J Immunol 1999;162(9):5511–5518.

59. Keane MP, Belperio JA, Burdick M, et al. ENA-78 is an important angiogenic factor in idiopathic pulmonary fibrosis. Am J Respir Crit Care Med 2001;164:2239–2242.

60. Renzoni EA, Walsh DA, Salmon M, et al. Interstitial vascularity in fibrosing alveolitis. Am J Respir Crit Care Med 2003;167(3):438–443.

61. Cosgrove GP, Brown KK, Schiemann WP, et al. Pigment epithelium-derived factor in idiopathic pulmonary fibrosis: a role in aberrant angiogenesis. Am J Respir Crit Care Med 2004;170:242–251.

62. Hyde DM, Henderson TS, Giri SN, et al. Effect of murine gamma interferon on the cellular responses to bleomycin in mice. Exp Lung Res 1988;14:687–704.

63. Raghu G, Brown KK, Bradford WZ, et al. A placebo-controlled trial of interferon gamma-1b in patients with idiopathic pulmonary fibrosis. N Engl J Med 2004;350(2): 125–133.

64. Strieter RM, Starko KM, Enelow RI, et al. Effects of interferon gamma-1b on biomarker expression in patients with idiopathic pulmonary fibrosis. Am J Respir Crit Care Med 2004;170:133–140.

65. Burdick MD, Murray LA, Keane MP, et al. CXCL11 attenuates bleomycin-induced pulmonary fibrosis via inhibition of vascular remodeling. Am J Respir Crit Care Med 2005;171(3):261–268.

66. Hamada N, Kuwano K, Yamada M, et al. Anti-vascular endothelial growth factor gene therapy attenuates lung injury and fibrosis in mice. J Immunol 2005;175(2):1224–1231.

67. Miller LJ, Kurtzman SH, Wang Y, et al. Expression of interleukin-8 receptors on tumor cells and vascular endothelial cells in human breast cancer tissue. Anticancer Res 1998;18(1A):77–81.

68. Richards BL, Eisma RJ, Spiro JD, et al. Coexpression of interleukin-8 receptors in head and neck squamous cell carcinoma. Am J Surg 1997;174(5):507–512.

69. Kitadai Y, Haruma K, Sumii K, et al. Expression of interleukin-8 correlates with vascularity in human gastric carcinomas. Am J Pathol 1998;152(1):93–100.

70. Singh RK, Gutman M, Radinsky R, et al. Expression of interleukin 8 correlates with the metastatic potential of human melanoma cells in nude mice. Cancer Res 1994; 54(12):3242–3247.

71. Cohen RF, Contrino J, Spiro JD, et al. Interleukin-8 expression by head and neck squamous cell carcinoma. Arch Otolaryngol Head Neck Surg 1995;121(2):202–209.

72. Chen Z, Malhotra PS, Thomas GR, et al. Expression of proinflammatory and proangiogenic cytokines in patients with head and neck cancer. Clin Cancer Res 1999;5(6): 1369–1379.

73. Smith DR, Polverini PJ, Kunkel SL, et al. IL-8 mediated angiogenesis in human bronchogenic carcinoma. J Exp Med 1994;179:1409–1415.

74. Arenberg DA, Kunkel SL, Burdick MD, et al. Treatment with anti-IL-8 inhibits non–small cell lung cancer tumor growth [abstr]. J Invest Med 1995;43(Suppl 3):479A.

75. Yatsunami J, Tsuruta N, Ogata K, et al. Interleukin-8 participates in angiogenesis in non–small cell, but not small cell carcinoma of the lung. Cancer Lett 1997;120(1): 101–108.

76. Arenberg DA, Keane MP, DiGiovine B, et al. Epithelial–neutrophil activating peptide (ENA-78) is an important angiogenic factor in non–small cell lung cancer. J Clin Invest 1998;102(3):465–472.

77. White ES, Flaherty KR, Carskadon S, et al. Macrophage migration inhibitory factor and CXC chemokine expression in non–small cell lung cancer: role in angiogenesis and prognosis. Clin Cancer Res 2003;9(2):853–860.

78. Chen JJ, Yao PL, Yuan A, et al. Up-regulation of tumor interleukin-8 expression by infiltrating macrophages: its correlation with tumor angiogenesis and patient survival in non–small cell lung cancer. Clin Cancer Res 2003;9(2): 729–737.

79. Keane MP, Belperio JA, Xue YY, et al. Depletion of CXCR2 inhibits tumor growth and angiogenesis in a murine model of lung cancer. J Immunol 2004;172(5): 2853–2860.

80. Gurtsevitch VE, O'Conor GT, Lenoir GM. Burkitt's lymphoma cell lines reveal different degrees of tumorigenicity in nude mice. Int J Cancer 1988;41(1):87–95.

81. Sgadari C, Angiolillo AL, Cherney BW, et al. Interferon-inducible protein-10 identified as a mediator of tumor necrosis in vivo. Proc Natl Acad Sci USA 1996;93(24): 13791–13796.

82. Arenberg DA, Kunkel SL, Polverini PJ, et al. Interferon-g–inducible protein 10 (IP-10) is an angiostatic factor that inhibits human non–small cell lung cancer (NSCLC) tumorigenesis and spontaneous metastases. J Exp Med 1996;184(3):981–992.

83. Feldman AL, Friedl J, Lans TE, et al. Retroviral gene transfer of interferon-inducible protein 10 inhibits growth of human melanoma xenografts. Int J Cancer 2002;99(1): 149–153.

84. Addison CL, Arenberg DA, Morris SB, et al. The CXC chemokine, monokine induced by interferon-gamma, inhibits non–small cell lung carcinoma tumor growth and metastasis. Hum Gene Ther 2000;11(2):247–261.

85. Semenza G. Signal transduction to hypoxia-inducible factor 1. Biochem Pharmacol 2002;64(5–6):993–998.

86. Semenza GL. Hypoxia-inducible factor 1: oxygen homeostasis and disease pathophysiology. Trends Mol Med 2001; 7(8):345–350.

87. Phillips RJ, Mestas J, Gharaee-Kermani M, et al. Epidermal growth factor and hypoxia-induced expression of CXC chemokine receptor 4 on non–small cell lung cancer cells is regulated by the phosphatidylinositol 3-kinase/PTEN/AKT/mammalian target of rapamycin signaling pathway and activation of hypoxia inducible factor-1alpha. J Biol Chem 2005;280(23):22473–22481.

88. Minet E, Michel G, Mottet D, et al. Transduction pathways involved in hypoxia-inducible factor-1 phosphorylation and activation. Free Radic Biol Med 2001;31(7):847–855.

89. Cramer T, Yamanishi Y, Clausen BE, et al. HIF-1alpha is essential for myeloid cell–mediated inflammation. Cell 2003;112(5):645–657.

90. Bonizzi G, Karin M. The two NF-kappaB activation pathways and their role in innate and adaptive immunity. Trends Immunol 2004;25(6):280–288.

91. Nakanishi C, Toi M. Nuclear factor-kappaB inhibitors as sensitizers to anticancer drugs. Nat Rev Cancer 2005;5(4): 297–309.

92. Mizukami Y, Jo WS, Duerr EM, et al. Induction of interleukin-8 preserves the angiogenic response in HIF-1alpha–deficient colon cancer cells. Nat Med 2005;11(9):992–927.

93. Richmond A. Nf-kappa B, chemokine gene transcription and tumour growth. Nat Rev Immunol 2002;2(9):664–674.

94. Yang JC, Haworth L, Sherry RM, et al. A randomized trial of bevacizumab, an anti-vascular endothelial growth factor antibody, for metastatic renal cancer. N Engl J Med 2003; 349(5):427–434.

95. Strieter RM. Masters of angiogenesis. Nat Med 2005;11(9): 925–927.

96. Garkavtsev I, Kozin SV, Chernova O, et al. The candidate tumour suppressor protein ING4 regulates brain tumour growth and angiogenesis. Nature 2004;428(6980):328–332.

97. Addison CL, Belperio JA, Burdick MD, Strieter RM. Overexpression of the Duffy antigen receptor for chemokines (DARC) by NSCLC tumor cells results in increased tumor necrosis. BMC Cancer 2004;4(1):28.

98. Arenberg DA, Kunkel SL, Polverini PJ, et al. Inhibition of interleukin-8 reduces tumorigenesis of human non–small cell lung cancer in SCID mice. J Clin Invest 1996;97(12): 2792–2802.

99. Moore BB, Arenberg DA, Stoy K, et al. Distinct CXC chemokines mediate tumorigenicity of prostate cancer cells. Am J Pathol 1999;154(5):1503–1512.

100. Shen H, Schuster R, Stringer KF, et al. The Duffy antigen/receptor for chemokines (DARC) regulates prostate tumor growth. FASEB J 2006;20(1):59–64.

101. Maione TE, Gray GS, Petro J, et al. Inhibition of angiogenesis by recombinant human platelet factor-4. Science 1990;247:77–79.

102. Bikfalvi A, Gimenez-Gallego G. The control of angiogenesis and tumor invasion by platelet factor-4 and platelet factor-4–derived molecules. Semin Thromb Hemost 2004; 30(1):137–144.

103. Eisman R, Surrey S, Ramachandran B, et al. Structural and functional comparison of the genes for human platelet factor 4 and PF4alt. Blood 1990;76(2):336–344.

104. Green CJ, Charles RS, Edwards BF, Johnson PH. Identification and characterization of PF4var1, a human gene variant of platelet factor 4. Mol Cell Biol 1989;9(4): 1445–1451.

105. Struyf S, Burdick MD, Proost P, et al. Platelets release CXCL4L1, a nonallelic variant of the chemokine platelet factor-4/CXCL4 and potent inhibitor of angiogenesis. Circ Res 2004;95(9):855–857.

106. Brandt E, Petersen F, Ludwig A, et al. The beta-thromboglobulins and platelet factor 4: blood platelet–derived CXC chemokines with divergent roles in early neutrophil regulation. J Leuk Biol 2000;67(4):471–478.

107. Gentilini G, Kirschbaum NE, Augustine JA, et al. Inhibition of human umbilical vein endothelial cell proliferation by the CXC chemokine, platelet factor 4 (PF4), is associated with impaired downregulation of p21(Cip1/WAF1). Blood 1999;93(1):25–33.

108. Sulpice E, Bryckaert M, Lacour J, et al. Platelet factor 4 inhibits FGF2-induced endothelial cell proliferation via the extracellular signal-regulated kinase pathway but not by the phosphatidylinositol 3-kinase pathway. Blood 2002;100(9):3087–3094.

109. Perollet C, Han ZC, Savona C, et al. Platelet factor 4 modulates fibroblast growth factor 2 (FGF-2) activity and inhibits FGF-2 dimerization. Blood 1998;91(9):3289–3299.

110. Dudek AZ, Nesmelova I, Mayo K, et al. Platelet factor 4 promotes adhesion of hematopoietic progenitor cells and binds IL-8: novel mechanisms for modulation of hematopoiesis. Blood 2003;101(12):4687–4694.

111. Shellenberger TD, Wang M, Gujrati M, et al. BRAK/CXCL14 is a potent inhibitor of angiogenesis and is a chemotactic factor for immature dendritic cells. Cancer Res 2004;64:8262–8270.

112. Frederick MJ, Henderson Y, Xu X, et al. In vivo expression of the novel CXC chemokine BRAK in normal and cancerous human tissue. Am J Pathol 2000;156(6):1937–1950.

113. Schwarze SR, Luo J, Isaacs WB, Jarrard DF. Modulation of CXCL14 (BRAK) expression in prostate cancer. Prostate 2005;13:13.

20
Lung Cancer Stem Cells

Timothy Craig Allen and Philip T. Cagle

Stem Cells

Germinal, embryonic, and somatic stem cells arise normally in human beings.[1] Adult germinal stem cells provide for the production of sperm and eggs.[1] Embryonic stem cells are self-renewing totipotent cells, derived from blastocysts, that can indefinitely propagate as undifferentiated cells and differentiate into most cell types under appropriate conditions in vitro and can differentiate into all cell lineages in vivo.[1-11] Embryonic stem cells have been isolated from human beings, but for ethical and other reasons their future use for research and treatment is uncertain.[1,3,5,12-14]

Telomeres, attached to the inner nuclear wall, determine the domain and stability of individual chromosomes—serve as "guardian of the genome"—and are essential for consistent segregation and maintenance of chromosomes during cell division.[2,15] Telomerase is an enzyme important for telomere maintenance.[2] Adult somatic stem cells, without sufficient telomerase activity to prevent telomere loss, do not have the capacity to replicate indefinitely.[1] Furthermore, unlike embryonic stem cells, which divide symmetrically, adult somatic stem cells are believed to maintain self-renewal and differentiation by asymmetric cell division, with one daughter cell retaining the parental stem cell properties and acting as a replacement for the parent stem cell and one transit cell daughter that either is differentiated or divides to produce a variety of differentiated cell types that form tissue.[1,8,16] Pluripotent adult somatic stem cells, with their limited self-renewal capacity, have been identified in mature hematopoietic, hepatic, mesenchymal, neural, epidermal, mammary, gastrointestinal, and pulmonary tissues and are responsible for tissue regeneration and repair.[1,8,17-20] Some authors believe that adult somatic stem cells are present in essentially every tissue in the body.[21,22] The concept of widespread distribution of adult somatic stem cells in all adult organs is uncertain, however.[8] The stem cells often localize in their respective tissues in a special microenvironment—the so-called stem cell niche.[23,24] It is hypothesized that these adult somatic stem cells, with their limited ability compared with embryonic stem cells to maintain their telomeres and prevent senescence, have an increased risk for malignant transformation.[1]

Cancer Stem Cells

The somatic stem cells of the hematopoietic system have been extensively studied, and the concept of cancer arising from hypothetical rare cells, with the stem cell properties of self-renewal and differentiation into progenitors, that exclusively maintain neoplastic clones—so-called cancer stem cells—is generally acknowledged for hematologic malignancies.[1,2,8,25-30] Bonnet et al. identified a common immunophenotype of leukemic stem cells.[1,25] Some leukemias have been shown to be composed of several clonal populations with heterogeneous proliferation and differentiation potential, and leukemia stem cells have been identified and shown to be necessary and sufficient for leukemia maintenance.[1,27,28] Bonnet et al. showed that leukemia, like the normal hematopoietic system, is organized as a hierarchy with only rare populations of stem cells retaining a clonogenic capacity.[8,25] Guan et al. found acute myeloid leukemia cells to be quiescent cells that were able to survive chemotherapeutic regimens directed toward dividing tumor cells.[1,31] Leukemia stem cells have also been identified with chronic myeloid leukemia.[1,32] Malignancies in solid tumors have been commonly thought to arise from differentiated organ- or tissue-specific somatic cells; however, the hypothesis exists that solid tumors also arise from cancer stem cells.[2,29,33] Specifically, it has been proposed that organ-specific cancers might originate from organ-specific stem cells.[2] Leukemia stem cells have been shown to be responsible for maintaining the tumor mass, and similar findings have been observed in human solid cancers such as breast cancer and brain tumors.[22,25,27,28,34-38]

213

The proposition for cancer stem cells is based on the principle that, in the multistep process of undergoing malignant transformation, a cell must have the capacity to self-renew in order to accumulate enough mutations to transform into a malignant cell.[3] These cells that are the origin of the cancer must either already have the capacity to self-renew or acquire that ability early in tumorogenesis.[3] Although better-differentiated cancer cells do not have this self-renewal capacity, a subset of tumor cells, the cancer stem cells, exists that does have the capacity to self-renew.[3,39] These cancer stem cells allow for the propagation of cancer cells that retain the primary tumor's diverse marker profile.[3,36] It follows that cancer therapy regimens that target the tumor mass but fail to have an influence on the cancer stem cells will allow for tumor recurrence and ultimately be unsuccessful.[3]

As the transformation of a normal cell into a cancer cell is considered to be a multistep process, cancer stem cells are likely to originate by a similar multistep transformation, with the cancer stem cell asymmetrically dividing to produce two cell populations—one retaining the cancer stem cell's self-renewing capacity and one with the ability to differentiate but lacking the ability to independently initiate tumor growth.[1] Alterations in the control of asymmetric division may cause aberrant self-renewal activity in the stem cells.[8] This hypothesis has been supported by studies utilizing *Drosophila*.[8,40] This hypothesis is supported by various findings, including (1) that not all cells in a tumor can maintain tumor growth; (2) that large numbers of tumor cells are required to successfully transplant a tumor into an immunologically competent animal; (3) that not all tumor cells are clonal despite their single-cell origin, consistent with a stem cell's ability to form various lineages; (4) that some tumor cells are morphologically reminiscent of the tissue of origin and retain some degree of biologic function; and (5) that some tumors appear dedifferentiated.[1,41] Cancer stem cells may be reactivated to duplicate the original tissue phenotype or may originate from genetically damaged somatic cells by redifferentiation to a progenitor-like state, acquiring self-renewal capacity de novo.[1] These rare clonogenic tumor cells, responsible for tumor growth and metastases, are termed *cancer stem cells* and have, like normal stem cells, both the capacity for self-renewal and the ability to produce heterogeneous differentiated cell types.[8,28] Cancer stem cells may arise from either stem cells or progenitor cells that have acquired self-renewal capacity; and multiple cancer stem cell populations might be formed during cancer progression or coexist in advanced malignancies.[8]

Cancer stem cells may be resistant to standard chemotherapeutic regimens and may therefore be a reservoir of tumor cells that can produce and expand populations of chemoresistant tumor cells.[22] Because cancer stem cells are highly resistant to chemotherapy, even small numbers of the immortal cells are sufficient to allow for recurrence.[1,42] It has been hypothesized that tumors derived from an early stem cell or its progenitor cell metastasize early and are phenotypically heterogeneous, whereas tumors derived from a later stem cell are less likely to metastasize and are more phenotypically homogeneous.[1,43]

Cancer Stem Cell Regulation

Alterations in self-renewal pathways are important in the formation of cancer stem cells.[8] A wide variety of cellular factors involved in the complex biology of normal adult stem cells, including self-renewal and differentiation, have been implicated in the development of cancer stem cells, including the Wingless (Wnt) signaling pathway, the Hh pathway, Oct-4, *Bmi-1*, the ecotropic viral integration site 1 (Evi1), Notch signaling pathways, Sonic hedgehog pathways, *HOX* genes, tumor suppressor genes, and oncogenes.[1,8,22,34,44–58] The Wnt signaling pathway is a critical regulatory component of both embryonic and adult stem cells.[22] The main cytoplasmic mediator of the Wnt signaling system is β-catenin.[22,47] The Wnt β-catenin pathway has been shown to play a role in the maintenance of stem cell self-renewal.[1,59,60] The Wnt signaling pathway is critical in the regulation of stem cell and progenitor cell biology, and Wnt signaling pathway activation has been identified in intestinal, epidermal, and hematopoietic cancers.[22,47] The Hh pathway is a critical regulator of hematopoietic and neuronal stem cell maintenance and has been found to be active in a variety of tumors.[22,50] The Pit-Oct-1/2-Unc86 domain transcription factor Octo4, identified in embryonic and adult stem cells, is not found in differentiated cells and is considered a marker of pluripotent stem cells.[22,51,61,62] Expression of Oct-4 has been observed in solid cancers, including colon, kidney, breast, gonadal, and brain cancers.[22,51,63] The protooncogene *Bmi-1*, a member of the Polycomb group *(PcG)* gene family, is involved with adult hematopoietic stem cell and neural stem cell self-renewal.[22,64–66] Glinsky et al. found that a conserved *Bmi-1*-driven gene expression pathway was engaged in normal adult stem cells and in 11 types of human cancers, including prostate, breast, ovarian, bladder, lung, glioma, medulloblastoma, mesothelioma, acute myeloid leukemia, mantle cell lymphoma, and lymphoma.[22,53] The ecotropic viral integration site 1 is an oncogenic transcription factor found in human and murine myeloid leukemia and has been identified in several mouse model embryonic tissues, suggesting that it plays an active role in normal mouse development.[22,34,67] It has also been found to be important in hematopoietic stem cell regulation.[22,34,68–70] *Bmi-1* and *SU(Z)12* are downstream targets of Sonic hedgehog and Wnt signaling, respectively, and provide a connection between epigenetic change regulators and developmental signaling pathways.[30]

Of the self-renewal regulators, the Polycomb family transcriptional repressor *Bmi-1* and the Wnt/β-catenin signaling pathway have been examined most closely with regard to cancer stem cell self-renewal regulation.[8,71,72] *Bmi-1* is necessary for self-renewal in adult hematopoietic stem cells and neural stem cells and is important in self-renewal of cancer stem cells.[8,65,66,73] Wnt/β-catenin signaling regulates *HOXB4* and Notch1, two important regulators of hematopoietic stem cell self-renewal.[8,74] Both the *Bmi-1* and the Wnt systems have been implicated in the regulation of metastases.[8] Brabletz et al. proposed that low-level β-catenin activation may confer self-renewal capacity, but higher level activation is required to trigger the epithelial-to-mesenchymal transition, or the dissemination process of primary tumors, essential for metastasis to occur.[8,75,76]

Future studies are needed to assess potential therapies using inhibitors acting on cancer stem cell populations, such as cyclopamine, a hedgehog signaling inhibitor; 6-bromoindirubin-3-oxime, which acts on GSK3; eisulind, an inhibitor of β-catenin signaling; and stI571/Gleevac/imatinib, a tyrosine kinase inhibitor.[30]

Clinical Implications of Cancer Stem Cells

A variety of clinical implications would arise from the continued support and advancement of the principle of cancer stem cells. Potentially, a significant reclassification of human cancers, no longer entirely based on pathologic characterization of the entire tumor, would be required, focusing instead on a method of identifying molecular signatures for altered self-renewal pathways such as *Bmi-1* and β-catenin in the cancer stem cells.[8] Another significant requirement would be the development of new therapeutic regimens targeting, and potentially eradicating, cancer stem cells, to supplement or potentially completely replace current treatments that target the tumor mass and most likely not destroying the entire cancer stem cell burden.[8] The recognition of rare cancer stem cells within the tumor mass would be a confounding factor in producing effective therapeutic regimens, as would the development of treatments that could, because the origins of cancer stem cells vary among cancers, target different cancer stem cell populations.[8]

Lung Cancer Stem Cells

Kondo et al. have identified cancer stem cells from several tumor cell lines, including C6 glioma, MCF-7 breast cancer, HeLa, and B104 neuroblastoma cell lines.[3,77]

Cancer stem cells have been identified in solid tumors such as breast cancer and pediatric brain tumors, and bronchioalveolar stem cells have been identified in normal human lung and lung tumors.[1,38,78–84] Pitt et al. observed that distal airway epithelial cells retain self-renewal capacity after pollution-derived injury, implying the presence of stem cells in the pool of neuroepithelial cells along the bronchial lining.[23,85]

Kim et al. identified bronchioalveolar stem cells that are precursors to Clara cells and type I and type II alveolar cells.[3,82] These cells show the capacity for self-renewal and in vitro differentiation. Oncogenic protein K-ras expression by these bronchioalveolar cells increases their proliferation.[3] These cells' capacity for self-renewal makes them likely to be capable of accumulating a variety of mutations and makes them candidates for non–small cell lung cancer precursor cells.[3]

Although cancer stem cells are generally considered to arise from mutated stem cells or progenitor cells of corresponding tissues, some originate from cells recruited from other tissues.[8] Bone marrow–derived mesenchymal stem cells have been suggested to give rise to gastric cancer stem cells in in vitro culture studies.[8,37] Haura hypothesized that bone marrow stem cells, recruited into the lung to respond to tobacco-induced epithelial injury, are the cancer stem cells responsible for lung cancer.[86] While this hypothesis is intriguing, the discovery of adult somatic stem cells within the lung negates the requirement that adult stem cells need to travel from the bone marrow in order for stem cell–driven repair to occur.

It has been hypothesized that the increase in lung adenocarcinomas relative to squamous cell carcinomas in about the past three decades is caused by changes in smoking behavior and cigarette design, specifically, the reduction of nicotine levels in cigarettes and the invention of efficient cigarette filters beginning about four decades ago.[87–90] Reduced nicotine in cigarettes causes smokers to increase puff frequency, volume, and/or duration.[89,91,92] The widespread use of effective cigarette filters has altered the composition of inhaled carcinogens so that particle-bound benzo(a)pyrene types have been generally replaced by gaseous nitrosamine and polyaromatic hydrocarbon types.[88,93] As a result, peripheral lung cancers have become more frequent.[92,94] As noted earlier, normal adult somatic stem cells may be found in stem cell niches, special microenvironments within which the stem cells reside.[23,24] Although the process of carcinogenesis is not fully understood, it seems that stem cells in this location already have undergone a cylindrical cell differentiation, thus provoking the development of atypical adenomatous hyperplasia, bronchiolar columnar cell dysplasia, and adenocarcinoma.[95–100] Further studies into stem cell dynamics in the lung, and their role, if any, in the development of lung cancer might lead to the development of new stem cell–targeted therapies that could improve the currently poor prognosis of lung cancer patients and potentially lead to a cure for lung cancers and even treatments to prevent lung cancer development.

References

1. Soltysova A, Altanerova V, Altaner C. Cancer stem cells. Minireview. Neoplasma 2005;52:435–440.
2. Pathak S, Multani AS. Aneuploidy, stem cells and cancer. In Bignoid LP, ed. Cancer: Cell Structures, Carcinogens, and Genomic Instability. Switzerland: Birkhauser Verlag; 2006:49–64.
3. Reyes M, Lund T, Lenvik T, et al. Purification and ex vivo expansion of postnatal marrow mesodermal progenitor cells. Blood 2001;98:2615–2625.
4. Martin GR. Isolation of a pluripotent cell line from early mouse embryos cultured in medium conditioned by teratocarcinoma stem cells. Proc Natl Acad Sci USA 1981;78:7634–7638.
5. Thomson JA, Itskovitz-Eldor J, Shapiro SS, et al. Embryonic stem cell lines derived from human blastocysts. Science 1998;282;114–117.
6. Shamblott M, Axelman J, Wang S, et al. Derivation of pluripotent stem cells from cultured human primordial germ cells. Proc Natl Acad Sci USA 1998;95:1326–1331.
7. Reubinoff BE, Pera MF, Fong CY, et al. Embryonic stem cell lines from human blastocysts: somatic differentiation in vitro. Nat Biotechnol 2000;287:399–404.
8. Guo W, Lasky JL, Wu H. Cancer stem cells. Pediatr Res 2006;59:59R–56R.
9. Dewey MJ, Martin DW, Martin GR, Mintz B. Mosaic mice with teratocarcinoma-derived mutant cells deficient in hypoxanthine phosphoribosyltransferase. Proc Natl Acad Sci USA 1977;74:5564–5568.
10. Evans MJ, Kaufman MH. Establishment in culture of pluripotential cells from mouse embryos. Nature 1981;292:154–156.
11. Martin GR. Teratocarcinomas as a model system or the study of embryogenesis and neoplasia. Cell 1975;5(3):229–243.
12. Frankel MS. In search of stem cell policy. Science 2000;287:1433–1438.
13. Snyder EY, Hinman LM, Kalichman MW. Can science resolve the ethical impasse in stem cell research? Nat Biotechnol 2006;24:397–400.
14. Vogel G. International standards proposed for stem cell work. Science 2006;313:26.
15. Pathak S. Telomeres in human cancer research. 10th All India Congress of Cytology and Genetics Award Lecture. Perspect Cytol Genet 2001;10:13–22.
16. Sherley JL. Asymmetric cell kinetics genes: the key to expansion of adult stem cells in culture. Stem Cells 2002;20:561–572.
17. Potten CS. Stem cells in gastrointestinal epithelium: numbers, characteristics and death. Philos Trans R Soc Lond B Biol Sci 1998;353:821–830.
18. Pittenger MF, Mackay AM, Beck SC, et al. Multilineage potential of adult human mesenchymal stem cells. Science 1999;284:143–147.
19. Gage FH. Mammalian neural stem cells. Science 2000;287:1433–1438.
20. Alison M, Sarraf C. Hepatic stem cells. J Hepatol 1998;29:676–682.
21. Romano G. The role of adult stem cells in carcinogenesis. Drug News Perspect 2005;18:555–559.
22. Romano G. Stem cell transplantation therapy: controversy over ethical issues and clinical relevance. Drug news Perspect 2004;17:637–645.
23. Meuwissen R, Berns A. Mouse models for human lung cancer. Genes Dev 2005;19:643–664.
24. Engelhardt JF. Stem cell niches in the mouse airway. Am J Respir Cell Mol Biol 2001;24:649–652.
25. Bonnet D, Dick JE. Human acute myeloid leukemia is organized as a hierarchy that originates from a primitive hematopoietic cell. Nat Med 1997;3:730–737.
26. Jaiswal S, Traver D, Miyamoto T, et al. Expression of BCR/ABL and BCL-2 in myeloid progenitors leads to myeloid leukemias. Proc Natl Acad Sci USA 2003;100:10002–10007.
27. Lapidot T, Sirard C, Vormoor J, et al. A cell initiating human acute myeloid leukemia after transplantation into SCID mice. Nature 1994;367:645–648.
28. Reya T, Morrison S, Clarke MF, Weissman IL. Stem cells, cancer, and cancer stem cells. Nature 2001;414:105–111.
29. Wang JCY, Dick JE. Cancer stem cells: lessons from leukemia. Trends Cell Biol 2005;15:494–501.
30. Galmozzi E, Facchetti F, La Porta CA. Cancer stem cells and therapeutic perspectives. Curr Med Chem 2006;13:603–607.
31. Guan Y, Gerhard B, Hogge DE. Detection, isolation, and stimulation of quiescent primitive leukemic progenitor cells from patients with acute myeloid leukemia (AML). Blood 2003;101:3142–3149.
32. Holyoake T, Jiang X, Eaves C, Eaves A. Isolation of a highly quiescent subpopulation of primitive leukemic cells in chronic myeloid leukemia. Blood 1999;2056–2064.
33. Berns A. Stem cells for lung cancer? Cell 2005;121:811–817.
34. Yuasa H, Oike Y, Iwama A, et al. Oncogenic transcription factor Evi1 regulates hematopoietic stem cell proliferation through GATA-2 expression. EMBO J 2005;24:1976–1987.
35. Singh SK, Clarke ID, Hide T, Dirks PB. Cancer stem cells in nervous system tumors. Oncogene 2004;23:7267–7273.
36. Singh SK, Hawkins C, Clarke ID, et al. Identification of human brain tumour initiating cells. Nature 2004;432:396–401.
37. Houghton J, Stoicov C, Nomura S, et al. Gastric cancer originating from bone marrow–derived cells. Science 2004;306:1568–1571.
38. Al-Hajj M, Wicha MS, Benito-Hernandez A, et al. Prospective identification of tumorigenic breast cancer cells. Proc Natl Acad Sci USA 2003;100:3983–3988.
39. Pardal R, Clarke MF, Morrison SJ. Applying the principles of stem-cell biology to cancer. Nat Rev Cancer 2003;3:895–902.
40. Causinus E, Gonzalez C. Induction of tumor growth by altered stem-cell asymmetric division in Drosophila melanogaster. Nat Genet 2005;37:1027–1029.

41. Nakagawara A, Ohira M. Comprehensive genomics linking between neural development and cancer: neuroblastoma as a model. Cancer Lett 2004;204:213–224.

42. Zhou S, Schuetz JD, Bunting KD, et al. The ABC transporter Bcrp1/ABCG2 is expressed in a wide variety of stem cells and is a molecular determinant of the side-population phenotype. Nat Med 2001;7:1028–1034.

43. Tu SM, Lin SH, Logothetis CJ. Stem-cell origin of metastasis and heterogeneity of solid tumours. Lancet Oncol 2002;3:508–513.

44. Miller SJ, Lavker RM, Sun TT. Interpreting epithelial cancer biology in the context of stem cells: tumor properties and therapeutic implications. Biochem Biophys Acta 2005;1756:25–52.

45. Woodward WA, Chen MS, Behbod F, Rosen JM. On mammary stem cells. J Cell Sci 2005;118:3585–3594.

46. Brickman JM, Burdon TG. Pluripotency and tumorigenicity. Nat Genet 2002;32:557–558.

47. Reya T, Clevers H. Wnt signaling in stem cells and cancer. Nature 2005;434:843–850.

48. Gregorieff A, Clevers H. Wnt signaling in the intestinal epithelium: from endoderm to cancer. Genes Dev 2005;19: 877–890.

49. Fukushima H, Yamamoto H, Itoh F, et al. Frequent alterations of the beta-catenin and TCF-4 genes, but not of the APC gene, in colon cancers with high-frequency microsatellite instability. J Exp Clin Cancer Res 2001;20:553–559.

50. Beachy PA, Karhadkar SS, Berman DM. Tissue repair and stem cell renewal in carcinogenesis. Nature 2004;432:324–331.

51. Tai MH, Chang CC, Kiupel M, et al. Oct4 expression in adult human stem cells: evidence in support of the stem cell theory of carcinogenesis. Carcinogenesis 2005;26: 495–502.

52. Lahad JP, Mills GB, Coombes KR. Stem cell-ness: a "magic marker" for cancer. J Clin Invest 2005;115:1463–1467.

53. Glinsky GV, Berezovska O, Glinskii AB. Microarray analysis identified a death-from-cancer signature predicting therapy failure in patients with multiple types of cancer. J Clin Invest 2005;115:1503–1521.

54. Austin TW, Solar GP, Ziegler FC, et al. A role for the Wnt gene family in hematopoiesis: expansion of multilineage progenitor cells. Blood 1997;89:3624–3635.

55. Bhardwaj G, Murdoch B, Wu D, et al. Sonic hedgehog induces the proliferation of primitive human hematopoietic cells via BMP regulation. Nat Immunol 2001;2: 172–180.

56. Spink KE, Polaski P, Weis WI. Structural basis of the Axin-adenomatous polyposis coli interaction. EMBO J 2000;19:2270–2279.

57. Taipale J, Beachy PA. The hedgehog and Wnt signaling pathways in cancer. Nature 2001;411:349–354.

58. Willert K, Brown JD, Danenberg E, et al. Wnt proteins are lipid-modified and can act as stem cell growth factors. Nature 2003;432:448–452.

59. Andl T, Reddy ST, Gaddapara T, Millar SE. WNT signals are required for the initiation of hair follicle development. Dev Cell 2002;2:643–653.

60. Jamora C, Dasgupta R, Kocieniewski P, Fuchs E. Links between signal transduction, transcription and adhesion in epithelial bud development. Nature 2003;422:317–322.

61. Donovan PJ. High Oct-ane fuel powers the stem cell. Nat Genet 2001;29:246–47.

62. Nichols J, Zevnik B, Anastassiadis K, et al. Formation of pluripotent stem cells in the mammalian embryo depends on the POU transcription factor Oct4. Cell 1998;95:379–91.

63. Hochedlinger K, Yamada Y, Beard C, Jaenisch R. Ectopic expression of Oct-4 blocks progenitor-cell differentiation and causes dysplasia in epithelial tissues. Cell 2005;121: 465–477.

64. Valk-Lingbeek ME, Bruggerman SW, van Lohuizen M. Stem cells and cancer; the polycomb connection. Cell 2004;118:409–418.

65. Park IK, Qian D, Kiel M, et al. Bmi-1 is required for maintenance of adult self-renewing haematopoietic stem cells. Nature 2003;425:962–967.

66. Molofsky AV, Pardal R, Iwashita T, et al. Bmi-1 dependence distinguishes neural stem cell self-renewal from progenitor proliferation. Nature 2003;425:962–967.

67. Perkins AS, Mercer JA, Jenkins NA, Copeland NG. Patterns of Evi-1 expression in embryonic and adult tissues suggest that Ev-1 plays an important regulatory role in mouse development. Development 1991;111:479–487.

68. Park LK, He Y, Lin F, et al. Differential gene expression profiling of adult murine hematopoietic stem cells. Blood 2002;99:488–498.

69. Phillips RL, Ernst RE, Brunk B, et al. The genetic program of hematopoietic stem cells. Science 2000;288:1635–1640.

70. Shimizu S, Nagasawa T, Katoh O, et al. EVI1 is expressed in megakaryocyte cell lineage and enforced expression of EVI1 in UT-7/GM cells induces megakaryocyte differentiation. Biochem Biophys Res Commun 2002;292:609–616.

71. Jamieson CH, Ailles LE, Dylla SJ, et al. Granulocyte-macrophage progenitors as candidate leukemic stem cells in blast-crisis CML. N Engl J Med 2004;351:657–667.

72. Lessard J, Sauvageau G. Bmi-1 determines the proliferative capacity of normal and leukaemic stem cells. Nature 2003;423:255–260.

73. Molofsky AV, He S, Bydon M, et al. Bmi-1 promotes neural stem cell self-renewal and neural development but not mouse growth and survival by repressing the p16Ink4a and p19Arf senescence pathways. Genes Dev 2005;19:1432–1437.

74. Reya T, Duncan AW, Ailles L, et al. A role for Wnt signaling in self-renewal from progenitor proliferation. Nature 2003;423:409–414.

75. Brabletz T, Jung A, Reu S, et al. Variable beta-catenin expression in colorectal cancers indicates tumor progression driven by the tumor environment. Proc Natl Acad Sci USA 2001;98:10356–10361.

76. Brabletz T, Jung A, Spaderna S, et al. Opinion: migrating cancer stem cells—an integrated concept of malignant tumour progression. Nat Res Cancer 2005;5:744–749.

77. Kondo T, Setoguchi T, Taga T. Persistence of a small subpopulation of cancer stem-like cells in the C6 glioma cell line. Proc Natl Acad Sci USA 2004;101:781–786.

78. Demirkazik A, Kessinger A, Lynch J, et al. Effect of prior therapy and bone marrow metastases on progenitor cell content of blood stem cell harvests in breast cancer patients. Biol Blood Marrow Transplant 2002;8:268–272.

79. Dick JE. Breast cancer stem cells revealed. Proc Natl Acad Sci USA 2003;100:3547–3549.

80. Pecora AL, Lazarus HM, Jennis AA, et al. Breast cancer cell contamination of blood stem cell products in patients with metastatic breast cancer: predictors and clinical relevance. Biol Blood marrow Transplant 2002;8:536–543.

81. Hemmati HD, Nakano I, Lazareff JA, et al. Cancerous stem cells can arise from pediatric brain tumors. Proc Natl Acad Sci USA 2003;100:15178–15183.

82. Kim CF, Jackson EL, Woolfenden AE, et al. Identification of bronchioalveolar stem cells in normal lung and lung cancer. Cell 2005;121:823–835.

83. Singh SK, Clark ID, Terasaki M, et al. Identification of a cancer stem cell in human brain tumors. Cancer Res 2003;63:5821–5828.

84. Ten Have-Opbroek AA, Benfield JR, Hammond WG, Dijkman JH. Alveolar stem cells in canine bronchial carcinogenesis. Cancer Lett 1996;101:211–217.

85. Pitt BR, Ortiz LA. Stem cells in lung biology. Am J Physiol Lung Cell Mol Physiol 2004;286:L621–L623.

86. Haura EB. Is repetitive wounding and bone marrow-derived stem cell mediated-repair an etiology of lung cancer development and dissemination? Med Hypothesis 2006;67:951–956.

87. Thun MJ, Lally CA, Flannery JT, et al. Cigarette smoking and changes in the histopathology of lung cancer. J Natl Cancer Inst 1997;89:1580–1586.

88. Cockburn MG, Wu AH, Bernstein L. Etiologic clues from the similarity of histology-specific trends in esophageal and lung cancers. Cancer Causes Contr 2005;16:1065–1074.

89. Wingo PA, Ries LAG, Giovino GA, et al. Annual report to the nation on the status of cancer, 1973–1996, with a special section on lung cancer and tobacco smoking. J Natl Cancer Inst 1999;91:675–690.

90. Levi F, Franceschi S, La Vecchia C, et al. Lung carcinoma trends by histologic type in Vaud and Neuchatel, Switzerland, 1974–1994. Cancer 1997;79:906–914.

91. National Cancer Institute. The FTC cigarette test method for determining tar, nicotine, and carbon monoxide yields of U.S. cigarettes. Report of the NCI expert committee. Smoking and Tobacco Control Monograph No. 7. Bethesda: U.S. Department of Health and Human Services, Public Health Service, National Institutes of Health, National Cancer Institute; NIH Publ No. 96-4028; 1996.

92. Brooks DR, Austin JHM, Heelan RT, et al. Influence of type of cigarette on peripheral versus central lung cancer. Cancer Epidemiol Biomarkers Prev 2005;14:576–581.

93. Popper HH. Bronchiolitis, an update. Virchows Arch 2000; 437:471–481.

94. Stellman SD, Muscat JE, Thompson S, et al. Risk of squamous cell carcinoma and adenocarcinoma of the lung in relation to lifetime filter cigarette smoking. Cancer 1997;80:382–388.

95. Ullmann R, Bongiovanni M, Halbwedl I, et al. Bronchiolar columnar cell dysplasia—genetic analysis of a novel preneoplastic lesion of peripheral lung. Virchows Arch 2003; 442:429–436.

96. Ullmann R, Bongiovanni M, Halbwedl I, et al. Is high-grade adenomatous hyperplasia an early bronchioloalveolar adenocarcinoma? J Pathol 2003;201:371–376.

97. Aoyagi Y, Yokose T, Minami Y, et al. Accumulation of losses of heterozygosity and multistep carcinogenesis in pulmonary adenocarcinoma. Cancer Res 2001;61:7950–7954.

98. Borczuk AC, Gorenstein L, Walter KL, et al. Non–small-cell lung cancer molecular signatures recapitulate lung developmental pathways. Am J Pathol 2003;163:1949–1960.

99. Copin MC, Buisine MP, Devisme L, et al. Normal respiratory mucosa, precursor lesions and lung carcinomas: differential expression of human mucin genes. Front Biosci 2001;6:D1264–D1275.

100. Mori M, Rao SK, Popper HH, et al. Atypical adenomatous hyperplasia of the lung: a probable forerunner in the development of adenocarcinoma of the lung. Mod Pathol 2001;14:72–84.

21
Gene Therapy Approaches for Lung Cancer

Jack A. Roth

Introduction

Lung cancers exhibit multiple genetic lesions that can be detected even in histologically normal bronchial mucosa from individuals with a smoking history. These genetic abnormalities provide an array of targets for therapy. Tobacco smoke has over 100 carcinogenic agents, and the specific interactions of specific carcinogens with genes that suppress tumors and repair DNA have been identified.[1] Dysfunctional tumor suppressor genes are the most common genetic lesions identified to date in human lung cancers. Functional copies of tumor suppressor genes can be introduced into cancer cells by gene transfer.

The *p53* tumor suppressor gene appears to play a central role in lung cancer development and was the initial focus of gene therapy approaches to lung cancer. This approach has been extensively studied in the clinic with intratumoral injection of a replication-defective adenovirus that expresses *p53* (Adp53). Overexpression of *p53* in cancer cells induces growth arrest and apoptosis. Injections of Adp53 have an excellent safety profile and have mediated tumor regression and growth arrest as monotherapy or have overcome resistance or increased the effectiveness of radiation therapy and chemotherapy. Expression of the *p53* transgene has occurred at high levels and is associated with activation of other genes in the p53 pathway. These studies indicate proof-of-principle for tumor suppressor gene therapy and represent a new paradigm in targeted therapy.

Mechanism of *p53* Tumor Suppression and Rationale for *p53* Gene Therapy

Expression of some gene products, including growth factors, oncogenes, cyclins, and cyclin-dependent kinases (Cdks) stimulate cell proliferation. Expression of tumor suppressor genes and other inhibitors of Cdks induce cell cycle arrest, thus limiting the cell proliferation. Two interconnected pathways, the retinoblastoma (Rb) pathway and the p53 pathway, which are both, in turn, regulated at the protein level by oncogenes and other tumor suppressor genes, contribute to the regulation of cell proliferation. The Rb protein regulates maintenance of, and release from, the G1 phase. The p53 protein monitors cellular stress and DNA damage, either causing growth arrest to facilitate DNA repair or inducing apoptosis if DNA damage is extensive.[2] When a cell is stressed by oncogene activation, hypoxia, or DNA damage, an intact p53 pathway may determine whether the cell will receive a signal to halt at the G1 stage of the cell cycle, whether DNA repair will be attempted, or whether the cell will self-destruct via apoptosis.

The *p53* gene is central in the processes of apoptosis, DNA repair following various cell stresses, and regulation of the cell cycle. Apoptosis plays a key role in numerous normal cellular mechanisms, from embryogenesis to DNA damage control due to random mutations, ionizing radiation, and DNA damaging chemicals, and has more recently been implicated as a major mechanism of cell death due to DNA-damaging cancer therapies such as chemotherapy and radiation. The observation that expression of a wild-type *p53* gene in a cancer cell triggers apoptosis was the seminal observation that lead to *p53* gene therapy approaches.[3] Prior to this it was thought that gene therapy could not replace all the damaged genes in a cancer cell and thus would not have an effect. The requirement for restoring only one of the defective genes to trigger apoptosis suggests that the DNA damage present in the cancer cell may prime it for an apoptotic event that can be activated through a single pathway.

The major functional role for the *p53* gene product is that of a transcription factor.[4] A group of genes whose expression is in part regulated by *p53* are the apoptosis genes. The balance between two proapoptotic versus pro-survival (antiapoptotic) signals, often compared to a rheostat, determines whether or not apoptosis will be induced. While these signals determine *p53*'s actions, expression of many of the genes that generate these critical signals is, in turn, regulated by the activation status of *p53*, forming a complex feedback loop. *p53* carries out its housekeeping duties by downregulating the "prosurvival" (or antiapoptotic) genes, including the antiapoptotic genes *Bcl-2* and *Bcl-xL* and upregulating the proapoptotic genes *Bax*, *Bad*, *Bid*, *Puma*, and *Noxa*.[5] Available transcripts of each of the pro- and antiapoptotic genes with *Bcl-2* homology-3 domains interact with one another to form heterodimers, and the relative ratio of proapoptotic to prosurvival proteins in these heterodimers determines activity of the resulting molecule, thereby determining whether the cell lives or dies. *p53* also targets the death-receptor signaling pathway, including DR5, and Fas/CD/95, the apoptosis machinery including caspase-6, Apaf-1, and PIDD, and may directly mediate cytochrome c release. Thus apoptosis is an important mechanism by which *p53* mediates its tumor suppressor function.

The p53 pathway is regulated at the protein level by other tumor suppressor genes and by several oncogenes.[2] For example, *MDM2* normally binds to the N-terminal transactivating domain of p53, prohibiting p53 activation and leading to its rapid degradation. Under normal conditions the half-life of p53 is only 20 min. In the event of genotoxic stress, resulting DNA damage causes phosphorylation of serines on p53, weakening binding to *MDM2* and destabilizing the p53/*MDM2* interaction and prolonging p53 half-life. The resulting increase in p53 DNA binding activity leads to an array of downstream signals that switch other genes on or off. In the normal cell, *MDM2* is inhibited by expression of *p14^ARF*, a tumor suppressor gene encoded by the same gene locus as *p16^INK4a* but read in an alternate reading frame.[6] Deletion or mutation of the tumor suppressor gene *p14^ARF*, which has been noted in some cancers, results in increased levels of *MDM2* and subsequent inactivation of p53, resulting in inappropriate progression through the cell cycle. The expression of *p14^ARF* is induced by hyperproliferative signals from oncogenes such as *ras* and *Myc*, thus indicating an important role for p53 in protecting the cell from oncogene activation. Importantly, p53 also plays a central role in mediating cell cycle arrest. This function is significant as prolonged tumor stability has often been observed in clinical trials of *p53* gene replacement, suggesting that this effect is predominate in some tumors over apoptosis. p53 is involved in regulating cell cycle checkpoints, and p53 expression can promote cell senescence through its control of cell cycle effectors such as *p21^Cip1/WAF1*.

Loss of function in the p53 pathway is the most common alteration identified in human cancer to date. About 50% of common epithelial cancers have *p53* mutations.[7–9] In some cancers, loss of *p53* also appears to be linked to resistance to conventional DNA damaging therapies that require functional cellular apoptosis to accomplish cell death.

Preclinical Studies of *p53* Gene Replacement

The studies described suggest that expressing a wild-type *p53* gene in cancer cells defective in *p53* function could mediate either apoptosis or cell growth arrest. Both results could be a therapeutic benefit in a cancer patient. Our initial studies showed that restoration of functional *p53* suppressed the growth of some, but not all, human lung cancer cell lines.[10] Because of limitations inherent in the use of retroviruses, subsequent studies of *p53* gene replacement in lung cancer made use of an adenoviral vector (Adp53).[11] The first published study of *p53* gene therapy showed suppression of tumor growth in an orthotopic human lung cancer model using a retroviral expression vector.[12]

Adp53 also induced apoptosis in cancer cells with defective *p53* function without significantly affecting normal cells.[13] Adp53 mediated inhibition of tumor growth in a mouse model of human orthotopic lung cancer[14] and induced apoptosis and suppression of proliferation in various other cancer cell lines.[15–18]

Although it was first thought that the inability to transduce every cell in a tumor might limit the effectiveness of gene therapy for cancer, studies[3,19] of three-dimensional cancer cell matrices and subcutaneous xenografts proved that therapeutic genes could penetrate beyond the injection site to nontransduced tumor cells and cause cell death via a "bystander effect." Bystander killing, now known to be an important phenomenon in the success of gene therapy, appears to involve regulation of angiogenesis,[20,21] immune upregulation,[22–24] and secretion of soluble proapoptotic proteins.[25]

Clinical Trials of *p53* Gene Replacement

The first clinical trial protocol for *p53* gene replacement was carried out with a retroviral vector expressing wild-type *p53* under control of a β-actin promoter.[26] The retroviral vector was injected into tumors of nine patients with unresectable non–small cell lung cancer (NSCLC) that had progressed on chemotherapy. Three of the nine patients demonstrated evidence of antitumor activity with no vector-related toxicity, demonstrating for the first time the feasibility and safety of *p53* gene therapy.[27,28]

In a phase I trial of 28 NSCLC patients whose cancers had progressed with conventional treatments, successful gene transfer using Adp53 was shown in 80% of evaluable patients.[29] Gene expression was detected in 46%, apoptosis was demonstrated in all but one of the patients expressing the gene, and no significant toxicity was observed. Greater than 50% reduction in tumor size was observed in two patients, with one patient remaining free of tumor more than a year after concluding therapy and another having a nearly complete regression of a chemotherapy and radiotherapy resistant upper lobe endobronchial tumor.

Gene Replacement in Combination with Conventional DNA-Damaging Agents in Non–Small Cell Lung Cancer

Many tumors are resistant to chemotherapy and radiation therapy and, therefore, progress after initial treatment. *p53*, often missing or nonfunctional in radiation- and chemotherapy-resistant tumors, is known to play a key role in detecting damage to DNA and either directing repair or inducing apoptosis. Once apoptosis was implicated as a mechanism of cell killing in response to these DNA-damaging agents, it followed that a defect in the normal apoptotic pathway might confer resistance to some tumor cells. Because of Adp53's low toxicity (less than a 5% incidence of serious adverse events) in initial trials, therapeutic strategies combining Adp53 gene replacement and conventional DNA-damaging therapies were logical extensions of earlier studies.[30]

Preclinical Studies

The fact that overexpression of *p53* in wild-type *p53* transfected cell lines could induce apoptosis in cancer cells was shown in several studies in vitro.[31–33] Subsequent studies that examined apoptosis in tumor cells treated with radiation or chemotherapeutic agents supported a link between apoptosis induction and functional *p53* expression.[34–39] Preclinical studies of *p53* gene therapy combined with cisplatin in cultured NSCLC cells and in human xenografts in nude mice showed that sequential administration of cisplatin and *p53* gene therapy resulted in enhanced expression of the *p53* gene product,[37,40] and similar studies of Adp53 gene transfer combined with radiotherapy indicated that delivery of Adp53 increased the sensitivity of *p53*-deficient tumor cells to radiation.[15]

Numerous additional studies have generated additional supporting evidence for a critical link between radiation sensitivity and the ability of a cell to induce apoptosis.[41–45] However, the radiosensitivity of some tumor types, for example, epithelioid tumors, does not appear to be correlated with *p53* status.[46–48]

Clinical Trials of Tumor Suppressor Gene Replacement Combined with Chemotherapy

Twenty-four NSCLC patients with tumors previously unresponsive to conventional treatment were enrolled in a phase I trial of *p53* combined with cisplatin.[49] Seventy-five percent of the patients had previously experienced tumor progression on cisplatin- or carboplatin-containing regimens. Up to six monthly courses of intravenous cisplatin, each followed 3 days later with intratumoral injection of Adp53, resulted in 17 patients remaining stable for at least 2 months, two patients achieving partial responses, four patients continuing to exhibit progressive disease, and one patient unevaluable because of progressive disease. Seventy-nine percent of tumor biopsy specimens showed an increase in number of apoptotic cells, 7% demonstrated a decrease in apoptosis, and 14% indicated no change.

A phase II clinical trial evaluated two comparable metastatic lesions in each NSCLC patient enrolled in the study.[50] All patients received chemotherapy, either three cycles of carboplatin plus paclitaxel or three cycles of cisplatin plus vinorelbine, and then Adp53 was injected directly into one lesion. Adp53 treatment resulted in minimal vector-related toxicity and no overall increase in chemotherapy-related adverse events. Detailed statistical analysis of the data indicated that patients receiving carboplatin plus paclitaxel, the combination of drugs providing the greatest benefit on its own, did not realize additional benefit from Adp53 gene transfer; however, patients treated with the less successful cisplatin and vinorelbine regimen experienced significantly greater mean local tumor regression, as measured by size, in the Adp53-injected lesion compared with the control lesion.

Clinical Trials of *p53* Gene Replacement Combined with Radiation Therapy

Preclinical studies suggesting that *p53* gene replacement may increase radiation sensitivity to some tumors[15,41,43–45] led to a phase II clinical trial of *p53* gene transfer combined with radiation therapy.[51] Nineteen patients with localized NSCLC were treated, with a complete response in 1 patient (5%), partial response in 11 patients (58%), stable disease in 3 patients (16%), and progressive disease in 2 patients (11%), while two patients (11%) were unevaluable because of tumor progression or early death. Three months following completion of therapy, biopsy specimens revealed no viable tumor in 12 patients (63%) and viable tumor in 3 (16%). Tumors of four patients (21%) were not biopsied because of tumor progression, early death, or weakness. The 1-year progression-free survival rate was 45.5%. Among 13 evaluable patients after 1 year, 5 (39%) had a complete response and 3 (23%) had a partial response or disease stabilization. Most treatment failures were caused by metastatic disease, not by local progression.

In this study, pre- and posttreatment biopsies of the tumor were performed for studies of gene expression. Adp53 vector-specific DNA was detected in biopsy specimens from 9 of 12 patients with paired biopsies (day 18 and day 19). The ratio of copies of Adp53 vector DNA to copies of actin DNA was 0.15 or higher in 8 of 9 patients (range, 0.05–3.85), with 4 patients having a ratio >0.5. For 11 patients with adequate samples for both vector DNA and mRNA analysis, 8 showed a postinjection increase in mRNA expression associated with detectable vector DNA. Postinjection increases in *p53* mRNA were detected in 11 of 12 paired biopsies obtained 24 hr after Adp53 injection, with 10 of 11 increasing threefold or greater. Preinjection biopsies that were negative for p53 protein expression by immunohistochemistry were stained for p53 protein expression after Adp53 injection. Staining results confirmed that the p53 protein was expressed in the posttreatment samples in the nuclei of cancer cells. Previous in vitro experiments in human NSCLC cell lines identified four genes (*p21* [*CDKN1A*], *MDM2*, *Fas*, and *Bak*) that showed the greatest increase in mRNA expression after induction of *p53* overexpression with Adp53. Therefore, in the current study, changes in mRNA levels for these four markers were determined at various time points before and during treatment using reverse transcriptase real-time polymerase chain reaction. The study was controlled by obtaining a pretreatment biopsy sample under the same conditions as the posttreatment biopsy sample. The inclusion of a time point during the radiation treatment allowed for a biopsy to be performed immediately before and 24 hr after Adp53 injection, thus allowing determination of the effects of the Adp53 on mRNA expression during treatment. For *p21* (*CDKN1A*) mRNA, increases of statistical significance were noted 24 hr after Adp53 injection and during treatment compared with the pretreatment biopsy. In the case of *MDM2* mRNA, increases were noted during treatment compared with the pretreatment biopsy. Levels of *Fas* mRNA did not show statistically significant changes during treatment. *Bak* mRNA expression increased significantly 24 hr after injection of Adp53, and thus Bak

appeared to be the protein most acutely upregulated by Adp53 injection.

Recently the first randomized clinical trial of *p53* gene therapy was reported. Ninety patients with squamous cell carcinoma of the head and neck were randomly allocated to receive intratumoral injection of Adp53 (10^{12} VP/dose/week for a total of 8 weeks) in combination with radiation therapy (70 GY/8 weeks) or radiation therapy alone. Complete remission was seen in 64.7% of patients receiving Adp53 combined with radiation therapy compared with 20% of patients receiving radiation therapy alone, which was highly significant statistically.[52]

Systemic Gene Therapy

Local control of cancers is important, but most patients with lung cancer die from systemic metastases. Thus gene delivery to distant sites of cancer is essential if cancer gene therapy is going to have an impact on survival. Recently, nanoscale synthetic particles that can encapsulate plasmid DNA and deliver it to cells after intravenous injections have been developed. This has been studied in mouse xenograft models of disseminated human lung cancer with delivery of *p53* and other tumor suppressor genes. Multiple *3p21.3* genes show different degrees of tumor suppressor function in various human cancers in vitro and in preclinical animal models. One of the tumor suppressor genes at this locus is *FUS1* which is not expressed in most lung cancers. When wild-type *FUS1* is expressed in a lung cancer cell, apoptosis occurs. To translate these findings to clinical applications for molecular cancer therapy, we recently developed a systemic treatment strategy by using a novel *FUS1*-expressing plasmid vector complexed with DOTAP:cholesterol (DOTAP:Chol) liposome, termed FUS1 nanoparticle, for treating lung cancer and lung metastases.[53,54] In a preclinical trial, we showed that intratumoral injection of FUS1 nanoparticles into subcutaneous NSCLC H1299 and A549 lung tumor xenografts resulted in significant inhibition of tumor growth. Intravenous injections of FUS1 nanoparticles into mice bearing experimental A549 lung metastasis caused a decrease in the number of metastatic tumor nodules. Treating lung tumor–bearing animals with DOTAP:Chol–FUS1 complexes resulted in prolonged survival (median survival time, 80 days) compared with control animals. These results demonstrate that the *FUS1* gene is a promising therapeutic agent for treatment of primary and disseminated human lung cancer.[53,54] Based on these studies, a phase I clinical trial with *FUS1*-mediated molecular therapy by systemic administration of FUS1 nanoparticles is now underway in stage IV lung cancer patients at the University of Texas M. D. Anderson Cancer Center in Houston, Texas.

Conclusion

Current cancer treatment, including radiation and chemotherapy, controls less than 50% of lung cancers, with an overall 5-year survival rate of approximately 15%. Combining existing treatments has reached a plateau of efficacy, and the addition of conventional cytoxic agents is limited because of toxicity. The clinical trials summarized in this chapter clearly demonstrate that, contrary to initial predictions that single gene therapy would not be effective for cancer because of multiple genetic lesions, gene replacement therapy targeted to a tumor suppressor gene can cause cancer regression by activation of multiple apoptotic and growth inhibitory pathways with minimal toxicity.

Gene expression has been documented and occurs even in the presence of an antiadenovirus immune response, clinical trials have demonstrated that direct intratumor injection can cause tumor regression or prolonged stabilization of local disease, and the low toxicity associated with gene transfer indicates that tumor suppressor gene replacement can be readily combined with existing and future treatments. Studies combining transfer of tumor suppressor genes in combination with conventional DNA-damaging treatments indicate that correction of a defect in apoptosis induction can restore sensitivity to radiation and chemotherapy in some resistant tumors, and indications that sensitivity to killing might be enhanced in already sensitive tumors may eventually lead to reduced toxicity from chemotherapy and radiation therapy from reduced doses. The most recent data from the laboratory showing damage to tumor suppressor genes in normal tissue and premalignant lesions even suggests that this treatment strategy may someday be useful in early intervention and even prevention of cancer. Preclinical studies have shown that systemic delivery can treat disseminated metastases. The ready availability of gene libraries, the ability to administer the genes without the extensive reformulation required of small molecules, and their specificity makes this an attractive therapeutic approach. Despite the obvious promise evident in the results of these studies though, it is critical to recognize that there are still gaps in knowledge and technology to address. The major issues for the future development of gene therapy include the following:

1. Developing more efficient and less toxic gene delivery vectors for systemic gene delivery
2. Identifying the optimal genes for various tumor types
3. Optimizing combination therapy
4. Monitoring gene uptake and expression by cancer cells
5. Overcoming resistance pathways

However, given the rapid progress in the field, it is likely that many of these technological problems will be solved in the near future.

References

1. Denissenko MF, Pao A, Tang M, et al. Preferential formation of benzo[a]pyrene adducts at lung cancer mutational hotspots in p53. Science 1996;274(5286):430–432.
2. Burns T, El-Deiry W. The p53 pathway and apoptosis. J Cell Physiol 1999;181:231–239.
3. Fujiwara T, Grimm EA, Mukhopadhyay T, et al. A retroviral wild-type p53 expression vector penetrates human lung cancer spheroids and inhibits growth by inducing apoptosis. Cancer Res 1993;53(18):4129–4133.
4. Raycroft L, Wu H, Lozano G. Transcriptional activation by wild-type but not transforming mutants of the p53 antioncogene. Science 1990;249:1049–1051.
5. Adams JM, Cory S. The Bcl-2 protein family: arbiters of cell survival. Science 1998;281(5381):1322–1326.
6. Kamijo T, Zindy F, Roussel MF, et al. Tumor suppression at the mouse INK4a locus mediated by the alternative reading frame product p19ARF. Cell 1997;91(5):649–659.
7. Isobe T, Hiyama K, Yoshida Y, et al. Prognostic significance of p53 and ras gene abnormalities in lung adenocarcinoma patients with stage I disease after curative resection. Jpn J Cancer Res 1994;85:1240–1246.
8. Quinlan DC, Davidson AG, Summers CL, et al. Accumulation of p53 protein correlates with a poor prognosis in human lung cancer. Cancer Res 1992;52:4828–4831.
9. Martin HM, Filipe MI, Morris RW, et al. p53 expression and prognosis in gastric carcinoma. Int J Cancer 1992;50(6):859–862.
10. Cai DW, Mukhopadhyay T, Roth JA. A novel ribozyme for modification of mutated p53 pre-mRNA in non–small cell lung cancer cell lines. 3rd Antisense Workshop, November 13, 1993.
11. Zhang WW, Fang X, Mazur W, et al. High-efficiency gene transfer and high-level expression of wild-type p53 in human lung cancer cells mediated by recombinant adenovirus. Cancer Gene Ther 1994;1(1):5–13.
12. Fujiwara T, Cai DW, Georges RN, et al. Therapeutic effect of a retroviral wild-type p53 expression vector in an orthotopic lung cancer model [commentary]. J Natl Cancer Inst 1994;86(19):1437–1438.
13. Wang JX, Bucana CD, Roth JA, et al. Apoptosis induced in human osteosarcoma cells is one of the mechanisms for the cytocidal effect of Ad5CMV-p53. Cancer Gene Ther 1995;2(1):9–17.
14. Georges RN, Mukhopadhyay T, Zhang Y, et al. Prevention of orthotopic human lung cancer growth by intratracheal instillation of a retroviral antisense K-ras construct. Cancer Res 1993;53(8):1743–1746.
15. Spitz FR, Nguyen D, Skibber J, et al. Adenoviral mediated p53 gene therapy enhances radiation sensitivity of colorectal cancer cell lines. Proc Am Assoc Cancer Res 1996;37:347.
16. Nielsen LL, Dell J, Maxwell E, et al. Efficacy of p53 adenovirus-mediated gene therapy against human breast cancer xenografts. Cancer Gene Ther 1997;4(2):129–138.
17. Bouvet M, Fang B, Ekmekcioglu S, et al. Suppression of the immune response to an adenovirus vector and enhancement of intratumoral transgene expression by low-dose etoposide. Gene Ther 1998;5:189–195.

18. Xu M, Kumar D, Srinivas S, et al. Parenteral gene therapy with p53 inhibits human breast tumors in vivo through a bystander mechanism without evidence of toxicity. Hum Gene Ther 1997;8:177–185.

19. Cusack JC, Spitz FR, Nguyen D, et al. High levels of gene transduction in human lung tumors following intralesional injection of recombinant adenovirus. Cancer Gene Ther 1996;3(4):245–249.

20. Miyashita T, Reed JC. Tumor suppressor p53 is a direct transcriptional activator of human bax gene. Cell 1995;80(2): 293–299.

21. Dameron KM, Volpert OV, Tainsky MA, et al. Control of angiogenesis in fibroblasts by p53 regulation of thrombospondin-1. Science 1994;265:1582–1584.

22. Molinier-Frenkel V, Le Boulaire C, Le Gal FA, et al. Longitudinal follow-up of cellular and humoral immunity induced by recombinant adenovirus-mediated gene therapy in cancer patients. Human Gene Ther 2000;11(13):1911–1920.

23. Yen N, Ioannides CG, Xu K, et al. Cellular and humoral immune responses to adenovirus and p53 protein antigens in patients following intratumor injection of an adenovirus vector expressing wild-type p53 (Ad-p53). Cancer Gene Ther 2000;7(4):530–536.

24. Carroll JL, Nielsen LL, Pruett SB, et al. The role of natural killer cells in adenovirus-mediated p53 gene therapy. Mol Cancer Ther 2001;1:49–60.

25. Owen-Schaub LB, Zhang W, Cusack JC, et al. Wild-type human p53 and a temperature-sensitive mutant induce Fas/APO-1 expression. Mol Cell Biol 1995;15(6):3032–3040.

26. Roth JA, Nguyen D, Lawrence DD, et al. Retrovirus-mediated wild-type p53 gene transfer to tumors of patients with lung cancer. Nat Med 1996;2(9):985–991.

27. Roth JA. Clinical Protocol: Modification of mutant K-ras gene expression in non–small cell lung cancer (NSCLC). Hum Gene Ther 1996;7(7):875–889.

28. Roth JA. Clinical Protocol: Modification of tumor suppressor gene expression and induction of apoptosis in non–small cell lung cancer (NSCLC) with an adenovirus vector expressing wildtype p53 and cisplatin. Hum Gene Ther 1996;7(8):1013–1030.

29. Swisher SG, Roth JA, Nemunaitis J, et al. Adenovirus-mediated p53 gene transfer in advanced non-small cell lung cancer. J Natl Cancer Inst 1999;91(9):763–771.

30. Yver A, Dreiling LK, Mohanty S, et al. Tolerance and safety of RPR/INGN 201, an adeno-viral vector containing a p53 gene, administered intratumorally in 309 patients with advanced cancer enrolled in phase I and II studies worldwide. Proc Am Soc Clin Oncol 1999;19:460a.

31. Yonish-Rouach E, Resnitzky D, Lotem J, et al. Wild-type p53 induces apoptosis of myeloid leukemic cells that is inhibited by interleukin-6. Nature 1991;352(6333):345–347.

32. Ramqvist T, Magnusson KP, Wang Y, et al. Wild-type p53 induces apoptosis in a Burkitt lymphoma (BL) line that carries mutant p53. Oncogene 1993;8:1495–1500.

33. Shaw P, Bovey R, Tardy S, et al. Induction of apoptosis by wild-type p53 in a human colon tumor-derived cell line. Proc Natl Acad Sci USA 1992;89(10):4495–4499.

34. Dewey WC, Ling CC, Meyn RE. Radiation induced apoptosis: relevance to radiotherapy. Int J Radiat Oncol Biol Phys 1995;33:781–796.

35. Roth JA. Review: Clinical protocol for modification of tumor suppressor gene expression and induction of apoptosis in non-small cell lung cancer (NSCLC) with an adenovirus vector expressing wildtype p53 and cisplatin. Hum Gene Ther 1995;6(2):252–255.

36. Meyn RE, Stephens LC, Hunter NR, et al. Apoptosis in murine tumors treated with chemotherapy agents. Anticancer Drugs 1997;6:443–450.

37. Fujiwara T, Grimm EA, Mukhopadhyay T, et al. Induction of chemosensitivity in human cancer cells in vivo by adenovirus-mediated transfer of the wild-type p53 gene. Surgical Forum 1994;45:524–526.

38. Nguyen DM, Spitz FR, Yen N, et al. Gene therapy for lung cancer: enhancement of tumor suppression by a combination of sequential systemic cisplatin and adenovirus-mediated p53 gene transfer. J Thorac Cardiovasc Surg 1996;112(5):1372–1377.

39. Hamada M, Fujiwara T, Hizuta A, et al. The p53 gene is a potent determinant of chemosensitivity and radiosensitivity in gastric and colorectal cancers. J Cancer Res Clin Oncol 1996;122(6):360–365.

40. Nguyen D, Spitz F, Kataoka M, et al. Enhancement of gene transduction in human carcinoma cells by DNA-damaging agents. Proc Am Assoc Cancer Res 1996;37:347.

41. Jasty R, Lu J, Irwin T, et al. Role of p53 in the regulation of irradiation-induced apoptosis in neuroblastoma cells. Mol Genet Metab 1998;65(2):155–164.

42. Akimoto T, Hunter NR, Buchmiller L, et al. Inverse relationship between epidermal growth factor receptor expression and radiocurability of murine carcinomas. Clin Cancer Res 1999;5(10):2884–2890.

43. Feinmesser M, Halpern M, Fenig E, et al. Expression of the apoptosis-related oncogenes bcl-2, bax, and p53 in Merkel cell carcinoma: can they predict treatment response and clinical outcome? Hum Pathol 1994;30(11):1367–1372.

44. Broaddus WC, Liu Y, Steele LL, et al. Enhanced radiosensitivity of malignant glioma cells after adenoviral p53 transduction. J Neurosurg 1999;91(6):997–1004.

45. Sakakura C, Sweeney EA, Shirahama T, et al. Overexpression of bax sensitizes human breast cancer MCF-7 cells to radiation-induced apoptosis. Int J Cancer 1996;67(1):101–105.

46. Brachman DG, Becket M, Graves D, et al. p53 mutation does not correlate with radiosensitivity in 24 head and neck cancer cells lines. Cancer Res 1993;53:3667–3669.

47. Slichenmyer WJ, Nelson WG, Slebos RJ, et al. Loss of a p53-associated G1 checkpoint does not decrease cell survival following DNA damage. Cancer Res 1993;53:4164–4168.

48. Danielsen T, Smith-Sorensen B, Gronlund HA, et al. No association between radiosensitivity and TP53 status, G(1) arrest or protein levels of p53, myc, ras or raf in human melanoma lines. Int J Radiat Biol 1994;75(9):1149–1160.

49. Nemunaitis J, Swisher SG, Timmons T, et al. Adenovirus-mediated p53 gene transfer in sequence with cisplatin to

tumors of patients with non–small-cell lung cancer. J Clin Oncol 2000;18(3):609–622.

50. Schuler M, Herrmann R, De Greve JL, et al. Adenovirus-mediated wild-type p53 gene transfer in patients receiving chemotherapy for advanced non–small-cell lung cancer: results of a multicenter phase II study. J Clin Oncol 2001;19(6):1750–1758.

51. Swisher S, Roth JA, Komaki R, et al. A phase II trial of adenoviral mediated p53 gene transfer (RPR/INGN 201) in conjunction with radiation therapy in patients with localized non–small cell lung cancer (NSCLC). Am Soc Clin Oncol 2000;19:461a.

52. Peng Z, Han D, Zhang S, et al. Clinical evaluation of safety and efficacy of intratumoral administration of a recombinant adenoviral-p53 anticancer agent (Genkaxin®). Mol Ther 2003;7:422–423.

53. Ito I, Ji L, Tanaka F, et al. Liposomal vector mediated delivery of the 3p FUS1 gene demonstrates potent antitumor activity against human lung cancer in vivo. Cancer Gene Ther 2004;11:733–739.

54. Uno F, Sasaki J, Nishizaki M, et al. Myristoylation of the FUS1 protein is required for tumor suppression in human lung cancer cells. Cancer Res 2004;64(9):2969–2976.

22
Response to Conventional Therapy and Targeted Molecular Therapy

Timothy Craig Allen, Anna Sienko, and Philip T. Cagle

Traditional Therapy

Currently, the standard chemotherapy regimen for non–small cell lung cancer (NSCLC) involves platinum-based anticancer drugs such as cisplatin, which functions by the formation of bulky platinum DNA adducts, along with a third-generation agent such as paclitaxel, gemcitabine, vinorelbine, or irinotecan.[1–4] Nonplatinum agents such as docetaxel, a taxane that functions by disrupting microtubule dynamics via β-tubulin binding, are also frequently used to treat NSCLC patients.[4,5] Vinorelbine, a vinca alkaloid, have also been used with some success in treating NSCLC patients.[1] The benefits of these standard systemic chemotherapeutic agents is limited for patients with advanced NSCLC, with half of those patients exhibiting an 8- to 11-month median survival despite cisplatin-based therapy.[2,6] Along with troubling cisplatin toxicity, the development of cisplatin resistance has become a serious concern.[1,3]

Future progress in NSCLC treatment may occur with the introduction of biologic agents that target highly specific intracellular pathways.[7] Specific genetic aberrations arising in NSCLC that are associated with chemotherapy response may be useful in the development of targeted therapy ("tailored therapy;" "customized therapy") for individual NSCLC patients.[2,7,8]

Predictors of Response to Traditional Therapy

Messenger RNA transcripts found in DNA repair pathways, including breast cancer protein 1 (BRCA1) and excision repair cross-complementing group 1 (ERCC1), bestow selective resistance to chemotherapeutic agents such as cisplatin and taxanes.[9] Low levels of BRCA1, a member of the ATM (mutated in ataxia telangiectasia) pathway for DNA damage repair during the cell cycle, has been shown to correlate with increased chemotherapy benefit for NSCLC patients with locally advanced disease receiving neoadjuvant gemcitabine/cisplatin chemotherapy.[10]

Thioredoxin-1 (TRX-1) overexpression activates hypoxia-inducible factor-1 (HIF-1), which in turn activates cyclooxygenase-2 (COX-2), causing increased vascular endothelial growth factor (VEGF).[11] Increased TRX-1 protects cells from apoptosis by inhibiting apoptosis signal-regulating kinase 1 and by activating nuclear factor-κB, causing resistance by chemotherapeutic agents such as cisplatin.[11]

The *ERCC1* gene, a part of the nucleotide excision repair pathway, is necessary for the repair of cisplatin DNA adducts in NSCLC treatment, and ERCC1 is a predictor of cisplatin sensitivity.[12] Low levels of ERCC1 have been associated with improved cisplatin response, thought to be due to decreased repair of platinum DNA adducts, and may be associated with improved survival in NSCLC patients.[12–15]

The 14-3-3 proteins bind many functionally diverse signaling proteins and help control the cell cycle and regulate apoptosis.[16] One 14-3-3 protein, 14-3-3σ, is associated with G2 cell cycle checkpoint control in response to DNA damage, and its methylation has been found to be an independent prognostic marker in NSCLC patients undergoing platinum-based chemotherapy.[16–18] De Las Penas et al. noted that, in NSCLC patients treated with cisplatin/gemcitabine, impaired DNA repair may correlate with better prognosis.[19] The authors studied the association of genetic polymorphisms in x-ray repair cross-complementing group 1 and group 3 (XRCC3) with survival and found XRCC3 241 MetMet to correlate favorably with survival in NSCLC patients given a cisplatin/gemcitabine regimen.[19]

Targeted Therapies

The generally late stage presentation and overall poor prognosis of NSCLC, along with the limited value of standard chemotherapeutic regimens, has prompted increased examination of molecular targeted therapies for NSCLC.[20] With its wide molecular heterogeneity, NSCLC has received extensive examination.[21] Agents that block epidermal growth factor receptor (EGFR) and inhibit angiogenesis are being studied intensely.[20] Some of these agents have shown improved treatment outcomes and improved response rates for patients with NSCLC, and their use, either alone or with standard chemotherapy regimens, may provide improved quality of life and increased survival for NSCLC patients.[20,21]

Epidermal Growth Factor Receptor-Targeted Therapies

Epidermal growth factor receptor is a receptor tyrosine kinase involved with cell proliferation, differentiation, migration, and cell survival.[22] It is upstream of several important targets, including COX-2, cyclin D1, phosphatidylinositol-3 kinase, and signal transducers and activators of transcription 3.[23] Its expression is associated with a poor prognosis in a variety of cancers.[7] Epidermal growth factor receptor is expressed in 80%–90% of NSCLC and is overexpressed in 45%–70%.[7,24,25] From 57% to 92% of squamous cell NSCLCs overexpress EGFR.[7,24,25] Molecular pathways involving EGFR that may be targeted for prognostic benefit have been intensely investigated in a large number of cancers, including NSCLC.[21] Epidermal growth factor receptor mutations in NSCLC patients have been shown to be associated with female sex, adenocarcinoma bronchoalveolar histology, and never-smokers.[26–29] Several anti-EGFR therapies have been studied, but currently two types predominate—tyrosine kinase inhibitors and monoclonal antibodies.[30] Several EGFR-targeted monoclonal antibodies and tyrosine kinase inhibitors have undergone clinical trials in NSCLC with advanced disease.[31]

Monoclonal Antibodies

The monoclonal antibody cetuximab (IMC-225; Erbitux), a chimeric human–mouse monoclonal immunoglobin (Ig)G1 antibody, blocks ligand binding, downstream signaling, and functional activation of the EGFR.[32–35] Cetuximab binds competitively to the extracellular domain of EGFR and prevents tyrosine kinase activation, leading to inhibited cell growth and, in some cases, apoptosis.[30,36] Its targeting of the extracellular domain allows it to block EGFR pathways in a highly specific manner.[37] It inhibits cell growth and, in some cases, induces apoptosis.[30] It is

generally well tolerated and is being studied in combination with chemotherapeutic agents in NSCLC patients.[30,38,39] Early studies show response rates with cetuximab of 29%–53% in untreated NSCLC patients with metastatic disease and a response rate of 28% in refractory or recurrent NSCLC patients given a combination of cetuximab and docetaxel.[40] Thienelt et al. studied 31 stage IV NSCLC patients treated with cetuximab along with paclitaxel and carboplatin in a phase I/II study and noted that response rate, time of progression, and median survival were slightly better than for historical controls of patients treated only with the paclitaxel/carboplatin regimen.[41] Robert et al. examined 35 chemotherapy-naive NSCLC patients with advanced disease treated with cetuximab along with gemcitabine and carboplatin in a phase I/IIa study and found 28.6% exhibited a partial response to therapy.[42] The authors noted that the combination was well tolerated.[42] Cetuximab/chemotherapy activity in patients who had previously progressed on the same therapeutic regimen suggests that some patients may have the ability to overcome resistance.[43]

Tyrosine Kinase Inhibitors

Tyrosine kinase inhibitors target the intracellular domain of EGFR in order to block signal transduction and inhibit the downstream effects of EGFR ligand binding.[7] These agents cause tumor regression by increasing apoptosis and inhibiting cell proliferation and angiogenesis.[30] Gefitinib and erlotinib are two selective tyrosine kinase inhibitors approved for treatment of advanced NSCLC.[44,45] These orally administered agents specifically act by competing with adenosine triphosphate (ATP) for the EGFR ATP binding site.[44] The characteristics associated with the presence of EGFR mutations in NSCLC—female sex, adenocarcinoma and bronchoalveolar histology, and never-smoking—are significantly related to tyrosine kinase receptor response in NSCLC.[26,46–49] About 10% of Caucasian and 25%–30% of Japanese NSCLC patients treated with them have shown objective responses.[44] Patients with NSCLC have shown responses to them even after proving to be refractory to conventional chemotherapy.[49] Another benefit of these drugs is that patient response is not substantially affected by the number of previous chemotherapy regimens, in contrast to traditional chemotherapy in which response rates decrease with each chemotherapy regimen used.[49]

Gefitinib (ZD1839), a specific inhibitor of EGFR tyrosine kinase, downregulates EGFR autophosphorylation and prevents its activation.[50] It was the first EGFR inhibitor to receive FDA approval.[21] In two large phase II trials (IDEAL 1 and 2), gefitinib was well tolerated and showed a modest overall response rate of 10%–20% with improved disease symptoms in about 40%; however, in two large Phase III trials (INTACT 1 and 2), gefitinib and platinum-based chemotherapy did not show a prognostic benefit compared with chemotherapy alone.[47,48,51–53] In the INTACT 1 study, Giaccone et al. examined 1,093 chemotherapy-naive NSCLC patients receiving a cisplatin/gemcitabine regimen alone or in association with gefitinib.[52] The authors found no significant difference in median survival times between the groups.[52] Herbst et al., in the INTACT 2 study, investigated 1,037 NSCLC patients receiving a paclitaxel/carboplatin regimen with or without gefitinib and found that gefitinib provided no additional benefit regarding survival, time to progression, or response rate.[53] Thatcher et al. studied 1,692 NSCLC patients and noted increased survival in never-smokers compared with smokers and in Asian patients compared with non-Asian patients.[51,54] Gefitinib benefit may therefore be limited in NSCLC patients, although studies using higher doses may be useful.[55]

Erlotinib, another EGFR inhibitor, inhibits EGFR phosphorylation and also interferes with signaling via the variant receptor EGFRvIII.[30] It induces cell cycle arrest in G1 and apoptosis.[30] It inhibits EGFR phosphorylation with a more than 1,000 times greater selectivity than other tyrosine kinase inhibitors.[30] Shepherd et al., in a phase III trial of NSCLC patients who had been treated with one or two previous chemotherapy regimens, found significantly improved overall survival and progression-free survival in patients treated with erlotinib compared with patients treated with placebo.[4,56] Symptomatic improvement and quality-of-life improvement were also associated with erlotinib treatment in the trial.[4,56]

Genes in the ErbB family encode receptor tyrosine kinases that mediate growth signal responses, and mutations in the tyrosine kinase domains of two ErbB genes, EGFR and HER2, occur in some lung adenocarcinomas. Lung adenocarcinomas may also contain mutations in downstream GTPases encoded by ras genes, with 15%–30% containing K-ras mutations.[57] EGFR and K-ras mutations are usually not identified in the same tumors, and, in contrast to fact that EGFR mutations are typically found in never-smokers, K-ras mutations generally are found in NSCLC patients with significant smoking histories.[57] Pao et al. examined 60 lung adenocarcinomas to determine whether K-ras mutations correlate with EGFR inhibitor (gefitinib or erlotinib) response and found that K-ras mutations correlated with lack of tumor cell sensitivity to either agent.[57] EGFR mutations are identified in 71%–100% of tumors responsive to tyrosine kinase inhibitors, and negative tumor testing for EGFR mutations does not preclude tyrosine kinase inhibitor treatment.[57] Identification of K-ras mutations might therefore be used to predict individual patient response to gefitinib or erlotinib—lung adenocarcinoma patients with K-ras mutations might not respond favorably to either tyrosine kinase inhibitor.[57]

The EGFR family includes HER2/neu (ErbB2), HER3 (ErbB3), and HER4 (ErbB4).[26] These receptors' roles in tumor proliferation make them potentially strong therapeutic targets.[26] The NSCLC response to tyrosine kinase inhibitors is associated with increased EGFR copy number, high EGFR protein expression, and/or specific EGFR mutations.[26] Cappuzzo et al., examining 102 NSCLC patients treated with gefitinib, found that EGFR-positive (as determined by fluorescence in situ hybridization) NSCLC patients who exhibit increased copy numbers of the HER2 gene had a better response rate, better disease control rate, longer time to progression, and improved survival.[26] The use of HER2 agents along with tyrosine kinase inhibitors should be investigated in future trials in order to evaluate any potential complementary therapeutic benefit from their use in NSCLC patients.

Antiangiogenesis Therapy

Neovascularization from preexisting blood vessels, termed angiogenesis, is generally required for NSCLC progression, and angiogenesis blockade is expected to prevent tumor cell growth and improve prognosis.[58] Angiogenesis regulation is complex and is controlled by a variety of angiogenesis-related molecules, including VEGF, a potent molecule that promotes tumor progression.[58] Bevacizumab (Avastin), an anti-VEGF antibody, has been shown to provide a significant prognostic benefit with tolerable toxicity when used in combination with standard first-line chemotherapeutic agents.[58] Bevacizumab is a recombinant humanized monoclonal antibody that blocks binding to the VEGF receptor (VEGFR)[59,60] and blocks the effects of VEGF.[60] Phase I trials showed it to be fairly well tolerated and without dose-limiting toxicity[61,62]; however, later trials showed serious bleeding risks with its use.[63] A Phase II trial with 99 patients with advanced NSCLC by Johnson et al. showed a modest survival benefit and suggested an increased time to progression in patients receiving bevacizumab and chemotherapy compared with patients receiving chemotherapy alone.[60,61] In that trial, there was a higher incidence of severe tumor-related bleeding in NSCLC patients with squamous histology and central tumors.[58] A phase III trial of 878 NSCC patients showed a significant prognostic benefit in patients receiving bevacizumab along with standard chemotherapy (12.5 months) compared with patients receiving standard chemotherapy alone (10.2 months).[58,63] The NSCLC patients receiving bevacizumab also had a significantly greater response rate (27%) compared with patients receiving only standard chemotherapy (10%) and had a significantly longer progression-free survival time (6.4 months vs. 4.5 months).[58,63,64] The trial patients had generally tolerable toxicity; however, a higher incidence of bleeding, including fatal bleeding, was identified in patients receiving bevacizumab.[58,63]

Other agents show potential use as antiangiogenesis agents in NSCLC patients. Early trials with the anti-EGFR drug erlotinib showed well-tolerated therapy with NSCLC activity, and preclinical studies with the anti-EGFR drug gefitinib showed it to induce apoptosis in *EGFR*-overexpressing tumor cells and to inhibit epithelial growth factor–induced angiogenesis.[58,65] Further randomized trials are needed to confirm and clarify the antiangiogenic effect of these EGFR inhibitors.[58] Other potential antiangiogenic agents, including the small-molecule receptor tyrosine kinase inhibitors sorafenib, AG-013736, sunitinib, and ZD6474, have been examined, some in phase I and phase II trials.[58,64,66–69] Their mode of action is via inhibition of VEGF receptor tyrosine kinase activity.[58,64]

Other Potential Targeted Therapies

Trastuzumab

Trastuzumab (Herceptin), a monoclonal antibody against HER2, is used to treat breast cancer.[70] Its effectiveness depends on immunohistochemically demonstrable high HER2 expression, which occurs uncommonly in NSCLC.[70,71] Lara et al., in a Phase II trial including 69 NSCLC patients, found disappointing results and closed the study to further accrual.[72] Other trials have found similar disappointing results.[73–75]

Pertuzumab

Pertuzumab is a humanized monoclonal antibody against the dimerization domain of HER2 and is the first in a new class of targeted therapeutic agents known as HER dimerization inhibitors.[76,77] Preclinical studies have shown it to inhibit breast, prostate, and NSCLC cell lines whether or not the cell lines overexpress HER2.[78] Friess et al. showed markedly inhibited serum tumor markers, correlating with decreased tumor volume, for NSCLC and breast cancer in human xenograft models with treatment with both pertuzumab and erlotinib.[76] Phase I and II clinical trials are in progress.[78]

Farnesyltransferase Inhibitor Sch66336

The nonpeptide farnesyltransferase inhibitor SCH66336, with other receptor tyrosine kinase inhibitors, inhibits NSCLC cell growth.[79] It possibly acts by decreasing hypoxia- or IGF-stimulated HIF-1α expression, thereby inhibiting angiogenic activity in NSCLC cells, and by inhibiting HIF-1α and heat shock protein 90 interaction, causing proteasomal degradation of HIF-1α.[79] Further investigation of SCH66336 regulation of HIF-1α is merited.

Retinoids and Rexinoids

Retinoids are natural and synthetic derivatives of vitamin A that act through nuclear retinoid receptors to activate target genes that signal biologic effects.[23,80] Retinoid effects are mediated through nuclear retinoid acid receptors and retinoid X receptors, each with three subtypes—α, β, and γ—that are downregulated in lung tumorigenesis.[23,81] Retinoids assist in regulating cell division, growth, differentiation, and proliferation and, while potentially useful for targeted therapy, have been associated with relatively harsh side effects, including skin reactions, severe headache, and hypertriglyceridemia.[82] Rexinoids are synthetic drugs that bind specifically to retinoid X receptors.[82] One of the rexinoids, bexarotene (Targretin), has been evaluated in phase I and II trials in NSCLC patients and found to be well tolerated alone and in combination with chemotherapy.[80,82,83] Hypertriglyceridemia and hypothyroidism occur but are generally manageable.[82] Studies have shown a survival benefit and phase III trials are ongoing.[82]

Antimethylation

Promoter hypermethylation of tumor suppressor genes occur frequently in cancers, and in NSCLC hypermethylation is an early event associated with tobacco carcinogen exposure.[84] Hypermethylation and deactivation occur frequently with p16, E-cadherin, and retinoic acid receptor-β, among other genes.[84] Two azanucleosides, decitabine and its ribonucleoside analog 5-azacytidine, inhibit methylation and have been shown in vitro to reactivate tumor suppressor genes and retard NSCLC in mouse models.[84] Its effect is amplified when it is combined with pharmacologic inactivation of histone acetylation by histone deacetylase inhibitors.[84] Future studies to evaluate appropriate dosage are required.[84]

Small Cell Lung Carcinoma

Small cell lung carcinoma (SCLC) is characterized by autocrine growth mechanisms, including stem cell factor and its receptor, c-Kit.[85,86] Imatinib mesylate (ST1571) is a tyrosine kinase inhibitor that selectively inhibits the ABL family, platelet-derived growth factor receptor, and Kit kinases.[86] In vitro treatment of small cell lung carcinoma with imatinib inhibits Kit activation, and imatinib induces growth inhibition in SCLC cell lines.[86] In a phase II study, Dy et al. studied 29 SCLC patients treated with imatinib and found that it did not show any clinical activity.[87] This was so even though patients were selected for c-Kit expression by their SCLCs.[87] Clinical trials of imatinib alone in SCLC patients have not shown any significant prognostic benefit.[88] Yokoyama et al. found inhibition of cell growth in SCLC cell lines that were treated with imatinib along with vitamin K2.[88] Maulik et al. noted that imatinib does not directly inhibit topoisomerase I and remarks that the combination of imatinib and topoisomerase I inhibition might provide therapeutic benefit for SCLC patients.[89] Further studies are needed to identify any prognostic benefits of combining imatinib with other therapies for patients with SCLC.

Conclusion

Conventional chemotherapy is currently of limited value in improving long-term survival of lung cancer patients. Expressions of DNA repair proteins may serve as predictors of individual response to conventional chemotherapy. Targeted molecular therapies, including kinase inhibitors and receptor antibodies, hold promise as cancer-specific therapies, alone or in combination with conventional therapies, but are limited to subpopulations of patients whose cancers possess the appropriate targets for these therapies.

References

 1. Pujol JL, Barlesi F, Daures JP. Should chemotherapy combinations for advanced non-small cell lung cancer be platinum-based? A meta-analysis of phase III randomized trials. Lung Cancer 2006;51:335–345.
 2. Rosell R, Cobo M, Isla D, et al. Applications of genomics in NSCLC. Lung Cancer 2005;2:S33–S40.
 3. Wang G, Reed E, Li QQ. Molecular basis of cellular responses to cisplatin chemotherapy in non-small cell lung cancer. Oncol Rep 2004;12:955–965.
 4. Silvestri GA, Rivera MP. Targeted therapy for the treatment of advanced non-small cell lung cancer. A review of the epidermal growth factor receptor antagonists. Chest 2005;128:3975–3984.
 5. Fanucchi M, Khuri FR. Taxanes in the treatment of non-small cell lung cancer. Treat Respir Med 2006;5:181–191.
 6. Belani CP. Optimizing chemotherapy for advanced non-small cell lung cancer: focus on docetaxel. Lung Cancer 2005;50:S3–S8.
 7. Rosell R, Fossella F, Milas L. Molecular markers and targeted therapy with novel agents: prospects in the treatment of non–small cell lung cancer. Lung Cancer 2002;38:S43–S49.
 8. Rosell R, Cecere F, Santarpia M, et al. Predicting the outcome of chemotherapy for lung cancer. Curr Opin Pharmacol 2006;6:1–9.
 9. Santarpia M, Altavilla G, Salazar F, et al. From the bench to the bed: individualizing treatment in non–small-cell lung cancer. Clin Transl Oncol 2006;8:71–76.
10. Taron M, Rosell R, Felip E, et al. BRCA1 mRNA expression levels as an indicator of chemoresistance in lung cancer. Hum Mol Genet 2004;13:2443–2449.
11. Csiki I, Yanagisawa K, Haruki N, et al. Thioredoxin-1 modulates transcription of cyclooxygenase-2 via hypoxia-inducible factor-1α in non-small cell lung cancer, Cancer Res 2006;66:143–150.
12. Seve P, Dumontet C. Chemoresistance in non–small cell lung cancer. Curr Med Chem Anticancer Agents 2005;5:73–88.
13. Garcia-Campelo R, Alonso-Curbera G, Anton Aparicio LM, Rosell R. Pharmacogenomics in lung cancer: an analysis of DNA repair gene expression in patients treated with platinum-based chemotherapy. Expert Opin Pharmacother 2005;6:2015–2026.
14. Simon GR, Sharma S, Cantor A, et al. Polymorphisms in ERCC1 and grade 3 or 4 toxicity in non–small cell lung cancer patients. Clin Cancer Res 2005;11:1534–1538.
15. Wachters FM, Wong LS, Timens W, et al. ERCC1, hRad51, and BRCA1 protein expression in relation to tumour response and survival of stage III/IV NSCLC patients treated with chemotherapy. Lung Cancer 2005;50:211–219.
16. Ramirez JL, Rosell R, Taron M, et al. 14-3-3s methylation in pretreatment serum circulating DNA of cisplatin-plus-gemcitabine-treated advanced non–small-cell lung cancer patients predicts survival: the Spanish lung cancer group. J Clin Oncol 2005;23:9105–9112.
17. Chan TA, Hermeking H, Lengauer C, et al. 14-3-3σ is required to prevent mitotic catastrophe after DNA damage. Nature 1999;401:616–620.
18. Osada H, Tatematsu Y, Yatabe Y, et al. Frequent and histological type-specific inactivation of 14-3-3σ in human lung cancers. Oncogene 2002;21:2418–2424.
19. de las Penas R, Sanchez-Ronco M, Alberola V, et al. Polymorphisms in DNA repair genes modulate survival in cisplatin/gemcitabine-treated non–small-cell lung cancer patients. Ann Oncol 2006;17:668–675.
20. Massarelli E, Herbst RS. Use of novel second-line targeted therapies in non–small cell lung cancer. Semin Oncol 2006;33:S9–S16.
21. Ramalingam S, Belani CP. Molecularly-targeted therapies for non–small cell lung cancer. Expert Opin Pharmacother 2005;6:2667–2679.
22. Lee SM. Is EGFR expression important in non-small cell lung cancer? Thorax 2006;66:98–99.
23. Hirsch FR, Lippman SM. Advances in the biology of lung cancer chemoprevention. J Clin Oncol 2005;23:3186–3197.
24. Rusch V, Klimstra D, Venkatraman E, et al. Overexpression of the epidermal growth factor receptor and its ligand transforming growth factor alpha is frequent in resectable non–small cell lung cancer but does not predict tumor progression. Clin Cancer Res 1997;3:515–522.
25. Fontanini G, Vignati S, Boldrini L, et al. Vascular endothelial growth factor is associated with neovascularization and influences progression of non-small cell lung carcinoma. Clin Cancer Res 1997;3:861–865.
26. Cappuzzo F, Varella-Garcia M, Shigematsu H, el al. Increased HER2 gene copy number is associated with response to gefitinib therapy in epidermal growth factor receptor-positive non–small-cell lung cancer patients, J Clin Oncol 2005;23:5007–5018.
27. Shigematsu H, Lin L, Takahashi T, et al. Clinical and biological features associated with epidermal growth factor receptor gene mutations in lung cancers. J Natl Cancer Inst 2005;97:339–346.

28. Pao W, Miller V, Zakowski M, et al. EGF receptor gene mutations are common in lung cancers from "never smokers" and are associated with sensitivity of tumors to gefitinib and erlotinib. Proc Natl Acad Sci USA 2004; 101:13306–13311.

29. Paez JG, Janne PA, Lee JC, et al. EGFR mutations in lung cancer: correlation with clinical response to gefitinib therapy. Science 2004;304:1497–1500.

30. Sridhar SS, Seymour L, Shepherd FA. Inhibitors of epidermal-growth-factor receptors: a review of clinical research with a focus on non–small-cell cancer. Lancet Oncol 2003;4: 397–406.

31. Raben D, Helfrich B, Chan DC, et al. The effects of cetuximab alone and in combination with radiation and/or chemotherapy in lung cancer. Clin Cancer Res 2005;11: 795–805.

32. Ciardiello F, De Vita F, Orditura M, et al. Epidermal growth factor receptor tyrosine kinase inhibitors in late stage clinical trials. Expert Opin Emerg Drugs 2003;8:501–514.

33. Ji H, Li D, Chen L, et al. The impact of human EGFR kinase domain mutations on lung tumorigenesis and in vivo sensitivity to EGFR-targeted therapies. Cancer Cell 2006;9: 485–495.

34. Humblet Y. Cetuximab: an IgG(1) monoclonal antibody for the treatment of epidermal growth factor receptor-expressing tumours. Expert Opin Pharmacother 2004;5: 1621–1633.

35. Harding J, Burtness B. Cetuximab: an epidermal growth factor receptor chimeric human–murine monoclonal antibody. Drugs Today (Barc) 2005;41:107–127.

36. Herbst RS, Langer CJ. Epidermal growth factor receptors as a target for cancer treatment: the emerging role of IMC-C225 in the treatment of lung and head and neck cancers. Semin Oncol 2002;29:S27–S36.

37. Kim ES, Vokes EE, Kies MS. Cetuximab in cancers of the lung and head and neck. Semin Oncol 2004;31:S61–S67.

38. Khalil MY, Grandis JR, Shin DM. Targeting epidermal growth factor receptor: novel therapeutics in the management of cancer. Expert Rev Anticancer Ther 2003;3:367–380.

39. Buter J, Giaccone G. EGFR inhibitors in lung cancer. Oncology (Williston Park) 2005;19:1667–1668.

40. Govindan R. Cetuximab in advanced non-small cell lung cancer. Clin Cancer Res 2004;10:S4241–S4244.

41. Thienelt CD, Bunn PA, Hanna N, et al. Multicenter phase I/II study of cetuximab with paclitaxel and carboplatin in untreated patients with stage IV non–small-cell lung cancer. J Clin Oncol 2005;23:8786–8793.

42. Robert F, Blumenschein G, Herbst RS, et al. Phase I/IIa study of cetuximab with gemcitabine plus carboplatin in patients with chemotherapy-naive advanced non–small-cell lung cancer. J Clin Oncol 2005;23:9089–9096.

43. Vokes EE, Chu E. Anti-EGFR therapies: clinical experience in colorectal, lung, and head and neck cancers. Oncology (Williston Park) 2006;20:S15–S25.

44. Giaccone G, Rodriguez JA. EGFR inhibitors: what have we learned from the treatment of lung cancer? Nat Clin Pract Oncol 2005;2:554–561.

45. Govindan R, Natale R, Wade J, et al. Efficacy and safety of gefitinib in chemonaive patients with advanced non-small cell lung cancer treated in an Expanded Access Program. Lung Cancer 2006; [Epub ahead of print]

46. Miller VA, Kris MG, Shah N, et al. Bronchioloalveolar pathologic subtype and smoking history predict sensitivity to gefitinib in advanced non–small-cell lung cancer. J Clin Oncol 2004;22:1103–1109.

47. Kris MG, Natale RB, Herbst RS, et al. Efficacy of gefitinib, an inhibitor of the epidermal growth factor receptor tyrosine kinase, in symptomatic patients with non-small cell lung cancer: a randomized trial. JAMA 2003;290:2149–2158.

48. Fukuoka M, Yano S, Giaccone G, et al. Multi-institutional randomized phase II trial of gefitinib for previously treated patients with advanced non–small-cell lung cancer (The IDEAL 1 Trial). J Clin Oncol 2003;21:2237–2246.

49. Amann J, Kalyankrishna S, Massion PP, et al. Aberrant epidermal growth factor receptor signaling and enhanced sensitivity to EGFR inhibitors in lung cancer. Cancer Res 2005;65:226–235.

50. Han SW, Kim TY, Hwang PG, et al. Predictive and prognostic impact of epidermal growth factor receptor mutation in non–small-cell lung cancer patients treated with gefitinib. J Clin Oncol 2005;23:2493–2501.

51. Maione P, Gridelli C, Troiani T, Ciardiello F. Combining targeted therapies and drugs with multiple targets in the treatment of NSCLC. Oncologist 2006;11:274–284.

52. Giaccone G, Herbst RS, Manegold C, et al. Gefitinib in combination with gemcitabine and cisplatin in advanced non–small-cell lung cancer: a phase III trial—INTACT 1. J Clin Oncol 2004;22:777–784.

53. Herbst RS, Giaccone G, Schiller JH, et al. Gefitinib in combination with paclitaxel and carboplatin in advanced non–small-cell lung cancer: a phase III trial—INTACT 2. J Clin Oncol 2004;22:785–994.

54. Thatcher N, Chang A, Parikh P, et al. Gefitinib plus best supportive care in previously treated patients with refractory advanced non–small-cell lung cancer: results from a randomized, placebo-controlled, muticentre study (Iressa Survival Evaluation in Lung Cancer). Lancet 2005;366: 1527–1537.

55. Lynch T, Kim E. Optimizing chemotherapy and targeted agent combinations in NSCLC. Lung Cancer 2005;50: S25–S32.

56. Shepherd FA, Rodriguez Pereira J, Ciuleanu T, et al. Erlotinib in previously treated non–small-cell lung cancer. N Engl J Med 2005;353:123–132.

57. Pao W, Wang TY, Riely GJ, et al. KRAS mutations and primary resistance of lung adenocarcinomas to gefitinib or erlotinib. PLoS Med 2005;2:e17.

58. Yano S, Matsumori Y, Ikuta K, et al. Current status and perspective of angiogenesis and antivascular therapeutic strategy: non–small cell lung cancer. Int J Clin Oncol 2006;11:73–81.

59. Lyseng-Williamson KA, Robinson DM. Spotlight on bevacizumab in advanced colorectal cancer, breast cancer, and non–small cell lung cancer. BioDrugs 2006;20:193–195.

60. Midgley R, Kerr D. Bevacizumab—current status and future directions. Ann Oncol 2005;16:999–1004.

61. Johnson DH, Fehrenbacher L, Novotny WF, et al. Randomized phase II trial comparing bevacizumab plus carboplatin

and paclitaxel with carboplatin and paclitaxel alone in previously untreated locally advanced or metastatic non–small-cell lung cancer. J Clin Oncol 2004;22:2184–2191.

62. Sandler AB, Johnson DH, Herbst RS. Anti-vascular endothelial growth factor monoclonals in non-small cell lung cancer. Clin Cancer Res 2004;10:S4258–S4262.

63. Belvedere O, Grossi F. Lung cancer highlights from ASCO 2005. Oncologist 2006;11:39–50.

64. de Castro G, Puglisi F, de Azambuja E, et al. Angiogenesis and cancer: a cross-talk between basic science and clinical trials (the "do ut des" paradigm). Crit Rev Oncol Hematol 2006;59:40–50.

65. Herbst RS, Johnson DH, Mininberg E, et al. A. Phase I/II trial evaluating the anti-vascular endothelial growth factor monoclonal antibody bevacizumab in combination with the HER-1/epidermal growth factor receptor tyrosine kinase inhibitor erlotinib for patients with recurrent non–small-cell lung cancer. J Clin Oncol 2005;23:2544–2555.

66. Morgensztern D, Govindan R. Clinical trials of antiangiogenic therapy in non–small cell lung cancer: focus on bevacizumab and ZD6474. Expert Rev Anticancer Ther 2006;6:545–551.

67. Lee D, Heymach JV. Emerging antiangiogenic agents in lung cancer. Clin Lung Cancer 2006;7:304–308.

68. Wakelee HA, Schiller JH. Targeting angiogenesis with vascular endothelial growth factor receptor small-molecule inhibitors: novel agents with potential in lung cancer. Clin Lung Cancer 2005;7:S31–S38.

69. Cascone T, Troiani T, Morelli MP, et al. Antiangiogenic drugs in non–small cell lung cancer treatment. Curr Opin Oncol 2006;18:151–155.

70. Krawczyk P, Chocholska S, Milanowski J. Anti-HER therapeutic agents in the treatment of non–small-cell lung cancer. Ann Univ Mariae Curie Sklodowska [Med] 2003;8:113–117.

71. Heinmoller P, Gross C, Beyser K, et al. HER2 status in non–small cell lung cancer: results from patient screening for enrollment to a phase II study of herceptin. Clin Cancer Res 2003;9:5238–5243.

72. Lara PN Jr, Laptalo L, Longmate J, et al. Trastuzumab plus docetaxel in HER2/neu-positive non–small-cell lung cancer: a California Cancer Consortium screening and phase II trial. Clin Lung Cancer 2004;5:231–236.

73. Hirsch FR, Langer CJ. The role of HER2/neu expression and trastuzumab in non–small cell lung cancer. Semin Oncol 2004;31:S75–S82.

74. Clamon G, Herndon J, Kern J, et al. Lack of trastuzumab activity in nonsmall cell lung carcinoma with overexpression of erb-B2: 39810: a phase II trial of Cancer and Leukemia Group B. Cancer 2005;103:1670–1675.

75. Gatzemeier U, Groth G, Butts C, et al. Randomized phase II trial of gemcitabine-cisplatin with or without trastuzumab

in HER2-positive non–small-cell lung cancer. Ann Oncol 2004;15:19–27.

76. Friess T, Scheuer W, Hasmann M. Combination treatment with erlotinib and pertuzumab against human tumor xenografts is superior to monotherapy. Clin Cancer Res 2005; 11:5300–5309.

77. Franklin MC, Carey KD, Vajdos FF, et al. Insights into ErbB signaling from the structure of the ErbB2–pertuzumab complex. Cancer Cell 2004;5:317–328.

78. Bianco AR. Targeting c-erbB2 and other receptors of the c-erbB family: rationale and clinical applications. J Chemother 2004;16:52–54.

79. Han JY, Oh SH, Morgillo F, et al. Hypoxia-inducible factor 1alpha and antiangiogenic activity of farnesyltransferase inhibitor SCH66336 in human aerodigestive tract cancer. J Natl Cancer Inst 2005;97:1272–1286.

80. Dragnev KH, Petty WJ, Ma Y, et al. Nonclassical retinoids and lung carcinogenesis. Clin Lung Cancer 2005;6:237–244.

81. Brabender J, Metzger R, Salonga D, et al. Comprehensive expression analysis of retinoic acid receptors and retinoid X receptors in non–small cell lung cancer: implications for tumor development and prognosis. Carcinogenesis 2005;26:525–530.

82. Rigas JR, Dragnev KH. Emerging role of rexinoids in non–small cell lung cancer: focus on bexarotene. Oncologist 2005;10:22–33.

83. Nandan, R. Promising results achieved with a combination of chemotherapy and two retinoids in patients with advanced non–small-cell lung cancer. Lung Cancer 2006;51:387–388.

84. Digel W, Lubbert M. DNA methylation disturbances as novel therapeutic target in lung cancer: preclinical and clinical results. Crit Rev Oncol Hematol 2005;55:1–11.

85. Wang WL, Healy ME, Sattler M, et al. Growth inhibition and modulation of kinase pathways of small cell lung cancer cell lines by the novel tyrosine kinase inhibitor STI 571. Oncogene 2000;19:3521–3528.

86. Johnson FM, Krug LM, Tran HT, et al. Phase I studies of imatinib mesylate combined with cisplatin and irinotecan in patients with small cell lung carcinoma. Cancer 2000;106:366–374.

87. Dy GK, Miller AA, Mandrekar SJ, et al. A phase II trial of imatinib (ST1571) in patients with c-kit expressing relapsed small-cell lung cancer: a CALGB and NCCTG study. Ann Oncol 2005;16:1811–1816.

88. Yokoyama T, Miyazawa K, Yoshida T, Ohyashiki K. Combination of vitamin K2 plus imatinib mesylate enhances induction of apoptosis in small cell lung cancer cell lines. Int J Oncol 2005;26:33–40.

89. Maulik G, Bharti A, Khan E, et al. Modulation of c-Kit/SCF pathway leads to alterations in topoisomerase-I activity in small cell clung cancer. J Environ Pathol Toxicol Oncol 2004;23:237–251.

23
Environmental Agents in Lung and Pleural Neoplasms

Steven R. Blumen and Brooke T. Mossman

Introduction

A number of chemical and other environmental pollutants, including noxious gases and metals, infectious agents, insoluble agents such as asbestos and wood dusts, and dietary factors, induce or promote lung cancers. Many of these agents are classified as "known" or "reasonably anticipated" carcinogens, including polycyclic aromatic hydrocarbons, metals such as cadmium, hexavalent chromium, and nickel compounds, and mineral fibers such as asbestos and erionite.[1] Others are "suspect" carcinogens based on inconclusive data from epidemiologic, animal, and mechanistic studies. The use of mechanistic studies to predict carcinogenicity of environmental and occupational agents in humans has been advocated recently as a critical component of risk analysis.[2] With the evolution and vast potential of new technologies such as microarray analysis and proteomics, our knowledge of the mechanisms of lung carcinogenesis has increased.

Because of the complexity of air pollution and cigarette smoke, as well as the long latency period necessary for development of lung neoplasms, it is naive to exclusively link the causation and development of lung cancers to a single compound. However, asbestos, a family of durable naturally occurring fibers, is clearly associated in epidemiologic studies with the development of lung cancers and malignant mesotheliomas, devastating tumors arising from serosal or mesothelial cells of the pleura, peritoneum, or pericardium.[3–5] Asbestos also can act additively or synergistically with components of cigarette smoke to cause increases in lung cancers[3,4] and may interact cooperatively with Simian virus 40 (SV40) in the causation of malignant mesothelioma.[5–7] In this chapter, we first review principles and mechanisms of action of environmental and occupational carcinogens in lung. We then focus on properties and mechanisms of action of asbestos fibers in the pathogenesis of lung cancers and mesotheliomas.

Mechanisms of Action of Environmental Carcinogens

Carcinogenesis is a multistep process that traditionally has been delineated into three phases: initiation, promotion, and progression. These phases in relationship to the sequential stages of epithelial alterations occurring during the development of lung carcinomas are illustrated in Figure 23.1.

Initiation is broadly defined as a heritable DNA alteration occurring from a genetic change caused by a carcinogen, and it is clear that a number of occupational and environmental agents cause mutations in genes that control DNA synthesis and repair, cell cycle regulation, and cell death. Some lung carcinogens, such as polycyclic aromatic hydrocarbons, must be metabolically activated by epithelial cells to form covalent adducts with DNA, whereas other agents such as metals and asbestos fibers may act primarily through epigenetic mechanisms whereby they do not directly alter DNA but modify the expression of genes that influence cell proliferation and cell death.

Epigenetic agents have been classically referred to as tumor *promoters*, which increase proliferation of *initiated*, that is, *preoplastic*, cells by a broad range of mechanisms, including changes in DNA methylation, stimulation of cell signaling pathways, elicitation of oxidative stress, and alteration of cell communication.[8] A rapidly dividing cell is more prone to subsequent genetic insults via ineffective DNA repair, and many genetic alterations occur in cells before they progress to invasive tumor cells, phenomena occurring over the long latency period of tumor development.[8]

Progression is broadly defined as the last phase of tumor development when cells acquire many genetic alterations, including activation of additional protooncogenes and/or inactivation of tumor suppressor genes. Critical protooncogenes and tumor suppressor genes

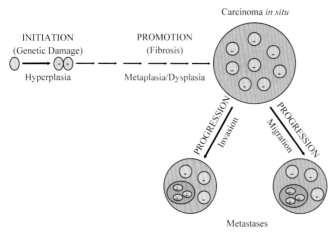

FIGURE 23.1. The stages of carcinogenesis in relation to the development of lung carcinomas. Genetic damage causes initiation of epithelial cells that subsequently undergo hyperplasia and become progressively more atypical during the process of tumor promotion. Lung fibrosis may be a promoting factor, causing a favorable environment for tumor development. During the progression phase of tumor development, additional mutations develop that may be critical to invasion, migration, and, eventually, tumor metastases.

have been elucidated in experimental models of lung cancers[9] and malignant mesothelioma.[10] However, their importance in the development of human tumors remains an open question, because not all tumors express consistent mutations in widely studied tumor suppressor genes (e.g., *p53*).

Asbestos: A Unique Carcinogen

Properties of Asbestos

Asbestos refers to a family of naturally occurring fibrous minerals, of which there are six distinct types: chrysotile ($Mg_3Si_2O_5[OH]_4$), the only member of the serpentine group, a curly and pliable fiber, and amosite, ($[Fe^{+2}]_2[Fe^{+2},Mg]_5Si_8O_{22}[OH]_2$), crocidolite ($[Fe^{+2}]_2[Fe^{+2},Mg]_5Si_8O_{22}[OH]_2$), anthophyllite ($Mg_7Si_8O_{22}[OH]_2$), tremolite ($Ca_2Mg_5Si_8O_{22}[OH]_2$), and actinolite ($Ca_2[Mg,Fe^{+2}]Si_8O_{22}[OH]_2$), all members of the amphibole family, which are more durable needle-like fibers (Figure 23.2). The increased durability of amphibole types of asbestos[11] and reactive properties of these fibers, including generation of reactive oxygen species (ROS),[12] have been linked to

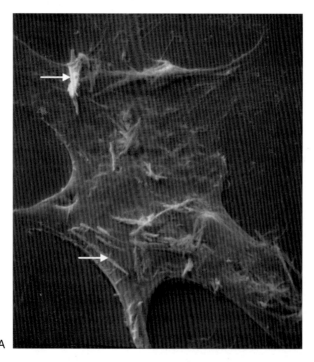
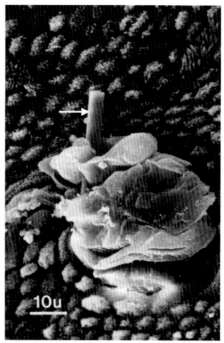

FIGURE 23.2. Scanning electron micrographs indicating the different morphologies and cell responses to chrysotile and amphibole types of asbestos. **(A)** Clumps of chrysotile fibrils (upper arrow) on the surface of a lung epithelial cell in culture. The lower arrow shows a fiber detected intracellularly. **(B)** Development of squamous metaplasia on the surface of a tracheal organ culture exposed for 4 weeks to amosite asbestos. Note the extracellular amosite fiber (arrow) protruding from the lesion.

the increased pathogenicity of crocidolite and amosite asbestos, compared with chrysotile, in lung cancers and malignant mesotheliomas.[3–5,13,14] The facts that amphibole asbestos fibers are insoluble, do not need to be metabolized to exert their effects, and can act during several stages of the carcinogenic process, as diagrammed in Figure 23.1, render them unique and durable carcinogens that can persist in lung epithelial and mesothelial cells, (i.e., target cells of lung carcinomas and mesotheliomas) during the long latency period of tumor development.

Asbestos-Associated Lung Cancers

Asbestos rarely causes tumors in nonsmoking asbestos workers, and it is considered less of a risk in the development of lung cancer than smoking.[3,4,13,15,16] However, the incidence of lung cancers increases additively or synergistically in asbestos workers who smoke. Several investigators report that adenocarcinomas and tumors developing in the lower, peripheral lung lobes are most commonly seen in asbestos-exposed lung cancer patients.[17,18] One hypothesis is that that pulmonary fibrosis (asbestosis) arises in the peripheral lung at sites of deposition of asbestos fiber and then creates a favorable and promoting environment for the development of lung cancers. Proliferating lung fibroblasts in these lesions may promote proliferation or metaplasia of lung epithelial cells through elaboration of growth factors or cell–cell communication.[19] Some studies suggest that there is an increased risk for lung cancer only in individuals who have clinical asbestosis, whereas critics argue that asbestosis and asbestos-induced lung cancer are independent processes.[20–22] As for lung cancer, cigarette smoke may also be a risk factor for asbestosis and may exacerbate the pathogenesis of asbestosis.[19,23] However, this is a subject of debate in the field.

Asbestos-Associated Mesothelioma

Malignant mesothelioma is a devastating cancer that typically originates from mesothelial cells of the pleura and, less commonly, the peritoneum or pericardium. Exposure to asbestos is believed to be the major risk factor for its development, as approximately 80% of mesothelioma patients have known exposure to asbestos.[3–5] Genetic predisposition, SV40, and other risk factors such as metals, rubber, pleural scarring, dietary factors, lung infections, and ionizing radiation have been implicated in the development of mesothelioma.[24–26] It has been suggested that differences between asbestos and nonasbestos-related malignant mesothelioma exist, with nonasbestos malignant mesothelioma occurring typically at younger ages.[6,7,27]

A large body of epidemiologic data shows that the amphiboles amosite and crocidolite are more carcinogenic than chrysotile in the development of malignant mesothelioma.[3–7,28,29] Furthermore, many asbestos workers are exposed to different types of asbestos, and analyses have shown that many individuals who have developed malignant mesothelioma following inhalation of supposedly "pure" chrysotile asbestos were also exposed to tremolite, a contaminant of certain Canadian chrysotile mines that is more persistent in lungs.[14]

Mechanisms of Asbestos-Induced Carcinogenesis

The fact that amphibole asbestos fibers persist in lung and pleura for many years compared with chrysotile asbestos, which dissolves or breaks down into shorter fibers over time due to leaching of magnesium,[30] suggests that they serve as a chronic stimulus for development of lung cancers or malignant mesotheliomas. Many studies show that long, thin fibers (>8 μm in length and <0.25 μm in diameter, as defined by Stanton and colleagues) are more tumorigenic after injection into the pleura or by inhalation when compared with shorter fibers (defined as a >3:1 length to diameter ratio) or nonfibrous particles.[3–5,29]

Mechanistic studies also suggest that the most pathogenic asbestos types, crocidolite and amosite, act at several stages in the carcinogenic process via elaboration of ROS.[12] These fibers have a high iron content that can drive Fenton-like reactions generating the hydroxyl radical (OH·), which is associated with mutagenicity and DNA damage. In contrast to long fibers of chrysotile that cause cell lysis and death, processes attributed to the positively charged magnesium on the fiber,[11] long rod-like amphibole fibers (>8 μm in length) are incompletely phagocytized by cells (see Figure 23.2B), causing elaboration of ROS by a prolonged oxidative burst. It is widely acknowledged that ROS are mutagenic and mitogenic.[12] In vitro studies have also demonstrated that long, thin asbestos fibers penetrate the nuclear membrane and physically interact with the mitotic spindle during cell division, an event linked to aneuploidy and other chromosomal changes.[31] Moreover, amphibole fibers cause oxidative DNA damage[12,32] and DNA breakage[33] in lung epithelial and mesothelial cells in vitro. Whether DNA damage by asbestos occurs in humans, especially people with compromised DNA repair pathways, remains to be proven.

Mechanisms of Asbestos-Induced Cell Signaling In Mitogenesis, Tumor Promotion, and Progression

A more plausible scenario for tumor promotion and progression by asbestos fibers during the long latency period of development of lung tumors and malignant mesotheliomas is the elicitation of multiple cell signaling path-

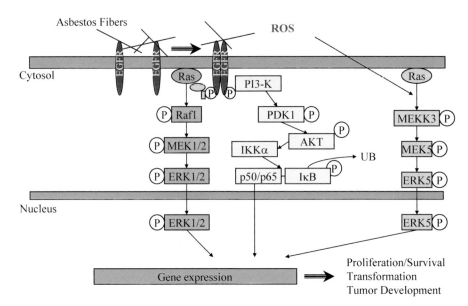

FIGURE 23.3. Multiple cell signaling and survival pathways are stimulated in epithelial and mesothelial cells after addition of fibers in vitro or inhalation of asbestos fibers. These pathways are stimulated by direct physical interaction of amphibole fibers with surface receptors such as the epidermal growth factor receptor (EGFR) and/or elaboration of reactive oxygen species (ROS) by fibers. These interactions then cause a cascade of phosphorylation events (P) that stimulate the Ras/ERK1/2, PI3K/Akt, NF-κB, and Ras/ERK5 pathways, leading to translo-

cation of respective complexes into the nucleus and their interaction with promoter regions of genes leading to proliferation, transformation, and tumor development. ERK, extracellular signal-regulated kinase; NF-κB, nuclear factor-κB; MEK, mitogen-activated protein/extracellular signal-regulated kinase; MEKK, MEK kinase;; PDK1 = 3-phosphoinositide-dependent protein kinase 1; PI3K, phosphatidylinositol-3 kinase; UB, ubiquitination.

ways either by direct interaction of asbestos fibers with the cell surface or by generation of ROS from fibers (Figure 23.3). These signaling pathways lead to activation of genes governing mitogenesis,[34] activation of growth factor receptors,[35] and cascades leading to autonomous dysregulation of tumor cell growth, escape from the normal cell cycle, and increased cell survival.[36] For example, antiapoptotic proteins are elevated in malignant mesothelioma cells, allowing cells to survive pro-apoptotic insults that normally would be lethal.[37]

Another feature of malignant mesotheliomas is increased production of vascular endothelial growth factor, which promotes angiogenesis and is regulated through a heparin growth factor/c-Met receptor-induced signaling pathway.[38] Our laboratory first showed that asbestos fibers cause activation of the mitogen-activated protein kinase (MAPK)[39,40] and the nuclear factor-κB (NF-κB)[36,41] survival pathways in mesothelial and lung epithelial cells. Most recently, we have also shown that the phosphatidylinositol-3-kinase(PI3K)/Akt pathway is activated by asbestos and is an important survival pathway in malignant mesothelioma.[42]

General Concepts of Mitogen-Activated Protein Kinase Signaling

Mitogen-activated protein kinases are families of serine-threonine kinases that phosphorylate specific proteins in

a cascade-like fashion and are checked by a series of phosphatases. Mitogen-activated protein kinase pathways are typically activated by extracellular stimuli and lead ultimately to the activation of nuclear transcription factors. There are at least three major families of MAPKs: the extracellular signal-regulated kinases 1, 2, and 5 (ERK1/2 and ERK5); the c-Jun N-terminal kinases (JNK1, JNK2, and JNK3), and the p38 kinases.[43] In general, activation of ERK cascades leads to increased cell division and survival, the JNKs (or stress-associated protein kinases) are thought to function in cell death and transcriptional regulation, and the p38 MAPKs are activated by certain cytokines and osmotic stress.

Mitogen-Activated Protein Kinase Signaling, Fos/Jun Proteins, and Activator Protein-1 Activation

An outcome of MAPK activation is transmission of a signal from the cell membrane to the nucleus, which promotes gene transcription. One of the transcription factors targeted for activation by the MAPKs is the activator protein-1 transcription factor, a dimeric protein complex composed of protein products of the *fos* and *jun* proto-oncogenes that are induced in a dose-dependent fashion by lower concentrations of crocidolite than chrysotile asbestos in mesothelial and tracheal epithelial cells.[34] The

Jun family of proteins includes c-Jun, JunB, and JunD, and these proteins can bind together in homodimeric fashion or with proteins of the Fos family (c-Fos, FosB, Fra-1, and Fra-2) to form heterodimers. The DNA binding specificity of different activator protein-1 complexes is highly conserved, and different Fos–Jun dimers have different DNA binding specificities that regulate transcription of discrete sets of genes governing cell proliferation, differentiation, and oncogenic transformation.

Asbestos and Mitogen-Activated Protein Kinase Signaling

As shown in Figure 23.3, crocidolite asbestos fibers directly cross-link and autophosphorylate the epidermal growth factor receptor (EGFR) in mesothelial cells which in turn leads to ERK1/2 activation.[39,40,44] Additionally, the initiation of the ERK1/2 response by asbestos involves the generation of ROS during phagocytosis of asbestos fibers or by redox reactions occurring on the surface of asbestos fibers. Addition of asbestos or hydrogen peroxide leads to ERK1/2 activation and apoptosis, which are prevented with the addition of the antioxidant N-acetyl-L-cysteine.[45] Apoptosis and cell proliferation are ongoing dynamic processes in mesothelial cells exposed to crocidolite asbestos and may be coupled in that apoptotic cell death leads to cell proliferation.

We have more recently shown that exposure of lung epithelial cells to asbestos leads to a protracted oxidant-induced activation of ERK5, which is Src kinase dependent but not EGFR dependent.[46] This study also shows that ERK1/2 activation by asbestos is EGFR dependent in these cells, providing strong evidence that cell signaling in response to asbestos is multifaceted and involves different MAPK cascades.

Nuclear Factor-κB Signaling by Asbestos

The NF-κB signaling pathway can be activated by a number of external and internal cell signals, including crocidolite asbestos and oxidants.[36,41] Normally NF-κB, a dimeric complex, is composed of subunits of Rel family proteins, commonly p50/p65 (RelA) dimers.[47] In resting cells, these dimeric complexes are bound to inhibitory κB (IκB) proteins, which maintain them in the cytoplasm (see Figure 23.3). Upon activation, the IκB complex becomes phosphorylated, allowing its dissociation from p50/p65 and ubiquitination and translocation of the freed NF-κB complex into the nucleus where it binds to specific κB sites on DNA, causing transcription of target genes. Nuclear factor-κB–dependent gene transcription leads to production of many proinflammatory cytokines and upregulation of cell adhesion molecules, growth factors, and immunoreceptors. In addition, NF-κB promotes cell survival through the induction of genes that cause inhibition of normal apoptotic mechanisms. Activation of NF-κB in malignant mesothelioma or lung tumors may govern resistance to anticancer drugs and therapeutic radiation. Because of the potential roles of NF-κB in inflammation, tumorigenesis, and tumor cell survival, chronic activation of NF-κB by amphibole asbestos fibers may be critical in both the development and maintenance of these tumors.

Phosphatidylinositol-3 Kinase/Akt Signaling by Asbestos

Akt (also known as protein kinase B [PKB]) is a cytoplasmic protein kinase that can be activated by PI3K via cell surface or growth factor receptors in response to various extracellular signals, including asbestos or SV40 T antigen.[27,38,48] The interactions between this pathway and the Ras signaling cascade are intensely studied because of their critical roles in cell survival and growth, malignant transformation, angiogenesis, and tumor invasion.[49,50] As shown in Figure 23.3, PI3K is phosphorylated or activated by both growth factor receptor tyrosine kinases and Ras, which leads to sequential phosphorylation of 3-phosphoinositide–dependent protein kinase 1 and Akt. Activation of Akt can lead to activation of the proapoptotic factors Bad and caspase-9, as well as stimulation of the prosurvival NF-κB signaling pathway via activation of IκB kinase α, positively affecting cell cycle progression.[51] Recent evidence has linked crocidolite asbestos and SV40 T antigen to activation of PI3K and Akt in human mesothelial cells, causing resistance to cell death by these agents.[38,48,52] Additionally, many human malignant mesotheliomas exhibit elevated constitutive levels of Akt, and it has been suggested that elevated Akt levels may be indicative of their resistance to anticancer drugs.[52] Pharmacologic inhibition of the Akt pathway inhibits malignant mesothelioma cell growth and increases their sensitivity to the chemotherapeutic agents cisplatin[42] and Onconase.[53] These data provide compelling evidence that the prosurvival protein Akt is involved in asbestos-mediated signaling in tumorigenesis; thus its pharmacologic targeting may be important in treating asbestos-mediated malignant mesothelioma and lung cancers.

Conclusion

Inhalation of asbestos fibers is associated with the development of lung tumors, primarily in asbestos workers who are smokers, and malignant mesotheliomas, which show no correlation with smoking history. The ability of asbestos fibers, particularly amphiboles, to act at multiple stages of the carcinogenic process and their persistence render them unique carcinogens in the lung and pleura. In malignant mesotheliomas, amphibole asbestos fibers appear to be complete carcinogens, whereas they are cocarcinogens as well as tumor promoters in the development of lung carcinomas.[54,55]

Although multiple mechanisms of interaction between components of cigarette smoke and asbestos have been reported, including impaired mucociliary clearance and increased cell transport and metabolism of polycyclic aromatic hydrocarbons by asbestos fibers, a recent review emphasizes the cooperativity of oxidants generated from cigarette smoke and asbestos fibers in the stimulation of MAPK signaling cascades, mucin hypersecretion, and epithelial cell transformation.[56] These events may account for the additive and synergistic effects on lung cancer development in asbestos workers who smoke. Targeting of the multiple signaling cascades initiated by asbestos fibers in lung epithelial and mesothelial cells may be critical in prevention and therapy of lung cancers and malignant mesotheliomas.

References

1. National Institute for Environmental Health Sciences (NTP). Tenth Report on Carcinogens. Washington, DC: National Institute for Environmental Health Sciences; 2002.
2. Mossman BT, Klein G, Zur Hausen H. Modern criteria to determine the etiology of human carcinogens. Semin Cancer Biol 2004;14(6):449–452.
3. Mossman BT, Gee JB. Asbestos-related diseases. N Engl J Med 1989;320(26):1721–1730.
4. Mossman BT, Bignon J, Corn M, et al. Asbestos: scientific developments and implications for public policy. Science 1990;247(4940):294–301.
5. Robinson BW, Lake RA. Advances in malignant mesothelioma. N Engl J Med 2005;353(15):1591–1603.
6. Vogelzang NJ. Emerging insights into the biology and therapy of malignant mesothelioma. Semin Oncol 2002;29(6 Suppl 18):35–42.
7. Powers A, Carbone M. The role of environmental carcinogens, viruses and genetic predisposition in the pathogenesis of mesothelioma. Cancer Biol Ther 2002;1(4):348–353.
8. Coleman W, Tsongalis G, eds. Molecular Basis of Human Cancer. Totowa, NJ: Humana Press; 2001.
9. Choy H, Pass HI, Rosell R, et al. Lung cancer. In Chang AE, Ganz PA, Hayes DF, et al., eds. Oncology: A Evidence-Based Approach. New York: Springer; 2006:545–621.
10. Murthy SS, Testa JR. Asbestos, chromosomal deletions, and tumor suppressor gene alterations in human malignant mesothelioma. J Cell Physiol 1999;180(2):150–157.
11. Guthrie GD, Mossman BT, eds. Health Effects of Mineral Dusts. Washington, DC: Mineralogic Society of America; 1993.
12. Shukla A, Gulumian M, Hei TK, et al. Multiple roles of oxidants in the pathogenesis of asbestos-induced diseases. Free Radic Biol Med 2003;34(9):1117–1129.

13. McDonald AD, McDonald JC. Epidemiology of malignant mesothelioma. In Antman K, Aisner J, eds. Asbestos-Related Malignancy. Orlando, FL: Grune & Stratton; 1987:31–55.
14. Churg A. Chrysotile, tremolite, and malignant mesothelioma in man. Chest 1988;93(3):621–628.
15. Saracci R. The interactions of tobacco smoking and other agents in cancer etiology. Epidemiol Rev 1987;9:175–193.
16. McDonald JC, McDonald JC. Epidemiology of asbestos-related lung cancer. In: Antman K, Aisner J, eds. Asbestos-Related Malignancy. Orlando, FL: Grune & Stratton; 1987:57–79.
17. Soutar CA, Simon G, Turner-Warwick M. The radiology of asbestos-induced disease of the lungs. Br J Dis Chest 1974;68:235–252.
18. Weiss W. Asbestosis and lobar site of lung cancer. Occup Environ Med 2000;57(5):358–360.
19. Mossman BT, Churg A. Mechanisms in the pathogenesis of asbestosis and silicosis. Am J Respir Crit Care Med 1998; 157(5 Pt 1):1666–1680.
20. Haus BM, Razavi H, Kuschner WG. Occupational and environmental causes of bronchogenic carcinoma. Curr Opin Pulm Med 2001;7(4):220–225.
21. Rom WN. Assessment of activation, differentiation, and carcinogenesis of lung cells by quantitative competitive RT-PCR. Am J Respir Cell Mol Biol 1998;19(1):3–5.
22. Kannerstein M, Churg J. Pathology of carcinoma of the lung associated with asbestos exposure. Cancer 1972;30(1):14–21.
23. Weiss W. Cigarette smoke, asbestos, and small irregular opacities. Am Rev Respir Dis 1984;130(2):293–301.
24. Hofmann J, Mintzer D, Warhol MJ. Malignant mesothelioma following radiation therapy. Am J Med 1994;97(4):379–382.
25. Hubbard R. The aetiology of mesothelioma: are risk factors other than asbestos exposure important? Thorax 1997;52(6):496–497.
26. Hillerdal G, Berg J. Malignant mesothelioma secondary to chronic inflammation and old scars. Two new cases and review of the literature. Cancer 1985;55(9):1968–1972.
27. Carbone M, Kratzke RA, Testa JR. The pathogenesis of mesothelioma. Semin Oncol 2002;29(1):2–17.
28. Hughes JM, Weill H. Asbestos exposure—quantitative assessment of risk. Am Rev Respir Dis 1986;133(1):5–13.
29. Health Effects Institute. Asbestos Research. Asbestos in Public and Commercial Buildings: A Literature Review and Synthesis of Current Knowledge. Cambridge, MA: Health Effects Institute;1991.
30. Jaurand MC, Gaudichet A, Halpern S, et al. In vitro biodegradation of chrysotile fibres by alveolar macrophages and mesothelial cells in culture: comparison with a pH effect. Br J Ind Med 1984;41(3):389–395.
31. Ault JG, Cole RW, Jensen CG, et al. Behavior of crocidolite asbestos during mitosis in living vertebrate lung epithelial cells. Cancer Res 1995;55(4):792–798.
32. Fung H, Kow YW, Van Houten B, et al. Patterns of 8-hydroxydeoxyguanosine formation in DNA and indications of oxidative stress in rat and human pleural mesothelial cells after exposure to crocidolite asbestos. Carcinogenesis 1997;18(4):825–832.

33. Nygren J, Suhonen S, Norppa H, et al. DNA damage in bronchial epithelial and mesothelial cells with and without associated crocidolite asbestos fibers. Environ Mol Mutagen 2004;44(5):477–482.

34. Heintz NH, Janssen YM, Mossman BT. Persistent induction of c-fos and c-jun expression by asbestos. Proc Natl Acad Sci USA 1993;90(8):3299–3303.

35. Gerwin BI, Lechner JF, Reddel RR, et al. Comparison of production of transforming growth factor-beta and platelet-derived growth factor by normal human mesothelial cells and mesothelioma cell lines. Cancer Res 1987;47(23):6180–6184.

36. Janssen YM, Barchowsky A, Treadwell M, et al. Asbestos induces nuclear factor kappa B (NF-kappa B) DNA-binding activity and NF-kappa B–dependent gene expression in tracheal epithelial cells. Proc Natl Acad Sci USA 1995;92(18):8458–8462.

37. Broaddus VC, Dansen TB, Abayasiriwardana KS, et al. Bid mediates apoptotic synergy between tumor necrosis factor-related apoptosis-inducing ligand (TRAIL) and DNA damage. J Biol Chem 2005;280(13):12486–12493.

38. Cacciotti P, Libener R, Betta P, et al. SV40 replication in human mesothelial cells induces HGF/Met receptor activation: a model for viral-related carcinogenesis of human malignant mesothelioma. Proc Natl Acad Sci USA 2001;98(21):12032–12037.

39. Zanella CL, Posada J, Tritton TR, et al. Asbestos causes stimulation of the extracellular signal-regulated kinase 1 mitogen-activated protein kinase cascade after phosphorylation of the epidermal growth factor receptor. Cancer Res 1996;56(23):5334–5338.

40. Zanella CL, Timblin CR, Cummins A, et al. Asbestos-induced phosphorylation of epidermal growth factor receptor is linked to c-fos and apoptosis. Am J Physiol 1999;277(4 Pt 1):L684–L693.

41. Janssen YM, Driscoll KE, Howard B, et al. Asbestos causes translocation of p65 protein and increases NF-kappa B DNA binding activity in rat lung epithelial and pleural mesothelial cells. Am J Pathol 1997;151(2):389–401.

42. Altomare DA, You H, Xiao GH, et al. Human and mouse mesotheliomas exhibit elevated AKT/PKB activity, which can be targeted pharmacologically to inhibit tumor cell growth. Oncogene 2005;24(40):6080–6089.

43. Johnson GL, Lapadat R. Mitogen-activated protein kinase pathways mediated by ERK, JNK, and p38 protein kinases. Science 2002;298(5600):1911–1912.

44. Pache JC, Janssen YM, Walsh ES, et al. Increased epidermal growth factor-receptor protein in a human mesothelial cell line in response to long asbestos fibers. Am J Pathol 1998;152(2):333–340.

45. Jimenez LA, Zanella C, Fung H, et al. Role of extracellular signal-regulated protein kinases in apoptosis by asbestos and H$_2$O$_2$. Am J Physiol 1997;273(5 Pt 1):L1029–L1035.

46. Scapoli L, Ramos-Nino ME, Martinelli M, et al. Src-dependent ERK5 and Src/EGFR-dependent ERK1/2 activation is required for cell proliferation by asbestos. Oncogene 2004;23(3):805–813.

47. Karin M, Greten FR. NF-kappaB: linking inflammation and immunity to cancer development and progression. Nat Rev Immunol 2005;5(10):749–759.

48. Cacciotti P, Barbone D, Porta C, et al. SV40-dependent AKT activity drives mesothelial cell transformation after asbestos exposure. Cancer Res 2005;65(12):5256–5262.

49. Kim D, Chung J. Akt: versatile mediator of cell survival and beyond. J Biochem Mol Biol 2002;35(1):106–115.

50. Shaw RJ, Cantley LC. Ras, PI(3)K and mTOR signalling controls tumour cell growth. Nature 2006;441(7092):424–430.

51. Karin M. Nuclear factor-kappaB in cancer development and progression. Nature 2006;441(7092):431–436.

52. Altomare DA, Vaslet CA, Skele KL, et al. A mouse model recapitulating molecular features of human mesothelioma. Cancer Res 2005;65(18):8090–8095.

53. Ramos-Nino ME, Vianale G, Sabo-Attwood T, et al. Human mesothelioma cells exhibit tumor cell–specific differences in phosphatidylinositol 3-kinase/AKT activity that predict the efficacy of Onconase. Mol Cancer Ther 2005;4(5):835–842.

54. Sabo-Attwood T, Ramos-Nino M, Mossman BT. Environmental carcinogens. In Chang AE, ed. Oncology: An Evidence-Based Approach. New York: Springer; 2006:233–243.

55. Mossman BT, Cameron GS, Yotti LP. Cocarcinogenic and tumor promoting properties of asbestos and other minerals in tracheobronchial epithelium. Carcinog Compr Surv 1985;8:217–238.

56. Mossman BT, Lounsbury KM, Reddy SP. Oxidants and signaling by mitogen-activated protein kinases in lung epithelium. Am J Respir Cell Mol Biol 2006;34(6):666–669.

24
Viral Oncogenesis

Cindy Noel Berthelot and Stephen K. Tyring

Introduction

For more than 100 years, researchers have suspected some tumors have an infectious etiology. In recent years, revelations regarding the origin of human cancers have come at an increasing pace. Infectious agents, mainly viruses, are among the few known causes of cancer and contribute to a variety of malignancies worldwide. In 1911, Peyton Rous successfully transmitted a malignancy from one chicken to another by injecting cell-free extracts from the tumor.[1] His work signaled a new era in cancer research, and ultimately the cancer was shown to be caused by an RNA virus, the Rous sarcoma virus. Although scientists sporadically demonstrated the transmissibility of other tumors, the majority of attempts were unsuccessful. A renaissance of the viral hypothesis occurred in 1950 when Ludwik Gross discovered the transmissibility of murine leukemias by infecting newborn mice with tumor extracts.[2] His work ushered in many additional studies, eventually leading to the discovery of several other viruses as causative factors of malignancy. In 1964, Epstein and colleagues observed herpesvirus-like particles in cells of Burkitt's lymphoma cell cultures.[3] Although virus particles were observed using electron microscopy, it was 1958 when Dennis Burkitt first speculated that this childhood tumor might have a viral origin.[4] His ideas were based on the observation that the tumor was endemic in certain geographic regions of equatorial Africa and coincided with regions affected by malaria. Although the particles were found in cultured Burkitt's lymphoma cells, designated as Epstein-Barr virus (EBV), it took almost 30 years before it was firmly identified as a human tumor virus.

As another viral infection emerged in the 1980s, it became evident that direct infection is not the sole mode by which viruses contribute to the development of human cancers. The acquired immunodeficiency syndrome (AIDS) epidemic, resulting from human immunodeficiency virus (HIV) infections and leading to severe immunosuppression, favors the development of B-cell lymphomas, Hodgkin's disease, Kaposi's sarcoma, and skin cancers.[5] Because HIV-DNA is not found in these cancer cells, the virus indirectly contributes to the emergence of these cancers by inducing profound immunosuppression and reducing host immune mechanisms. Other viral infections, including herpes simplex virus and cytomegalovirus, aid persisting tumor viruses (papillomaviruses and polyomaviruses) by amplifying the genomes of the latter in infected cells.[6,7] This mechanism emerges as a second indirect mode of interaction by which specific viruses may increase tumor formation. Chronic inflammation, due to infectious agents or other chronic stimuli of the immune system, may also increase the risk of malignancy.[8] It is estimated that chronic inflammation caused by infections account for approximately 21% of new cancer cases in developing countries and 9% in developed countries.[8]

In recent years, additional viruses associated with certain human tumors have been discovered. They include hepatitis C virus in a subset of hepatic cancers, human herpesvirus type 8 (HHV-8) in Kaposi's sarcoma, and approximately 50 novel papillomavirus genotypes in squamous and basal cell carcinomas of the skin.

Viruses account for several of the most common malignancies, up to 20% of all cancers. Several of these cancers are endemic, with a high incidence in certain geographic areas, whereas others have sporadic incidence. The specificity of a given association of a virus and an associated malignancy, depending on the virus, cancer, and geographic location, ranges from essentially 100% to as low as 15%. The mere presence within these tumors does not prove an etiologic relationship. Nevertheless, it provides a starting point for further investigation.

The agents considered here are EBV, HHV-8, human papillomavirus (HPV), hepatitis B and C viruses, human T-cell leukemia virus, human polyomavirus SV40, and jaagsiekte sheep retrovirus (Tables 24.1 and 24.2). Although viral oncogenesis is established in some human malignancies, viral oncogenesis in human lung cancer is

TABLE 24.1. Accepted and candidate human tumor viruses.

Virus	Human diseases	Human tumors
EBV	IM, oral hairy leukoplakia	BCL, BL, NPC, HD, TCL
HBV and HCV	Hepatitis, cirrhosis	Hepatocellular carcinoma
HPV	Skin warts, CA, intraepithelial neoplasias, LP	Cervical, skin, oropharynx, SCC, EV, and adenocarcinomas
HTLV-1	HAM/TSP	ATL
HHV-8	Unknown	KS, PEL, CD
SV40	Respiratory tract, cystitis	Mesothelioma, brain tumors, osteosarcomas, and non-HD

Note: ATL, acute T-cell leukemia; BCL, B-cell lymphomas; BL, Burkitt's lymphoma; CA, condyloma acuminata; CD, Castleman's disease; EBV, Epstein-Barr virus; EV, epidermodysplasia verruciformis; HAM, HTLV-1-associated myelopathy; HBV and HCV, hepatitis B and C viruses; HD, Hodgkin's disease; HHV-8, human herpesvirus type 8; HPV, human papillomavirus; HTLV-1, human T-cell leukemia virus; IM, infectious mononucleosis; KS, Kaposi's sarcoma; LP, laryngeal papillomas; NPC, nasopharyngeal carcinoma; PEL, primary effusion lymphoma; SCC, squamous cell carcinoma; SV40, Simian virus 40; TCL, T-cell lymphomas; TSP, tropical spastic paraparesis.

speculative and unproven at present; SV40 is under investigation as a possible factor in human mesothelioma.

Mechanisms of Tumorigenesis

The cellular mechanisms by which viral infections give rise to tumors may be considered in the context of the multistage theory of carcinogenesis. Tumor induction by viruses may be viewed as occurring by one of three general mechanisms. First, the genes of a virus may directly specify all the functional changes needed to convert a normal cell into a malignant one. Such viruses would induce tumorigenesis in a single step, and therefore malignancy would develop after a short latency period. The virus would supply all the abnormal functions

for the cell, and its continued presence would be required for malignant growth. Most DNA tumor viruses contain more than one viral oncogene, and each contributes to the oncogenic properties of the virus. In vitro studies show that some oncogenes, whether from DNA viruses or retroviruses, serve principally to prolong the lifespan of the cell, whereas others directly stimulate cell growth and division.[9] In the absence of a cooperating immortalizing gene, expression of an oncogene that stimulates abnormal cell growth usually induces the cell to undergo senescence or apoptosis. These are potent mechanisms to protect the organism from cancer. Immortalizing genes blunt apoptosis and thus account for the strong oncogenic activity when immortalizing and directly transforming genes are expressed together.

A second mechanism may be that viruses specify some, but not all, of the functional changes required for tumor development. The virus would contribute to the cell becoming a tumor cell, but certain additional cellular changes would be required for the cell to give rise to a tumor. Most frequently, the changes are alterations that complement the viral functions, and the continued presence of viral genetic material would be required. Alternatively, in some experimental tumors, changes are made in the tumor cell so that the persistence of the virus is no longer necessary.[10] Tumors that require cellular changes in addition to viral infection take longer to develop when compared with tumors in which the virus supplies all the abnormal functions required for tumorigenesis. This latency period may be a reflection of the requirement for accumulation of the additional genetic changes mediating malignant progression in a virally infected cell.

The third mechanism of viral oncogenesis is that viruses may induce tumors by an indirect process. Infection with the virus may simply increase the likelihood that the cellular changes required for tumorigenesis will occur. Tumor viruses that function by this mechanism typically induce malignancy after a long latency period.

TABLE 24.2. Properties of accepted and potential human tumor viruses.

Characteristic	HBV	HCV	EBV	HPV	HHV-8	SV40
Genome						
Nucleic acid	dsDNA	ssRNA	dsDNA	dsDNA	dsDNA	dsDNA
Size (kb/kbp)	3.2	9.4	172	8	165	5.2
No. genes	4	9	≈90	8–10	≈90	6
Cell tropism	HC, WBC	HC	OP, B cells, EC	SEC	VEC, LC	Kidney
Prevalence	Common (Asia, and Africa)	Common (Japan, and Caribbean)	Common	Common	Not ubiquitous	
Transmission	Vertical, parenteral, horizontal, venereal	Parenteral and horizontal	Saliva	Venereal, skin	Horizontal and venereal	Urine?
Transforming genes	*HBx?*	*NS3?*	*LMP-1*	*E6, E7*		Tag, tag

Note: EBV, Epstein-Barr virus; EC, epithelial cells; HBV and HCV, hepatitis B and C viruses; HC, hepatocytes; HHV-8, human herpesvirus type 8; HPV, human papillomavirus; LC, lymphocytes; OP, oropharynx; SEC, squamous epithelial cells; SV40, Simian virus 40; VEC, vascular endothelial cells; WBC, white blood cells.

Cell Proliferation and Carcinogenesis

In 1914, Boveri postulated that cancer was caused by mutations in cells arising from either germlines or the genetic material of somatic cells.[11] The discovery in 1953 of the structure of DNA and its transmission of genetic information to daughter cells implied that alterations related to carcinogenesis ultimately involved changes in DNA. During the past few decades, considerable evidence has accumulated supporting the hypothesis that cancer is caused by alterations in specific genes. These genes have been identified and belong to two different classes: those that act in a dominant manner, called *oncogenes*, and those that require damage of both alleles of a given gene, consistent with a recessive mode of action, called *tumor suppressor genes*.[12,13]

It has also become apparent not only that damage to DNA is the basis for carcinogenesis but also that more than one genetic mistake is required. A two-hit genetic model for carcinogenesis was originally postulated by Knudson based on his examination of sporadic and hereditary retinoblastomas in children.[14] Knudson demonstrated that, based on spontaneous mutations occurring during normal retinoblast DNA replication, DNA alterations could occur in sufficient numbers to explain the rate of retinoblastoma occurrence under sporadic and hereditary means.

Based on the strongly supported assumptions that cancer is caused by multiple alterations in DNA and that DNA replication does not have 100% fidelity, there are two ways in which any agent (chemical, radiation, or infectious organism) can increase the chance of a cell becoming malignant.[15,16] The agent can either damage DNA directly (DNA-reactive chemicals and radiation) or increase the number of DNA replications (hormones and infectious agents).

A significant feature of tumor viruses is that they can induce morphologic transformation of some cells in culture.[17] The ability of these viruses to transform cells in vitro typically corresponds with their ability to induce tumors in animals. In vitro studies have shown that the capacity of tumor viruses to directly transform cells is due to the expression of viral oncogenes. Although not closely related to cellular genes, the oncogenes of retroviruses are actually derived from a class of cellular genes that are highly conserved in evolution.[18] Most of the oncogenic activities of their encoded proteins fall into one of three categories. Some proteins, such as the epidermal growth factor homologs of poxviruses, mimic activities of proteins encoded by cellular protooncogenes.[19] Others, such as the middle T antigen of polyomavirus, activates proteins encoded by protooncogenes.[20] The E6 and E7 proteins of some HPV, the large T antigen of SV40 virus, and the E1A and E1B proteins of adenoviruses bind to and functionally inactivate cellular proteins encoded by tumor suppressor genes.[21,22] Most genes of this class inhibit growth of the target cell so that the loss of this inhibitory activity contributes to transformation by these viral oncoproteins. Functional inactivation of tumor suppressor genes, usually by genetic alteration, has been identified in many nonviral tumors in animals and humans.[23]

Viruses in Human Tumors

In humans, members of several different virus families are associated with the development of malignancy (see Tables 24.1 and 24.2). As previously mentioned, EBV was originally isolated from biopsy tissue samples of the childhood malignancy African Burkitt's lymphoma. An association with EBV was subsequently discovered in nasopharyngeal carcinoma, which develops with high incidence among Cantonese Chinese, Alaskan Inuits, and in Mediterranean Africa.[24] Epstein-Barr virus is also accepted as a cause of posttransplantation lymphomas.[25] In addition, it is also implicated to cause a subset of Hodgkin's lymphoma, gastric carcinomas, T-cell lymphomas, and rare smooth muscle sarcomas in children with AIDS.[26-28]

The association of EBV with these malignancies is quite persuasive. The first link to EBV was demonstrated as patients with these malignancies had significantly elevated antibody titers to viral antigens, including viral capsid antigen and early antigen.[29] Similarly, early seroepidemiologic studies revealed that patients with nasopharyngeal carcinoma had elevated immunoglobulin A antibody titers to the same antigens.[30] Appearance of immunoglobulin A antibodies to EBV preceded the development of nasopharyngeal carcinoma by several years and correlates with tumor burden and recurrence. In EBV-associated tumors, the viral antigen Epstein-Barr nuclear antigen 1 is detected in all the tumor cells. Moreover, the EBV genome is located in the malignant epithelial cells and not the infiltrating lymphocytes in the nasopharyngeal tissue.[29]

An additional compelling factor is that all the malignancies associated with EBV contain homogenous episomal genomes detected with use of the EBV terminal assay.[31] A key biologic property of EBV that underlies its clear association with malignancy is its ability to alter B-cell growth regulation and induce permanent growth transformation. This ability of EBV to cause neoplastic growth is most clearly demonstrated by the development of B-cell lymphoproliferation in immunocompromised patients.[32,33] Lymphoproliferative diseases associated with EBV may develop in patients with congenital immune impairment, including the X-linked lymphoproliferative syndrome, severe combined immunodeficiency, adenosine deaminase deficiency, patients with Wiscott-Aldrich syndrome, organ transplant recipients, and those with AIDS.

Human herpesvirus 8 is a double-stranded DNA virus belonging to the γ-subfamily of herpesviruses. Similar to other γ-Herpesvirinae, HHV-8 establishes a life-long latent infection in the B lymphocytes of its host. Human herpesvirus 8 encodes a diverse array of genes involved in transformation, signaling, prevention of apoptosis, and immune evasion. Human herpesvirus 8 has been linked to several malignancies in humans, including Kaposi's sarcoma, primary effusion lymphomas, and multicentric Castleman's disease. The evidence linking HHV-8 to Kaposi's sarcoma, primary effusion lymphomas, and multicentric Castleman's disease is substantial and has been confirmed in multiple studies. Human herpesvirus 8 has also been linked to multiple myeloma, angiosarcomas, and malignant skin tumors in posttransplantation patients, such as Bowen's disease, squamous cell carcinoma, actinic keratosis, and extramammary Paget's disease. However, these disease associations are controversial and not well established.[34]

Because of evidence of high levels of cytokines and growth factors in lesions of Kaposi's sarcoma and multicentric Castleman's disease, it is believed that HHV-8 transforms cells through a paracrine mechanism. Human herpesvirus 8 has been shown to immortalize primary bone marrow–derived endothelial cells, and the virus induces proliferation, anchorage independence, and survival of these cells.[35] Furthermore, several of the HHV-8 gene products, including viral G protein–coupled receptor and K1, are transforming in vitro and in transgenic mice.[36,37] The K1 protein can transform rodent fibroblasts in vitro, and, when injected into nude mice, these cells induce multiple and disseminated tumors. Transgenic animals expressing K1 also develop sarcomas and lymphomas. Viral G protein–coupled receptor immortalizes primary endothelial cells, and transgenic mice expressing it develop angioproliferative Kaposi's sarcoma-like lesions. Viral G protein–coupled receptor also activates phospholipase C and phosphatidylinositol 3-kinase pathways, it and upregulates several cytokines and paracrine factors. Thus, this protein may contribute to malignancy by inducing and sustaining cell proliferation.[38,39]

Human herpesvirus 8 also encodes several viral homologs of cellular chemokines and cytokines, including viral interleukin-6, the antiapoptotic viral Bcl-2, viral Fas-associated death domain-like interleukin-1 converting enzyme inhibitory protein (vFLIP/Orf71), and viral inhibitor of apoptosis (vIANP/K7). Human herpesvirus 8 contains several immune evasion genes, including K3 and K5 proteins, that downregulate major histocompatibility complex I expression. In summary, the functions of the HHV-8 proteins ensure life-long viral persistence in the host, contributing to HHV-8–associated malignancy.

Human papillomavirus has been consistently associated with cancer of the cervix. Virtually 100% of cervical cancers contain HPV; however, only some types of HPV have this association. Of the approximately 130 HPV types distinguished thus far, 30 are labeled anogenital types, and only a subset of these are considered high-risk (HPV-16 and HPV-18). Human papillomaviruses 31 and 45 are also found in these cancers and, when combined with HPV-16 and HPV-18, account for 80% of cervical and anal cancers. Some vulvar, vaginal, and penile cancers are associated with HPV, as well as several grades of cervical dysplasia.

Recently, multivalent prophylactic HPV vaccines, currently in the late stages of clinical testing, were found to be safe, immunogenic, and efficacious.[40] Phase III tests of a quadrivalent vaccine have shown 100% effectiveness at preventing HPV-16–associated and HPV-18–associated cervical intraepithelial neoplasia grades 2 and 3, adenocarcinoma in situ, and cervical cancer through 2 years of postvaccination follow-up. Prophylactic HPV vaccines have the potential to block the acquisition of HPV and hence subsequent development of anogenital neoplasia.

Other low-risk types of HPV are associated with condyloma acuminata. Finally, numerous HPV types, including HPV-5 and HPV-8, may cause the rare genodermatosis epidermodysplasia verruciformis. An autosomal recessive inheritance pattern has been suggested; however, X-linked and autosomal dominant inheritance patterns have also been reported. Epidermodysplasia verruciformis may be caused by mutations of the genes *EVER1* and *EVER2*, which are located on the EV1 locus, 17q25.[41,42] These lesions may undergo malignant transformation in 30%–70% of cases, usually involving the sun-exposed areas.[43] Therefore, sun protection and sun avoidance are key to preventing further skin cancers. The central mechanism of HPV oncogenesis is the disruption of tumor suppressor genes, resulting in dysregulation of cell growth and inhibition of apoptosis. The HPV genes *E6* and *E7* are overexpressed as a consequence of the deletion of the E2 region in integrated HPV genomes. *E7* causes proteasomal degradation of retinoblastoma protein and related proteins so that cellular growth is dysregulated. *E6* causes degradation of p53 so that the abnormally growing cells are spared from apoptosis. In general, *E6* and *E7* of high-risk strains of HPV are more efficient at inactivating tumor suppressor proteins. Cofactors in anogenital HPV oncogenesis include smoking, oral contraceptive use, the presence of other sexually transmitted diseases (e.g., chlamydia, herpes simplex virus), chronic inflammation, immunosuppressive conditions including HIV infection, parity, dietary factors, and polymorphisms in the human leukocyte antigen system.[44]

Hepatocellular carcinoma is among the most common cancers in the world. Most cases of hepatocellular carcinoma are due to hepatitis B virus (HBV), but the incidence of hepatitis C virus (HCV)–associated hepatocellular carcinoma is increasing. This association of HBV as a major etiologic agent of hepatocellular carcinoma has been firmly established, with an estimated 10- to 15-fold increase risk for chronic HBV carriers.[45–47] The epidemiologic evidence for HCV as a cause of hepatocellular carcinoma is less established, but estimates of the lifetime risk of hepatocellular carcinoma in patients chronically infected with HCV are between 5% and 20%.[47] There is an exponential relationship between hepatocellular carcinoma and age, indicating that, as in other human cancers, multiple steps are required. The long latency between HBV or HCV infection and hepatocellular carcinoma may signify indirect action of these viruses, perhaps through long-term toxic effects of the immune response against hepatocytes. This may trigger ensuing chronic inflammation, continuous cell death, and consequent cell proliferation.[48] Cofactors, such as aflatoxins and alcohol, may also potentiate the action of viruses.

A role for viral proteins in hepatocellular carcinoma oncogenesis might be sensitization of liver cells to mutagens. In transgenic mice models, unregulated expression of the HBV X and S proteins is associated with hepatocarcinogenesis.[49,50] The HBx protein behaves as a transactivator of cellular genes such as oncogenes, growth factors, and cytokines and binds and inactivates p53. It also interacts with the DNA protein DDB1, which may affect repair functions and allow the accumulation of genetic changes. Rearrangement of integrated HCV sequences in hepatocellular carcinoma may lead to abnormal expression of the S gene protein. Specific activation of c-Raf-1/ERK2 signaling by the truncated pre-S2S protein leads to increased proliferation of hepatocytes.

Human T-cell lymphoma/leukemia virus (HTLV) is the first human retrovirus discovered in the context of malignancy, namely, certain acute T-cell leukemias (ATLs), endemic to southern Japan. Type 1 HTLV (HTLV-1) causes ATL in 3%–5% of infected persons over their lifetime.[51] Unlike other retroviruses that cause cancers in animals and humans, HTLV-1 does not contain a classic oncogene. However, the virus induces expression of cellular protooncogenes. In nonendemic areas, including the United States, England, some parts of the Caribbean islands, South America, and Africa, the virus is also associated with ATL, some forms of T-cell lymphomas, and mycosis fungoides. Human T-cell lymphoma/leukemia virus can also cause a progressive myelopathy in 1%–5% of infected people. Certain human leukocyte antigen alleles increase the risk of ATL. Route of exposure may also determine outcome. Mucosal exposure may lead to an impaired immune response that may affect pathogenesis of the disease and further leukemogenesis.

A second retrovirus, HTLV-2, was isolated from a case of hairy cell leukemia; however, it has yet to be firmly established as a causative factor. The virus is T-cell trophic, and in found in transformed CD4+ T cells and CD8+ T cells.

Type 1 HTLV infects B and T lymphocytes, dendritic cells, fibroblasts, and rodent cells. Human T-cell lymphoma/leukemia virus 1 proviral DNA integrates in a common chromosomal site in all ATL cells in a given patient, producing a state of clonality.[51] However, the integration site is not unique but differs in different cases of ATL, and it does not produce insertional mutagenesis. Unlike many other known retroviruses, HTLV1 encodes the trans-acting factor Tax that causes cellular transformation and induces and interacts with specific cellular genes.[52]

There are three primate polyomaviruses with a role in malignancy for each: JC virus, BK virus, and SV40. This discussion focuses on SV40, a DNA virus discovered as 1 of 40 or more viruses infecting *Macacus rhesus* and *Macacus cynomolgus* monkey kidney cells. Between 1955 and 1963, SV40 was introduced to the human population by contaminated inactivated and early live attenuated polio vaccines, produced in SV40-infected monkey cells.[53] Conservative estimates suggest more than 98 million children and adults in the United States were inadvertently exposed to the contaminated vaccines. These vaccines were also distributed to many other countries. In addition, different adenovirus vaccines used on a limited scale for U.S. military personnel from 1961 to 1965 also contained live SV40. There is also evidence that SV40 may be contagiously transmitted in humans by horizontal infection, independent of early administration of the contaminated vaccines. Simian virus 40 in its natural host, the rhesus monkey, replicates without producing lesions. However, it is a potent agent for cell cultures from species that are nonpermissive for viral replication, including hamster, mouse, rat, bovine, and guinea pig.[54] Simian virus 40 replicates in human diploid fibroblasts and transforms them.

An association of primary polyomavirus infection with mild respiratory tract disease, mild pyrexia, and transient cystitis has been reported. The first report of SV40 in human cancer was in 1974 when the virus and T antigen were detected in metastases from a malignant melanoma. However, there have been no further reports of this association. Simian virus 40 has been closely linked to malignant mesothelioma, a rare but aggressive cancer of mesothelial cells. Exposure to asbestos is the major factor identified in the development of mesothelioma; however, evidence suggests that SV40 may be a nonessential cofactor in its development.[55] In cell culture, human mesothelial cells are nonpermissive for SV40 replication, and asbestos could serve as a synergistic element for transformation. Simian virus 40 is also associated with some brain tumors, osteosarcomas, non-Hodgkin's lymphoma, and thyroid, pituitary, and parotid gland tumors.[56]

The site of latent infection in humans is not known, but the presence of SV40 in urine suggests the kidneys as a site of possible latency, as it occurs in its natural monkey host.[56] The mechanism of SV40 tumorigenesis in humans is related to the properties of two oncoproteins, the large T antigen (Tag) and the small t antigen (tag). The large T antigen acts mainly by blocking the functions of p53 and retinoblastoma tumor suppressor proteins. Simian virus 40 also induces chromosomal aberrations in host cells, generating genetic instability in the tumor cell. Large T antigen fixes these chromosomal damages in the infected cell, which may explain how low viral loads of SV40 may cause human tumors. The small t antigen has a mitogenic role by binding protein phosphatase 2A, leading to constitutive activation of the Wingless pathway resulting in continuous cell proliferation.

The possibility that SV40 is implicated in mesothelioma and other human cancers has stimulated interest in the development of a recombinant vaccine against SV40.[57] A recombinant vaccine vector containing a modified SV40 large T antigen sequence was constructed, which excluded the p53 and retinoblastoma binding sites.[58] The vaccine also excluded the aminoterminal oncogenic CRI and J domains.[59] This vector can efficiently prime the immune response to provide antigen-specific prophylactic and therapeutic protection against SV40 tumors. Such vaccines may represent useful immunoprophylactic and immunotherapeutic intervention against human tumors associated with SV40.

Jaagsiekte sheep retrovirus (JSRV) causes sheep pulmonary adenomatosis, a contagious ovine pulmonary adenocarcinoma. The host range of JSRV is in part limited by species-specific differences in the virus entry receptor hyaluronidase 2, which is not functional as a receptor in mice but is functional in humans.[60] One of the unique features of this virus is that in infected animals the only tissues that show expression of the virus are the tumor cells in the lung.[61] Sheep are immunotolerant of JSRV because of the expression of closely related endogenous retroviruses, which are not present in humans and most other species, and this may facilitate oncogenesis. Bronchoalveolar adenocarcinoma in humans morphologically resembles sheep pulmonary adenomatosis. Previously, positivity for JSRV by immunostaining, reverse transcription polymerase chain reaction, and Western blot was reported in most nonmucinous bronchoalveolar adenocarcinomas. Although the possibility of a JSRV with bronchoalveolar adenocarcinoma cannot be excluded, several published reports have shown that the association with JSRV is probably very weak, if present at all.[62,63]

As mentioned previously, HIV indirectly contributes to the emergence of some cancers by inducing profound immunosuppression and reducing host immune mechanisms. Several studies have shown that lung cancer risk was substantially elevated in HIV-infected individuals.[64,65] However, the incidence was unrelated to HIV-induced immunosuppression, and incidence remains high after adjustment for smoking, suggesting the involvement of additional factors. The prognosis of lung cancer is poorer in HIV-infected patients than in the general population, and data on the efficacy and toxicity of chemotherapy in these patients is scant. Surgery is the preferred treatment for localized disease in patients with adequate functional status and general health, regardless of their immune status. Prospective clinical trials are needed to define the optimal lung cancer treatment strategies in HIV-infected patients.

Several studies have searched for the role of EBV and HPV in human lung cancer. However, no evidence for an etiologic role for these two viruses in the development of pulmonary adenocarcinoma or pleural mesothelioma have been found.[66–68] Although data suggest that the conventional human oncogenic viruses (HPV, EBV) are unlikely to play a role in the development of lung carcinomas, studies should be conducted to establish any causative viruses and develop treatment options (vaccines).

Conclusion

After more than 100 years of intense research, the role of infectious agents in a substantial subset of human tumors has been clearly established. At present, an etiologic relationship of virus infections to tumor development can be linked to approximately 20% of cancer burden. Viruses should be regarded as the second most important risk factor for cancer development in humans, exceeded only by tobacco consumption.[69] Although often necessary, some infections are not sufficient for the induction of their respective cancers. It is now widely accepted that human carcinogenesis is a multistep process, and phenotypic changes during cancer progression reflect the sequential accumulation of genetic alterations in cells.[70,71] Additional modifications need to occur within the genome of the infected host cell, or secondary events must take place to dampen the host's immune system. The identification of viral infections as a major risk factor for cancer development should pave the way for new strategies in cancer prevention, particularly the development of new vaccines. Although viral oncogenesis is established in some human malignancies, viral oncogenesis in human lung cancer is, at present, speculative. Simian virus 40 is under investigation as a possible factor in human mesothelioma, and JSRV is unproven as a causative agent for lung cancer in humans. Further studies and examination are needed to determine the roles of viruses in lung malignancies.

References

1. Rous P. Transmission of a malignant new growth by means of a cell-free filtrate. Conn Med 1973;37(10):526.

2. Gross L. Susceptibility of newborn mice of an otherwise apparently "resistant" strain to inoculation with leukemia. Proc Soc Exp Biol Med 1950;73:246–248.

3. Epstein MA, Achong BG, Barr YM. Virus particles in cultured lymphoblasts from Burkitt's lymphoma. Lancet 1964 Mar 28;15:702–703.

4. Burkitt D. A sarcoma involving the jaws in African children. Br J Surg 1958;46(197):218–223.

5. Biggar RJ, Rabkin CS. The epidemiology of AIDS-related neoplasms. Hematol Oncol Clin North Am 1996;10(5):997–1010.

6. Schlehofer JR, Gissmann L, Matz B, et al. Herpes simplex virus–induced amplification of SV40 sequences in transformed Chinese hamster embryo cells. Int J Cancer 1983;32(1):99–103.

7. Schmitt J, Schlehofer JR, Mergener K, et al. Amplification of bovine papillomavirus DNA by N-methyl-N′-nitro-N-nitrosoguanidine, ultraviolet irradiation, or infection with herpes simplex virus. Virology 1989;172(1):73–81.

8. Pisani P, Parkin DM, Munoz N, et al. Cancer and infection: estimates of the attributable fraction in 1990. Cancer Epidemiol Biomarkers Prev 1997;6(6):387–400.

9. Hunter T. Cooperation between oncogenes. Cell 1991;64(2):249–270.

10. Grunwald DJ, Dale B, Dudley J, et al. Loss of viral gene expression and retention of tumorigenicity by Abelson lymphoma cells. J Virol 1982;43(1):92–103.

11. Wunderlich V. JMM—past and present. Chromosomes and cancer: Theodor Boveri's predictions 100 years later. J Mol Med 2002;80(9):545–548.

12. Munger K, Hayakawa H, Nguyen CL, et al. Viral carcinogenesis and genomic instability. EXS 2006;96:179–199.

13. Knudson AG Jr. Antioncogenes and human cancer. Proc Natl Acad Sci USA 1993;90(23):10914–10921.

14. Knudson AG Jr. Mutation and cancer: statistical study of retinoblastoma. Proc Natl Acad Sci USA 1971;68(4):820–823.

15. Cohen SM, Ellwein LB. Cell proliferation in carcinogenesis. Science 1990;249(4972):1007–1011.

16. Cohen SM, Ellwein LB. Genetic errors, cell proliferation, and carcinogenesis. Cancer Res 1991;51(24):6493–6505.

17. Bignold LP, Coghlan BL, Jersmann HP. Cancer morphology, carcinogenesis and genetic instability: a background. EXS 2006;96:1–24.

18. Temin HM. Evolution of cancer genes as a mutation-driven process. Cancer Res 1988;48(7):1697–1701.

19. Buller RM, Chakrabarti S, Moss B, et al. Cell proliferative response to vaccinia virus is mediated by VGF. Virology 1988;164(1):182–192.

20. Courtneidge SA. Further characterisation of the complex containing middle T antigen and pp60. Curr Top Microbiol Immunol 1989;144:121–128.

21. Huibregtse JM, Beaudenon SL. Mechanism of HPV E6 proteins in cellular transformation. Semin Cancer Biol 1996;7(6):317–326.

22. Jones DL, Munger K. Interactions of the human papillomavirus E7 protein with cell cycle regulators. Semin Cancer Biol 1996;7(6):327–337.

23. Hanahan D, Weinberg R. The hallmarks of cancer. Cell 2000;100(1):57–70.

24. Wei WI, Sham JS. Nasopharyngeal carcinoma. Lancet 2005;365(9476):2041–2054.

25. Capello D, Rossi D, Gaidano G. Post-transplant lymphoproliferative disorders: molecular basis of disease histogenesis and pathogenesis. Hematol Oncol 2005;23(2):61–67.

26. Takada K. Epstein-Barr virus and gastric carcinoma. Mol Pathol 2000;53(5):255–261.

27. Mueller N, Evans A, Harris NL, et al. Hodgkin's disease and Epstein-Barr virus. Altered antibody pattern before diagnosis. N Engl J Med 1989;320(11):689–695.

28. McClain KL, Leach CT, Jenson HB, et al. Association of Epstein-Barr virus with leiomyosarcomas in children with AIDS. N Engl J Med 1995;332(1):12–18.

29. Raab-Traub N. Epstein-Barr virus and nasopharyngeal carcinoma. Semin Cancer Biol 1992;3(5):297–307.

30. Henle G, Henle W. Epstein-Barr virus-specific IgA serum antibodies as an outstanding feature of nasopharyngeal carcinoma. Int J Cancer 1976;17(1):1–7.

31. Raab-Traub N, Flynn K. The structure of the termini of the Epstein-Barr virus as a marker of clonal cellular proliferation. Cell 1986;47(6):883–889.

32. Hamilton-Dutoit SJ, Pallesen G, Karkov J, et al. Identification of EBV-DNA in tumour cells of AIDS-related lymphomas by in-situ hybridisation. Lancet 1989;1(8637):554–552.

33. Katz BZ, Raab-Traub N, Miller G. Latent and replicating forms of Epstein-Barr virus DNA in lymphomas and lymphoproliferative diseases. J Infect Dis 1989;160(4):589–598.

34. Ablashi DV, Chatlynne LG, Whitman JE Jr, et al. Spectrum of Kaposi's sarcoma–associated herpesvirus, or human herpesvirus 8, diseases. Clin Microbiol Rev 2002;15(3):439–464.

35. Flore O, Rafii S, Ely S, et al. Transformation of primary human endothelial cells by Kaposi's sarcoma–associated herpesvirus. Nature 1998;394(6693):588–592.

36. Moore PS, Chang Y. Kaposi's sarcoma-associated herpesvirus immunoevasion and tumorigenesis: two sides of the same coin? Annu Rev Microbiol 2003;57:609–639.

37. Damania B. Modulation of cell signaling pathways by Kaposi's sarcoma–associated herpesvirus (KSHVHHV-8). Cell Biochem Biophys 2004;40(3):305–322.

38. Cesarman E, Mesri EA, Gershengorn MC. Viral G protein–coupled receptor and Kaposi's sarcoma: a model of paracrine neoplasia? J Exp Med 2000;191(3):417–422.

39. Nicholas J. Human herpesvirus-8–encoded signalling ligands and receptors. J Biomed Sci 2003;10(5):475–489.

40. Dekker AH. Fostering acceptance of human papillomavirus vaccines. J Am Osteopath Assoc 2006;106(3 Suppl 1):S14–S18.

41. Sun XK, Chen JF, Xu AE. A homozygous nonsense mutation in the EVER2 gene leads to epidermodysplasia verruciformis. Clin Exp Dermatol 2005;30(5):573–574.

42. Ramoz N, Rueda LA, Bouadjar B, et al. Mutations in two adjacent novel genes are associated with epidermodysplasia verruciformis. Nat Genet 2002;32(4):579–581.

43. Lane JE, Bowman PH, Cohen DJ. Epidermodysplasia verruciformis. South Med J 2003;96(5):613–615.

44. Trottier H, Franco EL. The epidemiology of genital human papillomavirus infection. Vaccine 2005 Dec 13; [Epub ahead of print].

45. Beasley RP, Hwang LY, Lin CC, et al. Hepatocellular carcinoma and hepatitis B virus. A prospective study of 22,707 men in Taiwan. Lancet 1981;2(8256):1129–1133.
46. Szmuness W. Hepatocellular carcinoma and the hepatitis B virus: evidence for a causal association. Prog Med Virol 1978;24:40–69.
47. Sun CA, Wu DM, Lin CC, et al. Incidence and cofactors of hepatitis C virus–related hepatocellular carcinoma: a prospective study of 12,008 men in Taiwan. Am J Epidemiol 2003;157(8):674–682.
48. Nakamoto Y, Guidotti LG, Kuhlen CV, et al. Immune pathogenesis of hepatocellular carcinoma. Exp Med 1998;188(2): 341–350.
49. Chisari FV, Klopchin K, Moriyama T, et al. Molecular pathogenesis of hepatocellular carcinoma in hepatitis B virus transgenic mice. Cell 1989;59(6):1145–1156.
50. Kim CM, Koike K, Saito I, et al. HBx gene of hepatitis B virus induces liver cancer in transgenic mice. Nature 1991; 351(6324):317–320.
51. Gallo R. Human retroviruses after 20 years: a perspective from the past and prospects for their future control. Immunol Rev 2002;185:236–265.
52. Chu ZL, DiDonato JA, Hawiger J, et al. The tax oncoprotein of human T-cell leukemia virus type 1 associates with and persistently activates IkappaB kinases containing IKKalpha and IKKbeta. J Biol Chem 1998;273(26):15891– 15894.
53. Vilchez RA, Kozinetz CA, Arrington AS, et al. Simian virus 40 in human cancers. Am J Med 2003;114(8):675–684.
54. Arrington AS, Butel JS. SV40 and human tumors. In Khalili K, Stoner GL, eds. Human Polyomaviruses: Molecular and Clinical Perspectives. New York: Wiley-Liss Inc; 2001:431– 460.
55. Cerrano PG, Jasani B, Filiberti R, et al. Simian virus 40 and malignant mesothelioma [review]. Int J Oncol 2003;22(1): 187–194.
56. Barbanti-Brodano G, Sabbioni S, Martini F, et al. Simian virus 40 infection in humans and association with human diseases: results and hypotheses. Virology 2004;318(1): 1–9.
57. Imperiale MJ, Pass HI, Sanda MG. Prospects for an SV40 vaccine. Semin Cancer Biol 2001;11(1):81–85.
58. Xie YC, Hwang C, Overwijk W, et al. Induction of tumor antigen-specific immunity in vivo by a novel vaccinia vector encoding safety-modified simian virus 40 T antigen. J Natl Cancer Inst 1999;91(2):169–175.
59. Saenz-Robles MT, Sullivan CS, Pipas JM. Transforming functions of Simian virus 40. Oncogene 2001;20(54):7899– 7907.
60. Wootton SK, Halbert CL, Miller AD. Sheep retrovirus structural protein induces lung tumours. Nature 2005; 434(7035):904–907.
61. McGee-Estrada K, Palmarini M, Hallwirth C. A Moloney murine leukemia virus driven by the jaagsiekte sheep retrovirus enhancers shows enhanced specificity for infectivity in lung epithelial cells. Virus Genes 2005;31(3):257–263.
62. Yousem SA, Finkelstein SD, Swalsky PA, et al. Absence of jaagsiekte sheep retrovirus DNA and RNA in bronchioloalveolar and conventional human pulmonary adenocarcinoma by PCR and RT-PCR analysis. Hum Pathol 2001; 32(10):1039–1042.
63. Hiatt KM, Highsmith WE. Lack of DNA evidence for jaagsiekte sheep retrovirus in human bronchioloalveolar carcinoma. Hum Pathol 2002;33(6):680.
64. Engels EA, Brock MV, Chen J, et al. Elevated incidence of lung cancer among HIV-infected individuals. J Clin Oncol 2006;24(9):1383–1388.
65. Lavole A, Wislez M, Antoine M, et al. Lung cancer, a new challenge in the HIV-infected population. Lung Cancer 2006;51(1):1–11.
66. Brouchet L, Valmary S, Dahan M, et al. Detection of oncogenic virus genomes and gene products in lung carcinoma. Br J Cancer 2005;92(4):743–746.
67. Conway EJ, Hudnall SD, Lazarides A, et al. Absence of evidence for an etiologic role for Epstein-Barr virus in neoplasms of the lung and pleura. Mod Pathol 1996;9(5):491– 495.
68. Coissard CJ, Besson G, Polette MC, et al. Prevalence of human papillomaviruses in lung carcinomas: a study of 218 cases. Mod Pathol 2005;18(12):1606–1609.
69. zur Hausen H. Viruses in human cancers. Science 1991; 254(5035):1167–1173.
70. Butel JS. Viral carcinogenesis: revelation of molecular mechanisms and etiology of human disease. Carcinogenesis 2000;21(3):405–426.
71. Yokota J, Nishioka M, Tani M, Kohno T. Genetic alterations responsible for metastatic phenotypes of lung cancer cells. Clin Exp Metastasis 2003;20(3):189–193.

Section 4
Molecular Pathology of Pulmonary and Pleural Neoplasms: Specific Histologic Types

25
Adenocarcinoma and Its Precursor Lesions

Helmut H. Popper

Why Is Adenocarcinoma Now the Most Common Lung Carcinoma?

In the 1940s and 1950s, squamous cell carcinomas and small cell carcinomas (SCLCs) were regarded as the cigarette smoke–associated carcinomas, whereas adenocarcinomas were not. Even in the mid-1980s squamous cell carcinomas and SCLCs were the leading carcinomas in Europe, the United States, and southeast Asia. In an autopsy survey performed at the Medical University of Graz from 1980 to 1986, there were 35% lung cancer deaths from squamous cell carcinoma, 25% from SCLC, and only 12% adenocarcinomas (in Austria all patients dying in hospitals can be autopsied, the decision being made by the pathologist). In a second survey from the same institution from 1990 to 1996 adenocarcinoma was the most common at 37% of all lung cancer deaths (personal observation). In a combined survey of lung cancer biopsy tissue and resected lung cancer, adenocarcinoma further increased to 42% in 2001 and now is the leading lung cancer in most industrialized countries.

In 1950, the first large-scale epidemiologic studies demonstrated that lung cancer is causatively associated with cigarette smoking. Although cigarette consumption has gradually decreased in most industrialized countries, death from lung cancer has reached a high among males and females. In the younger cohorts, the lung cancer death rate is decreasing in both men and women in parallel with the relative increase of lung adenocarcinoma. Contributors to this change in the histologic types of lung cancer are a decrease in average nicotine and tar content of cigarettes from about 2.7 and 38mg in 1955 to 1.0 and 13.5mg in 1993, respectively, and the use of "light" cigarettes. Other major factors relate to changes in the composition of the cigarette tobacco blend and to a general acceptance of cigarettes with filter tips. However, smokers compensate for the lowered nicotine content, especially of "light" cigarettes by inhaling the smoke more deeply and by smoking more intensely. Under these conditions, the peripheral lung is exposed to increased amounts of carcinogens in the tobacco smoke, which then is suspected to lead to lung adenocarcinoma.

Importantly, because of the efficacy of the filters, particulate matter with bound carcinogens are withheld in the filters, but vaporized toxins and carcinogens are enriched in the tobacco smoke and delivered to the alveolar periphery. Among the significant changes in the composition of the tobacco blend is a significant increase in nitrate content (from 0.5% to 1.2%–1.5%), which raises the yields of nitrogen oxides and N-nitrosamines in the smoke. Furthermore, the more intense smoking by the consumers of low-yield cigarettes increases N-nitrosamines in the smoke two- to threefold. Among the N-nitrosamines is 4-(methylnitrosamino)-1-(3-pyridyl)-1-butanone (NNK), a powerful lung carcinogen in animals that is exclusively formed from nicotine. This organ- and tobacco-specific nitrosamine is capable of inducing adenocarcinoma in the lung.[1] Given the long latency of approximately 20–25 years for clinical manifestations of lung cancer, it is understandable why we started seeing more adenocarcinoma in the 1990s, 25 years after filtered cigarettes were introduced. The effect of using filters has been evaluated in animal experiments. Mice were exposed to either full tobacco smoke or to filtered tobacco smoke devoid of particulate matter. Analysis of the filtered smoke showed reduced concentrations of polycyclic aromatic hydrocarbons and tobacco smoke–specific nitrosamines below 18%. Aldehydes and other volatile organic compounds such as 1,3-butadiene, benzene, and acrolein were not as much reduced (about 50% to 90%). Some potentially carcinogenic metals reached levels in filtered smoke ranging from 77% to less than 1%. However, mice exposed to the filtered tobacco smoke atmosphere had practically identical lung tumor yield and incidence as had the animals being exposed to unfiltered smoke. Witschi therefore concluded that 1,3-butadiene might be an important contributor to lung tumorigenesis in this mouse model of tobacco smoke carcinogenesis.[2]

Cigarette Smoke, Filtered Versus Unfiltered Cigarettes, and Their Carcinogens

Some of the toxic effects of tobacco substances discussed here are also covered in Chapter 49, with redundancy avoided as much as possible. The protective system of the respiratory tract is discussed only in Chapter 49.

Tobacco smoking results in inhalation of various amounts of toxins that can induce a wide variety of effects on different cell systems in the respiratory tract. The toxins are acidic as well as basic; heat is also harmful to the respiratory tract. The most toxic substances are within the vapor phase of tobacco sidestream smoke and cause respiratory epithelial damage.[3] Many tobacco smoke constituents are potent inducers of oxygen radicals and thus cause DNA strand breaks, DNA adducts, oxidative DNA damage, chromosome aberrations, and micronucleus formation.[4] In addition, they also can affect the mitotic spindle apparatus and influence the methylation of promoter regions of tumor suppressor genes.[5-8] In addition, many metal oxides, such as chromium, cadmium, and arsenic oxides, are generated during tobacco burning. Many of these can either generate oxygen radicals or act as catalyzing agents in concert with nitroso compounds in generating these radicals. A comprehensive list of tobacco constituents can be found in articles published by Zaridze et al.[9] and Stabbert et al.[10] as well as in publications by the International Agency for Cancer Research (http://www.iarc.fr/IARCPress/index.php).

For some of these components the mechanisms of their toxic and carcinogenic action has been elucidated. The nitrosamine 4-(methylnitrosamino)-1-(3-pyridyl)-1-butanone is formed by nitrosation of nicotine. It simultaneously stimulates Bcl-2 and c-Myc phosphorylation through activation of both extracellular signal-regulated kinases (ERK) 1 and 2 and protein kinase C (PKC)-α, which is required for NNK-induced survival and proliferation. Phosphorylation of Bcl-2 promotes a direct interaction between Bcl-2 and c-Myc in the nucleus and on the outer mitochondrial membrane that significantly enhances the half-life of the c-Myc protein. Thus, NNK induces a functional cooperation of Bcl-2 and c-Myc in promoting cell survival and proliferation.[11]

Nicotine and NNK also activate the Akt pathway and increase cell proliferation and survival. Nicotinic activation of Akt increases phosphorylation of multiple downstream substrates of Akt in a time-dependent manner, including glycogen synthase kinase-3, forkhead in rhab-

domyosarcoma, tuberin, the molecular target of rapamycin, and p70S6K1. In addition, nicotine decreased apoptosis. Tsurutani and colleagues thus demonstrated tobacco component–induced, Akt-dependent proliferation, and nuclear factor (NF)-κB–dependent survival of cancer cells.[12]

Herzog and coworkers showed that NNK-induced cervical intraepithelial neoplasia in mice and found that a genotoxic metabolite of this carcinogen causes numerous karyotypic changes in lung epithelial cells and modulates the evolutionary pathway of mouse adenocarcinomas. Each of these chromosomes contains sites of orthology with those altered in human lung adenocarcinomas, suggesting similar roles in human lung cancer.[13] From the studies on mutations of the *TP53* gene in normal-appearing epithelial cells, which usually precede the development of dysplasia, it has become clear that many of the different tobacco carcinogens leave their specific "fingerprint" by interacting specifically with some genes within the cell cycle.[14]

The Architecture of Bronchi, Bronchioles, and Alveoli and Their Cellular Constituents

The architecture of the human bronchial system and the composition of the epithelial lining system highlight another aspect of the modification of inhaled substances, especially tobacco smoke. In humans as in primates, the branching of the bronchial tree is asymmetric. A bronchus divides into a main branch with a diameter of two thirds and a smaller one with one third of the diameter. This gives rise to air flow turbulences at the bifurcations, causing a deposition of particulates according to their respective sizes: the larger particles will be deposited at larger bronchial bifurcations, and the smaller (<2.5 μm) will reach the alveolar periphery.

The particle phase in tobacco smoke is composed of ash but also contains incompletely combusted particles from tobacco plants, such as nitrosamines and polycyclic aromatic hydrocarbons, and metal oxides. Coal and incompletely combusted plant particles have the tendency to bind polycyclic aromatic hydrocarbons and nitrosylated hydrocarbons either chemically or physically and thus prolong the time of contact of the harmful chemicals with the respiratory epithelium. This results in a toxin- and carcinogen-rich particle fraction acting at larger bifurcations during the era of the filterless cigarettes.

Regeneration and Its Implications

After an acute inflammatory reaction, normally the epithelium is restored to its full function. However, when the inhalation of toxic substances persists, adaptive changes will take place. This is dependent on the location of the lesion. Whereas columnar cell hyperplasia followed by goblet cell hyperplasia, and finally transitional and squamous cell metaplasia are the main steps of repair and protection in the large bronchi,[15] proliferation of Clara cells, secretory and goblet cell hyperplasia as well as pneumocyte type II proliferation, resulting in the so-called cuboidal transformation of the epithelium, can be found in the bronchioles and the bronchoalveolar region. This results in different types of dysplasia, such as bronchiolar columnar cell dysplasia in bronchioles[16] and atypical adenomatous hyperplasia in alveoli.[17] Rarely squamous cell metaplasia can be encountered in the peripheral lung, most often associated with the effects of cytotoxic drugs.

The effects of tobacco smoke on the DNA repair system have been investigated in recent years.[18–20] Another important mechanism especially investigated in lung cancer is gene silencing by methylation. Promoter methylation of several tumor suppressor genes is an early event in tobacco smoke–induced carcinogenesis and occurs long before dysplastic changes of the epithelium take place and thus might also influence the remodeling of the architecture.[6,8,21–24]

Atypical Adenomatous Hyperplasia, Bronchiolar Columnar Cell Dysplasia, Atypical Goblet Cell Hyperplasia, and Other Lesions?

Given the wide spectrum of differentiation of adenocarcinomas, not much is known about the precursor lesions. Atypical adenomatous hyperplasia (AAH) is regarded as the precursor of bronchoalveolar adenocarcinoma.[17,25,26] It usually consists of an atypical proliferation of pneumocyte and Clara cell-like elements, covering the alveolar septa in a lepidic fashion. However, given the variants of bronchoalveolar carcinoma, AAH just represents the classic variant, whereas the precursors for mucinous, tall columnar, and sclerosing bronchoalveolar carcinoma are unknown. Expanding these thoughts further, what are the precursor lesions for mixed, papillary, colloid, and solid adenocarcinomas?

Recently, bronchiolar columnar cell dysplasia (BCCD) was described as a precursor for adenocarcinomas arising from bronchioles[16] and bronchial epithelial dysplasia for adenocarcinomas arising from larger bronchi.[15] In BCCD an increase in chromosomal aberrations was demonstrated from 2.6 in BCCD to 14.7 in concomitant adenocarcinomas. Among the aberrations were losses of 3p, 9, 13, and 14 and gains of 1q, 17, 19q, and 20q.[16] In congenital cystic adenomatous malformations in children, a proliferation of atypical goblet cells and development of tumors have been described.[27,28] Stacher et al. presented data

confirming the preneoplastic nature of these goblet cell proliferations, which might give rise to mucinous adenocarcinomas.[29] In both atypical goblet cell hyperplasia and the concomitant adenocarcinomas gains of chromosomes 2 and 4 were found. This fits well with the predominance of gains reported in adenocarcinomas of nonsmokers. In addition, Stacher et al. found nuclear expression of interleukin (IL)-13, IL-4Rα, and MUC2. This likely reflects an association with goblet cell differentiation, but it also drives proliferation in atypical goblet cell hyperplasia.[29]

The Role of Cancer Stem Cells

The most common theory for cancer development is mutations caused by carcinogens acting on the genomic integrity of local stem cells within the lung. An alternate theory has been proposed, that lung cancer is a bone marrow stem cell–derived disease. Chronic cigarette smoking results in lung inflammation and epithelial damage that activates a chronic wound repair program. Recent studies have demonstrated that bone marrow–derived stem cells can respond to epithelial wounding and contribute to epithelial repair. The identification of cancer stem cells that are distinct from the bulk tumor cells through their ability to self-renew may suggest that such cells are important in the development of lung cancer. Confirmation of the hypothesis would suggest that the transition time from a normal cell to overt cancer cell may be much shorter than that based on the multistep cancer progression model. This theory also implies that bone marrow–derived lung cancer stem cells would require stem cell poisons for cure.[30]

Injury models have suggested that the lung contains anatomically and functionally distinct epithelial stem cell populations. Identified at the bronchoalveolar duct junction, bronchoalveolar stem cells were resistant to bronchiolar and alveolar damage and proliferated during epithelial cell renewal. Bronchoalveolar stem cells expanded in response to oncogenic K-ras in culture and in precursors of lung tumors in vivo. These data support the hypothesis that bronchoalveolar stem cells are a stem cell population that maintains the bronchiolar Clara cells and alveolar cells of the distal lung and that their transformed counterparts give rise to adenocarcinoma.[31] In the central portion of the lung other stem cells might reside that are supposed to give rise to small cell carcinoma.

The stem cell theory and all its implications with respect to organ stem cell–based lung carcinogenesis are now widely accepted. However, the theory that bone marrow–derived stem cells might also be capable of giving rise to lung cancer needs more research and support before being accepted as an alternative cell pool for cancer cells. In addition, the origin of tumor–associated stroma cells is still an enigma. While most investigators believe that these cells represent a host reaction toward the invading cancer cells, there is accumulation of data that indicate in some cases this might be true, but in others the stroma cells are also genetically modified by the carcinogens and thus may be part of the tumor.

The Bronchoalveolar Carcinoma Story: Is There Room for a Noninvasive Adenocarcinoma?

In the 1999 and 2004 WHO classifications, bronchoalveolar carcinoma was defined as a noninvasive adenocarcinoma arising from the bronchoalveolar region and growing along alveolar septa with no or minimal inflammation.[32] This has decreased the numbers of bronchoalveolar carcinomas dramatically. Arguments for this new definition were the much better prognosis and the observation that in the invasive portion there is no longer a bronchoalveolar pattern.

This new definition has increased the problem of sampling error or the workload, because ideally bronchoalveolar carcinoma cases now should be sampled completely to avoid missing the invasive portion. In addition, this definition suffers from two problems: In all other organ systems carcinomas are defined by their ability to invade the stroma. A mucinous adenocarcinoma anywhere in the body does not change its name. It starts as in situ carcinoma and invades. Not surprisingly, if a bronchoalveolar carcinoma invades, it has to change its shape, because within the stroma there are no alveoli to be covered. A round shape is the most efficient structure to nurture all cells equally; the distance to the nearest blood vessel is optimal for all cells. Therefore, most bronchoalveolar carcinomas acquire a tubular architecture when invading the lung stroma. In the present classification a bronchoalveolar carcinoma that invades the lung is reclassified into mixed adenocarcinoma, because it usually presents itself with tubular structures in its invasive portion. In this respect in lung pathology there is a special adenocarcinoma for a peripheral in situ adenocarcinoma. The other problem is distinction from AAH. In the present classification bronchoalveolar carcinoma is separated from AAH by a higher grade of atypia and a size ≥5 mm in diameter. Grade of atypia is a subjective criterion generally with low interobserver agreement. At present no criteria exist for atypia grading. Size, on the other hand, is an unreliable factor. Highly aggressive adenocarcinomas may invade even when they are 3 mm, whereas slowly proliferating adenocarcinomas may reach considerable size before invading the stroma.

However, there are unique features that make bronchoalveolar carcinoma an unusual variant of adenocarcinoma. In contrast to all the other adenocarcinomas, bronchoalveolar carcinoma does not induce a desmoplastic stroma reaction, and there is no angioneogenesis as seen in any other pulmonary carcinoma. This highlights a unique way of nutrition in bronchoalveolar carcinoma. Bronchoalveolar carcinoma most probably uses the available vascular network extensively. This aspect has not been looked at scientifically and may contain many interesting aspects of the biology of this unique variant of adenocarcinoma.

Genomic Aberrations in Adenocarcinoma

Aberrations of the tumor DNA in adenocarcinomas have been described in several studies. Generally adenocarcinomas have less balanced chromosomal aberrations then other non–small cell carcinomas (NSCLCs). With array comparative genomic hybridization, several types of chromosomal aberrations can be seen, from simple to more complex types (Figure 25.1). This may be relevant prognosis, metastasis, or survival and needs further investigation.

In loss of heterozygosity (LOH) studies, losses have been found at 9p in the earliest stage of lung cancer development.[33] Within the chromosomal loss described on 9q, the well-known tumor suppressor gene *TSC1* (tuberous sclerosis gene 1) is found, whereas *TSC2* is located on the short arm of chromosome 16. Loss of heterozygosity on 9q34 (the *TSC1* position) is frequently found in adenocarcinomas. A partial LOH at *TSC*1 and/or *TSC2* was observed more frequently in cases of well-differentiated adenocarcinoma and associated AAH. *TSC1* and *TSC2* thus might be involved in the development of lung adenocarcinoma.[34]

In another study, Kitaguchi et al. confirmed these findings and added losses on 3p and 17p.[35] They also analyzed AAH and concomitant adenocarcinomas. Loss of heterozygosity was found in a few AAH lesions, usually those with pronounced atypia, while marked LOH was seen in the corresponding carcinomas. These results indicated for the first time that AAH could be the preneoplastic stage of lung adenocarcinoma.[35]

Similarly, Takamochi et al. found LOH on 9q with increasing frequency in AAH and adenocarcinomas. Less frequently LOH was seen on 16p. This again points to a causal relationship of the *TSC1* and *TSC2* genes or another neighboring tumor suppressor gene on 9q for early stages of lung adenocarcinoma.[36]

In a comparative study of squamous cell carcinoma and adenocarcinomas, Petersen et al. have found chromosomal losses in both on chromosomes 1p, 3p, 4q, 5q, 6q, 8p, 9p, 13q, 18q, and 21q and gains for chromosomes 5p, 8q, 11q13, 16p, 17q, and 19q.[37] However, they also found differences. Adenocarcinomas more frequently showed gains of chromosome 1q and losses on chromosomes 3q, 9q, 10p, and 19, whereas squamous cell carcinomas were characterized by gains of chromosome 3q and 12p as well as deletions of 2q. In particular, the overrepresentation of the chromosomal band 1q23 and the deletion at 9q22 were significantly associated with adenocarcinoma differentiation.[37] *FHIT*, a well known gene (on 3p) deleted in almost all small cell carcinomas, was less frequently deleted in adenocarcinomas and occurred at a relatively late developmental stage.[38] Similarly, Wong et al. reported gains in decreasing order from 16p followed by gain of 20q, with overlapping regions at 16p13.1–p13.2 and 20q13.2, respectively[39]. Other overrepresented loci were observed at 5p, 7p, 8q, 12q 17q, and 19q; DNA underrepresentation was observed less commonly and included 8p, 9p, 13q, and 18q[39] The investigative group headed by Sy focused on differences between adenocarcinomas and squamous cell carcinomas and found common gains of 1q21–q24, 5p15–p14, and 8q22–q24.1 and losses of 17p13–p12 in both carcinomas, whereas gains of 2p13–p11.2, 3q25–q29, 9q13–q34, 12p, 12q12–q15, and 17q21 and loss of 8p were preferentially associated with squamous cell carcinoma. As determined with spectral karyotyping analysis, rearrangements involved t(1;13), t(1;15), t(7;8), t(8;15), t(8;9), t(2;17) and t(15;20) translocations. The t(8;12) translocation was exclusively found in adenocarcinomas.[40]

The chromosomal region 17p was studied in detail by Tsuchiya and colleagues.[41] They found allelic losses on D17S379 to be associated with advanced lesions of adenocarcinomas, while D17S513 was more frequently deleted in poorly differentiated tumors. Therefore, a new tumor suppressor gene was proposed on chromosome 17p13.3 distal to the *p53* gene, with a probable role in progression and differentiation of adenocarcinomas.[41]

Aoyagi et al. have published a very useful study that covers the progression from AAH to invasive bronchioloalveolar adenocarcinomas.[42] Their stepwise progression model starts with AAH and progresses to noninvasive bronchoalveolar carcinoma with atelectasis (type B) and finally to invasive bronchoalveolar carcinoma (type C). It was shown that from type A to type C a significant rise in allelic losses of 3p, 17p, 18q, and 22q occurred.[42]

This view was also confirmed by data from the study of Ullmann et al., who showed an increasing number of chromosomal aberrations from low-grade AAH, via high-grade AAH, to invasive adenocarcinoma and noninvasive bronchoalveolar adenocarcinoma.[26] A high degree of overlap among genetic changes was found in high-grade AAH, bronchoalveolar carcinoma, and adenocarcinoma within individual patients.

In another investigation, genetic aberrations were compared between smokers and never-smokers. Losses or gains at chromosomal arms 3p, 6q, 9p, 16p, 17p, and 19p were present more often in adenocarcinomas from smokers than from nonsmokers. Allelic imbalances in adenocarcinomas from nonsmokers were rare but occurred more often at 19q, 12p, and 9p. In general, aberrations in chromosomes 1–5 were rare in adenocarcinomas from never-smokers but common in smokers (Figure 25.2). These observations support the idea that lung cancers in nonsmokers arise through genetic alterations distinct from the common events observed in tumors from smokers.[43]

Specific Gene Loci in Adenocarcinomas

Different genes and gene loci were investigated in several studies. Mucin genes such as *MUC5AC* and *MUC5B* are related to mucus formation in adenocarcinomas. Mucinous bronchoalveolar carcinoma has a particular pattern of mucin gene expression, indicating that it has sustained a well-differentiated phenotype similar to the goblet cell. *MUC4* is the earlier mucin gene expressed in the foregut, before epithelial differentiation, and is expressed independently of mucous secretion in both normal adult airways and carcinomas. In addition to their function in differentiation, these genes are also associated with proliferation.[44,45]

p16 is located on chromosome 9p21, a region with frequent LOH in lung cancer. However, more frequent than loss is aberrant methylation of the p16 promoter region resulting in negative p16 protein expression. Alterations of the *p16* gene were associated with poor prognosis, and in particular the prognosis of patients with aberrant p16 methylation was significantly worse than that of patients without aberrant methylation. These alterations were associated with bronchoalveolar carcinoma and non–bronchoalveolar carcinoma.[46]

Yokota et al. confirmed the frequent inactivation of the $p16^{INK4A}/Rb$ and *p53* genes in adenocarcinomas.[47] In addition, the authors identified *MYO18B* on chromosome 22q12.1 as a novel myosin family gene. This gene is inactivated in approximately 50% of lung cancers by deletions, mutations, and methylation. The restoration of *MYO18B* suppressed anchorage-independent growth of lung cancer cells, making the *MYO18B* gene a strong candidate for a metastasis suppressor gene of human lung cancer.[47]

The gene most frequently studied in squamous and adenocarcinomas is epidermal growth factor receptor (*EGFR*). Epidermal growth factor receptor protein overexpression was observed more frequently in squamous cell carcinomas but also in 80% of the bronchoalveolar carcinomas. The prevalent fluorescence in situ hybridization patterns were balanced disomy and trisomy for the

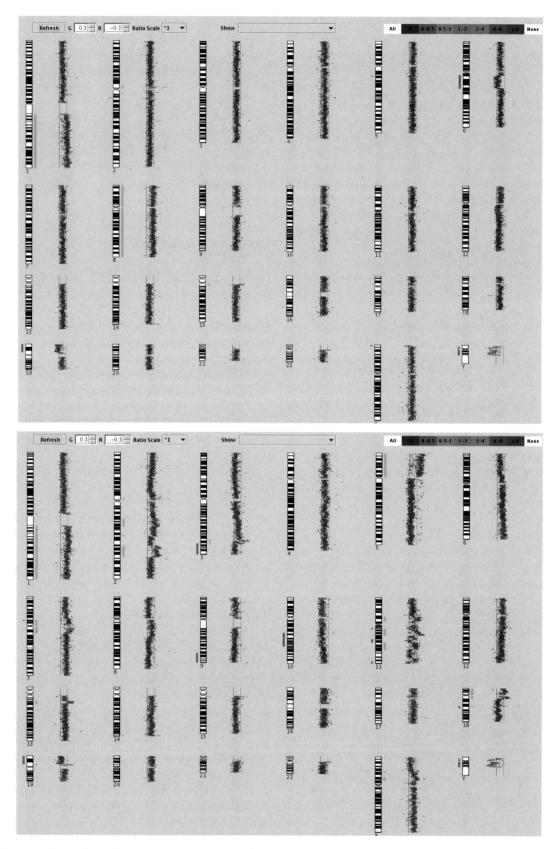

FIGURE 25.1. Complex and simple aberrations in adenocarcinomas. Array comparative genomic hybridization of two cases. (Presented at the United States and Canadian Academy of Pathology meeting, San Antonio, March 2005.)

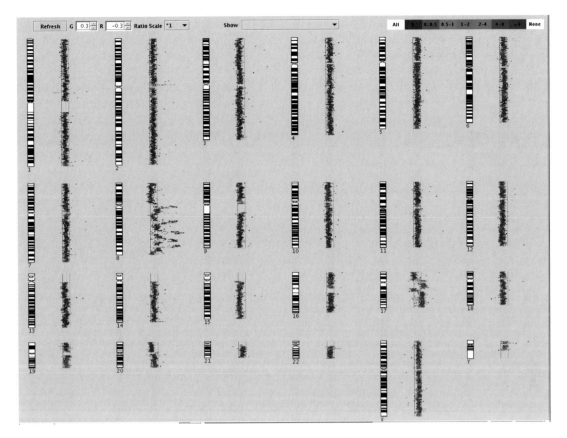

FIGURE 25.1. *Continued*

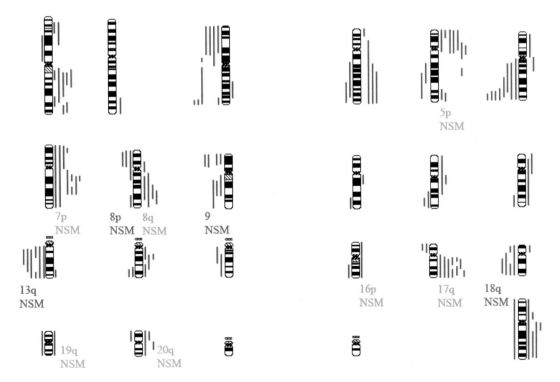

FIGURE 25.2. Chromosomal aberrations in adenocarcinomas of smokers and never-smokers based on personal investigations and literature data.

EGFR gene, whereas balanced polysomy and gene amplification were less frequently seen in the patients. Gene copy number correlated with protein expression. Overexpression of EGFR and high gene copy numbers had no significant influence on prognosis.[48] This gene and its signaling cascade are discussed in more detail later.

The K-*ras* oncogene has long been associated with adenocarcinoma histology. K-*ras* mutations were detected at codon 12 in approximately 40% of adenocarcinomas and large cell carcinomas. Interestingly, all of the lung adenocarcinomas and large cell carcinomas containing a K-*ras* mutation exhibited allelic loss of the wild-type K-*ras* allele when a correlation between LOH of the region on chromosome 12p and K-*ras* mutation was made. These results provide strong evidence that the wild-type K-*ras* is a tumor suppressor.[49]

The finding of an association between K-*ras* mutation and loss of wild-type allele was not confirmed in another study. Uchiyama et al.[50] showed more mutated K-*ras* than wild-type mRNA expression in cell lines. By immunohistochemical analysis, positive staining for K-*ras* was found in the vast majority of NSCLCs, indicating a wild-type K-*ras* expression. These findings indicate that the wild-type K-*ras* allele is occasionally lost in human lung cancer and that the oncogenic activation of mutant K-*ras* is more frequently associated with an overexpression of the mutant allele than with a loss of the wild-type allele in human NSCLC development.[50]

Yanagitani et al. identified a new gene locus at chromosome 19q13.3.[51] The results of this study suggest that the chromosome 19q13.3 region contains a gene or genes associated with lung adenocarcinoma risk. The specific gene or genes have not been identified thus far.

RNA Expression in Adenocarcinoma

In general, cDNA expression arrays have not fulfilled what has been expected from this fascinating technology. Moreover, many of these initial reports have not been expanded into functional analyses of the identified RNAs. However, in these reports there is still a wealth of information hidden, waiting to be explored.

Mutations of *EGFR*, *HER2/neu*, and K-*ras* are frequently found in pulmonary adenocarcinomas. Methylation percentages of the genes ranged from 13% to 54%. Mutations of the three genes were never found to be present simultaneously, whereas methylation tended to be present synchronously. *CRBP1* and *CDH13* methylation were good indicators of CpG methylation phenotype in NSCLC and were correlated with a poorer prognosis in adenocarcinomas. An *EGFR* mutation had an inverse correlation with methylation of SPARC (secreted protein acidic and rich in cysteine), an extracellular Ca^{2+}-binding

matricellular glycoprotein associated with the regulation of cell adhesion and growth, and the *p16^INK4A* gene.[52] K-*ras* mutations occurred in adenocarcinoma and were associated with smokers, men, and poorly differentiated adenocarcinoma. Regression analysis showed smoking history was the significant determinant for *EGFR* and K-*ras* mutations, whereas gender was a confounding factor. *EGFR* mutations are prevalent in lung adenocarcinoma and plays a prominent oncogenic role in never-smokers,[53] whereas K-*ras* mutations are associated with cigarette smoking status.[54] The high-risk predicting role of *p185^c-erbB2* expression and a K-*ras* mutation in lung adenocarcinoma was confirmed by the study of Kern et al.[55]

K-*ras* codon 12 mutations were detected in 39% of the AAHs and 42% of the adenocarcinomas. In patients with both an AAH and a synchronous lung adenocarcinoma, one third had a K-*ras* mutation in the adenocarcinoma but not in the AAH, another one third had mutations in the AAH but not in the adenocarcinoma, and the rest did not harbor mutations in either the AAH or the adenocarcinoma or had mutations in both. In just one patient the same K-*ras* mutation was present in the AAHs and adenocarcinoma of the patient. The detection of independent activating point mutations in a cancer-causing gene points to the neoplastic nature of AAH and suggests that glandular neoplasm of the lung arises from a background of field cancerization.[56]

Several array studies tried to identify novel genes and also compared different subtypes of NSCLC. An investigation using a large cDNA microarray recapitulated morphologic classification of squamous, large cell, small cell, and adenocarcinoma based on gene expression patterns. Not surprisingly, genes associated with bronchiolar and alveolar cell proteins such as Clara cell proteins and surfactant apoproteins were found to be upregulated in adenocarcinomas. A subclassification of adenocarcinomas correlating with the degree of tumor differentiation as well as patient survival was proposed.[57] In another array study. Singhal and colleagues identified 40 genes differentially expressed in lung adenocarcinomas.[58] For several genes, such as *cyclin B1, cyclin D1, p21, and MDM2*, the data available from other reports were confirmed. In addition, 19 novel genes were identified, among them many cell cycle regulating genes such as *Cdc2, Cdc20, cyclin F, cullin 4A, cullin 5, ZAC, p57, DP-1, p34, GADD45*, and *PISSLRE*.

Endoh et al. separated adenocarcinomas by hierarchical clustering into three major groups, one of them with significant poor survival. *PTK7, CIT, SCNN1A, PGES, ERO1L, ZWINT*, and two *EST*s were identified as having particular predictive value.[59] Thus far these genes have not been confirmed by an independent study.

In another cDNA array study using 308 apoptotic genes, 24 genes, including *Akt*, *Bcl-xL*, *PTEN*, and *Fas* were predicted to be differentially expressed in lung adenocarcinomas. In addition, *RIP*, *caspase-1*, and *PDK-1* were identified as novel genes.[60] Expanding the importance of antiapoptotic mechanisms, Chen and colleagues showed in a cell culture study that overexpression of *p-FADD* leads to an increase in NF-κB activity and a decrease in the number of cells in the G2 phase of the cell cycle.[61] With cDNA microarray analysis increased levels of *FADD* transcripts were significantly correlated with an overexpression of cyclins D1 and B1. The induction of NF-κB activity might facilitate cell cycle progression and be the underlying molecular basis for aggressive tumor behavior of lung adenocarcinoma.[61] Another group of antiapoptotic proteins were identified in NSCLC: the isoforms β, γ, σ, and τ of the antiapoptotic protein 14-3-3; 14-3-3ε and ζ were present in abundance.[62]

Two studies stressed the importance of angiogenesis and vascular endothelial growth factor (VEGF) expression. In the study by Su et al., cyclooxygenase-2 (COX-2) expression or prostaglandin E_2 treatment activated the HER2/neu receptor and induced VEGF-C. The Src kinase was involved in the VEGF-C upregulation by prostaglandin E_2. In immunohistochemical investigations, the COX-2 level in lung adenocarcinoma was highly correlated with VEGF-C and lymphatic vessels density. This means that COX-2 upregulates VEGF-C and promotes lymphangiogenesis via the EP1/Src/HER2/neu signaling pathway.[63] In the study by Saad et al., coexpression for p53 and HER2/neu predicted the worst outcome in adenocarcinomas. In bronchoalveolar carcinoma HER2/neu, p53, and VEGF were significantly less expressed. Vascular epithelial growth factor was associated with angiolymphatic invasion in conventional adenocarcinoma.[64] In another study a correlation of tumor microvessel count with IL-8 mRNA expression was demonstrated. Interleukin-8 mRNA expression was not only associated with angiogenesis but also tumor progression, survival, and time to relapse.[65] How this correlated with VEGF induction is not clear yet.

Another protein with the regulation of VEGF was recently described. The reversion-inducing cysteine-rich protein with Kazal motifs (*RECK*) was isolated as a transformation suppressor gene and encodes a membrane-anchored regulator of the matrix metalloproteinases. The *RECK gene* can suppress tumor invasion, metastasis and angiogenesis. Expression of *RECK* and tumor angiogenesis were inversely correlated in adenocarcinomas. *RECK* most probably suppresses VEGF induced angiogenesis[66].

Overexpression of hepatocyte growth factor receptor (c-Met) was frequently detected in adenocarcinoma cells, and overexpression of hepatocyte growth factor (HGF) was detected in pneumocytes type II. Overexpression of HGF was correlated with cigarette smoking and tumor stages. Nicotine activated HGF expression in pneumocytes type II cells and in lung cancer cells.[67] Ma et al. demonstrated RNA for *c-Met* and c-Met protein especially in adenocarcinoma.[68] Phosphorylated c-Met was preferentially observed at the invasive front. *c-Met* alterations were identified within the semaphorin domain and the juxtamembrane domain. Downregulation of c-Met by small interfering RNA inhibited c-Met and subsequently phospho-Akt.[68]

The LKB1 kinase forms a complex with LMO4, GATA-6, and Ldb1 and enhances GATA-mediated transactivation. It has the potential to induce p21 expression in collaboration with LMO4, GATA-6, and Ldb1 through the p53-independent mechanism. This may be one of its important functions as a tumor suppressor.[69] In addition, LKB1 can activate the expression of *TSC1* and *TSC2* genes and activate the cyclic adenosine monophosphate-kinase α (AMPKα). *TCS1* and *TSC2* as well as AMPKα can inhibit directly or indirectly the activation of the Akt/mTOR pathway, probably another important tumor suppressor function.[70,71]

Silencing of the *RUNX3* gene may play an important role in the pathogenesis of lung adenocarcinoma. *RUNX3* methylation was significantly found more frequently in nonsmokers with adenocarcinoma histology.[72] *RUNX* genes are transcription factors within the transforming growth factor (TGF)-β signaling pathway and have been implicated in cell cycle regulation, differentiation, apoptosis, and malignant transformation.[24] *RUNX* genes also interact with *S100* genes, but this interaction is not clear yet. Borczuk et al. showed the importance of TGF-β.[73] Transforming growth factor-β receptor II downregulation seems to be an early event in lung adenocarcinoma metastasis. Repression of TGF-β receptor II in lung cancer cells increased tumor cell invasiveness and activated p38 mitogen-activated protein kinases.[73]

Hofmann et al. used an oligo-array and identified the transcription factors TTF1, DAT1, and TF-2 as being exclusively upregulated in adenocarcinomas.[74] In addition, matrix metalloproteinase-12 and urokinase plasminogen activator-α were associated with metastasis and thus predicted global survival of the patients.[74]

Field and colleagues looked for DNA methylation in squamous cell carcinomas and adenocarcinomas.[75] In squamous cell carcinomas, the *ARHI*, *MGMT*, *GP1β*, *RARβ*, and *TMEFF2* genes were methylated, whereas *TMEFF2*, *MGMT*, and *CDKNIC* genes were methylated in adenocarcinomas. Therefore, histologic types of lung cancer may be distinguished based on their specific methylation profiles.[75]

MicroRNA has been shown to play a major role in carcinogenesis. MicroRNAs regulate mRNA expression as well as translation into proteins. Yanaihara et al. studied miRNA expression profiles and correlated these with survival of lung adenocarcinomas.[76] High *hsa-mir-155* and low *hsa-let-7a-2* expression correlated with poor survival.

Proteomics of Adenocarcinoma

Proteomics is still in its infancy. Most important, many studies have analyzed protein expression only in non–small cell carcinomas and have not further subcategorized the different entities within NSCLC. Because the protein expression in adenocarcinomas differs from that in squamous cell carcinomas, these studies cannot be included in our focus. In other reports different NSCLCs were included and mentioned in the methods sections but not further separated in the results sections. Again, these studies, although interesting, cannot be evaluated. Probably similar to the situation in cDNA array studies, the study authors could only analyze a few cases and thus avoided discussing these entities separately because of statistical limitations. Proteomics, however, is more important than RNA expression, because proteins such as phosphorylated kinases will exert their effects, and a proof of an activated protein can be taken as evidence for functional signaling.

In one of the first two-dimensional fluorescence differential gel electrophoresis investigations, 32 protein spots were identified by hierarchical clustering and principal component analysis. The proteins corresponding to the spots were identified by mass spectrometry. Based on the expression profiles of the 32 spots, cancer cells were categorized into three histologic groups: the squamous cell carcinoma group, the adenocarcinoma group, and a group of carcinomas with other histologic types. These corresponded very well to the histologic classification, showing that there is a differential protein profile for each of these types.[77] Not surprisingly, many proteins, such as surfactant proteins, which are specifically expressed in peripheral lung tissue, belong to spatially expressed profiles. Because the majority of adenocarcinomas, in contrast to squamous cell carcinomas, arise in peripheral locations, these spatially expressed proteins are specific for one or the other group.

In a similar investigation, Keshamouni et al. identified 51 differentially expressed proteins by two-dimensional liquid chromatography tandem mass spectrometry.[78] Twenty-nine proteins were upregulated, and 22 proteins were downregulated. Downregulated proteins were predominantly enzymes involved in regulating nutrient or drug metabolism. The majority of the TGF-β–induced proteins (tropomyosins, filamins A and B, β$_1$-integrin, heat shock protein 27, transglutaminase 2, cofilin, 14-3-3 zeta, ezrin-radixin-moesin) are involved in the regulation of cell migration, adhesion, and invasion, suggesting the acquisition of an invasive phenotype.[78] In another study, four genes out of 42 proteins were identified, *PRDX1*, *EEF1A2*, *CALR*, and *KCIP-1*, in which elevated protein expression correlated with both increased DNA copy number and transcript levels. Specific inhibition of *EEF1A2* and *KCIP-1* expression in cell lines showed suppression of proliferation and induction of apoptosis. Immunohistochemical analysis of *EEF1A2* and *KCIP-1* in tissue microarrays showed that gene amplification was associated with high protein expression and that protein overexpression was related to tumor grade, disease stage, Ki-67 expression, and a shorter survival of patients with lung adenocarcinoma.[79]

In an immunohistochemical study, 86 proteins were evaluated, and the results were analyzed by nonparametric tests, hierarchical clustering, and principal component analysis. By the same statistical approach, it was possible to distinguish adenocarcinomas from squamous cell carcinomas with 98% accuracy. It was also possible to separate adenocarcinomas into three groups that significantly differed in survival. Cathepsin E and heat shock protein 105 were identified as previously unknown predictors of survival in lung adenocarcinoma.[80]

Out of these studies an interesting aspect evolved. Messenger RNA expression sometimes is and in other studies is not correlated with protein expression and synthesis. For example, mRNA coding for the important transcription factor eIF-5A was significantly increased in lung adenocarcinomas, but eIF-5A protein expression was not correlated to its mRNA levels, indicating that eIF-5A protein expression is posttranscriptionally regulated. Interestingly, high eIF-5A protein expression was correlated with poor survival.[81] From these findings it is evident that gene amplification needs to be accompanied by mRNA and protein overexpression. Furthermore, proteins need to be activated and modified to gain function.

Tsuta and coworkers compared pulmonary signet ring cell carcinomas, solid adenocarcinomas with mucin production, and mucinous variants of bronchoalveolar adenocarcinomas for the expression of MUC1, MUC5AC, MUC6, cytokeratin 7, and thyroid transcription factor TTF1.[82] Signet ring cell carcinomas and solid adenocarcinomas showed high expression of MUC1, cytokeratin 7, and TTF1 and low expression of MUC5AC and MUC6. In contrast, mucinous bronchoalveolar carcinoma showed high expression of MUC5AC, MUC6, and CK7 but low expression of MUC1 and TTF-1. Hierarchical clustering showed that signet ring cell and solid adenocarcinomas belong to the same category as alveolar lining cells, whereas mucinous bronchoalveolar adenocarcinomas clustered together with gastric foveolar cells and bronchial goblet cells, supporting the view that pulmonary signet ring cell carcinomas belong to another peripheral differentiation spectrum than mucinous bronchoalveolar carcinoma.[82]

Regulatory Pathways in Adenocarcinoma

From discussed results of genomic, expression, and proteomic studies it can easily be deduced that not a single gene or protein might be responsible for the development and progression of pulmonary adenocarcinomas, but instead one or even several deregulated signaling systems are responsible. Furthermore, not only might deregulation of just growth signaling cascades be responsible to adenocarcinoma development but also a concomitant deregulation of apoptosis.[83] Those signaling cascades that are well characterized and have been associated with pulmonary adenocarcinomas are discussed here.

The Epidermal Growth Factor Receptor System

The EGF/EGFR system is activated by homo- or heterodimer of ligands as well as the receptor tyrosine kinase EGFR. Epidermal growth factor can associate with another EGF or with HER2/neu (ErbB2), ErbB3, or Erb34. Even a heterodimer with TGF-α is possible and activates EGFR.[84] In addition, the EGF receptor can also dimerize and in this conformation seems to be more effective in downstream signaling.[85,86] Downstream signaling goes via Ras and Raf activation further downstream into ERK and mitogen-activated protein (MAP) kinase phosphorylation. Several binding proteins such as Gab1 or Grb2 might modulate the activation of different MAP and ERK kinases, but this has not been clarified yet. Finally, ERK can further activate a multitude of transcription factors downstream, such as cAMP response element binding (CREB), Elk-1, p90S6 kinase 1, c-Fos, and c-Jun. However, instead of targeting the nuclear transmission machinery, ERK can also signal back into the cytoplasm by activating mTOR via p90S6K (RSK) and thus acting into another pathway (Figure 25.3). The mechanism that induces the selection of the different transcription factors is not clear.

A good example and a first insight into these mechanisms are provided by the study of Sithanandam et al.[87] Two carcinoma cell lines expressed ErbB3 and TGF-α and responded to TGF-α stimulation with an increase of the p85 regulatory subunit of PI3K, activation of Akt, phosphorylation of glycogen synthase kinase-3β, increase of cyclin D1 protein, and activation of the cell cycle,

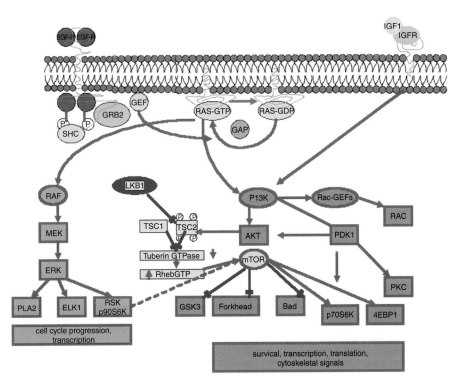

FIGURE 25.3. The epidermal growth factor receptor/extracellular signal-regulated kinase pathway. Simplified schema based on published data. (Reproduced with permission from Pirker R, Popper H. New concepts in pulmonary oncology. Eur Respir Mono 2007;39:63–87.)

resulting in cell growth. The effector pathway from the EGFR to PI3K in these nontransformed cells included the adaptor protein Grb2, the docking protein Gab1, and the phosphatase Shp2. Thus, alternate pathways downstream of EGFR can regulate mitosis[87].

Overexpression of EGFR is one of the earliest and most consistent abnormalities in the bronchial epithelium of high-risk smokers, it is found in basal cell hyperplasia, and it persists through squamous metaplasia, dysplasia, and carcinoma in situ.[88] Epidermal growth factor receptor and HER2/neu are highly expressed in bronchial preneoplasia. In invasive tumors, EGFR is expressed predominantly in squamous cell carcinomas, but also in adenocarcinomas and large cell carcinomas, whereas Her2/neu is more often expressed in adenocarcinomas. The genetic mechanisms responsible for overexpression of EGFR and HER2 proteins might include gene dosage (over-representation or amplification), as well as translational and posttranslational mechanisms. Gene amplification for EGFR and HER2 is demonstrated in only a minority of carcinomas.[89]

The EGFR mutations were more frequent in well to moderately differentiated adenocarcinomas tumors, independent of age, disease stages, or survival. The EGFR mutations never occurred in tumors with K-ras mutations, whereas EGFR mutations were independent of TP53 mutations. The EGFR mutations define a distinct subset of pulmonary adenocarcinomas without K-ras mutations not caused by tobacco carcinogens.[90] In tumors with EGFR mutations, an enhanced tyrosine kinase activity was demonstrated in response to epidermal growth factor. An increased sensitivity to inhibition by gefitinib was also seen.[91]

Shigematsu and coworkers analyzed EGFR mutations within the tyrosine kinase domain mutations in detail in 617 NSCLCs.[92] In NSCLC patients, EGFR tyrosine kinase domain mutations were significantly more frequently found in never-smokers than in smokers, more often in adenocarcinomas than in other histologies, in patients of East Asian ethnicity versus other ethnicities, and more often in females. K-ras gene mutations were present in a minority of the 617 NSCLCs but not in any tumor with an EGFR tyrosine kinase domain mutation.[92]

The Platelet-Derived Growth Factor System

Platelet-derived growth factor (PDGF) and its receptors are well known in normal peripheral lung epithelia. Platelet-derived growth factor was demonstrated in cases of squamous cell carcinoma (64%) and adenocarcinoma (55%) and in all cases of large cell carcinoma and adenosquamous carcinoma. Platelet-derived growth factor receptor was detected in the tumor stroma. Positive PDGF staining was associated with a poor prognosis in patients with lung carcinoma, independent of age, sex,

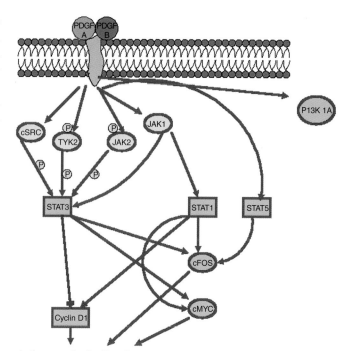

Antiapoptosis, Proliferation

FIGURE 25.4. The platelet-derived growth factor pathway. Simplified schema based on published data.

stage, and degree of cell differentiation. Platelet-derived growth factor B mRNA was detected in all squamous cell carcinomas and in 85% of adenocarcinomas.[93]

The PDGF system can directly signal into the different signal transducers and activators of transcription (STAT) and via STAT1 activate cyclin D1, or it can indirectly activate STATs via the activation/phosphorylation of Janus kinase (JAK) 1, JAK2, tyrosine kinase 2, or Src. Downstream molecules are the transcription factors c-Myc and c-Fos. However, PDGF receptor activation can also cause an activation of PI3K (regulatory and catalytic subunits 1A) and thus transactivate the Akt/mTOR pathway (Figure 25.4). However, these different activation pathways have not been analyzed in lung carcinomas.

The Histone Deacetylase System

Packing and unwinding of DNA for translational repression is tightly regulated by histone deacetylases (HDACs). Cooperation among acetylases NF-κB, STAT, CREB, and RNA polymerase 2 opens coiled DNA by histone acetylation and makes chromatin easily accessible for transcription. On the contrary, HDAC together with methyl CpG binding protein 2 and other factors methylate DNA, deacetylate histones, and thus tightly pack the DNA,

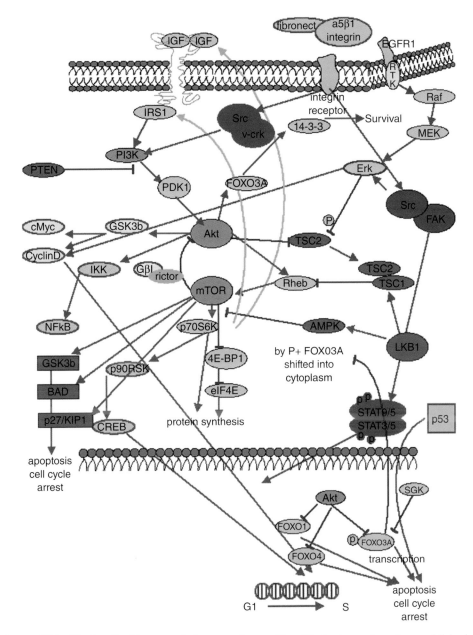

FIGURE 25.5. The insulin-like growth factor pathway. Simplified schema based on published data.

making it inaccessible for transcription. Hierarchical clustering analysis showed that lung cancer tissues could be divided into three groups based on the expression level of class I and class II HDAC genes. The group with reduced expression of class II HDACs showed poor prognosis. These results suggest that class II HDACs may repress critical genes and that low expression of these genes may play a role in lung cancer progression.[94]

Insulin-Like Growth Factor System

Transgenic overexpression of insulin-like growth factor (IGF)-2 in lung epithelium induced lung tumors in 69%

of mice older than 18 months of age. These tumors displayed morphologic characteristics of human pulmonary adenocarcinoma (tubuloacinar architecture, expression of thyroid transcription factor 1, surfactant protein B, and surfactant protein C propeptide). Insulin-like growth factor I receptor can activate the downstream signaling molecules ERK12 or alternatively the p38 MAP kinase pathways (Figure 25.5). Interestingly, both the ERK1/2 and p38 MAP kinase pathways converge on the transcription factor CREB. Insulin-like growth factor II receptor induced proliferation and CREB phosphorylation in human lung cancer cell lines, suggesting that IGF-II and CREB contribute to the growth of human lung tumors.[95] Despite its common expression in pulmonary adenocarcinomas, this pathway and its impact on proliferation and survival of tumor cells has not been explored.

The Vascular Endothelial Growth Factor and Angiogenesis System

Vascular endothelial growth factor is a frequently expressed protein in NSCLC. Vascular endothelial growth factor and its receptors play a major role in lung development as signaling mechanisms for the development of large-, medium-, and small-sized blood vessels and lymphatics. This system also plays an important part in lung cancer development and progression. In addition, VEGF and VEGF receptors (VEGFRs) are connected with many other pathways in a fore- and backward signaling manner (Figure 25.6). Frequent positive reactions for VEGF-C were found in NSCLC, especially in patients with adenocarcinoma, whereas VEGFR-3 expression significantly correlated with age, gender, and squamous cell carcinoma. Staining of VEGF-C showed significantly less favorable survival rates. The survival rates for positive VEGFR-3 staining were also significantly lower. Positive staining for both VEGF-C and VEGFR-3 was associated with the most unfavorable prognosis. Multivariate analysis demonstrated that VEGFR-3 expression was the only independent negative prognostic factor.[96]

A high expression of VEGF was observed in 75% and 73% of squamous cell carcinomas and adenocarcinomas, respectively, and in all cases of large cell carcinomas. High vascularity was associated with high VEGF expression. Vascular epithelial growth factor and microvessel density were correlated with low tumor differentiation. A simultaneous high expression of VEGF and reduced expression of E-cadherin was correlated with tumor dedifferentiation.[97] The *VEGF-C* gene expression was significantly elevated in cells overexpressing COX-2. Prostaglandin EP1 receptor was involved in this COX-2–mediated VEGF-C upregulation. Cyclooxygenase-2 or prostaglandin E_2 treatment could activate the HER2/neu tyrosine kinase receptor and further on VEGF-C. The Src kinase was positively involved in HER2/neu transactivation. Cyclooxygenase-2 levels were highly correlated with VEGF-C and lymphatic vessels density.[63]

Vascular endothelial growth factor and IGF binding protein 3 (IGFBP-3) mRNA were found to be overexpressed in differentiated pulmonary adenocarcinomas. Vascular endothelial growth factor can be regulated by the hypoxia-inducible factor 1 (HIF-1) pathway. Insulin-like growth factor binding protein 3 is also regulated by HIF1 but modulates the activities of IGFs and induces apoptosis. Forty genes were identified as the most significantly associated with VEGF expression, 17 of which were also associated with IGFBP-3, and 12 were known to be induced through the HIF-1 pathway. Bradykinin receptor B2 was one of these highly correlated genes associated with VEGF expression in lung adenocarcinoma.[98]

A new protein, connective tissue growth factor (CTGF), was shown to inhibit the metastatic activity of human lung cancer cells. Xenograft tumors derived from CTGF transfectants grew more slowly than those from controls and had reduced expression of HIF-1α and VEGF-A, vascularization, and metastasis. Xenograft tumors derived from CTGF-overexpressing cells that were additionally transfected with HIF-1α had higher VEGF-A expression. Tumors of patients with the same disease stage but with high CTGF protein expression had reduced microvessel density. Connective tissue growth factor inhibition of metastasis involves the inhibition of VEGF-A–dependent angiogenesis, possibly by promoting HIF-1α protein degradation.[99]

The Nuclear Factor-κB Pathway

The NF-κB pathway is quite complex and interconnected with several other pathways. It not only can signal into the nucleus but also can activate other factors in the

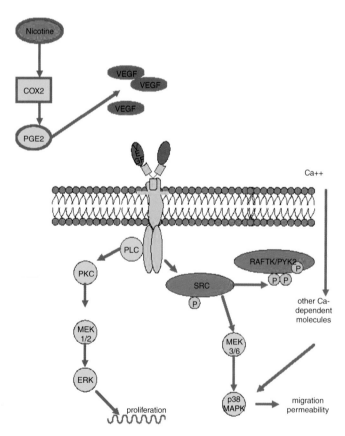

FIGURE 25.6. The vascular endothelial growth factor pathway. Simplified schema based on published data.

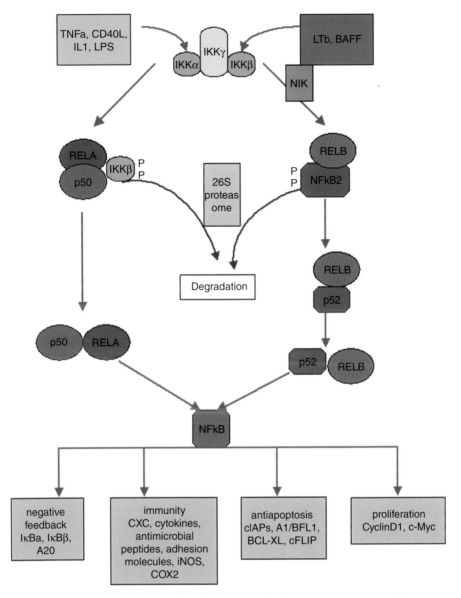

FIGURE 25.7. The nuclear factor-κB pathway. Simplified schema based on published data.

cytoplasm (Figure 25.7). Nuclear factor-κB is highly expressed in SCLC and some variants of large cell carcinomas but rarely in adenocarcinomas. However, cigarette smoke condensate can induce NF-κB activation up to 24 hours, and thus a final conclusion about the NF-κB pathway in adenocarcinomas cannot be drawn. Celecoxib, a chemopreventive drug, abrogated p65 phosphorylation, nuclear translocation, and NF-κB–dependent reporter gene expression and induced the expression of COX-2, cyclin D1, and matrix metalloproteinase-9. The chemopreventive effects may in part be mediated through suppression of NF-κB and NF-κB–regulated gene expression, which may contribute to its ability to suppress proliferation and angiogenesis.[100]

The Hepatocyte Growth Factor Pathway

In contrast to squamous cell carcinomas, the expression of c-Met mRNA and its protein product in adenocarcinoma and large cell carcinoma is more heterogeneous. Overexpression was demonstrated in approximately 35% of adenocarcinomas. In adenocarcinoma intermediate to high levels of c-Met, immunoreactivity correlated with better tumor differentiation. Furthermore, an accentuation of c-Met immunoreactivity was often noted in cancer cells at the advancing edge of tumors, supporting a role for Met in lung cancer invasion and differentiation.[101] In contrast to SCLC, the c-Met signaling cascade has not been explored in adenocarcinomas.

From Invasion to Metastasis

As in all other carcinomas, the neoplastic process progresses in a stepwise fashion. There is an expansion of the noninvasive carcinoma cell within the mucosa, followed by invasion and finally metastasis. Each of these processes is accompanied by several genetic changes and adaptations. For invasion, carcinoma cells have to develop mechanisms of matrix degradation, have to downregulate intercellular adhesion, but also have to evolve mechanisms of orientation along matrix proteins similar to what leukocytes use. Metastasis requires not only the ability to migrate toward high oxygen gradients and blood vessels and invade the vessels but also to survive within the circulation, adhere to endothelia, emigrate, and establish a metastatic focus and induce neoangiogenesis. Each of these steps might be based on several genetic or epigenetic changes or modifications of genes and proteins.

In the study by Beer et al., 50 genes were identified for low and high-risk stage I lung adenocarcinomas, significantly differing with respect to survival.[102] They included genes not previously associated with survival, such as *IGFBP-3*, *heat shock protein 70*, *cystatin C (cysteine protease inhibitor)*, *ErbB2 (Her2/neu)*, *Crk*, *Grb7*, and *VEGF*. Goeze and coworkers compared primary pulmonary adenocarcinomas and metastases for differences in chromosomal imbalances.[103] The generation of a case-by-case histogram for the comparison of primary tumors and corresponding metastases suggested that deletions on chromosomes 3p12–p14, 3p22–p24, 4p13–15.1, 4q21-qter, 6q21-qter, 8p, 10q, 14q21, 17p12–p13, 20p12, and 21q and overrepresentations on chromosomes 1q21–q25, 7q11.2, 9q34, 11q12–q13, 14q11–q13, and 17q25 are associated with the metastatic phenotype. In contrast, losses on chromosome 19 and gains on 3p, 4q, 5p, and 6q were preferentially found in nonmetastasizing tumors.[103]

In lung cancer, both the *p16^{INK4A}/Rb* and *p53* genes are frequently inactivated and are critical determinants for the regulation of cell growth and apoptosis. However, it still remains unclear whether these genes are also involved in the regulation of metastatic potential in lung cancer cells. Yokota and coworkers identified a novel myosin family gene *MYO18B* (chromosome 22q12.1) that showed frequent LOH in advanced lung cancer.[47] This gene was found to be inactivated in approximately 50% of lung cancers by deletions, mutations, and methylation. Restoration of *MYO18B* expression suppressed anchorage-independent growth of lung cancer cells, making it a candidate for a metastasis suppressor gene.[47] In another interesting investigation, an association of several genes with metastatic adenocarcinoma was established. Matrix metalloproteinase-2, plasminogen activator inhibitor-1, and interleukin-1α were upregulated, whereas the expression of carcinoembryonic antigen, caspase-5, Fas ligand, Prk/FNK, cyclin E, cyclin B1, Ki-67, proliferating cell nuclear antigen, Smad4, macrophage proinflammatory human chemokine-3α/LARC, c-Met, and CD44 were downregulated.[83]

These findings are important but preliminary steps toward our understanding of early lung carcinogenesis. Much remains to be done. Proteins associated with the metastatic phenotype and regulatory mechanisms for metastasis need to be identified.

References

1. Wynder EL, Muscat JE. The changing epidemiology of smoking and lung cancer histology. Environ Health Perspect 1995;103Suppl 8:143–148.
2. Witschi H. Carcinogenic activity of cigarette smoke gas phase and its modulation by beta-carotene and N-acetylcysteine. Toxicol Sci 2005;84:81–87.
3. Schick S, Glantz S. Philip Morris toxicological experiments with fresh sidestream smoke: more toxic than mainstream smoke. Tob Control 2005;14:396–404.
4. Husgafvel-Pursiainen K. Genotoxicity of environmental tobacco smoke: a review. Mutat Res 2004;567:427–445.
5. Dopp E, Saedler J, Stopper H, et al. Mitotic disturbances and micronucleus induction in Syrian hamster embryo fibroblast cells caused by asbestos fibers. Environ Health Perspect 1995;103:268–271.
6. Harden SV, Tokumaru Y, Westra WH, et al. Gene promoter hypermethylation in tumors and lymph nodes of stage I lung cancer patients. Clin Cancer Res 2003;9:1370–1375.
7. Lu C, Soria JC, Tang X, et al. Prognostic factors in resected stage I non–small-cell lung cancer: a multivariate analysis of six molecular markers. J Clin Oncol 2004;22:4575–4583.
8. Toyooka S, Maruyama R, Toyooka KO, et al. Smoke exposure, histologic type and geography-related differences in the methylation profiles of non-small cell lung cancer. Int J Cancer 2003;103:153–160.
9. Zaridze DG, Safaev RD, Belitsky GA, et al. Carcinogenic substances in Soviet tobacco products. IARC Sci Publ 1991:485–488.
10. Stabbert R, Voncken P, Rustemeier K, et al. Toxicological evaluation of an electrically heated cigarette. Part 2: Chemical composition of mainstream smoke. J Appl Toxicol 2003;23:329–339.
11. Jin Z, Gao F, Flagg T, Deng X. Tobacco-specific nitrosamine NNK promotes functional cooperation of Bcl2 and c-Myc through phosphorylation in regulating cell survival and proliferation. J Biol Chem 2004;279:40209–40219.
12. Tsurutani J, Castillo SS, Brognard J, et al. Tobacco components stimulate Akt-dependent proliferation and NFkappaB-dependent survival in lung cancer cells. Carcinogenesis 2005;26:1182–1195.
13. Herzog CR, Desai D, Amin S. Array CGH analysis reveals chromosomal aberrations in mouse lung adenocarcinomas induced by the human lung carcinogen 4-(methylnitrosamino)-1-(3-pyridyl)-1-butanone. Biochem Biophys Res Commun 2006;341:856–863.
14. Norppa H. Cytogenetic biomarkers and genetic polymorphisms. Toxicol Lett 2004;149:309–334.

15. Wang GF, Lai MD, Yang RR, et al. Histological types and significance of bronchial epithelial dysplasia. Mod Pathol 2006;19:429–437.

16. Ullmann R, Bongiovanni M, Halbwedl I, et al. Bronchiolar columnar cell dysplasia—genetic analysis of a novel preneoplastic lesion of peripheral lung. Virchows Arch 2003; 442:429–436.

17. Mori M, Rao SK, Popper HH, et al. Atypical adenomatous hyperplasia of the lung: a probable forerunner in the development of adenocarcinoma of the lung. Mod Pathol 2001;14:72–84.

18. Hu Z, Ma H, Lu D, et al. A promoter polymorphism (−77T > C) of DNA repair gene XRCC1 is associated with risk of lung cancer in relation to tobacco smoking. Pharmacogenet Genomics 2005;15:457–463.

19. Matullo G, Dunning AM, Guarrera S, et al. DNA repair polymorphisms and cancer risk in non-smokers in a cohort study. Carcinogenesis 2005;27(5):997–1007.

20. Zienolddiny S, Campa D, Lind H, et al. Polymorphisms of DNA repair genes and risk of non–small cell lung cancer. Carcinogenesis 2006;27:560–567.

21. Forgacs E, Zochbauer-Muller S, Olah E, Minna JD. Molecular genetic abnormalities in the pathogenesis of human lung cancer. Pathol Oncol Res 2001;7:6–13.

22. He B, You L, Uematsu K, et al. SOCS-3 is frequently silenced by hypermethylation and suppresses cell growth in human lung cancer. Proc Natl Acad Sci USA 2003;100: 14133–14138.

23. Lamy A, Sesboue R, Bourguignon J, et al. Aberrant methylation of the CDKN2a/p16[INK4a] gene promoter region in preinvasive bronchial lesions: a prospective study in high-risk patients without invasive cancer. Int J Cancer 2002; 100:189–193.

24. Li QL, Kim HR, Kim WJ, et al. Transcriptional silencing of the RUNX3 gene by CpG hypermethylation is associated with lung cancer. Biochem Biophys Res Commun 2004; 314:223–228.

25. Miller RR. Alveolar atypical hyperplasia in association with primary pulmonary adenocarcinoma: a clinicopathological study of 10 cases. Thorax 1993;48:679–680.

26. Ullmann R, Bongiovanni M, Halbwedl I, et al. Is high-grade adenomatous hyperplasia an early bronchioloalveolar adenocarcinoma? J Pathol 2003;201:371–376.

27. Granata C, Gambini C, Balducci T, et al. Bronchioloalveolar carcinoma arising in congenital cystic adenomatoid malformation in a child: a case report and review on malignancies originating in congenital cystic adenomatoid malformation. Pediatr Pulmonol 1998;25:62–66.

28. MacSweeney F, Papagiannopoulos K, Goldstraw P, et al. An assessment of the expanded classification of congenital cystic adenomatoid malformations and their relationship to malignant transformation. Am J Surg Pathol 2003;27: 1139–1146.

29. Stacher E, Ullmann R, Halbwedl I, et al. Atypical goblet cell hyperplasia in congenital cystic adenomatoid malformation as a possible preneoplasia for pulmonary adenocarcinoma in childhood: a genetic analysis. Hum Pathol 2004;35:565–570.

30. Haura EB. Is repetitive wounding and bone marrow–derived stem cell mediated-repair an etiology of lung cancer development and dissemination? Med Hypotheses 2006;67:951–956.

31. Kim CF, Jackson EL, Woolfenden AE, et al. Identification of bronchioalveolar stem cells in normal lung and lung cancer. Cell 2005;121:823–835.

32. Kerr KM, Fraire AE, Pugatch B, et al. Atypical adenomatous hyperplasia. In Travis WD, Brambilla E, Müller-Hermelink HK, Harris CC, eds. Pathology and Genetics of Tumours of the Lung, Pleura, Thymus and Heart. Lyon, France: IARC Press; 2004:73–75.

33. Kishimoto Y, Sugio K, Hung JY, et al. Allele-specific loss in chromosome 9p loci in preneoplastic lesions accompanying non–small-cell lung cancers. J Natl Cancer Inst 1995; 87:1224–1229.

34. Suzuki K, Ogura T, Yokose T, et al. Loss of heterozygosity in the tuberous sclerosis gene associated regions in adenocarcinoma of the lung accompanied by multiple atypical adenomatous hyperplasia. Int J Cancer 1998;79:384–389.

35. Kitaguchi S, Takeshima Y, Nishisaka T, Inai K. Proliferative activity, p53 expression and loss of heterozygosity on 3p, 9p and 17p in atypical adenomatous hyperplasia of the lung. Am J Clin Pathol 1999;111:610–622.

36. Takamochi K, Ogura T, Suzuki K, et al. Loss of heterozygosity on chromosomes 9q and 16p in atypical adenomatous hyperplasia concomitant with adenocarcinoma of the lung. Am J Pathol 2001;159:1941–1948.

37. Petersen I, Bujard M, Petersen S, et al. Patterns of chromosomal imbalances in adenocarcinoma and squamous cell carcinoma of the lung. Cancer Res 1997;57:2331–2335.

38. Fong KM, Biesterveld EJ, Virmani A, et al. FHIT and FRA3B 3p14.2 allele loss are common in lung cancer and preneoplastic bronchial lesions and are associated with cancer-related FHIT cDNA splicing aberrations. Cancer Res 1997;57:2256–2267.

39. Wong MP, Fung LF, Wang E, et al. Chromosomal aberrations of primary lung adenocarcinomas in nonsmokers. Cancer 2003;97:1263–1270.

40. Sy SM, Wong N, Lee TW, et al. Distinct patterns of genetic alterations in adenocarcinoma and squamous cell carcinoma of the lung. Eur J Cancer 2004;40:1082–1094.

41. Tsuchiya E, Tanigami A, Ishikawa Y, et al. Three new regions on chromosome 17p13.3 distal to p53 with possible tumor suppressor gene involvement in lung cancer. Jpn J Cancer Res 2000;91:589–596.

42. Aoyagi Y, Yokose T, Minami Y, et al. Accumulation of losses of heterozygosity and multistep carcinogenesis in pulmonary adenocarcinoma. Cancer Res 2001;61:7950–7954.

43. Sanchez-Cespedes M, Ahrendt SA, Piantadosi S, et al. Chromosomal alterations in lung adenocarcinoma from smokers and nonsmokers. Cancer Res 2001;61:1309–1313.

44. Copin MC, Buisine MP, Devisme L, et al. Normal respiratory mucosa, precursor lesions and lung carcinomas: differential expression of human mucin genes. Front Biosci 2001;6:D1264–D1275.

45. Moniaux N, Escande F, Porchet N, et al. Structural organization and classification of the human mucin genes. Front Biosci 2001;6:D1192–D1206.

46. Tanaka R, Wang D, Morishita Y, et al. Loss of function of p16 gene and prognosis of pulmonary adenocarcinoma. Cancer 2005;103:608–615.

47. Yokota J, Nishioka M, Tani M, Kohno T. Genetic alterations responsible for metastatic phenotypes of lung cancer cells. Clin Exp Metastasis 2003;20:189–193.

48. Hirsch FR, Varella-Garcia M, Bunn PA Jr, et al. Epidermal growth factor receptor in non–small-cell lung carcinomas: correlation between gene copy number and protein expression and impact on prognosis. J Clin Oncol 2003;21:3798–3807.

49. Li J, Zhang Z, Dai Z, et al. LOH of chromosome 12p correlates with Kras2 mutation in non–small cell lung cancer. Oncogene 2003;22:1243–1246.

50. Uchiyama M, Usami N, Kondo M, et al. Loss of heterozygosity of chromosome 12p does not correlate with KRAS mutation in non–small cell lung cancer. Int J Cancer 2003; 107:962–969.

51. Yanagitani N, Kohno T, Kim JG, et al. Identification of D19S246 as a novel lung adenocarcinoma susceptibility locus by genome survey with 10-cM resolution microsatellite markers. Cancer Epidemiol Biomarkers Prev 2003;12:366–371.

52. Suzuki M, Shigematsu H, Iizasa T, et al. Exclusive mutation in epidermal growth factor receptor gene, HER-2, and KRAS, and synchronous methylation of nonsmall cell lung cancer. Cancer 2006;106:2200–2207.

53. Tam IY, Chung LP, Suen WS, et al. Distinct epidermal growth factor receptor and KRAS mutation patterns in non–small cell lung cancer patients with different tobacco exposure and clinicopathologic features. Clin Cancer Res 2006;12:1647–1653.

54. Bongiorno PF, Whyte RI, Lesser EJ, et al. Alterations of K-ras, p53, and erbB-2/neu in human lung adenocarcinomas. J Thorac Cardiovasc Surg 1994;107:590–595.

55. Kern JA, Slebos RJ, Top B, et al. C-erbB-2 expression and codon 12 K-ras mutations both predict shortened survival for patients with pulmonary adenocarcinomas. J Clin Invest 1994;93:516–520.

56. Westra WH, Baas IO, Hruban RH, et al. K-ras oncogene activation in atypical alveolar hyperplasias of the human lung. Cancer Res 1996;56:2224–2228.

57. Garber ME, Troyanskaya OG, Schluens K, et al. Diversity of gene expression in adenocarcinoma of the lung. Proc Natl Acad Sci USA 2001;98:13784–13789.

58. Singhal S, Amin KM, Kruklitis R, et al. Alterations in cell cycle genes in early stage lung adenocarcinoma identified by expression profiling. Cancer Biol Ther 2003;2:291–298.

59. Endoh H, Tomida S, Yatabe Y, et al. Prognostic model of pulmonary adenocarcinoma by expression profiling of eight genes as determined by quantitative real-time reverse transcriptase polymerase chain reaction. J Clin Oncol 2004;22:811–819.

60. Singhal S, Amin KM, Kruklitis R, et al. Differentially expressed apoptotic genes in early stage lung adenocarcinoma predicted by expression profiling. Cancer Biol Ther 2003;2:566–571.

61. Chen G, Bhojani MS, Heaford AC, et al. Phosphorylated FADD induces NF-kappaB, perturbs cell cycle, and is associated with poor outcome in lung adenocarcinomas. Proc Natl Acad Sci USA 2005;102:12507–12512.

62. Qi W, Liu X, Qiao D, Martinez JD. Isoform-specific expression of 14-3-3 proteins in human lung cancer tissues. Int J Cancer 2005;113:359–363.

63. Su JL, Shih JY, Yen ML, et al. Cyclooxygenase-2 induces EP1- and HER-2/Neu–dependent vascular endothelial growth factor-C up-regulation: a novel mechanism of lymphangiogenesis in lung adenocarcinoma. Cancer Res 2004;64:554–564.

64. Saad RS, Liu Y, Han H, et al. Prognostic significance of HER2/neu, p53, and vascular endothelial growth factor expression in early stage conventional adenocarcinoma and bronchioloalveolar carcinoma of the lung. Mod Pathol 2004;17:1235–1242.

65. Yuan A, Yang PC, Yu CJ, et al. Interleukin-8 messenger ribonucleic acid expression correlates with tumor progression, tumor angiogenesis, patient survival, and timing of relapse in non–small-cell lung cancer. Am J Respir Crit Care Med 2000;162:1957–1963.

66. Takenaka K, Ishikawa S, Kawano Y, et al. Expression of a novel matrix metalloproteinase regulator, RECK, and its clinical significance in resected non–small cell lung cancer. Eur J Cancer 2004;40:1617–1623.

67. Chen JT, Lin TS, Chow KC, et al. Cigarette smoking induces overexpression of hepatocyte growth factor in type II pneumocytes and lung cancer cells. Am J Respir Cell Mol Biol 2006;34:264–273.

68. Ma PC, Jagadeeswaran R, Jagadeesh S, et al. Functional expression and mutations of c-Met and its therapeutic inhibition with SU11274 and small interfering RNA in non–small cell lung cancer. Cancer Res 2005;65:1479–1488.

69. Setogawa T, Shinozaki-Yabana S, Masuda T, et al. The tumor suppressor LKB1 induces p21 expression in collaboration with LMO4, GATA-6, and Ldb1. Biochem Biophys Res Commun 2006;343:1186–1190.

70. Mak BC, Yeung RS. The tuberous sclerosis complex genes in tumor development. Cancer Invest 2004;22:588–603.

71. Lizcano JM, Goransson O, Toth R, et al. LKB1 is a master kinase that activates 13 kinases of the AMPK subfamily, including MARK/PAR-1. EMBO J 2004;23:833–843.

72. Sato K, Tomizawa Y, Iijima H, et al. Epigenetic inactivation of the RUNX3 gene in lung cancer. Oncol Rep 2006;15:129–135.

73. Borczuk AC, Kim HK, Yegen HA, et al. Lung adenocarcinoma global profiling identifies type II transforming growth factor-beta receptor as a repressor of invasiveness. Am J Respir Crit Care Med 2005;172:729–737.

74. Hofmann HS, Bartling B, Simm A, et al. Identification and classification of differentially expressed genes in non–small cell lung cancer by expression profiling on a global human 59.620-element oligonucleotide array. Oncol Rep 2006;16:587–595.

75. Field JK, Liloglou T, Warrak S, et al. Methylation discriminators in NSCLC identified by a microarray based approach. Int J Oncol 2005;27:105–111.

76. Yanaihara N, Caplen N, Bowman E, et al. Unique microRNA molecular profiles in lung cancer diagnosis and prognosis. Cancer Cell 2006;9:189–198.

77. Seike M, Kondo T, Fujii K, et al. Proteomic signatures for histological types of lung cancer. Proteomics 2005;5: 2939–2948.

78. Keshamouni VG, Michailidis G, Grasso CS, et al. Differential protein expression profiling by iTRAQ-2DLC-MS/MS of lung cancer cells undergoing epithelial-mesenchymal transition reveals a migratory/invasive phenotype. J Proteome Res 2006;5:1143–1154.

79. Li R, Wang H, Bekele BN, et al. Identification of putative oncogenes in lung adenocarcinoma by a comprehensive functional genomic approach. Oncogene 2006;25:2628–2635.

80. Ullmann R, Morbini P, Halbwedl I, et al. Protein expression profiles in adenocarcinomas and squamous cell carcinomas of the lung generated using tissue microarrays. J Pathol 2004;203:798–807.

81. Chen G, Gharib TG, Thomas DG, et al. Proteomic analysis of eIF-5A in lung adenocarcinomas. Proteomics 2003;3: 496–504.

82. Tsuta K, Ishii G, Nitadori J, et al. Comparison of the immunophenotypes of signet-ring cell carcinoma, solid adenocarcinoma with mucin production, and mucinous bronchioloalveolar carcinoma of the lung characterized by the presence of cytoplasmic mucin. J Pathol 2006;209:78–87.

83. Gemma A, Takenaka K, Hosoya Y, et al. Altered expression of several genes in highly metastatic subpopulations of a human pulmonary adenocarcinoma cell line. Eur J Cancer 2001;37:1554–1561.

84. Mulet A, Garrido G, Alvarez A, et al. The enlargement of the hormone immune deprivation concept to the blocking of TGFalpha-autocrine loop: EGFR signaling inhibition. Cancer Immunol Immunother 2006;55:628–638.

85. Fernandes A, Hamburger AW, Gerwin BI. ErbB-2 kinase is required for constitutive stat 3 activation in malignant human lung epithelial cells. Int J Cancer 1999;83:564–570.

86. Boulougouris P, Elder J. Epidermal growth factor receptor structure, regulation, mitogenic signalling and effects of activation. Anticancer Res 2001;21:2769–2775.

87. Sithanandam G, Smith GT, Fields JR, et al. Alternate paths from epidermal growth factor receptor to Akt in malignant versus nontransformed lung epithelial cells: ErbB3 versus Gab1. Am J Respir Cell Mol Biol 2005;33:490–499.

88. Franklin WA, Veve R, Hirsch FR, et al. Epidermal growth factor receptor family in lung cancer and premalignancy. Semin Oncol 2002;29:3–14.

89. Hirsch FR, Scagliotti GV, Langer CJ, et al. Epidermal growth factor family of receptors in preneoplasia and lung cancer: perspectives for targeted therapies. Lung Cancer 2003;41(Suppl 1):S29–S42.

90. Kosaka T, Yatabe Y, Endoh H, et al. Mutations of the epidermal growth factor receptor gene in lung cancer: biological and clinical implications. Cancer Res 2004;64:8919–8923.

91. Lynch TJ, Bell DW, Sordella R, et al. Activating mutations in the epidermal growth factor receptor underlying responsiveness of non–small-cell lung cancer to gefitinib. N Engl J Med 2004;350:2129–2139.

92. Shigematsu H, Lin L, Takahashi T, et al. Clinical and biological features associated with epidermal growth factor receptor gene mutations in lung cancers. J Natl Cancer Inst 2005;97:339–346.

93. Kawai T, Hiroi S, Torikata C. Expression in lung carcinomas of platelet-derived growth factor and its receptors. Lab Invest 1997;77:431–436.

94. Osada H, Tatematsu Y, Saito H, et al. Reduced expression of class II histone deacetylase genes is associated with poor prognosis in lung cancer patients. Int J Cancer 2004;112: 26–32.

95. Moorehead RA, Sanchez OH, Baldwin RM, Khokha R. Transgenic overexpression of IGF-II induces spontaneous lung tumors: a model for human lung adenocarcinoma. Oncogene 2003;22:853–857.

96. Arinaga M, Noguchi T, Takeno S, et al. Clinical significance of vascular endothelial growth factor C and vascular endothelial growth factor receptor 3 in patients with nonsmall cell lung carcinoma. Cancer 2003;97:457–464.

97. Stefanou D, Goussia AC, Arkoumani E, Agnantis NJ. Expression of vascular endothelial growth factor and the adhesion molecule E-cadherin in non–small cell lung cancer. Anticancer Res 2003;23:4715–4720.

98. Gharib TG, Chen G, Huang CC, et al. Genomic and proteomic analyses of vascular endothelial growth factor and insulin-like growth factor-binding protein 3 in lung adenocarcinomas. Clin Lung Cancer 2004;5:307–312.

99. Chang CC, Lin MT, Lin BR, et al. Effect of connective tissue growth factor on hypoxia-inducible factor 1alpha degradation and tumor angiogenesis. J Natl Cancer Inst 2006;98:984–995.

100. Shishodia S, Aggarwal BB. Cyclooxygenase (COX)-2 inhibitor celecoxib abrogates activation of cigarette smoke-induced nuclear factor (NF)-kappaB by suppressing activation of IkappaBalpha kinase in human non–small cell lung carcinoma: correlation with suppression of cyclin D1, COX-2, and matrix metalloproteinase-9. Cancer Res 2004; 64:5004–5012.

101. Tsao MS, Liu N, Chen JR, et al. Differential expression of Met/hepatocyte growth factor receptor in subtypes of non–small cell lung cancers. Lung Cancer 1998;20:1–16.

102. Beer DG, Kardia SL, Huang CC, et al. Gene-expression profiles predict survival of patients with lung adenocarcinoma. Nat Med 2002;8:816–824.

103. Goeze A, Schluns K, Wolf G, et al. Chromosomal imbalances of primary and metastatic lung adenocarcinomas. J Pathol 2002;196:8–16.

26
Molecular Pathology of Squamous Cell Carcinoma and Its Precursors

Soon-Hee Jung, Bihong Zhao, Li Mao, and Jae Y. Ro

Introduction

The normal respiratory mucosal epithelium at birth may undergo histologic changes during life due to exposure to a variety of environmental irritants, including tobacco smoke, radon exposure, and occupational toxins. Long-term carcinogenic insults may result in the development of multiple premalignant or malignant lesions in the respiratory epithelium. There is a wide spectrum of histopathologic changes in the respiratory epithelium, including hyperplastic lesions (basal cell hyperplasia/reserve cell hyperplasia), metaplastic lesions (primarily squamous metaplasia), dysplasia (mild, moderate, and severe), squamous cell carcinoma in situ, and invasive squamous cell carcinoma.[1] The precursor lesions are also described as preneoplastic, premalignant, or preinvasive and are defined as epithelial abnormalities that are cytologically neoplastic but do not penetrate the basement membrane.[2] These lesions have the capacity to progress to invasive carcinoma, to regress toward normal, or to remain indolent.[3]

Based on recent molecular findings, lung cancer is not the result of a sudden transforming event in the bronchial epithelium but rather is a multistep process of phenotypic changes in which gradual, both spatially and temporally, genetic and cellular changes occur.[4,5] First, development of preinvasive lesions and/or carcinoma is associated with a substantial and sequential accumulation of mutations from even remote events. At least a 4- to 5-year interval is required before a dysplastic lesion in the large airways progresses to squamous cell carcinoma in situ. These sequential molecular changes are the genetic drive that transforms the normal epithelium into hyperplasia, squamous metaplasia, dysplasia, carcinoma in situ, and eventually to invasive carcinoma (Figure 26.1). Second, it is clear that exposure of the whole airway mucosa to tobacco smoke or other mutagens is necessary to cause the entire bronchial tree to be at risk of developing lung cancer;

therefore, the concept of "field cancerization" was introduced.

Numerous recent studies have reported that multifocal distribution of preinvasive lesions should be present in keeping with the "field cancerization" effect of cigarette smoke, supporting a model in which a field with genetically altered cells plays a central role.[4,5] The induction of field cancerization is similar to the proposed model of head and neck squamous cell carcinoma (HNSCC) carcinogenesis.[6] The carcinogen exposure forms a "field" of altered cells in the following hypothetical order: (1) initiation, in which DNA damage occurs; (2) promotion, in which genetic and epigenetic changes confer additional genomic damage; and (3) progression to locally invasive or metastatic disease.

There are numerous well-documented genetic alterations in lung carcinogenesis taking place at different levels of gene expression regulation. For example, on a small genetic scale (i.e., at the DNA level), there are deletions, insertions, and point mutations of dominant oncogenes such as the *ras* gene, tumor suppressor genes such as *p53* gene, the retinoblastoma (*Rb*) gene, and the *p16* gene. On a larger genetic scale (i.e., at the chromosomal level), there is loss of heterozygosity (LOH) of the *p53* and *Rb* genes and DNA aneuploidy. Finally, at an epigenetic level there is gene silencing through promoter hypermethylation or histone deacetylation. All the molecular and cellular alterations ultimately result in aberrant expression of genes involved in the control of cell proliferation, differentiation, and apoptosis,[7–9] causing accelerated cell proliferation, dedifferentiation, and elimination/decrease in apoptosis.

The purpose of this chapter is to briefly summarize the recently described molecular abnormalities in carcinogenesis of squamous cell carcinoma of the lung. These abnormalities include altered expression and gain of function of oncogenes, loss of tumor suppressor gene function, and epigenetic alterations such as tumor acquired aberrant promoter methylation.

FIGURE 26.1. Sequential histologic and molecular changes during the multistage pathogenesis of squamous cell carcinoma of the lung and its precursors. CIS, carcinoma in situ; LOH, loss of heterozygosity. (Modified from Hirsch et al.[5])

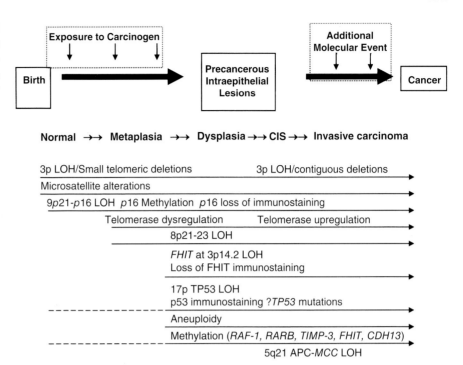

Chromosomal Abnormalities: Loss of Heterozygosity

Loss of heterozygosity is a very common phenomenon in carcinogenesis. Loss of heterozygosity in a *cell* represents the loss of a single parent's contribution to part of the cell's *genome*, which often indicates the presence of a *tumor suppressor gene* in the lost region. Often, the remaining copy of the tumor suppressor gene will be inactivated by a *point mutation* or an epigenetic change.

The chromosomal abnormalities of squamous cell carcinoma of the lung are very similar to the proposed model of HNSCC carcinogenesis.[6] However, the allelic losses of squamous cell lung carcinoma are slightly different from those of HNSCC.

At the earliest initiation step of carcinogenesis of squamous cell carcinoma, a clonal patch (40,000–360,000 cells), consisting of *p53*-mutated cells, is formed. This process is similar to HNSCC; however, the additional deletions of 3p and 13q are predominant in squamous cell carcinoma of the lung, which lead to the conversion of a patch of clonal cells to a field of cells, expanding the molecular alterations at the expense of normal tissue. Allelotyping studies on precisely microdissected tissues, including lung cancer, preneoplastic lesions, and normal respiratory epithelium, showed that LOH on chromosome 3p is the important early molecular event in the development of lung cancer, and it is observed in more than 90% of small cell and squamous cell lung cancers and in 50% of adenocarcinomas (Figure 26.2).[10] Several distinct regions are frequently lost, including 3p12, 3p14.2,

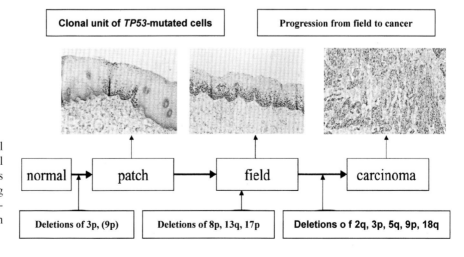

FIGURE 26.2. Immunohistochemical tissue *p53* expression and chromosomal abnormalities during the carcinogenesis of squamous cell carcinoma of the lung compared with head and neck squamous cell carcinoma. (Modified from Braakhuis et al.[6])

TABLE 26.1. Progressive increase in chromosomal abnormalities and mutations in squamous cell carcinoma of the lung and its precursors.

Histologic lesions	Abnormality frequently present
Hyperplasia/metaplasia	Small areas of loss of heterozygosity (LOH) in 3p (3p21.3 [RASSF1A and SEMA3B], 3p22–24, 3p25, 3p21.4, 3p14.2 [FHIT]), del 9p, aneuploidy
Dysplasia	LOH in 8p21–23, 17p13 (p53), 13q (Rb), 9p, aneuploidy (p53 mutations)
Carcinoma in situ	LOH in 3p, 5q21 (APC-MCC), 9p, aneuploidy, p53 mutations, ras mutations
Invasive or metastatic carcinoma	del 3p, del 9p, aneuploidy, p53 mutations, ras mutations, multiple other mutations

Source: Kerr[1] and Gazdar et al.[16]

3p21.3, 3p24, and 3p25; it is believed that these regions contain multiple tumor suppressor genes.

During field progression, a number of genetic alterations take place. The specific parental allelic loss in chromosomal deletions in preneoplastic lesions is referred to as *allele-specific mutations*. Allele-specific mutations are detected in smoking-related damaged epithelium and are likely to be phenomena of major biologic significance.[9,11,12] In addition to chromosome 3p deletion, LOH occurs at other chromosomes, including 2q, 9p21, 8p21–23, 11q13, 22q, 13q14 (Rb) and 17p13 (p53). The allelic losses of 2q, 3p, and 22q play an important role in the development of squamous cell carcinoma of the lung, and deletions of 9p and 18q are also important. Deletions at 5q21 (the adenomatous polyposis coli (APC) and mutated in colorectal cancer (MCC) region) have been detected in carcinoma in situ (Table 26.1).[1,13,14] Recently many chromosome 3p genes have been identified, including the fragile histidine triad (FHIT), CACNA2D2, 101F6, NPRL2, Ras association domain family 1A (RASSF1A), SEMA3B, SEMA3F, FUS1, DLEC1, RBSP3A, RBSP3B, and retinoid acid receptor β (RARβ).[15]

p53 Mutations

The p53 family of genes includes p53, p73, and p63. The p53 gene, located on chromosome 17p13, encodes a 53-kD nuclear transcription factor that activates the transcription of the downstream target genes, including p21, MDM2, GADD45, and Bax. By binding to the promoter of the p21 gene, p53 induces p21 expression, hence executing the inhibitive function of p21 in cell cycle at the G1/S checkpoint. p53 also binds to MDM2, a protein that also affects the cell cycle, apoptosis, and tumorigenesis through interactions with other proteins, including Rb and ribosomal protein L-1. GADD45, another p53-responsive stress protein, modifies DNA accessibility on damaged chromatin; and Bax forms a heterodimer with

Bcl-2 and plays an important role in apoptosis. Thus, p53 has multiple roles in maintaining the stability of the genome during cellular stress from DNA damage, hypoxia, and activated oncogenes.

Dysfunction of p53 is the most frequent and important genetic alteration in carcinogenesis of the lung. Loss of p53 functions occurs when mutations inactivate the p53 gene; hundreds of p53 mutations occur at variable times, and/or there is LOH at 17p13. The site of the p53 locus may be lost hemizygously in small cell lung carcinoma (SCLC) (90%) and non–small cell lung carcinoma (NSCLC) (65%). Among NSCLCs, squamous carcinomas and large cell carcinomas present a higher frequency of p53 mutation than adenocarcinomas.[17] Mutant p53 cannot activate p21 and causes a subsequent loss of tumor suppression function, promoting cellular proliferation.[18] Missense p53 mutations could result in accumulation of high levels of mutant p53 protein. Bronchial epithelium with a single point mutation consisting of a G:C to T:A transversion in codon 245 reveals morphologic abnormalities, including squamous metaplasia and mild to moderate atypia.[19] Mutations of p53 correlate with cigarette smoking and are mostly composed of the G to T transversion that is expected in tobacco smoke–related carcinogenesis.[20] Mutations in p53 in lung cancer are clustered in the middle of the gene at codons 157, 245, 248, and 273. These mutational sites correlate with the tobacco smoke carcinogen benzo[α] pyrene diol-epoxide–induced adducts that form at CpG sites at codons 157, 248, and 273 in bronchial epithelial cells in vitro. Codon 157 mutations appear to be unique to lung cancer.[21]

The theory of field carcinogenesis can be supported by the widespread presence of a single somatic p53 point mutation in the bronchi of a smoker. Inactivating p53 mutations are detected in over 50% of smokers and can be found very early in the carcinogenesis of squamous cell carcinoma as well as adenocarcinoma.[22,23] The p53 mutations occur in about one third of mild and moderate dysplasia and in two thirds of severe dysplasia, carcinoma in situ, and invasive carcinoma, which suggests that the majority of p53 mutations occur before the onset of invasion (Table 26.2).[23]

TABLE 26.2. Frequency of p53 protein accumulation at multiple stages of bronchial carcinogenesis.

Mucosal pattern	No. positive/No. total	% Positive
Normal	0/23	0
Squamous metaplasia	1/15	6.7
Mild dysplasia	4.25/16	26.6
Moderate dysplasia	5.58/19	29.4
Severe dysplasia	24.8/36	68.9
Carcinoma in situ	15.6/28	55.7
Microinvasive carcinoma	6.75/10	67.5
Invasive carcinoma	27.8/37	75.1

Source: Bennett et al.[23]

The *p16*/Cyclin D1/Cyclin-Dependent Kinase 4/Retinoblastoma Pathway and Aberrant Methylation

$p16^{INK4}$ is a kinase inhibitor of cyclin-dependent kinase 4 (Cdk4) and inhibits phosphorylation of Rb, making it also a tumor suppressor gene. Disruption of *p16* function results in inappropriate hyperphosphorylation and inactivation of Rb, which makes Rb dissociate with transcription factor E2F (a transcription factor that activates S-phase genes), leading to a no-brake cell cycle in cell proliferation. Although inactivation of the Rb pathway occurs through inactivation of the Cdk4 inhibitor $p16^{INK4}$ and/or upregulation of cyclin D1, the loss of Rb alleles at chromosomal region 13q14 can also occur, but less common (15%) in NSCLC. Abnormalities of cyclin D1, Cdk4, and p16 are more common (70%) in NSCLC. The $p16^{INK4a}$ gene is most commonly altered in NSCLC by aberrant promoter methylation (25%) and homozygous deletions or point mutations (10%–40%). Inactivation of $p16^{INK4}$ by DNA methylation especially has been found in early stages of squamous cell precursor lesions—17% of reserve cell hyperplasia, 24% of squamous metaplasia, and 50% of carcinoma in situ—whereas homozygous deletions and/or mutations may occur more frequently in later stages of NSCLC development (see Figure 26.1).

The $p16^{INK}$ locus at 9p21 has two RNA transcripts (E1A and E1B). *p16* arises from the E1A-containing transcript, while $p14^{ARF}$ (alternate reading frame) contains the E1B transcript. $p14^{ARF}$ binds to the MDM2–p53 complex and prevents p53 degradation. Blocking of p53 degradation links the E2F/Rb pathway to prolongation of activation of p53 and cell cycle arrest.[24,25] In addition to $p16^{INK4}$ methylation, abnormal gene methylation of RARβ, H-cadherin, APC, and RASFF1 is relatively frequent in bronchial brushing and sputum and oropharyngeal epithelial cells of heavy smokers. Methylation is less frequent in the bronchoalveolar lavage fluid and hence the distal lung parenchyma.[26] Aberrant methylation of multiple genes in the upper aerodigestive tract epithelium of heavy smokers is also frequently seen.[6,24,27–32]

The *PTEN/MMAC1* Tumor Suppressor Gene

The tumor suppressor gene *PTEN* (phosphatase and tensin homolog deleted on chromosome 10), also called *MMAC1* (mutated in multiple advanced cancers) is located on chromosome 10q23.[33,34] *PTEN* has been reported to play a role in apoptosis, cell cycle arrest, cell migration, and cell spreading.[35–37] Homozygous deletion and mutation of *PTEN* rarely occurs in NSCLC

(11%).[38,39] On the other hand, LOH has been reported in 91% of SCLC and in 41% of NSCLC.[40] In squamous cell carcinoma of the lung, *PTEN* loss occurs significantly more often in the early stages (stage I or II) of the disease. PTEN protein loss also occurs more frequently in tumors with low or no aberrant *p53* staining. Therefore, PTEN loss may be a favorable prognostic marker.[40]

Telomerase Dysregulation and Upregulation

Telomerase is a cellular reverse transcriptase that stabilizes telomere length by adding hexameric TTAGGG repeats onto the telomeric ends of the chromosomes, thus compensating for the continued erosion of telomeres that occurs in its absence. The core catalytic subunit of telomerase, hTERT, is expressed in embryonic cells and in adult male germline cells, but it is undetectable in normal somatic cells except for proliferative cells of renewal tissues (e.g., hematopoietic stem cells, activated lymphocytes, basal cells of the epidermis, proliferative endometrium, and intestinal crypt cells). In contrast, germ cells and cancer cells maintain telomere length using the enzyme telomerase and are able to divide indefinitely.[41–43]

Telomere dysfunction activates a *p53*-dependent checkpoint. The loss of telomere function and *p53* deficiency may accelerate carcinogenesis.[44] Telomerase is expressed in most human cancers, including lung carcinomas. Increased telomerase activity (80%) was reported in primary lung cancer samples compared with the adjacent normal lung tissue samples (4%) by using a polymerase chain reaction–based telomeric repeat amplification protocol (TRAP assay).[45] The increased telomerase activity in primary lung cancers was associated with increased cell proliferation rates and advanced pathologic stage.[46] Reactivation of telomerase expression is essential for the continuous proliferation of cancer cells to reach immortality. Telomerase dysregulation may also occur in preneoplastic bronchial epithelial dysplasia. Telomerase positivity was found in basal epithelial cells of normal bronchial epithelium (26%) and in the epithelium of small bronchi and bronchioles of peripheral lung samples (23%). The abnormal bronchial epithelial cells have shown much increased telomerase activity (i.e., 71% in hyperplasia, 80% in metaplasia, 82% in dysplasia, and 100% in carcinoma in situ).[47] Therefore, telomerase appears to be increasingly expressed from normal epithelium to squamous metaplasia, dysplasia, and carcinoma in situ but is decreased in invasive carcinoma with a direct correlation between protein and mRNA levels of expression.

Telomere shortening represents an early genetic abnormality in bronchial carcinogenesis (predominantly in high-grade, preinvasive lesions), preceding telomerase expression and p53/Rb inactivation. A direct correlation between hTERT and p53 expression was found.[48] The telomerase protein expression has recently been shown to be present in noncancerous epithelia before secondary cancer development, and the authors concluded that detection of telomerase protein in noncancerous bronchial epithelia might become a useful marker in detecting patients at high risk for lung cancer development.[49] Why telomerase is reexpressed in lung cancer cells is currently unknown.

Amplification of Oncogenes

Although the amplification of mutant *ras* genes is common in adenocarcinoma (50%) and amplification of *c-Myc* genes is common in small cell carcinoma (80%–90%), they are less common or absent in squamous cell carcinoma.[50,51] Small percentages of NSCLC have been shown to have amplifications of several other genes, including *c-erbB2 (HER2/neu)*[52] and *Bcl-2*,[53–55] and MDM,[56] a multidrug resistance-associated protein.[57–59]

The frequency of *c-erbB2* overexpression in NSCLC is approximately 25%.[52] Patients with squamous cell carcinoma showing *Bcl-2* positivity greater than 50% have been shown to have a survival advantage. However, none of these abnormal gene amplifications has been shown to be useful screening tools for preneoplastic genetic changes or for elucidation of premalignant biology.

Epidermal Growth Factor Receptor and Tyrosine Kinase Inhibitors

The epidermal growth factor receptor (EGFR) is a tyrosine kinase receptor that is commonly altered in epithelial tumors. Structurally, each receptor is composed of an extracellular ligand binding domain, a transmembrane domain, and an intracellular domain that possesses tyrosine kinase activity. The EGFRs exist as inactive monomers. Upon binding to ligands, such as epidermal growth factor (EGF) or transforming growth factor-α, the receptors undergo conformational changes that facilitate homo- or heterodimerization. The EGFR induces cancer via at least three major mechanisms: overexpression of EGFR ligands, amplification of EGFR, and mutational activations of EGFR. The majority of NSCLCs overexpress EGFR, and EGFR is also frequently overexpressed in preneoplastic bronchial lesions.[60] Also, overexpression of EGFR is associated with adverse prognosis of NSCLC. Thus, EGFR is an excellent potential target for prevention and therapy.

Recent reports of lung cancers showing mutations in the *EGFR* gene have generated considerable interest, because such mutations are associated with an increased

sensitivity to the therapeutic drug gefitinib. Gefitinib, marketed as Iressa (ZD1839), is a small tyrosine kinase inhibitor molecule that inhibits the protein kinase activity of EGFR.[61] The tyrosine kinase domain *EGFR* mutations are more commonly found in adenocarcinoma of lung, in females, in patients from Asian nations including Japan, Korea, and China, and in nonsmokers.[62–66] However, the overexpression or amplification of *EGFR* is frequently found in squamous cell carcinoma of the lung, oropharynx, and skin as well as other NSCLCs.[67] Although *EGFR* positivity as determined by fluorescence in situ hybridization represented by high polysomy and gene amplification is higher in adenocarcinoma (33%) and NSCLCs (30.2%), it is also expressed in squamous cell carcinoma (26.7%; Figure 26.3).[68]

Erlotinib HCl (Tarceva™) is the HER1/EGFR tyrosine kinase inhibitor that has demonstrated a survival benefit in all subsets of patients, both female and male—including adenocarcinoma and squamous cell carcinoma, both current smokers and exsmokers, and both Asians and non-Asians—evaluated in a randomized phase III trial of Tarceva (BR.21). The presence of the *EGFR* mutation among patients with NSCLC treated with erlotinib may also increase the responsiveness to the erlotinib, but it is not indicative of a survival benefit.[69,70]

There are several methods with which to predict tyrosine kinase inhibitor sensitivity, such as immunohistochemistry or proteomic profiles to detect the amplification of the *EGFR* gene and measurement of the presence of phosphorylated Akt, which is a downstream target of the EGFR pathway, but not phosphorylated mitogen-activated protein kinase.[71] The correlations among *EGFR* gene amplification, gene mutation, phosphorylation of

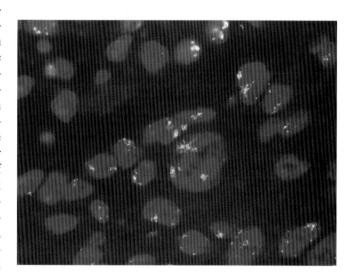

FIGURE 26.3. *EGFR* gene amplification with a clustered pattern determined by fluorescence in situ hybridization in a squamous cell carcinoma patient. (Courtesy of Dr. Sung-Hye Park, Seoul National University Hospital, Seoul, South Korea.)

TABLE 26.3. Epidermal growth factor overexpression, mutation, and amplification in lung cancer.

	Overexpression	Mutation	Amplification
Squamous cell carcinoma	70%	0%	10%–27%
Adenocarcinoma	50%	20%–55% (deletion in exon 19, point mutation in exons 18 and 21, duplication in exon 20)	10%–33%
Non-small cell lung carcinoma	50%–80%	13%	33%–45%

Source: Shigematsu et al.,[62] Paez et al.,[65] Jeon et al.,[68] Cappuzzo et al.,[71] Hirsh et al.,[73] Kosaka et al.,[74] and Reissmann et al.[75]

EGFR protein, and activation of its downstream molecules and extracellular signal-related protein kinase 1/2 (ERK1/2) reveal its downstream molecular function in a reciprocal and/or complementary manner in the maintenance and/or progression of carcinomas in the majority of NSCLC patients (Table 26.3).[72]

Autocrine Growth Factors

Autocrine growth factors, including neuropeptides and gastrin-releasing peptides, have been demonstrated in SCLC. Bombesin-like peptides, which have also been elevated in bronchoalveolar lavage and urine specimens of smokers, may play a role in tumor progression.[75-78] Neuropeptide antagonists, such as substance P and bradykinin derivatives, also induce apoptosis of both SCLC and NSCLC.[79] The autocrine and paracrine effects of multiple neuropeptides, growth factors, and chemokines, which are induced by smoking and are shown to be elevated in lung tumors, could induce angiogenesis, tissue invasion, homing of metastases, and immune modulation.[80] However, the exact role of autocrine growth factors in squamous cell carcinoma of the lung and preinvasive lesions has not been described.

Conclusion

Lung cancer is still the number one cause of death in cancer-related mortalities for both men and women in the Western countries. There is still lack of reliable means to screen early lesions, and the patients with symptoms or patients with lesions detected by chest x-ray already have advanced disease. Recent advances in molecular biology and pathology, through implementation of many newly advanced technologies in molecular biology, have led to better understanding of the carcinogenesis in the lung and morphologic and molecular changes in early preinvasive lesions. For squamous cell carcinoma, cumulative genetic damages seem to correspond with the different grades of morphologic changes, from low- to

high-grade dysphasia. Morphologically, normal mucosa may already contain genetic abnormalities. Stepwise histologic changes are believed to occur from normal through the various grades of squamous metaplasia, mild, moderate, and severe dysplasia, and carcinoma in situ before the lesion becomes microinvasive. However, currently not a single set of biomarkers has emerged that can be used for accurate prediction of the development of lung cancer in any particular individual.[81]

Some authors propose that ectopic expression of telomerase in bronchial epithelia may precede transformation in human hung cancer development and that detection of telomerase protein in noncancerous bronchial epithelia will become a useful marker for detecting patients at high risk for lung cancer development,[49] and the polyclonal antibodies against hTERT and EGFR are available for paraffin-embedded sections. Serum hTERT mRNA and EGFR mRNA are also useful as tumor markers for lung cancer,[82] and there is a linear relationship between increasing marker expression and severity of bronchial dysplastic change for p53, EGFR, and Ki-67.[23,62,83] However, more data are needed before a definite conclusion could be made.

Detection of genetic lesions in preneoplastic tissues combined with new radiographic screening methods, such as spiral computed tomography scans, will open new doors for early diagnosis, identifying individuals at high risk of developing lung cancer and directing intervention with chemoprevention. Laser-induced fluorescence endoscope bronchoscopy may help to localize preinvasive and early-invasive bronchial lesions. Early detection of precursors of lung cancer may provide an opportunity to treat disease early. Most radiographically occult cancers are histopathologically squamous cell carcinoma and are located in relatively large central bronchi without evidence of invasion beyond the bronchial cartilage.

Some authors suggested that if the patient is a surgical candidate, surgery is still the first option and yields good 5-year survival and recurrent rates.[84,85] For patients who are not surgical candidates, photodynamic therapy would be an option.[84] Other alternatives for early superficial squamous cell carcinoma include electrocautery, cryotherapy, and brachytherapy. Following treatment, patients should be closely monitored for recurrent diseases and development of metachronous lesions.

The new findings of molecular pathology will lead to new treatment strategies, including drugs designed to inhibit enzyme activity, monoclonal antibodies against growth factors and their receptors, vaccines against tumor specific mutant peptides, or gene therapy to replace the defective tumor suppressor genes. These new tools will lead to a new era in the diagnosis, prevention, and treatment of lung cancer. Gefitinib is a good example of this kind of treatment. More developments will follow.

References

1. Kerr KM. Morphology and genetics of preinvasive pulmonary disease. Curr Diagn Pathol 2004;10:259–268.
2. Travis WD, Colby TV, Corrin B, et al., eds. Histological Typing of Lung and Pleural Tumors. WHO International Histological Classification of Tumours, 3rd ed. Berlin: Springer; 1999.
3. Rocha AT, McCormack M, Montana G, Schreiber G. Association between lower lobe location and upstaging for early-stage non–small cell lung cancer. Chest 2004;25:1424–1430.
4. Miller YE. Pathogenesis of lung cancer; 100 year report. Am J Respir Cell Mol Biol 2005;3:216–223.
5. Hirsch FR, Franklin WA, Gazdar AF, Bunn Jr PA. Early detection of lung cancer: clinical perspectives of recent advances in biology and radiology. Clin Cancer Res 2001;7: 5–22.
6. Braakhuis BJ, Tabor MP, Kummer JA, et al. A genetic explanation of Slaughter's concept of field cancerization: evidence and clinical implications. Cancer Res 2003;3: 1727–1730.
7. Yokota J, Takashi K. Molecular footprints of human lung cancer progression. Cancer Sci 2004;95:197–204.
8. Rom WN, Tchou-Wong KM. Molecular and genetic aspects of lung cancer. Methods Mol Med 2003;75:3–26.
9. Wistuba II, Gazdar AF. Characteristic genetic alterations in lung cancer. In: Driscoll B, ed. Lung Cancer: Molecular Pathology Methods and Reviews, vol 1. Los Angeles: Humana Press; 2003:3–28.
10. Forgacs E, Zochbauer-Muller S, Olah E, Minna JD. Molecular genetic abnormalities in the pathogenesis of human lung cancer. Pathol Oncol Res 2001;7(1):6–13.
11. Hung J, Kishimoto Y, Sugio K, et al. Allele-specific chromosome 3p deletions occur at an early stage in the pathogenesis of lung carcinoma. JAMA 1995;273:558–563.
12. Kishimoto Y, Sugio K, Hung JY, et al. Allele-specific loss in chromosome 9p loci in preneoplastic lesions accompanying non-small-cell lung cancers. J Natl Cancer Inst 1995;87:1224–1229.
13. Chung GTY, Sundaresan V, Hasleton P, et al. Clonal evolution of lung tumors. Cancer Res 1996;56:1609–1614.
14. Thiberville L, Payne P, Vielkinds J, et al. Evidence of cumulative losses with progression of premalignant epithelial lesions to carcinoma of the bronchus. Cancer Res 1995;55: 5133–5139.
15. Zavorovsky ER, Lerman MI, Minna JD. Chromosome 3 abnormalities in lung cancer. In Pass HI, Carbone DP, Johnson DH, et al, eds. Lung Cancer, 3rd ed. Philadelphia: Lippincott Williams & Wilkins; 2005:118–134.
16. Gazdar AF, Bader S, Hung J, et al. Molecular genetic changes found in human lung cancer and its precursor lesions. Cold Spring Harb Symp Quant Biol 1994;109:565–572.
17. Vincenzi B, Schiavon G, Silletta M, et al. Cell cycle alterations and lung cancer. Histol Histopathol 2006;21:423–435.
18. Greenblatt MS, Benett WP, Hollstein M, Harris CC. Mutations in the p53 tumor suppressor gene: clues to cancer etiology and molecular pathogenesis. Cancer Res 1994;54: 4855–4878.
19. Franklin WA, Gazdar AF, Haney J, et al. Widely dispersed p53 mutation in respiratory epithelium. A novel mechanism for field carcinogenesis. J Clin Invest 1997;100:2133–2137.
20. Harris CC. p53 tumor suppressor gene: from the basic research laboratory to the clinic—an abridged historical perspective. Carcinogenesis 1996;17:1187–1198.
21. Ramet M, Casten K, Jarvinen K, et al. p53 protein expression is correlated with benzo[a]pyrene-DNA adducts in carcinoma cell lines. Carcinogenesis 1996;16:2117–2124.
22. Pfeifer GP, Denissenko MF, Olivier M, et al. Tobacco smoke carcinogens, DNA damage and p53 mutations in smoking-associated cancers. Oncogene 2002;21:7435–7451.
23. Bennett WP, Colby TV, Travis WD, et al. p53 protein accumulates frequently in early bronchial neoplasia. Cancer Res 1993;53:4817–4822.
24. Gorgoulis VG, Zacharatos P, Kotsinas A, et al. Alterations of the p16–pRb pathway and the chromosome locus 9p21–22 in non–small-cell lung carcinomas. Relationship with p53 and MDM2 protein expression. Am J Pathol 1998;153: 1749–1765.
25. Bates S, Phillips AC, Clark PA, et al. p14[ARF] links the tumour suppressors RB and p53. Nature 1998;395:124–125.
26. Zochbauer-Muller S, Lam S, Toyooka S, et al. Aberrant methylation of multiple genes in the upper aerodigestive tract epithelium of heavy smokers. Int J Cancer 2003;107: 612–616.
27. Belinsky SA, Nikula KJ, Palmisano WA, et al. Aberrant methylation of p16[INK4a] is an early event in lung cancer and a potential biomarker for early diagnosis. Proc Natl Acad Sci USA 1998;95:11891–11896.
28. Brambilla E, Moro D, Gazzeri S, Brambilla C. Alterations of expression of Rb, p16(INK4A) and cyclin D1 in non–small cell lung carcinoma and their clinical significance. J Pathol 1999;188:351–360.
29. Park MJ, Shimizu K, Nakano T, et al. Pathogenetic and biologic significance of TP14[ARF] alterations in nonsmall cell lung carcinoma. Cancer Genet Cytogenet 2003;141:5–13.
30. Gazzeri S, Gouyer V, Vour'ch C, et al. Mechanisms of p16INK4A inactivation in non small-cell lung cancers. Oncogene 1998;16:497–504.
31. Sato M, Horio Y, Sekido Y, et al. The expression of DNA methyltransferases and methyl-CpG-binding proteins is not associated with the methylation status of p14(ARF), p16(INK4a) and RASSF1A in human lung cancer cell lines. Oncogene 2002;21:4822–4829.

32. Bates S, Phillips AC, Clark PA, et al. p14ARF links the tumour suppressors RB and p53. Nature 1998;395:124–125.

33. Li J, Yen C, Liaw D, et al. PTEN, a putative protein tyrosine phosphates gene mutated in human brain, breast, and prostate cancer. Science 1997;275:1943–1947.

34. Steck PA, Pershouse MA, Jasser SA, et al. Identification of a candidate tumour suppressor gene, MMAC1, at chromosome 10q23.3 that is mutated in multiple advanced cancers. Nat Genet 1997;15:356–362.

35. Weng L, Brown J, Eng C. PTEN induces apoptosis and cell cycle arrest through phosphoinositol-3-kinase/Akt-dependent degradation and –independent pathways. Hum Mol Genet 200;10:237–242.

36. Mamllapalli R, Gavrilova N, Mihaykiva VT, et al. PTEN regulates the ubiquitin-dependent degradation of the CDK inhibitor p27(KIP1) through the ubiquitin E3 ligase SCF(SKP2). Curr Biol 2001;11:23–27.

37. Tamura M, Gu J, Matsumoto K, et al. Inhibition of cell migration, spreading, and focal adhesions by tumor suppressor PTEN. Science 1998;280:1614–1617.

38. Forgacs E, Biesterveld EJ, Sekido Y, et al. Mutation analysis of the PTEN/MMAC1 gene in lung cancer. Oncogene 1998;17:1557–1565.

39. Petersen S, Rudolf J, Bockmuhl U, et al. Distinct regions of allelic imbalance on chromosome 10q22–q26 in squamous cell carcinomas of the lung. Oncogene 1998;17:449–454.

40. Marsit CJ, Zheng S, Aldape K, et al. PTEN expression in non–small cell lung cancer: evaluating its relation to tumor characteristics, allelic loss, and epigenetic alteration. Hum Pathol 2005;36:768–776.

41. de Lange T. Activation of telomerase in a human tumor. Proc Natl Acad Sci USA 1994;91:2882–2885.

42. Harley CB, Villeponteau B. Telomere and telomerase in aging and cancer. Curr Opin Genet Dev 1995;5:249–255.

43. Kiyono T, Foster SA, Koop JI, et al. Both Rb/p16^{INK4a} inactivation and telomerase activity are required to immortalize human epithelial cells. Nature 1998;396:84–88.

44. Chin L, Artandi SE, Shen Q, et al. p53 deficiency rescues the adverse effects of telomere loss and cooperates with telomere dysfunction to accelerate carcinogenesis. Cell 1999;97:527–538.

45. Hiyama K, Hiyama E, Ishioka S, et al. Telomerase activity in small-cell and non–small-cell lung cancers. J Natal Cancer Inst 1995;87:895–902.

46. Albanell J, Lonardo F, Rusch V, et al. High telomerase activity in primary lung cancers: association with increased cell proliferation rates and advanced pathologic stage. J Natl Cancer Inst 1997;89:1609–1615.

47. Yashima K, Litzky LA, Kaiser L, et al. Telomerase expression in respiratory epithelium during the multistage pathogenesis of lung carcinomas. Cancer Res 1997;57:2373–2377.

48. Lantuejoul S, Soria JC, Morat L, et al. Telemerase shortening and telomerase reverse transcriptase expression in preinvasive bronchial lesions. Clin Cancer Res 2005;11:2074–2082.

49. Miyazu YM, Miyazawa T, Hiyama K, et al. Telomerase expression in noncancerous bronchial epithelia is a possible marker of early development of lung cancer. Cancer Res 2005;65:9623–9627.

50. Mills NE, Fishman CL, Rom WN, et al. Increased prevalence of K-ras oncogene mutations in lung adenocarcinoma. Cancer Res 1995;55:1444–1447.

51. Viallet J, Minna J. Dominant oncogenes and tumor suppressor genes in the pathogenesis of human lung cancer. Am J Respir Cell Mol Biol 1990;2:225–232.

52. Kern JA, Robinson RA, Gazdar AF, et al. Mechanisms of p185HER2 expression in human non–small cell lung cancer cell lines. Am J Respir Cell Mol Biol 1992;6:359–363.

53. Pazzella F, Turley H, Kuzu I, et al. bcl-2 protein in non–small cell lung carcinoma. N Engl J Med 1993;329:690–694.

54. Walker C, Robertson L, Myskow M, Dixon G. Expression of the BCL-2 protein in normal and dysplastic bronchial epithelium and in lung carcinomas. Br J Cancer 1995;72:164–169.

55. Uren AG, Vaux DL. Molecular and clinical aspects of apoptosis. Pharmacol Ther 1996;72:37–50.

56. Marchetti A, Buttitta F, Pellegrini S, et al. mdm2 gene amplification and overexpression in non–small cell lung carcinomas with accumulation of the p53 protein in the absence of p53 gene mutations. Diagn Mol Pathol 1995;4:93–97.

57. Cole SP, Bhardwaj G, Gerlach JH, et al. Overexpression of a transporter gene in a multidrug-resistant human lung cancer cell line. Science 1992;258:1650–1654.

58. Eijdems EW, De Haas M, Coco-Martin JM, et al. Mechanisms of MRP overexpression in four human lung cancer cell lines and analysis of the MRP amplicon. Int J Cancer 1995;60:676–684.

59. Ray ME, Guan XY, Slovak ML, et al. Rapid detection, cloning and molecular cytogenetic characterization of sequences from an MRP-encoding amplicon by chromosome microdissection. Br J Cancer 1994;70:85–90.

60. Brunn PA Jr, Franklin W. Epidermal growth factor receptor expression, signal pathway, and inhibitors in non–small cell lung cancer. Semin Oncol 2002;29:38–44.

61. Kris MG, Natale RB, Herbst RS, et al. Efficacy of gefitinib, an inhibitor of the epidermal growth factor receptor tyrosine kinase, in symptomatic patients with non–small cell lung cancer: a randomized trial. JAMA 2003;290:2149–2158.

62. Shigematsu H, Lin L, Takahashi T, et al. Clinical and biological features associated with epidermal growth factor receptor gene mutations in lung cancers. J Natl Cancer Inst 2005;97:339–346.

63. Cohen MH, Williams GA, Sridhara R, et al. United States Food and Drug Administration drug approval summary: gefitinib (ZD1839; Iressa) tablets. Clin Cancer Res 2004;10:1212–1218.

64. Lynch TJ, Bell DW, Sordella R, et al. Activating mutations in the epidermal growth factor receptor underlying responsiveness of non–small cell lung cancer to gefitinib. N Engl J Med 2004;350:2129–2139.

65. Paez JG, Janne PA, Lee JC, et al. EGFR mutations in lung cancer: correlation with clinical response to gefitinib therapy. Science 2004;304:1497–1500.

66. Pao W, Miller V, Zakowski M, et al. EGF receptor gene mutations are common in lung cancers from "never smokers" and are associated with sensitivity of tumor to

gefitinib and erlotinib. Proc Natl Acad Sci USA 2004;101: 13306–13311.

67. Borczuk AC, Gorenstein L, Walter K, et al. Non–small cell lung cancer molecular signatures recapitulate lung developmental pathways. Am J Pathol 2003;163:1949–1960.

68. Jeon YK , Sung SW, Chung J-H, et al. Clinicopathologic features and prognostic implications of epidermal growth factor receptor (EGFR) gene copy number and protein expression in non–small cell lung cancer. Lung Cancer 2006;54:387–398

69. Shepherd FA, Pereira JR, Ciuleanu T, et al. Erlotinib in previously treated non–small cell lung cancer. N Engl J Med 2005;353:123–132.

70. Tsao M-S, Sakurada A, Cutz J-C, et al. Erlotinib in lung cancer—molecular and clinical predictors of outcome. N Engl J Med 2005;353:133–144.

71. Cappuzzo F, Magrini E, Ceresoli GL, et al. Akt phosphorylation and gefitinib efficacy in patients with advanced non–small cell lung cancer. J Natl Cancer Inst 2004;96:1133–1141.

72. Suzuki S, Igarashi S, Hanawa M, et al. Diversity of epidermal growth factor receptor–mediated activation of downstream molecules in human lung carcinomas. Mod Pathol 2006;28:1–13.

73. Hirsh F, Scagliotti GV, Langer CJ, et al. Epidermal growth factor family of receptors in preneoplasia and lung cancer: perspectives for targeted therapies. Lung Cancer 2003;41: S29.

74. Kosaka T, Yatabe Y, Endoh H, et al. Mutations of the epidermal growth factor receptor gene in lung cancer. Biological and clinical implications. Cancer Res 2004;64: 8919–8923.

75. Reissmann PT, Koga H, Figlin RA, et al. Amplification and overexpression of the cyclin D1 and epidermal growth factor receptor genes in non–small cell lung cancer. J Cancer Res Clin Oncol 2004;125:61–70.

76. Kelly MJ, Linnoila RI, Avis IL, et al. Antitumor activity of a monoclonal antibody directed against gastrin-releasing peptide in patients with small cell lung cancer. Chest 1997;112:256–261.

77. Aguayo SM, Kane MA, King TE Jr, et al. Increased levels of bombesin-like peptides in the lower respiratory tract of asymptomatic cigarette smokers. J Clin Invest 1989;84: 1105–1113.

78. Aguayo SM, King TE Jr, Kane MA, et al. Urinary levels of bombesin-like peptides in asymptomatic cigarette smoker: a potential risk marker for smoking-related diseases. Cancer Res 1992;52:2727s–2731s.

79. Chan D, Gera L, Stewart J, et al. Bradykinin antagonist dimer, CU201, inhibits the growth of human lung cancer cell lines by a "biased agonist" mechanism. Proc Natl Acad Sci USA 2002;99:4608–4613.

80. Strieter RM, Belperio JA, Burdick MD, et al. CXC chemokines: angiogenesis, immunoangiostasis, and metastases in lung cancer. Ann NY Acad Sci 2004;1078:351–360.

81. Sutedja G. New techniques for early detection of lung cancer. Eur Respir J 2003;21:57s–66s.

82. Miura N, Nakamura H, Sato R, et al. Clinical usefulness of serum telomerase reverse transcriptase (hTERT) mRNA and epidermal growth factor receptor (EGFR) mRNA as a novel tumor marker for lung cancer. Cancer Science 2006;97:1366–1373.

83. Merrick DT, Kittelson J, Winterhalder R, et al. Analysis of cErbB1/epidermal growth factor receptor and c-ErbB2/HER-2 expression in bronchial dysplasia: evaluation of potential targets for chemoprevention of lung cancer. Clin Cancer Res 2006;12:2281–2288.

84. Mathur PN, Edell E, Sutedja T, et al. Treatment of early stage non–small cell lung cancer. Chest 2003;123:176–180.

85. Koike T, Terashima M, Takizawa T, et al. Surgical results for centrally-located early stage lung cancer. Ann Thorac Surg 2000;70:1176–1179.

27
Molecular Pathology of Large Cell Carcinoma and Its Precursors

Jennifer A. Eleazar and Alain C. Borczuk

Introduction

The classification of lung carcinomas remains primarily morphologic with individual instances in which immunohistochemistry can serve as an adjunctive test. In the case of large cell carcinoma, the current WHO classification system remains partly one of exclusion; that is, the tumor should lack morphologic features that are generally associated with small cell lung carcinoma (SCLC), adenocarcinoma, and squamous cell carcinoma (Figure 27.1A).[1] For example, a poorly differentiated carcinoma with demonstrable mucin (more than five mucin-positive cells in at least two high-power fields) by special stains would be designated as solid adenocarcinoma with mucin rather than as large cell carcinoma.

It is known that ultrastructural evidence of squamous and glandular differentiation can be recognized within large cell carcinomas.[2,3] As a result, exclusionary criteria require cut-off values such as the one indicated earlier for solid adenocarcinoma with mucin. Although not explicitly stated in the WHO classification, it has been suggested that 10% of squamous cell carcinoma or adenocarcinoma within a tumor that is otherwise undifferentiated is sufficient to diagnose the tumor as either squamous cell carcinoma or adenocarcinoma rather than large cell carcinoma.

There are notable subcategories within large cell carcinoma. Perhaps the most significant subset is the large cell neuroendocrine carcinoma (LCNEC; see also Chapter 29). Large cell neuroendocrine carcinoma was described in 1991 and included in the 1999 WHO classification.[4] These tumors have histologic features that are associated with neuroendocrine differentiation ("carcinoid-like"), including organoid/nesting morphology, trabecular growth, and rosette formation. Large cell neuroendocrine carcinoma cells are generally larger than those of SCLC, have more cytoplasm, and have nuclear features that include frequent nucleoli and vesicular chromatin. Necrosis is common. Documentation of neuroendocrine dif-

ferentiation by immunohistochemical stains such as chromogranin, synaptophysin, or CD56 is required (Figure 27.1B).

A second subcategory of large cell carcinoma is basaloid carcinoma.[5] The histology of this tumor is notable for its solid nodular pattern with necrosis that resembles the organoid pattern of LCNEC. In contrast to LCNEC, the nuclei in basaloid carcinoma are smaller and more fusiform and generally do not show prominent nucleoli. Both tumors share peripheral palisading within the nodular nests (Figure 27.1C). Neuroendocrine markers are generally negative in basaloid carcinoma. This growth pattern can be seen in squamous cell carcinomas, but in these instances the tumors are classified as a basaloid variant of squamous cell carcinoma. Basaloid carcinomas lack squamous differentiation. This observation justifies a large cell carcinoma categorization, along with studies indicating a poor prognosis.[6]

A third variant is the lymphoepithelioma-like carcinoma (LELC).[7,8] In contrast to other tumors within this category, this type is not smoking associated and is associated with Epstein-Barr virus (EBV) infection in Asian populations.[9,10] Tumor cells are large, have vesicular nuclei with prominent nucleoli, and have indistinct cellular borders imparting a syncytial growth pattern. Most important to this diagnosis is an associated lymphocytic/lymphoplasmacytic infiltrate around tumor nests and intermingled between tumor cells (Figure 27.1D). The inflammatory population is reactive but is present in both primary and metastatic sites.

Two additional categories of large cell carcinoma include clear cell carcinomas and large cell carcinoma with rhabdoid phenotype. Clear cell carcinoma shows no squamous or glandular differentiation and demonstrates cytoplasmic clearing. This clearing can be due to glycogen accumulation, but this is not always the case. Large cell carcinoma with rhabdoid phenotype features cells with large eosinophilic cytoplasmic inclusions, with >10% of the cells exhibiting this morphologic finding (Figure 27.1E).[11]

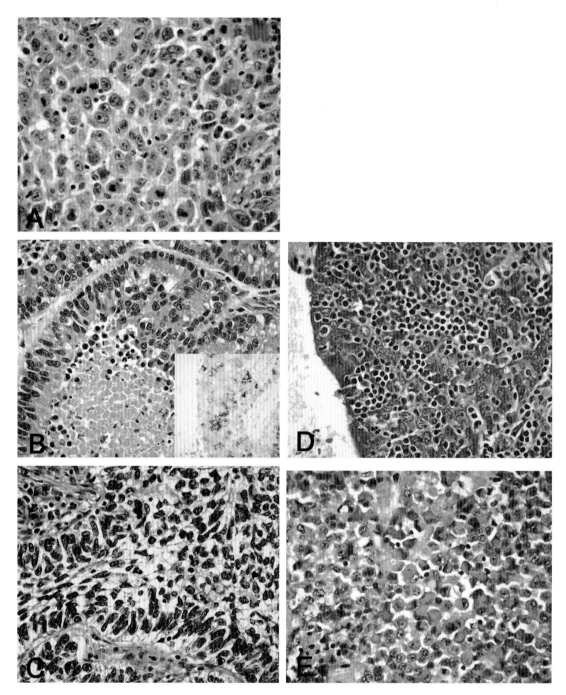

FIGURE 27.1. Histologic features of large cell carcinomas. **(A)** Large cell carcinoma. **(B)** Large cell neuroendocrine carcinoma, with inset showing synaptophysin immunoreactivity. **(C)** Basaloid carcinoma. **(D)** Lymphoepithelioma-like carcinoma. **(E)** Large cell carcinoma with rhabdoid phenotype. (Hematoxylin and eosin, original magnification, ×150).

The WHO classification seems straightforward at first glance, but in practice there are some complexities. For example, spindle or giant cell elements in a large cell carcinoma would place it in the sarcomatoid carcinoma class as a pleomorphic carcinoma, as the spindle/giant cell component is the most recognizable. A combined LCNEC with spindle/giant cell elements is classified as a large cell carcinoma, in this case because the LCNEC component is readily identifiable and immunohistochemically confirmable. Another area of difficulty involves large cell tumors that have neuroendocrine morphology but are negative for neuroendocrine markers by immunohistochemistry (LCCNM). Although it has been proposed that they may be similar to LCNEC,[12] it remains unclear whether this category of tumors resembles large cell carcinoma or LCNEC more closely.

The purpose of this introduction is to review the current classification of large cell carcinomas. These definitions are likely to improve interobserver reliability but also underscore the complexities of lung tumor classification. Molecular studies may assist in this classification process, but there remain many unanswered questions within this subgroup of tumors.

Molecular Studies: Immunohistochemical Markers

Lineage Specific Markers

Tumor classification is enhanced by immunohistochemistry, and many of our speculations regarding the cellular origin of tumors are based on this technique. Markers currently in use for lung tumors that have been studied in large cell carcinomas are summarized in Table 27.1[3–5,9–11,13–22]

Large Cell Carcinoma

The specific cell of origin for large cell carcinoma is not known. Large cell carcinomas represent poorly differentiated carcinomas, not completely undifferentiated tumors. For example, the majority of large cell carcinomas and subtypes express pan-cytokeratin (pan-CK), a marker of epithelial differentiation. Overall, approximately 65% of large cell carcinomas stain positively for pan-CK or epithelial membrane antigen,[3,13–15] whereas a higher percentage stain for cytokeratin 7 (CK7), a subtype expressed in lung epithelium, although not exclusively so.[15,16] A marker with relative specificity to Clara cells and type II pneumocytes is thyroid transcription factor 1 (TTF-1).[23] Thyroid transcription factor 1 immunoreactivity is seen in 50% of cases of large cell carcinoma.[16,17] Approximately 30% of large cell carcinomas are positive for peripheral airway cell markers such as surfactant protein A (SP-A) or 10-kD Clara cell protein as well.[24,25]

Rossi et al.[17] subdivided 45 cases of large cell carcinoma into adenocarcinomas (60%), squamous cell carcinomas (22%), and large cell carcinoma with neuroendocrine differentiation (LCCND) (9%) based on their expression of CK7, high-molecular-weight CK, TTF-1 and CD56/neural cell adhesion molecule. Using a similar strategy, Au et al.[18] demonstrated hierarchical clustering of large cell carcinoma based on immunohistochemistry of 18 markers (including pan-CK, p63, TTF-1 and CK5/6, chromogranin, and synaptophysin) into four groups. Of the large cell carcinomas, 29 tumors (53%) clustered within a group composed of predominantly adenocarcinomas and 15 tumors (27%) clustered within a group composed of squamous cell carcinoma. The remaining 11 large cell carcinomas formed two smaller mixed clusters in which large cell carcinoma were about half the cases. This suggests that some morphologic large cell carcinoma may have immunohistochemically detectable differentiation but that some do not.

In summary, large cell carcinomas have ultrastructural features and immunohistochemical phenotypes similar to those observed in adenocarcinomas, coexpressing TTF-1 and CK7 as well as other markers of adenocarcinoma such as carcinoembryonic antigen, secretory component, SP-A, and B72.3 (see Table 27.1). A smaller group of large cell carcinomas have squamous cell features.

Large Cell Neuroendocrine Carcinoma

Approximately 75% of LCNEC stain positive for chromogranin, with 84%–100% and 90%–100% of cases positive for synaptophysin and CD56, respectively.[4,15,19,20] In contrast to large cell carcinoma, LCNECs are less frequently high-molecular-weight CK positive and less frequently CK7 positive (see Table 27.1; LCNECs are also discussed in detail in Chapter 29).[15,19,21] Similar to large cell carcinoma, TTF-1 positivity is seen in approximately 30%–75% of cases of LCNEC.[17,19,21,22]

It is important to note a caveat regarding TTF-1 as a marker linking tumor type to origin in lung type II cells or Clara cells. Thyroid transcription factor 1 staining in cases of SCLC is not limited to SCLCs of pulmonary origin. Whereas pulmonary SCLC is positive for TTF-1 in over 80% of cases, extrapulmonary SCLCs are positive as well (between 30% and 50%).[26] The expression of TTF-1 in SCLC may not reflect its transcriptional control of surfactant-related genes. In this setting, TTF-1 reactivity may reflect significant transcriptional dysregulation in an undifferentiated tumor or a relationship to primitive neuroendocrine differentiation. Therefore, it is unclear whether TTF-1 immunoreactivity in LCNEC and large cell carcinoma should be interpreted as evidence of common origin with adenocarcinoma. In the case of large cell carcinoma, staining for other surfactant proteins has been described. It remains to be determined whether TTF-1 staining in LCNEC reflects type II or Clara cell origin, a relation to adenocarcinoma, or an as yet not understood relationship with neuroendocrine differentiation.

Basaloid Carcinoma

Basaloid carcinomas are frequently positive for CKs KL1 and high-molecular-weight CK (34BE12). Thyroid transcription factor 1 is negative, and reactivity for neuroendocrine markers is infrequent.[5,19]

Lymphoepithelioma-Like Carcinoma

The carcinoma cells in these tumors are positive for CK, whereas the accompanying lymphoid infiltrate stains for leukocyte common antigen, ubiquitin carboxyl-terminal esterase L1, and CD8.[9,10] Studies of patients from western countries do not demonstrate evidence of EBV, with rare exceptions described in case reports.[27] These tumors often express the oncoprotein Bcl-2 but typically show low detection rates for latent membrane protein 1 (LMP-1).[9,10] One series demonstrated LMP-1 in 16 of 30 cases, but showed no survival difference for LMP-1–positive tumors.[28]

Large Cell Carcinoma with Rhabdoid Phenotype

Large cell carcinomas with rhabdoid phenotype are positive for vimentin and often positive for pan-CK and epithelial membrane antigen.[11,29,30] Positive staining for CK7 and neuroendocrine markers can be seen.[11,29] None of the cases studied showed TTF-1 immunoreactivity.[29]

Molecular Pathway and Prognostic Markers

In addition to markers of cell lineage/cell of origin, large cell carcinomas have been studied for a variety of markers that may have prognostic significance (Table 27.2).[13,15,24,31–41]

Large Cell Carcinoma and Large Cell Neuroendocrine Carcinoma

Overall, tumors with higher rates of apoptosis have poorer survival.[42] Although Bcl-2 expression is associated with longer survival in studies of non–small cell lung carcinoma (NSCLC),[43] this was not shown in the large cell carcinoma subgroup.[31] Large cell neuroendocrine carcinoma showed higher frequencies of Bcl-2 and Bak immunoreactivities than did large cell carcinoma; in LCNEC, loss of Bcl-2 expression was associated with poorer survival.[42]

Epidermal growth factor receptor (EGFR) immunoreactivity has been reported in 56% of large cell carcinomas. In one series, elevated EGFR immunoreactivity was associated with more aggressive clinical behavior and shorter survival.[33] For HER2/neu, overexpression is not commonly detected, and this has been studied in large cell carcinoma, LCNEC, and LELC.[10,18,34] In LCNEC, c-Kit immunoreactivity was seen in 57% of cases, but no association with survival was detected.[34]

Increased nuclear p53 immunoreactivity was seen in LCNEC (65%), with only 35% of large cell carcinomas having significant immunoreactivity. p21 immunoreactivity was associated with poorer survival. Matrix metalloproteinase-9 (MMP-9), important in invasion and metastasis, was found at a higher frequency in LCNEC.[44] These markers were also examined in LCCNMs, that is, large cell tumors with neuroendocrine morphology only. It is of note that for p53, p21, and MMP-9 staining the LCCNM had more similarity to large cell carcinoma than to LCNEC in frequency of staining. In fact, while overall survival was poor, the large cell carcinoma and LCCNM survival curves were similar, with poorer survival for LCNEC.

In keeping with frequent 3p deletion and loss of heterozygosity (LOH) at 3p14 (Figures 27.2 and 27.3), fragile histidine triad (FHIT) immunostaining was negative in 16 cases of LCNEC studied.[25,39,45–52] Silencing of FHIT has been attributed to promoter hypermethylation. Although this has been studied in NSCLC collectively and determined to be a poor prognosis marker, data for a significant number of large cell carcinoma have not been reported.[35]

Large cell neuroendocrine carcinomas show an inverse relationship between expression of retinoblastoma (Rb) and p16.[22,36] Increased staining for cyclin D1 is seen in about 25% of cases. The most common pattern is p16 positive, Rb negative, cyclin D1 negative.[37] Either Rb loss, p16 loss, or cyclin D1 overexpression was seen in 37 of 40 LCNEC. The subgroup of p16-negative, Rb-negative LCNEC showed poorer survival than p16-positive, Rb-negative LCNEC. Overall, an inverse relationship between Rb and p16 is seen in 65% of NSCLC, and this is consistent with what has been reported for LCNEC.[38] Immunoreactivity for p16 was retained in SCLC but more frequently lost in large cell carcinoma and LCNEC. p16 promoter hypermethylation was reported in 33% of large cell carcinomas and 48% of LCNEC but was not observed in SCLC; this mechanism was proposed for p16 loss[39] in large cell carcinomas and LCNEC.

Basaloid Carcinoma

The examination of 48 basaloid carcinomas for p16, Rb, and cyclin D1 abnormalities revealed 50% with p16 loss and one third with immunoreactivity for cyclin D1.[40] This tumor type shows an inverse relationship with Rb and p16 and a direct relationship with Rb and cyclin D1, as in other tumors studied. For basaloid carcinoma, the poorest prognosis is associated with combined a Rb-negative, p16-positive, cyclin D1–positive pattern.

TABLE 27.1. Summary of immunohistochemistry studies focusing on differentiation markers commonly used in tumor diagnosis.

	CK (KL1)	EMA	HMWCK	CK7	TTF-1	CEA	B72.3	Chromogranin	Synaptophysin	CD56	Vimentin	p63
Large cell carcinoma	77/122 (63%)	34/52 (65%)	27/63 (43%)	46/64 (72%)	32/64 (50%)	31/61 (51%)	11/44 (25%)	2/98 (2%)	10/61 (16%)	4/45 (9%)		20/54 (37%)
LCNEC	23/26 (88%)		16/140 (11%)	2/6 (33%)	54/124 (44%)	9/16 (56%)	3/6 (50%)	63/85 (74%)	45/55 (82%)	72/79 (91%)	1/16 (6%)	4/8 (50%)
Basaloid	32/38 (84%)		28/28 (100%)		0/28 (0%)			0/28 (0%)	1/28 (4%)	3/28 (11%)		
LELC	31/31 (100%)	2/2 (100%)									0/2 (0%)	
Rhabdoid	17/23 (74%)	5/6 (83%)		2/3 (67%)	0/3 (0%)			3/6 (50%)	3/6 (50%)		23/23 (100%)	

Note: CEA, carcinoembryonic antigen; CK, cytokeratin; EMA, epithelial membrane antigen; HMWCK, high-molecular-weight cytokeratin; LCNEC, large cell neuroendocrine carcinoma; LELC, lymphoepithelioma-like carcinoma; TTF-1, thyroid transcription factor 1.
Source: Data are compiled from references 3–5, 9–11, and 13–22.

TABLE 27.2. Summary of Immunohistochemistry Markers Focusing on Molecular Pathways and Prognosis.

	Apoptosis related				HER2/neu	c-Kit	p53	p21	FHIT	Cyclin B1	MMP-9	Cyclin D1	p16	Rb
	Bcl-2	Bax	Mcl-1	Bak										
Large cell carcinoma	13/37 (35%)	11/15 (73%)	28/35 (80%)	3/15 (20%)	0/52 (0%)		9/26 (35%)	9/26 (35%)			10/26 (38%)	6/43 (8%)	9/18 (50%)	5/10 (50%)
LCNEC	11/20 (55%)	18/20 (90%)	19/20 (95%)	13/20 (65%)	3/40 (8%)	32/56 (57%)	26/40 (65%)	24/40 (60%)	0/16 (0%)	37/44 (84%)	17/24 (71%)	24/102 (24%)	74/94 (79%)	41/99 (41%)
Basaloid												16/48 (33%)	24/48 (50%)	38/48 (79%)
LELC	27/28 (96%)				0/23 (0%)		4/23 (17%)							
Rhabdoid							1/1 (100%)							

Note: FHIT, fragile histidine triad; LCNEC, large cell neuroendocrine carcinoma; LELC, lymphoepithelioma-like carcinoma; MMP-9, matrix metalloproteinase-9; Rb, retinoblastoma.
Source: Data are compiled from references 13, 15, 24, and 31–41.

Large Cell Carcinoma vs. NSCLC and Adenocarcinoma

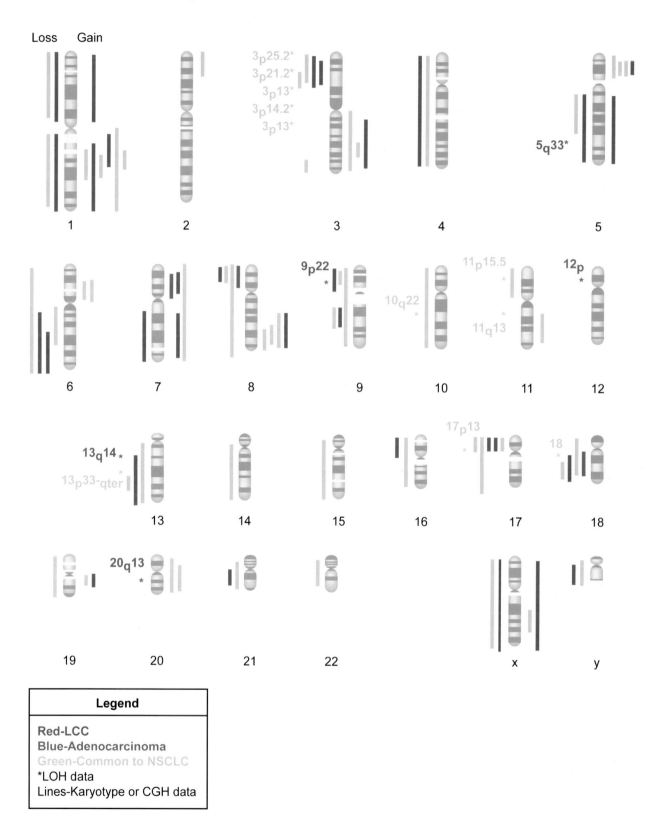

FIGURE 27.2. Summary of cytogenetic studies comparing adenocarcinoma, non–small cell lung carcinoma and large cell carcinoma (LCC), including classic cytogenetics, comparative genomic hybridization (CGH), and loss of heterozygosity (LOH) studies. Lines indicate cytogenetic or CGH studies, and asterisks indicate LOH studies.[39,45–50]

Large Cell Neuroendocrine Carcinoma vs. Small Cell Carcinoma

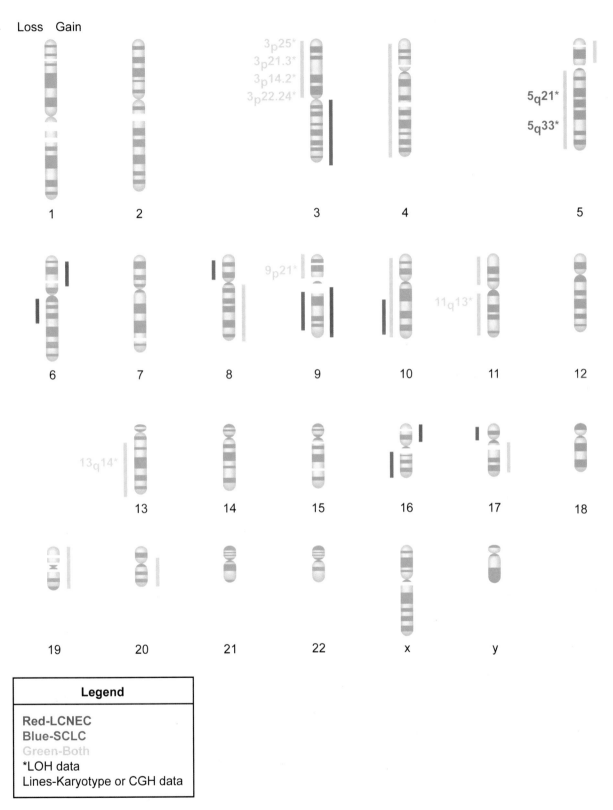

FIGURE 27.3. Summary of cytogenetic studies comparing small cell lung carcinoma (SCLC) and large cell neuroendocrine carcinoma (LCNEC), including classic cytogenetics, comparative genomic hybridization (CGH), and loss of heterozygosity (LOH) studies. Lines indicate cytogenetic or CGH studies, and asterisks indicate LOH studies.[22,39,51,52]

Studies of Single Genes

Large cell carcinomas have been studied for expression and mutation of single genes that are known to be relevant to carcinogenesis, including oncogenes and cell cycle genes. These studies are of interest in the context of understanding the relationship between large cell carcinoma and other NSCLCs, as well as the spectrum of neuroendocrine carcinomas.

Large Cell Carcinoma

Studies of *c-Myc* in large cell carcinoma demonstrate a high rate of overexpression.[41] Examination of *c-Myc* copy number showed that the frequency of amplification and the actual copy number were high among all lung carcinomas (SCLC and NSCLC) and did not differ among histologic subtypes, although all six large cell carcinomas had 6–12 copies.[53] It has also been shown that *cyclin B1* expression is frequently detected in LCNEC (84%)[36]; the identification of *cyclin B1* as a *c-Myc* target gene[54] and increased gene expression of *c-Myc* and *cyclin B1* as poor prognosis markers in NSCLC[55] are possibly related observations.

p53 is frequently mutated in large cell carcinoma. In one series of NSCLC, four of four (100%) large cell carcinomas showed mutated *p53*—two in exon 7 and one each in exon 5 and exon 8. In this series, *p53* mutation was seen with higher frequency in smokers and with poorer differentiation. The overall rate of *p53* mutation was 49% in squamous cell carcinoma and 22% in adenocarcinoma. The focus of that study, *topoisomerase IIα*, was not overexpressed in large cell carcinoma[56] In a metaanalysis comparing *p53* mutation and immunohistochemistry in resected lung cancers, Tammemagi et al. found the highest rate of *p53* mutation in large cell carcinoma (54%, n = 105) among NSCLCs, and the lowest rate was in adenocarcinoma (35%, n = 693).[57] Immunohistochemistry studies of abnormal p53 protein accumulation showed similar findings. Although concordance between immunohistochemistry results and mutation status was not high (κ = 0.33), it was noted that most *p53*-mutated tumors showed positive immunoreactivity, with discordant cases having immunoreactive tumor without *p53* mutation. Whether this excess number of positive cases detected with immunohistochemistry represents underdetection by mutation analysis because of contamination of nonneoplastic tissue remains unclear. Overall, *p53* mutations are common in large cell carcinoma and are seen at a comparable rate in other NSCLCs of moderate to poor differentiation.

Inactivation of *p16* has also been studied in large cell carcinoma.[58] In a study of seven large cell carcinomas, 71% showed *p16* promoter hypermethylation, along with about one third of squamous cell carcinoma and adenocarcinomas. Hypermethylation of *p16* promoter and *p53* mutations was seen in large cell carcinoma, but higher rates of *p16* promoter hypermethylation and *p53* mutations were seen in former smokers than in current smokers and nonsmokers. Promoter hypermethylation was a more frequent mechanism of inactivation than mutation. Only one of five large cell carcinoma had *cyclin D1* reactivity detected by immunohistochemistry.[59] This low frequency of *cyclin D1* expression in large cell carcinoma was confirmed in another series of 33 large cell carcinomas studied with Northern blot analysis and immunohistochemistry,[60] although the results in large cell carcinoma are somewhat lower than in LCNEC.

K-*ras* mutation is an important mechanism for carcinogenesis in lung adenocarcinoma, seen in about one third of these tumors. Various studies have examined K-*ras* mutations in large cell carcinoma, with some variation in results. In a series of 24 large cell carcinomas, only 1 showed a K-*ras* mutation, while 41 of 141 adenocarcinomas were mutated.[61] In a series of 12 large cell carcinomas,[62] 3 showed a K-*ras* mutation at codon 12 or 13, while 10 of 33 adenocarcinomas were mutated. In that series, 25% of large cell carcinoma had *RASSF1A* promoter (3p gene) hypermethylation, while only 7% had both K-*ras* mutation and *RASSF1a* promoter hypermethylation. Fifty percent of large cell carcinomas had neither *RASSF1A* nor K-*ras* mutation. Interestingly, only 5% of squamous cell carcinomas had activating K-*ras* mutations.

With regard to tumor classification, studies of pleomorphic carcinomas (tumors with a spindle cell or giant cell component) for *p53* and K-*ras* may shed light on the relationships among squamous cell carcinoma, adenocarcinoma, and large cell carcinoma components in pleomorphic/sarcomatoid carcinoma. In one series,[63] 9% of pleomorphic carcinomas had K-*ras2* point mutations in contrast to 36% of adenocarcinomas and 0% squamous cell carcinomas. Mutations in *p53* were seen in 14% of pleomorphic carcinomas (3 of 22, 2 of 3 exon 7), 27% of adenocarcinomas, and 43% of squamous cell carcinomas (exon 8 being the most common site). In a second series,[64] 6 of 27 (22%) pleomorphic carcinomas had a K-*ras* mutation in both spindled and nonspindled populations. This rate was higher than in prior studies but was determined with laser capture microdissection, perhaps eliminating normal tissue contamination. Of the pleomorphic carcinomas, 2 of 12 with large cell carcinoma as the carcinomatous component had a mutated K-*ras* (17%) compared with 4 of 12 (33%) with adenocarcinoma and 0 of 3 with squamous cell carcinoma as the carcinomatous component. The differences in rates of K-*ras* mutation may reflect the histology of the epithelial component in pleomorphic carcinomas.

Large Cell Neuroendocrine Carcinoma

In LCNEC, a *MEN-1* mutation was seen in 1 of 13 cases, while none were seen in SCLC.[65] This is relevant because 67% of carcinoids show *MEN* inactivation, indicating differences between low- and high-grade neuroendocrine carcinoma. In a study of 83 LCNEC, no mutations for *kit*, *PDGFR-α*, *PDGFR-β*, or *c-Met* were seen. By immunohistochemistry, however, 63% were *kit* positive, 60% *PDGFR-α* positive, 82% *PDGFR-β* positive, and 47% *c-Met* positive.[66]

K-*ras* mutations were detected in codon 13 in 1 of 18 cases of LCNEC studied. Overall, few K-*ras* mutations have been described in neuroendocrine lung tumors of any kind. A *p53* mutation was detected in 10 of 18 cases studied; LOH at the *p53* locus occurred in 9 cases in that series. Overall, 13 of 18 LCNEC cases in that study showed a *p53* abnormality.[67] In a study of 23 high-grade neuroendocrine carcinomas (15 LCNEC, 8 SCLC), 4 cases of LCNEC and 3 cases of SCLC showed point mutations in *p53*. No *c-raf1* or K-*ras* mutations were seen in any of the cases.[68]

Lymphoepithelioma-Like Carcinoma

Examination of 11 LELCs showed one tumor with an *EGFR* mutation and none with K-*ras* mutations. *EGFR* mutations were associated with nonsmokers in adenocarcinoma, but the same association was not found in LELCs.[69] In a series of 23 LELCs, in situ hybridization detected EBV in all cases.[10] It is also notable that EBV detected with in situ hybridization has been reported in Asian populations with squamous cell carcinomas (6 of 43) that were not histologically LELCs. No large cell carcinomas (n = 12) or adenocarcinomas (n = 67) in the same series were EBV positive; all 5 LELCs were positive.[32]

An interesting aspect of this tumor type is the infiltration of mononuclear cells. Monocyte chemoattractant protein-1 (MCP-1) has been demonstrated in 86% of LELC cases, and it has been suggested that expression of this protein is an important mechanism contributing to the distinctive morphologic features of this tumor. MCP-1 expression was studied by reverse transcriptase polymerase chain reaction and in situ hybridization. All the informative tumors showed MCP-1 by polymerase chain reaction, but only the LELC were positive by in situ hybridization within the tumor cells; non-LELC cases were positive by in situ hybridization in nonneoplastic stromal cells,[70] indicating different cells of origin for the MCP-1 in LELC compared with non-LELC.

Chromosomal Studies and Large Cell Carcinoma

Several studies have examined chromosomal alterations in NSCLC. Other studies have focused specifically on large cell carcinoma and LCNEC.

Cytogenetic Studies of Large Cell Carcinoma

Johansson et al. examined 26 pulmonary large cell carcinomas using classic cytogenetics techniques and compared their results with previously published data on NSCLCs.[45] The majority of tumors, 20 of 26, showed clonal aberrations. Of these 20, 17 tumors showed complex karyotypes. The most frequent aberrations involved losses of 1p, 1q, 3p, 6q, 7q, and 17p and gains of 5q, 7p, and regions of chromosomes 11, 1, and 7. The authors suggested that the combination of 17p loss and abnormalities of chromosomes 1 and 6 in large cell carcinoma resembles the karyotypic pattern of adenocarcinoma more closely than that of squamous cell carcinoma.

Many of the karyotypic changes in large cell carcinoma are common to NSCLC,[46] including losses of 9p, 3p, 6q, 8p, 9q, 13q, 17p, 18q, 19p, 21q, and 22q and gains of chromosome 7 (7p and q), 1q, 3q, and 5p. Loss of 3p, which includes the *RASSF1A* and *FHIT* loci, is a common finding. Loss of 9p may involve the *p16* gene, and loss of 17p involves the *p53* gene (see Figure 27.2).

Comparative Genomic Hybridization

Large Cell Carcinoma

Comparative genomic hybridization (CGH) analysis of 10 large cell carcinomas and 20 lung adenocarcinomas showed 26 of 30 cases with DNA copy number alterations.[47] Examination of specific abnormalities showed similar DNA gains in 8q, 1q, 6pcen-21, and 5p14 and losses in 6qcen-23 and 17 in both adenocarcinomas and large cell carcinoma. Gains of 7pcen-p21 and losses of 8p and 18 were more often seen in adenocarcinoma in that study; overall, 8p and 18p losses as well as 7p gains have been reported in NSCLCs and large cell carcinomas (see Figure 27.2). Examination of two large cell carcinoma cell lines by CGH revealed similar findings, with gains in 5p, 8q 15q, 6p, 20 q, 1q21–11, 2p, and 3q and losses in 5q12–q32, 18q, 6q, 9, and 13q.[48]

Large Cell Neuroendocrine Carcinoma

Ullmann et al. performed CGH on 13 LCNECs and compared them to previously published SCLC CGH profiles.[51] The losses in 3p, 4q, 5q, and 13q and the gain in 5p were common to both tumor types; these aberrations are common features of lung carcinomas. Gains in 3q, commonly seen in SCLCs (66%), were found in only 1of 13 LCNECs. A 16q deletion was seen in 50% of SCLCs, but only rarely in LCNECs and adenocarcinomas. A 17p deletion was seen in 75% of SCLCs but in less than 25% of other tumor subtypes. Other findings included a 10q deletion in SCLCs and squamous cell carcinomas but not in LCNECs and adenocarcinomas, and a 6p gain was seen in LCNECs, squamous cell carcinomas, and adenocarcinomas but not in SCLCs. While it is clear that certain aberrations are common to all high-grade lung carcinomas, the differences are of interest. There are features that suggest similarities between LCNECs and SCLCs (see Figure 27.3) and that within NSCLCs LCNEC has features in common with adenocarcinoma.

Loss of Heterozygosity Studies

Large Cell Carcinoma

Although both large cell carcinomas and LCNECs show 3p LOH, more frequently 3p LOH is found in LCNECs and SCLCs than in large cell carcinomas.[22] Loss of heterozygosity at 5q33 is more often a feature of large cell carcinoma than LCNEC. LCNECs and SCLCs were more similar to each other than to large cell carcinoma, with 3p14.2 (FHIT), 3p21, and 5q21 seen more frequently in LCNECs and SCLCs than in classic large cell carcinoma. TP53 and 13q14 LOH were seen in all tumor types.

In a study of 23 squamous cell carcinomas, 23 adenocarcinomas, and 8 large cell carcinomas, LOH was most frequent in squamous cell carcinomas. Loss of heterozygosity at 17p was more frequent in squamous cell carcinoma than in adenocarcinoma or large cell carcinoma, and this was accompanied by LOH at 11p (11p15.4 and 11p13). When adenocarcinoma demonstrated 11p deletions, these were in the same regions as in squamous cell carcinoma, only in fewer cases.[49]

Examination of LOH in 22 adenocarcinomas and 8 large cell carcinomas demonstrated 12p LOH in 46% of adenocarcinomas and 50% of large cell carcinomas. Activating K-ras mutations were identified in the majority of the adenocarcinomas and large cell carcinomas that showed 12p LOH. This suggested that the wild-type allele may serve a tumor suppressor role and that LOH at 12p is needed as a second hit to an activating mutation in K-ras.[50] Once again, a similarity was found between large cell carcinoma and adenocarcinoma.

Large Cell Neuroendocrine Carcinoma

Shin et al. studied 13 LCNECs for 5q LOH.[52] The following results were obtained: 91% with 5q14.3–q21 LOH, 54% with 5q22.2–q23 LOH, 30% with 5q23–q33 LOH,

and 84% with 5q35.1–35.2. This suggests possible loci for tumor suppressor genes. The 5q22.2 region was near APC but did not usually involve APC. The 5q23 region included interferon regulatory factor 1 (IRF-1), a transcription factor that may play a tumor suppressor role.[52] Upregulation of IRF-1 causes apoptosis,[71] and loss is associated with cell growth in various neoplasms.[72]

Loss of heterozygosity at 3p was present at a high rate in LCNEC and SCLC when compared with carcinoids. Loss of heterozygosity at 5q21 was seen at the highest rate in SCLC and then in LCNEC, but both tumors showed more frequent 5q21 LOH than carcinoids. A high frequency of LOH was seen at 13q14 and 9p21 in SCLCs and LCNECs. All neuroendocrine tumors studied had a high rate of 11q LOH. Abnormalities in p53 were frequent in LCNEC, with LOH in 9 of 18 cases and mutation in 10 of 18 cases; of these, 6 cases had both LOH and a mutation in p53. Therefore, within the class of neuroendocrine tumors, LOH for TP53 and p53 point mutations and losses at 3p14.2 (FHIT), 3p21, 3p22, 5q21, 9p21 (p16), and 13q14.2 (Rb) were associated with high-grade neuroendocrine carcinomas (SCLCs and LCNECs) and therefore were associated with poor prognosis.[67]

Gene Expression Profiling Studies

Gene expression profiling is a high throughput method that uses high-density cDNA/oligonucleotide microarrays to analyze the relative expressions of genes within a particular tissue type. Several studies have focused on lung tumors, and a subset of large cell carcinomas has been studied, including cell lines and human tumors. What these studies have in common is analysis of a set of samples, clustering of cases using statistical algorithms to indicate which cases have common gene expression profiles, validation to confirm the gene expression profiles, and sorting of genes by functional categories in each class.

In an expression profiling study of 25 primary NSCLCs of the lung, 7 large cell carcinomas studied did not cluster together. In fact, large cell carcinomas clustered with both adenocarcinomas and squamous cell carcinomas. This did not suggest a similarity among large cell carcinomas but did suggest that perhaps they were poorly differentiated squamous cell carcinomas or adenocarcinomas.[73]

Garber et al. studied 67 lung tumors, 4 of which were large cell carcinoma.[74] Three of these tumors clustered within a group of six tumors, the remainder of which were adenocarcinomas. One large cell carcinoma clustered in a subgroup of adenocarcinomas. Interestingly, the large cell group was on a branch of the tree adjacent to the SCLC group. In supervised analysis, several genes were noted to be upregulated in large cell carcinoma, including HMGI(Y), fos-related antigen 1, pleckstrinA1, tissue plasminogen activator, and Fra-1. Perhaps of greater interest

28
Small Cell Carcinoma

Elisabeth Brambilla

Introduction

Small cell carcinoma is defined as a malignant epithelial tumor consisting of small cells with scant cytoplasm, defined cytoplasmic border, typical finely granular "salt and pepper" nuclear chromatin pattern, and inconspicuous or absent nucleoli. Small cell carcinoma is characterized by extensive necrosis, a high mitosis rate, and conspicuous nuclear molding. The criteria of the definition of small cell carcinoma have not changed from the original World Health Organization classification to the revised ones.[1,2] The definition is based essentially on cytologic criteria, and the most discriminating criteria probably are the chromatin pattern and the very high nuclear to cytoplasmic ratio (8 to 9/10) beyond cell size. Fortunately, the definition of small cell lung carcinoma (SCLC) did not change so that the literature on clinical behavior, molecular biology, molecular pathology, and drug sensitivity are still relevant. The only major change between the recent and previous classifications resides in the abandonment of the variant intermediate cell type of oat cell carcinoma, essentially because of a lack of clinical and therapeutic differences. (It is likely that oat cell lung carcinoma was an "artifact" due to poor preservation of cells in small biopsy specimens.)

On surgical samples, 28% of SCLCs are combined with a variable component of non small cell carcinoma. In this chapter, it is recommended that least 10% of the lesion be small cell to qualify for SCLC, combined.[3]

No precursor lesion for SCLC has been recognized thus far. When preinvasive lesions are discovered in the lung surrounding SCLC surgical samples, they have the appearance of squamous dysplasia and carcinoma in situ but do not contain neuroendocrine cells. However, pagetoid-type migration of small cells arising from the tumor may give the impression of preinvasive SCLC. Replacement of bronchial epithelium by neuroendocrine cells of small size looking like a preinvasive lesion for SCLC has occasionally been seen, but this has been very rare.

Diffuse neuroendocrine hyperplasia is not considered a preinvasive lesion for SCLC. It occurs in the setting of carcinoid, single or multiple, but has never been shown associated with SCLC.

Molecular Pathology

The discussion of molecular pathology is divided into two parts: the molecular signature reflecting cell differentiation with diagnostic potential and the molecular pathology related to SCLC pathogenesis.

Signature of Cell Differentiation

The phenotypic traits constitute immunohistochemical features that are distinctive of SCLC and are useful in the clinical diagnosis. Small cell lung carcinomas commonly show all three specific neuroendocrine markers: chromogranin, synaptophysin, and CD56/neural cell adhesion molecule (NCAM). The last one is believed to be the most sensitive marker for SCLC.[4] Less than 2% of SCLCs have none of these three neuroendocrine markers, providing adequate sensitivity. Small cell lung carcinomas are known for their high mitotic rate, but this can be difficult sometimes to appreciate because of the high level of apoptotic features: necrosis and the density of chromatin. In a number of bronchial biopsies with crush artifact, Ki-67 may be of great help in demonstrating that the rate of proliferation is extremely high, ruling out the alternative diagnoses of tumorlets, carcinoids, and lymphoid aggregates. By definition, SCLC is a proliferation arising from basal bronchial cells and express low-molecular-weight cytokeratins.

Eighty-five percent of SCLC are positive for thyroid transcription factor 1 (TTF-1). According to previous studies, only high-grade neuroendocrine carcinomas, and

293

not carcinoid, express TTF-1 although this has been debated in the literature.[5] Expression of TTF-1 in SCLC is useful in the differential diagnosis with basaloid carcinoma from which they are distinguished by TTF-1 and the presence of neuroendocrine marker in contrast to basaloid carcinomas. The differential diagnosis of an SCLC includes other small cell tumors potentially arising in the lung and in the thorax, such as primitive neuroectodermal tumors, that are less mitotically active than SCLC but also mark for CD99 (MIC2) and not for cytokeratin and TTF-1.[6,7] Unfortunately, CD99 does not discriminate between SCLC and primitive neuroectodermal tumors, as 25% of SCLC express MIC2 according to recent studies.[8]

The Molecular Genetics Alterations Related to Small Cell Lung Carcinoma Pathogenesis: Proliferation and Progression

Chromosomal Imbalances

Small cell lung carcinomas are invariably aneuploid neoplasms, and a more than diploid chromosomal number is typical of SCLC. Small cell lung carcinomas are characterized by chromosomal imbalances with a high incidence of deletions on chromosome 3p, 4q, 5q, 10q, 13q, and 17p along with DNA gains on 3q, 5p, 6p, 8q, 17q, 19q, and 20q.[9,10] Chromosome duplication can be demonstrated in the vast majority of SCLCs associated with 3q isochromosome formation. In addition, gain of chromosome 17q24–q25 is proposed as a potential marker for brain metastasis formation.[11]

The Sonic Hedgehog Pathway

Small cell lung carcinomas express Sonic Hedgehog (Shh) at least in cell lines. Sonic Hedgehog binding to its receptor Patch leads to activation of the transcription factor Gli1. This signaling pathway is characterized by elaboration and reception of Shh signals in the epithelial compartment of stem cells and induces neuroendocrine differentiation. This pathway is activated in SCLC and involved in the maintenance of the malignant phenotype. The Shh pathway may be blocked by the chemical compound cyclopamine (an extract of *Veratrum*), which also blocks cell proliferations.[12]

Human Achaete-Scute Homolog 1 Expression

Human achaete-scute homolog 1 (hASH1) is a member of the basic helix-loop-helix family of transcription factor and is known to play a crucial role in neuronal/endocrine determination and differentiation in the normal development of the nervous system and endodermal endocrine cells.[13,14] A high level of hASH1 is uniformly present in

classic SCLC, in non–small cell lung carcinoma (NSCLC) with neuroendocrine features, and in bronchial carcinoid tumors and cell lines.[15] In transgenic mice, hASH1 expression induces progressive airway hyperplasia and metaplasia and increases the tumorigenicity in distal airways. However, the resulting tumors are adenocarcinoma exhibiting frequent neuroendocrine differentiation but not SCLC. In the spectrum of lung neuroendocrine tumors, hASH1 has been shown to be virtually absent in differentiated typical carcinoids but is expressed in atypical carcinoids in large cell neuroendocrine carcinoma and SCLC.[16] No relation has been shown between hASH1 expression and neural cell adhesion molecule expression. The data acquired strongly suggest that hASH1 expression in pulmonary neuroendocrine tumors imitates its early and transient expression pattern during development and is instrumental in establishment of the neuroendocrine phenotype but not necessary for its maintenance.

p53 Pathway Alterations

Mutation of the *p53* gene is the most frequent genetic abnormality identified in human cancers and is more common in SCLC than in NSCLC. *p53* mutation occurs in 80% of SCLC through missense point mutations that increase the half-life of the protein, enabling immunohistochemical detection of a stabilized p53 mutant protein. However, 20% of SCLC display atypical mutations such as an intronic splicing site mutation leading to unstable mRNA and absence of protein expression. Nonstabilized p53 mutant forms explain most of the discrepancies between mutation detected by sequencing of p53 (80%) and overexpression of p53 protein using immunohistochemical determination (70%).[17] The frequency, type, and pattern of mutation in SCLC is strongly related to cigarette smoking, with a high prevalence of G to T transversions.

Downstream of the p53 pathway, several target genes of p53 are deregulated, the most common being *Bcl-2* and *Bax* and their ratio.[18,19] *Bcl-2* is negatively transcriptionally regulated by p53, whereas Bax is positively regulated by p53. Indeed, upregulation of *Bcl-2* (antiapoptotic) and downregulation of *Bax* (inducer of apoptosis) is more frequent in SCLC than in NSCLC and reflects resistance to apoptosis in SCLC.

Fas, a member of the tumor necrosis factor (TNF) transmembrane protein superfamily, is a transcriptional target gene of p53. Upon contact with its ligand (*FasL*), *Fas* induces apoptosis by way of intracellular signaling pathways, including FADD (Fas-associated death domain) and caspase-8. Fas pathway alterations leading to resistance to apoptosis have been reported in a wide variety of human solid tumors, including lung carcinoma.[20,21] The loss of cell surface expression of *Fas* in neuroendocrine lung tumor cell lines correlates with cell resistance to *Fas*-mediated apoptosis in vitro.[22] In immunohistochemistry studies, *Fas* expression was low or absent in SCLC compared with normal epithelial cells (94% below normal, 16% negative). In contrast, *FasL*, which was underexpressed compared with normal in the majority of adenocarcinomas and squamous cell carcinomas (70%), was strongly overexpressed in 90% of SCLC on frozen sections. This strong change in the ratio of *Fas* to *FasL* (>1 in SCLC) was correlated with the *Bax* to *Bcl-2* ratio (<1). *FasL* overexpression in the context of *Fas* downregulation in SCLC suggests escape from suicidal activation of tumor cells. This alteration most likely enables SCLC cells to induce paracrine killing of *Fas*-expressing cytotoxic T cells, explaining why SCLCs have a paucity of a lymphocytic infiltrate and specifically of cytotoxic CD8 T cells. Although caspase-8 is reported to be consistently methylated in lung cancer cell lines,[23] the caspase-8–independent cell death pathway via receptor-interacting protein kinase is proposed as an effector molecule of *Fas*-derived apoptosis.[24]

Retinoblastoma Alterations in Lung Cancer

Downstream from the p53 pathway, retinoblastoma (Rb) is the main effector of the cell cycle checkpoint at G1, according to its phosphorylation state, which is regulated partially by p53. Indeed, one of the main p53 target genes, *p21*, is a cyclin-dependent kinase (Cdk) inhibitor that prevents Rb phosphorylation (allowing G1 arrest) and inactivation of Rb function, an essential step in SCLC carcinogenesis. G1 arrest is achieved by the hypophosphorylated form of Rb, which binds E2F1 and represses its transcriptional activities. Cyclin D1 in complex with Cdk4 and Cdk6 achieves phosphorylation of Rb with release of E2F1 transcription followed by G1 to S transition. In tumors, Rb loss, cyclin D1 overexpression, and loss of Cdk4 inhibitors (p16[INK4]) induces persistent Rb, resulting in evasion of cell cycle checkpoint G1. The most dramatic alteration is Rb *loss*, which is characteristic of SCLC.[25–27]

The mechanism of *Rb* gene activation in SCLC (82%–100%) is poorly understood. Mutations have been described in SCLC lines and less frequently in tumors.[28] Only 25% of mutations in SCLC tumors in exons 13–18 or 20–24 of the *Rb* gene were detected, and reverse transcriptase polymerase chain reaction analysis revealed a low level or absence of Rb mRNA in 58% without methylation of the CpG island in the 5' end of the *Rb* gene. In lung carcinoma there is a strong inverse relationship between Rb and p16 in SCLC ($p < 0.001$) as well as a direct relationship between cyclin D1 and Rb ($p < 0.001$), showing that Rb is the major targeted pathway of cell cycle regulation. In NSCLC the alternative mechanism of Rb loss is via Rb hyperphosphorylation through p16 loss

or cyclin D1 overexpression.[29–31] Intact Rb protein expression occurs in only 10% of SCLC. Cyclin D1 overexpression occurs in only 1.3% of SCLC and p16 loss in 7% of SCLC.[32] In contrast, cyclin E overexpression may be seen more frequently in SCLC (30%–40%) with concomitant Rb loss (personal observation).

Alteration of Upstream Regulators of p53: p14[ARF] and MDM2

p14[ARF] was previously known to mediate the p53/MDM2–dependent cell cycle checkpoint in response to oncogenic hyperproliferative signals.[33] We and others have recently identified a new p53- and/or MDM2-independent function of p14[ARF].[34–36] In light of these data, it is now recognized that p14[ARF] can delay cell cycle progression and induce apoptosis in a p53-dependent as well as a p53-independent manner. Evidence was recently provided that p14[ARF] activates both ATM/ATR and Chk1/Chk2 kinases to trigger its antiproliferative function via G2 arrest, regardless of the p53 status by an original mechanism requiring the histone acetylase Tip60.[37] Consistent with p14 function independent of the pP53 pathway, we have observed the concomitant inactivation of p14 and p53 in 40% of high-grade neuroendocrine lung tumors, especially SCLC.[38] Indeed, we demonstrated lack of p14[ARF] protein expression in 60% of SCLC on frozen section with polyclonal homemade antibody. A reevaluation of p14 loss in SCLC with a commercial antibody yielded a 40% loss of p14. We recently documented the role of p14[ARF] in response to DNA damage through activation of ATM/ATR leading to Chk2 phosphorylation.[39] A mutual exclusion between p14[ARF] loss and lack of Chk2 phosphorylation ($p < 0.003$) and a mutual exclusion between p14[ARF] loss and/or Chk2 loss ($p < 0.0006$) was found.

MDM2, initially identified as an amplified gene on a murine double minute chromosome, is a transcriptional target of p53. MDM2 also antagonizes p53-dependent transcriptional activities by directly binding its N-terminal region.[40–42] Furthermore, MDM2 can promote the degradation of p53, acting as an ubiquitin-protein ligase to ubiquitinate p53[43] and triggering its nuclear export and degradation by cytoplasmic proteasome. The inhibitory effect of MDM2 toward p53 is counteracted by human p14[ARF]. Direct binding of p14[ARF] to MDM2 inhibits p53 degradation by blocking p53–MDM2 nuclear export,[44] sequestration of MDM2 into the nucleolus,[45] and inhibition of its ubiquitin ligase activity. So doing, p14[ARF] prevents the negative feedback regulation of p53 by MDM2.

Conversely, high levels of MDM2 allow relocalization of endogenous p14[ARF] from nucleolus to nucleoplasm, suggesting that a balance between both proteins' levels and their respective subcellular locations is important to regulate their effects. Abnormalities of MDM2 expression have been reported in human tumors, especially in sarcomas.[46] With immunohistochemistry and western blotting to detect the various MDM2 isoforms, one of the isoforms of MDM2 was overexpressed in 31% of all neuroendocrine lung tumors and in 30% of SCLCs with a strong mutual exclusion of p14 loss of expression ($p < 0.0001$). Furthermore the MDM2:p14 >1 ratio was correlated with a high-grade phenotype among neuroendocrine tumors overexpressing MDM2 ($p = 0.002$), suggesting that MDM2 overexpression and p14^{ARF} are exclusive of each other and act on common pathways to regulate p53- and/or Rb-dependent or -independent functions. Indeed, MDM2 is at the crossroad of p53 and Rb function. Interaction of MDM2 with Rb inhibit growth regularly function of Rb through an unknown mechanism. Therefore, MDM2 overexpression and/or p14 loss in SCLC disrupt both p53 and Rb functions and allow for consistent inactivation of the p53/Rb pathway in SCLC with evasion of G1 and G2 arrest.

E2F1 Overexpression

The transcription factor E2F1 is a key component of the cell cycle that acts to transactivate genes required for S phase, entry such as *DNA polymerase-α, thymidine kinase, dihydrofolate reductase, methylmalonyl-CoA mutase, Cdc6, cyclin A, cyclin E, Cdc2, c-Myc,* and *E2F1* itself. E2F1 is potentially implicated in human carcinogenesis and is released by pRb phosphorylation. A distinct pattern of E2F1 expression in human NSCLC and SCLC has been demonstrated.[47] As determined with both immunohistochemistry and Northern blot analysis, E2F1 product is overexpressed in 92% of SCLCs and is undetectable in 90% of NSCLCs. Although no amplification was found, there is a strong increase in E2F1 mRNA expression and protein upregulation with nuclear accumulation as well as overexpression of E2F1 target genes. E2F1 overexpression in high-grade neuroendocrine lung tumors (large cell neuroendocrine carcinoma and SCLC) is associated with a high Ki-67 index and a Bcl-2:Bax ratio >1. E2F1 upregulation in SCLC is probably responsible for an unexpected cyclin E upregulation in SCLC in the context of Rb loss, because cyclin E is one of the transcription targets of E2F1.[47]

Chromosome 3p Deletion

Most SCLCs as well as the majority of squamous cell carcinomas demonstrates large 3p segments of allelic loss. These regions are gene rich, and the genes identified with loss of heterozygosity are potential tumor suppressor genes. Putative tumors genes have been identified at four widely separated regions on the chromosome arms susceptible for LOH: 3p12.13 (*ROBO1/DUTT1*), 3p14.2

(*FHIT*), 3p21.3 (*RASSF1, Fus1, SEMA3B, SEMA3F, β-catenin*), and 3p24.6 (*VHL, RARβ*).[48]

Interestingly, the *FHIT* gene is downregulated with loss of protein expression in more than 80% of SCLCs.[49] The *FHIT* gene is involved in regulation of apoptosis and in cell cycle control.[50] Loss of *FHIT* function therefore results in proliferation in SCLC. It is probably *SEMA3F* (class 3 semaphorin) that causes the most frequent alterations in lung cancer and especially in SCLC with regard to lack of function of candidate tumor suppressor genes on 3p deletion sites. Of the tumor suppressor genes present on 3p21.3, *RASSF1* and *SEMA3B* are candidate tumor suppressor genes. Indeed, *RASSF1* (Ras-associated domain family 1A) is frequently inactivated in lung cancer by methylation, and particularly in 90% of SCLC, and has growth suppressive and antitumorigenesis properties on lung cancer cell lines.[51,52] *RASSF1* has been shown to interfere with cell cycle progression through interaction with the Rb pathway. Another member of semaphorin family, *SEMA3B*, is present on 3p21 and is a potential tumor suppressor gene. Methylation of *SEMA3B* promoter has been found in NSCLC but not in SCLC. Another candidate tumor suppressor gene on 3p is *RARβ* at 3p24.26 Retinoic acid plays an important role in lung development and differentiation through its interaction with retinoid nuclear receptors encoded by the *RARβ* gene and others such as *RAR-XR*. Epigenetic inactivation by methylation of *RAR-XR* has been reported in 72% of SCLCs.[53]

Telomerase Expression

Telomeres, which represent the ends of the eukaryotic chromosomes, shorten at each cell division. Telomere shortening leads to chromosome degradation, end fusion, and cellular senescence and acts as a mitotic clock. In germline cells as well as in tumor cells, telomerase, a ribonucleoprotein complex composed of a reverse transcriptase catalytic subunit (hTERT), synthesizes telomeric DNA, allowing cells to proliferate indefinitely.[54] The hTERT synthesizes telomeric DNA by copying a template region of an RNA subunit (hTERC), hTERC being the only limiting factor. Expression of hTERT is confined to cells expressing telomerase activity. This can be evaluated by a sensitive polymerase chain reaction–based telomere repeat amplification protocol (TRAP assay), hTERT mRNA can be detected by in situ hybridization or reverse transcriptase polymerase chain reaction, and telomerase (hTERT level) relies on Western blot or immunohistochemistry using a specific antibody (44F12 from Novocastra).[55] Almost all SCLCs display substantial telomerase activity.[56–59] Consistent expression of hTERT using 44F12 monoclonal antibody was found in SCLC in complete concordance with in situ hybridization and TRAP results. In contrast to some nuclear staining occurring in a portion of NSCLCs, hTERT always displays a diffuse intense nuclear staining in SCLCs.

Angiogenic Factors

Vascular endothelial growth factor (VEGF) is a key factor of tumor angiogenesis and is upregulated in numerous benign and malignant tumors. The effect of $VEGF_{165}$ is mediated by two tyrosine kinase receptors : VEGF-R1 (Flt-1) and VEGF-R2 (KDR/Flk-1). The prevailing concept is that VEGF is secreted by tumor cells, whereas its receptors are expressed by endothelial cells enhancing cell proliferation and migration in a paracrine manner. However, this dogma of VEGF secretions by tumor cells entirely devoted to tumor angiogenesis has been ruled out. The receptors VEGF-R1 and VEGF-R2 are also expressed on tumor cells as well as accessory important VEGF receptors.

The discovery of two coreceptors of VEGF-KDR, neuropilin 1 (NP1) and neuropilin 2 (NP2), which were initially identified in neuronal cells and on endothelial cells and expressed in a number of tumor cells of different origin (breast, prostate, and lung), suggest that VEGF might be involved in an autocrine loop directly or through its neuropilin receptors. Several tumor cells, including lung cancer cells, express VEGF-R1 and VEGF-R2[60,61] and NP1 and NP2[62] as well as demonstrate the role of VEGF-R1 and VEGF-R2 in normal lung development and notably in alveolar epithelial cells maturation.[63]

Another ligand of neuropilin, an antagonist to VEGF, is SEMA3F. SEMA3F was previously isolated in SCLC cell lines from recurring homozygous deletion at 3p21.3, a region that also undergoes loss of heterozygosity in lung tumors, with a very high frequency in SCLCs. SEMA3F binds both NP1 and NP2 and shares these receptors with $VEGF_{165}$ in endothelial and tumor cells. Competition between SEMA3A and $VEGF_{165}$ has been demonstrated in vitro, suggesting SEMA3F and VEGF competition for binding to a common receptor. Loss of SEMA3F and gain of VEGF would confer a growth advantage to tumors. Recently a proapoptotic role and an antimigration role of SEMA3F were demonstrated.[64] SEMA3F was negative or delocalized from membrane (normal localization) to cytoplasm in all SCLCs studied. Therefore, SEMA3F plays an important role in cell adhesion and apoptosis, and its loss in SCLC is appears to be significant and contributory in its pathogenesis.

Cadherin–Catenin Complex Proteins

The invasive growth of tumor cells and the tendency to early metastasis are major impediments to curative surgical resection of SCLC. Among the transmembrane glycoproteins, E-cadherin, a member of the cadherin family that mediates homotypic calcium-dependent cell–cell adhesion, plays a critical role in carcinogenesis and in tumor invasion. β-Catenin is a cytoplasmic protein that interacts directly with E-cadherin and links this molecule to the actin cytoskeleton via α-catenin. The full adhesive function of E-cadherin depends therefore on the integrity of the entire E-cadherin/catenin/actin network. Not only may E-cadherin downregulation decrease differentiation and increase tumor aggressiveness and metastasis, but also free cytoplasmic β-catenin can enter the nucleus and function as transcriptional activator with activating TCF/LEF (T-cell factor/lymphoid enhancer factor) target genes such as *Myc* and *cyclin D1*. E-cadherin and β-catenin losses have been associated with a poor survival in NSCLC. A study of the E-cadherin–β-catenin complex in neuroendocrine lung tumors showed that impaired expression of E-cadherin and β-catenin was observed with a higher frequency in high-grade neuroendocrine tumors (90 %). β-Catenin nuclear staining was not found in SCLC in contrast with β-catenin activation in colorectal carcinogenesis.[65-67] Interestingly, the *β-catenin* gene maps at a classic site for 3p deletion in SCLC, 3p21.3, consistent with its tumor suppressor function rather than oncogene function.

Tyrosine-Kinase Growth Factor and Receptors

Tyrosine-kinase receptors are key molecules in normal cellular differentiation, and they are commonly deregulated or mutated in human cancers and represent attractive molecular targets for alternative therapies using effective and safe selective inhibitors.[68] The Kit receptor tyrosine kinase is a transmembrane type III tyrosine kinase encoded by the *c-Kit* gene and with high homology with platelet-derived growth factor (PDGF) receptor.[68-73] When inactivated, Kit and PDGF receptors promote a cascade of intracytoplasmic signals leading to cell growth in several cell lines.

Tamborini et al. recently discovered an autocrine loop between Kit overexpression and phosphorylation in the cerebrospinal fluid in SCLC.[74] Very little has been reported about PDGF and relevant receptors in tumor cells of SCLC. Met, the product of the protooncogene *c-Met*, is a tyrosine kinase receptor intimately involved in epithelial/mesenchymal transition and interaction. Aberrant Met activation through binding with a high-affinity ligand hepatocyte growth factor/scatter factor or through autophosphorylation as a result of *c-Met* mutation provokes a cytoplasmic signal cascade resulting in activation of multiple signal transducers, including phosphatidylinositol-3 kinase, signal transducers and activators of transcriptions, extracellular signal-regulated kinases 1 and 2, focal adhesion kinase, and phospholipase C-γ.[75-77] The hepatocyte growth factor/Met pathway is functional in SCLC and could be opposed by chemical compounds such as Geldanamycin to induce apoptosis by interference with Met.[78] Recently the presence of *c-Met* mutations on the juxtamembrane domain of SCLC cell lines and tumor tissues was demonstrated.[79] Signaling through the hepatocyte growth factor/Met pathway has been shown to lead to tumor growth angiogenesis and to the development of an invasive phenotype in several malignancies, thus having a definitive role in SCLC oncogenesis for which clinical investigations based on tyrosine kinase receptor inhibitors have been promising.[78,80–85]

References

1. Travis WD, Colby TV, Corrin B, et al. WHO Histological Classification of Tumours. Histological Typing of Lung and Pleural Tumours, 3rd ed. Berlin: Springer-Verlag; 1999.
2. Travis WD, Brambilla E, Muller-Hemerlink HK, Harris CC, eds. World Health Organization Classification of Tumours. Pathology and Genetics of Tumours of the Lung, Pleura, Thymus and Heart. Lyon: IARC Press; 2004.
3. Nicholson SA, Beasley MB, Brambilla E, et al. Small cell lung carcinoma (SCLC): a clinicopathologic study of 100 cases with surgical specimens. Am J Surg Pathol 2002;26:1184–1197.
4. Lantuejoul S, Moro D, Michalides RJ, et al. Neural cell adhesion molecules (NCAM) and NCAM-PSA expression in neuroendocrine lung tumors. Am J Surg Pathol 1998;22:1267–1276.
5. Sturm N, Rossi G, Lantuejoul S, et al. Expression of thyroid transcription factor-1 (TTF-1) in the spectrum of neuroendocrine cell lung proliferations with special interest in carcinoids. Hum Pathol 2002;33(2):175–182.
6. Halliday BE, Slagel DD, Elsheikh TE, et al. Diagnostic utility of MIC-2 immunocytochemical staining in the differential diagnosis of small blue cell tumors. Diagn Cytopathol 1998;19:410–416.
7. Lumadue JA, Askin FB, Perlman EJ. MIC2 analysis of small cell carcinoma. Am J Clin Pathol 1994;102:692–694.
8. Pelosi G, Leon ME, Veronesi G, et al. Decreased immunoreactivity of CD99 is an independent predictor of regional lymph node metastases in pulmonary carcinoid tumors. J Thorac Oncol 2006;1(5):468–477.
9. Balsara BR, Testa JR. Chromosomal imbalances in human lung cancer. Oncogene 2002;21:6877–6883.
10. Petersen I, Langreck H, Wolf G, et al. Small-cell lung cancer is characterized by a high incidence of deletions on chromosomes 3p, 4q, 5q, 10q, 13q and 17. Br J Cancer 1997;75(1):79–86.
11. Petersen I, Hidalgo A, Petersen S, et al. Chromosomal imbalances in brain metastases of solid tumors. Brain Pathol 2000;10:395–401.
12. Watkins DN, Berman DM, Burkholder SG, et al. Hedgehog signaling within airway epithelial progenitors and in small cell lung cancer. Nature 2003;422:313–317.
13. Borges M, Linnoila RI, van de Velde HJ, et al. An achaete-scute homologue essential for neuroendocrine differentiation in the lung. Nature 1997;386:852–855.
14. Ito T, Udaka N, Yazawa T, et al. Basic helix-loop-helix transcription factors regulate the neuroendocrine differentiation of fetal mouse pulmonary epithelium. Development 2000;127:3913–3921.
15. Linnoila RI, Zhao B, DeMayo JL, et al. Constitutive achaete-scute homologue-1 promotes airway dysplasia and lung neuroendocrine tumors in transgenic mice. Cancer Res 2000;60:4005–4009.
16. Jiang SX, Kameya T, Asamura H, et al. hASH1 expression is closely correlated with endocrine phenotype and differentiation extent in pulmonary neuroendocrine tumors. Mod Pathol 2004;17:222–229.
17. Gazzeri S, Brambilla E, Caron De Fromentel C, et al. p53 genetic abnormalities and myc activation in human lung carcinomas. Int J Cancer 1994;58:24–32.
18. Brambilla E, Negoescu A, Gazzeri S, et al. Apoptosis-related factors P53, Bcl2, and Bax in neuroendocrine lung tumors. Am J Pathol 1996;149:1941–1952.
19. Jiang SX, Kameya T, Sato Y, et al. Bcl2 protein expression in lung cancer and close correlation with neuroendocrine differentiation. Am J Pathol 1996;148:837–846.
20. Gastman BR, Atarshi Y, Reichert TE, et al. Fas ligand is expressed on human squamous cell carcinomas of the head and neck, and it promotes apoptosis of T lymphocytes. Cancer Res 1999;59:5356–5364.
21. Ungefroren H, Voss M, Jansen M, et al. Human pancreatic adenocarcinomas express Fas and Fas ligand yet are resistant to Fas-mediated apoptosis. Cancer Res 1998;58:1741–1749.
22. Viard-Leveugle I, Veyrenc S, French LE, et al. Frequent loss of Fas expression and function in human lung tumors with overexpression of FasL in small cell lung carcinoma. J Pathol 2003;(201)2:268–277.
23. Shivapurkar N, Toyooka S, Eby MT, et al. Differential inactivation of caspase-8 in lung cancer. Cancer Biol Ther 2002;1(1):54–58.
24. Holler N, Zaru R, Micheau O, et al. Fas triggers an alternative caspase 8–independent cell death pathway using kinase RIP as effector molecule. Nat Immunol 2000;1:489–495.
25. Cagle PT, El-Naggar AK, Xu HJ, et al. Differential retinoblastoma protein expression in neuroendocrine tumors of the lung. Am J Pathol 1997;150:393–400.
26. Gouyer V, Gazzeri S, Bolon I, et al. Mechanism of retinoblastoma gene inactivation in the spectrum of neuroendocrine lung tumors. Am J Respir Cell Mol Biol 1998;18:188–196.
27. Yuan J, Knorr J, Altmannsberger M, et al. Expression of p16 and lack of pRB in primary small cell lung cancer. J Pathol 1999;189:358–362.
28. Harbour JW, Lai SL, Whang-Peng J, et al. Abnormalities in structure and expression of the human retinoblastoma gene in SCLC. Science 1988;241:353–357.
29. Dosaka-Akita H, Cagle PT, Hiroumi H, et al. Differential retinoblastoma and p16(INK4) protein expression in neuroendocrine tumors of the lung. Cancer 2000;88:550–556.
30. Kratzke RA, Greatens TM, Rubins JB, et al. Rb and p16^{INK4} expression in resected non small cell lung tumors. Cancer Res 1996;56:3415–3420.
31. Gazzeri S, Gouyer V, Vour'ch C, et al. Mechanism of p16^{INK4A} inactivation in non small-cell lung cancers. Oncogene 1998;16(4):497–505.

32. Beasley MB, Lantuejoul S, Abbondanzo S, et al. The p16/cyclin D1/Rb pathway in neuroendocrine tumors of the lung. Hum Pathol 2003;34(2):136–142.

33. Sherr CJ. Tumour surveillance via the ARF-p53 pathway. Genes Dev 1998;12:2984–2991.

34. Eymin B, Leduc C, Coll JL, et al. P14^{ARF} induces G2 arrest and apoptosis independently of p53 leading to regression of tumors established in nude mice. Oncogene 2003;22:1822–1835.

35. Hemmati PG, Gillissen B, von Haefen C, et al. Adenovirus-mediated overexpression of p14(ARF) induces p53 and Bax-independent apoptosis. Oncogene 2002;21:3149–3161.

36. Weber JD, Jeffers JR, Rehg JE, et al. p53-independent functions of the p19(ARF) tumor suppressor. Genes Dev 2000;14:2358–2365.

37. Eymin B, Claverie P, Salon C, et al. p14^{ARF} activates a Tip60-dependent ATM/ATR/CHK pathway in response to genotoxic stresses. Mol Cell Biol 2006;26(11):4339–4350.

38. Gazzeri S, Della Valle V, Chaussade L, et al. The human p19^{ARF} protein encoded by the β transcript of the p16^{INK4} gene is frequently lost in small cell lung tumors. Cancer Res 1998;58:3926–3931.

39. Eymin B, Claverie P, Salon C, et al. P14^{ARF} triggers G2 arrest through ERK-mediated Cdc25C phosphorylation, ubiquitination and proteasomal degradation. Cell Cycle 2006;5(7):759–765.

40. Chen J, Marechal V, Levine AJ. Mapping of the p53 and mdm-2 interaction domains. Mol Cell Biol 1993;13:4107–4114.

41. Momand J, Zambetti GP, Olson DC, et al. The mdm-2 oncogene product forms a complex with the p53 protein and inhibits p53-mediated transactivation. Cell 1992;69:1237–1245.

42. Oliner JD, Pietenpol JA, Thiagalingam S, et al. Oncoprotein MDM2 conceals the activation domain of tumour suppressor p53. Nature 1993;362:857–860.

43. Haupt Y, Maya R, Kazaz A, et al. Mdm2 promotes the rapid degradation of p53. Nature 1997;387:296–299.

44. Tao W, Levine AJ. Nucleocytoplasmic shuttling of oncoprotein Hdm2 is required for Hdm2-mediated degradation of p53. Proc. Natl Acad Sci USA 1999;96:3077–3080.

45. Weber JD, Taylor LJ, Roussel MF, et al. Nucleolar Arf sequesters Mdm2 and activates p53. Nat Cell Biol 1999;1:20–26.

46. Cordon-Cardo C, Latres E, Drobnjak M, et al. Molecular abnormalities of mdm2 and p53 genes in adult soft tissue sarcomas. Cancer Res 1994;54:794–799.

47. Eymin B, Gazzeri S, Brambilla C, et al. Distinct pattern of E2F1 expression in human lung tumors: E2F1 is upregulated in small cell lung carcinoma. Oncogene 2001;20:1678–1687.

48. Zabarovsky ER, Lerman MI, Minna JD. Tumor suppressor genes on chromosome 3p involved in the pathogenesis of lung and other cancers. Oncogene 2002;21:6915–6935.

49. Sozzi G, Pastorino U, Moiraghi L, et al. Loss of FHIT function in lung cancer and preinvasive bronchial lesions. Cancer Res 1998;58:5032–5037.

50. Sard L, Accornero P, Tornielli S, et al. The tumor suppressor gene FHIT is involved in the regulation of apoptosis and cell cycle control. Proc Natl Acad Sci USA 1999;96:8489–8492.

51. Dammann R, Li C, Yoon JH, et al. Epigenetic inactivation of a RAS association domain family protein from the lung tumour suppressor locus 3p21.3. 52. Nat Genet 2000;25:315–319.

52. Burbee DG, Forgacs E, Zochbauer-Muller S, et al. Epigenetic inactivation of RASSF1A in lung and breast cancers and malignant phenotype suppression. J Natl Cancer Inst 2001;93:691–699.

53. Virmani AK, Rathi A, Zöchbauer-Müller S, et al. Promoter methylation and silencing of the retinoic acid receptor-β gene in lung carcinomas. J Natl Cancer Inst 2000;92:1303–1307.

54. Holt SE, Shay JW. Role of telomerase in cellular proliferation and cancer. J Cell Physiol 1999;180:10–18.

55. Lantuejoul S, Soria JC, Lorimier P, et al. Differential expression of telomerase reverse transcriptase (hTERT) in lung tumors. Br J Cancer 2004;90:1222–1229.

56. Hiyama K, Hiyama E, Ishioka S, et al. Telomerase activity in small cell and non small cell lung cancers. J Natl Cancer Inst 1995;87:895–902.

57. Albanell J, Lonardo F, Rush V, et al. High telomerase activity in primary lung cancers: association with increased cell proliferation rates and advanced pathologic stage. J Natl Cancer Inst 1997;89:1609–1615.

58. Gomez-Roman JJ, Fontalba Romero A, Sanchez Castro L, et al. Telomerase activity in pulmonary neuroendocrine tumours. Am J Surg Pathol 2000;24:417–421.

59. Lantuejoul S, Salon C, Soria JC, et al. Telomerase expression in lung preneoplasia and neoplasia. Int J Cancer 2007;120:1835–1841.

60. Decaussin M, Sartelet H, Robert C, et al. Expression of vascular endothelial growth factor (VEGF) and its receptors (VEGF-R1-Flt1 and VEGF-R2-Flk1/KDR) in non small cell lung carcinoma (NSCLC): correlation with angiogenesis and survival. J. Pathol 1999;188:369–377.

61. Tian X, Song S, Wu J, et al. Vascular endothelial growth factor: acting as an autocrine growth factor for human gastric adenocarcinoma cell MGC803. Biochem Biophys Res Commun 2001;286:505–512.

62. Lantuejoul S, Constantin B, Drabkin H, et al. Expression of VEGF, semaphorin SEMA3F and their common receptors neuropilins NP1 and NP2 in preinvasive bronchial lesions, lung tumors and cell lines. J Pathol 2003;200:336–347.

63. Compernolle V, Brusselmans K, Acker T, et al. Loss of HIF-2α and inhibition of VEGF impair fetal lung maturation, whereas treatment with VEGF prevents fatal respiratory distress in premature mice. Nature Med 2002;(8)7:702–710.

64. Kusy S, Nasarre P, Chan D, et al. Selective suppression of in vivo tumorigenicity by semaphoring SEMA3F in lung cancer cells. Neoplasia 2005;7(5):457–465.

65. Salon C, Moro D, Lantuejoul S, et al. The E-cadherin/β-catenin adhesion complex in neuroendocrine tumors of the lung : a suggested role upon local invasion and metastasis. Hum Pathol 2004;35(9):1148–1155.

66. Salon C, Lantuejoul S, Eymin B, et al. The E-cadherin–β-catenin complex and its implication in lung cancer progression and prognosis. Future Oncol 2005;1(5):649–660.

67. Clavel CE, Nollet F, Berx G, et al. Expression of the E-cadherin-catenin complex in lung neuroendocrine tumours. J Pathol 2001;194:20–26.
68. Heldin CH, Ostman A, Ronnstrand L. Signal transduction via platelet-derived growth factor receptors. Biochim Biophys Acta 1998;1378:F79–F113.
69. Pelosi G, Fasullo M, Leon ME, et al. CD117 immunoreactivity in high-grade neuroendocrine tumors of the lung: a comparative study of 39 large-cell neuroendocrine carcinomas and 27 surgically resected small-cell carcinomas. Virchows Arch 2004;445:449–455.
70. Rossi G, Cavazza A, Marchioni A, et al. Kit expression in small cell carcinomas of the lung: effects of chemotherapy. Mod Pathol 2003;16:1041–1047.
71. Hibi K, Takahashi T, Sekido Y, et al. Coexpression of stem cell factor and the c-kit genes in small-cell lung cancer. Oncogene 1991;6:2291–2296.
72. Rygaard K, Nakamura T, Spang-Thomsen M. Expression of the protooncogene c-met and c-kit and their ligands, hepatocyte growth factor/scatter factor and stem cell factor in SCLC cell lines and xenografts. Br J Cancer 1993;67:137–146.
73. Krystal GW, Hines SJ, Organ CP. Autocrine growth of small cell lung cancer mediated by coexpression of c-kit and stem cell factor. Cancer Res 1996;56:370–376.
74. Tamborini E, Bonadiman L, Negri T, et al. Detection of overexpression and phosphorylation wild-type Kit receptor in surgical specimens of small cell lung cancer. Clin Cancer Res 2004;10:8214–8219.
75. Maulik G, Shrikhande A, Kijima T, et al. Role of the hepatocyte growth factor receptor, c-Met, in the oncogenesis and potential for therapeutic inhibition. Cytokine Growth Factor Rev 2002;13:41–59.
76. Ma PC, Maulik G, Christensen J, et al. c-Met: structure, functions and potential for therapeutic inhibition. Cancer Metastasis Rev 2003;22:309–325.
77. Trusolino L, Comoglio PM. Scatter-factor and semaphorin receptors: cell signalling for invasive growth. Nature Rev 2002;2:289–300.
78. Maulik G, Kijima T, Ma PC, et al. Modulation of the c-met/hepatocyte growth factor pathway in small cell lung cancer. Clin Cancer Res 2002;8:620 627.
79. Ma PC, Kijima T, Maulik G, et al. C-MET mutational analysis in small cell lung cancer: novel juxtamembrane domain mutations regulating cytoskeletal functions. Cancer Res 2003;63:6272–6281.
80. Wang WL, Healy ME, Sattler M, et al. Growth inhibition and modulation of kinase pathways on small cell lung cancer cell lines by the novel tyrosine kinase inhibitor STI571. Oncogene 2000;19:3521–3528.
81. Krystal GW, Honsawek S, Litz J, et al. The selective tyrosine kinase inhibitor STI571 inhibits small cell lung cancer growth. Clin Cancer Res 2000;6:3319–3326.
82. Krystal GW, Honsawek S, Kiewlich D, et al. Indolinone tyrosine kinase inhibitors block Kit activation and growth of small cell lung cancer cells. Cancer Res 2001;61:3660–68.
83. Abrams TJ, Lee LB, Murray LJ, et al. SU11248 inhibits KIT and platelet-derived growth factor receptor β in preclinical models of human small cell lung cancer. Mol Cancer Ther 2003;2:471–478.
84. Buchdunger E, Cioffi CL, Law N, et al. Abl protein-tyrosine kinase inhibitor STI571 inhibits in vitro signal transduction mediated by c-kit and platelet-derived growth factor receptors. J Pharmacol Exp Ther 2000;295:139–145.
85. Bondzi C, Litz J, Dent P, et al. Src family kinase activity is required for Kit-mediated mitogen-activated protein (MAP) kinase activation; however, loss of functional retinoblastoma protein makes MAP kinase activation unnecessary for growth of small cell lung cancer cells. Cell Growth Differ 2000;11:305–314.

29
Neuroendocrine Carcinomas and Precursors

Elisabeth Brambilla

Introduction

Neuroendocrine lung tumors are usually classified into four histologic types that were shifted in the World Health Organization classification into three entities: small cell lung carcinoma (SCLC), large cell neuroendocrine carcinoma (LCNEC), and carcinoids (typical and atypical).[1,2] This subset of tumors shares morphologic, ultrastructural, immunohistochemical, and molecular characteristics. The four main types neuroendocrine lung tumors show varying degrees of neuroendocrine morphologic features, and they behave according to three grades of clinical aggressivity, the low-grade typical carcinoids, the intermediate-grade atypical carcinoids, and the high-grade LCNECs and SCLCs, which share many features including epidemiologic growth factor and oncogenic pathways. However, the concept of a continuous spectrum from carcinoid to SCLC has no other scientific basis than a common neuroendocrine differentiation.

There is increasing evidence that typical carcinoids and atypical carcinoids are closely related to each other, whereas LCNECs and SCLCs are very close entities. Epidemiologically, patients with typical and atypical carcinoids are significantly younger than those with SCLCs and LCNECs. Within the high-grade neuroendocrine tumors, LCNECs and SCLCs are morphologically distinct, but this is their main difference because chemotherapy used for SCLC has been recently shown effective in LCNEC. Clinically, approximately 20%–40% of patients with typical and atypical carcinoids are nonsmokers, and virtually all patients with LCNEC are heavy cigarette smokers. Patients with the hereditary disease multiple endocrine neoplasia type 1 (MEN1) are prone to the development of carcinoids more often atypical. The same applies for the sporadic somatic mutation of *MEN1*, which has been described in atypical carcinoids[3] A large mutation analysis of the *MEN1* gene did not show any mutation in SCLC and LCNEC.[4] According to genetic and epigenetic abnormalities, typical and atypical carcinoids are closely related whether or not LCNEC strongly mimics SCLC (see Chapter 25).

No precursor lesion has been acknowledged and recognized for SCLC and LCNEC. Carcinoids may arise in the context of diffuse idiopathic pulmonary neuroendocrine hyperplasia, believed to be a precursor or predisposing background.

Histopathologic Definitions

Carcinoid tumors are characterized by organoid growth patterns suggesting neuroendocrine differentiation. Tumor cells are uniform and have a finely eosinophilic granular cytoplasm and nuclei with a regularly granulated chromatin pattern. Typical carcinoid is characterized by fewer than 2 mitoses per $2\,mm^2$ and lack necrosis; atypical carcinoid is characterized by 2–10 mitoses per $2\,mm^2$ and/or foci of necrosis. Thus, the distinction between typical and atypical carcinoids relies on objective criteria of mitoses and necrosis.

Large cell neuroendocrine carcinoma is a variant of large cell carcinoma characterized by proliferation of large cells with low nuclear to cytoplasmic ratio that have histologic features suggesting neuroendocrine differentiation, such as organoid nesting pattern, trabecular growth, rosettes, and perilobular palisading.[1,5] The tumor is made of large cells with abundant cytoplasm, the nuclear chromatin is granular and sometimes vesicular, and the nucleoli are frequently prominent. The mitotic count is typically more than 11 per $2\,mm^2$, which allows the differential diagnosis with atypical carcinoids (which have a lower mitotic count), and large zones of necrosis are common in contrast to focal necrosis in atypical carcinoids. The demonstration of at least one well-documented and obvious neuroendocrine differentiation marker is required for the diagnosis of LCNEC. The specific neuroendocrine markers are chromogranin, synaptophysin, and CD56/neural cell adhesion molecule.[6] It is stressed that these neuroendocrine markers are necessary for diagnosis of only LCNECs, not for diagnosis of carcinoids and SCLCs.

Molecular Pathology: Differentiation Signs

Carcinoids typically display all neuroendocrine markers. Most carcinoid tumors stain for cytokeratin, and the patchy globular Golgi pattern is frequent. All carcinoid tumors express neurofilaments of low and high molecular weights. The neuroendocrine markers chromogranin, synaptophysin, Leu-7 (CD57), and neural cell adhesion molecule (CD56) are strongly positive.[7] Besides regular cytokeratin expression, expressions of cytokeratins 1, 5, 10, and 14 collectively represented in the 34βE12 antibody, which is typical of NSCLC, are typically negative in both carcinoids and LCNEC. In contrast, combined LCNECs, which represent 30% of LCNECs and are characterized by a mixture of any combination of LCNEC components and a conventional NSCLC, express cytokeratins 1, 5, 10, and 14 (revealed by 34βE12) in their NSCLC-associated component. Sustentacular cells, which are S100 positive as they are seen in paraganglioma, are present in half the carcinoids. Varying results have been observed for thyroid transcription factor 1 (TTF-1) expression in carcinoids. We strongly support the absence of TTF-1 expression in proximal carcinoids, typical or atypical, although this concept is not completely clear for the moment and debate is still open.[8,9]

It is important to realize that entrapped normal alveolar type II cells strongly express TTF-1, unlike carcinoids. In addition, sclerosing hemangioma, which enters in the differential diagnosis of carcinoids, expresses TTF-1.[9-11] In carcinoids and in LCNECs, CD99/MIC2 is often positive.[12,13] In contrast with absence of TTF-1 in carcinoids, about 50% of LCNECs express TTF-1 with a typical nuclear pattern that is of great help for their distinction from basaloid carcinoma, which do not express TTF-1.[10,14,15]

Molecular Alterations Reflecting Malignant Proliferation

The molecular alterations discussed here are the ones believed to drive proliferation and malignancy in neuroendocrine tumors other than SCLC.

Carcinoids (Typical and Atypical)

Somatic Genetics: Cytogenetics and Comparative Genomic Hybridization

An imbalance in gene copy number is relatively rare in carcinoids compared with high-grade neuroendocrine tumors.

Allelic loss of the 11p13 locus of *MEN1* occurs not only in the carcinoids in the context of MEN1 disease but also as a sporadic genetic event in nonfamilial carcinoid tumors. The same feature is encountered in gastrointestinal carcinoids. The *MEN1* gene encodes the protein menin,[3,16] which is believed to act as a tumor suppressor protein in the JunD activation pathway. According to comparative genomic hybridization studies, loss of 11p13 material occurs in 0%–50% of typical carcinoids and in 50%–70% of atypical carcinoids.[17,18] Atypical carcinoids, but not typical carcinoids, may display loss of 10q and 13q material.[18]

Loss of heterozygosity in high-grade neuroendocrine carcinoma occurs at 3p (involving five candidate tumor suppressor genes), 13q (location of the retinoblastoma [*Rb*] gene), 9p21 (*p16*), and 17p (*p53*) and are rare in typical carcinoids but more frequent in atypical carcinoids, although at a lower rate than in SCLCs.[16] Loss of heterozygosity at 3p14.2 and 21.3 has been found in 40% of atypical carcinomas with a significantly lower rate than in NSCLC or the high-grade neuroendocrine tumors LCNEC and SCLC. Loss of heterozygosity at 13q14 (location of the *Rb* gene) is exceptional in typical carcinoids but may occur in 20% of atypical carcinoids.[19]

p53 Pathway Alterations

Mutations of *p53* are extremely rare in typical carcinoids and occur in about 10% of atypical carcinoids.[20,21] The *p53* mutation seen in atypical carcinoids is of an unusual type (G:C to A:T transition or nonsense mutations rather than G:T transversion).[16] Accordingly, aberrant p53 overexpression reflecting a *p53* mutation and stabilization detected by immunohistochemistry have not been reported in carcinoids or in atypical carcinoids.[20]

Downstream alterations of the target genes of p53 are typically absent in carcinoids, with no deregulation of the Bcl-2:Bax ratio. Carcinoids are characterized by a low level of Bcl-2 and a high level of Bax.

The Retinoblastoma Pathway

Retinoblastoma inactivation and loss are typical of high-grade neuroendocrine tumors. In contrast, typical carcinoids retain Rb expression and 20% of atypical carcinoids show loss of Rb expression compared with internal controls (normal epithelial cells, fibroblasts, and endothelial cells). In carcinoids displaying Rb loss, cytokine-dependent kinase inhibitor p16[INK4] loss and/or cyclin D1 upregulation may be observed. These two abnormalities are found in less than 10% of typical carcinoids and a in maximum of 30% of atypical carcinoids.[19] A mutual exclusion between Rb loss and p16/cyclin D1 alterations is observed in these low-grade neuroendocrine tumors, showing that cyclin D1 and p16 coordinate the level of Rb phosphorylation and loss of control of G1 arrest. In contrast, cyclin E overexpression, which is observed in

25% of typical carcinoids and 40% of atypical carcinoids, may be concomitant with Rb loss, suggesting that cyclin E participates in phosphorylation of targets other than Rb or carries other functions independent of Rb in G1 arrest and cell cycle control.

Upstream p53 Pathway Alterations

The p14^{ARF} protein is a member of the p53 pathway and functions independent of p53. In response to oncogenic stimuli and DNA damage, p14^{ARF} sequesters MDM2 in the nucleoli, preventing p53/MDM2-dependent proteolysis, allowing its function in cell cycle arrest and/or apoptosis. Expression of the p14^{ARF} protein, which is lost in 40% of atypical carcinoids and in SCLC, is lost in only 5% of typical carcinoids.[22] Abnormalities of MDM2 have been rarely reported in carcinoids.[23] Thirty percent of carcinoids (typical and atypical) show overexpression of MDM2 compared with normal epithelial cells.

In carcinoids as well as in other neuroendocrine tumors, MDM2 overexpression and p14 loss are inversely correlated (p < 0.0001),[23] suggesting that the MDM2:p14^{ARF} ratio acts as a rheostat in modulating the activity and function of both downstream tumor suppressor genes *p53* and *Rb*.

The Fas Pathway of Apoptosis

Fas (CD95) is another p53 transcriptional target gene strongly downregulated in all types of neuroendocrine lung tumors, whereas overexpression of its ligand FasL is characteristic of SCLC. In carcinoids, low Fas expression is seen in 80% of the cases as compared to normal basal epithelial cells. No evidence has been provided of whether normal bronchial neuroendocrine cells express Fas and Fas ligand (FasL). Carcinoid tumors express FasL in 40% of the cases.

A downstream effector of the Fas/FasL pathway of apoptosis is caspase-8, which is located on chromosome 2q33 and is frequently lost and but sometimes methylated in SCLC cell lines. Caspase-8 was shown to be silenced by methylation in 18% of bronchial carcinoids (7/40 cases) and in the vast majority of SCLC.. Fas abrogation of the tumor necrosis factor receptor pathway may also be present in carcinoids.[24]

Telomerase Inactivation

Several recent studies have reported telomere activity and telomere lengths in carcinoids compared with other neuroendocrine lung tumors.[25,26] Typical carcinoids as well as atypical carcinoids show telomerase activation and present with long telomeres.[26] We could confirm that only 20% of typical and atypical carcinoids show telomerase activation using immunohistochemistry (personal data, S. Lantuejoul 2006, submitted).

Angiogenic Factors, Growth Factors, and Migration Factors

Twenty-five percent of carcinoids express high levels of vascular endothelial growth factor (VEGF) as do normal neuroendocrine cells in the lung.[27] A ligand of VEGF receptor 2, SEMA3F, is expressed at intermediate or high levels in carcinoids, in contrast to its loss in high-grade neuroendocrine tumors. In addition, the vast majority express SEMA3F at the normal membrane location, so that the ratio of SEMA3F to VEGF, two competitive ligands of VEGF receptor 2, is quite normal in carcinoids.[28] The majority of typical and atypical carcinoids (54% and 81%) express intermediate or low levels of the two coreceptors of VEGF receptor 2 neuropilins 1 (NP1) and 2 (NP2). Levels of NP1 and NP2 are significantly lower in all histological types of neuroendocrine lung tumors, including high grade and low grade, when compared with NSCLCs.

The VEGF/SEMA3F/NP pathway appears to be characterized by the preservation of SEMA3F expression in carcinoid tumors in favor of low level of invasiveness of this tumor type and by a reasonable conservation of apoptosis. Indeed, recent studies indicate that SEMA3F suppressed tumor formation and tumor migration in mice and reduced apoptosis.[29] The balance between SEMA3F and VEGF predicts a low cell mobility and preserved apoptotic process in low-grade neuroendocrine tumors.

The tyrosine kinase pathway represented by c-Kit, c-Met, and platelet-derived growth factor is rarely activated in carcinoids. The adhesion molecule complex E-cadherin–β-catenin has been reported recently.[30] The vast majority of carcinoids maintain a normal E-cadherin and β-catenin expression with membranous pattern, although 30% of carcinoids show impairment of one of these molecule (loss or cytoplasmic delocalization). This is in agreement with a single previous study of E-cadherin expression in neuroendocrine tumors including 12 carcinoids.[31] It should be noted that half of carcinoids have a dissociated expression between β-catenin preserved and membranous and impaired cytoplasmic delocalization of E-cadherin. Similar results have been reported in gastrointestinal tumors.[32] β-Catenin nuclear expression has not been shown in carcinoids. Also interesting is that impaired E-cadherin expression correlated with extensive disease in typical and atypical carcinoids. The E-cadherin expression pattern in neuroendocrine tumors may indicate aggressiveness.

Large Cell Neuroendocrine Carcinoma

Somatic Genetics: Cytogenetics and Comparative Genomic Hybridization

Large cell neuroendocrine carcinomas demonstrate very similar chromosomal imbalances to those found in SCLC,[17,33,34] including frequent 3p deletions.

Molecular Pathology: The p53 and Retinoblastoma Pathways

Large cell neuroendocrine carcinomas share genetic alterations commonly seen in SCLC: a high rate of *p53* mutation,[16,20,21,35,36] Bcl-2 overexpression with Bax downregulation,[20] and a high telomerase activity. However, lower frequencies of loss of Rb protein expression and of E2F1 overexpression are observed in LCNEC than in SCLC.[37,38] Loss of p14^{ARF} occurs with the same frequency of 40% as in SCLC. E2F1 is abnormally overexpressed in 50% of LCNECs compared with 80% of SCLCs and none in carcinoids. Retinoblastoma loss is less frequent in LCNEC (68%) than in SCLC (78%).[19] p16 is lost in 20% of LCNEC, and cyclin D1 is overexpressed in 10% of them. All together, 35% of LCNEC retaining Rb expression have cytokine-dependent kinase inhibitor p16^{INK4} loss and/or cyclin D1 upregulation.

Cyclin E overexpression is similar in LCNEC than in SCLC (50%) and can be seen concomitantly with Rb loss. This might be the result of E2F1 upregulation, which is observed in 50% of the cases, unlike NSCLC, in which it is undetectable. Indeed, one of the E2F1-related transcriptional targets is cyclin E. Consequently cyclin E overexpression closely correlates with upregulated E2F1. A high level of MDM2 is observed in about 30% of LCNECs with an inverse relation between MDM2 overexpression and p14 loss.[23] Both alterations of MDM2 overexpression and Rb loss can be seen concurrently in high-grade neuroendocrine carcinomas, especially LCNEC. Upstream to p53, MDM2 and p14 display the same picture in LCNEC and in SCLC. Downstream to p53, and at the level of G1 arrest, the only difference between them resides in the higher frequency of Rb expression maintenance in LCNEC than SCLC.

Apoptotic Factors

Bcl-2 is an antiapoptotic protein in the downstream pathway transcriptionally inhibited by p53 and is activated with a high frequency in LCNEC and in SCLC. Ninety percent of LCNEC have a high expression of Bcl-2 (score >50) and a low Bax expression (score < 50) with a Bcl-2:Bax ratio >1. In this regard, LCNEC also imitates SCLC.

Fas and Fas Ligand

Fas, another targeted gene for positive transcription by p53, has been studied in a small series of LCNEC.[39] Large cell neuroendocrine carcinomas have a strong downregulation of Fas and a very low Fas expression score compared with normal lung tissue, and half of them are completely negative. The Fas ligand was found to be upregulated in 40% of the cases with a high level result-

ing in the vast majority (95%) having a Fas:FasL ratio of <1, the same frequency as SCLC. Actually, the Fas:FasL score ratio was quite constantly low as was the Bax:Bcl2 score ratio. This reflects a strong downregulation of apoptosis in LCNEC mitochondrial as well as death receptor pathways.

Angiogenic Factors

A small number of cases have been studied for VEGF, semaphorin, and neuropilin expression in LCNEC and showed overexpression of VEGF in all cases, loss of SEMA3F in 40%, and increased expression of NP1 and NP2 compared with normal epithelial cells in 70% and 90%, respectively. In this regard, LCNECs show the same pattern of moderate expression of VEGF and neuropilins as SCLCs.

Growth Factors and Receptors

Tyrosine kinase receptors and related growth factors in LCNEC were studied in a large series of LCNEC.[40] Platelet-derived growth factor receptor-β (PDGF-Rβ) was strongly expressed in 80% of LCNECs, c-Kit in 63%, PDGF-Rα in 60%, Met in 47%, and scatter factor in 56%. Interestingly, the only prognostic factor in LCNEC was Met expression, which significantly correlated with overall survival ($p = 0.03$). There was no mutation observed in Met or tyrosine kinase receptor–positive LCNECs. Met-positive LCNEC patients who underwent NSCLC-based adjuvant chemotherapy had the worst overall survival ($p < 0.0001$). This disadvantage for survival for chemotherapy-treated patients was maintained in a Cox analysis ($p = 0.01$). The most important positive survival variable was the SCLC-based chemotherapy for LCNEC.

Adhesion Molecule of E-Cadherin–β-Catenin Complex

Two pertinent studies were performed for LCNEC.[30,41] Eighty-four percent of LCNECs had impaired E-cadherin staining (loss of membranous staining and/or aberrant cytoplasmic staining), and 73% had impaired β-catenin expression, so the vast majority of LCNECs have lost the normal expression of this adhesion molecule complex. The correlation between these impairments ($p = 0.01$) was strong. The one case was detected with β-catenin nuclear staining in contrast with the previous study using electron microscopy. No β-catenin or E-cadherin mutation was detected in LCNEC. The patterns of E-cadherin and β-catenin expression are common in LCNECs and SCLCs, implying that E-cadherin and β-catenin adhesion complex deregulation plays a role in the pathogenesis of these high-grade neuroendocrine tumors. Correlations between impaired E-cadherin and

305

extended stage III–IV ($p = 0.04$) and between impaired E-cadherin and the presence of nodal metastasis ($p = 0.01$) have been shown in LNECs.[30]

Diffuse Idiopathic Pulmonary Neuroendocrine Cell Hyperplasia and Tumorlets

Tumorlets are defined as microscopic peribronchiolar nodular aggregates of uniform, round, oval, or spindle-shaped cells with a moderate amount of cytoplasm and a morphology similar to the cells of carcinoid tumors (according to the World Health Organization 1999 definition). These are most of the time multiple and found in fibrosed lung, such as in tuberculosis and bronchiectasis, and around scars. The differential diagnosis between tumorlets (<0.5 cm diameter) and carcinoids (≥0.5 cm diameter) is arbitrary. Most of the tumorlets encountered in scarred lung are sporadic and not considered as primary.

The rare idiopathic form of diffuse pulmonary neuroendocrine cell hyperplasia (diffuse idiopathic pulmonary neuroendocrine cell hyperplasia) occurs when the tumorlets are frequent and multiple in the lung. In the idiopathic form, the tumorlets have the same histologic appearance, are marked consistently with the neuroendocrine markers and cytokeratins, and express the same profile as carcinoid tumors, including expression of ASH1 and absence of TTF-1. Thyroid transcription factor 1 has been shown as absent in large series of tumorlets,[10] although this finding is controversial. There has been no genetic study of tumorlets and other hyperplastic neuroendocrine conditions.

Diffuse idiopathic pulmonary neuroendocrine cell hyperplasia is defined as a generalized proliferation of hyperplastic neuroendocrine cells as scattered single cells, small nodules (neuroendocrine bodies), or linear proliferation of pulmonary neuroendocrine cells that may be confined to the bronchial and bronchiolar epithelium (suprabasal), can proliferate into the bronchial lumina and create bronchial obstruction, or may proliferate in extraluminal subbasal localization in the form of tumorlets. Their expansion gives rise to one or multiple carcinoids.

There is nothing known about the molecular pathology of diffuse idiopathic pulmonary neuroendocrine cell hyperplasia. It is considered as a preinvasive lesion for carcinoids but not for high-grade neuroendocrine tumors. There has been no description of a context of diffuse idiopathic pulmonary neuroendocrine cell hyperplasia in SCLC or LCNEC patients. It is of interest that an allelic imbalance at the 11q13 chromosomal location of the *MEN1* tumor suppressor gene was rarely detected in tumorlets and was not searched for in diffuse idiopathic pulmonary neuroendocrine cell hyperplasia, although it was present in a high percentage of carcinoid tumors.[42]

References

1. Travis WD, Colby TV, Corrin B, et al. WHO Histological Classification of Tumours. Histological Typing of Lung and Pleural Tumours, 3rd ed. Berlin: Springer-Verlag; 1999.
2. Travis WD, Brambilla E, Muller-Hemerlink HK, Harris CC, eds. World Health Organization Classification of Tumours. Pathology and Genetics of Tumours of the Lung, Pleura, Thymus and Heart. Lyon: IARC Press; 2004.
3. Debelenko LV, Brambilla E, Agarwal SK, et al. Identification of MEN1 gene mutations in sporadic carcinoid tumors of the lung. Hum Mol Genet 1997;6:2285–2290.
4. Debelenko LV, Swalwell JI, Kelley MJ, et al. MEN1 gene mutation analysis of high-grade neuroendocrine lung carcinoma. Genes Chromosomes Cancer 2000;28:58–65.
5. Travis WD, Linnoila RI, Tsokos MG, et al. Neuroendocrine tumors of the lung with proposed criteria for large-cell neuroendocrine carcinoma. An ultrastructural, immunohistochemical, and flow cytometric study of 35 cases. Am J Surg Pathol 1991;15:529–553.
6. Lantuejoul S, Moro D, Michalides RJ, et al. Neural cell adhesion molecules (NCAM) and NCAM-PSA expression in neuroendocrine lung tumors. Am J Surg Pathol 1998;22:1267–1276.
7. Travis WD, Rush W, Flieder DB, et al. Survival analysis of 200 pulmonary neuroendocrine tumors with clarification of criteria for atypical carcinoid and its separation from typical carcinoid. Am J Surg Pathol 1998;22:934–944.
8. Folpe AL, Gown AM, Lamps LW, et al. Thyroid transcription factor-1: immunohistochemical evaluation in pulmonary neuroendocrine tumors. Mod Pathol 1999;12:5–8.
9. Oliveira AM, Tazelaar HD, Myers JL, et al. Thyroid transcription factor-1 distinguishes metastatic pulmonary from well-differentiated neuroendocrine tumors of other sites. Am J Surg Pathol 2001;25:815–819.
10. Sturm N, Rossi G, Lantuejoul S, et al. Expression of thyroid transcription factor-1 in the spectrum of neuroendocrine cell lung proliferations with special interest in carcinoids. Hum Pathol 2002;33:175–182.
11. Wick MR. Immunohistology of neuroendocrine and neuroectodermal tumors. Semin Diagn Pathol 2000;17:194–203.
12. Pelosi G, Fraggetta F, Sonzogni A, et al. CD99 immunoreactivity in gastrointestinal and pulmonary neuroendocrine tumours. Virchows Arch 2000;437:270–274.
13. Pelosi G, Leon ME, Veronesi G, et al. Decreased immunoreactivity of CD99 is an independent predictor of regional lymph node metastases in pulmonary carcinoid tumors. J Thorac Oncol 2006;1(5):468–477.
14. Lyda MH, Weiss LM. Immunoreactivity for epithelial and neuroendocrine antibodies are useful in the differential diagnosis of lung carcinomas. Hum Pathol 2000;31:980–987.
15. Sturm N, Lantuejoul S, Laverriere MH, et al. Thyroid transcription factor 1 and cytokeratins 1, 5, 10, 14 (34betaE12)

expression in basaloid and large-cell neuroendocrine carcinomas of the lung. Hum Pathol 2001;32:918–925.

16. Onuki N, Wistuba II, Travis WD, et al. Genetic changes in the spectrum of neuroendocrine lung tumors. Cancer 1999; 85:600–607.

17. Ullmann R, Schwendel A, Klemen H, et al. Unbalanced chromosomal aberrations in neuroendocrine lung tumors as detected by comparative genomic hybridization. Hum Pathol 1998;29:1145–1149.

18. Walch AK, Zitzelsberger HF, Aubele MM, et al. Typical and atypical carcinoid tumors of the lung are characterized by 11q deletions as detected by comparative genomic hybridization. Am J Pathol 1998;153:1089–1098.

19. Beasley MB, Lantuejoul S, Abbondanzo S, et al. The p16/cyclin D1/Rb pathway in neuroendocrine tumors of the lung. Hum Pathol 2003;34:136–142.

20. Brambilla E, Negoescu A, Gazzeri S, et al. Apoptosis-related factors p53, Bcl2, and Bax in neuroendocrine lung tumors. Am J Pathol 1996;149:1941–1952.

21. Przygodzki RM, Finkelstein SD, Langer JC, et al. Analysis of p53, K-ras-2, and C-raf-1 in pulmonary neuroendocrine tumors. Correlation with histological subtype and clinical outcome. Am J Pathol 1996;148:1531–1541.

22. Eymin B, Claverie P, Salon C, et al. p14^{ARF} activates a Tip60-dependent ATM/ATR/CHK pathway in response to genotoxic stresses. Mol Cell Biol 2006;26(11):4339–4350.

23. Eymin B, Gazzeri S, Brambilla C, et al. Mdm2 overexpression and p14^{ARF} inactivation are two mutually exclusive events in primary human lung tumors. Oncogene 2002;21: 2750–2761.

24. Shivapurkar N, Toyooka S, Eby MT, et al. Differential inactivation of caspase-8 in lung cancers. Cancer Biol Ther 2002;1:54–58.

25. Zaffaroni N, De Polo D, Villa R, et al. Differential expression of telomerase activity in neuroendocrine lung tumours: correlation with gene product immunophenotyping. J Pathol 2003;201:127–133.

26. Zaffaroni N, Villa R, Pastorino U, et al. Lack of telomerase activity in lung carcinoids is dependent on human telomerase reverse transcriptase transcription and alternative splicing and is associated with long telomeres. Clin Cancer Res 2005;11(8):2832–2839.

27. Sartelet H, Decaussin M, Devouassoux G, et al Expression of vascular endothelial growth factor (VEGF) and its receptors (VEGF-R1 (Flt-1) and VEGF-R2 (KDR/Flk-1) in tumorlets and in neuroendocrine cell hyperplasia of the lung. Hum Pathol 2005;35(10):1210–1217.

28. Brambilla E, Constantin B, Drabkin H, et al. Semaphorin SEMA3F localization in malignant human lung and dividing cells: a suggested role in cell adhesion and cell migration. Am J Pathol 2000;156(3):939–950.

29. Kusy S, Nasarre P, Chan D, et al. Selective suppression of in vivo tumorigenicity by semaphoring SEMA3F in lung cancer cells. Neoplasia 2005;7(5):457–465.

30. Salon C, Moro D, Lantuejoul S, et al. The E-cadherin/β-catenin adhesion complex in neuroendocrine tumors of the lung: a suggested role upon local invasion and metastasis. Hum Pathol 2004;35(9):1148–1155.

31. Clavel CE, Nollet F, Berx G, et al. Expression of the E-cadherin–catenin complex in lung neuroendocrine tumours. J Pathol 2001;194:20–26.

32. Sanders DS, Perry I, Hardy R, et al. Aberrant E-cadherin expression in a feature of clonal expansion in the gastrointestinal tract associated with repair and neoplasia. J Pathol 2000;190:526–530.

33. Institute of Pathology "Rudolf-Virchow-Haus." Comparative Genomic Hybridization (CGH). 2003. University Hospital Charité Humboldt-University of Berlin. http://amba.charite.de/cgh/. Accessed February 12, 2007.

34. Ullmann R, Petzmann S, Sharma A, et al. Chromosomal aberrations in a series of large-cell neuroendocrine carcinomas: unexpected divergence from small-cell carcinoma of the lung. Hum Pathol 2001;32:1059–1063.

35. Brambilla E, Gazzeri S, Moro D, et al. Immunohistochemical study of p53 in human lung carcinomas. Am J Pathol 1993;143:199–210.

36. Brambilla E, Moro D, Gazzeri S, et al. Alterations of expression of Rb, p16(INK4A) and cyclin D1 in non-small cell lung carcinoma and their clinical significance. J Pathol 1999; 188:351–360.

37. Eymin B, Karayan L, Seite P, et al. Human ARF binds E2F1 and inhibits its transcriptional activity. Oncogene 2001;20: 1033–1041.

38. Eymin B, Gazzeri S, Brambilla C, et al. Distinct pattern of E2F1 expression in human lung tumors: E2F1 is upregulated in small cell lung carcinoma. Oncogene 2001;20:1678–1687.

39. Viard-Leveugle I, Veyrenc S, French LE, et al. Frequent loss of Fas expression and function in human lung tumors with overexpression of FasL in small cell lung carcinoma. J Pathol 2003;(201)2:268–277.

40. Rossi G, Cavazza A, Marchioni A, et al. Role of the chemotherapy and the receptor tyrosine kinases KIT, PDGFRα, PDGFRβ and Met in large-cell neuroendocrine carcinoma of the lung. J Clin Oncol 2005;23(34):8774–8785.

41. Nawrocki B, Polette M, Van Hengel J, et al. Cytoplasmic redistribution of E-cadherin–catenin adhesion complex is associated with down-regulated tyrosine phosphorylation of E-cadherin in human bronchopulmonary carcinomas. Am J Pathol 1998;153:1521–1530.

42. Finkelstein SD, Hasegawa T, Colby T, et al. 11q13 allelic imbalance discriminates pulmonary carcinoids from tumorlets. A microdissection-based genotyping approach useful in clinical practice. Am J Pathol 1999;155:633–640.

30
Pulmonary Lymphomas

Candice C. Black, Norman B. Levy, and Gregory J. Tsongalis

Introduction

Cancer continues to be a major public health problem throughout the world. It is estimated that one in four individuals in the United States will succumb to malignant disease. For 2006, the American Cancer Society has estimated that there will be 66,670 new cases of lymphoma, including 7,800 cases of Hodgkin's lymphoma and 58,870 cases of non-Hodgkin's lymphoma.[1] Approximately 52% of these cases will be male and 48% female. In addition, lymphoma will account for approximately 20,000 deaths in 2006, with equal affliction in males and females.[1] Primary pulmonary lymphoma is rare, representing only 3%–4% of cases of extranodal non-Hodgkin's lymphoma and 0.5%–1% of primary pulmonary malignancies.[2]

Both benign and malignant lymphoid proliferations may involve the lung. The benign disorders include follicular bronchitis, localized/nodular lymphoid hyperplasia (formerly referred to as *pseudolymphoma*), and lymphoid interstitial pneumonia.[3] The gastrointestinal tract, skin, and thyroid are among the more common sites for the occurrence of extranodal lymphoma. The lung is not considered one of the more common sites for these malignant occurrences.

Lymphoma can occur in the lung via three main routes: primary lymphoma arising in the lung parenchyma, secondary lymphoma spreading from the circulation, and direct invasion of mediastinal and hilar lymph nodes or thymic primary lymphomas. Primary pulmonary lymphoma is defined as a clonal lymphoid proliferation that affects either one or both lungs in the absence of detectable extrapulmonary involvement at diagnosis or during the subsequent 3 months.[4] The most common subtypes of primary pulmonary lymphoma are marginal zone B-cell lymphoma of the mucosa-associated lymphoid tissue (MALT) type, primary pulmonary diffuse large B-cell lymphoma, lymphomatoid granulomatosis, and pulmonary Langerhans cell histiocytosis. The latter is part

of a larger family of congenital and acquired histiocytic proliferations, a few of which are clonal and possibly neoplastic. Langerhans cell histiocytosis is not further discussed here.

Clinically, primary pulmonary lymphoma may be divided into four large categories that reflect different treatment paradigms: de novo primary lymphoma of the lung, recurrent or secondary lymphoma of the lung, lymphoma arising after solid organ transplantation, and acquired immunodeficiency syndrome (AIDS)–related primary pulmonary lymphoma.[5,6]

Mucosa-Associated Lymphoid Tissue Lymphoma

More than 80% of all pulmonary lymphomas are of the marginal zone B-cell type or MALT. This diagnosis represents the most common de novo primary lung lymphoma. Histologically, these lymphomas resemble MALT lymphomas that occur in other extranodal sites.[7,8]

The MALT lymphomas are malignancies that appear to arise from acquired mucosal lymphoid tissue that accumulates secondary to an inflammatory stimulus. Mucosal lymphoid tissue serves an immunologic function that is absent or minimal in normal physiologic conditions. It has been well studied in the human gastrointestinal tract, especially in the Peyer's patches of the ileum. In Peyer's patches, the MALT tissue is architecturally similar to a reactive lymphoid follicle except that the marginal B zone is expanded, the lamina propria contains T lymphocytes and immunoglobulin A–secreting plasma cells, and CD8⁺ T cells are present in mucosal epithelium. Whereas direct antigenic stimulation with certain inflammatory antigens, such as *Helicobacter pylori* gastritis, and Hashimoto thyroiditis are associated with MALT lymphomas elsewhere, no direct antigenic trigger has been correlated with pulmonary MALT lymphomas.[8] Certain autoimmune disorders such as systemic lupus erythematosis and

Gougerot-Sjogren syndrome may also be associated with the acquisition of MALT and subsequent neoplastic transformation to pulmonary MALT lymphoma.

Most MALT lymphomas are discovered incidentally on chest radiographs. When present, symptoms include cough, dyspnea, chest pain, and hemoptysis. Most patients are adults, 50–70 years old, with a slight female predominance.[9] The most common radiologic appearance of primary non-Hodgkin's lymphoma is an area of opacification with poorly defined margins and air bronchograms.[10] The air bronchograms correlate with the location of the MALT tissue, cuffing epithelial lined airways. Less common radiographic patterns include nodules, diffuse air space consolidation, and segmental or lobar atelectasis.[10]

Case 30.1

A 51 year-old nonsmoking female presented to her primary care doctor with complaint of persistent cough. Her past medical history was noncontributory, and she did not take any medications. Her husband was a cigarette smoker. After a failed trial of antibiotics, a chest x-ray was obtained. Her right upper lobe showed patchy opacification with numerous air bronchograms. No distinct masses were identified. An open lung wedge biopsy specimen was obtained of an area that was palpably firmer to the surgeon. The biopsy tissue showed expanded interstitium, septae, and pleura with nodular uniform small lymphocyte aggregates. In the firmer areas, the lymphoid tissue formed a confluent mass, and in the sur-

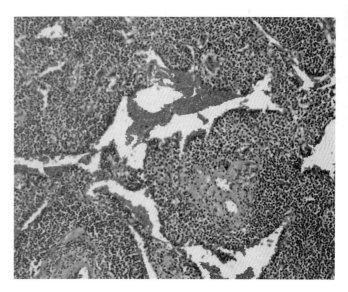

FIGURE 30.2. Pulmonary mucosa-associated lymphoid tissue lymphoma showing diffuse infiltration and widening of the interstitium with nodular aggregates of lymphocytes.

rounding lung the lymphoid tissue cuffed small airways. In the alveolar spaces, pneumocytes were obliterated by the lymphoid tissue. In larger airways, subtle lymphoepithelial lesions were identified. The lesional cells were immunoreactive for pan–B-cell markers and negative for CD10, CD5, Bcl-6 and CD23. The Ki-67 proliferative rate was 1%–2%. No nodal involvement was detected by computed tomography. The diagnosis of low-grade B-cell MALT lymphoma was rendered (Figures 30.1 to 30.3).

Microscopically, the presence of a dense monomorphic lymphoid infiltrate with tumefactive and/or lymphangitic growth patterns and the formation of architecture-obscuring nodules is consistent with this diagnosis. The lymphoid infiltrate tracks along bronchovascular bundles, through interlobular septa, and along pleura. Scattered nodules and secondary vascular infiltration/angiitis may be present. Lymphoepithelial complexes, neoplastic lymphoid cells within the epithelium, are also common, although not pathognomonic. The cells are uniform and appear similar to centrocytes with irregular nuclear contours and scant or clear cytoplasm. Plasma cell differentiation is associated with up to one third of cases. These cases may be associated with a monoclonal gammopathy and may show cytoplasmic secretory immunoglobulin with immunohistochemical stains.[9] The MALT lymphomas are low grade with predominately small cells and low proliferative rates, including low Ki-67 proliferation fractions (<10%).[9] If sheets of large cells are present, the diagnosis of focal diffuse large B-cell lymphoma should

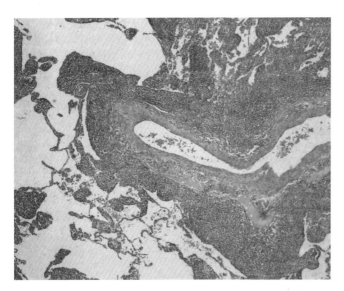

FIGURE 30.1. Pulmonary mucosa-associated lymphoid tissue lymphoma showing nodular lymphoid aggregates surrounding a pulmonary artery.

be rendered. High-grade MALT lymphoma is no longer recognized in the World Health Organization classification. Based on studies of serial biopsies, it has been estimated that up to 15% of MALT lymphomas may progress to diffuse large B-cell lymphoma.[11]

The differential diagnosis for MALT lymphoma includes other low-grade small B-cell lymphocytic proliferations as well as nonneoplastic lymphoid hyperplasias. In fewer than 10% of cases, a low-grade B-cell lymphoma does not meet the criteria for MALT-type lymphoma. These cases are a mix of follicular lymphomas, mantle cell lymphomas, and B-cell chronic lymphocytic leukemia/lymphoma.[4] Helpful features for distinguishing neoplastic from benign lymphoid proliferations are the tumefactive lymphangitic and nodular patterns of growth, the monomorphic clonal B-cell population, periodic acid-Schiff–positive intranuclear inclusions (Dutcher bodies), and lymphoepithelial complexes. Dutcher bodies can rarely be identified in benign conditions but are much more commonly associated with lymphomas or myeloma. Secondary organizing pneumonitis or granulomatous inflammation can sometimes obscure the neoplastic nature of the lymphoid population, which can be a potential diagnostic pitfall. Recognizing the tumefactive growth pattern and lymphangitic spread of the lymphoid cells is critical. The majority of MALT cases are CD20 positive and CD5, Bcl-6, CD10, and CD23 negative. Although there is no characteristic marker for MALT lymphoma, more recent molecular genetic developments may help in the identification of this disease.

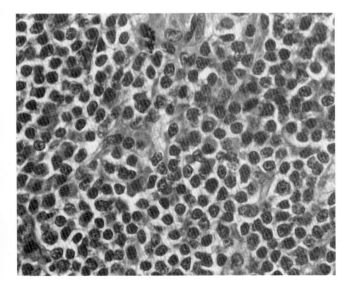

FIGURE 30.3. Pulmonary mucosa-associated lymphoid tissue lymphoma showing sheets of uniform low-grade nuclei, a few with a vague plasmacytoid appearance and a few wrinkled nuclei with centrocyte-like features.

TABLE 30.1. Translocations identified in mucosa-associated lymphoid tissue lymphoma.

Translocation	Genes involved
t(1;2)(p22;p12)	*Bcl-10* and *IgK*
t(1;14)(p22;q32)	*Bcl-10* and *IgH*
t(3;14)(p14;q32)	*FOXP1* and *IgH*
t(11;18)(q21;q21)	*API2* and *MALT1*
t(14;18)(q32;q21)	*IgH* and *MALT1*

Source: Data are from references 7–12.

Significant advances in our understanding of this entity have been made since the first description of MALT lymphoma in 1983.[12] Several chromosomal changes in MALT lymphomas have been identified and include translocations as well as quantitative changes in chromosome number (aneuploidy). The known translocations in pulmonary MALT lymphomas are listed in Table 30.1.[12–17] There are two important points of interest with respect to these translocations: (1) the translocations appear to be specific for MALT lymphoma and (2) the translocations occur in more than 50% of pulmonary MALT lymphoma. The most common aneuploidies described in MALT lymphomas include trisomies 3, 12, and 18.[18,19]

The translocations identified in MALT lymphomas affect pathways critical in antigen-mediated T- and B-cell activation via the nuclear factor (NF)-κB transcription factor family. Members of this family are crucial for the expression of genes associated with lymphocyte activation, proliferation, and generation of immune responses. BCL10 and MALT1 translocations are thought to induce NF-κB activation which in turn results in activation of the necessary genes for lymphocyte function. Using fluorescence in situ hybridization or reverse transcription polymerase chain reaction technologies, the identification of a translocation or aneuploidy may be more useful than gene rearrangement studies because they can identify a clonal population of cells and simultaneously characterize the disease process.

The majority of patients with MALT lymphoma present with localized stage I or II extranodal disease.[11] Dissemination occurs in up to 30% of cases, usually to other extranodal sites. If the disease is local, local treatment such as surgery may be curative. When disseminated, the lesions are indolent, although not usually curable. Because of the unique antigen-driven nature of MALT lymphomas, treatment directed at the antigen may result in regression of the lymphoma, usually in early lesions.[11] Dissemination to lymph nodes also occurs, although rarely no primary extranodal site can be found clinically. The provisional category of *nodal marginal zone lymphoma* has been suggested within the REAL classification system for these cases.[11] The patient population and disease course are the same.

Diffuse Large B-Cell Lymphoma

Diffuse large B-cell lymphoma accounts for 11%–19% of primary pulmonary lymphomas.[5,20] Half of these cases coexist with MALT lymphoma, suggesting possible transformation. Diffuse large B-cell lymphoma represents the most common type of primary pulmonary lymphoma associated with AIDS and is also the most common type associated with immunosuppressed patients such as those with organ transplants.[4] These two populations are further discussed below. Excluding these populations, the mean age of onset is 60 years without gender predisposition. Patients are often symptomatic with fever and weight loss. Radiographically, a single noncavitary mass is the most common finding.

Histologically, the malignant cells are large and blast-like with frequent mitoses and necrosis (Figure 30.4). The cells form a confluent tumor mass and involve septae, pleura, vessels, and airways.[2,20,21] The cells express B-cell phenotype (CD20[+], CD79a[+]) with a variable reactive T-cell background. The malignant B cells are Epstein-Barr virus (EBV) negative in immunocompetent hosts.[22] The differential diagnosis includes poorly differentiated carcinoma, amelanotic melanoma, and other large cell lymphomas such as anaplastic large cell lymphoma and mediastinal large B-cell lymphoma invading lung. The immunoprofile of the tumor aids distinction. Lymphomatoid granulomatosis must also be distinguished, especially if the latter shows angiotropism. A negative EBV immunostain or in situ hybridization can help distinguish these. Lymphomatoid granulomatosis also shows a more pronounced T-cell infiltrate.

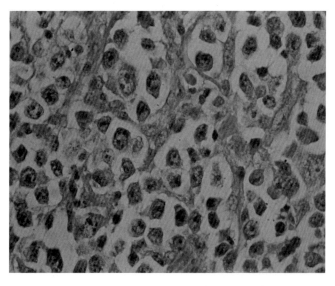

FIGURE 30.4. Diffuse large B-cell lymphoma showing sheets of large pleomorphic cells with frequent mitoses.

The prognosis of non-AIDS and nontransplant diffuse large B-cell lymphoma is poor, with a mean survival of 8–10 months. Surgical resection followed by chemotherapy is standard treatment.[2,21,23]

Posttransplantation Lymphoma

Organ transplant patients are a unique population. Diffuse large B-cell lymphoma is most common, although T-cell lymphomas account for up to 14%. No clinical differences are seen between the disease courses of the T- and B-cell types. The lymphoma appears to be driven by unrestrained proliferation of EBV-infected B cells. This is caused by suppression of normal immunosurveillance from the therapeutic drugs intended to prevent transplant rejection.[24] Continued immunostimulation from the transplanted organ may also play a role. Certain therapeutic drugs such as FK506, OKT3, and ATG, while effective at preventing rejection, are associated with increased risk of transplant-associated lymphoma.[24] The risk also appears to be associated with the type of organ transplanted. Lung transplant patients are at greater risk than other organ recipients, with the exception of combined heart–lung transplants. The theory is that greater immunosuppression is given to these patients because of the catastrophic effect acute rejection would cause. Posttransplantation lymphomas preferentially occur in the anatomic region of the transplant or in the transplant organ proper. Young transplant patients (<10 years) and older patients (>60 years) are at the greatest risk.[24]

Radiographically, lung involvement with posttransplantation lymphoma presents as multiple nodules scattered throughout the lung. Rare solitary nodules or reticulonodular patterns have also been described. The nodules range in size from 5 to 20 mm and are circumscribed and without cavitation.[10] Pleural effusions are common, although no pleural masses are present.[10]

The treatment of this group of patients is also unique, as reduction in immunosuppressive antirejection medication may be effective. Early-onset lymphomas are usually EBV positive and responsive to therapeutic drug alterations. Late-onset lymphomas tend to be EBV negative. This group of lymphomas may be EBV negative, and, because they are less responsive to therapeutic alterations, have a worse prognosis.

Pulmonary Lymphoma in Acquired Immunodeficiency Syndrome

Pulmonary lymphoma in AIDS is another unique population worth separate mention. Following Kaposi's sarcoma, lymphoma is the second most common tumor occurring in AIDS patients. Primary pulmonary lymphoma is rare, accounting for 0.3% per 100 patients per year.[25] Up to 40% of AIDS patients present with a thoracic tumor, and primary pulmonary lymphoma accounts for 8%–15% of these.[26,27] Diffuse large B-cell lymphoma is the most common type. The patients are usually at later stages of the disease with very low CD4 counts (<50/μL). EBV infection of tumor cells can be demonstrated in nearly every case.[25–27]

The radiographic appearance is that of one or multiple well-circumscribed rapidly enlarging pulmonary nodules. Unlike posttransplantation lymphomas, cavitation is commonly present.[10,25] Regional lymph node enlargement is either absent or less than that in posttransplantation lymphoma cases.[25–27] The prognosis of AIDS-related primary pulmonary lymphoma is poor, with survival means of 4 months despite chemotherapy.[25]

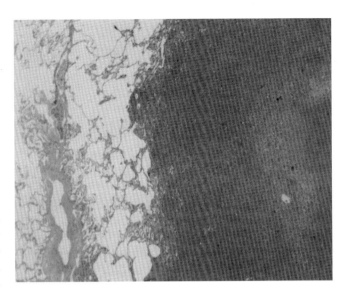

FIGURE 30.6. Lymphomatoid granulomatosis, showing a more advanced lesion with palisading granulomatous inflammation with central necrosis.

Case 30.2

A 57-year-old male presented to his primary care doctor with complaint of fevers, night sweats, fatigue, and swelling. He required hospital admission for new-onset renal failure and pulmonary infiltrates. He was given a trial of prednisone for presumed pulmonary–renal syndrome, and a renal biopsy was performed. The biopsy tissue showed interstitial nephritis. His creatinine normalized with the prednisone for 4 months. He began to have worsening breathlessness and bilateral pulmonary infiltrates, greater in the lower lung fields. A transbronchial biopsy specimen was obtained and showed mild nonspecific inflammation. Cultures were negative. His prednisone was increased.

His conditioned continued to worsen for approximately 4 months. His chest x-rays began to show nodular masses with evidence of focal central cavitation. A second transbronchial biopsy specimen was obtained. This showed inflammation with necrosis and and a small arteriole with vasculitis. Although his antineutrophil cytoplasmic antibody test was negative, he was presumed to have Wegener's granulomatosis. He was given oral and intravenous Cytoxan. Despite this, his pulmonary lesions progressed, and new lesions appeared. An open lung biopsy specimen was obtained, which showed extensive lymphoid infiltrate accompanied by necrosis. Angiocentricity was focally noted. The majority of lymphocytes were small cells with condensed chromatin. A second, minor population of larger cells, some multinucleate, with vesicular chromatin and prominent mitoses, was also present. The majority of small lymphocytes were EBV-negative T cells. The larger irregular cells were CD20-positive, EBV-positive B cells. A final diagnosis of grade II lymphomatoid granulomatosis was rendered. In light of the diagnosis, the prior renal and second transbronchial biopsy specimens were reviewed, and the opinion that these likely represented grade I lymphomatoid granulomatosis was offered (Figures 30.5 to 30.7).

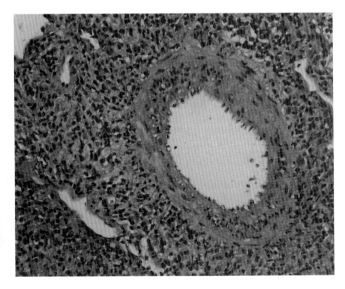

FIGURE 30.5. Lymphomatoid granulomatosis, an early manifestation showing arteriolar infiltration by lymphocytes and a lymphoid cuff.

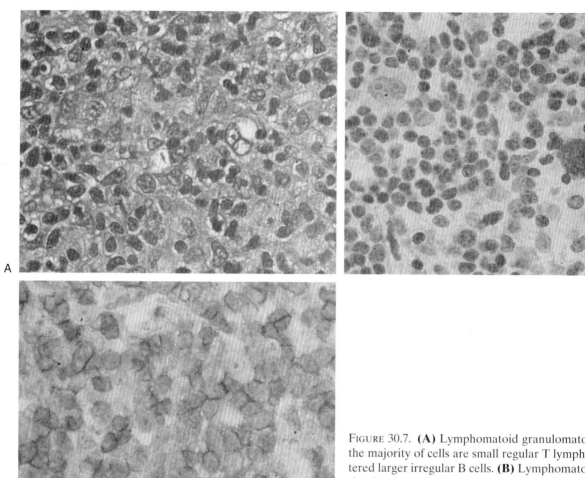

FIGURE 30.7. **(A)** Lymphomatoid granulomatosis showing that the majority of cells are small regular T lymphocytes with scattered larger irregular B cells. **(B)** Lymphomatoid granulomatosis showing cytoplasmic immunoreactivity for Epstein-Barr virus (latent membrane protein by immunohistochemistry) within large atypical B cells. **(C)** Lymphomatoid granulomatosis showing the dominant cell marking for T-cell marker UCHL.

Lymphomatoid Granulomatosis

Lymphomatoid granulomatosis historically was distinguished from the Wegener family of pulmonary angiitis and granulomatoses by Liebow.[28] It is an angiocentric destructive granulomatous lymphoreticular infiltrate.[28] Although it is very rare (500–600 cases reported in the literature), it seems to have a male predominance (1:6.5) with an age range of 30–50 years. Although >90% of patients have lung involvement, other organs are usually also involved, including skin (36%–53% of cases), brain, and kidney.[4]

Most patients are symptomatic at diagnosis, and most symptoms are respiratory. Neurologic symptoms include blindness, confusion, ataxia, convulsions, and sensorimotor neuropathies.[4,29] Skin involvement includes erythema,

nodules, and rarely ulceration.[4,29] In >80% of cases, the radiographs show multiple bilateral poorly defined nodular opacities. The lower lung fields are affected more than the upper lung fields.[30] The nodules follow a bronchovascular distribution and converge to form masses that can spontaneously excavate, migrate, or regress.[30] Excavation and migration likely correspond to infarction, necrosis, and remodeling.

Lymphomatoid granulomatosis is an EBV-driven B-cell lymphoma with a variable disease course. Spontaneous remissions have occurred. The lesions appear as angiocentric polymorphic infiltrates of atypical or activated lymphoid cells mixed with varying degrees of plasma cells and macrophages. With more advanced or necrotic lesions, connective tissue and elastic stains may be needed to demonstrate the angiocentricity. Varying degrees of organizing fibrosis may be present in the surrounding lung parenchyma. Viral proteins for EBV or viral genomic sequences have been found within the lymphoid infiltrate in up to 70% of cases. Although early studies suggested that this may be a T-cell lymphoproliferative disorder associated with EBV, subsequent studies determined that the EBV-infected cells were in fact B cells.[31] These cells expressed the EBV viral proteins lysosome-associated membrane protein (LMP) and EBV-associated nuclear antigen (EBNA). In addition, the EBR1 and EBR2 viral genomic sequences have been detected in these cell types by colorimetric in situ hybridization. The grading of these lesions has been described based on the number of EBV-infected cells per high power field (Table 30.2).[31] The infected cells also express B-cell markers. These cells appear large and atypical or activated, although they may be the minority cell within the T-cell–rich background population. Although the T cells may be the major cell type, they are polyclonal and reactive.

Lesions are graded from I to III based on proportions of atypical and inflammatory cells.[4,29] Grade III lesions have a worse prognosis that more closely resembles that of diffuse large B-cell lymphoma. Lymphomatoid granulomatosis may also progress to diffuse large B-cell lymphoma. The differential diagnosis includes necrotizing granulomatous infection and Wegener's or other autoimmune vasculitis and angiocentric T-cell lymphoma. The T cells of T angiocentric T-cell lymphoma are CD3 positive.[32] Clinical, radiographic, and microbiologic correlations may be necessary to understand the patient's entire disease course.

Prognosis is dependent on grade. Patients with low-grade disease confined to the lung or skin tend to waxing and waning courses, with 14%–27% spontaneous remission. Overall, for all grades, prognosis is poor, with a mean survival of 4 years.[4] One third of patients with grade I disease will progress to grade III lymphoma. Two thirds of patients with grade II disease will progress to grade III lymphoma.[32]

Conclusion

A significant amount of progress has been made in our understanding of the etiology and pathophysiology of pulmonary lymphoma because of advances in immunohistochemistry and molecular biology techniques. The association of EBV-infected cells with lymphomatoid granulomatosis identified the role of an infectious agent with this lymphoproliferative disorder and has raised the question as to what roles other infectious agents may play in such disorders. As our breadth of knowledge increases with respect to the underlying mechanisms involved in the development of these disorders, it is hopeful that this will give rise to new therapeutics.

References

1. Jemal A, Siegel R, Ward E, et al. Cancer statistics 2006. CA Cancer J Clin 2006;56:106–130.
2. L'Hoste RJ Jr, Filippa DA, Leiberman PH, Bretsky S. Primary pulmonary lymphomas. A clinicopathologic analysis of 36 cases. Cancer 1984;54:1397–1406.
3. Campo E, Chott A, Kinney MC, et al. Update on extranodal lymphomas. Conclusions of the workshop held by the EAHP and the SH in Thessaloniki, Greece. Histopathology 2006;48:481–504.
4. Cadranel J, Wislez M, Antoine M. Primary pulmonary lymphoma. Eur Respir J 2002;20:750–762.
5. Li G, Hansmann ML, Zwinggers T, Lennert K. Primary lymphomas of the lung: morphologic, immunohistochemical, and clinical features. Histopathology 1990;16:519–531.
6. Turner RR, Colby TV, Doggett RS. Well-differentiated lymphocytic lymphoma: a study of 47 patients with primary manifestation in the lung. Cancer 1984;54:2088–2096.
7. Isaacson PG, Spencer J. Malignant lymphoma of mucosa-associated lymphoid tissue. Histopathology 1987;11:445–462.
8. Isaacson PG, Spencer J. The biology of low grade MALT lymphoma. J Clin Pathol 1995;48:395–397.
9. Nicholson AG, Harris NL. Marginal zone B-cell lymphoma of the mucosa associated lymphoid tissue (MALT) type. In Travis WD, Brambilla E, Muller-Hermelink HK, Harris CC, eds. World Health Organization Classification of Tumors. Tumors of the Lung, Pleura, Thymus and Heart. Lyon, France: World Health Organization;2004:88–90.
10. Lee KS, Kim Y, Primack SL. Imaging of pulmonary lymphomas. Am J Roentgenol 1997;168:339–345.
11. Harris NL, Jaffe ES, Stein H, et al. A revised European-American classification of lymphoid neoplasms: a proposal from the International Lymphoma Study Group. Blood 1994;84(5):1361–1392.
12. Willis TG, Jadayel DM, Du MQ, et al. Bcl10 is involved in t(1;14)(p22;q32) of MALT B cell lymphoma and mutated in multiple tumor types. Cell 1999;96:35–45.
13. Dierlamm J, Baens M, Wlodarska I, et al. The apoptosis inhibitor gene API2 and a novel 18q gene, MLT, are recurrently rearranged in the t(11;18)(q21;q21) associated with

TABLE 30.2. Grades of lymphomatoid granulomatosis.

Grade I	Few or no EBV-infected cells (<5/hpf)
	No necrosis
	Polymorphous
Grade II	Scattered EBV-infected cells (15–20/hpf)
	Foci of necrosis
	Polymorphous
Grade III	Sheets of EBV-infected cells
	Necrosis
	Cellular monomorphism

Note: EBV, Epstein Barr virus; hpf, high power field.
Source: Data are from references 31 and 32.

mucosa-associated lymphoid tissue lymphomas. Blood 1999;93:3601–3609.

14. Streubel B, Lamprecht A, Dierlamm J, et al. T(14;18) (q32;q21) involving IGH and MALT1 is a frequent chromosomal aberration in MALT lymphoma. Blood 2003;101: 2335–2339.

15. Wotherspoon AC, Finn TM, Isaacson PG. Trisomy 3 in low-grade B-cell lymphomas of mucosa-associated lymphoid tissue. Blood 1995;85:2000–2004.

16. Dierlamm J, Pittaluga S, Wlodarska I, et al. Marginal zone B-cell lymphomas of different sites share similar cytogenetic and morphologic features. Blood 1996;87:299–307.

17. Streubel B, Vinatzer U, Lamprecht A, et al. T(3;14) (p14.1;q32) involving IGH and FOXP1 is a novel recurrent chromosomal aberration in MALT lymphoma. Leukemia 2005;19:652–658.

18. Streubel B, Simonitsch-Klupp I, Mullauer L, et al. Variable frequencies of MALT lymphoma-associated genetic aberrations in MALT lymphomas of different sites. Leukemia 2004;18:1722–1726.

19. Remstein ED, Kurtin PJ, Einerson RR, et al. Primary pulmonary MALT lymphomas show frequent and heterogeneous cytogenetic abnormalities, including aneuploidy and translocations involving API2 and MALT1 and IGH and MALT1. Leukemia 2004;18:156–160.

20. Fitch M, Caprons F, Berger F, et al. Primary pulmonary non-Hodgkin's lymphomas. Histopathology 1995;26:529–537.

21. Kennedy JL, Nathwani BN, Burke JS, et al. H. Pulmonary lymphomas and other pulmonary lymphoid lesions. A clinicopathologic and immunologic study of 64 patients. Cancer 1985;56:539–552.

22. Nicholson AG, Harris NL. Primary pulmonary diffuse large B cell lymphoma. In Travis WD, Brambilla E, Muller-Hermelink HK, Harris CC, eds. World Health Organization Classification of Tumors. Tumors of the Lung, Pleura,

Thymus and Heart. Lyon, France: World Health Organization; 2004:91.

23. Cordier JF, Chailleux E, Lauque D, et al. Primary pulmonary lymphomas. A clinical study of 70 cases in nonimmunocompromised patients. Chest 1993;103:201–208.

24. Opelz G, Dohler B. Lymphomas after solid organ transplantation: a Collaborative Transplant Study report. Am J Transplant 2003;4:222–230.

25. Ray P, Antoine M, Mary-Krause M, et al. AIDS-related primary pulmonary lymphoma. Am J Respir Crit Care Med 1998;158:1221–1229.

26. Polish LB, Cohn DL, Ryder JW, et al. Pulmonary non-Hodgkin's lymphoma in AIDS. Chest 1986;96:1321–1326.

27. Ioachim HL, Dorsett B, Cronin W, et al. Acquired immunodeficiency syndrome-associated lymphomas: clinical, pathologic, immunologic and viral characteristics of 111 cases. Hum Pathol 1991;22:659–673.

28. Leibow AA, Carrington CR, Friedman PJ. Lymphomatoid granulomatosis. Hum Pathol 1972;3:457–558.

29. Katzenstein AL, Leibow AA. Lymphomatoid granulomatosis. A clinicopathologic study of 152 cases. Cancer 1979;43:360–373.

30. Wechsler RJ, Steiner RM, Israel HL, Patchefsky AS. Chest radiograph in Lymphomatoid granulomatosis: comparison with Wegener granulomatosis. Am J Roentgenol 1984;142:79–83.

31. Wilson WH, Kingma DW, Raffeld M, et al. Association of lymphomatoid granulomatosis with Epstein-Barr viral infection of B lymphocytes and response to interferon-α2b. Blood 1996;87:4531–4537.

32. Koss MN, Harris NL. Lymphomatoid granulomatosis. In Travis WD, Brambilla E, Muller-Hermelink HK, Harris CC, eds. World Health Organization Classification of Tumors. Tumors of the Lung, Pleura, Thymus and Heart. Lyon, France: World Health Organization; 2004: 92–94.

31
Posttransplantation Lymphoproliferative Disorder

Aamir Ehsan and Jennifer L. Herrick

Introduction

Lymphoproliferative disorders are known complications of congenital and acquired immunodeficiency and/or iatrogenic-induced immunosuppression. A lymphoplasmacytic proliferation or lymphoma developing as a consequence of continuous iatrogenic immunosuppression following solid organ transplantation and hematopoietic stem cell transplantation (HSCT) is called posttransplantation lymphoproliferative disorder (PTLD). Posttransplantation lymphoproliferative disorders are a morphologically and clinically heterogenous group of disorders, many of which are associated with the Epstein-Barr virus (EBV). Morphologically the spectrum ranges from polyclonal lymphoplasmacytic proliferations resembling infectious mononucleosis to frankly neoplastic lymphomas. These lymphomas are commonly EBV positive B cell and less commonly EBV negative (B or T cell) in origin. Clinically, some of these disorders regress after reduction of the immunosuppressive regimen, and others progress to serious and potentially fatal lymphomas requiring chemotherapy.

Like other allograft transplant patients, PTLDs arising in lung transplant recipients are infrequent and share similar etiologies, morphologies, and clinical outcomes, therefore requiring an analogous therapeutic approach. Lungs are commonly the primary site of PTLD involvement as a consequence of lung and lung–heart transplantation and are also secondarily involved in PTLD suffered by other allograft recipients. Because the consideration of PTLD involvement of the lung is similar to PTLD as a whole, this chapter mainly addresses the general features of this disease as we understand it presently.

Classification

Posttransplantation lymphoproliferative disorders have been recognized as a complication of transplantation for more than 35 years.[1] Because the behavior of these lesions is widely disparate with very different therapeutic considerations, many histologic classifications have been actively proposed to guide management.[2–4] Two morphologic patterns seen in PTLD are (1) a polymorphic pattern in which the lymphoid population is composed of a spectrum of cell types, including small lymphocytes, plasmacytoid lymphocytes, plasma cells, small and large cleaved cells, small and large noncleaved cells, and immunoblasts; and (2) a monomorphic pattern in which the neoplastic population is composed of monomorphic cells with cytologic atypia and can be of B, T, or plasma cell origin. The initial classification scheme proposed that the polymorphous pattern encompasses polymorphic B-cell hyperplasia and polymorphic B-cell lymphoma, with the presence of necrosis and lymphoid atypia as a predictor of a more aggressive lesion requiring cytotoxic therapy.[2] Subsequent studies demonstrated that the lesions containing a monomorphic lymphoid pattern were most likely to have a clonal cell population and lead to a more aggressive outcome.[3,4] The same study could not correlate necrosis or atypical lymphoid cells with clinical behavior or monoclonality. The monomorphic pattern of PTLDs morphologically resembles the de novo lymphomas seen in nontransplantation settings and may be of any subtype of lymphoma. Both polymorphic and monomorphic patterns can be seen in the same biopsy specimen, and the distinction between the two may be problematic as both patterns can have either polyclonal or monoclonal lymphoid populations. At present, most PTLD lesions are

TABLE 31.1. WHO classification of posttransplantation lymphoproliferative disorder (PTLD).

Early lesions	
Reactive plasmacytic hyperplasia	
Infectious mononucleosis-like	
Polymorphic	
Monomorphic	
B-cell neoplasms	T-cell neoplasms
Diffuse large B-cell lymphoma	Peripheral T-cell lymphoma
(immunoblastic, centroblastic,	Other types
anaplastic)	
Burkitt's/Burkitt's-like lymphoma	
Plasma cell myeloma	
Plasmacytoma-like lesions	
Hodgkin lymphoma and Hodgkin lymphoma–like PTLD	

Source: WHO Classification of Tumours. Tumours of Haematopoietic and Lymphoid Tissues. Post-transplant Lymphoproliferative Disorders. NL Harris, SH Swerdlow, G Frizerra, DM Knowles. Page 264, IARC Press, Lyon 2001, with permission.

classified according to the World Health Organization (WHO) Classification of Hematopoietic Tumors (Table 31.1).[5] Unfortunately, even using the current WHO classification to standardize the subtyping of PTLD, neither morphology nor clonality can be used consistently to predict the clinical behavior of these lesions.

Incidence and Risk Factors

Many factors affect the occurrence of PTLD. These include allograft types (different types of solid organ, as well as bone marrow transplants), type of immunosuppression regimen, age of the patient, EBV serostatus (EBV-negative recipients of EBV-positive allografts are at higher risk), donor–recipient human leukocyte antigen (HLA) mismatch, and T-cell–depleted stem cell allografts. The overall risk of PTLD varies from 1% in HSCT recipients to 10% in heart and combined heart–lung transplant recipients (liver transplant, 2%–8%; renal transplant, 1%–2%).[6,7]

The incidence of PTLD is four times higher in pediatric than adult transplant recipients, most likely due to the seronegative EBV status of many pediatric patients.[8] The pretransplantation EBV status is considered one of the most important risk factors for developing PTLD[9] and is also important in rare EBV-negative adult patients. In addition, the PTLD risk was found to be four- to sixfold higher in a group of patients with simultaneous cytomegalovirus (CMV) disease.[10] It is presumed that CMV can modify EBV replication through the manipulation of inflammatory cytokines such as tumor necrosis factor (TNF)-α.[11] As mentioned earlier, the type of allograft confers varying risk, according to the amount of immunosuppression needed for

graft acceptance. The type of immunosuppressive drug has long been implicated in increased risk (e.g., azathioprine, tacrolimus, and OKT3); however, with additional clinical experience allowing smaller dosages, the incidence of PTLD assigned to a particular drug has decreased. This area is difficult to objectively study because of the practice of multidrug therapy, but some regimens show a two- to fivefold increased risk. Although HSCT patients have an overall lower risk of PTLD, those who receive T-cell–depleted donor cells in an effort to minimize graft-versus-host disease have a significantly higher incidence of subsequent PTLD. This observation aided in the link between T-cell competency and PTLD development. Patients requiring HSCT due to a primary immunodeficiency state, such as a congenital white cell derangement disorder, are also at increased risk. An HLA-mismatched donor becomes a more significant risk factor that increases with the degree of unmatched antigens. Also, the risk rises substantially if more than one risk factor is present. Male gender, white race, younger age at transplantation, and hepatitis C infection have been suggested as potential risk factors for PTLD.[12] Except for the possibility of hepatitis C, the underlying condition necessitating transplantation does not appear to have an association.

Lung Transplantation and Posttransplantation Lymphoproliferative Disorder

Posttransplantation lymphoproliferative disorder is an infrequent complication after lung transplantation, but the reported incidence varies widely between 1.8% and 20%,[13–15] with most reports approximating 5%. The variability in the incidence may be secondary to the type of immunosuppression regimen, age of population studied, EBV serostatus, and CMV prophylaxis. A high incidence of PTLD has been observed in pediatric patients with cystic fibrosis.[16] Other underlying diseases requiring transplantation do not appear to have a correlation with the development of PTLD.

Epstein-Barr virus–seronegative patients prior to lung transplantation carry approximately a sevenfold increased risk in developing PTLD. However, this group of patients is not commonly influenced by pretransplantation EBV serostatus, as most lung transplantations are performed on middle-aged patients (median age, 55 years) who are overwhelmingly EBV seropositive.

Posttransplantation lymphoproliferative disorder after lung transplantation presents as a thoracic lesion (pulmonary nodule), detected on imaging studies, or less commonly as an extrathoracic mass. It has an interesting propensity to involve the transplanted organ, in contrast to other solid organ–associated PTLD. It also is more likely to arise earlier and behave more aggressively, with the median time of onset reported as 7 months (compared with 40 months seen in other solid organ transplant PTLDs). In lung transplant patients, the more commonly seen PTLD arises early (<1 year after transplantation) and is more often confined to the thorax, and the less common cases arise late (>1 year after transplantation) which are more often confined to the extrathoracic organs. Posttransplantation lymphoproliferative disorder after lung transplantation is composed of recipient cells and are almost always B cells disorders (polymorphic or monomorphic), the majority of which are EBV driven (77%). The clinical and morphologic features are heterogeneous as seen with any other solid organ transplant or HSCT recipients. Monitoring, treatment, and prophylaxis options are similar to those for other allograft recipients.

Pathogenesis

The majority of PTLDs are EBV driven, and an impaired EBV-specific cytotoxic T-lymphocyte (CTL) response is the most common etiology in these disorders.[3,17] With the use of more sensitive in situ methods, EBV-negative cases have been estimated at approximately 20% of all cases (interestingly, up to 50% of PTLDs in renal allograft recipients are EBV negative), and the incidence may be increasing. The etiology of this is unclear because of the failure to link other common infectious agents.[17–19] As opposed to EBV-positive PTLD that most often is B cell in origin, the EBV-negative PTLD may be either B cell or T cell in origin. The PTLD arising in a solid organ transplant setting is usually of host origin (less often of donor origin), suggesting the lack of control of host EBV-infected cells by iatrogenically dampened T cells. In HSCT patients, the transplantation regimen essentially destroys all recipient immune cells, and the engrafted stem cells result in an immune system that is of donor origin—hence the PTLD in the HSCT setting is of donor origin.

The exact pathogenesis of PTLD is not fully known; however, recent studies have begun to explore the causative role of EBV, mode of B-cell infection, and the molecular histogenesis of PTLD. Our understanding of the molecular basis of these disorders is limited, and the study of pathogenesis at the genetic level is in its infancy. To understand the pathogenesis, it is important to know the virology, mode of infection, and latency phases of EBV; the normal biology of B cells; the molecular histogenesis of PTLD; and the mechanisms utilized in evasion of immune surveillance. In the following sections, we discuss the pathogenesis, molecular histogenesis, diagnosis, prognosis, and therapy of PTLD.

Virology of Epstein-Barr Virus

Epstein-Barr virus is a ubiquitous lymphotropic herpesvirus that infects more than 90% of humans worldwide. The virus was discovered by Epstein, Achong, and Barr in 1964 employing an electron microscope to visualize cells cultured from Burkitt lymphoma tissue.[20] Infection with EBV occurs during early childhood through intimate contact via oral secretions, with the majority of primary infections having only subclinical symptoms. In healthy carriers the virus persists in the latent form. Recently, resting memory B lymphocytes have been shown to be the main reservoir cells. The number of EBV-infected B lymphocytes in a healthy carrier remains relatively stable over many years (range, from 1 to 50 B lymphocytes per 1 million in the circulation).[21,22]

The EBV genome is a linear, 184-kbp, double-stranded DNA that has been cloned and sequenced (Figure 31.1). Infection of B lymphocytes by EBV occurs when the major envelope glycoprotein gp350/220 of the virus binds to the viral receptor, the CD21 molecule that functions as the C3d complement receptor (Figure 31.2). CD21-like receptors are also present on T cells, natural killer cells, and monocytes. Approximately 500 bp of variable number tandem repeat segments are present at both termini of EBV. Different isolates differ in their variable number of tandem repeats, and an individual isolate tends to contain a constant number of repeats even through serial passage. This attribute can be exploited for use to identify the clonality of the virus within a B-cell population.

Prior to infection, the EBV genome is present in a linear form. Following infection, there are three possible cellular responses: (1) a latent persistence of the EBV genome, (2) a replicative production of new virions, or (3) cell death secondary to the host response to infection. To establish as a latent infection the genome becomes circular to form an episome. It is during this process that random deletions of the variable number of tandem repeats occur, creating a unique virion fingerprint differing from the virion that infected the next lymphocyte by 500-bp intervals. After establishing itself within the cellular DNA as an episome, the EBV DNA is exactly replicated in all cell progeny, and, as previously stated, this principle can be used to determine the origin of neoplastic cells when evaluating EBV-driven disorders. Within the host cell the EBV genome is predominantly present as multiple extrachromosomal double-stranded episomes organized as nucleosomes. Some viral DNA can be integrated into the chromosomal DNA; however, this process does not have the capacity for reinfection. The replication of viral genome occurs by cellular DNA polymerases.

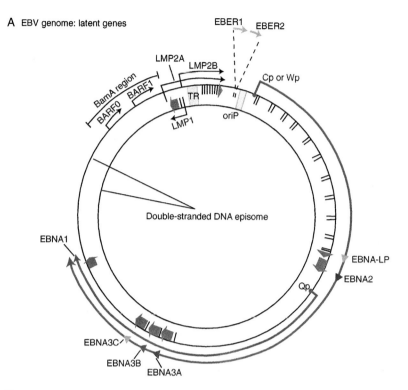

A EBV genome: latent genes

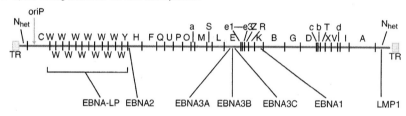

B Open reading frames for the EBV latent proteins

The Epstein—Barr virus (EBV) genome

FIGURE 31.1. The episomal viral genome encodes the latent phase proteins as well as Epstein-Barr virus (EBV)–encoded RNA (EBERs). Both ends of the open frame genome contain terminal repeat segments that undergo random deletions that create a unique fingerprint for each virus. EBNA, Epstein-Barr nuclear antigen; ICAM, intercellular cell adhesion molecule; LFA, leukocyte function–associated antigen; LMP, latent membrane protein; LP, leader protein. (From Murray PG, Young LS. Epstein-Barr virus infection: basis of malignancy and potential for therapy. Expert Rev Mol Med 2001;15:1–20, with permission of Cambridge University Press.)

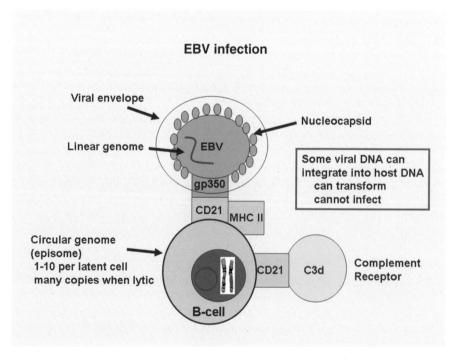

FIGURE 31.2. Schematic diagram of the virus interaction with B lymphocytes through the C3d complement receptor CD21. The viral nuclear capsid induces an antibody response detectable in serologic tests. The linear genome becomes a circular episome within the lymphocyte. Integration into the host cell DNA does occur; however, only the episomal form is available to infect other cells. EBV, Epstein-Barr virus; MHC, major histocompatibility complex. (Courtesy of Jennifer L. Herrick, MD.)

In Vitro Epstein-Barr Virus Infection

In vitro EBV exclusively infects B lymphocytes and transforms them into an immortalized B-lymphoblastoid cell line. The in vitro infection of B cells by EBV results in a latent infection. The EBV genome encodes approximately 100 viral proteins. Most of these proteins are used for regulating the replicating viral DNA, forming structural proteins of the virion and modulating the host immune response. Of these 100 genes, only 10 are expressed during the latent phase[23]: six nuclear proteins, Epstein-Barr nuclear antigens (EBNAs 1, 2, 3A, 3B, 3C) and leader protein (LP); three latent membrane proteins (LMP-1, -2A, and -2B); and small nonpolyadenylated RNAs termed Epstein-Barr virus encoded RNA (EBER-1 and -2). The EBERs have been observed to be the most abundantly transcribed RNA during latency (10^4–10^5 copies/cell), although they are not translated and are not well understood. Because these EBERs are so plentiful, an in-situ procedure is commonly utilized as a sensitive method to identify the presence of EBV infection in paraffin-embedded tissue sections.

Table 31.2 lists the latent protein functions. Epstein-Barr nuclear antigen-1 maintains and replicates the episomal EBV genome in the B cell by sequence-specific binding to the plasmid origin of viral replication[19] and is expressed in all latent phase cells. Many times, EBNA-1 is the only viral protein expressed. Epstein-Barr nuclear antigen-1 acts in concert with other viral promoters and contributes to the transcriptional regulation of EBNAs and LMP-1. Epstein-Barr nuclear antigen-2 upregulates the expression of LMP-1 and LMP-2. Epstein-Barr nuclear antigen-2 and EBNA-3 (A and C) proteins also regulate the expression of cellular proteins responsible for growth and transformation of B lymphocytes. Epstein-Barr nuclear antigen-LP interacts with EBNA-2 and is essential for the effective growth of virus-transformed B lymphocytes in vitro.

The goal of EBV infection is to immortalize the cell, and, to accomplish this, the cell must first be transformed (activated). The main transforming protein of EBV is LMP-1. There are many important effects of this protein: (1) It acts as an oncogene, and transgenic mice with expression of LMP-1 have been shown to develop B-cell lymphomas.[24,25] (2) It upregulates expression of antiapoptotic proteins such as bcl-2 and A20.[26,27] (3) It acts as a functional homolog of CD40. The CD40 receptor activates the cell when T helper cells send a signal. LMP-1 bypasses the dependence on T-cells and activates the virally infected B cell as a homologue of CD40. Latent membrane protein-1 binds to many TNF receptor–associated factors that interact with nuclear factor-κB, and regional cytokines resulting in additional B-cell proliferation. (4) It upregulates cellular adhesion molecules such as leukocyte function-associated antigens 1 and 3

TABLE 31.2. Functions of Epstein-Barr virus (EBV) proteins expressed during latent infection.

EBNA-1	Required for episome replication and maintenance of the viral genome Only EBV protein expressed in latent phase; protects latent genome
EBNA-2	Essential for B-cell immortalization and expression of EBNA-1 and EBNA-3. Upregulates activation receptors CD21 and CD23 Upregulates LMP-1 and LMP-2 expression Transactivates cellular and EBV genes
EBNA-3	EBNA-3A and EBNA-3C (not EBNA-3B) are essential for transformation/immortalization
EBNA-LP	Upregulates autocrine factors critical to B-cell growth Possible role in RNA processing
LMP-1	Second most abundant EBV RNA in latently infected B cells Essential for transformation of B cells into immortalized cells LMP-1 promoter contains an EBNA-2 response element that upregulates LMP-1 expression; LMP-1 can be expressed in the absence of EBNA-2 Blocks apoptosis, in part via activation of the bcl-2 oncogene Induction of adhesion molecules LFA-1, LFA-3, and ICAM-1, which promote interaction between B and T lymphocytes
LMP-2	Colocalizes with LMP-1 Prevents reactivation of EBV-infected B cells Not essential for virus-induced transformation
EBER-1, -2	EBV-encoded nonpolyadenylated RNAs (most abundant RNA in latently infected B cells); function unknown/not required for transformation

Note: The following are required for transformation in vitro: EBNA-1, EBNA-2, EBNA-3A, EBNA-3C, and LMP-1.
EBER, Epstein-Barr virus–encoded RNA; EBNA, Epstein-Barr nuclear antigen; ICAM, intercellular cell adhesion molecule; LFA, leukocyte function–associated antigen; LMP, latent membrane protein; LP, leader protein.

and intracellular adhesion molecule type 1, which promote interaction between B and T lymphocytes.

Although not required for B-cell transformation in vitro, LMP-2 serves the virus by blocking tyrosine kinase phosphorylation, which prevents the reactivation of latently infected EBV cells.[28] This function allows the cell to generate less attention from the immune surveillance. Normally, expression of B-cell receptor is required for B-cell maturation, and a loss of B-cell receptor leads to apoptosis.[29] Latent membrane protein-2 is a functional homolog of B-cell receptor, allowing for the survival of B-cell receptor–deficient immature B cells in transgenic mouse models.[30,31] In addition, LMP-2 also rescues human B-cell receptor–deficient B cells after infection by EBV.

In Vivo Epstein-Barr Virus Infection

Primary infection with EBV in vivo results from intimate contact via oral secretions. Recent studies indicate that intraepithelial B cells rather than oropharyngeal epithelial cells are the primary site of infection and the origin of infectious virions shed in saliva. When infection is delayed until at least adolescence, the resultant clinical condition is called *infectious mononucleosis*. The primary EBV infection is controlled by both humoral and cellular (cytotoxic) immune systems. The humoral response against viral proteins is important for the serologic diagnosis of different phases of infection. The CTL response constitutes the atypical lymphocytosis seen in primary EBV infection. In healthy carriers most of the infected B lymphocytes generated in the initial infection are cleared through immune surveillance. However, circulating resting memory B cells serve as the reservoir for lifelong latent infection.

Persistence of Infection

During an acute primary infection, the EBV-infected cells transform and express all 10 viral proteins, resulting in recognition and elimination by the CTLs and natural killer cells of the immune system. The main mechanism of surveillance of viral infection is through the HLA class I–restricted CD8-positive lymphocytes, with limited activity by CD4-positive HLA class II–restricted cells. In an immunocompetent state, the memory CTL activity is maintained and manages to keep the infection under control; however, it is unable to completely eradicate it because of the evasive mechanisms the virus employs. The limited expression of viral genes (*EBNA-1* and *LMP-2*) in latently infected memory B cells prevents them from being noticed and subsequently destroyed by CTLs. The CTLs have the ability to target all of the EBV encoded viral proteins except EBNA-1, which they cannot recognize. In addition, LMP-2A prevents the reactivated state, which would subject the cell to additional undesired immune surveillance.

Serologically, the healthy EBV carrier state following a primary EBV infection is demonstrated by the presence of antiimmunoglobulin G to EBV viral capsid antigen (VCA) toward the gp350 protein complex, low titers of anti-EA (early antigen), and EBNA-1 antibodies. During the lifespan of the immunocompetent host, the titers of these antibodies remain stable, consistent with a latent infection. In an immunocompetent person, any infected cell entering a lytic phase expresses many viral proteins

recognizable to CTLs, and the infected cells are effectively removed. Hence, there is a dynamic equilibrium during the lifespan of the host, with CTL cells controlling the random EBV-infected cells that enter the lytic phase and spew many infective viral particles, adding to the circulating virion pool (viral load). In a carrier state, the intraepithelial B cells of the oropharynx are thought to be not only the site of infection but also the reservoir for the infectious virions shed in saliva. If the population of CTLs is compromised (e.g., in acquired or congenital immunosuppression), the balance of viral control can be tipped in favor of the infected cell population being allowed to live as a transformed cell or enter the lytic phase. As one can imagine, this would result in a higher viral load and has the potential to spawn lymphoproliferative disorders such as PTLD.

Before we explore the model of in vivo EBV infection of the B cells, it is important to review what is known about normal B-cell activation and maturation. Naïve B cells are small, round lymphocytes some of which organize into primary follicles within tissue. Immunophenotypically, they are CD20-positive B cells that also express immunoglobulin (Ig) M and IgD. Because they function as guardsmen waiting for any future passing antigen, they need to be long lived and therefore are Bcl-2 positive. Upon presentation of antigen by dendritic and antigen-specific T cells (through CD40), the naïve B cell transforms to become a large activated cell. The conglomeration of these cells forms the germinal center that pushes the residual primary follicle naïve B cells into a mantle formation cuffing the newly formed germinal center. The large activated cells within the germinal centers are called *centroblasts*. These cells enter into the survival of the fittest competition in which the majority of the population loses Bcl-2 expression and most express c-Myc, CD10, Bcl-6, and CD77. During this step, the variable region of the immunoglobulin genes, as well as the *Bcl-6* gene, undergoes somatic hypermutation and isotype switching. This results in marked intraclonal diversity and alters the affinity of the antibody to various antigens. Centroblasts differentiate into smaller cells called *centrocytes*. The Bcl-6 protein is a nuclear zinc finger transcription factor that is expressed by centroblasts and centrocytes. The Bcl-6 protein is not expressed by naïve B cells, memory cells, and plasma cells. The centrocytes express proapoptotic genes such as *Fas, Bax*, and *p53*. The least fit centrocytes (with decreased affinity for antigen) lose Bcl-2 and undergo apoptosis, while only those few centrocytes with increased affinity for the specific antigen retain Bcl-2 and avoid apoptosis. These rescued centrocytes interact with T cells through the CD40 ligand, which detects the cell's superior fit to the antigen and allows it to differentiate into a memory B cell or plasma cell. This system provides for only the B cell with the blueprint for

TABLE 31.3. Transcription programs used by Epstein-Barr virus to establish and maintain infection.

Type of infected B cell	Program	Genes expressed	Function of the program
Naïve B cell	Growth	*EBNA-1—EBNA-6 LMP-1, LMP-2*	Activates B cells
Germinal center cell	Default	*EBNA-1, LMP-1/2*	Differentiates activated B cells into memory B cells
Peripheral blood memory B cell	Latency	None	Allows lifetime persistence
Dividing peripheral blood memory B cell	EBNA-1	*EBNA-1*	Allows viral DNA in latency program cell to divide
Plasma cell	Lytic	All lytic genes	Replicates virus in plasma

Source: Thorley-Lawson and Gross,[32] with permission.

the best matching antibody to be chosen to differentiate into a plasma cell or a memory cell and prevents a deluge of mediocre antibodies within the plasma.

A model for viral-induced transcription programs to establish and maintain infection has been outlined by Thorley-Lawson and Gross, consisting of the growth, default, latency, division, and lytic programs, and is helpful in the discussion of the pathogenesis of EBV infection.[32] Intraepithelial B lymphocytes are resting cells that are either IgM-positive memory B cells or naïve B cells. The present model for in vivo EBV infection holds that the virus enters the oropharyngeal epithelium and targets resting B cells, most likely naïve B cells (Table 31.3 and Figure 31.3).[32] These infected naïve B cells initiate a transcription program to become centroblasts through the germinal center reaction, some of which eventually are chosen to become memory B cells. What happens when EBV infects naïve B cells in vivo is not precisely known

but is assumed to reiterate the well-studied similar mechanism in vitro. The virus infects B cells through CD21, which is a receptor for the C3d component of the complement system. The viral gp350/220 receptor binds to CD21 and its coreceptor major histocompatibility complex (MHC) class II molecule. This changes the B cell from a resting to an activated state using the same motif as if it were activated by complement. The resting naïve B cells enter a program of proliferation, called the *growth program*, as centroblasts. During this time, the infected B cells express all 10 of the latent proteins. These EBV-infected centroblasts are morphologically and phenotypically similar to normal B cells activated by antigen and T-cell priming and parallels this activation in the sequence of cell maturation. The activation of naïve B cells under the influence of antigen and T cells occurs through the CD40 ligand and associated lymphokines. To avoid reliance on the tightly controlled T-cell system, EBV pro-

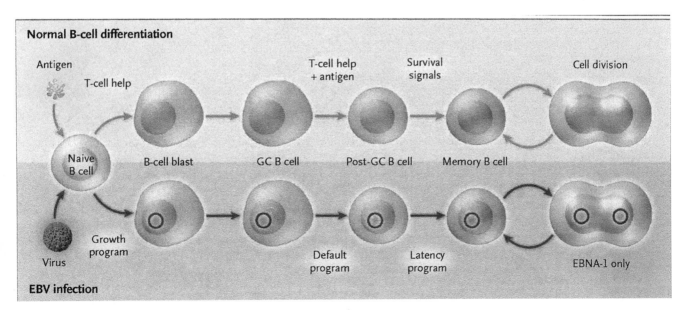

FIGURE 31.3. In vivo model of Epstein-Barr virus (EBV) infection paralleling the normal B-cell pathway with a virally infected (antigen and T-cell independent) pathway ending with a persistent infection in memory B cells. EBNA, Epstein-Barr nuclear antigen; GC, germinal center. (From Thorley-Lawson and Gross,[32] with permission.)

vides its own functional homolog of CD40 in the form of LMP-1 (as discussed earlier). Latent membrane protein-1 contains a carboxy-terminal domain that is functionally similar to the cytoplasmic domain of CD40. This provides a constitutive surrogate T-cell signal to infected B cells. Thus EBV does not need the help of T cells to activate B cells. When B cells are activated through antigen-specific T cells, they undergo a limited set of divisions before they either undergo apoptosis or differentiate to memory cells. In contrast, when EBV infects naïve B cells, the proliferating lymphoblasts continue to proliferate indefinitely rather than differentiate or die. This is called *immortalization*, a term most often used for in vitro infection. In a pure sense, they are not transformed cells (like other DNA viruses such as adenoviruses) because there are no true mutations. They are better considered to be lymphoid cells with the ability to proliferate indefinitely and, with continued unchecked continuation, can acquire DNA mutations that may result in a malignant cell line.

In contrast to the in vitro process of immortalization, the in vivo proliferation in a healthy state does not proliferate unchecked because of the recognition of the expressed latent proteins by CTLs. A more covert cell population is the memory cell, and, because the virus has a brief window of time to establish a persistent infection, there is a switch from the growth program to differentiation into a memory B cell (called the *default program*) while within the germinal centers. Later the memory cells exit the cell cycle and enter the peripheral blood, where expression of all latent proteins is turned off. This is known as the *latency program* and provides for lifetime persistence of the viral pool. To maintain a consistent circulating pool, rare divisions of memory B cells occur. These dividing memory cells transiently express only the EBNA-1 protein, which is unrecognizable to CTLs, and therefore are undetected. Under unknown mechanisms, a few memory B cells differentiate into plasma cells and produce antibody responsible for producing antibodies to EBV proteins. The presence of virus within these antibody-producing plasma cells reactivates viral replication, and infectious virions are produced in these cells.

Summarizing the model discussed, EBV presence in memory B cells is a result of differentiated naïve B-cell infection and not direct memory cell infection. The difference between the immune-activated B-cell–driven reaction and the EBV-driven reaction is that in the latter the viral genes activate the growth program (in place of antigen) and provide transcription signals that transition the cell to become a memory B cell. Thus, EBV utilizes normal B-cell development but without the requirement of antigen or T cell activation and uses the following strategies: (1) The LMP-1 protein functions as a T cell/CD40 homolog. The EBV LMP-1 protein, by acting as

CD40 ligand, drives the germinal center cell reaction independently. (2) Normally, the expression of B-cell receptor provides proliferative and survival signals to B cells, and the ablation of this protein leads to death within a few hours. In its quest for prolonged survival of infected cells, viral LMP-2A contains functional homology to B-cell receptor and has been shown not only to replace the receptor in the development of B cells but also to rescue immunoglobulin negative B cells from death.

Normally memory B cells, when exposed to new antigens and antigen-specific T cells, undergo a secondary response and eventually differentiate into plasma cells, while some remain as memory B cells. This mechanism is tightly regulated so that not all cells become only plasma cells. The circulating latently EBV-infected memory B cells have potential to undergo activation (like a secondary response) in mucosal lymphoid tissue. This activation may come from some cellular ligand–receptor interactions (e.g., CD40 ligand by LMP-1, B-cell receptor by LMP-2A and lymphokines such as interleukin (IL)-10 and transforming growth factor-β). Whatever the mechanism, the infected memory B cells may undergo lytic replication in the mucosal sites, such as oropharynx, by differentiating into plasma cells. The new virions produced can infect more naïve B cells and subsequently form new memory B cells or spread to infect other individuals via shared oral secretions. Because, as was previously mentioned, the latently infected EBV pool of approximately 1–50 B cells per 1 million in the peripheral circulation remains stable over years, a steady-state production and killing of infected cells is obviously in effect.[33] The mechanisms of this tight regulation in vivo are not well understood.

Cellular Signaling Pathway

As discussed earlier, LMP-1 is a viral analog of the family of TNF receptors in human cells. Like the cellular TNFs, LMP-1 has a cytoplasmic domain that binds to intracellular proteins called *TNF-receptor–associated factors*, which in turn activate nuclear factor-κB transcription factor, resulting in cellular proliferation. Another EBV-encoded protein that is important for B-cell transformation is LMP-2A. Also, as discussed earlier, the loss of B-cell receptor leads to apoptosis of B cells. As a safeguard against abnormal B-cell proliferation, the germinal center cells found to have a dysfunctional B-cell receptor while undergoing somatic hypermutation are prone to apoptosis. In a proportion of PTLD cases a somatic *V* gene mutation has been identified that results in a nonfunctional immunoglobulin molecule. Despite this, B cells are rescued from apoptosis by the expression of B-cell receptor mimicking LMP-2A, which leads to the cell survival. The latter supports the role of EBV in the pathogenesis of PTLD.

Immunosurveillance and Evasion of the Immune System

There are two basic principles of the immune system. First is the presence of an effective and functionally capable surveillance mechanism (such as the cellular response, ligands, cytokines, lymphokines), and second is the need for effective processing of antigens or peptides by antigen-presenting cells so that threats may be recognized and eliminated by the immune system. In a healthy physiologic state there is a constant dynamic equilibrium between these two. In vivo infection with EBV results in a potent humoral and cellular response. The cellular response, composed of CTLs (CD8-positive cells), is the most important for control of EBV infection. This CTL response, although strong, is not fully capable of clearing all EBV-infected cells, demonstrated by the greater than 90% carrier state. Hence, EBV-infected B cells persist in an immunocompetent host and can undergo reactivation if the immunity is dampened. The virus, by minimizing its pathogenic effects, has evolved the following strategies to evade the immune system:

1. Restricting gene expression during latent infection
2. Interfering with cytokines
3. Affecting cytotoxic activity

Restricted Gene Expression During Latent Infection

In vivo infection with EBV results in an interaction between viral evasion strategies and host immune response. An intense T-cell response includes high levels of EBV-specific CD4- and CD8-positive lymphocytes. During an acute EBV infection, only a small number of infected B cells express many viral genes, produce virions, and undergo lytic infection. These cells are immediately recognized and destroyed by cytotoxic T cells. However, in immunocompromised individuals, there is an absence of effective CTL function, and the growth-transforming properties of EBV may act in conjunction with genetic and environmental factors to result in various malignancies (e.g., lymphoproliferative disorders). The persistence of EBV in memory B cells by averting the body's immune surveillance (CTLs) and the mechanism of maintaining the pool of EBV-infected memory B cells in a carrier state are not fully understood. It is accepted that in an EBV-seropositive healthy state, the memory B cells have a restricted viral gene expression, although there is no agreement regarding which viral proteins are expressed in memory cells. It has been postulated that no proteins are expressed; however, some studies show the presence of EBNA-1 and LMP-2A, as well as EBER transcripts, in these cells. Epstein-Barr virus nuclear antigen-1 is required for maintenance of the viral genome; therefore, the expression of this protein in memory B cells is a projected postulate that seems logical. Also, the EBNA-1 protein protects the genome from cellular proteasomal processing, thereby preventing the presentation of viral proteins to CTLs. However, the search for cells expressing solely EBNA-1 in vivo has not been successful despite continued effort. Additionally, LMP-2A is a known CTL target, and LMP-2A mRNA has been demonstrated in memory B cells. However, it should be noted that the LMP-2A protein is not expressed in these cells, which may aid in avoiding recognition by CTLs.

Interference with Cytokines

Interference with cytokines is another mechanism used by EBV to evade immunosurveillance (Figure 31.4).[34] One of the gene products of EBV, BCRF1, has more than 80% homology to human IL-10,[35] the cytokine that inhibits the synthesis of interferon-γ (IFN-γ) by mononuclear cells in vitro.[36] The IFN-γ produced by lymphocytes and natural killer cells inhibits the outgrowth of EBV-transformed B lymphocytes. Thus IFN-γ inhibition by BCRF1 or IL-10 is advantageous to the survival of the virus. The BCRF1 also impairs T-cell proliferation, thus affecting the immune system's ability to clear the virus. Hence BCRF1 or IL-10 promotes B-cell growth, differentiation, and transformation. Another EBV protein, BARF1, functions as a soluble receptor for colony-stimulating factor-1 (CSF-1). Colony-stimulating factor-1 normally enhances the expression of IFN-α by monocytes that in turn inhibit the growth of EBV-infected B cells in vitro. The BARF1 protein functions as a decoy receptor so the CSF-1 will bind to it instead of its normal receptor, thereby blocking the upregulation of IFN-α.[37] As IFN-γ and IFN-α inhibit the growth of EBV-infected B cells in vitro; the BCRF1 and BARF1 proteins help the virus to survive and evade the immune system. In addition, LMP-1 and BHRF1 contribute to longer cell survival through Bcl-2–related mechanisms. Latent membrane protein-1 upregulates the expression of Bcl-2 and other proteins, such as A20, that inhibit apoptosis,[21] and the BHRF1 protein directly functions as a homolog of the Bcl-2 protein, both utilizing the cellular mechanisms to prevent infection.[38]

Cytotoxic Activity

Cytotoxic T lymphocytes are predominantly CD8-positive T lymphocytes that, in concert with MHC class I molecules, recognize viral peptides on the cell surface. The binding of CTLs to infected cells is enhanced by intercellular cell adhesion molecule-1 and leukocyte function–associated antigen-3 and results in the eventual killing of a targeted cell by the CTLs' cytotoxic proteins.

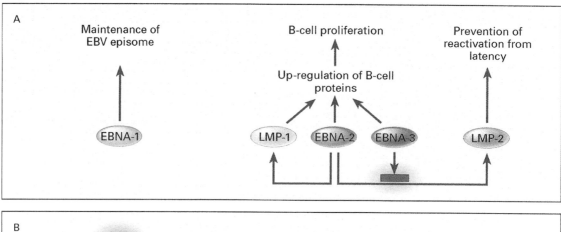

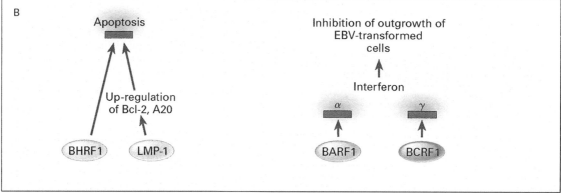

FIGURE 31.4. **(A)** Mechanisms of maintenance, proliferation, and differentiation by Epstein-Barr virus (EBV) latent proteins. **(B)** Mechanisms of host immune response evasion by EBV. EBNA, Epstein-Barr virus nuclear antigen; LMP, latent membrane protein. (From Cohen,[34] with permission.)

When the immune status is compromised, the activity of CTLs is reduced, leading to increased numbers of EBV-infected B cells and setting the stage for the development of lymphoproliferative disorders.

Aside from the aforementioned EBNA-1 linked blockage of proteosomal degradation in the cell that prevents the presentation of viral antigens to CTLs,[39] other mechanisms of CTL evasion are evident. Epstein-Barr virus–positive Burkitt lymphoma cells avoid recognition by expressing only EBNA-1, which, as stated earlier, is not recognized by CTLs.[40] In addition, Burkitt lymphoma cells have low expression of transporter proteins needed for antigen processing, have a reduced amount of cellular adhesion molecules that allow cells to contact each other, and also less MHC class I molecules, which affects CTL activity.[41] Burkitt lymphoma cells grown in cell culture, in contrast, usually express all of the transformation-associated genes and high levels of MHC class I and adhesion molecules on the surface.[41,42] Population-based genetic differences have demonstrated the influence of HLA variations in CTL effectiveness. Many CTL responses are directed against the viral EBNA-3 protein, and this recognition is HLA-A11 restricted.[43] However, EBV may undergo antigen variation to evade CTL killing. For example, B cells infected by EBV isolates from Southeast Asia are often resistant to killing by HLA-A11–restricted CTLs. The HLA-A11 phenotype is common in Southeast Asia, and the EBV in this region has a mutation of the EBNA-3 epitope recognized by CTLs. On the contrary, in Europe and Africa, where HLA-A11 is infrequent, the virus is not mutated in this region.

Patterns of Epstein-Barr Virus Latency and Related Diseases

In vitro EBV infection transforms resting B cells into permanent latently infected lymphoblastoid cells lines. In these cell lines, every cell carries multiple extrachromosomal copies of the episomal form of the virus and expresses all 10 latent proteins (described previously). The infection of B cells results in three different patterns of EBV protein expression categorized as latency I, latency II, and latency III. In latency I, EBNA-1 and EBER are expressed, whereas in latency II EBNA-1, EBER, LMP-1, and LMP-2 are expressed. In latency III, all the latent genes are expressed. Therefore, lymphoblastoid cell lines are an example of a latency III infection.

TABLE 31.4. Types of Epstein-Barr virus latency in various disease states.

EBNA-1	EBNA-2	EBNA-3	LMP-1	LMP-2	EBER	Latency	Disease
+	−	−	−	−	+	I	Burkitt lymphoma
+	−	−	+	+	+	II	CHL, NPCA, PTCL
+	+	+	+	+	+	III	PTLD, IM, XLPD

Note: CHL, classical Hodgkin lymphoma; EBER, Epstein-Barr virus–encoded RNA; EBNA, Epstein-Barr nuclear antigen; IM, infectious mononucleosis; LMP, latent membrane protein; NPCA, nasopharyngeal carcinoma; PTCL, peripheral T-cell lymphoma; PTLD, posttransplantation lymphoproliferative disorder; XLPD, X-linked lymphoproliferative disorder.
Source: Cohen.[34] with permission.

Another nomenclature of latency programs have been developed based on the behavior of the virus in normal B cells during persistent in vivo infection. According to this hypothetical model, EBV infection of the naïve B cells (IgD positive, CD27 negative) express all latent proteins and undergo proliferation to become centroblasts. This is called the *growth program* or *latency III infection*. The EBV-infected cells undergo a germinal center reaction in which somatic mutation of V region genes and differentiation to centroblasts and centrocytes occur. During this differentiation process, the pattern of EBV gene expression is called the *default program* or *latency II infection*. Mutated B cells expressing antigen receptors with high affinity for the immunizing antigen subsequently differentiate into plasma cells or are selected into the pool of memory B cells. The memory B cells show another type of latency called *latency program* or *latency I* during which EBER and EBNA-1 (and perhaps LMP-2A) are expressed. This type of latency results in the evasion of the immune surveillance. Neoplastic cells seen in EBV-associated malignancies can have different patterns of latency, indicating the cell of origin of these disorders (see Table 31.4). Latency I type is seen in Burkitt lymphoma, whereas Hodgkin lymphoma, peripheral T-cell lymphoma, and nasopharyngeal carcinoma are the latency II type. Latency III is seen in PTLDs, infectious mononucleosis, and X-linked lymphoproliferative disorders.

Molecular Histogenesis

Under the current WHO classification of hematopoietic neoplasms, PTLDs are divided into four broad categories (see Table 31.1).[5] These lesions are morphologically, molecularly, and clinically heterogenous disorders (Table 31.5). Most are B cell in origin and EBV positive (Figure 31.5) and express type III latency (growth program). Based on correlative studies of morphologic and molecular features, specific categories of PTLD have been shown to be of clinical relevance.[44–46] In recent years, our greater

TABLE 31.5. Immunoglobulin H (IgH) gene rearrangement and Epstein-Barr virus (EBV) clonality patterns of B-cell posttransplantation lymphoproliferative disorder (PTLD).

	Early lesions	Polymorphic PTLD	Monomorphic PTLD
Morphology	IM-like Plasmacytic	B-cell population with full range of maturation	Monomorphic B-cell population
IgH rearrangement	Polyclonal	Oligoclonal or monoclonal	Monoclonal
EBV clonality	Polyclonal	Clonal	Clonal
Genes	None	None	c-Myc, p53 or N-ras
Clinical response	Regress	Can regress or progress	Progress

Note: The monoclonal subtype often has alterations of oncogenes and tumor suppressor genes. It is notable that synchronous lesions can have variable subtypes by morphology. It is uncertain whether these subtypes progress or evolve from one another. In myeloma and plasmacytoma-like monomorphic PTLD it may be difficult to demonstrate IgH or EBV clonality; therefore, monotypic light chain demonstration by immunophenotypic methods is most useful in this setting. Hodgkin lymphoma-like PTLD is rare and the response to reduced immunosuppression alone is unknown. IM, infectious mononucleosis.

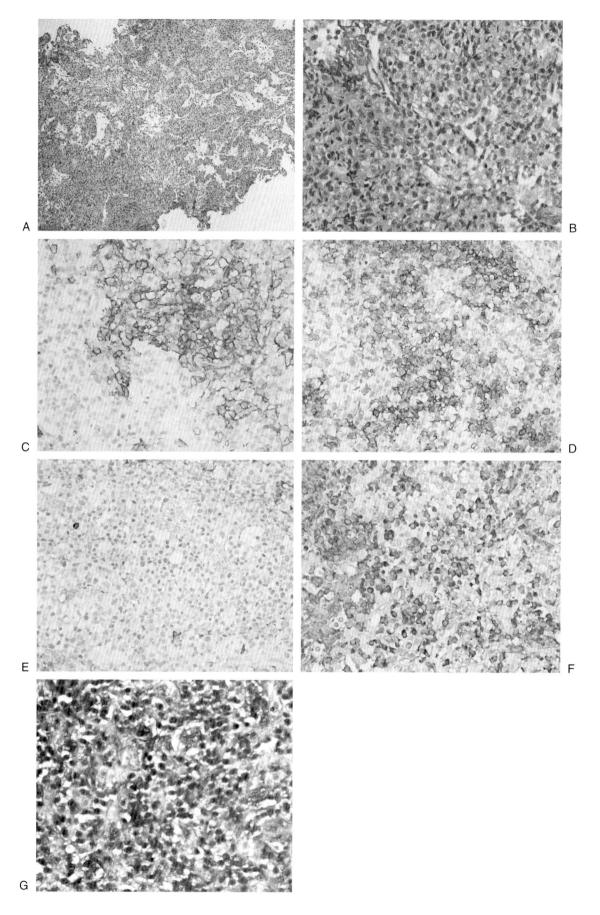

understanding of the histogenesis of B-cell lymphomas has resulted in categorizing them as arising from various B-cell compartments that include naïve B cells, germinal center B cells, and post–germinal center B cells.[47–49] We know that somatic hypermutation of immunoglobulin variable (IgV) genes occurs within the germinal center B cells under the influence of T-cell–dependent immune reactions. Thus, the absence of an IgV mutation suggests an origin from naïve B cells, whereas the presence of IgV mutation indicates a germinal center or post–germinal center origin of lymphoma. Furthermore, the presence of ongoing IgV mutations with intraclonal heterogeneity suggests the neoplastic cells' origin from centroblasts, whereas the absence of intraclonal heterogeneity is consistent with a derivation from late centrocytes or post–germinal center cells.[47–49] In addition, a mutation of the *Bcl-6* protooncogene occurs at the time of germinal center transit.[50,51] De novo cases of diffuse large B-cell lymphomas using gene array technology have shown two major patterns (i.e., germinal center B-cell-like and activated B-cell-like). Patients with the germinal center B-cell-like array pattern had a significantly better overall survival than those with the activated B-cell profile.[52]

Phenotypic markers by immunohistochemistry have been identified that correlate well with genotype markers of B-cell histogenesis. These include CD10, Bcl-6, multiple myeloma oncogene-1 protein (MUM-1), and CD138. The expression of CD10 and Bcl-6 correlates with the germinal center stage of B-cell differentiation; MUM-1 expression correlates with B cells exiting the germinal center and with post–germinal center cells, and CD138 is a marker of preterminal B-cell differentiation.[53–55]

When studied with the immunohistochemical panel (CD10, Bcl-6, CD138, MUM-1) and IgV mutations, PTLD can arise from the broad range of B-cell differentiation and not solely from the pool of memory cells that harbor EBV in healthy carriers. The first molecular histogenetic category of PTLD shows IgV mutations with the Bcl-6$^+$/MUM-1$^{-/+}$/CD138$^-$ phenotype, suggesting germinal center B-cell derivation. A second category shows the Bcl-6$^-$/MUM-1$^+$/CD138$^-$ phenotype, indicating an origin from B cells that have concluded the germinal center reaction (late germinal center). A third category of PTLD shows the BCL-6$^-$/MUM-1$^+$/CD138$^+$ phenotype consistent with post–germinal center B-cell derivation. Most PTLDs have a late germinal center phenotype (second category) followed by a post–germinal center phenotype (third category) and, rarely, a germinal center phenotype (first category).[56]

Both polymorphic and monomorphic subtypes can fall into any of these categories. It is uncertain whether these categories have any affect on prognosis and clinical behavior. One recent small study has suggested a correlation between the histogenetic phenotype of B-cell PTLD and the allograft type, with HSCT-associated PTLD showing a post–germinal center phenotype more frequently than solid organ transplant–associated PTLD.[57] This post–germinal center phenotype has been suggested to explain the poorer prognosis with HSCT-associated PTLD, although in this study the phenotype did not correlate with prognosis. Other studies have not validated these results.

Genetic Profile

Several genetic features have been studied in PTLD cases. These include immunoglobulin and T-cell gene rearrangement clonality, EBV clonality, cytogenetic analysis, and oncogenes such as *Myc, ras, p53, and Bcl-6*. In early lesions of PTLD, the immunoglobulin genes are in the germline, and no mutations of *Myc, ras, p53,* and *Bcl-6* are seen. In polymorphic PTLD, immunoglobulin genes are clonally rearranged along with clonal EBV genomes; however *Myc, ras, p53,* and *Bcl-6* show no mutation. Monomorphic lesions of PTLD often show clonal immunoglobulin rearrangement with mutation of *Myc, ras, p53,* and *Bcl-6* oncogenes. Mutations of the *Bcl-6* oncogene are seen in 40% of polymorphic and 90% of monomorphic PTLD cases and have been associated with a poor response to reduced immunosuppression. Therefore, it has been demonstrated that the classification of PTLD into separate morphologic and genetic categories is clinically relevant.[4]

Some studies have evaluated deletions and mutations of the *LMP-1* oncogene in EBV-positive PTLD cases. A small 30-bp deletion in the carboxy-terminal domain of LMP-1 has been described. However, no significant differ-

---

FIGURE 31.5. Images from a 58-year-old patient with a history of lung transplantation for chronic obstructive pulmonary disease 18 months prior to presentation with multiple lung nodules. **(A)** Hematoxylin and eosin–stained sections (×200) of dense atypical large monomorphic lymphoid cells. **(B)** Hematoxylin and eosin–stained (×400) sheets of large atypical lymphoid cells admixed with plasma cells—polymorphic posttransplantation lymphoproliferative disorder (PTLD). **(C)** CD20 immunostain (×400) shows atypical cells are B cells strongly positive for CD20. **(D)** CD138 immunostain (×400) shows plasma cells are strongly positive for CD138. **(E)** Kappa light chain immunostain (×400) shows most cells are negative. **(F)** Lambda light chain immunostain (×400) shows plasma cells are predominantly positive for lambda stain, indicating lambda light chain restriction or a clonal process. **(G)** Epstein Barr–encoding RNA in situ hybridization with strong positivity, confirming an Epstein-Barr–driven PTLD of polymorphic but monoclonal type.

ences in morphologic features, clinical outcomes, or prognoses have been demonstrated in the deleted cases when compared to patients with wild-type *LMP-1* genes.[58,59]

Diagnosis and Evaluation

The early clinical manifestation of PTLD is usually nonspecific, including such symptoms as fever, weight loss, and malaise. In the pediatric population, infectious mononucleosis may be the initial presentation. The highest incidence of PTLD is in the first year after any allograft transplantation. Although PTLD has been reported as early as 1 week and as late as 9 years posttransplantation, the median onset of disease is 6 months after solid organ transplantation and approximately 10–13 months after HSCT. Because early diagnosis and treatment affect the prognosis, serial monitoring of EBV DNA viral load (whole blood, peripheral blood mononuclear cells, or plasma), EBV serology and diagnostic imaging are routinely used to monitor transplant recipients.

Epstein-Barr virus serology includes the detection of antibodies to VCA (IgG and IgM), EBV-EA, and EBNA (Table 31.6). Only in a primary infection are IgM antibodies to VCA present, and a reactivated infection causes a fourfold or higher increase in anti-VCA IgG and anti-EA. A chronic infection is defined as a combination of low titers of anti-VCA IgG and anti-EBNA. Although some studies have suggested the clinical utility of using EBV serology in predicting PTLD (perhaps in conjunction with EBV viral load), other studies have demonstrated its limitations.[60,61] Transplant recipients are immunosuppressed, and their humoral immune system is not capable of reacting like that of immunocompetent individuals. Thus, the pattern of EBV serology may not be an optimal assay for predicting or confirming the diagnosis of PTLD.

Quantitative polymerase chain reaction (PCR) is commonly used in monitoring the EBV viral load in transplant recipients.[62–64] It has been demonstrated that EBV transcripts are increased significantly in immunosuppressed individuals. Many PCR-based assays are clinically available, such as the EBV viral load assay performed on whole blood/peripheral blood mononuclear cells as the analyte or an EBV viral load assay using serum or plasma.[65] In evaluating PCR-based assays and to assess the positive or negative predictive value, it becomes important to understand the methodology (e.g., primer set used, sensitivity, and specificity) and define the threshold limit deemed as a positive result in the patient population tested. For example, increased specificity can be seen when evaluating EBV viral load results from a cohort of patients in whom PTLD is clinically suspected and compared with results obtained from patients undergoing surveillance in the absence of the disease. The EBV serostatus may affect both the sensitivity and specificity of the assay. Pediatric patients becoming seropositive after transplantation are most likely to become chronic asymptomatic carriers with high baseline EBV viral load than patients who are seropositive before transplantation. Conversely, adult patients who are seropositive prior to transplantation are most likely to have low baseline EBV viral load. Therefore, a subsequent measurement of a high EBV viral load reflects a greater change in the latter patients and is more predictive of the development of PTLD.

Common assays are those using peripheral blood mononuclear cells and plasma for EBV viral load assessment. Although PCR assays are very sensitive in detecting EBV transcripts, they lack the clinical specificity in predicting the development of PTLD. Also, as one might expect, the EBV viral load has limitations in predicting the occurrence of EBV-negative PTLD cases. Recently, the role if IL-10 has been emphasized in PTLDs, and high levels of IL-10 have been detected in the plasma of PTLD patients. Some studies have suggested the IL-10 assay in conjunction with the EBV viral load has clinical diagnostic utility for the early diagnosis of PTLD. Unfortunately, this assay also has a limitation in EBV-negative cases, as IL-10 levels are not elevated in EBV-negative cases. This assay is not currently routinely used.

A definitive diagnosis of PTLD is rendered on a tissue biopsy. Tissue sections show whether the lesion is polymorphic or monomorphic, which may predict the clinical course and help guide therapy. Epstein-Barr virus–encoded RNA in situ hybridization can be performed on paraffin-embedded tissue sections, as EBER transcripts

TABLE 31.6. Patterns of Epstein-Barr virus (EBV) serology in different phases of infection.

EBV serostatus	Anti-VCA (total)	VCA IgM	Anti-EA	Anti-EBNA
Naïve	−	−	−	−
Early infection	+	+	−/+	−
Convalescent infection	+	+/−	−/+	−/+
Recent past infection	+	+/−	−/+	−/+
Remote infection	+	−	Low level/−	+ (EBNA > EA)
Reactivation	≥4-fold increase	−/Weak +	≥4-fold increase	No increase

Note: EA, early antigen; EBNA, Epstein-Barr nuclear antigen; VCA, viral capsid antigen.

are seen in almost all EBV-positive cases of PTLD. Clonality of the lesion can be assessed by demonstrating kappa or lambda light chain restriction using either flow cytometric or immunohistochemical methods. Molecular genetic studies can be performed for B-cell or T-cell clonality by IgH and T-cell receptor rearrangements. In addition, EBV clonality can be performed on fresh or frozen tissue using Southern blot analysis.

Treatment and Management

Because PTLD is a clinically heterogeneous disorder, it is a major challenge for treating physicians. At present, there is no consensus in managing patients with PTLD due to many reasons. First, the pathogenesis of PTLD is not well understood; second, there is an absence of large randomized controlled treatment trials; and third, as mentioned in the previous discussion, there is an absence of reliable assays to predict the development of PTLD. Identifying the population at risk and prevention by immunosurveillance play important roles in the management of these disorders.[62,66,67] Advances in the morphologic and molecular genetic categorization of PTLD with clinical relevance has been useful in predicting the clinical outcome in patients.[46] As an example, the category of early lesions, which are not clonal, have been shown to present with localized disease and frequently respond to reduced immunosuppression alone. On the other hand, monomorphic lesions that are monoclonal, especially those with Bcl-6 mutations, are unlikely to respond to reduced immunosuppression alone and usually require aggressive therapy, including conventional lymphoma chemotherapy.[45,68]

The therapeutic options fall into five major categories: (1) reduction of immunosuppression, (2) conventional chemotherapy, (3) anti–B-cell monoclonal antibodies (e.g., rituximab), (4) antiviral drugs, and (5) adoptive immune therapy. The initial treatment of PTLD, irrespective of the morphologic subtype, is to reduce immunosuppression with the hope of partially restoring the host CTL function, which could result in the elimination of infected cells. Also, if the patient needs conventional chemotherapy, reduced immunosuppression helps decrease infectious complications. This needs to be carefully individualized, as reducing the immunosuppression poses a risk of allograft rejection. The guidelines for reducing immunosuppression are not well established, and common dilemmas concerning the amount and length of time required are still not well established. The response to reduced immunosuppression is typically seen in 2–4 weeks and is usually monitored by following the reduction in the EBV viral load and/or tumor size by imaging studies.[62,63,69] It is interesting to note that some cases of EBV-negative PTLD respond to reduced immunosuppression alone. The mortality rate is 50%–80% in cases

of PTLD that failed to respond to reduced immunosuppression alone. In some studies, the regression of polyclonal and monoclonal lesions after a reduction of the immunosuppressive dose ranges from 23% to 50%.[70–72] In solid organ transplant recipients, a reduction of immunosuppression has been beneficial; however, the withdrawal of immunosuppression in HSCT recipients is precarious, as these patients are dependent on donor engraftment to restore immune competence.

Conventional chemotherapy is used for patients who do not respond to reduced immunosuppression alone or for patients who have a higher stage of disease with monomorphic or monoclonal PTLD lesions. When chemotherapy is administered, it is always in combination with reduced immunosuppression. Although a clinical response to chemotherapy is usually observed, the duration of remission is unpredictable.[73,74] Rituximab, a monoclonal anti-CD20 (mature B-cell) antibody, has been used relatively successfully as an adjunct to reduced immunosuppression with and without chemotherapy. As most PTLD lesions are B cell in origin, the use of rituximab may be a rational treatment approach. The results of patients treated with rituximab are promising, and the response rate can be as high as 90%, with a durable remission lasting several months. However, the experience of using rituximab in the PTLD setting has been less than 10 years in duration, and more studies are needed to evaluate the long-term remission rate. Rituximab may be given along with lower doses of chemotherapy to avoid the toxic side effects of higher doses, especially in the pediatric population. It is important to understand that rituximab essentially depletes all mature B cells (normal and tumor cells) and does not have any known effect on CTL function. Thus long-term EBV control and late relapse could be a potential problem.[75–78]

Transfused EBV-specific CTLs have been used in clinical trials with some success. This therapeutic approach is also called *adoptive T-cell therapy*. Epstein-Barr virus–specific CTLs can be harvested from the donor (allogeneic) or from the recipient (autologous). Posttransplantation lymphoproliferative disorders arising in an HSCT setting are often donor in origin, and allogeneic EBV-specific CTLs has been used successfully.[79–83]

Autologous EBV-specific CTLs can be generated from EBV-seropositive recipients prior to transplantation. This approach is helpful for solid organ transplant recipients, because PTLDs arising in this setting are mostly recipient in origin. However, this approach cannot be taken for patients who are EBV seronegative at the time of solid organ transplantation, precisely the population with an increased risk of PTLD. Closely HLA-matched allogeneic EBV-specific CTLs have been used in these cases with variable success.[84] In contrast to stem cell transplant recipients, the allogeneic EBV-specific CTLs do not survive long enough in recipients of solid organ transplans.[85,86]

A retroviral gene transfer methodology (introducing EBV viral product–specific T-cell receptors) is another interesting approach to generate autologous EBV-specific CTLs from seronegative recipients.[87] Surgical resection or local radiation has also been used in PTLD cases with a goal to relieve local symptoms and/or reduce the tumor burden. In rare cases of a localized lesion, a surgical excision may be curative. Other adjunct therapeutic modalities include cytokine-based therapies such as IFN-α and anti–IL-6. At present, there is insufficient evidence to support their use.

Prophylaxis

Because EBV infection is often the etiology of PTLD, prophylaxis should be focused on prevention of reactivation in seropositive individuals and controlling and/or minimizing the clinical consequences of primary infection in seronegative recipients. Several approaches have been used, including avoidance of overimmunosuppression, continuous immunosurveillance, the use of prophylactic antiviral medications, an EBV vaccine and in vitro–generated EBV-specific CTLs.

The incidence of PTLD varies even among institutions, probably because of the amount and type of immunosuppression regimen used, the type of allograft transplanted, and the patient population (pediatric vs. adult) at a particular transplant facility. Pediatric patients (who are seronegative at the time of transplantation) who undergo liver transplantation or seronegative patients who undergo heart–lung transplantation are most likely to receive a more intensive immunosuppressive regimen than are patients who are EBV seropositive and undergo renal transplantation. Thus the degree of immunosuppression needs to be carefully considered when treating different patient populations. There are no standard protocols/guidelines for reducing immunosuppression, and the clinical judgment depends on the patient's clinical status, the EBV viral load, graft function, and the histology and clonality of the lesion. Continuous immunosurveillance means prospective monitoring of the EBV viral load in transplant recipients and commencing therapy when a predetermined threshold is reached. A legitimate concern is that only a fraction of patients with a high EBV viral load develop PTLD, and some patients with EBV-positive PTLD have a low viral load.[88,89]

Antiviral agents are often given along with reduced immunosuppression; however, the clinical efficacy of this approach is undetermined. These agents have no effect on latently infected EBV-positive B cells but do limit the lytic replication of EBV-infected cells.[90,91] An EBV vaccine using the gp350 EBV protein is currently under development with the hope that a vaccine given to EBV-seronegative individuals prior to transplantation will induce seroconversion and the formation of EBV-specific antibodies. Preliminary data have shown success with a good immune response in healthy EBV seronegative individuals[92]; however, the antibody responses in EBV seronegative immunosuppressed individuals need to be evaluated.

Epstein-Barr Viral Load in Immunocompromised Hosts

As mentioned above, the CTL response is important for the control of EBV infection, and in healthy carriers most infected B lymphocytes are cleared through immunosurveillance. However, 1–50 B lymphocytes per 1 million remain infected and serve as the reservoir for lifelong latent infection. In immunocompromised individuals or transplant patients receiving immunosuppressive therapy, the balance between EBV replication, latency, and CTL control is deranged, and decreased EBV-specific CTL activity results in increased virus replication and increased numbers of circulating latently infected B cells. Therefore, immunosuppressed patients have an increased EBV viral load, but all these patients do not necessarily develop PTLD and retain the restricted transcription pattern seen in healthy carriers (EBER, EBNA-1, and LMP-2A). As EBNA-2 and LMP-1 proteins are not expressed, the increased viral load is not due to cellular proliferation but rather to the increased number of EBV-infected cells gaining entry to the B-cell memory compartment. Therefore, the presence of high EBV viral load in transplant recipients is a very sensitive but not a very specific assay for the diagnosis of PTLD. In other words, as mentioned previously, the presence of a high EBV viral load does not always mean the person has PTLD; however, the absence of a high viral load argues against the development of PTLD. Of course, the EBV-negative PTLD cases would also have either negative or low EBV viral load. Therefore, an increased EBV viral load and the presence of a slight increase in the number of EBER-positive cells on the tissue sections needs to be interpreted with caution and morphologic features need to be correlated with clinical manifestations.

Epstein-Barr Virus–Negative Disease

About 15%–20% of PTLD are EBV negative and are often seen in renal transplant recipients (up to 50% of renal allograft recipients developing PTLD are EBV negative). Knowledge of the etiology, behavior, and optimal treatment for EBV-negative PTLD remains limited, partly because of the rarity of these lesions. It is uncertain whether EBV-negative PTLD represents a

distinct entity. In one study, the morphologic, immunophenotypic, genotypic, and clinical features of the EBV-
negative and EBV-positive PTLD cases were compared.[23,93]
Epstein-Barr virus–negative PTLD occurred a median of
50 months posttransplantation compared with 10 months
for EBV-positive cases.

Although any morphologic subtype of PTLD can be
seen, the EBV-negative cases are often monomorphic
and can demonstrate B-cell and less often T-cell clonality.
Some of the B-lineage monomorphic lesions have *c-Myc*
and/or *Bcl-2* rearrangements. The EBV-negative PTLD
cases often require chemotherapy and are typically more
aggressive than the EBV-positive cases; however, some
cases do respond to reduced immunosuppression alone.
Irrespective of their morphologic pattern, reduced immunosuppression should always be considered before starting chemotherapy.

Prognosis

Prognosis is variable given the heterogeneity of the clinical and morphologic features. The data about prognosis
are mainly based on case reports and retrospective studies.
Most of the early lesions and some cases of polymorphic
PTLD tend to regress with reduced immunosuppression;
however, most cases of polymorphic and monomorphic
subtypes fail to regress and require conventional chemotherapy. Although the overall survival rates range between 25% and 35%, the prognosis varies with many
factors, such as the age of the patient, extent of the disease,
performance status of the patient, morphologic diagnosis,
presence of clonality, and involvement of allograft by the
disease. The mortality caused by PTLD in solid organ
transplant recipients can be as high as 60% and in HSCT
recipients as high as 80%. Monoclonal PTLDs, T-cell
lymphomas and EBV- negative PTLD cases have the
worse prognosis. The International Prognostic Index,
which is useful for determining the prognosis of patients
with de novo non-Hodgkin lymphoma, is less useful in
this setting.[94]

References

1. Penn I, Hammon W, Brettschneider L, et al. Malignant lympho-mas in transplantation patients. Transplant Proc 1969;1:106.
2. Frizerra G, Hanto DW, Gajl-Peczalska KJ, et al. Polymor-phic diffuse B-cell hyperplasia and lymphomas is renal transplant recipients. Cancer Res 1981;41:4262–4279.
3. Nalesnik MA, Jaffe R, Starzl TE, et al. The pathology of PTLDs occurring the setting of cyclosporine A–prednisone immunosuppression. Am J Pathol 1988;133:173–192.
4. Knowles DM, Cesarman E, Chadburn A, et al. Correlative morphologic and molecular genetic analysis demonstrates three distinct categories of post transplantation lymphopro-liferative disorders. Blood 1995;85:552–565.
5. Harris NL, Swerdlow SH, Frizerra G, et al. Post transplant lymphoproliferative disorders in Tumours of Haematopoi-etic and Lymphoid Tissues. In Jaffe ES, Harris NL, Stein H, Vardiman JW, eds. WHO Classification of Tumours. Lyon, France: IARC Press; 2001:264–269.
6. Levine SM, Angel L, Anzueto A, et al. A low incidence of posttransplant lymphoproliferative disorder in 109 lung transplant recipient. Chest 1999;116:1273–1277.
7. Montone KT, Litzky LA, Wurster A, et al. Analysis of Epstein-Barr virus associated posttransplantation lympho-proliferative disorder after lung transplantation. Surgery 1996;119:544–551.
8. Shapiro R, Nalesnik M, McCauley J, et al. PTLD in adult and pediatric renal transplant recipients receiving tacroli-mus based immunosuppression. Transplantation 1999;68:1851–1854.
9. Walker RC, Paya CV, Marshall WF, et al. Pretransplantation seronegative Epstein-Barr virus status is the primary risk factor to posttransplantation lymphoproliferative disorder in adult heart, lung, and other solid organ transplantations. J Heart Lung Transplant 1995;14:214–221.
10. Newell KA, Alonso EM, Kelly SM. Association between liver transplantation for Langerhans cell histiocytosis, rejec-tion and development of PTLD in children. J Pediatr 1999;131:98–103.
11. Ho M, Jaffe R, Miller G. The frequency of EBV infection and associated lymphoproliferative disease after transplan-tation and its manifestations in children. Transplantation 1988;45:719–724.
12. Shpilberg O, Wilson J, Whiteside TL. Pre-transplant immu-nological profile and risk factor analysis of PTLD develop-ment: the results of a nested matched case–control study: The University of Pittsburg PTLD study group. Leuk Lym-phoma 1999;36:109–113.
13. Levine SM, Angel L, Anzueto A, et al. A low incidence of PTLD in 109 lung transplant recipient. Chest 1999;116:1273–1277.
14. Aris RM, Maia DM, Neuringer IP, et al. PTLD in EBV naïve lung transplant recipients. Am J Respir Crit Care Med 1996;154:1712–1717.
15. Montone KT, Litzky LA, Wurster A, et al. Analysis of EBV associated PTLD after lung transplantation. Surgery 1996;119:544–551.
16. Cohen AH, Sweet SC, Mendeloff E, et al. High incidence of PTLD in pediatric patients with cystic fibrosis. Am J Resp Crit Care Med 2000;161:1252–1255.
17. Ferry JA, Jacobson JO, Conti D, et al. Lymphoproliferative disorders and hematologic malignancies following organ transplantation. Mod Pathol 1989;2:583–592.
18. Leblond V, Davi F, Charlotte F, et al. Post transplant lym-phoproliferative disorders not associated with EpsteinBarr virus: a distinct entity? J Clin Oncol 1998;16:2052–2059.
19. Nelson BP, Nalesnik MA, Bahler DW, et al. Epstein-Barr virus negative post transplant lymphoproliferative disor-ders: a distinct entity? Am J Surg Pathol 2000;24:375–385.
20. Epstein MA, Achong BG, Barr YM. Virus particles in cul-tured lymphoblasts from Burkitt's lymphoma. Lancet 1964;15:702–703.
21. Babcock GJ, Decker LL, Volk M, et al. EBV persistence in memory B cells in-vivo. Immunity 1998;9:395–404.

22. Joseph AM, Babcock GJ, Thorley-Lawson DA. EBV persistence involves strict selection of latently infected B cells. J Immunol 2000;165:2975–2981.

23. Kieff E, Rickinson AB. EBV and its replication. In Knipe DM, Howley PM, eds. Fields Virology, 4th ed, vol 2. Philadelphia: Lippincott Williams & Wilkins; 2001:2511–2574.

24. Wang D, Liebowitz D, Kieff E. An EBV membrane protein expressed in immortalized lymphocytes transforms established rodent cells. Cell 1985;43:831–840.

25. Kulwichit W, Edwards RH, Davenport EM, et al. Expression of the EBV LMP-1 induces B-cell lymphoma in transgenic mice. Proc Natl Acad Sci USA 1998;95:11963–11968.

26. Henderson S, Rowe M, Gregory C, et al. Induction of bcl-2 expression by EBV LMP-1 protects infected B cells form programmed cell death. Cell 1991;65:1107–1115.

27. Laherty CD, Hu HM, Opipari AW, et al. The EBV LMP-1 gene product induces A20 zinc finger protein expression by activating nuclear factor kappa B. J Biol Chem 1992;267:24157–24160.

28. Miller CL, Burkhardt AL, Lee JH, et al. Integral membrane protein 2 of EBV regulates reactivation from latency through dominant negative effects on protein tyrosinase kinases. Immunity 1995;2:155–166.

29. Lam KP, Kuhn R, Rajewsky K. In vivo ablation of surface immunoglobulin on mature B cells by inducible gene targeting results in rapid cell death. Cell 1997;90:1073–1083.

30. Caldwell RG, Wilson JB, Anderson SJ, et al. EBV LMP2A drives B cell development and survival in the absence of normal B cell receptor signals. Immunity 1998;9:405–411.

31. Casola S, Otipoby KL, Alimzhanov M, et al. B cell receptor signal strength determines B cell fate. Nat Immunol 2004; 5:317–327.

32. Thorley-Lawson DA, Gross A. Persistence of the EBV and the origins of associated lymphomas. N Engl J Med 2004; 350(13):1328–1337.

33. Babcock GJ, Decker LL, Volk M, et al. EBV persistence in memory B cells in-vivo. Immunity 1998;9:395–404.

34. Cohen JI. EBV Infection. N Eng J Med 2000;343(7):481–492.

35. Moore KW, Vieira P, Fiorentinio DF, et al. Homology of cytokine synthesis inhibitory factor (IL-10) to the EBV gene BCRF1. Science 1990;248:1230–1234.

36. Hsu D-H, de Waal Malefyt R, Fiorentino DF, et al. Expression of IL-10 activity by EBV protein BCRF1. Science 1990;250:830–832.

37. Cohen JI, Lekstrom K. EBV BARF1 protein is dispensable for B-cell transformation and inhibits alpha interferon secretion form mononuclear cells. J Virol 1999;73:7627–7632.

38. Henderson S, Huen D, Rowe M, et al. EBV coded BHRF1 protein, a viral homolog of bcl-2, protects human B cells form programmed cell death. Proc Natl Acad Sci USA 1993;90:8479–8483.

39. Levitskaya J, Shapiro A, Leonchiks A, et al. Inhibition of ubiquitin/proteosome-dependent protein degradation by the Gly-Ala repeat domain of the EBAN-1. Proc Natl Acad Sci USA 1997;94:12616–12621.

40. Rooney CM, Rowe M, Wallace LE, et al. EBV positive Burkitt's lymphoma cells not recognized by virus-specific T-cell surveillance. Nature 1985;317:629–631.

41. Gregory CD, Muraay RJ Edwards CF, et al. Down regulation of cell adhesion molecules LFA-3 and ICAM-1 in EBV⁺ Burkitt's lymphoma underlies tumor cell escape form virus-specific T cell surveillance. J Exp Med 1988;167:1811–1824.

42. Rowe M, Khanna R, Jacob CA, et al. Restoration of endogenous antigen processing in Burkitt's lymphoma cells by EBV LMP-1: coordinate up regulation of peptide transporters and HLA-class I antigen expression. Eur J Immunol 1995;25:1374–1384.

43. DeCampos-Lima PO, Levitsky B, Brooks J, et al. T cell responses and virus evolution: loss of HLA A11-restricted CTL epitopes in EBV isolates for highly A11-positive populations by selective mutation of anchor residues. J Exp Med 1994;179:1297–1305.

44. Knowles DM, Cesarman E, Chadburn A, et al. Correlative morphologic and molecular genetic analysis demonstrates three distinct categories of PTLDs. Blood 1995;85:552–565.

45. Cesarman E, Chadburn A, Liu YF, et al. BCL-6 gene mutations in PTLD predict response to therapy and clinical outcome. Blood 1998;92:2294–2302.

46. Chadburn A, Chen JM, Hsu DT, et al. The morphologic and molecular genetic categories of PTLDs are clinically relevant. Cancer 1998;82:1978–1987.

47. Muller-Hermelink HK, Greiner A. Molecular analysis of human immunoglobulin heavy chain variable genes (IgVH) in normal and malignant B cells. Am J Pathol 1998;153:1341–1346.

48. Kuppers R, Klein U, Hansman ML, et al. Cellular origin of human B-cell lymphoma. N Engl J Med 1999;341:1520–1529.

49. Stevenson FK, Sahota SS, Ottensmeier CH, et al. The occurrence and significance of V gene mutations in B cell–derived human malignancy. Adv Cancer Res 2001;83:81–116.

50. Pasqualucci L, Migliazza A, Fracchiolla N, et al. BCL-6 mutations in normal germinal center B cells: evidence of somatic hypermutation acting outside Ig loci. Proc Natl Acad Sci USA 1998;95:11816–11821.

51. Shen HM, Peters A, Baron B, et al. Mutation of BCL-6 gene in normal B cells by the process of somatic hypermutations of Ig genes. Science 1998;280:1750–1752.

52. Alizadeh AA, Eisen MB, Davis RE, et al. Distinct types of diffuse large B cell lymphoma identified by gene expression profiling. Nature 2000;403:503–511.

53. Catoretti G, Chang C-C, Cechova C, et al. BCL-6 protein is expressed in germinal-center B cells. Blood 1995;86:45–53.

54. Falini B, Fizzotti M, Pucciarini A, et al. A monoclonal antibody (MUM1p) detects expression of the MUMI/IRF1 protein in a subset of germinal center B cells, plasma cells, and activated T cells. Blood 2000;95:2084–2092.

55. Carbone A, Gloghini A, Larocca LM, et al. Expression profile of MUMi/IRF-4, BCL-6, and CD138/syndecan-1 defines novel histogenetic subsets of human immunodeficiency virus-related lymphomas. Blood 2001;97:744–751.

56. Capello D, Cerri M, Muti G, et al. Molecular histogenesis of PTLDs. Blood 2003;102(10):3775–3785.

57. Novoa-Takara L, Perkins SL, Qi D, et al. Histogenetic phenotypes of B cells in PTLDs by immunohistochemical analysis correlate with transplant type. Solid organ vs hematopoietic stem cell transplantation. Am J Clin Pathol 2005; 123:104–112.

58. Smir BN, Hauke RJ, Bierman PJ, et al. Molecular epidemiology of deletions and mutations of the LMP1 oncogene of the EBV in PTLD. Lab Invest 1996;75(4):575–588.

59. Scheinfeld AG, Nador RG, Cesarman E, et al. EBV LMP-1 oncogene deletion in PTLDs. Am J Pathol 1997;151(3):805–812.

60. Carpentier L, Tapiero B, Alvarez F, et al. EBV EA serologic testing in conjunction with peripheral blood EBV DNA load as a marker for risk of PTLD. J Infect Dis 2003;188:1853–1863.

61. Henle W, Henle G. EBV specific serology in immunologically compromised individuals. Cancer Res 1981;41:4222–4225.

62. Green M, Reyes J, Weber S, et al. The role of viral load in the diagnosis, management and possible prevention of EBV associated PTLD following solid organ transplantation. Curr Opin Organ Transplant 1999;4:292–296.

63. Tsai D, Nearey M, Hardy C, et al. Use of EBV PCR for the diagnosis and monitoring of PTLD in adult solid organ transplant recipients. Am J Transplant 2002;2:946–954.

64. Green M, Caccuarelli TV, Mazareigos GV, et al. Serial measurements of EBV load in peripheral blood in pediatric liver transplant recipient for PTLD. Transplantation 1998;66:1641–1644.

65. Wagner HJ, Wessel M, Jabs W, et al. Patients at the risk for development of PTLD: plasma versus peripheral blood mononuclear cells as material for quantification of EBV loads by using real-time quantitative PCR. Transplantation 2001;72(6):1012–1019.

66. Cockfiled SM. Identifying the patient at risk for PTLD. Transplant Infect Dis 2001;3:70–78.

67. Preiksaitis JK. New developments in the diagnosis and management of PTLDs in solid organ transplant recipients. Clin Infect Dis 2004;39(7):1016–1023.

68. Penn I. The role of immunosuppression in lymphoma formation. Springer Semin Immunopathol 1998;20(34):343–355.

69. Oertel S, Trappe RU, Zeidler K, et al. Epstein-Barr viral load in whole blood of adults with post transplant lymphoproliferative disorder after solid organ transplantation does not correlate with clinical course. Ann Hematol 2006;85(7):478–484.

70. Orjuela M, Gross TG, Cheung YK, et al. A pilot study of chemoimmunotherapy (cyclophosphamide, prednisone, rituximab) in patients with PTLD following solid organ transplantation. Clin Cancer Res 2003;9(10 Pt 2):3945S–3952S.

71. Penn I. Immunosuppression—a contributory factor in lymphoma formation. Clin Transplant 1992;6:214.

72. Benkerrow MD, Randy A, Fischer A. Therapy for transplant-related lymphoproliferative diseases. Hemat Oncol Clin North Am 1993;7:467.

73. Muti G, Cantoni S, Oreste P, et al. PTLDs: improved outcome after clinico-pathologically tailored treatment. Haematologica 2002;87(1):67–77.

74. McCarthy M, Ramage J, McNair A, et al. The clinical diversity and role of chemotherapy in lymphoproliferative disorder in liver transplant recipients. J Hepatol 1997;27(6):1015–1021.

75. Milpied N, Vasseur B, Parquet N, et al. Humanized anti-C20 monoclonal antibody (Rituximab) in post transplant B lymphoproliferative disorder: a retrospective analysis on 32 patients. Ann Oncol 2000;11(Suppl 1):113–116.

76. Ganne V, Siddiqi N, Kamaplath B, et al. Humanized anti-C20 monoclonal antibody (rituximab) in PTLD. Clin Transplant 2003;17(5):417–422.

77. Ifthikharuddin JJ, Mieles LA, Rosenblatt JD, et al. Co-expression in PTLD; treatment with rituximab. Am J Hematol 2000;65(2):171–173.

78. Reynaud-Gaubert M, Stoppa AM, Gaubert J, et al. Anti-CD20 monoclonal antibody therapy in EBV associated B-cell lymphoma following lung transplantation. J Heart Lung Transplant 2000;19(5):492–495.

79. Rooney CM, Smith CA, Ng CY, et al. Use of gene modified virus specific T lymphocytes to control EBV related lymphoproliferations. Lancet 1995;345(8941):9–13.

80. Rooney CM, Smith CA, Ng CY, et al. Infusion of cytotoxic T cells for the prevention and treatment of EBV induced lymphoma in allogeneic transplant recipients. Blood 1998;92(5):1549–1555.

81. Wagner HJ, Cheng YC, Huls MH, et al. Prompt versus preemptive intervention for EBV lymphoproliferative disease. Blood 2004;103(10):3979–3981.

82. Liu Z, Savoldo B, Huls H, et al. EBV specific cytotoxic T lymphocytes for the prevention and treatment of EBV associated post transplant lymphomas. Recent Results Cancer Res 2002;159:123–133.

83. Heslop HE, Ng CY, Li C, et al. Long term restoration of immunity against EBV infection by adoptive transfer of gene-modified virus-specific T lymphocytes. Nat Med 1996;2(5):551–555.

84. Haque T, Wilkeie GM, Taylor C, et al. Treatment of EBV positive PTLD with partly HLA-matched allogeneic cytotoxic T cells. Lancet 2002;360(9331):436–442.

85. Gottschalk S, Rooney CM, Heslop HE. Post transplant lymphoproliferative disorders. Annu Rev Med 2005;56:29–44.

86. Comoli P, Labirio M, Basso S, et al. Infusion of autologous EBV specific cytotoxic T cells for prevention of EBV related lymphoproliferative disorder in solid organ transplant recipients with evidence of active virus replication. Blood 2002;99(7):2592–2598.

87. Feng S, Buell JF, Chari RS, et al. Tumors and transplantation. The 2003 third annual ASTS state of the art winter symposium. Am J Transplant 2003;3(12):1481–1487.

88. Leblond V, Choquet S. Lymphoproliferative disorders after liver transplantation. J Hepatol 2004;40(5):728–735.

89. Scheenstra R, Verschuuren EA, de Hann A, et al. The value of prospective monitoring of EBV DNA in blood samples of pediatric liver transplant recipients. Transplant Infect Dis 2004;6(1):15–22.

90. Green M, Michaels MG, Webber SA, et al. The management of EBV associated PTLD in pediatric solid organ transplant recipients. Pediatr Transplant 1999;3(4):271–281.

91. Davis CL. The antiviral prophylaxis of PTLD. Springer Semin Immunopathol 1998;20(34):437–453.

92. Gu SY, Huang TM, Ruan L, et al. First EBV vaccine trial in humans using recombinant vaccinia virus expressing the major membrane antigen. Dev Biol Stand 1995;84:171–177.

93. Dotti G, Fiocchi R, Motta T, et al. EBV negative lymphoproliferative disorders in long-term survivors after heart, kidney, and liver transplant. Transplantation 2000;69(5):827–833.

94. Ghobrial IM, Habermann TM, Maurer MJ, et al. Prognostic analysis for survival in adult solid organ transplant recipients with post-transplantation lymphoproliferative disorders. J Clin Oncol 2005;23(30):7574–7582.

32
Unusual Benign and Malignant Neoplasms of Lung: Molecular Pathology

Dongfeng Tan, Guoping Wang, and Sadir Alrawi

Sclerosing Hemangioma

Pulmonary sclerosing hemangioma is a unique lung neoplasm. It occurs sporadically in middle-aged patients, although cases have been reported in the pediatric population and may be associated with familial adenomatous polyposis.[1,2] Sclerosing hemangiomas are typically peripheral and involve lung parenchyma. However, they rarely present as endobronchial polypoid masses resulting in clinical symptoms of bronchial obstruction.[3] The lesions have sclerosis and hemorrhagic cystic spaces lined by surface/cuboidal cells thought to be reactive and solid areas consisting of round/polygonal cells thought to be neoplastic. For many years sclerosing hemangioma was thought to be a vascular tumor because of its microscopic appearance, hence the name.

The histogenesis and origin of sclerosing hemangioma of lung were uncertain for many years. Many immunohistochemical, ultrastructural, and recent molecular studies provide interesting insights. One of the largest cohort studies of sclerosing hemangioma study was performed by the investigators at the Armed Forces Institute of Pathology.[4] The authors studied 100 cases of pulmonary sclerosing hemangioma that presented as peripheral (95%), solitary (96%) masses of less than 3 cm in diameter (74%) in asymptomatic patients who were mostly women (83%) with a mean age of 46.2 years. Immunohistochemistry for multiple epithelial, mesothelial, pneumocyte, neuroendocrine, and mesenchymal markers was performed on 47 cases to investigate the histogenesis of this neoplasm. Both surface/cuboidal and round/polygonal cells stained with epithelial membrane antigen and thyroid transcription factor-1 (TTF-1) in more than 90% of cases. However, the round cells were uniformly negative for pan-cytokeratin and positive for cytokeratin-7 and CAM 5.2 in only 31% and 17% of cases respectively. Surfactant proteins A and B as well as Clara cell antigen were positive in varying numbers of surface cells, but they were negative in the round tumor cells. Neuroendocrine cells either as isolated scattered cells or as nodules within the center of sclerosing hemangioma were detected (chromogranin, Leu-7, synaptophysin positive) in three cases. The expression of TTF-1 in the absence of surfactant proteins A and B and Clara cell antigens in the round cells of sclerosing hemangioma suggests that they are derived from primitive respiratory epithelium. The alveolar pneumocytes and neuroendocrine cells may either represent phenotypic differentiation of a primitive respiratory epithelial component or they correspond to nonneoplastic entrapped or hyperplastic elements. The latter is favored. The concomitant positivity of both cell types in sclerosing hemangioma for TTF-1 and epithelial membrane antigen, and the negativity of round cells for pancytokeratin and neuroendocrine markers, provide useful clues for histogenesis. It also provides a panel of immunophenotypic markers aiding in the diagnosis of this lung neoplasm in small biopsy or fine-needle aspiration specimens. The round cells/polygonal tumor cells in sclerosing hemangioma coexpress TTF-1 and epithelial membrane antigen without cytokeratin immunoreactivity.[3,5]

Ultrastructural and immunophenotypic studies[6] have demonstrated that cuboidal cells of sclerosing hemangioma resemble reactive proliferating type II pneumocytes, which can fuse into multinuclear giant cells. On the other hand, polygonal cells, which are true tumor cells, likely originate from multipotential primitive respiratory epithelium and possess the capability for multipotential differentiation.

A recent study suggested that neoplastic cells of sclerosing hemangioma are undifferentiated "stromal cells."[5] The nuclei of the tumor cells stained positive for hepatocyte nuclear factor-3α and -3β as well as TTF-1; the latter was further confirmed by in situ hybridization staining.

In summary, pulmonary sclerosing hemangioma is a proliferation of fetal/primitive type II pneumocytes. Therefore, *pneumocytoma* or *pneumoblastoma* appears to be a more appropriate name for this lesion.

Recent loss of heterozygosity (LOH) studies have postulated that sclerosing hemangioma may be a neoplasm originating from the cells of the terminal lobular unit, similar to the nonmucinous variant of bronchoalveolar carcinoma. In this study, a number of overlapping features of sclerosing hemangioma and bronchoalveolar carcinoma were noted. Dacic et al. examined a potential relationship between the two entities.[7] They analyzed the patterns of allelic loss of tumor suppressor genes in sclerosing hemangioma and bronchoalveolar carcinoma by microdissection-based LOH analysis using a panel of seven polymorphic microsatellite markers located on 1p, 5q, 9p, 10q, and 17p. They showed similar patterns of allelic loss between bronchoalveolar carcinoma and sclerosing hemangioma. A statistically significant difference in allelic loss between sclerosing hemangioma and bronchoalveolar carcinoma was located only on chromosomal arm 5q ($p = 0.04$). Microsatellite marker D5S615 was significantly more frequently affected in sclerosing hemangioma than in bronchoalveolar carcinoma (66.7% vs. 28.6%; $p = 0.04$). The new molecular data support the hypothesis of a common origin of sclerosing hemangioma and bronchoalveolar carcinoma. A putative tumor suppressor gene that might play a role in tumorigenesis of sclerosing hemangioma may be located on the chromosomal arm 5q.

Sclerosing hemangioma of the lung shows a predilection for middle-aged women. This prompted investigators to examine sclerosing hemangioma for the expression of ERα (human estrogen receptor) and ERβ (a second isoform of estrogen receptor). To investigate the staining patterns of these tumors, Wu et al. stained lung tissues from patients with non–small cell lung carcinomas and nonneoplastic type II pneumocytes for comparison. In their study, 37 pulmonary sclerosing hemangiomas and 301 non–small cell lung cancer specimens were examined immunohistochemically. There was no ERα expression. The overall frequency of overexpression for ERβ was 91.9%. It was detected in both female (in 91.4% of 35 cases) and male (in 100.0% of 2 tumors from men) patients. There was ERβ overexpression in all 9 tumors of solid pattern, 6 of 7 tumors of papillary pattern, all 4 tumors of sclerotic pattern, 12 of 13 tumors of hemorrhagic pattern, and 3 of 4 tumors of mixed pattern. The staining pattern of the neoplastic cells of the sclerosing hemangioma was similar to that of type II pneumocytes adjacent to the tumor rather than that of non–small cell lung cancers, in which the frequency of ERβ overexpression was 45.8%.

like cells (lymphangioleiomyomatosis cells, perivascular epithelioid cells) around airways, vessels, and lymphatics that leads to cystic lung lesions and lymphatic abnormalities.[9] Lymphangioleiomyomatosis presents insidiously with progressive breathlessness or dramatically with recurrent pneumothorax, chylothorax, or sudden abdominal hemorrhage. Computed tomography scans show numerous thin-walled cysts throughout the lungs with no air trapping and abdominal angiomyolipomas in up to 35% of cases. Pulmonary function tests show reduced flow rates (forced expiratory volume in 1 sec) and diffusing capacity for carbon monoxide. Exercise testing shows gas-exchange abnormalities, ventilatory limitation, and hypoxemia that may occur with near-normal lung function. Tissue biopsy material with immunoreactivity for HMB-45 positivity establishes the diagnosis. There is no effective treatment for lymphangioleiomyomatosis, but on-going therapeutic trials with rapamycin appear promising, and, finally, lung transplantation is available.

Lymphangioleiomyomatosis occurs sporadically. However, a significant minority of cases are associated with tuberous sclerosis complex, an autosomal dominant syndrome characterized by hamartoma-like tumor growths. Rarely, lymphangioleiomyomatosis is associated with multiple soft tissue tumors, including a large solitary fibrous tumor of the lung, a huge cavernous hemangioma of the liver, a meningioma of the right pontocerebellar angle, and a focus of nodular stromal hyperplasia of the ovary, in addition to endocrine tumors, including a papillary carcinoma of the thyroid gland and a parathyroid adenoma, indicating a possible tumor syndrome.[10] However, no familiar cases have been reported thus far.

At the molecular level, the tumor suppressor genes TSC1 and TSC2 (tuberous sclerosis complex 1 and 2) have been implicated in the pathogenesis of lymphangioleiomyomatosis, with mutations and LOH in TSC2 in lymphangioleiomyomatosis cells. TSC1 encodes hamartin, with a postulated role in actin cytoskeleton reorganization.[9] TSC2, which may play a central role as a tumor suppressor gene in tumorigenesis of lymphangioleiomyomatosis, encodes tuberin, a protein with roles in cell growth and proliferation, transcriptional activation, and endocytosis. Lymphangioleiomyomatosis cells, as defined by TSC2 LOH, have been detected in blood and body fluids and can metastasize. Studies have further indicated that TSC2 may play a putative tumor suppressor role in aberrant growth of smooth muscle-like cells in lymphangioleiomyomatosis.[11]

Lymphangioleiomyomatosis

Lymphangioleiomyomatosis is a rare progressive disease of women predominantly of child-bearing age that is characterized by a proliferation of abnormal smooth muscle-

Solitary Fibrous Tumor

Solitary fibrous tumors are rare neoplasms that typically develop in the pleura but have been reported in lung parenchyma as well[12] and at a variety of other locations.

A rare familial case has been documented.[13] The tumor was first described by Klemperer and Rabin in 1931.[14] It was initially termed *localized mesothelioma*, because the tumor was believed to arise from mesothelial cells and were circumscribed. However, immunohistochemical evidence reveals that these fibrous lesions originate from the submesothelial mesenchyme rather than from mesothelial cells. Solitary fibrous tumors of the pleura express vimentin, which is a marker of mesenchymal cells, and do not express cytoplasmic keratins, which are found in mesotheliomas. Electron microscopy has confirmed that these tumors are of mesenchymal rather than mesothelial origin.[15] Solitary fibrous tumors of the pleura typically present in the sixth and seventh decades of life, and occasionally in the pediatric population.[16] Clinically, benign solitary fibrous tumors of the pleura may be associated with paraneoplastic syndromes, especially clubbing and hypoglycemia. Although a solitary fibrous tumor is usually a slow-growing tumor with favorable prognosis, recurrence with malignant progression after complete resection rarely occurs; a small number of de novo malignant cases have been reported. Histologically, all the tumors are characterized by a proliferation of patternless bland spindle cells with variable amounts of thick, often hyalinized or keloid-like collagen bundles. Highly cellular areas may be focally observed and accompanied by frequent mitoses and cellular pleomorphism. Most if not all tumors show characteristic immunoreactivity for CD34. Immunoreactivity to Bcl-2 protein is also common. The labeling indices of p53, MDM2 protein, and Ki-67 are generally low. Although most benign solitary fibrous tumors of the pleura are small, some are huge pedunculated tumors.[17] These tumors may be present for many years and do not cause symptoms until they are quite large. The malignant tumors are often >10cm on presentation.

A recent report documented the presence of solitary fibrous tumors of the pleura in a mother and daughter.[13] The event may be due to chance, exposure to a common environmental agent, or a germline mutation that was genetically transmitted. The gene or chromosome responsible for solitary fibrous tumors of the pleura has not yet been identified. Different cytogenetic studies of solitary fibrous tumors of the pleura have been reported,[18-20] including trisomies 8, 21, and 5. Miettinen and coworkers, using comparative genomic hybridization (CGH), showed that changes in DNA copy number occurred more commonly in those solitary fibrous tumors that were >10cm and in those with greater mitotic activity.[17] We analyzed 15 solitary fibrous tumors and 11 hemangiopericytomas by CGH, a powerful molecular cytogenetic tool that can be applied to DNA extracted from formaldehyde-fixed and paraffin-embedded tissue. All of these tumors were immunohistochemically similar and showed reactivity for CD34 antigen but not for keratins, desmin, or muscle actins. Only one solitary fibrous tumor <10cm showed

DNA copy number changes (a single loss in chromosome 13), but seven of eight solitary fibrous tumors >10cm (including all four tumors with more than 4 mitoses per 10 high power fields) showed changes, mostly chromosomal gains in 5q 7, 8, 12, and 18. Four cases showed losses, two of them in chromosome 13 and two others in 20q. These findings suggest that CGH might be useful in the evaluation of malignant transformation of solitary fibrous tumors. The most common change, gain of the entire chromosome 8, seen in two cases as the only change, suggests trisomy 8 and parallels a similar finding previously described in other fibrous tumors, such as subsets of desmoid fibromatosis and infantile fibrosarcoma. In contrast, hemangiopericytomas, including large and mitotically active tumors, showed no DNA copy number changes on CGH. This suggests that hemangiopericytomas are genetically different from solitary fibrous tumors.

Other complex translocations in solitary fibrous tumors have been identified. A breakpoint in chromosome 4 was found in case reports of solitary fibrous tumors in both pleural and peritoneal locations.[20] Debiec-Rychter et al. reported a malignant solitary fibrous tumor with a 47,XY,t(4;9)(q13;p23), +5 karyotype.[18] This chromosome 4q13 breakpoint and pleural solitary fibrous tumor with a 46,XY,t(4;15)(q13;q26) karyotype was further characterized by fluorescence in situ hybridization analysis and localized within the 5-cm interval that was flanked by regions specific to YAC clones 761A7 and 886C11. Chromosome translocations involving chromosome 4q13 may characterize a separate cytogenetic subgroup of solitary fibrous tumors. Dal Cin et al. have also reported a special chromosome abnormality in a solitary fibrous tumor.[19] They found trisomy 21 as the sole chromosome abnormality in a solitary fibrous tumor. Nevertheless, these are individual case studies that need confirmation. Given that no consistent chromosomal abnormality has been reported, further cytogenetic or molecular genetic investigations of solitary fibrous tumors are in order.

In a polymerase chain reaction–single strand conformational polymorphism analysis of solitary fibrous tumors and a subsequent sequence analysis of the *p53* gene disclosed a point mutation at codon 161 in exon 5 in 1 of the 13 cases analyzed. According to follow-up information, none of the patients had developed local recurrence or distant metastasis even in a higher histologic grade group. Complete surgical excision and long-term follow-up are advisable for patients with solitary fibrous tumors.

Lipomatous Neoplasms

Various morphologic features of lipomatous neoplasms are associated with specific chromosomal patterns and clinical features such as age, sex, and tumor site, location, and size. Simple lipomas are known to be karyotypically heterogeneous, but this has not been correlated with clinicopathologic features. Willen and coworkers, in the Soft Tissue Tumor Study Group, systemically examined 165 cases of solitary soft tissue lipomas; short-term cultures were analyzed cytogenetically.[21] The karyotypes were divided into the following groups: normal karyotype; 12q13–15 aberrations; 6p rearrangements; 13q rearrangements, 8q11–13 aberrations; and ring or giant marker chromosomes or both. An abnormal chromosomal pattern was observed in 129 of 165 cases (78%). Apart from the finding that normal karyotypes were more common in patients younger than 30 years, there was no significant association between cytogenetic pattern and patient sex or age or tumor localization, size, or depth. Although the pathogenetic basis and clinicopathologic relevance (if any) of the cytogenetic subtypes among benign lipomas remain unexplained, more evidence suggests that a 12q13–15 aberration may play a role in tumorigenesis of lipomatous lesions.

Chromosome segment 12q13→q15 recombines with many different chromosome bands in lipomas, and a dozen recurrent translocations have been identified. The HMGA2 gene is often rearranged. Fusion genes between HMGA2 (12q14→q15) and LPP (3q27→q28), LHFP (13q12), and CMKOR1 (2q37) have been reported. Most recently, Nilsson and colleagues systematically studied eight lipomas with rearrangements involving chromosome bands 12q14→q15 and 5q32→q33.[22] They demonstrated that in chromosome 5, five of the cases had a breakpoint in the 5′ part of EBF in 5q33, while three cases had breakpoints located about 200 kb 3′ of EBF. In chromosome 12, the breakpoints clustered to the region of HMGA2. Four cases had breaks within the gene and four had breaks 5′ to HMGA2, where the gene BC058822 is located. Two versions of an HMGA2/EBF fusion transcript were detected in one case; one transcript was in frame and the other out of frame. Identical EBF/BC058822 fusion transcripts, seen in two cases, one of which also had the HMGA2/EBF transcript, were out of frame and resulted in truncation of EBF. Because EBF and HMGA2 have different orientations, the findings must be explained by complex aberrations including multiple breaks. The combined data indicate that the pathogenetically significant event that contributes to the tumor development is fusion, truncation, or transcriptional activation of HMGA2.

Myxoid Liposarcoma

Myxoid liposarcomas are characterized cytogenetically by a t(12;16)(q13;p11).[23] It is reasonable to assume that this translocation corresponds to the consistent rearrangement of one or two genes in 12q13 and/or 16p11

and that the loci thus affected are important in the normal control of fat cell differentiation and proliferation. An elegant study was performed with the Southern blot technique to test whether a gene of the CCAAT/enhancer binding protein (C/EBP) family, CHOP, which maps to 12q13 and is assumed to be involved in adipocyte differentiation, could be the 12q gene in question.[24] Using a cDNA probe that spans the CHOP coding region, Aman et al. detected one rearranged and one wild-type allele in nine of nine myxoid liposarcomas with t(12;16).[23] With polymerase chain reaction–generated, site-specific probes corresponding to the noncoding exons 1 and 2 and intron 2 of CHOP, rearrangements in five of seven tumors mapped to the 2.4 and 1.6 kbp PstI fragments that contain the first two exons and introns of the gene and the upstream promoter region. In contrast to the findings in myxoid liposarcomas, no tumor without a t(12;16) exhibited aberrant CHOP restriction digest patterns.

Chondroma and Chondrosarcoma

Myxoid chondrosarcoma is a soft tissue neoplasm cytogenetically characterized by the translocations t(9;22)(q22;q11–12) or t(9;17)(q22;q11), generating EWS/CHN or RBP56/CHN fusion genes, respectively.[25] However, genetic aberrations in other cartilaginous tumors have not yet been well characterized. Early data showed that nonrandom chromosome loci are aberrantly affected in cartilaginous lesions and that these abnormalities may be of significant histopathogenetic consequence.[26]

A recent study performed by Ozaki and associates showed some interesting results and advanced our understanding of the tumorigenesis of cartilaginous tumors.[27] Particularly, the authors analyzed the molecular–chromosomal aberrations in 10 chondrosarcomas (4 grade III tumors, 4 grade II tumors, and 2 grade I tumors) and in three benign cartilaginous tumors. Genomic imbalances were detected in 9 of 10 cases of chondrosarcomas. The median number of changes was 7.0 per tumor (range 0–23) and the gain-to-loss ratio was 1:1.4. The most frequent gains involved 7q, 5p, or 21q and the most frequent losses were 17p, 13q, 16p, or 22q. The three benign cartilaginous tumors each had two (zero gains and two losses), six (one gain and five losses), and eight (one gain and seven losses) chromosomal aberrations. Both of the gains occurred on 13q21, and losses were frequently observed on chromosomes 19 and 22q in all three cases. Losses of chromosome 16p, 17p, 22q, or 19 were common in both chondrosarcomas and benign cartilaginous tumors. However, aberrations from chromosomes 2 to 11, 14, 15, 18, or 21 were detected only in chondrosarcomas. Therefore, although the number of aberrations between benign and malignant cartilaginous tumors appears to be similar, these two entities may be differentiated by determining which chromosomes are affected. In addition, these chromosome abnormalities appear to be diagnostically and prognostically valuable in classifying and grading chondromatous neoplasms.

Vascular Lesions

Many vascular lesions represent intriguing examples of developmental dysmorphogenesis. Their diversity reflects the multiple factors involved in the proper regulation of vasculogenesis and angiogenesis. Molecular discoveries have indicted genes expressed in endothelial cells and involved in receptor signaling. These mutated genes encode tyrosine kinase receptors and intracellular signaling molecules. It is clear that derangements in transforming growth factor-β signaling are involved in formation of arteriovenous malformations, but only in hereditary hemorrhagic telangiectasia. There may also be a role for extracellular matrix components in the evolution of vascular anomalies. For example, endothelial-to-smooth muscle cell signaling could occur via extracellular matrix. This is corroborated by the fact that there are differences in supporting cells for venous and capillary–venous anomalies.[28]

Traditional strategies for treatment of vascular anomalies are based on destroying the vascular spaces, using laser or intralesional injection of sclerosing agents, and surgical resection. Identification of causative genes opens the door to biologic therapy. Transgenic animal models could be used to identify modifying factors, evaluate novel treatments, and devise ways to prevent evolution of a vascular malformation. Animal models of vascular anomalies will also facilitate the study of molecular pathways controlling vasculogenesis and angiogenesis. Already, vascular epithelial growth factor and angiopoietin are known to be associated with developmental as well as tumor-induced angiogenesis. Other common disorders involving dysregulation of vascular growth could be due to deranged signaling. Thus, identification of these genes could expose therapeutic targets for a wide range of angiogenic disorders.

Using linkage analysis, Boon et al. established that some families with inherited venous malformations show linkage to chromosome 9p21; the mutation causes ligand-independent activation of an endothelial cell-specific receptor tyrosine kinase, TIE-2.[29] The authors have demonstrated that vascular malformations with glomus cells (known as glomangiomas), inherited as an autosomal dominant trait in five families, are not linked to 9p21 but, instead, link to a new locus, on 1p21–p22, called VMGLOM (lod score 12.70 at recombination fraction). It is likely that venous tumors (i.e., glomangiomas) are caused by mutations in a novel gene that may act to regulate angiogenesis, in concert with the TIE-2 signaling pathway.

Glomus Tumors

Glomus tumors typically have a solid pattern of sharply demarcated, round glomus cells with prominent, mildly dilated pericytoma-like vessels. Vascular invasion and focal atypia are relatively common, and low mitotic activity (less than 4 mitoses per 50 high power fields) is occasionally seen. Immunohistochemically, tumors are typically positive for α-smooth muscle actin and calponin, and nearly all had a net-like pericellular laminin and collagen type IV positivity. Tumors are usually negative for desmin and S100 protein. Miettinen et al. studied 34 gastric glomus tumors and found that all tumors lacked Kit expression and the gold-intensified staining technique–specific mutations in the c-Kit gene.[30]

Epithelioid Hemangioendothelioma and Angiosarcoma

Pulmonary epithelioid hemangioendothelioma is an intermediate-grade vascular tumor with a distinctive epithelioid character and intraalveolar and intravascular growth. Epithelioid angiosarcoma is high-grade epithelioid vascular malignancy. Epithelioid hemangioendotheliomas arise from endothelial cells. They are readily immunoreactive with endothelial markers such as CD31, CF34, and factor VIII. Ultrastructurally, conspicuous 100–150 μm thick cytofilaments are present, and Weibel-Palade bodies are usually seen. However, little is known regarding the genetics of epithelioid hemangioendothelioma. In two cases, an identical chromosomal translocation involving chromosomes 1 and 3 (t 1:3) was noted.

Other Sarcomas

Pulmonary Synovial Sarcoma

Pulmonary synovial sarcoma is a malignant mesenchymal tumor that displays varied epithelial differentiation. Although it is commonly seen as a metastatic tumor, it rarely occurs in the lung. The histogenesis of pulmonary synovial sarcoma is unknown. It is postulated that it arises from a totipotential stromal cell. The cytogenetic characteristics of synovial sarcoma is the t(X,18)(p11;q11) translocation.[31] This translocation, identified by fluorescence in situ hybridization or reverse transcriptase polymerase chain reaction using paraffin-embedded tissue, gives rise to the fusion of the SYT gene on 18p11 to the SSX1/SSX2 gene on Xq11.

Pulmonary Artery Sarcoma

Pulmonary artery sarcoma is a sarcoma arising from the large pulmonary arteries. It can display fibroblastic, myofibroblastic, or smooth muscle differentiation. Com-

33
Primary Versus Metastatic Cancer: Gene Expression Profiling

Jaishree Jagirdar and Philip T. Cagle

General Comments

Accurate identification of the primary site of a cancer is important to predict prognosis and select appropriate therapy. Approximately 10%–15% of cancers initially present as metastases to solid organs, body cavities, or lymph nodes. However, the primary site of the metastatic cancer is not always clinically apparent. About 3%–5% of all cancers are carcinomas of unknown primary, making this type of tumor one of the 10 most frequent cancers in the world.[1–9] Even with autopsy, in a series published in 2005 by Al-Brahim et al., a primary site was identified in only 51% of 53 cases of metastatic cancer of unknown origin.[9]

Primary lung carcinoma is a common cancer and the most frequent cause of cancer death, but the lung is also rich in vasculature through which the entire systemic blood supply flows for oxygenation. As a result, metastatic carcinoma is even more common in the lung than is primary lung carcinoma. In most cases, the primary site is already known clinically when a metastasis appears in the lung, and biopsy and histopathologic diagnosis of the metastatic tumor are not necessary. However, the patient with a cancer of unknown primary in the lung is a classic and relatively common diagnostic dilemma in clinical pulmonary medicine, clinical oncology, surgical pathology, and cytopathology.[10–15]

The combination of clinical, radiologic, and histopathologic findings have been traditionally used to assess whether a mass or masses in the lung are from a primary lung cancer or nonpulmonary metastatic cancer and, if the latter, to assess the probable primary site of the metastasis. However, a metastatic cancer can potentially mimic a primary carcinoma of the lung in all of these traditional evaluations and vice versa, and many cases remain of unknown or equivocal origin based with these modalities.

Background: Value of Immunohistochemistry

Immunohistochemistry has proven useful for many cases of lung masses of unknown primary. Specific markers such as thyroid transcription factor 1 (TTF-1) for lung or thyroid primary and prostate-specific antigen for metastatic prostate cancer are the most useful if positive. Cytokeratins 7 (CK7) and 20 (CK20) have been useful in distinguishing primary lung carcinoma (CK7 positive, CK20 negative) from common metastatic colon carcinoma (CK7 negative, CK20 positive). The exception to this is that a primary mucinous carcinoma of the lung assumes the same CK7 and CK20 profile as the colonic carcinoma. Immunohistochemistry is also very valuable when the morphology is ambiguous in small fine-needle aspiration specimens. We have found a combination of TTF-1, renal cell carcinoma Ma (RCC Ma), and CD10 very valuable in distinguishing metastatic renal cell carcinoma to the lung from a lung primary.[16,17] Renal cell carcinoma Ma is a monoclonal antibody generated against a fraction of normal human renal proximal tubule. Renal cell carcinomas are RCC Ma and CD10 positive, whereas only a small fraction of lung tumors are positive for CD10 and none are positive for RCC Ma. Conversely, all renal cell carcinomas are negative for TTF-1, whereas 75% of lung non–small cell carcinomas are positive for TTF-1. However, even with immunohistochemistry, the primary site is not identified in many cases.[10–15] Using an algorithm and a panel first with 27 immunohistochemical markers and then with 10 immunohistochemical markers, some 12% of primary and paired metastatic carcinomas were still not correctly identified.[15]

341

Molecular Markers in the Differential Diagnosis of Primary Versus Metastatic Tumor to the Lung: Are We There?

Similar to the phenotypic markers detected by immunohistochemistry, hypothetically, some molecular genetic markers might differentiate between primary sites of tumors provided that the genetic markers are unique to a specific primary site. Many common abnormalities of the genes and gene products of the cell cycle, signaling pathways, and transcription factors are similar or the same in primary carcinomas of the lung and in metastatic carcinomas from various sites and therefore are not useful in differentiating the primary site of a tumor. Only those molecular genetic markers that are specific or relatively restricted to specific primary sites are candidates for identification of a primary site.[12,13]

Microarray platforms allow investigation of the expression of thousands of genes at one time to identify molecular genetic markers of potential diagnostic utility. Examples of molecular markers that have been reported to be specific or restricted for a primary site of an adenocarcinoma are listed in Table 33.1.[18,19] Diagnostic genes detectable by reverse transcription polymerase chain reaction (RT-PCR) are recognized for several sarcomas that might metastasize to the lung and are only rarely primary in the lung, including the *SYT/SSX* fusion genes in synovial sarcomas and the *EWS/ETS* fusion genes in the Ewing family of sarcomas (see Chapters 32 and 35).[20,21] The testing for a specific molecular marker on rare occasion requiring extended times to obtain results is not a practical approach for most pathology or molecular diagnostics laboratories. As molecular diagnostics has grown into a regular participant in routine clinical diagnostics, platforms for rapid, high throughput molecular diagnoses of the sites of origin of cancers have been explored.

TABLE 33.1. Markers for specific primary sites of adenocarcinomas.

Primary site	Marker
Prostate	Prostate-specific antigen, lipophilin B
Breast	Mammoglobin 1, lipophilin B
Pancreas	thyroid transcription factor 2, prostate stem cell antigen, metallothionein-IL, glutathione peroxidase 2
Stomach	Pepsinogen C
Bladder	Uroplakin II
Colon	Mucin 2, A33, glutathione peroxidase 2
Ovary	Lipophilin B
Lung	Thyroid transcription factor 1 (provided thyroid primary excluded)

Gene expression profiling, using microarray platforms (cDNA or oligonucleotide) as described in Chapter 12, is a new approach to the molecular diagnosis of the primary sites of cancers.[18,22–30] In theory, gene expression profiling involves detecting a pattern of gene expressions from a tumor sample of unknown type and site of origin that matches the expected gene expression pattern of a known type of tumor from a known primary site. The investigator collects tumors that can be classified as being from a known primary site, for example, adenocarcinomas of the lung, colon, breast, and prostate. These groups of tumors representing the different primary sites are used as a "training set." Genes that correlate with tumors from each of the primary sites are known as *informative genes* or *predictor genes*, and identification of a threshold number of these informative genes in a tumor indicates the probable primary site of the tumor. Simplistically, one can think of this as follows: if a tumor expresses 8 out of 10 genes for lung cancer and only 1 or 2 for colon, breast, or prostate, that tumor has a higher probability of being a lung cancer. A computer is trained to recognize the gene profiles that correspond to a particular primary site using the training set of tumors, and the patterns are validated using a "test set" of tumors, which are of unknown primary site ("blinded") to the computer. Because the investigator knows the primary site of the tumors in the test set, the accuracy of prediction by gene expression profiling can be calculated. In reality, the number of potential informative/predictor genes examined, determination of the relative weight to give to each of these many genes, and the calculations of the probable primary site from this information for each of many tumors are complex.

Recently, an expression profile of lung adenocarcinomas showed two distinct subgroups of primary lung adenocarcinomas. One group had a specific profile of terminal respiratory unit and was associated with higher incidence of *EGFR* (epidermal growth factor) mutations, while the other group was classified as a nonterminal respiratory unit type of adenocarcinoma associated with nonspecific cell cycling and proliferation markers. The former group with the lung-specific profile related to normal lung function and could be exploited in distinguishing primary lung from metastatic carcinoma.[31] The process involves the use of algorithms, statistics, software programs, and sophisticated "site of origin classifiers" such as support vector machines and artificial neural networks, as discussed later.

Because many thousands of genes can now be probed with microarray technology, the number of data points to be evaluated is extremely large in each experiment. For example, Su et al. hybridized RNA from 100 tumors from 10 different primary sites in their training set to oligonucleotide microarrays containing probe sets for 12,533 genes, which resulted in 1.25×10^6 data points from which they selected 110 genes that most accurately predicted origin from 1 of the 10 primary sites.[18]

Several investigators have reported on the feasibility of gene expression profiling as a molecular diagnostic tool. In 1999, Golub et al. reported success in differentiating between acute myeloid leukemia and acute lymphoblastic leukemia based on global gene expression analysis of patient samples using DNA microarrays.[23] From 6,817 genes, they found that 1,100 genes were more highly correlated with distinguishing between acute myeloid leukemia and acute lymphoblastic leukemia class than would be expected by chance. They selected 50 informative genes that they thought were the best predictors of diagnosis on the basis of 38 samples with known diagnosis of acute myeloid leukemia or acute lymphoblastic leukemia. This was applied to an independent collection of 34 leukemia samples and made strong predictions for 29 of the 34 samples, reporting an accuracy of 100%. Their work demonstrated the feasibility of cancer classification based solely on gene expression.

Khan et al. used gene expression profiles or "signatures" and artificial neural networks (ANNs) to classify cancers in specific diagnostic categories.[24] Artificial neural networks are computer-based algorithms that imitate the behavior of neurons in the brain that can closely approximate any nonlinear function and are trained to recognize and classify complex patterns. Beginning with a cDNA microarray containing 6,567 genes, they found that they could correctly classify small, round, blue cell tumors into one of four diagnoses with 96 genes and ANN. They used the ANN models calibrated with the 96 genes on 25 "blinded" samples and were able to correctly classify all 20 samples of small, round, blue cell tumors and rejected 5 samples that were not in this category.

In their test set, Su et al., as mentioned earlier, predicted the correct site of origin in 71 of 75 cases, including 11 of 12 metastases.[18] Ramaswamy et al. used microarrays containing 16,063 oligonucleotide probe sets to identify the gene expression profiles of 144 primary tumors from 14 common cancer categories.[25] They reported an overall classification accuracy of 78% with gene expression profiling compared with an accuracy of 9% by random classification. However, poorly differentiated cancers were not accurately classified according to their site of origin, suggesting that poorly differentiated cancers have significantly different gene expression patterns compared with better differentiated cancers from the same site. Giordano et al. used oligonucleotide microarrays with 7,129 gene probe sets to obtain gene expression profiles of 57 pulmonary, 51 colonic, and 46 ovarian adenocarcinomas.[26] Using statistical analyses, they state that they were able to correctly classify the site of origin of 152 of 154 of the adenocarcinomas. These early studies demonstrate the feasibility of gene expression profiling for diagnosing the site of origin of a cancer of unknown origin.

Bloom et al. reported high levels of accuracy that they thought were acceptable for clinical application by using an ANN-based classification technique that was capable of classifying both cDNA platform and oligonucleotide platform data as well as mixed platform data, derived from multiple tumor types.[27] They constructed a cDNA-based tumor classifier, an oligonucleotide-based tumor classifier, and a mixed platform, multitissue classifier to exploit both types of data. They reported that their classifiers were capable of evaluating 21 different tumor types with up to an 88% accuracy rate using as few as 400 genes.

Rather than a complex classifier based on support vector machines and ANNs, Shedden et al. proposed a simplified method for the molecular classification of primary sites using a tree-based framework based on tumor morphology, progressing sequentially from coarse to fine classification with each sequential decision using a nearest neighbor predictor.[28] This approach is very familiar to surgical pathologists and, indeed, resembles how histopathologic diagnoses are made routinely. These investigators used microarray data sets from three previous studies mentioned earlier, those of Ramaswamy et al.,[25] Giordano et al.,[26] and Su et al.[18] The authors stated that they were able to correctly classify 157 of 190 cancers using as few as 45 genes, comparable to the results obtained with sophisticated site of origin classifiers using thousands of genes.

In 2005, Tothill et al. reported generating gene expression data using both a quantitative PCR platform and a microarray platform.[29] These were used to train and validate a cross-platform support vector machine. They indicated that their microarray support vector machine classifier was able to make high confidence predictions of site of origin in 11 of 13 cancers of unknown origin.

In 2006, Ma et al. investigated an RT-PCR–based expression assay involving 92 genes using routine formalin-fixed, paraffin-embedded tissue samples to accurately and objectively identify the sites of origin of cancers.[30] They measured expressions of 22,000 genes in a microarray database of 466 frozen and 112 formalin-fixed, paraffin-embedded samples of both primary and metastatic cancers. Using an algorithm, they determined gene combinations that were optimal for multitumor classification. They designed a 92-gene RT-PCR assay to generate a database for 481 frozen and 119 formalin-fixed, paraffin-embedded tumor samples. Their microarray-based classifier showed 84% accuracy in classifying the site of origin for 39 tumor types via cross-validation and 82% accuracy in predicting the site of origin for 112 independent formalin-fixed, paraffin-embedded samples. Ma et al. were able to successfully translate the microarray database to the RT-PCR platform, permitting an overall success rate of 87% in correctly classifying the site of origin for 32 different tumor classes in the validation set of 119 tumor samples.[30] Because their system uses RT-PCR and formalin-fixed, paraffin-embedded tissues, the authors concluded that their platform was suitable for rapid clinical adoption.

Molecular Markers in the Differentiation of Synchronous and Metachronous Lung Lesions Versus Recurrence/Metastases

Patients with pulmonary neoplasms are at an increased risk for a second tumor in the lung either at the same time or later in their life.[32–34] The incidence of multiple separate primary tumors of the lung has been reported to range from 0.2% to 2.0% of patients with lung carcinomas.[35,36] It is important to determine whether the second tumor represents a true independent primary or recurrence/metastasis, because it will significantly change the staging of the tumor and therefore management and prognosis of the patient. Histology is often the same in the two tumors, which makes it difficult to distinguish the two possibilities based on morphologic examination alone.[37–39] More than 30 years ago, Martini and Melamed proposed criteria for the diagnosis of independent primary tumors of the lung (the so-called synchronous and metachronous tumors).[38] These criteria have been widely used for patient management. In 1995, Antakli et al. proposed modified criteria for distinguishing synchronous/metachronous primaries from recurrence or metastases.[40] These criteria included anatomically distinct lesions with associated premalignant lesions, with no systemic metastases, mediastinal spread, and a different DNA ploidy. However, the survival for these patients with supposedly stage I diseases (especially synchronous tumors) showed large variations in different series,[36,41–43] which may be explained by the arbitrary nature of the conventional criteria and their lack of biologic and molecular basis. In addition, the criteria proposed include parameters such as morphology, location, presence or absence of in situ lesion, and vascular invasion, which can only be applied to resection or autopsy specimens but not at the time of biopsy when this information would be most useful clinically. Technical advances have been made in recent years that allow microdissection of nearly pure populations of tumor cells. As a result, we can analyze tumor cells in detail to determine their clonality. Molecular study of oncogenes and tumor suppressors and X-chromosome inactivation are some of the commonly used methods for clonality analysis.[44–55]

Loss of heterozygosity (LOH) analysis in tumor cells has been widely used with success.[56–62] Tumor cells that are clonal often show similar patterns of LOH when multiple genes and chromosomal loci are analyzed.[56,59–62]

Using microdissection and LOH analysis, we studied specimens from patients with multiple pulmonary neoplasms to determine if modern techniques can help us distinguish true independent primary from recurrence/metastasis.[63] We approached this problem by microdissecting malignant cells and comparing patterns of LOH of multiple genes and chromosomal loci between paired tumors. We found that primary tumors of the lung and their metastasis share nearly identical patterns of LOH. In contrast, most synchronous and metachronous tumors as defined by the current arbitrary criteria appeared to be genetically different; therefore, they likely represented independent primary tumors. Rare synchronous tumors had similar genetic profiles, raising the possibility of recurrence/metastasis. Our data suggest that molecular analysis can help fingerprint tumors and has the potential to significantly impact management and prognosis of patients.[63] The LOH studies need to be further investigated and confirmed by more elaborate gene profiling.

Although the use of gene expression profiling to identify a primary lung cancer from a nonpulmonary metastasis, and, if the latter, to identify the site of origin is promising, it has not yet received clinical application. The use of platforms that are established and readily available in the clinical laboratory and that provide meaningful turnaround time in the clinical setting will make molecular classification of cancers of unknown or equivocal origin much more practical in the future.

References

1. Nystrom JS, Weiner JM, Heffelfinger-Juttner J, et al. Metastatic and histologic presentations in unknown primary cancer. Semin Oncol 1977;4:53–58.
2. Burton EC, Troxclair DA, Newman WP 3rd. Autopsy diagnoses of malignant neoplasms: how often are clinical diagnoses incorrect? JAMA 1998;280:1245–1248.
3. Hillen HFP. Unknown primary tumours. Postgrad Med J 2000;76:690–693.
4. Levi F, Te VC, Erler G, et al. Epidemiology of unknown primary tumours. Eur J Cancer 2002;38:1810–1812.
5. van de Wouw AJ, Janssen-Heijnen ML, Coebergh JW, Hillen HF. Epidemiology of unknown primary tumours; incidence and population-based survival of 1285 patients in Southeast Netherlands, 1984–1992. Eur J Cancer 2002;38:409–413.
6. Pavlidis N, Briasoulis E, Hainsworth J, Greco FA. Diagnostic and therapeutic management of cancer of an unknown primary. Eur J Cancer 2003;39:1990–2005.
7. Varadhachary GR, Abbruzzese JL, Lenzi R. Diagnostic strategies for unknown primary cancer. Cancer 2004;100:1776–1785.
8. Pavlidis N, Fizazi K. Cancer of unknown primary (CUP). Crit Rev Oncol Hematol 2005;54:243–250.
9. Al-Brahim N, Ross C, Carter B, Chorneyko K. The value of postmortem examination in cases of metastasis of unknown origin-20-year retrospective data from a tertiary care center. Ann Diagn Pathol 2005;9:77–80.

parative genomic hybridization revealed frequent gains or amplification of 12q13–q15 with amplification of SAS/CDK4, MDM2 and GLI. In addition, there was amplification of platelet-derived growth factor receptor A on 4q12. Less consistent alterations have been identified, including losses on 3p, 3q, 4q, 9p, 5p, 6p, and 11q.[32]

Alveolar Soft Part Sarcoma

Alveolar soft part sarcoma is a rare soft tissue tumor of unknown origin and pathogenesis. Alveolar soft part sarcoma was first described by Christophersen in 1952. It frequently occurs in people aged 15–35 years and shows a female preponderance. The most common site is in the lower extremities. These tumors are usually indolent in behavior but have a high propensity to recur locally after excision and to metastasize early. The lungs, brain, and bone are common sites of metastatic disease. The characteristic histopathologic features of an alveolar pattern and diastase-resistant periodic acid–Schiff positivity and rhomboid crystals are diagnostic. Renal cell carcinoma occasionally mimics alveolar soft part sarcoma but often shows a focal tubular pattern of growth and lacks the crystals. Extraadrenal paraganglioma can also simulate alveolar soft part sarcoma because of its organoid pattern, but it too lacks the characteristic crystals. There are no pathognomonic molecular markers for alveolar soft part sarcoma to date, although recent studies have shown that the crystals are immunoreactive to protein MCT1 (monocarboxylate transporter) and to CD147.[33] However, the significance of this finding is not known. The histogenesis of this tumor is the subject of extensive research, which has yielded results varying from skeletal muscle to neural origin. To date, none of the histogenetic hypotheses has been accepted.

Investigators clinicopathologically analyzed 16 cases of alveolar soft part sarcoma. They examined the expression of *hMSH2/hMLH1* of DNA mismatch repair genes by immunohistochemistry and the promoter hypermethylation of these DNA mismatch repair genes by methylation-specific polymerase chain reaction to elucidate any possible association between mutation status of these genes and inactivation of the *hMSH2/hMLH1* genes.[34] Furthermore, microsatellite instability analysis and LOH on chromosome 5q analysis were used for some cases of alveolar soft part sarcoma in which DNA derived from normal tissue was available. Three of eight (37.5%) alveolar soft part sarcomas showed low microsatellite instability, and two of these three cases showed immunohistochemical lack of expression for either *hMSH2* or *hMLH1*. Loss of heterozygosity on 5q was present in two of six (33.3%) informative cases, and both cases showed LOH on the D5S346 marker, a microsatellite marker near the *APC* locus. Thus, inactivation of *hMSH2/hMLH1* of DNA mismatch repair genes seems to have an impor-

tant role to play in the mutagenesis of the tumor-suppressor genes in alveolar soft part sarcoma.

References

1. Batinica S, Gunek G, Raos M, et al. Sclerosing haemangioma of the lung in a 4-year-old child. Eur J Pediatr Surg 2002;12(3):192–194.
2. Hosaka N, Sasaki T, Adachi K, et al. Pulmonary sclerosing hemangioma associated with familial adenomatous polyposis. Hum Pathol 2004;35(6):764–768.
3. Devouassoux-Shisheboran M, de la Fouchardiere A, Thivolet-Bejui F, et al. Endobronchial variant of sclerosing hemangioma of the lung: histological and cytological features on endobronchial material. Mod Pathol 2004;17(2):252–257.
4. Devouassoux-Shisheboran M, Hayashi T, Linnoila RI, et al. A clinicopathologic study of 100 cases of pulmonary sclerosing hemangioma with immunohistochemical studies: TTF-1 is expressed in both round and surface cells, suggesting an origin from primitive respiratory epithelium. Am J Surg Pathol 2000;24(7):906–916.
5. Yamazaki K. Type-II pneumocyte differentiation in pulmonary sclerosing hemangioma: ultrastructural differentiation and immunohistochemical distribution of lineage-specific transcription factors (TTF-1, HNF-3 alpha, and HNF-3 beta) and surfactant proteins. Virchows Arch 2004;445(1):45–53.
6. Wang E, Lin D, Wang Y, et al. Immunohistochemical and ultrastructural markers suggest different origins for cuboidal and polygonal cells in pulmonary sclerosing hemangioma. Hum Pathol 2004;35(4):503–508.
7. Dacic S, Sasatomi E, Swalsky PA, et al. Loss of heterozygosity patterns of sclerosing hemangioma of the lung and bronchioloalveolar carcinoma indicate a similar molecular pathogenesis. Arch Pathol Lab Med 2004;128(8):880–884.
8. Wu CT, Chang YL, Lee YC. Expression of the estrogen receptor beta in 37 surgically treated pulmonary sclerosing hemangiomas in comparison with non–small cell lung carcinomas. Hum Pathol 2005;36(10):1108–1112.
9. Steagall WK, Taveira-DaSilva AM, Moss J. Clinical and molecular insights into lymphangioleiomyomatosis. Sarcoidosis Vasc Diffuse Lung Dis 2005;22(Suppl 1):S49–S66.
10. Cagnano M, Benharroch D, Geffen DB. Pulmonary lymphangioleiomyomatosis. Report of a case with associated multiple soft-tissue tumors. Arch Pathol Lab Med 1991;115(12):1257–1259.
11. Goncharova EA, Goncharov DA, Spaits M, et al. Abnormal growth of smooth muscle-like cells in lymphangioleiomyomatosis: role for tumor suppressor TSC2. Am J Respir Cell Mol Biol 2006;34(5):561–572.
12. Patsios D, Hwang DM, Chung TB. Intraparenchymal solitary fibrous tumor of the lung: an uncommon cause of a pulmonary nodule. J Thorac Imaging 2006;21(1):50–53.
13. Jha V, Gil J, Teirstein AS. Familial solitary fibrous tumor of the pleura: a case report. Chest 2005;127(5):1852–1854.
14. Tagliabue F, Vertemati G, Confalonieri G, et al. Benign solitary fibrous tumour of the pleura: a clinical review and report of six cases. Chir Ital 2005;57(5):649–653.
15. Morimitsu Y, Nakajima M, Hisaoka M, Hashimoto H. Extrapleural solitary fibrous tumor: clinicopathologic study

of 17 cases and molecular analysis of the p53 pathway. APMIS 2000;108(9):617–625.

16. Kanamori Y, Hashizume K, Sugiyama M, et al. Intrapulmonary solitary fibrous tumor in an eight-year-old male. Pediatr Pulmonol 2005;40(3):261–264.

17. Miettinen MM, el-Rifai W, Sarlomo-Rikala M, et al. Tumor size-related DNA copy number changes occur in solitary fibrous tumors but not in hemangiopericytomas. Mod Pathol 1997;10(12):1194–1200.

18. Debiec-Rychter M, de Wever I, Hagemeijer A, Sciot R. Is 4q13 a recurring breakpoint in solitary fibrous tumors? Cancer Genet Cytogenet 2001;131(1):69–73.

19. Dal Cin P, Sciot R, Fletcher CD, et al. Trisomy 21 in solitary fibrous tumor. Cancer Genet Cytogenet 1996;86(1):58–60.

20. Travis WD, Churg A, Aubry MC, Ordonez NG. Mesenchymal tumors. In Travis WD, Brambilla E, Muller-Hermelink HK, Harris CC, eds. Pathology and Genetics. Tumours of the Lung, Pleura, Thymus and Heart. Lyon, France: IARC Press; 2004:141–144.

21. Willen H, Akerman M, Dal Cin P, et al. Comparison of chromosomal patterns with clinical features in 165 lipomas: a report of the CHAMP study group. Cancer Genet Cytogenet 1998;102(1):46–49.

22. Nilsson M, Mertens F, Hoglund M, et al. Truncation and fusion of HMGA2 in lipomas with rearrangements of 5q32→q33 and 12q14→q15. Cytogenet Genome Res 2006; 112(1–2):60–66.

23. Aman P, Ron D, Mandahl N, et al. Rearrangement of the transcription factor gene CHOP in myxoid liposarcomas with t(12;16)(q13;p11). Genes Chromosomes Cancer 1992; 5(4):278–285.

24. Yousem SA, Tazelaar HD, Manabe T, Dehner LP. Inflammatory myofibroblastic tumor. In Travis WD, Brambilla E, Muller-Hermelink HK, Harris CC, eds. Pathology and Genetics. Tumours of the Lung, Pleura, Thymus and Heart. Lyon, France: IARC Press; 2004:105–106.

25. Panagopoulos I, Mertens F, Isaksson M, et al. Molecular genetic characterization of the EWS/CHN and RBP56/CHN fusion genes in extraskeletal myxoid chondrosarcoma. Genes Chromosomes Cancer 2002;35(4):340–352.

26. Bridge JA, Bhatia PS, Anderson JR, Neff JR. Biologic and clinical significance of cytogenetic and molecular cytogenetic abnormalities in benign and malignant cartilaginous lesions. Cancer Genet Cytogenet 1993;69(2):79–90.

27. Ozaki T, Wai D, Schafer KL, et al. Comparative genomic hybridization in cartilaginous tumors. Anticancer Res 2004;24(3a):1721–1725.

28. Vikkula M, Boon LM, Mulliken JB. Molecular genetics of vascular malformations. Matrix Biol 2001;20(5–6):327–335.

29. Boon LM, Brouillard P, Irrthum A, et al. A gene for inherited cutaneous venous anomalies ("glomangiomas") localizes to chromosome 1p21–22. Am J Hum Genet 1999;65(1): 125–133.

30. Miettinen M, Paal E, Lasota J, Sobin LH. Gastrointestinal glomus tumors: a clinicopathologic, immunohistochemical, and molecular genetic study of 32 cases. Am J Surg Pathol 2002;26(3):301–311.

31. Essary LR, Vargas SO, Fletcher CD. Primary pleuropulmonary synovial sarcoma: reappraisal of a recently described anatomic subset. Cancer 2002;94:459–469.

32. Yi JE, Tazelaar HD, Burke A, Manabe T. Pulmonary artery sarcoma. In Travis WD, Brambilla E, Muller-Hermelink HK, Harris CC, eds. Pathology and Genetics. Tumours of the Lung, Pleura, Thymus and Heart. Lyon, France: IARC Press; 2004:109–110.

33. Saito T, Oda Y, Kawaguchi K, et al. Possible association between tumor-suppressor gene mutations and hMSH2/hMLH1 inactivation in alveolar soft part sarcoma. Hum Pathol 2003;34(9):841–849.

34. Ladanyi M, Antonescu CR, Drobnjak M, et al. The precrystalline cytoplasmic granules of alveolar soft part sarcoma contain monocarboxylate transporter 1 and CD147. Am J Pathol 2002;160(4):1215–1221.

10. Brown RW, Campagna LB, Dunn JK, Cagle PT. Immuno-histochemical identification of tumor markers in metastatic adenocarcinoma: A diagnostic adjunct in the determination of primary site. Am J Clin Pathol 1997;107:12–19.
11. Cagle PT. Differential diagnosis between primary and metastatic carcinomas. In Brambilla C, Brambilla E, eds. Lung Tumors: Fundamental Biology and Clinical Management. New York: Marcel Dekker; 1999:127–137.
12. Dail D, Cagle P, Marchevsky A, et al. Tumours of the lung: metastases to the lung. In Travis WD, Brambilla E, Harris CC, Muller-Hermelink HK, eds. World Health Organization Classification of Tumours, Pathology and Genetics: Tumours of the Lung, Pleura, Thymus and Heart. Lyon, France: IARC; 2004.
13. Cagle PT. Carcinoma of the lung. In Churg AM, Myers JL, Tazelaar HD, Wright JL, eds. Pathology of the Lung, 3rd ed. New York: Thieme; 2005:413–479.
14. Laga AC, Allen T, Bedrossian C, et al. Metastatic carcinoma. In Cagle PT, ed. The Color Atlas and Text of Pulmonary Pathology. New York: Lippincott Williams & Wilkins; 2005:77–79.
15. Dennis JL, Hvidsten TR, Wit EC, et al. Markers of adenocarcinoma characteristic of the site of origin: development of a diagnostic algorithm. Clin Cancer Res 2005;11:3766–3772.
16. McGregor DK, Khurana KK, Cao C, et al. Diagnosing primary and metastatic renal cell carcinoma: the use of the monoclonal antibody "renal cell carcinoma marker." Am J Surg Pathol 2001;25(12):1485–1492.
17. Butnor KJ, Nicholson AG, Allred DC, et al. Expression of renal cell carcinoma-associated markers erythropoietin, CD10, and renal cell carcinoma marker in diffuse malignant mesothelioma and metastatic renal cell carcinoma. Arch Pathol Lab Med 2006;130(6):823–827.
18. Su AI, Welsh JB, Sapinoso LM, et al. Molecular classification of human carcinomas by use of gene expression signatures. Cancer Res 2001;61:7388–7393.
19. Dennis JL, Vass JK, Wit EC, et al. Identification from public data of molecular markers of adenocarcinoma characteristic of the site of origin. Cancer Res 2002;62:5999–6005.
20. Sekido Y, Fong KM, Minna JD. Molecular genetics of lung cancer. Annu Rev Med 2003;54:73–87.
21. Sorensen PH, Triche TJ. Gene fusions encoding chimeric transcription factors in solid tumors. Semin Cancer Biol 1996;7:3–14.
22. Hill DA, O'Sulivan MJ, Zhu X, et al. Practical application of molecular genetic testing as an aid to the surgical pathologic diagnosis of sarcomas: a prospective study. Am J Surg Pathol 2002;26:965–977.
23. Golub TR, Slonim DK, Tamayo P, et al. Molecular classification of cancer: class discovery and class prediction by gene expression monitoring. Science 1999;286:531–537.
24. Khan J, Wei JS, Ringner M, Saal LH, et al. Classification and diagnostic prediction of cancers using gene expression profiling and artificial neural networks. Nat Med 2001;7:673–679.
25. Ramaswamy S, Tamayo P, Rifkin R, et al. Multiclass cancer diagnosis using tumor gene expression signatures. Proc Natl Acad Sci USA 2001;98:15149–15154.
26. Giordano TJ, Shedden KA, Schwartz DR, et al. Organ-specific molecular classification of primary lung, colon, and ovarian adenocarcinomas using gene expression profiles. Am J Pathol 2001;159:1231–1238.
27. Bloom G, Yang IV, Boulware D, et al. Multi-platform, multi-site, microarray-based human tumor classification. Am J Pathol 2004;164:9–16.
28. Shedden KA, Taylor JM, Giordano TJ, et al. Accurate molecular classification of human cancers based on gene expression using a simple classifier with a pathological tree-based framework. Am J Pathol 2003;163:1985–1995.
29. Tothill RW, Kowalczyk A, Rischin D, et al. An expression-based site of origin diagnostic method designed for clinical application to cancer of unknown origin. Cancer Res 2005;65:4031–4040.
30. Ma XJ, Patel R, Wang X, et al. Molecular classification of human cancers using a 92-gene real-time quantitative polymerase chain reaction assay. Arch Pathol Lab Med 2006;130:465–473.
31. Takeuchi T, Tomida S, Yatabe Y, et al. Expression profile-defined classification of lung adenocarcinoma shows close relationship with underlying major genetic changes and clinicopathologic behaviors. J Clin Oncol 2006;24(11):1679–1688.
32. Martini N, Bains MS, Burt ME, et al. Incidence of local recurrence and second primary tumors in resected stage I lung cancer. J Thorac Cardiovasc Surg 1995;109:120–129.
33. Pairolero PC, Williams DE, Bergstrahl EL, et al. Postsurgical stage I bronchogenic carcinoma: morbid implications of recurrent disease. Ann Thorac Surg 1984;38:331–338.
34. Rosengart TK, Martini N, Ghosn P, et al. Multiple primary lung carcinomas: prognosis and treatment. Ann Thorac Surg 1991;52:773–778.
35. Carey FA, Donnelly SC, Walker WS, et al. Synchronous primary lung cancers: prevalence in surgical material and clinical implications. Thorax 1993;48:344–346.
36. Rohwedder JJ, Weatherbee L. Multiple primary bronchogenic carcinoma with a review of the literature. Am Rev Respir Dis 1974;109:435–445.
37. Hida T, Ariyoshi Y, Sugiora T, et al. Synchronous lung cancer presenting with small cell carcinoma and adenocarcinoma. Chest 1993;104:1602–1604.
38. Martini N, Melamed MR. Multiple primary lung cancers. Thorac Cardiovasc Surg 1975;70:606–612.
39. Neugut AI, Sherr D, Robinson E, et al. Differences in histology between first and second primary lung cancer. Cancer Epidemiol Biomarkers Prev 1992;1:109–112.
40. Antakli T, Schefer RF, Rutherford JE, et al. Second primary lung cancer. Ann Thorac Surg 1995;59:863–867.
41. Deschamps C, Pairolero PC, Trastek VF, et al. Multiple primary lung cancers. Results of surgical treatment. J Thorac Cardiovasc Surg 1990;99:769–777.
42. Wu SC, Lin ZQ, Xu CW, et al. Multiple primary lung cancers. Chest 1987;92:892–896.
43. Cunha JD, Herndon JE II, Herzan DL, et al. Poor correspondence between clinical and pathologic staging in stage 1 non–small cell lung cancer: results from CALGB 9761, a prospective trial. Lung Cancer 2005;48:241–246.

44. Yang HK, Linnoila RI, Conrad NK, et al. TP53 and RAS mutations in metachronous tumors from patients with cancer of the upper aerodigestive tract. Int J Cancer 1995;64:229–233.

45. Szych C, Staebler A, Connolly DC, et al. Molecular genetic evidence supporting the clonality and appendiceal origin of *Pseudomyxoma peritonei* in women. Am J Pathol 1999;154: 1849–1855.

46. Fujita M, Enomoto T, Wada H, et al. Application of clonal analysis. Differential diagnosis for synchronous primary ovarian and endometrial cancers and metastatic cancer. Am J Clin Pathol 1996;105:350–359.

47. Cuatrecasas M, Matias-Guiu X, Prat J, et al. Synchronous mucinous tumors of the appendix and the ovary associated with pseudomyxoma peritonei. A clinicopathologic study of six cases with comparative analysis of c-Ki-ras mutations. Am J Surg Pathol 1996;20:739–746.

48. Koness RJ, King TC, Schechter S, et al. Synchronous colon carcinomas: molecular-genetic evidence for multicentricity. Ann Surg Oncol 1996;3:136–143.

49. Lau DH, Yang B, Hu R, et al. Clonal origin of multiple lung cancers: K-ras and p53 mutations determined by nonradioisotopic single-strand conformation polymorphism analysis. Diagn Mol Pathol 1997;6:179–184.

50. Yamamoto S, Tada M, Lee CC, et al. p53 status in multiple human urothelial cancers: assessment for clonality by the yeast p53 functional assay in combination with p53 immunohistochemistry. Jpn J Cancer Res 2000;91:181–189.

51. Goto K, Konomoto T, Hayashi K, et al. p53 mutations in multiple urothelial carcinomas: a molecular analysis of the development of multiple carcinomas. Mod Pathol 1997;10: 428–437.

52. Werness BA, DiCioccio RA, Piver MS. Identical, unique p53 mutations in a primary ovarian mucinous adenocarcinoma and a synchronous contralateral ovarian mucinous tumor of low malignant potential suggest a common clonal origin. Hum Pathol 1997;28:626–630.

53. Lyda MH, Noffsinger A, Belli J, et al. Multifocal neoplasia involving the colon and appendix in ulcerative colitis: pathological and molecular features. Gastroenterology 1998;115: 1566–1573.

54. Eguchi K, Yao T, Konomoto T, et al. Discordance of p53 mutations of synchronous colorectal carcinomas. Mod Pathol 2000;13:131–139.

55. Ribeiro U, Safatle-Ribeiro AV, Posner MC, et al. Comparative p53 mutational analysis of multiple primary cancers of the upper aerodigestive tract. Surgery 1996;120:45–53.

56. Takahashi T, Habuchi T, Kakehi Y, et al. Clonal and chronological genetic analysis of multifocal cancers of the bladder and upper urinary tract. Cancer Res 1998;58:5835–5841.

57. Emmert-Buck MR, Chuaqui R, Zhuang Z, et al. Molecular analysis of synchronous uterine and ovarian endometrioid tumors. Int J Gynecol Pathol 1997;16:143–148.

58. Krebs PA, Albuquerque A, Quezado M. The use of microsatellite instability in the distinction between synchronous endometrial and colonic adenocarcinomas. Int J Gynecol Pathol 1999;18:320–324.

59. Lin WM, Forgacs E, Warshal DP, et al. Loss of heterozygosity and mutational analysis of the PTEN/MMAC1 gene in synchronous endometrial and ovarian carcinomas. Clin Cancer Res 1998;4:2577–2583.

60. Scholes AG, Woolgar JA, Boyle MA, et al. Synchronous oral carcinomas: independent or common clonal origin? Cancer Res 1998;58:2003–2006.

61. Shimizu S, Yatabe Y, Koshikawa T. High frequency of clonally related tumors in cases of multiple synchronous lung cancers as revealed by molecular diagnosis. Clin Cancer Res 2000;6:3994–3999.

62. Hiroshima K, Toyozaki T, Kohno H. Synchronous and metachronous lung carcinomas: molecular evidence for multicentricity. Pathol Int 1998;48:869–876.

63. Huang J, Behrens C, Dimopulo O, et al. Molecular analysis of synchronous and metachronous tumors of the lung: impact on management and prognosis. Ann Diagn Pathol 2001;5(6):321–329.

34
Diffuse Malignant Mesothelioma: Genetic Pathways and Mechanisms of Oncogenesis of Asbestos and Other Agents That Cause Mesotheliomas

Françoise Galateau-Sallé and Jean Michel Vignaud

Introduction

Malignant mesothelioma (MM) is an aggressive neoplasm caused by exposure to asbestos fibers in 80% of cases.[1,2] Although asbestos has been banned in most developed countries, the incidence of mesothelioma is still rising because of the long latency period from the time of exposure to development of the disease (20–40 years). Asbestos fibers interact with the mesothelial cells from which these tumors arise in several different ways and generate reactive oxygen species (see Chapter 44), cytokines, and growth factors secondary to inflammatory responses from the host, resulting in DNA damage. Protooncogenes may be activated, leading to cell proliferation and susceptibility to mutations. Over time, structural alterations and numerical losses and gains to chromosomes occur, producing genomic instability and alteration of the role of tumor suppressor genes. These complex cytogenetic and molecular events in MM development attest to the multistep process from a benign proliferation to a malignant neoplasm.

During the past several years, evolving molecular techniques have yielded insight into mesothelioma oncogenesis, diagnosis, prognosis, and potential therapy. This chapter reviews the mechanisms of asbestos-induced oncogenesis, the abnormal expression of oncogenes and growth factors, the chromosomal damage including chromosomal deletion and polysomy (both reflecting genomic instability), and the roles of three well-established tumor suppressor genes ($p16^{INK4A}$, $p53$, and $NF2$) and their interactions with Simian virus (SV) 40. The profile of methylation of other tumor suppressor genes possibly involved, the role of metabolic polymorphisms, and the results of microarray gene profiling are also considered.

Mechanisms of Oncogenesis in Mesothelioma

Asbestos-Induced Oncogenesis

Asbestos is a generic name for fibers belonging to the family of fibrous silicates, which have different carcinogenicities. Animal model experiments have shown that the long and thin asbestos fibers (>8 μm in length and <0.25 μm in width) are strongly carcinogenic, inducing pleural MM, whereas shorter and thicker fibers are at low or no risk of causing MM, according to the Stanton hypothesis.[3] The concept that the pathogenicity of fibers is based on their length has recently raised some controversy and has been the subject of several publications suggesting that it is not prudent to take the position that short asbestos fibers convey little risk of disease.[4] More recent studies have proposed the classification of fibers according to their biopersistence. Long fibers cannot be phagocytosed by alveolar macrophages, whereas short fibers are easily engulfed and removed from the lung but can also be retained if the dosage exposure is high enough. Specific physiochemical characteristics of fibers, such as surface charge and structure, and their in situ biopersistence are also suspected to have a role in the transformation of mesothelial cells.

The early molecular events induced by asbestos in the pleura that ultimately lead to mesothelioma are unclear. We know that asbestos may cause damage to macromolecules by direct physical interaction or by the indirect action of reactive oxygen species produced by inflammatory cells in response to asbestos. Studies of animal models and cell cultures have demonstrated that, in situ, asbestos fibers generate reactive oxygen and reactive nitrogen species, both of which target critical biologic macromolecules such as DNA, signal transduction proteins, and lipid membranes.[5] Types of asbestos-induced DNA damage identified thus far include altered DNA bases, DNA single-strand breaks,[6] chromosomal alterations, and sister chromatid exchanges.[7]

Additionally, reactive oxygen species and asbestos DNA damage, through phosphorylation of the epidermal growth factor receptor, can trigger signal transduction cascades. Asbestos can activate mitogen-activated protein kinase signaling pathways,[2,8] and crocidolite more specifically triggers the extracellular-regulated kinase cascade. Several of the transcription factors in these pathways, such as nuclear factor (NF)-κB, activator protein-1, (c-fos, c-Jun), and c-Myc, are highly expressed in mesothelioma and encode transcription factors that activate various genes critical in the initiation of DNA synthesis.[9] In contrast, hydroxyl radicals and asbestos fibers, unlike nonfibrogenic particles, induce apoptosis in normal mesothelial cells, whereas mesothelioma cell lines are highly resistant to apoptosis. The mechanisms leading to this resistance are unclear but not linked to a Bax/Bcl-2 imbalance. Recently, aberrant regulation of the phosphatidylinositol-3 kinase (PI3K)/Akt signaling pathway has been shown to be responsible for resistance to cell death in human mesothelial cells after exposure to amphibole fibers (amosite).[10] Akt signaling regulates cell proliferation and survival, cell growth, glucose metabolism, cell motility, and angiogenesis.[11] Caciotti et al. have also reported that the PI3K/Akt pathway is activated in response to growth factors in the presence of Tag (large T antigen of the SV40 virus), conferring progressive resistance to apoptosis.[10] Recently, Yang et al. demonstrated that, in human mesotheliomas, tumor necrosis factor (TNF)-α released by macrophages activates NF-κB and that NF-κB activation leads to mesothelioma cell survival and resistance to the cytotoxic effects of asbestos.[12] Further investigations are necessary for a better understanding of the balance between proliferation and apoptosis in mesothelial cells. Finally, it has also been suggested that the net balance of the lymphokines and cytokines produced by macrophages after phagocytosis of asbestos fibers creates local immunosuppression.[13] Although 80% of MM develop in individuals with high levels of exposure to asbestos, only a fraction of those exposed to asbestos develop mesothelioma, suggesting that additional factors play a role in individual susceptibility.

Viruses

Simian virus 40 was implicated in the etiology of MM in 1993, when Ciccala et al. reported that 100% of mesotheliomas developed in hamsters after intracardial injection.[14] Despite a large body of data suggesting that SV40 is implicated in different human tumors, there is still controversy regarding the exact role of SV40 in mesothelioma development (see later discussion). It has been reported that the transforming potency of SV40 results from the activity of two viral proteins, Tag and small t antigen (tag). However, a recent statement by the British Thoracic Society characterized the evidence in favor of SV40 as a cofactor for mesothelioma as "weak."[15]

Radiation

There have been several reports implicating either radiation (Thorotrast) or thoracic and abdominal radiotherapy as causes contributing to the development of mesothelioma.[16] Recently a European and North American cohort of 40,576 patients who underwent radiotherapy for testicular cancer were assessed for incidence of second solid tumors. For the first time, among 10-year survivors, a statistically significantly elevated risk was observed for cancer of the pleura (MM; relative risk [RR] = 3.4, 95% confidence interval [CI] = 1.7–5.9) that interestingly was higher when compared with cancers from other sites.[17,18]

Other Etiologic Factors

Other etiologic factors, such as chronic pleural irritation (chronic empyema, plombage therapy for tuberculosis), for which the degree of proof is weak, have been suggested as causes of MM. Genetic susceptibility has been recently reported.[2]

Cytogenetics, Deletion Mapping, and Gene Profiling in Mesothelioma

Karyotypic Analysis Studies

Karyotypic analysis studies performed during the past several decades failed to identify a specific karyotypic change that may prove to be of diagnostic value and showed the complexity of the karyotypes in this malignancy. Most MMs display multiple clonal chromosomal abnormalities.[19,20] However, a number of recurrent anomalies have been found. These include deletions at multiple sites or loss of one entire copy of chromosomes 4 and, particularly, 22; polysomy for chromosomes 5, 7, and 20; and losses at 1p21–2, 3p21, 6q15–21, 9p21–22, 15q11.1–q15, and 22q12, suggesting that tumor suppressor genes critical to MM tumorigenesis may reside at these loci.[19,21-24] Many of the tumors have several chromosomal losses in combination.

Comparative Genomic Hybridization Studies

Comparative genomic hybridization studies have confirmed the karyotype findings and identified even more chromosomal losses and gains than either conventional cytogenetics or fluorescence in situ hybridization.[25] Although considerable variability was reported from one laboratory to another, some recurrent imbalances were noted in most studies: underrepresentation of 1p21 (21%), 6q22 (16%), 9p21 (34%), 13q12–14 (19%), 14q12–24 (23%), and 22q (32%) and overrepresentation of 7p14–15 (14%), 7q(19, 26–28), and 5p, which encodes SKP2(5p13), a protein involved in control of the cell cycle.

Statistically significant correlations have been found between a high content of asbestos fibers in lung tissue from MM patients and partial or total loss of chromosomes 1 and 4 as well as a breakpoint at locus 1p11–22 ($p = 0.009$). This supports a role for high asbestos burden in mesothelial mutagenesis.[29]

Deletion Mapping

Recurrent losses from specific chromosomal regions are consistent with a recessive mechanism of oncogenesis and can be viewed as indicators of relevant tumor suppressor genes. Deleted regions, defined in cytogenetic studies, have been mapped at the molecular genetic level by loss of heterozygosity (LOH) analysis using polymorphic DNA markers.

Allelic losses at 1p21–22 were observed in more than 70% of MM cases.[26] The shorter region of overlap (SRO) localized deletions to a 4 cM segment within 1p22. Losses at 1p36 were also detected, although with a lesser incidence (46%).

The highest frequency of allelic losses on chromosome 3p occurs at the 3p21.3 locus D3F15S2 (69%) and the 3p21.1 locus D3S2 (62%). The 3p21 region is a site of frequent deletions in lung carcinoma, and a region where the search for candidate tumor suppressor genes identified RASSF1, β-catenin, and semaphorins SEM3A and SEM3F genes.[26]

Loss of heterozygosity studies at multiples sites on chromosome 4 detected losses at 4q33–34 (80%), 4q25–26 (60%), and 4p15.1–15.3 (50%) regions,[30] confirming comparative genomic hybridization and cytogenetic studies.

Deletions of chromosome 6q fell into four discrete regions involving markers mapped within the 6q14–q21, 6q16.6–21, 6q21–q23.2, and 6q25 regions.[31] Altogether, allelic losses of 6q were observed in 61% of the cases. These genomic losses have also been described in breast cancer, ovarian cancer, and non-Hodgkin's lymphoma. Suppression of tumorigenicity of breast cancer cells was obtained by microcell transfer of deleted 6q regions, suggesting that tumor suppressive gene(s) are present in these regions.[32]

Loss of part or all of 9p, particularly the 9p21–22 region, is a frequent event in MM. The 9p21 region is homozygously deleted in 43% of cell lines and in 22% of tumor samples.[33] The SRO of this homozygous deletion is a 1 Mb segment that contains two tumor suppressor genes: p16/CDKN2 and the alternatively spliced p14^{ARF}.

Loss of heterozygosity on chromosome 13 was observed in 66% of cases with the SRO (7 cM) located at 13q13.3–q14.2, which was found deleted in 42% of MM cases. This region is the site of the BRCA2 gene. Allelic losses at 14q (32%) in three distinct regions were also reported (14q11.2–13.2, 14q22.3–24.3, 14q32.12).[34]

Underrepresentation of 15q was demonstrated by comparative genomic hybridization. The minimal region of deletion involved 15q11.1–q15. Losses overlapping this region have been observed in other types of malignancy such as prostate and ovarian cancer, suggesting that this region contains a tumor suppressor gene. The RAD51 gene, located at 15q15.1, participates in the repair of double-stranded DNA breaks and is potentially a candidate tumor suppressor gene.[35]

Gene Profiling and Mesothelioma

Gene profiling studies of MM[36–42] have yielded confusing results, with many studies showing a myriad of known and unknown genes that are overexpressed and underexpressed in mesothelioma. It is not possible here to comprehensively address all of the genes and associated molecular pathways discovered in this manner. We highlight select studies pertaining to microarray analysis in MM.

A typical analysis by Singhal et al. reveals genes that participate in glucose metabolism, mRNA translation, and cytoskeletal remodeling and identifies upregulated genes that have potential diagnostic, therapeutic, and prognostic implications for patients.[39] Some of these upregulated genes are discussed. Adenotin (gp96) is closely related to Hsp90. This gene is considered to be an important factor in inducing tumor-specific immunity. Lung-related resistance protein gene may be partially responsible for resistance to chemotherapy. This protein acts as a transporter and removes cytotoxic drugs from the cell. Galectin-3 binding protein is a β-galactoside binding protein that participates in cell growth, differentiation, adhesion, and malignant transformation. Increased expression in tumors has been linked to advanced tumor stage, progression, metastases, and poor outcome. The laminin receptor plays a role in tumor development, progression, and metastasis. It has been associated with decreased survival in breast, lung, and ovarian cancers. Voltage-dependent anion channel genes VDAC1 and VDAC2 participate in the apoptotic pathway through interactions with the Bcl-2 family of proteins. Mesotheliomas express high levels of Bax and Bcl-xL, and VDAC overexpression may be an attempt to suppress the anti-apoptotic effects of Bax and Bcl-xL. The Ku80 gene participates in DNA double-stranded break repair, and the protein from this gene opposes anticancer drug-induced apoptosis.

A comparison (based on a series of 99 tumor samples) by Lopez-Rios et al. of the expression profile of epithelioid versus sarcomatous MM identified many genes significantly overexpressed among the former, including previously unrecognized ones such as uroplakins and kallikrein 11.[40] The top genes specifically expressed in *p16/CDNK2A*–deleted cases were *RHOBT3, SHOX2*, and *DLC1*, and in nondeleted cases they were *B-factor* (properdine) and *MTAP* (methylthioadenosine phosphorylase). More aggressive MM expressed higher levels of Aurora kinases A and B and functionally related genes involved in mitosis and cell cycle control (including *CCDN1*, encoding cyclin D1, *BIRC5/survivin, CDC25C phosphatase*, and *BTG2*, a transcriptional repressor of *CCDN1*). It is noteworthy that all these genes participate in a network of genes linked directly or indirectly to each other.

Several studies also reported that genes involved in intracellular signaling pathways are upregulated: the mitogen-activated protein kinase cascade (*JNK1, NIK, PAK1, ERK5*, and *TRAF2* genes), notch signaling pathway (*JAGGED1* and *JAGGED2* genes), and Wnt-frizzled signaling pathway (*SARP1, FRIZZLED, Dickkopf-1, β-catenin*, and *n-cadherin* genes), and the cell cycle (*cyclin D1, cyclin D3, CDK phosphatase*), cellular growth (*FGF3*), and drug resistance (*Ku80*) genes.

The gene profiling study by Gordon et al. illustrates the role of gene expression in predicting outcome with mesotheliomas, regardless of histologic type.[41] From a total of 46 genes that were identified as being of prognostic value, four upregulated genes that had the highest statistically significant values for a favorable outcome group (median survival of 35 months) and for a poor outcome group (median survival 7 months) were selected. Genes that were overexpressed in the favorable outcome group, as compared to the poor outcome group, were selenium-binding protein, KIAA0977 protein, an expressed sequence tag similar to the L6 tumor antigen, and leukocyte antigen-related protein. The upregulated genes in the poor outcome group, as compared to the favorable outcome group, were cytosolic thyroid hormone-binding protein, calgizzarin, insulin-like growth factor-binding protein-3, and GDP-dissociation inhibitor 1. Five expression ratios were identified (level of expression of one gene overexpressed in the favorable outcome group/level of expression of one gene overexpressed in the poor outcome group) that independently placed the mesothelioma cases into the correct favorable and poor outcome groups. However, Lopez-Rios et al.[40] (40) evaluated three recently published microarray-based outcome prediction models[37,40,41] and showed that their accuracies, about 65%, were consistently lower than the estimates in the original publication. Moreover, microarray-based prediction of prognosis was inferior to prediction of prognosis based on standard clinicopathologic variables and *p16/CDNK2A* status. The very limited overlap between prognostic gene lists obtained by the three groups emphasizes that such lists are "noisy," and the significance of individual genes on these lists should be viewed with great caution. (Differences in array platforms, data analysis packages, or modifications in the filtering of the genes may result in differences in classifier genes among reports). Nonetheless, supervised analyses of microarray data provide leads for new diagnostic markers and potential therapeutic targets.

Certain gene profiling studies have also compared expression between mesothelioma and lung cancer.[43] Results obtained with such methods have been encouraging in differentiating between mesothelioma and lung cancer. Using 15 ratios between genes overexpressed in mesotheliomas (five genes, *calretinin, VAC-β, MRX OX-2, PTGIS*, hypothetical protein *KIAA0977*) and in adenocarcinomas of the lung (*TACSTD1, claudin-7, TTF-1*), it was possible to accurately categorize the tumors as mesotheliomas or lung cancers in over 90% of cases using just a single expression ratio. When using a two or three gene expression ratio, it was possible to accurately classify mesotheliomas and adenocarcinomas of the lung in 95% and 99% of the cases, respectively.

Polymorphisms in Genes as Risk Factors for Asbestos-Related Malignant Mesothelioma

The role of xenobiotic metabolizing gene polymorphisms in the risk of MM from asbestos exposure has been reported in a few studies. Two studies of MM risk associated with glutathione-S-transferase *(GSTM1)* and N-acetyltransferase 2 *(NAT2)* produced contradictory results. Hirvonen et al.[44] showed an increased risk of MM in subjects occupationally exposed to asbestos and carrying a homozygous deletion of the *GSTM1* gene or the *NAT2* slow acetylator genotype (individuals with either defect had a twofold risk of developing MM, and those with combined defects had a fourfold risk of developing MM), whereas Neri et al.[45] did not observe any association with the *GSTM1* gene and found an increased risk of developing MM for *NAT2* fast acetylators. These investigators also found that combination of *GSTT1* null and *GSTM1* null genotypes determined an increased risk of MM and reported an association of MM with microsomal epoxide hydrolase (mEH). Reduced activity of mEH, an enzyme involved in the detoxification of oxidative compounds, might increase susceptibility to oxidative stress. They also found that mEH interacted with both *NAT2* and *GSTM1* genes, according to a multiplicative model. These preliminary results favor the hypothesis that metabolic gene polymorphisms involved in oxidation processes have a role in modulating individual susceptibility to MM in subjects with different degrees of asbestos exposure.

Dianzani et al.[46] studied the relationship between seven genetic polymorphisms of DNA repair genes, including *XRCC1-R399Q*, *XRCC3-T241M*, *XPD*, and *OGG1*, and the development of MM in a population-based study conducted in an area with high asbestos exposure. Data showed an association between the *XRCC1-399Q* variant and MM among subjects with asbestos exposure, the risk increasing as a function of the number of Q alleles.

Tumor Suppressor Gene Inactivation in Mesothelioma

With the completion of the human genome project, it has been possible to identify many different oncogenes and tumor suppressor genes that are proposed to be involved in the multistep process from mesothelial proliferation to mesothelioma development. The oncogenes that have been identified are not exclusive to mesothelioma but are shared with many other malignant human tumors. Similarly, tumor suppressor genes that are deleted, altered, or inactivated in mesothelioma are those seen in other tumors as well. However, current knowledge confirms a pathogenic role for cyclin-dependent kinase (Cdk) inhibitor *p16^{INK4A}*, *p53*, and *NF2*.

Loss of Cyclin-Dependent Kinase Inhibitor Function

A recurrent genetic abnormality in the development of cancer is the loss of the G1 to S checkpoint control locus. An important moderator of this control is the presence of pRb in an underphosphorylated state.[47] (47). The phosphorylation of the retinoblastoma protein (pRb) is mediated by Cdk4 and Cdk6, with the corresponding inhibition of the kinase activity regulated by the family of Cdk inhibitors (see Chapter 2). A high frequency of mesothelioma cell lines exhibit homozygous deletion of the 9p21 region. The *CDKN2A* locus, which encodes the alternative *p16^{INK4A}* and *p14^{ARF}* gene products, is located in this region, also encoding the Cdk inhibitor *p15^{INK4B}*. The p16 protein is an inhibitor of Cdk4/6. Thus loss/inactivation of *p16^{INK4A}* would lead to cell cycle deregulation through the loss of a key inhibitor of G1/S progression. The most frequent modes of inactivation of p16 are homozygous deletions and methylation, whereas missense mutations are rare. More than 80% of mesothelioma cell lines have homozygous deletions of one or more *p16^{INK4A}* exons, but only 22% of tumor specimens have these deletions.[47–50] Fluorescence in situ hybridization analysis has revealed a reduced copy number of the *p16^{INK4A}* gene in most mesotheliomas, and immunohistochemistry studies

suggest that loss of *p16^{INK4A}* expression is a universal finding in mesotheliomas.[47] Hirao et al. found that 8.8% of tumor specimens (4 out of 45) exhibited a methylated promoter region of the gene.[49] Taken collectively, these data allow the conclusion that homozygous deletions and methylation of p16 occurs in MM in vivo and in vitro.

p14^{ARF} is another tumor suppressor gene encoded at the same locus. The product of *p14^{ARF}* is required for activation of *p53* in response to the activation of oncogenes such as *ras* and *Myc* and for loss of *Rb*. *p14^{ARF}* rarely has independent loss of function from *p16^{INK4A}*.[49,51] Thus homozygous loss of *p16^{INK4A}* and *p14^{ARF}* would collectively affect both the p53 and pRb-dependant growth regulatory pathways and particularly permit evasion of G1 arrest. The burden of asbestos exposure and the loss of *p16^{INK4A}* have been tied to development of mesothelioma. Potentially, *p16^{INK4A}* deletion allows for development of mesothelioma with less asbestos exposure.[49] Moreover, the homologous Cdk inhibitor *p15^{INK4B}* is absent in mesothelioma as well. *p15^{INK4B}* has been found to be deleted in addition to *p16^{INK4A}* in a high percentage of mesotheliomas.[52] Experiments involving the reintroduction of *p16^{INK4A}* and *p14^{ARF}* into mesothelioma cell lines and xenografts were successful. The expression of *p16^{INK4A}* in transfected mesothelioma cells correlated with decreased phosphorylation of pRb and resulted in cell cycle arrest and apoptosis, as well as inhibition of tumor formation and diminished tumor size.[53] Similarly, after transduction of *p14^{ARF}*, overexpression of *p14^{ARF}* in mesothelioma leads to increased levels of both *p53* and *p21* and inhibition of mesothelioma growth in culture.[54]

The *p53* Gene

Loss of heterozygosity at the 17p13 locus, where *p53* maps, is very rare in MM, and *p53* mutations are rarely found.[51,55] However, *p53* stabilization as determined by immunohistochemistry was reported in 25%–70% of MM cases.[56,57] This suggests the role of a protein partner that may associate with *p53* to stabilize it. This lack of *p53* mutations fails to explain the effect of *p53* on the development of MM. Indeed, frequent loss of *p14^{ARF}* (an in-hibitor of *p53* and *MDM2* interaction) leads to *MDM2*-mediated inactivation of *p53*. *MDM2* induces proteasome-mediated ubiquitination of *p53* and was found to be overexpressed in about 30% of MM cases.[58–60] However, it has been shown, using MM cell lines, that *p53*-induced apoptosis may occur in the absence of *p14^{ARF}*.[61] In this model, inhibition of *MDM2* using nutlin (an imidazoline compound that disrupts the interaction between *p53* and *MDM2*) induces G1 arrest but not apoptosis. Furthermore, *SV40Tag* complexes with *p53*, as well as with pRb, disrupting normal cell cycle control and antagonizing *p53*-induced apoptosis.[62] A downstream target of *p53* activation is the induction of *p21* expression. *p21*, a multifunctional Cdk inhibitor, plays a critical role in the G2/M cell cycle checkpoint. Increased expression of $p21$ in mesothelioma is associated with patients having an improved survival, whereas decreased expression of $p21$ has been associated with decreased patient survival.[63]

The NF2 Gene

Population studies have linked the autosomally dominant disease neurofibromatosis type 2 to the loss of the function of the NF2 gene located on the long arm of chromosome 22. NF2 encodes a protein called *schwannomin* or *merlin* (meosin ezrin radixin-like protein) that connects the cytoskeleton to the plasma membrane. Merlin inactivation is very frequent in sporadic vestibular schwannomas, meningiomas, and MM. Extensive LOH analysis of chromosome 22 losses in MM has not been performed because an entire copy of chromosome 22 is lost in most cases, but LOH studies have documented allelic losses at the NF2 locus in more than 70% of MM cases. NF2 somatic mutations were found in 55% of mesothelioma cell lines and in 41% of tumors.[64,65] All mutations resulted in in-frame deletions or truncation of merlin and a nondetectable protein by Western blot analysis, suggesting that truncated forms of the protein are unstable. All cases exhibiting mutations of NF2 showed allelic losses, implying that inactivation of NF2 in MM occurs via the classic Knudson "two-hit" model of tumor suppressor gene inactivation.[33] Re-expression of merlin in NF2-deficient MM cells strongly inhibits mobility, migration, and invasiveness of the cells. This could be related in part to upregulation of focal adhesion kinase activity, which is a key component of cellular pathways affecting migration and invasion. Expression of merlin attenuated focal adhesion kinase phosphorylation, and restoration of merlin expression in NF2 null MM cells overexpressing focal adhesion kinase resulted in significantly decreased invasiveness.[66] Interestingly, an animal model (Nf2+/− knockout mice exposed to asbestos) recapitulating many of the molecular features of human mesothelioma has been recently described[67,68] and is useful for preclinical testing of novel therapies.

Tumor Suppressor Gene Methylation in Mesothelioma

In addition to the well-characterized tumor suppressor gene $p16^{INK4A}$, investigations have shown that many other confirmed or putative suppressor genes potentially involved in MM oncogenesis display a promoter hypermethylation with a high frequency. Suzuki et al. investigated the methylation of 12 tumor suppressor genes by methylation-specific polymerase chain reaction in 63 MMs and MM cell lines.[69] Methylation of eight promoter genes

occurred in over 20% of tumor samples: HIC1 (22%), RASSF1A (32%), cyclin D2 (35%), HPP1 (35%), DcR2 (41%), RRAD (56%), DRM/gremlin (60%), and DcR1 (74%). HIC1 (hypermethylated in cancer 1), a zinc-finger transcription factor gene, has a p53-binding site by which the gene is activated. HPP1 is silenced in hyperplastic colon polyps, colorectal carcinoma, and lung cancers. DcR1 and DcR2 are antiapoptotic decoy receptors that bind the tumor necrosis factor–related apoptosis-inducing ligand. RRAD, a GTPase gene, plays a role in tumor growth in breast cancer. DRM/gremlin is silenced in many types of cancers and is a homolog to the rat *drm* gene. Interestingly, the frequencies of HPP1, RASSF1A, cyclin D2, and RRAD methylation and the value of the methylation index were significantly higher in SV40 sequence-positive MM than in SV40-negative MM.[69] Methylation of TMS1 (a gene encoding a caspase recruitment domain [CARD] aberrantly methylated in breast and lung cancers) and HIC1 was associated with shortened survival. Of interest is the finding that SV40-infected human mesothelial cells showed progressive aberrant methylation of several genes—HIC1, RASSF1A, HPP1, DcR1, TMS1, CRBP1 (this gene participates in the retinoid signaling pathway and is silenced by methylation in several cancers), and RRAD—during serial passages.

Recently Fischer et al. reported modest methylation frequencies for APC1A (14.3%), RASSF1A (19.5%), and DAPK (20.0%) in MM, whereas hypermethylation of E-cadherin (71.4%) and FHIT (78.0%) occurred at a high frequency.[70] Intermediate frequency values were seen for $p16^{INK4A}$ (28.8%), APC1B (32.5%), $p14^{ARF}$ (44.2%), and RARβ (55.8%). Combining RARβ status with either DAPK or RASSF1A status showed a significantly shorter survival of those patients versus those with only one or no epigenetic alterations ($p = 0.025$ and 0.040, respectively).

The ability of SV40 infection to silence genes is shown by mammalian cell cultures infected with SV40. An SV40 infection induces expression of methyltransferase enzymes (DNMT1, DNMT3b) that lead to global genomic DNA methylation.[71] Thus SV40 may inactivate tumor suppressor genes through epigenetic changes, suggesting a transformation mechanism more complex than simple inactivation of the p53 and Rb gene products by Tag antigen.

Simian Virus 40 and Human Mesothelioma

During the past three decades more than 60 original studies have reported the detection of SV40 in MM, primary brain tumors, and osteosarcomas, although with geographic differences. DNA sequence analyses and Tag protein detection have ruled out laboratory contamina-

tion of tumor samples and have shown Tag protein in
52%–90% of patients with mesothelioma from the United
States, Germany, Italy, and France.[72–74] The purpose of the
metaanalysis of controlled studies by Vilchez and Butel
was to analyze the extent to which SV40 may be associated with human MM.[75] The analysis included 15 studies;
the combined odds ratio (OR) of analysis was 16.8 (95%
CI, 10.3–27.5) and was based on 528 patients with malignant MM and 468 controls. Modifiers detected were
the type of control tissue and the method of detection
of SV40. The adjusted OR was 15.1 (95% CI, 9.2–25).
Finally, these results were confirmed by an independent
multilaboratory study organized by the International
Mesothelioma Interest Group.[76]

There is only one known serotype of SV40, but genetic
strains exist,[77] and further studies are necessary to determine whether SV40 strains differ in pathogenic and/or
oncogenic capacities. SV40 Tag is an essential replication
protein that is required for initiation of viral DNA synthesis and that also stimulates host cells to enter S phase
and undergo DNA synthesis.[75,78] Because of this ability to
subvert cell cycle control, Tag represents the major transforming protein of SV40. Human mesothelial cells are
highly susceptible to SV40 infection and transformation
(1,000 times higher than human fibroblasts), and addition
of asbestos fibers enhances their transformation.[79,80]
Microdissection of human mesothelial samples followed
by polymerase chain reaction analysis detected SV40 Tag
only in cancer cells and not in adjacent stromal cells.[81,82]
The Tag antigens bind and block important tumor suppressor proteins, which include p53, pRb, p107, and p130/
Rb2.[83] Simian virus 40 Tag sequesters p53, abolishing its
function and allowing cells with genetic damage to survive
and enter S phase, leading to an accumulation of Tag-
expressing cells with genomic mutations that may promote
tumorigenic growth. Experiments have shown that Tag
and p53 are often coexpressed.[62] In addition, tumor cells
expressing Tag failed to induce p21, indicating that p53
was inactivated by its interaction with Tag.[62]

Finally, treatment of SV40-positive mesothelioma cell
lines with Tag antisense restored the p53 pathway and
induced p21 expression and growth arrest (84). Retinoblastoma protein normally binds transcription factor
E2F; Tag causes dissociation of pRb/E2F complexes,
releasing E2F to activate expression of growth-stimulatory genes.[83,85] Furthermore, the finding that SV40 infection induces telomerase activity in human mesothelial
cells indicates that the presence of SV40 may result in
cells prone to develop into malignancies when genetic
damage is induced.[86] Recent studies also showed that
Notch-1, the hepatocyte growth factor, and insulin-like
growth factor 1 are upregulated in infected human mesothelial cells, and the tumour suppressor gene RASSF1A
is inhibited.[79,81,87] Although in vitro studies have established that SV40 disrupts critical cell cycle control path-

ways, definitive proof that in vivo Tag can inactivate
p53 and Rb family genes is still missing, and it remains
unknown whether these perturbations are sufficient for
the virus to induce the development of malignancies in
humans. This explains the conclusion of the Institute of
Medicine[88] that "the biological evidence is of moderate
strength that SV40 exposure could lead to cancer in
humans under natural conditions."

Wilms' Tumor 1 Susceptibility Gene

The Wilms' tumor 1 gene (WT1), originally described as
a protooncogene in mouse mammary tumors, has been
identified as a tumor suppressor gene involved in the
etiology of Wilm's tumor, 10% of which carry mutations
in the gene. Expression of the WT1 gene has also been
observed in other tumor types such as MM and leukemia.
WT1 is expressed in almost all MM but has not been
found to be mutan.[89] WT1 maps at locus 11p13. Exons
5 and 9 alternatively spliced give rise to four different
protein isoforms.

The WT1 proteins seem to perform two main functions.
They regulate the transcription of a variety of target
genes and may be involved in posttranscriptional processing of RNA. Depending on the tumor type, WT1
proteins might function as either tumor suppressor proteins or survival factors. The WT1 protein represses transcription from promoters of several growth response
genes, including insulin-like growth factor (IGF) receptor
(IGFR) and epidermal growth factor (EGF) receptor
(EGFR), and it is known to bind to several other proteins
(notably p53, p63, and p73).

In agreement with a role for WT1 in transcription regulation, many of these proteins are also transcription
factors that may alter the transcription regulation properties of WT1. For instance, binding of WT1 stabilizes p53,
enhances binding of p53 to consensus sequence, and
inhibits p53-mediated apoptosis.[90] Association between
WT1 and p73 diminishes their respective transcriptional
activation properties, and p73 inhibits DNA binding by
WT1.[91] However, although WT1 is expressed in almost all
MM and in most reactive mesothelial cells, no correlation
between WT1 immunostaining and EGFR or IGFR
expression was found, and no significant correlation with
p53 expression was found as well.[92] Uematsu et al. suggested that, in MM, WT1 signaling is activated through
Disheveled overexpression and downstream β-catenin
signaling.[93] Inhibition of this signaling leads to significant
antitumor effects in mesothelioma cell lines. Recently, it
has been shown that WT1 signaling inhibits apoptosis
through β-catenin and that cells expressing WT1 resist
apoptosis induction by chemotherapy.[94,95] Thus the role
of WT1 in mesothelioma development is still to be
clarified.

Abnormal Expression of Growth Factors and Cytokines

By connecting stromal cells with tumor cells, the intra-tumoral network of growth factors and cytokines produced by both types of cells tightly regulates tumor cell proliferation and migration and angiogenesis. Although rapid progress has been made in the understanding of how growth factors act in a complex environment, caution must be exerted in interpreting data, especially from in vitro experiments, because the overall growth factor–cytokine balance is likely to strongly vary within and between tumors. However, among the multiple growth factors associated with mesothelial cell proliferation and migration, IGF, platelet-derived growth factor (PDGF). and EGF are important.[96]

Insulin-like growth factor, in an autocrine or paracrine fashion, can stimulate tumor growth and extracellular matrix development.[97] Expression of the two tyrosine kinase IGF receptors IGFR1 and IGFR2 has been found to be present in all MM cell lines. In an array analysis with confirmatory polymerase chain reaction testing, IGF-1, IGF-2, IGFR1, and IGFR2 were found to be overexpressed in mesothelioma. Insulin-like growth factor 1 was overexpressed 43.3-fold and the corresponding IGFR over 2.6-fold.[98] Interestingly, the presence of a functioning IGFR has been shown to be necessary for SV40-induced transformation of mesothelial cells, arguing for an important role of the IGFR in the development of mesothelioma.[99] Moreover, inhibition of the IGFR1, using an antisense expression plasmid, resulted in decreased mesothelioma proliferation in hamsters. However, the IGF pathway needs further elucidation before the associations can be confirmed.

Overexpression of PDGF proteins (A and B chains) and PDGF receptors (α and β) has also been reported, suggesting an autocrine loop of growth control in mesothelioma.[100,101] However, this has not been confirmed. Antisense oligonucleotides against PDGF A chain inhibit growth of some mesothelial cells, whereas antisense oligonucleotides against PDGF B chain do not, and at least some mesotheliomas do not express β-receptor.

The EGFR was found to be overexpressed in most MMs, mainly in the epithelioid variant, as well as in reactive pleuritis.[102] Surprisingly, EGFR expression appeared to be a prognostic factor indicating better survival.[103,104] The ligand for this receptor is transforming growth factor-α, which is often time overexpressed in mesothelioma.[104] Epidermal growth factor receptor has been associated with increased proliferation and angiogenesis and thus has been considered as a target for EGFR inhibitors. Interference with the autocrine loop may reduce cell proliferation significantly in mesotheliomas. However, treatment of the patients with gefitinib (an EGFR receptor tyrosine kinase inhibitor) had no effect on the relapse-free survival, but the overall survival was more than doubled (from 3.64 to 8.1 months).[102,105] Cortese et al., screening a series of 66 MMs, failed to detect the most common EGFR tyrosine kinase inhibitor mutations identified in gefitinib-responsive non–small cell lung carcinoma (no size polymorphisms in EGFR exon 19 were detected, and no point mutations were found in any of the evaluated codons [858, 861, and 719]).[106]

Conclusion

We have described the current views on the genetics and molecular abnormalities of MM, showing multiple and complex connections between the deregulated pathways that contribute to the outcome of mesothelioma. Malignant mesothelioma may be a cancer in which genetics, radiation, viruses, and environmental carcinogens such asbestos and erionite interact to cause malignancy. Future investigations are needed for a more advanced understanding of the stepwise process leading from increased mesothelial cell proliferation to mesothelioma, providing new effective therapeutics for curing this deadly disease.

References

1. Goldberg M, Imbernon E, Rolland P, et al. The French National Mesothelioma Surveillance Program. Occup Environ Med 2006 Feb 9; [Epub ahead of print].
2. Galateau-Salle F, Brambilla E, Cagle PT, et al. Pathology of malignant mesothelioma, an update of the International Mesothelioma Panel. In Galateau-Sallé F, ed. London: Springer Verlag; 2006:1–10.
3. Stanton MF, Layard M, Tegeris A, et al. Relation of particles dimension to carcinogenicity in amphibole asbestoses and fibrous minerals. J Natl Cancer Inst 1981;67:965–975.
4. Dodson RF, Atkinson MA, Levin JL. Asbestos fiber length as related to potential pathogenicity: a critical review. Am J Ind Med 2003;44:291–297.
5. Kamp DW, Graceffa P, Prior WA, Weitzman SA. The role of free radicals in asbestos-induced diseases. Free Radic Biol Med 1992;4:293–315.
6. Jaurand MC. Mechanisms of fiber-induced genotoxicity. Environ Health Perspect 1997;105:1073–1084.
7. Sukla A, Gulumian M, Hei TK, et al. Multiple role of oxidants in the pathogenesis of asbestos-induced diseases. Free Radic Biol Med 2003;34:1117–1129
8. Zanella CL, Posada J, Tritton TR, Mossman BT. Asbestos causes stimulation of the extracellular signal-regulated kinase 1 mitogen-activated protein kinase cascade after phosphorylation of the epidermal growth factor receptor. Cancer Res 1996;56:5334–5338.
9. Robledo R, Mossmann D. Cellular and molecular mechanism of asbestos induced fibrosis. J Cell Physiol 1999;180: 158–166.

10. Caciotti P, Barbone D, Altomare A, et al. SV40–dependant AKT activity drives mesothelial cell transformation after asbestos exposure. Cancer Res 2005;65:5256–5262.

11. Altomare DA, You H, Xiao GH, et al. Human and mouse mesotheliomas exhibit elevated AKT/PKB activity, which can be targeted to inhibit tumor cell growth. Oncogene 2005;24:6080–6089.

12. Yang H, Bochetta M, Kroczynski B, et al. TNF-alpha asbestos-induced cytotoxicity via NF-Kappa B dependant pathway mechanism for asbestos oncogenesis. Proc Natl Acad Sci USA 2006;103:10397–10402.

13. Rosenthal GJ, Simeonova P, Corsini E. Asbestos toxicity: an immunologic perspective. Rev Environ Health 1999;14: 11–19.

14. Ciccala C, Pompetti F, Carbone M. SV40 induces mesothelioma in hamsters. Am J Pathol 1993;142:1524–1533.

15. Statement on malignant mesothelioma in the United Kingdom: British Thoracic Society Standards of Care Committee. Thorax 2001;56:250–265.

16. Roggli VL, Oury TD, Sporn TA. Mesothelioma. In Roggli VL, Oury TD, Sporn TA, eds. Asbestos Associated Diseases. New York: Springer-Verlag; 2003:109–110.

17. Travis LB, Fossa SD, Schonfeld SJ, et al. Second cancers among 40,576 testicular cancer patients: focus on long-term survivors. J Natl Cancer Inst 2005;97:1354–1365.

18. Allan JM, Travis LB. Mechanisms of therapy-related carcinogenesis. Nat Rev Cancer 2005;5:943–955.

19. Sandberg AA, Bridges J. Updates on the cytogenetics and molecular genetics of bone and soft tissue tumors. Mesothelioma. Cancer Genet Cytogenet 2001;127:93–110.

20. Sandberg AA, Bridge JA. The Cytogenetics of Bone and Soft Tissue Tumors. Austin: RG Landes; 1994.

21. Taguchi T, Jhanwar SC, Siegfried JM, et al. Recurrent deletions of specific chromosomal sites in 1p, 3p, 6q, and 9p in human malignant mesothelioma. Cancer Res 1993;53:4349–4355.

22. Lee WC, Testa JR. Somatic genetic alterations in human malignant mesothelioma [review]. Int J Oncol 1999;14:181–188.

23. Popescu NC, Chahinian AP, DiPaolo JA. Nonrandom chromosome alterations in human malignant mesothelioma. Cancer Res 1988;48:142–147.

24. Ribotta M, Rosco F, Salvio M, et al. Recurrent chromosome 6 abnormalities in malignant mesothelioma. Monaldi Arch Chest Dis 1998;53:228–235.

25. Segers K, Ramael M, Singh SK, et al. Detection of numerical chromosomal aberrations in paraffin embedded malignant pleural mesothelioma by non-isotopic in situ hybridization. J Pathol 1995;175:219–226.

26. Murthy S, Testa JR. Asbestos, chromosomal deletions and tumor suppressor gene alterations in human malignant mesothelioma. J Cell Physiol 1999;199:150–157.

27. Björkqvist AM, Tammilehto L, Anttila S, et al. Recurrent DNA copy number changes in 1q, 4q, 6q, 9p, 13q, 14q and 22q detected by comparative genomic hybridization in malignant mesothelioma. Br J Cancer 1997;75:523–527.

28. Balsara BR, Bell DW, Sonoda G, et al. Comparative genomic hybridization and loss of heterozygosity analyses identify a common region of deletion at 15q11.1–15 in human malignant mesothelioma. Cancer Res 1999;59:450–454.

29. Tiainen M, Tammilehto L, Rautonen JK, et al. Chromosomal abnormalities and their correlations with asbestos exposure and survival in patients with mesothelioma. Br J Cancer 1989;60:618–626.

30. Shivapurkar N, Virmani AK, Wistuba II, et al. Deletions of chromosome 4 at multiple sites are frequent in malignant mesothelioma and small cell lung carcinoma. Clin Cancer Res 1999;5:17–23.

31. Bell DW, Jhanwar SC, Testa JR. Multiple regions of allelic loss from chromosome arm 6q in malignant mesothelioma. Cancer Res 1997;57:4057–4062.

32. Negrini M, Sabbioni S, Possati L, et al. Suppression of tumorigenicity of breast cancer cells by microcell-mediated chromosome transfer: studies on chromosomes 6 and 11. Cancer Res 1994;54:1331–1336.

33. Cheng JQ, Lee WC, Klein MA, et al. Frequent mutations of NF2 and allelic loss from chromosome 22q12 in malignant mesothelioma: evidence for a two-hit inactivation. Genes Chromosome Cancer 1999;24:238–242.

34. De Rienzo A, Jhanwar SC, Testa JR. Loss of heterozygosity analysis of 13q and 14q in human malignant mesothelioma. Genes Chromosome Cancer 2000;28:337–341.

35. Lim D, Hasty P. A mutation in mouse rad51 results in early an embryonic lethal that is suppressed by a mutation in p53. Mol Cell Biol 1996;16:7133–7143.

36. Mohr S, Keith G, Galateau-Salle F, et al. Cell protection, resistance and invasiveness of two malignant mesotheliomas as assessed by 10k-microarray. Biochim Biophys Acta 2004;1688:43–60.

37. Pass HI, Liu Z, Wali A, et al. Gene expression profiles predict survival and progression of pleural mesothelioma. Clin Cancer Res 2004;10:849–859.

38. Hoang C, D'Cunha J, Kratzke M, et al. Gene expression profiling identifies matriptase overexpression in malignant mesothelioma. Chest 2004;125:1843–1852.

39. Singhal S, Wiewrodt R, Malden LD, et al. Gene expression profiling of malignant mesothelioma. Clin Cancer Res 2003;9:3080–3097.

40. Lopez-Rios F, Chuai S, Flores R, et al. Global gene expression profiling of pleural mesotheliomas: overexpression of aurora kinases and P16/CDKN2A deletion as prognostic factors and critical evaluation of microarray-based prognostic prediction. Cancer Res 2006;66:2970–2979.

41. Gordon GJ, Jensen RV, Hsial LL, et al. Using gene expression ratios to predict outcome among patients with mesothelioma. J Natl Cancer Inst 2003;95:598–605.

42. Hicks J. Biologic, cytogenetic, and molecular factors in mesothelial proliferations. Ultrastruct Pathol 2006;30:19–30.

43. Gordon GJ, Jensen RV, Hsial LL, et al. Translation of microarray data into clinically relevant cancer diagnostic tests using gene expression ratios in lung cancer and mesothelioma. Cancer Res 2002;62:4963–4967.

44. Hirvonen A, Pelin K, Tammilehto L, et al. Inherited GSTM1 and NAT2 defects as concurrent risk modifiers in asbestos related human malignant mesothelioma. Cancer Res 1995;55:2981–2983.

45. Neri M, Filiberti R, Taioli E, et al. Pleural malignant meso-thelioma, genetic susceptibility and asbestos exposure. Mutat Res 2005;592:36–44.

46. Dianzani I, Gibello L, Biava A, et al. Polymorphisms in DNA repair genes as risk factors for asbestos-related malignant mesothelioma. Mutat Res 2006;599:124–134.

47. Kratzke RA, Otterson GA, Lincoln CE, et al. Immunohis-tochemical analysis of the p16INK4 cyclin-dependent kinase inhibitor in malignant mesothelioma. J Natl Cancer Inst 1995;87:1870–1875.

48. Wong L, Zhou J, Anderson D, Kratzke RA. Inactivation of p16INK4a expression in malignant mesothelioma by methylation. Lung Cancer 2002;38:131–136.

49. Hirao T, Bueno R, Chen CJ, et al. Alterations of the p16 (INK4) locus in human malignant mesothelial tumors. Carcinogenesis 2002;23:1127–1130.

50. Prins JB, Williamson KA, Kamp MM, et al. The gene for the cyclin-dependent-kinase-4 inhibitor, CDKN2A, is preferentially deleted in malignant mesothelioma. Int J Cancer 1998;75:649–653.

51. Papp T, Schipper H, Pemsel H, et al. Mutational analysis of N-ras, p53, p16INK4a, p14ARF and CDK4 genes in primary malignant mesothelioma. Int J Oncol 2001;18: 425–433.

52. Xio S, Li D, Vijg J, et al. Codeletion of p15 and p16 in primary malignant mesothelioma. Oncogene 1995;11:511–515.

53. Frizelle SP, Grim J, Zhou J, et al. Re-expression of p16INK4a in mesothelioma cells results in cell cycle arrest, cell death, tumor suppression and tumor regression. Onco-gene 1998;16:3087–3095.

54. Yang CT, You L, Yeh CC, et al. Adenovirus-mediated p14ARF gene transfer in human mesothelioma cells. J Natl Cancer Inst 2000;92:636–641.

55. Metcalf RA, Welsh JA, Bennet WP, et al. p53 and K-ras mutations in human mesothelioma cell lines. Cancer Res 1992;52:2610–2615.

56. Ramael M, Lemmens G, Eerdekens C, et al. Immunoreac-tivity for p53 protein in malignant mesothelioma and non-neoplastic mesothelium. J Pathol 1992;168:371–375.

57. Kafiri G, Thomas DM, Shepherd NA, et al. p53 expression is common in malignant mesothelioma. Histopathology 1992;21:331–334.

58. Segers K, Backhovens H, Singh SK, et al. Immunoreactiv-ity for p53 and mdm2 and the detection of p53 mutations in human malignant mesothelioma. Virchows Arch 1995; 427:431–436.

59. Mor O, Yaron P, Huszar M, et al. Absence of p53 mutations in malignant mesothelioma. Am J Respir Cell Mol Biol 1997;16:9–13.

60. Ungar S, Van De Meeren A, Tammilehto L, et al. High levels of MDM2 are not correlated with the presence of wild-type p53 in human malignant mesothelioma cell lines. Br J Cancer 1996;74:1534–1540.

61. Hopkins-Donaldson S, Belyanskaya LL, Simoes-Wurst AP, et al. p53-induced apoptosis occurs in the absence of p14[ARF] in malignant pleural mesothelioma. Neoplasia 2006;7:551–559.

62. Carbone M, Rizzo P, Grimley PM, et al. Simian virus 40 large T antigen binds p53 in human mesotheliomas. Nature Med 1999;8:908–912.

63. Baldi A, Groeger AM, Esposito V, et al. Expression of p21 in SV40 large T antigen positive human pleural mesothelioma: relationship with survival. Thorax 2002;57: 353–356.

64. Sekido Y, Pass HI, Bader S, et al. Neurofibromatosis type 2 (NF2) gene is somatically mutated in mesothelioma but not in lung cancer. Cancer Res 1995;55:1227–1231.

65. Bianchi AB, Mitsunaga SI, Cheng JQ, et al. High frequency of inactivating mutations in the neurofibromatosis type 2 gene (NF2) in primary malignant mesotheliomas. Proc Natl Acad Sci USA 1995;92:10854–10858.

66. Poulikakos PI, Xiao GH, Gallagher R, et al. Re-expression of the tumor suppressor NF2/merlin inhibits invasiveness in mesothelioma cells and negatively regulates FAK. Oncogene 2006;25:5960–8.

67. Lecomte C, Andujar P, Renier A, et al. Similar tumor sup-pressor gene alteration profiles in asbestos-induced murine and human mesothelioma. Cell Cycle 2005;12:1862–1869.

68. Altomare DA, Vaslet CA, Skele KL, et al. A mouse model recapitulating molecular features of human mesothelioma. Cancer Res 2005;65:8090–8095.

69. Suzuki M, Toyooka S, Shivapurkar N, et al. Aberrant meth-ylation profilc of human malignant mesotheliomas and its relationship to SV40 infection. Oncogene 2005;24:1302–1308.

70. Fischer JR, Ohnmacht U, Rieger N, et al. Promoter meth-ylation of RASSF1A, RARβ, and DAPK predict poor prognosis of patients with malignant mesothelioma. Lung Cancer 2006;54(1):109–116.

71. Toyooka S, Pass HI, Shivapurkar N, et al. Aberrant meth-ylation and simian virus 40 tag sequences in malignant mesothelioma. Cancer Res 2001;61:5727–5730.

72. Jasani B, Cristaudo A, Emri SA, et al. Association of SV40 with human tumors. Seminar Cancer Biol 2001;11:49–61.

73. Carbone M, Pass HI, Rizzo P, et al. Simian virus 40-like DNA sequences in human pleural mesothelioma. Onco-gene 1994;9:1781–1790.

74. Galateau-Salle F, Bidet P, Iwatsubo Y, et al. SV40-like DNA sequences in pleural mesothelioma, bronchopulmo-nary carcinoma, and non-malignant pulmonary diseases. J Pathol 1998;184:252–257.

75. Vilchez RA, Butel JS. Emergent human pathogen simian virus 40 and its role in cancer. Clinical Microbiol Rev 2004;17:495–508.

76. Testa JR, Carbone M, Hirvonen A, et al. A multi-institu-tional study confirms the presence and expression of simian virus 40 in human malignant mesotheliomas. Cancer Res 1998;58:4505–4509.

77. Lednicky JA, Butel JS. Simian virus 40 regulatory region structural diversity and the association of viral archetypal regulatory regions with human brain tumors. Semin Cancer Biol 2001;11:39–47.

78. Carbone M, Kratzke RA, Testa JR. The pathogenesis of mesothelioma. Semin Oncol 2002;29:2–17.

79. Bocchetta M, Di Resta I, Powers A, et al. Human meso-thelial cells are unusually susceptible to simian virus 40-mediated transformation and asbestos cocarcinogenicity. Proc Natl Acad Sci USA 2000;97:10214–10219.

80. Burmeister B, Schwerdtle T, Poser I, et al. Effects of asbes-tos on initiation of DNA damage, induction of DNA-strand breaks, p53 expression and apoptosis in primary SV40-

transformed and malignant human mesothelioma cells. Mutation Res 2004;558:81–92.

81. Gazdar AF, Butel JS, Carbone M. SV40 and human tumours: myth, association or casualty? Nat Rev Cancer 2002;2:957–964.

82. Shivapurkar N, Wiethege T, Wistuba II, et al. Presence of simian virus 40 sequences in malignant mesotheliomas and mesothelial cell proliferations. J Cell Biochem 1999;76: 181–188.

83. Saenz-Robles MT, Sullivan CS, Pipas JM. Transforming functions of simian virus 40. Oncogene 2001;20:7899–7907.

84. Khalili K, Stoner G, editors. Human Polyomaviruses: Molecular and Clinical Perspectives. New York: Wiley-Liss; 2001.

85. Sullivan CS, Pipas JL. T antigens of simian virus 40: molecular chaperones for viral replication and tumorigenesis. Microbiol Mol Biol 2002;66:179–202.

86. Foddis R, De Rienzo A, Broccoli D, et al. SV40 infection induces telomerase activity in human mesothelial cells. Oncogene 2002;21:1434–1442.

87. Cacciotti P, Libener R, Betta F, et al. SV40 replication in human mesothelial cells induces HGF/MET receptor activation: a model for viral-related mesothelioma. Proc Natl Acad Sci USA 2001;98:12032–12037.

88. Stratton K, Almario DA, McCormik MC. Immunization Safety Review: SV40 Contamination of Polio Vaccine and Cancer. Washington, DC: The National Academic Press; 2003.

89. King JE, Thatcher N, Pickering CA, Hasleton PS. Sensitivity and specificity of immunohistochemical markers used in the diagnosis of epithelioid mesothelioma: a detailed systematic analysis using published data. Histopathology 2006;48:223–232.

90. Maheswaran S, Englen C, Bennet P, et al. The WT1 gene product stabilizes p53 and inhibits p53-mediated apoptosis Genes Dev 1995;9:2143–2156.

91. Scharnhorst V, Dekker P, van der Eb AJ, Jochemsen AG. Physical interaction between WT1 and p73 proteins modulates their functions. J Biol Chem 2000;275:10202–10211.

92. Amin KM, Litzky LA, Smythe WR, et al. Wilms' tumor 1 susceptibility (WT1) gene products are selectively expressed in malignant mesothelioma. Am J Pathol 1995; 186:300–305.

93. Uematsu K, Kanazawa S, You L, et al. Wnt pathway activation in mesothelioma: evidence of disheveled overexpression and transcriptional activity of beta-catenin. Cancer Res 2003;63:4547–4551.

94. You L, He B, Uematsu K, et al. Inhibition of wnt-1 signaling induces apoptosis in beta-catenin deficient mesothelioma cells. Cancer Res 2004;64:3474–3478.

95. Chen S, Guttridge DC, You Z, et al. Wnt-1 signaling inhibits apoptosis by activating beta-catenin/T-cell factor-mediated transcription. J Cell Biol 2001;152:87–96.

96. Liu Z, Klominek J. Chemotaxis and chemokinesis of malignant mesothelioma cells to multiple growths factors. Anticancer Res 2004;24(3a):1625–1630.

97. Syrokou A, Tzanakakis GN, Hjerpe A, Karamanos NK. Proteoglycans in human malignant mesothelioma. Stimulation of their synthesis induced by epidermal, insulin and platelet-derived growth factors involves receptor with tyrosine kinase activity. Biochimie 1999;81:733–744.

98. Hoang CD, Zhang X, Scott PD, et al. Selective activation of insulin receptor substrate-1 and -2 in pleural mesothelioma cells: association with distinct malignant phenotypes. Cancer 2004;64:7479–7485.

99. Porcu P, Ferber A, Pietrzkowski Z, et al. The growth-stimulatory effect of simian virus 40 T antigen requires the interaction of insulin like growth factor 1 with its receptor. Mol Cell Biol 1992;11:5069–5077.

100. Gerwin BI, Lechner JF, Reddel RR, et al. Comparison of production of transforming growth factor-beta and platelet-derived growth factor by normal human mesothelial cells and mesothelioma cells lines. Cancer Res 1987;47: 6180–6184.

101. Versnel MA, Hagemeijer A, Bouts MJ, et al. Expression of c-sis (PDGF B-chain) and PDGF A-chain genes in ten human malignant mesothelioma cell lines derived from primary and metastatic tumors. Oncogene 1988;2:601–605.

102. Jänne PA, Taffaro M, Salgia R, Johson B. Inhibition of epidermal growth factor signaling in malignant pleural mesothelioma. Cancer Res 2002;62:5242–5247.

103. Dazzi H, Hasleton P, Thatcher N, et al. Malignant pleural mesothelioma and epidermal growth factor 5EGF-R). Relashionship of EGF-R with histology and survival using paraffin embedded tissue and the F4 monoclonal antibody. Br J Cancer 1990;61:924–926.

104. Cai Y, Roggli V, Mark E, et al. Transforming growth factor alpha and epidermal growth factor receptor in reactive and malignant mesothelial proliferations. Arch Pathol Lab Med 2004;128:68–70.

105. Govindan R, Kratzke RA, Herndon JE 2nd, et al. Cancer and leukemia group B. Clin Cancer Res 2005;11:2300–2304.

106. Cortese JF, Gowda AL, Wali A, et al. Common EGFR mutations conferring sensitivity to gefitinib in lung adenocarcinoma are not prevalent in human malignant mesothelioma. Int J Cancer 2006;118:521–552.

35
Molecular Pathology of Pediatric Tumors of the Lung

Josefine M. Heim-Hall

Introduction

Primary lung tumors, both benign and malignant, are overall rare in the pediatric population. Among 166 cases seen at the Armed Forces Institute between 1950 and 1989, malignant tumors were more frequent than benign tumors, with a ratio of 1:1.68. Inflammatory myofibroblastic tumor, also known as inflammatory pseudotumor or plasma cell granuloma, is the most common benign pediatric lung tumor and is discussed later. Epithelial lung malignancies are rare in childhood. Although histologic subtypes are similar to those that occur in adults, the frequencies of types differ, with carcinoid tumors being the most common.[1] There is no known association of environmental or genetic factors and the development of epithelial malignancies in children. Pleuropulmonary blastoma, discussed later, is truly a tumor of childhood and never occurs in adults. Thoracopulmonary small round cell tumor, also called Askin's tumor, is not restricted to childhood but is most common in adolescents and young adults and will therefore be discussed here as well.

Pleuropulmonary Blastoma

Pleuropulmonary blastoma (PPB) is an aggressive and rare dysontogenetic tumor of childhood. The term *dysontogenetic* denotes a lesion that resembles the developmental anatomy of the organ of origin. Such lesions include PPB, Wilms' tumor, hepatoblastoma, and pancreatoblastoma and are characterized by the proliferation of both mesenchymal and epithelial elements. Pleuropulmonary blastoma is frequently associated with a predisposition to develop other childhood neoplasms as well as with dysplasias and developmental abnormalities, occurring either in the same patients or in their family members. This association has been found in about 25% of cases of PPB and includes other PPBs, pulmonary cysts, cystic

nephroma, sarcomas, medulloblastoma, thyroid dysplasias and neoplasias, malignant germ cell tumors, Hodgkin's disease, leukemia, and Langerhans cell histiocytosis.[2]

Although originally regarded as a variant of the adult pulmonary blastomas, PPB is now considered to be an entirely distinct entity with only a superficial resemblance. The most significant difference between the childhood and the adult types is the complete absence of a malignant epithelial component in PBB, while the adult-type pulmonary blastomas are either biphasic tumors composed of malignant glands and malignant mesenchyme (the so-called biphasic pulmonary blastoma) or tumors composed of malignant tubules with benign mesenchyme (the well-differentiated fetal adenocarcinoma).

In contrast to the adult types, PPB occurs exclusively in childhood, and most cases are diagnosed in the first 4 years of life. Tumors are intrapulmonary, mediastinal, or pleural-based masses ranging in size from 2 to 28 cm.[3,4] Clinical presentation is with respiratory difficulty, fever, pain, and cough. The clinical course is aggressive, with high recurrence rates and frequent metastases to the brain, bones, and liver.[5]

In the largest study of this tumor (50 cases), patients' ages ranged from newborn to 146 months, with the majority being diagnosed in the first 4 years of life.[4] Tumors have been subclassified into three types.[6] Type I is exclusively cystic without a grossly detectable solid component, type II exhibits both solid and cystic areas, and type III is completely solid. Type I is the least common and occurs on average in the youngest group (median age, 9 months).[5] It is composed of peripherally located thin-walled cysts. The neoplastic component is only recognized by microscopic examination and consists of a layer of primitive tumor cells beneath a benign epithelial surface. This layer may be discontinuous and subtle, making the distinction from a benign cyst difficult. Type II is the most common type and is diagnosed at a median age of 34 months, whereas type III, which is slightly less common

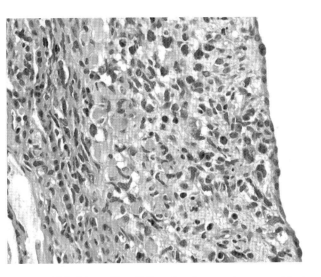

FIGURE 35.1. Type II solid/cystic pleuropulmonary blastoma with benign epithelial surface surrounded by primitive blastema and sarcomatous elements with rhabdomyoblastic features. Hematoxylin and eosin stain; magnification, ×40. (Courtesy of Dr. Teresa Hayes.)

than type II, is diagnosed at a median age of 42 months. The solid areas of the types II and III tumors have mixed blastematous and sarcomatous features. Blastematous cells are small and primitive in appearance with little cytoplasm and oval nuclei with inconspicuous nucleoli and numerous mitotic figures. The sarcomatous areas are composed of spindle cells arranged in a fascicular pattern resembling fibrosarcoma. Foci of rhabdomyoblastic differentiation are evident with hematoxylin and eosin stain in the form of rhabdomyoblasts and cross striations (Figure 35.1) or by immunohistochemistry and are identified in the majority of cases, including all subtypes. Cartilaginous differentiation and cellular anaplasia are frequently associated with types II and III.

Immunohistochemistry

Vimentin diffusely stains the spindle cell areas and focally blastematous areas. Staining with S100 is limited to foci of cartilaginous differentiation. Muscle-specific markers (desmin, myogenin) are positive in the cells with obvious rhabdomyoblastic features and less consistently in small primitive cell areas. Cytokeratin is positive in the epithelium of cystic spaces but negative in tumor cells.

Cytogenetic and Molecular Studies

Cytogenetic analysis has been reported to date for at least 25 cases of PPB. A summary listing of the karyotypes of 23 previously published cases and of 2 additional cases is provided by Quilichini et al.[7] Most cases analyzed by cytogenetics had complex numerical and structural chromosomal abnormalities (Figure 35.2). The main recurrent abnormality was numerical gains of chromosome 8 (22 cases), and it has been speculated that this represents a primary event in the genesis of PPB.[8] Structural abnormalities of chromosome 8 have been described in several cases (rearrangements of the long arm in three cases and of either the long, short or both arms in two cases). A candidate gene has not been identified to date.

Two cases showed structural rearrangement of the short arm of chromosome 11. Given the reported occurrence of 11p alterations in other embryonal/dysontogenetic tumors (deletions of 11p in Wilms' tumor, loss of heterozygosity at 11p13 in embryonal rhabdomyosarcoma), a possible common genetic pathway involving the 11p region has been suggested.[2]

In addition to conventional cytogenetics, other molecular techniques have been employed in some cases of PPB. Multicolor spectral karyotyping was used in one case,[9] and it showed trisomy 8 and unbalanced translocations between chromosomes 1 and X. Comparative genomic hybridization performed in one case[10] showed multiple gains and losses, with a profile overlapping that of embryonal rhabdomyosarcoma (gains of chromosomes 2, 7, and 8 and loss on chromosome 10).[11] Multiplex fluorescence in situ hybridization (FISH) was performed in two cases mentioned earlier[7] and confirmed a structural aberration of chromosome 8 and also a *TP53* deletion on der (17) in one of the two cases.

The nonneoplastic nature of the epithelial component of PPB has been demonstrated by FISH studies that showed chromosome 8 gains in all mesenchymal elements (Figure 35.3), including undifferentiated blastematous, rhabdomyoblastic, fibroblastic, and chondroblastic areas, whereas the epithelium did not show such alterations.[12]

Relationship of Pleuropulmonary Blastoma to Congenital Cystic Adenomatoid Malformation

One of the important differential diagnoses when considering PPB is congenital cystic adenomatoid malformation. Congenital cystic adenomatoid malformation has been classified into four types,[13] with type 4 being characterized by large cysts lined by flattened epithelium resting on loose mesenchymal tissue. It is this type that is most easily confused with the purely cystic form of PPB, given the histologic similarities and a similar age range. Both congenital cystic adenomatoid malformation type 4 and PPB type 1 contain cystic spaces lined by benign epithelium, and both contain mesenchymal tissue that may show skeletal muscle differentiation. A careful search for areas of dense subepithelial or septal spindle cell proliferation with or without thickening of the septum is necessary in such cases to prompt a diagnosis of PPB.[5]

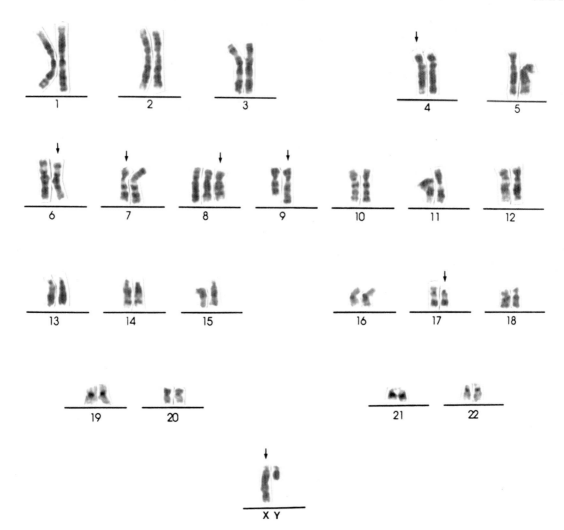

FIGURE 35.2. Giemsa-banded karyotype in an example of pleuropulmonary blastoma. Arrows indicate clonal aberrations, including trisomy 8. (From Vargas et al.,[12] with permission of Springer.)

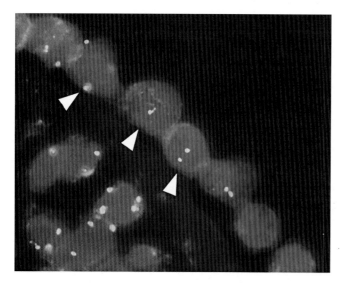

FIGURE 35.3. Fluorescence in situ hybridization. Epithelial cell nuclei (arrowheads) show one or two fluorescent signals for chromosome 8 per cell. Underlying primitive mesenchymal cells show multiple signals per nuclei, indicating polysomy. (From Vargas et al.,[12] with permission of Springer.)

A recent cytogenetic analysis comparing 11 cases of congenital cystic adenomatoid malformation to 2 cases of PPB showed normal karyotypes in all congenital cystic adenomatoid malformations and clonal abnormalities in both PPB, therefore emphasizing the biologic distinctiveness of these two lesions.[14]

Inflammatory Myofibroblastic Tumor

Inflammatory myofibroblastic tumor has been known in the literature under a number of designations, including inflammatory pseudotumor, plasma cell granuloma, and inflammatory fibrosarcoma. In adults, the lung is the most frequent site. In children, extrapulmonary sites including liver, spleen, mediastinum, central nervous system, and soft tissues are more common than the lungs.

Most inflammatory myofibroblastic tumors behave in a benign fashion, but malignant behavior due to recurrences with local invasion and metastatic spread does occur. Inflammatory myofibroblastic tumor is therefore considered a tumor of low malignant potential (of intermediate malignant behavior in the 2002 WHO classification of soft tissue tumors). Clinical features when the lung is involved include cough, dyspnea, fever, chest pain, and hemoptysis. Some cases are asymptomatic and are discovered incidentally. Most tumors are peripheral, well circumscribed, and solitary, but endobronchial growth with formation of a polypoid mass or penetration through the pleura has also been observed.

Histologically, inflammatory myofibroblastic tumor is composed of fibroblastic/myofibroblastic spindle cells, growing in fascicles set against a background of a plasma cell–rich inflammatory infiltrate (Figure 35.4). Mitotic

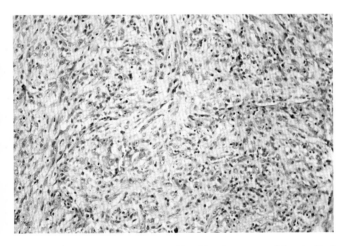

FIGURE 35.4. Inflammatory myofibroblastic tumor with spindled myofibroblasts in a loose myxoid and inflammatory background containing lymphocytes and plasma cells. (Courtesy of Dr. Cheryl Coffin.)

activity is variable, but there are no atypical mitoses nor is there significant nuclear pleomorphism. Immunohistochemical stains are consistent with a myofibroblastic phenotype (muscle-specific actin/smooth muscle actin positive, and less frequently desmin and cytokeratin positive).

Cytogenetic and Molecular Studies

The question whether inflammatory myofibroblastic tumor is a reactive or a neoplastic process had been a matter of controversy until the detection of recurrent cytogenetic abnormalities in inflammatory myofibroblastic tumor, lending support to its neoplastic nature. Clonal aberrations involving the short arm of chromosome 2p23 were originally described in anaplastic large cell lymphoma, but subsequently similar abnormalities were found in inflammatory myofibroblastic tumor.[15] Chromosome 2p23 is the site of a tyrosine kinase receptor gene, the human *ALK* (anaplastic lymphoma kinase) gene, that belongs to the insulin growth factor superfamily.[16] Under normal circumstances, ALK expression is limited to rare neural cells in human tissues, implying a role in neural development and differentiation.[17] ALK is abnormally expressed in translocations involving the *ALK* gene at 2p23. Antibodies to the protein products of the *ALK* gene (ALK1 and p80) detect ALK expression associated with these gene rearrangements and correlate well with the results of FISH and reverse transcriptase polymerase chain reaction (RT-PCR). Monoclonal antibody ALK1 and polyclonal antibody p80 are the most commonly used immunohistochemical markers for detection of ALK deregulation in formalin-fixed, paraffin-embedded tissues.

In anaplastic large cell lymphoma, ALK clonal abnormalities are associated with the characteristic t(2;5)(p23q35) resulting in the NPM/ALK fusion protein in the majority of cases.[18] Several variant translocations have also been described in a smaller proportion resulting in fusion of alternate partner proteins with the ALK protein.[19–25] The immunohistochemical ALK or p80 staining pattern is typically nuclear and cytoplasmic with the classic t(2;5)(p23q35) translocation, whereas variant translocations are associated with a predominantly cytoplasmic staining pattern.[17]

In inflammatory myofibroblastic tumor, ALK rearrangements and/or ALK1 and p80 positivity have been reported in variable proportions ranging from 36% to 60%.[26,27] In one study of 47 inflammatory myofibroblastic tumors,[28] immunoreactivity for ALK1 and/or p80 was detected in 36% of cases and FISH was positive for ALK rearrangement in 47%. The ALK abnormalities occurred in both pediatric and adult patients.

Several fusion oncogenes partnering with the *ALK* gene have been identified in inflammatory myofibroblastic tumor. The partner proteins thus far identified are TPM3 at 1p23,[29] TPM4 at 19p13,[28] ATIC at 2q35,[30] CARS at 11p15,[31] CLTC at 17q23,[32] RANBP2 at 2q13,[33] and SEC31L1 at 4q21.[34]

Rearrangements of the 2p23 region can be detected with FISH methods.

An NPM/ALK two-color FISH probe is used to specifically detect the t(2;5)(p23;q35) translocation, and it detects the characteristic translocation of anaplastic large cell lymphoma. In inflammatory myofibroblastic tumor, the alternative rearrangements involving the *ALK* gene can be detected with a dual break-apart ALK probe that flanks the *ALK* gene region at 2p23.[16]

Immunohistochemical markers ALK1 and p80 with a cytoplasmic staining pattern correlate with the results of RT-PCR and FISH methods and are an easy way to detect ALK rearrangements in suspected inflammatory myofibroblastic tumor (Figures 35.5 and 35.6). One limitation in the use of ALK1/p80 immunohistochemistry is its lack of specificity among mesenchymal tumors. Among such neoplasms, abnormalities of ALK1 and p80 expression were found in malignant peripheral nerve sheath tumor, rhabdomyosarcoma, leiomyosarcoma, and malignant fibrous histiocytoma.[16] On the other hand, several benign fibroblastic lesions in the differential diagnosis with inflammatory myofibroblastic tumor, including nodular fasciitis, desmoid tumor, myofibromatosis, and leiomyoma, were negative for these markers. Some malignant mesenchymal tumors, such as synovial sarcoma, infantile fibrosarcoma, and myofibroblastic sarcoma, were likewise negative. Previous studies had shown similar results with the addition of neuroblastoma, which was also positive in a few cases.[35]

In summary, the demonstration of ALK expression by immunohistochemical or molecular methods is of diagnostic utility when inflammatory myofibroblastic tumor

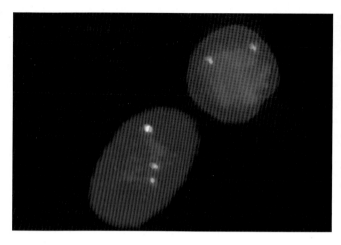

FIGURE 35.6. Fluorescence in situ hybridization with the ALK probe showing a split probe signal in the cell on the left. (Courtesy of Dr. Cheryl Coffin.)

is a consideration. A positive result has to be interpreted with caution in the context of histologic and clinical data and after exclusion of anaplastic large cell lymphoma. Conversely, a negative result does not rule out inflammatory myofibroblastic tumor, given that a considerable proportion of histologically indistinguishable tumors are ALK negative.

Prognostic Significance of ALK Expression

Although ALK expression has been associated with a better prognosis in anaplastic large cell lymphoma, its prognostic significance in inflammatory myofibroblastic tumor is less certain. Some studies[36,37] have shown ALK-positive inflammatory myofibroblastic tumor to occur at a younger age and to have a better prognosis, whereas others[38] did not show this advantage. Given the small number of cases in these studies, the role of ALK expression in inflammatory myofibroblastic tumor as a prognostic marker remains unclear.

Etiologic Role of Infectious Agents

Various infectious agents have been suspected to play a role in the pathogenesis of inflammatory myofibroblastic tumor. This is not surprising given the overlap of clinical features of inflammatory myofibroblastic tumor with those of infectious processes such as fever, anemia, increased erythrocyte sedimentation rate, and malaise.

Human herpesvirus 8 (HHV-8) DNA sequences with a spectrum of expressed viral genes different from those observed in Kaposi's sarcoma have been reported in adult pulmonary inflammatory myofibroblastic tumor.[39] Subsequent studies, including pediatric pulmonary inflammatory myofibroblastic tumor, did not confirm this association. Specifically, HHV-8 immunostaining against

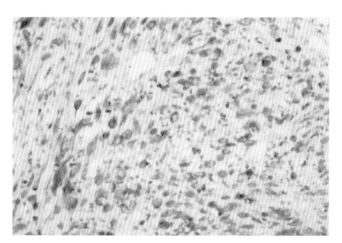

FIGURE 35.5. Staining of ALK in an inflammatory myofibroblastic tumor showing a strong cytoplasmic pattern. (Courtesy of Dr. Cheryl Coffin.)

latent ORF73, which is usually present in other HHV-8–associated diseases, was negative in that study.[35]

Epstein-Barr virus (EBV) has also been implicated in inflammatory myofibroblastic tumor pathogenesis. Positive in situ hybridization results with the EBV–encoded RNA (EBER) probe were seen in several studies, mostly in splenic inflammatory myofibroblastic tumor and a few cases of lymph node and hepatic inflammatory myofibroblastic tumor[40,41] Only one of the four pediatric lung inflammatory myofibroblastic tumors studied was positive in a recent study.[35] The number of EBER-positive spindled tumor cells in this study was much greater inside the tumor than in the surrounding tissue, making a role of EBV in tumorigenesis more likely.

Malignant Small Round Cell Tumor of the Thoracopulmonary Region

Originally described by Askin et al.,[42] the malignant small round cell tumor of the thoracopulmonary region is now considered a member of the Ewing family of tumors (EFTs), which encompasses osseous and extraosseous Ewing's sarcoma and peripheral primitive neuroectodermal tumor. Primitive neuroectodermal tumor is a highly aggressive primitive round cell tumor of uncertain histogenesis with variable degrees of neural differentiation. Despite its name, there is no evidence of neural crest origin. Given its most common occurrence in mesenchyme-rich organs (bone, soft tissue, visceral parenchyme), a mesenchymal origin appears most plausible.

Primitive neuroectodermal tumor of the thoracopulmonary region, like those arising in other sites, affects all

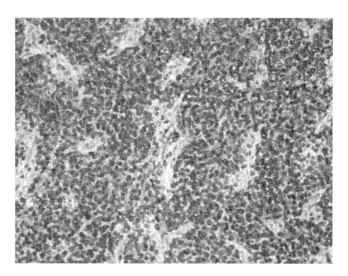

FIGURE 35.8. Askin's tumor diffusely positive for CD99 with membranous staining pattern.

ages, with a predilection for the second to third decade. It typically originates in the chest wall with secondary infiltration of the pleura and lungs, but purely intrapulmonary examples also exist.

Histologic features are those of a primitive small round cell tumor with uniform undifferentiated tumor cells growing in patternless sheets (Figure 35.7). Hemorrhage and necrosis are common. Neural differentiation may be apparent in the form of Homer-Wright-like neural rosettes, but many tumors have a completely undifferentiated phenotype.

Immunohistochemical stains are negative with most mesenchymal markers with the exception of vimentin. Neural markers S100, CD56, chromogranin, and synaptophysin may be positive but often only focally or weakly. Cytokeratin positivity is rarely seen.

The most helpful marker is CD99 (O13, HBA71), which is positive in >90% of primitive neuroectodermal tumor with a characteristic membranous staining pattern (Figure 35.8). Given the lack of specificity of CD99, it has to be interpreted in the context of a comprehensive panel of immunohistochemical stains aimed at ruling out tumors with a similar histologic phenotype, in particular the small round cell tumors of childhood. These include leukemia/lymphoma, solid variant of alveolar rhabdomyosarcoma, mesenchymal chondrosarcoma, desmoplastic round cell tumor, poorly differentiated synovial sarcoma, metastatic neuroblastoma, and Wilms' tumor.

Cytogenetic and Molecular Studies in Ewing's Family of Tumors

The discovery of consistent genetic alterations in EFTS has made cytogenetic and molecular techniques an invaluable adjunct in the diagnosis of these tumors. In contrast

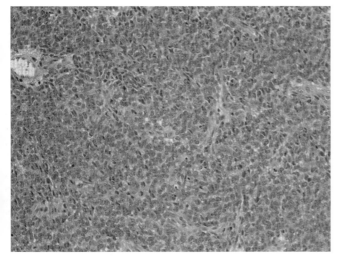

FIGURE 35.7. Askin's tumor with sheet-like arrangement of primitive tumor cells. Hematoxylin and eosin stain; magnification, ×20.

to adult epithelial malignancies, in which similar mutations can be found in a variety of different tumor types, the *EWS/ETS* fusion gene appears to be specific for ESFT.[43] In fact, these nonrandom translocations are currently considered to be the defining feature of ESFT. They are characterized by fusion of the *EWS* gene with one of the several members of the ETS family of transcription factors.[44]

Because the *EWS* gene was only discovered in the context of fusion to *FLI1*, the normal function of *EWS* is still under investigation.[43] A current hypothesis is that *EWS* gene products act as adapters between transcription and mRNA processing by interacting with components of the transcription apparatus and splicing factors.[45,46] The *ETS* fusion partner belongs to the family of transcription factors that is defined by a conserved ETS domain that recognizes a certain DNA motif.[47] Within this family, at least 30 different genes have been identified and several of these (i.e., *FLI1, ERG, E1AF, FEV,* and *ZSG*) are involved in cancer-associated gene fusions. The EWS/ETS fusion proteins appear to modulate the expression of target genes in a sequence-specific manner that is determined by the ETS component coming under the control of the EWS component.[48] The most frequent gene fusion in ESFT is *EWS/FLI1*. It is found in up to 95% of ESFT and results from a t(11;22)(q24;q12) translocation. At a genomic level, different *EWS/FLI1* fusions have been described, each with variable combinations of exons flanking the fusion point.[49–51] Results of a few recent studies suggest prognostic significance of differences in fusion type,[49,52] but confirmation of these results through prospective studies is still required.

Although considered a traditional oncogene ("promoting the proliferation and blocking differentiation of a committed neural crest cell"), *EWS/FLI1* has been shown to not only inhibit tissue specific differentiation but also to promote Ewing's-specific neuroectodermal differentiation. This has been nicely demonstrated in an experiment using a rhabdomyosarcoma cell line transfected with a tetracycline-inducible expression vector that induces expression of *EWS/FLI1*. The cell lines underwent a change in phenotype from myogenic to primitive neuroectodermal as demonstrated by light microscopic features and immunohistochemical profile of cultured cells and xenograft tumors.[53]

At a cytogenetic level, the t(11;22)(q24;q12) translocation leads to fusion of *EWS* at 22q12 to *FLI1* at 11q24 and the formation of *EWS/FLI1* on der (22) comprising the 5′ end of *EWS* and the 3′ end of *FLI1*.[54] The fusion gene encodes an oncoprotein consisting of the N-terminal domain of *EWS* and the DNA-binding domain of *FLI1*[55]. The second most common translocation is t(12;22)(q22;q12), found in approximately 5% of cases,[56] which leads to the fusion of *EWS* to *ERG* at 21q22. Other translocations are seen in less than 1% of cases

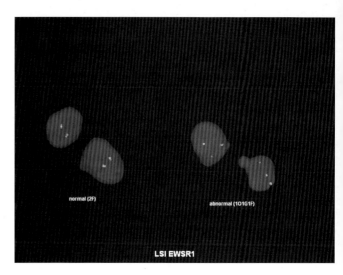

FIGURE 35.9. FISH-EWSR1 (22q12) dual color break apart probe shows split signals in this example of Ewing's sarcoma/PNET (Courtesy of Dr. Siddharth Adhvaryu.)

and include t(7;22)(p22;q12),[57] t(17;22)(q12;q12),[58,59] t(2;22)(q33;q12),[60] and inv (22),[61] leading to fusion of *EWS* with the *ETS* genes *ETV1, E1AF, FEV,* and *ZSG,* respectively.

Detection of translocations involving the *EWS* gene has become an important tool in the differential diagnosis of small round cell tumors. Both RT-PCR- and FISH-based methods are available and offer certain advantages and disadvantages. The advantage of RT-PCR is its ability to identify precise fusion transcripts and specific chromosomal breakpoints involved in the translocation. Therefore, this technique allows distinction between fusion types, which, as mentioned earlier, may be of prognostic significance. Although RT-PCR works well with fresh frozen tissue, it is considerably less sensitive with paraffin-embedded, formalin-fixed tissue.[62] Fluorescence in situ hybridization probes, on the other hand, are highly sensitive and specific in fixed tissue. Both "home brew" fusion probes and commercial break-apart probes can be used, and both are relatively easy to interpret. Fusion probes are typically designed to detect the *EWS/FLI1* fusion and would miss any of the variant *ETS* gene family rearrangements, whereas break-apart probes offer the advantage of detecting *EWS* fusion with different *ETS* genes (Figure 35.9).

References

1. Lal DR, Clark I, Shalkow J, et al. Primary epithelial lung malignancies in the pediatric population. Pediatr Blood Cancer 2005;45(5):683–686.
2. Priest JR, Watterson J, Strong L, et al. Pleuropulmonary blastoma: a marker for familial disease. J Pediatr 1996; 128(2):220–224.

3. Manivel CJ, Priest JR, Watterson J, et al. Pleuropulmonary blastoma: the so-called pulmonary blastoma of childhood. Cancer 1988;62(8):1516–1526.

4. Priest JR, McDermott MB, Bhatia S, et al. Pleuropulmonary blastoma: a clinicopathologic study of 50 cases. Cancer 1997;80(1):147–161.

5. Hill DA. USCAP Specialty Conference: case 1-type I pleuropulmonary blastoma. Pediatr Dev Pathol 2005;8(1):77–84.

6. Dehner LP, Watterson J, Priest J. Pleuropulmonary blastoma. A unique intrathoracic neoplasm of childhood. Perspect Pediatr Pathol 1995;18:214–226.

7. Quilichini B, Andre N, Bouvier C, et al. Hidden chromosomal abnormalities in pleuropulmonary blastomas identified by multiplex FISH. BMC Cancer 2006;6:4.

8. Kelsey AM, McNally K, Birch J, et al. Case of extra pulmonary, pleuro-pulmonary blastoma in a child: pathological and cytogenetic findings. Med Pediatr Oncol 1997;29(1):61–64.

9. Barnard M, Bayani J, Grant R, et al. Use of multicolor spectral karyotyping in genetic analysis of pleuropulmonary blastoma. Pediatr Dev Pathol 2000;3(5):479–486.

10. Roque L, Rodrigues R, Martins C, et al. Comparative genomic hybridization analysis of a pleuropulmonary blastoma. Cancer Genet Cytogenet 2004;149(1):58–62.

11. Bridge JA, Liu J, Qualman SJ, et al. Genomic gains and losses are similar in genetic and histologic subsets of rhabdomyosarcomas, whereas amplification predominates in embryonal with anaplasia and alveolar subtypes. Genes Chromosomes Cancer 2002;33(3):310–321.

12. Vargas SO, Nose V, Fletcher JA, et al. Gains of chromosome 8 are confined to mesenchymal components in pleuropulmonary blastoma. Pediatr Dev Pathol 2001;4(5):434–445.

13. Stocker JT. Congenital and developmental diseases. In Dail DH, Hammar SP, eds. Pulmonary Pathology. Berlin: Springer-Verlag; 1994:155–181.

14. Vargas SO, Korpershoek E, Kozakewich HP, et al. Cytogenetic and p53 profiles in congenital cystic adenomatoid malformation: insights into its relationship with pleuropulmonary blastoma. Pediatr Dev Pathol 2006;9:190–195.

15. Griffin CA, Hawkins AL, Dvorak C, et al. Recurrent involvement of 2p23 in inflammatory myofibroblastic tumors. Cancer Res 1999;59(12):2776–2780.

16. Cessna MH, Zhou H, Sanger WG, et al. Expression of ALK1 and p80 in inflammatory myofibroblastic tumor and its mesenchymal mimics: a study of 135 cases. Mod Pathol 2002;15(9):931–938.

17. Pulford K, Morris SW, Turturro F. Anaplastic lymphoma kinase proteins in growth control and cancer. J Cell Physiol 2004;199(3):330–358.

18. Falini B, Bigerna B, Fizzotti M, et al. ALK expression defines a distinct group of T/null lymphomas ("ALK lymphomas") with a wide morphological spectrum. Am J Pathol 1998; 153(3):857–886.

19. Nakamura S, Shiota M, Nakagawa A, et al. Anaplastic large cell lymphoma: a distinct molecular pathologic entity: a reappraisal with special reference to p80(NPM/ALK) expression. Am J Surg Pathol 1997;21(12):1420–1432.

20. Shiota M, Fujimoto J, Takenaga M, et al. Diagnosis of t(2;5)(p23;q35)-associated Ki-1 lymphoma with immuno-histo-chemistry. Blood 1994;84(11):3648–3652.

21. Pittaluga S, Wiodarska I, Pulford K, et al. The monoclonal antibody ALKI identifies a distinct morphological subtype of anaplastic large cell lymphoma associated with 2p23/ALK rearrangements. Am J Pathol 1997;151(2):343–51.

22. Pulford K, Lamant L, Morris SW, et al. Detection of anaplastic lymphoma kinase (ALK) and nucleolar protein nucleo-phosmin (NPM)-ALK proteins in normal and neoplastic cells with the monoclonal antibody ALKI. Blood 1997;89(4):1394–1404.

23. Falini B, Bigerna B, Fizzotti M, et al. ALK expression defines a distinct group of T/null lymphomas ("ALK lymphomas") with a wide morphological spectrum. Am J Pathol 1998;153: 875–886.

24. Cataldo KA, Jalal SM, Law ME, et al. Detection of t(2;5) in anaplastic large cell lymphoma: comparison of immunohistochemical studies, FISH, and RT-PCR in paraffin-embedded tissue. Am J Surg Pathol 1999;23(11):1386–1392.

25. Lamant L, Pulford K, Bischof D, et al. Expression of the ALK tyrosine kinase gene in neuroblastoma. Am J Pathol 2000;156(5):1711–1721.

26. Coffin CM, Patel A, Perkins S, et al. ALK1 and p80 expression and chromosomal rearrangements involving 2p23 in inflammatory myofibroblastic tumor. Mod Pathol 2001;14(6): 569–576.

27. Cook JR, Dehner LP, Collins M, et al. Anaplastic lymphoma kinase (ALK) expression in the inflammatory myofibroblastic tumor: a comparative immunohistochemical study. Am J Surg Pathol 2001;25(11):1364–1371.

28. Coffin CM, Patel A, Perkins S, et al. ALK1 and p80 expression and chromosomal rearrangements involving 2p23 in inflammatory myofibroblastic tumor. Mod Pathol 2001; 14(6):569–576.

29. Lawrence B, Perez-Atavde A, Hibbard MK, et al. TPM3-ALK and TPMA4-ALK oncogenes in inflammatory myofibroblastic tumors. Am J Pathol 2000;157(2):377–384.

30. Debiec-Rychter M, Marynen P, Hagemeijer A, et al. ALK-ATIC fusion in urinary bladder inflammatory myofibroblastic tumor. Genes Chromosomes Cancer 2003;38(2):187–190.

31. Debelenko LV, Arthur DC, Pack SD, et al. Identification of CARS-ALK fusion in primary and metastatic lesions of an inflammatory myofibroblastic tumor. Lab Invest 2003;83(9): 1255–1265.

32. Bridge JA, Kanamori M, Ma Z, et al. Fusion of the ALK gene to the clathrin heavy chain gene. CLTC, in inflammatory myofibroblastic tumor. Am J Pathol 2001;159(2):411–415.

33. Ma Z, Hill DA, Collins MH, et al. Fusion of ALK to the Ran-binding protein 2 (RANBP2) gene in inflammatory myofibroblastic tumor. Genes Chromosomes Cancer 2003; 37(1):98–105.

34. Panagopoulos I, Nilsson T, Domanski HA, et al. Fusion of the SEC31L1 and ALK genes in an inflammatory myofibroblastic tumor. Int J Cancer 2006;118(5):1181–1186.

35. Lamant L, Pulford K, Bischof D, et al. Expression of the ALK tyrosine kinase gene in neuroblastoma. Am J Pathol 2000;156(5):1711–1721.

36. Mergan F, Jaubert F, Sauvat F, et al. Inflammatory myofibroblastic tumor in children: clinical review with anaplastic lymphoma kinase, Epstein-Barr virus, and human herpesvirus 8 detection analysis. J Pediatr Surg 2005;40(10):1581–1586.

37. Chan JK, Cheuk W, Shimizu M. Anaplastic lymphoma kinase expression in inflammatory pseudotumors. Am J Surg Pathol 2001;25(6):761–768.

38. Coffin CM, Watterson J, Priest JR, et al. Extrapulmonary inflammatory myofibroblastic tumor (inflammatory pseudotumor). A clinicopathologic and immunohistochemical study of 84 cases. Am J Surg Pathol 1995;19(8):859–872.

39. Gomez-Roman JJ, Ocejo-Vinyals G, Sanchez-Velasco P, et al. Presence of human herpesvirus -8 DNA sequences and overexpression of human II-6 and cyclin D1 in inflammatory myofibroblastic tumor (inflammatory pseudotumor). Lab Invest 2000;80(7):1121–1126.

40. Arber DA, Kamel OW, van de Rijn M, et al. Frequent presence of the Epstein-Barr virus in inflammatory pseudotumor. Hum Pathol 1995;26(10):1093–1098.

41. Neuhauser TS, Derringer GA, Thompson LD, et al. Splenic inflammatory myofibroblastic tumor (inflammatory pseudotumor): a clinicopathologic and immunophenotypic study of 12 cases. Arch Pathol Lab Med 2001;125(3):379–885.

42. Askin FB, Rosai J, Sibley RK, et al. Malignant small cell tumor of the thoracopulmonary region in childhood: a distinctive clinicopathological entity of uncertain histogenesis. Cancer 1997;43:2438–2451.

43. Arvand A, Denny CT. Biology of EWS/ETS fusions in Ewing's family tumors. Oncogene 2001; 20(40):5747–5754.

44. Delattre O, Zucman J, Melot T, et al. The Ewing family of tumors a subgroup of small-round-cell tumors defined by specific chimeric transcripts. N Engl J Med 1994;331(5):294–299.

45. Ohno T, Ouchida M, Lee L, et al. The EWS gene, involved in Ewing family of tumors, malignant melanoma of soft parts and desmoplastic small round cell tumors, codes for an RNA binding protein with novel regulatory domains. Oncogene 1994;9(10):3087–3097.

46. Yang L, Embree LJ, Tsai S, et al. Oncoprotein TLS interacts with serine-arginine proteins involved in RNA splicing. J Biol Chem 1998;273(43):27761–27764.

47. Sementchenko VI, Watson DK. Ets target genes: past, present and future. Oncogene 2000;19(55):6533–6548.

48. Khoury J. Ewing sarcoma family of tumors. Adv Anat Pathol 2005;12(4):212–220.

49. Zoubek A, Dockhorn-Dworniczak B, Delattre O, et al. Does expression of different EWS chimeric transcripts define clinically distinct risk groups of Ewing tumor patients? J Clin Oncol 1996;14(4):1245–1251.

50. Zoubek A, Pfleiderer C, Salzer-Kuntschik M, et al. Variability of EWS chimaeric transcripts in Ewing tumours: a comparison of clinical and molecular data. Br J Cancer 1994;70(5):908–913.

51. Zucman J, Melot T, Desmaze C, et al. Combinatorial generation of variable fusion proteins in the Ewing family of tumours. EMBO J 1993;12(12):4481–4487.

52. De Alava E, Kawai A, Healey JH, et al. EWS-FLI1 fusion transcript structure is an independent determinant of prognosis in Ewing's sarcoma. J Clin Oncol 1998;16(4):1248–1255.

53. Hu-Lieskovan S, Zhang J, Wu L, et al. EWS-FL11 Fusion protein up-regulates critical genes in neural crest development and is responsible for the observed phenotype of Ewing's family of tumors. Cancer Res 2005;65(11):4633–4644.

54. Delattre O, Zucman J, Plougastel B, et al. Gene fusion with an ETS DNA-binding domain caused by chromosome translocation in human tumours. Nature 1992;359(6391):162–165.

55. May WA, Gishizky ML, Lessnick SL, et al. Ewing sarcoma 11;22 translocation produces a chimeric transcription factor that requires the DNA-binding domain encoded by FL11 for transformation. Proc Natl Acad Sci USA 1993;90(12):5752–5756.

56. Sorensen PH, Lessnick SL, Lopez-Terrada D, et al. A second Ewing's sarcoma translocation, t(21:22), fuses the EWS gene to another ETS-family transcription factor, ERG. Nat Genet 1994;6(2):146–151.

57. Jeon IS, Davis JN, Braun BS, et al. A variant Ewing's sarcoma translocation (7;22) fuses EWS gene to the ETS gene ETV1. Oncogene 1995;10(6):1229–1234.

58. Kaneko Y, Yoshida K, Handa M, et al. Fusion of an ETS-family gene, E1AF, to EWS by t(17;22)(q12;q12) chromosome translocation in an undifferentiated sarcoma of infancy. Genes Chromosomes Cancer 1996;15(2):115–121.

59. Urano F, Umezawa A, Hong W, et al. A novel chimera gene between EWS and E1A-F, encoding the adenovirus E1A enhancer-binding protein in extraosseous Ewing's sarcoma. Biochem Biophys Res Commun 1996;219(2):608–612.

60. Peter M, Couturier J, Pacquement H, et al. A new member of the ETS family fused t EWS in Ewing tumors. Oncogene 1997;14(10):1159–1164.

61. Mastrangelo T, Modena P, Tornielli S, et al. A novel zinc finger gene is fused to EWS in small round cell tumor. Oncogene 2000;19(33):3799–3804.

62. Bridge RS, Rajaram V, Dehner LP, et al. Molecular diagnosis of Ewing sarcoma/primitive neuroectodermal tumor in routinely processed tissue: a comparison of two FISH strategies and RT-PCR in malignant round cell tumors. Mod Pathol 2006;19(1):1–8.

Section 5
Molecular Pathology of Pulmonary Infections

36
Basis of Susceptibility to Lung Infection

Frank C. Schmalstieg and Armond S. Goldman

Introduction

The myriad microbial pathogens encountered by the lung presents a daunting challenge to the human immune system. Nowhere else in the body is such a vast surface area (approximately $100\,m^2$)[1] directly exposed to airborne pathogens at about 20 times per minute. Not only is the area and exposure extreme, but the underlying blood circulation is only two cell layers, of about $0.5\,\mu m$ each, removed from the alveolar surface. Furthermore, gravity and manifold branching of bronchioles and bronchi interfere with the expulsion of these organisms and tissue debris that occurs during lung infection. It is not surprising, then, that pneumonias are among the most common infectious diseases in the United States.[2]

Understanding the susceptibility to lung infection requires a comprehension of (1) the anatomy and function of the lung, (2) environmental exposures, (3) systemic and mucosal immune functions, (4) virulence of pathogens, and (5) genetic variabilities of the host defenses. Numerous "experiments of nature" and identification of the molecular mechanisms of pathogen entry into lung cells especially have provided unique insights into understanding immune aspects of host susceptibility. More recently, rapid, high volume methods of analyzing potential genetic determinants for host susceptibility to specific pathogens have shown considerable promise. These considerations and their results are explored in some detail in this chapter.

Lung Anatomy and Function

Unique Aspects of the Lung Microcirculation

Three distinct circulations supply the lung and airways with blood. They are the tracheal, bronchial, and pulmonary circulations. The tracheal arteries branch from the superior and inferior thyroid arteries and drain to the inferior thyroid venous plexus. More importantly, the bronchial arterial supply is from the thoracic aorta, and the venous drainage from this artery is largely (~70%) anastomosed to the pulmonary circulation in a precapillary location[3] in the sheep. This also likely occurs in humans. These anastomoses are significant because neutrophils may be influenced by mediators from airway epithelium and then interact directly with the pulmonary capillaries, thus providing a connection with inflammation in the airway and in the alveolar capillaries. In this regard, the capillary diameter in the bronchial microcirculation is about $8.5\,\mu m$ but only approximately $5.5\,\mu m$ in the pulmonary capillaries.[4] Neutrophils have to deform during passage through the pulmonary capillaries (Figure 36.1) because of their relatively large diameter (10–$15\,\mu m$). In contrast, erythrocytes pass through those capillaries more readily because of their smaller diameters. Delay in the passage of neutrophils results in a relative increase in neutrophil concentration in the pulmonary capillaries.[5] This may be an adaptive modification for better control of any organisms breaching the extensive and exposed surfaces of the alveoli. The slowing and momentary stopping of neutrophils in the pulmonary capillaries under certain stimuli may allow selectin- and integrin-independent migration of these cells from the capillaries.[6,7]

The bronchial circulation is also unique in that airway injury can stimulate a fivefold increase in bronchial blood flow in sheep.[8] Although the increased blood flow during injury amounts to less than 3% of the cardiac output, neutrophils activated in the bronchial microcirculation may be directly delivered to the pulmonary capillaries to produce damage. In fact, bronchial artery ligation decreases lung edema in a sheep model of smoke and burn injury.[9] The anatomy of the lung then potentially allows damage in the airway to produce inflammatory changes in the lung that may enhance lung protection or lead to further damage under some circumstances.

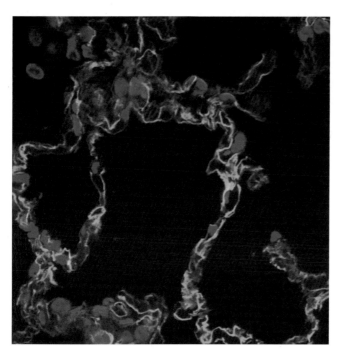

FIGURE 36.1. Confocal image of neutrophils in pulmonary alveolar capillaries in a sheep with a traumatic lung injury and criteria for acute respiratory distress syndrome. Green is type IV collagen, red is myeloperoxidase, and blue is the nuclear stain DAPI. Many neutrophils are seen in the pulmonary capillaries, of which many demonstrate the extensive deformability necessary to pass through the capillaries. (Magnification, ×630.)

Epithelial Cilia and Airway Surface Fluid

The lumen of the airways of the human is lined with fluid 5–20 μm thick.[10] Electron microscopy studies suggest that the fluid is in two phases, a low-viscosity aqueous layer in contact with the tips of the cilia of respiratory epithelial cells and a second layer above this consisting of a mucous gel. The cilia beat semisynchronously to create a "conveyor" effect from the lower to the upper airways. Consequently, secretions of airway epithelial cells and glands as well as debris may be expelled by coughing. The importance of ciliary motion is underscored by primary ciliary dyskinesia, an autosomal recessive heterogeneous disorder of ciliary function and movement.[11] Approximately half of these individuals have Kartagener's syndrome with situs inversus of the heart and abdominal organs likely caused by the necessity of ciliary motion in determining the asymmetric placement of those organs during embryologic development. Individuals with ciliary dysfunction may develop bronchiectasis if pulmonary toilet and control of infection are not maintained. Recurrent and chronic otitis media and sinusitis are also common.

An additional consequence of ciliary dysfunction is a deficiency of airway nitric oxide. Although the specific mechanism for this deficiency is not known, endothelial nitric oxide synthase (*NOS3*) is located in close proximity to the basal, intracellular portion of the cilia, suggesting that interaction of endothelial nitric oxide synthase with the ciliary body is necessary for production of airway nitric oxide.[12] It is likely that control of ciliary motion is through nitric oxide–dependent effects on guanyl cyclase.[12] Furthermore, nasal nitric oxide concentration was correlated with impaired ciliary clearance in the upper airways of patients with recurrent sinusitis and pneumonia,[13] providing further support for the importance of mucociliary clearance and infection.

Cough Reflex

Cough reflex is a complex neural event that begins with activation of nonadrenergic, noncholingeric nerve fibers utilizing neural transmitters such as neurokinins in the laryngopharyngeal area and larger upper airways. The afferents involved in the neural pathways are within the vagus nerve. This is consistent with observations that cough may be produced also by certain stimulations of the external ear, esophagus, and abdominal organs.[14] The central controls of the cough reflex, including voluntary and involuntary aspects, remain poorly understood. Although it seems obvious that this reflex is important in protection of the airway, there are few studies to objectively document this view. However, Addington et al. found that pneumonia in stroke victims with defective cough reflex had significantly more complications than did patients with an intact cough reflex.[15]

Innate Immunity

Parsing immunity into innate and adaptive components is useful only if it is understood that the division is artificial and that there are numerous perturbations by each component on the other. This will be obvious in the following discussion.

Complement

The three known pathways that activate complement, the alternative, classic, and lectin pathways, converge at the C3 component. The serum proteins comprising the complement system not only support opsonization by the activation of C3, chemotaxis by the activation of C5, and direct killing of microorganisms through the terminal lysis sequence but also are capable of modifying both T- and B-cell immunity.[16,17] The general view is that the most important role of complement is as an opsonin supporting enhanced phagocytosis in the blood. However, in the murine lung the clearance of pneumococci was complement dependent for both blood-borne and aerosolized bacteria.[18] The source of the C3 in the lung appeared to be from the serum rather than local production. It is not clear whether the clearance was from increased phagocytosis or by direct killing. Interestingly, C3-deficient animals do not have decreased entry of neutrophils into the lung but do have increased inflammation. The last point is important because it suggests that C3 may have an antiinflammatory effect in the lung. A possible explanation for this effect may relate to the observation that phagocytosis of apoptotic neutrophils by alveolar macrophages results in less cytokine production by these macrophages and less alveolar inflammation.[19] The C3 in the lung may increase phagocytosis of apoptotic neutrophils with the consequence of decreased cytokine production by the macrophages.

Therefore, the complement system may have inflammatory and antiinflammatory effects in the lung. Also, decreased concentrations of C3 are likely clinically relevant for diseases such as systemic lupus erythematosus in which low C3 concentrations may lead to increased susceptibility to bacterial pathogens.

Surfactant

Surfactant proteins A and D (SP-A and SP-D) belong to a protein family known as *collectins*. These proteins have a collagen-like sequence in the N-terminal portion of the molecule and a C-type lectin moiety at the C-terminal end. These proteins are produced by alveolar type II cells and serve not only as surfactants to reduce surface tension and allow expansion of alveoli without excessive pressures but also recognize pathogen-associated molecular patterns. They bind to oligosaccharide-containing proteins (galactosylceramide for SP-A and glucosylceramide for SP-D) on pathogen surfaces and produce aggregation and arrest of these infecting organisms. Surfactant protein A binds to *Staphylococcus aureus*[20] and *Herpes simplex*.[21] Opsonization is accomplished by interaction of the collagen domain of SP-A and the C1q receptor on the alveolar macrophage surface. Surfactant protein A oligomerizes into six trimeric subunits, which greatly resemble the overall topography of C1q. In addition to *Staph. aureus* and *H. simplex*, it is now clear that a wide range of both Gram-positive and Gram-negative organisms associate with SP-A and SP-D. In addition to opsonic activity, these molecules also have the ability to directly interfere with the growth and viability of certain microorganisms and viruses.[22] In part this is accomplished through the ability of these molecules to permeabilize the membranes of microorganisms through interaction of the collagen domain with membrane lipids.[23] Both SP-A and SP-D are able to increase the phagocytosis of apoptotic neutrophils by alveolar macrophages.[24] As previously mentioned, alveolar macrophages that ingest apoptotic neutrophils produce less inflammatory cytokines. The physiologic importance of these molecules is underscored by recognition of decreases in these proteins by severe viral and bacterial pneumonia. Individuals with cystic fibrosis (CF) exhibit a correlation between collectin deficiencies and lung inflammation.[25] In addition, immunosuppressed mice deficient in SP-A have increased susceptibility to *Pneumocystis jiroveci* pneumonia compared with SP-A-competent controls.[26]

Lung Epithelial Cells

Lung epithelium is directly exposed to air containing significant quantities of microorganisms and viruses. Not surprisingly, these cells and their pathogen counterparts have evolved numerous attack and defense mechanisms. For example, rhinovirus enters airway epithelium by binding to the intercellular adhesion molecule-1. The epithelium responds with the synthesis of an array of cytokines, including interferon-α and -β, proinflammatory cytokines, interleukin (IL)-1β and tumor necrosis factor (TNF)-α, acute phase reactants IL-6 and IL-16, chemokines including IL-8, Gro-α, epithelial cell-derived neutrophil-activating peptide (ENA) 78, macrophage inflammatory protein (MIP)-1α, RANTES, monocyte chemoattractant protein (MCP)-1, eotaxin, and granulocyte-macrophage colony-stimulating factor (GM-CSF; reviewed by Message and Johnston[27]). More recently, IL-17, which is necessary for the coordinated release of GM-CSF and the CXC chemokines and subsequent defense against Gram-negative bacteria, was found in airway epithelial cells.[28] These mediators are able to attract and activate T cells, natural killer (NK) cells, macrophages, eosinophils, and neutrophils. Moreover, certain of these cells may remain in the systemic circulation to have actions distant from the airway as was discussed earlier for neutrophils. Although these actions may aid in killing pathogens, they also may injure lung tissue by producing a cycle of defense, inflammation, destruction, and repair.

It has been suggested that internalization of *Pseudomonas aeruginosa* occurs through the CF transmembrane conductance regulator (CFTR), which is deficient in CF patients.[29,30] This now seems largely discounted.[31] Rather than acting as a portal of entry for *Pseud. aeruginosa*, it appears that this organism penetrates bronchial epithelial cells lacking the CFTR more easily and is able to replicate within these cells. Thus, epithelial cells with an intact CFTR are more resistant to *Pseud. aeruginosa* uptake and produce more IL-8 upon challenge with these bacteria. Therefore, the CFTR is an infection resistance factor for *Pseud. aeruginosa* in bronchial epithelial cells. A plausible explanation for the persistence of *Pseud. aeruginosa* pulmonary infections in CF patients may be the failure to initially clear infections with this organism and the consequent development of a chronic infection and inflammation characterized by intense neutrophil accumulations and damage to the host defense mechanisms of the lung.

Alveolar Macrophages

Alveolar macrophages are the first-line defense of the lung against inhaled pathogens. Not surprisingly, they play a prominent role in the further orchestration of the ensuing inflammatory response against these pathogens. In accomplishing this task, alveolar macrophages must assume a complex role of initiating the inflammatory reaction and modulating the reaction to limit damage and aid in repair. Consistent with the role, these cells are much longer lived and more resistant to apoptosis than are blood monocytes. In part, these characteristics stem from a decrease in the phosphatase PTEN (phosphatase and tensin homolog, deleted on chromosome 10).[32] This relative deficiency compared with blood monocytes results in increased activity of the Akt pathway and subsequent resistance to apoptosis through the action of AFX, a member of a subfamily of forkhead transcription factors.[33] Furthermore, pneumonia induced by tracheal instillation of pneumococci in mice deficient in one of the class A macrophage scavenger receptors have increased mortality.[34] These pattern recognition receptors are trimeric glycoproteins with multiple functions (e.g., bacterial adherence and opsonization[35]) and possible participation in phagocytosis of apoptotic cells. In this regard, knowledge of the alveolar macrophage surface molecules that promote phagocytosis of apoptotic neutrophils is incomplete. However, CD44[36] and SP-A[37] appear to play important roles. Not only do alveolar macrophages remove apoptotic neutrophils and thereby limit inflammation but also the process of phagocytosis of these apoptotic neutrophils decreases proinflammatory cytokine production by alveolar macrophages.[38,39]

Another series of pattern recognition molecules, the Toll-like receptors (TLRs), are present on alveolar macrophages, and, in concert with CD14 (ligand for lipopolysaccharides and lipoproteins), they transduce signals resulting from the binding of these bacterial products to later components of the cell signaling pathway (Figure 36.2). Signaling of TLR-4 also upregulates the receptor for vitamin D3 and the products of the vitamin D1-hydroxylase genes, which in turn signals the induction of cathelicidin, an antibacterial peptide that kills mycobacteria,[40] when vitamin D3 is present. Also, MyD88, an adaptor protein that mediates TLR signaling, appears to be very important in host defense against airway bacteria. The essential function of MyD88 in clearance of *Pseud. aeruginosa* in mice was recently demonstrated by MyD88 knockout mice and bone marrow reconstitution experiments.[41]

Experiments to quantitate the role of alveolar macrophages in in vivo infections have been problematic. However, numerous careful experiments with airway inoculation of *Streptococcus pneumonia* have begun to clarify the role of alveolar macrophages in airway-related infections. Instillation of large numbers of pneumococci result in severe disease, and survival depends on neutrophil clearance of the bacteria.[19] Furthermore, depletion of alveolar macrophages in this model delayed removal of apoptotic neutrophils with resultant increased inflammation. In contrast, when small numbers of pneumococci are administered, clearances of these bacteria occur within the first 6 hr before neutrophil recruitment.[42] Depletion of alveolar macrophages delayed this process. Finally, in established pneumonia, neutrophils play a predominant role, and alveolar macrophages play a role in directing neutrophil recruitment.[19] Therefore, alveolar macrophages contribute to bacterial clearance and killing of low concentrations of pathogens, whereas larger numbers of organisms and established lung infection require neutrophils. However, in these latter cases, regulation of neutrophil influx and clearance of apoptotic neutrophils by alveolar macrophages are essential.

Neutrophils

"Experiments of nature" provide valuable insights into the role of neutrophils in host defense. The two congenital disorders that are most instructive are chronic granulomatous disease (CGD) and leukocyte adherence deficiency-1 (LAD-1). In the first case, the defect is in one of the known subunits of the neutrophil NADPH oxidase. It results in an inability of the neutrophils to produce superoxide anion and subsequent reactive oxygen species. The failure to produce superoxide anion greatly inhibits the ability of the neutrophils to kill phagocytosed catalase-positive bacteria and fungi.[43] These patients characteristically have "deep" tissue infections, including lung abscesses. The reason for this tissue location of infection is related to the life cycle of this cell. Mature neutrophils are produced in the bone marrow in about 2 weeks. They remain in the circulation for 6 to 12 hr and then exit the microcirculation into the tissues. Because neutrophils are on an apoptotic program from the time they leave the bone marrow, these potentially toxic cells are disposed of once they become apoptotic by directed phagocytosis by resident tissue macrophages. This is an especially active process in liver sinusoids by Kupffer cells.[44] Because phagocytosis by neutrophils is unaffected by defects in the NADPH oxidase complex, these neutrophils retain live catalase-positive bacteria or fungi they have ingested. Resident and elicited macrophages have the same defect in oxidative metabolism and are also defective in their ability to kill these organisms. The persistence of organisms deposited by neutrophils and macrophages in deep tissue locations provides an explanation for the granulomatous reactions seen in various organs including the lung. These patients are especially susceptible to *Staph. aureus* and *Aspergillus* sp. (both catalase-positive organisms) infections in the lung. Other troublesome infections

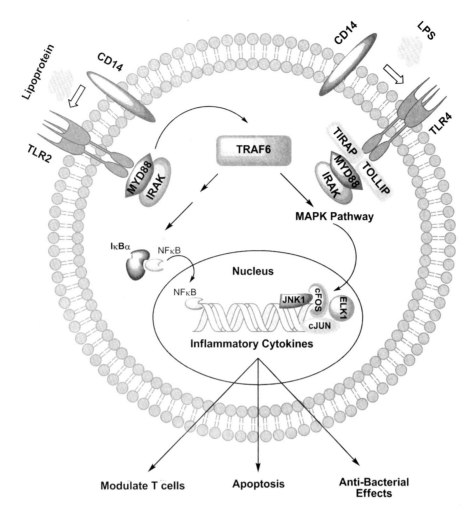

FIGURE 36.2. Schematic representation of Toll-like receptor (TLR) signaling. This diagram indicates the necessary role of CD14 in the interaction of bacterial lipoprotein (TLR2) and bacterial lipopolysaccharide (TLR4). The central role of MyD88 protein (myeloid differentiation primary response gene 88), IRAK (interleukin-1 receptor–associated kinase), and TRAF6 (tumor necrosis factor [TNF] receptor-associated factor 6) in subsequent signaling is indicated. Several intermediate signaling events are not shown for clarity. However, the signaling through this pathway results in nuclear factor (NF)-κB, c-Jun and c-Fos (constituents of the activator protein-1 transcription factor complex), JNK1, and Elk-1. These nuclear transcription factors result in inflammatory cytokines, including interleukin (IL)-2, IL-8, interferon-γ, and TNF-α. These mediators can modulate T cells, influence their polarization, cause apoptosis in various cell types, and produce direct antibacterial effects. These signaling pathways are active in macrophages, epithelial cells, and dendritic cells. IκBα, inhibitor κBα; LPS, lipopolysaccharide; MAPK, mitogen-activated protein kinase; TIRAP, Toll-interleukin 1 receptor domain-containing adapter protein; TOLLIP, Toll-interacting protein.

include the opportunistic organisms *Nocardia* sp. and *Serratia marcescens*. These observations implicate oxidative metabolism in defense of the lung and provide insight into the mechanism of protection.

A second experiment of nature involving leukocyte function is also instructive. Leukocyte adherence deficiency (type 1) is caused by defects in the common β-subunit of β$_2$-integrin.[45] This defect results in greatly decreased emigration of neutrophils from the microcirculation. Study of this defect greatly clarified the mechanism by which neutrophils move from the circulation into tissues utilizing sequential selectin-mediated slowing of cells followed by activation of these cells by chemokine(s) with subsequent conformational change of neutrophil β$_2$-integrins to allow binding to their counter structures. Finally, these cells emigrate into the interstitium in response to a chemokine(s) gradient (Figure 36.3). The same general paradigm pertains to other cells as well, including lymphocytes.[46] Patients with these defects have frequent skin infections, perirectal abscesses, and severe gingivitis. More serious infections including pneumonia may occur but are less common. Death may

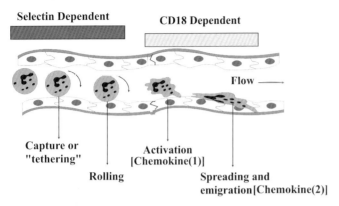

Selectin Dependent   **CD18 Dependent**

Flow ⟶

Capture or "tethering"   Activation [Chemokine(1)]

Rolling   Spreading and emigration [Chemokine(2)]

FIGURE 36.3. Emigration paradigm for neutrophils. This illustration demonstrates the necessary steps of capture of neutrophils from a rapidly flowing microcirculation through interaction of selectin molecules and their ligands supporting rolling of the leukocytes along the vessel wall. Subsequently, an activation event mediated through a chemokine and its receptor occurs that results in "inside-out" signaling that causes a conformational change in the neutrophil integrins. The "activated" integrins bind to their receptors on the endothelial cell, allowing spreading of the neutrophils to occur. Finally, the neutrophils move through the vessel wall in response to a chemotactic gradient that may or may not involve the same chemokine creating the initial activation event. Although neutrophils are highlighted here, the same general steps apply to other migrating cell types, including lymphocytes.

result in these patients because of overwhelming bacterial invasion of the trachea and upper airway sometimes associated with a viral respiratory infection. Even a minor infection may cause an extraordinary number of neutrophils (>200,000/mm³) to appear in the peripheral blood with consequent obstruction of the mesenteric arteries and infarction of the bowel.

Why are there not more lung infections in LAD? A probable reason is the nature of the pulmonary microcirculation. Because neutrophil diameters exceed those of pulmonary capillaries, they must deform to pass through this circulation.[4] Direct observations of these cells indicate that they frequently stop completely. Immobile neutrophils might be predicted to emigrate from vessels in a selectin-independent and β₂-integrin–independent fashion. There is considerable evidence to indicate that this occurs in pneumococcal pneumonia but not in certain Gram-negative bacterial pneumonias.[47] This behavior may also be part of the explanation why emigration of neutrophils in the pulmonary microcirculation occurs in the capillaries rather than in the postcapillary venules, as is the case with most microcirculations. Of course, the ability to emigrate from pulmonary capillaries is highly useful for the defense of the alveolus (and occasionally deleterious when neutrophils damage these structures).

It is of interest that the neutrophils also express TLRs (with the exception of TLR3) and CD14. Signaling through these receptors can elicit both pro- and antiinflammatory changes in neutrophils.[48]

In summary, both neutrophils and alveolar macrophages are central to the defense of the lung. In general, small airborne inoculums of pathogens are likely disposed of by alveolar macrophages. However, when the inoculum is larger from either hematogenous or airway sources, the neutrophil is essential for clearance of the infection. It is also clear that the alveolar macrophage has evolved to direct and terminate much of the neutrophil activity that occurs in the alveolus.

Adaptive Immunity

Congenital defects in adaptive immunity again provide important clues to the mechanisms of host defense in the lung. X-linked severe combined immunodeficiency is the most common inherited form of combined T- and B-cell immunodeficiencies. Patients with this disease have viral, fungal, and bacterial pneumonias with organisms that are usually cleared without difficulty. *Pneumocystis jiroveci* (formerly *Pneumocystis carinii*), often in concert with parainfluenza virus type 3 and/or adenovirus pneumonia, is especially troublesome for these patients.[49] In contrast, patients with defects in humoral immunity, such as Bruton's agammaglobulinemia (see later), have a more limited repertoire of troublesome infections that are principally respiratory bacterial pathogens that invade the upper and lower respiratory tracts.

It is also helpful to consider a unique form of X-linked severe combined immunodeficiency secondary to a single missense mutation in the common γ-chain that allows some association of this signaling component of the IL-2 receptor with its target Janus kinase 3.[50-53] These patients have less difficulty with *Pneum. jiroveci* pneumonia and other fungal infections of the lung, but do have difficulty with viruses, especially human *H. simplex*. Although they have substantial quantities of immunoglobulins, these immunoglobulins do not exhibit specific affinity for pathogens. Consideration of Bruton's tyrosine kinase deficiency (see later) and this variant of X-linked severe combined immunodeficiency suggests that lung infections with *Pneumocystis*, fungal organisms, and human herpesviruses are chiefly defended through T lymphocytes.

Another instructive human immunodeficiency is the Mendelian determined susceptibility to weakly pathogenic mycobacteria syndrome. This syndrome may be caused by deficiencies in either a subunit of the interferon (IFN)-γ receptor, the p40 subunit of IL-12, the β₂-subunit of the IL-12 and IL-23 receptors, and defects in signal transducers and activators of transcription (STAT) protein 1. Individuals with these defects have increased susceptibility to weakly pathogenic mycobacteria or *Salmonella typhi*. Significantly, humans with these deficiencies appear to have intact immune systems except for these lacunar defects.[54] This is in stark contrast to the situation with mice in which IFN-γ–related defects result in widespread difficulty in clearance of many intracellular organisms and resistance to lymphoma.[55] The significance of these observations is that the ideas of T-cell polarization (i.e., Th1/Tc1 and Th2/Tc2 cells) in the mouse draw heavily from these observations. Interferon-γ is a major factor in mice in producing CD4+ Th1 cells, whereas IL-4 is a major influence for production of Th2 cells. An analogous situation exists for CD8+ cytotoxic T cells. Although this paradigm has aided the past three decades of immunologic discovery, the ability of the human to develop a near-normal immune system in the face of severe defects in IFN-γ indicate that the mechanism of polarization in the human may be considerably different from that in the mouse. Nevertheless, there is little doubt that T-cell polarization is of great importance in both mice and humans. Some caution then must be exercised in the following discussion of human T-cell polarization with regard to host defense of the lung because parallels will be drawn from work with murine systems.

T Lymphocytes

T-cell function in the lung is interwoven with NK T cells, NK cells, and dendritic cells. For example, the initial driving forces for production of Th1 in vivo requires initial and rapid production of IFN-γ (or in the human perhaps other signals as well) that may be provided by NKT and NK cells. Dendritic cells may induce polarization of naïve αβ T cells to either Th1 or Th2 effector cells.[56] In this regard, it is interesting that activated neutrophils adhere to naïve dendritic cells through a Mac-1 and carcinoembryonic antigen–related cell adhesion molecule 1/dendritic cell–specific C-type lectin mechanism to strongly promote Th1 responses,[57,58] further blurring the boundaries between innate and adaptive immunity. Th1 cells produce IFN-γ, IL-2, TNF-α, and GM-CSF, whereas Th2 cells produce IL-4, IL-5, IL-9, IL10, and IL-13. The mediators from these two polarized phenotypes are capable of antagonizing the activities of each other, further driving polarization of each phenotype. Th1 responses typically activate tissue macrophages to kill intracellular pathogens by a STAT1-dependent pathway involving nitric oxide. Macrophages require an exogenous source of interferons to effectively stimulate this pathway. Not surprisingly, Th1 responses are critical for lung defense against mycobacteria and to some extent viruses. T helper 2 responses may antagonize Th1 responses and serve as a dampening mechanism to limit lung damage in these processes. Th2 responses favor IgE and IgG4 class switching, mechanisms important in para-

sitic infections. It is not difficult to envision genetic influences on these processes by certain antigenic stimulation that might result in inappropriate polarization affecting host defense adversely. Experimental examples of this putative behavior using inbred mouse strains are numerous. One such example is the poor ability of the BALBc strain of mice to defend against *Leishmania*.[59]

Major histocompatibility complex I (MHC I)–restricted activities of CD8+ Tc1 or Tc2 cells are specialized and different from those of MHC 2 restricted function of CD4+ Th1 or Th2 cells. Tc1 and Tc2 cells must recognize molecular targets on pathogens through interaction of the αβ T-cell receptor in context with class I MHC, which results in cytolytic attack by these cells utilizing perforin and/or granzyme pathways. In general, Tc1 cells have the more vigorous cytolytic activity of the two cell types. These cytolytic T cells are of obvious importance in killing of virally infected cells in the lung. In addition to these effector T cells, a smaller population of long-lived memory cells exists (as reviewed by Moser and Willimann[60]). These cells are less well characterized than their effector counterparts. They consist of central memory cells that are associated with lymph nodes and bear the lymph tissue address code of CCR7, CD62L, and α4β7, which determines their continuous recirculation among lymph nodes, spleen, and Peyer's patches (Table 36.1). Effector T-cell memory cells lack CCR7 but retain receptors for inflammatory cytokines, allowing them to circulate in the blood and to be excluded from lymph nodes and prepared to participate in inflammatory lesions (see Table 36.1). A third category of memory T cells, designated peripheral immune surveillance T cells, is characterized by chemokine receptors matching those cytokines produced by the specific tissues they occupy. Consequently, those cells remain in the tissues. The extent that these subsets of memory T cells can change to other types of memory T cells is not clear. However, it is known that effector T-cell memory cells may reacquire CCR7 expression, suggesting that there may be some interchange among these subtypes of memory T cells.[61] It is then clear that chemokines along with adhesion molecules define migration patterns of T cells, some of which are specific for tissue locations.

In addition to the T-cell subsets previously discussed, a fundamentally different class of T cells characterized by CD4+CD25+ and by the presence of the forkhead, winged-helix transcription factor Foxp3, must be included (reviewed by Gavin and Rudensky[62]). These cells differ from the other polarized T cells in that they arise from the thymus and are present without further antigenic manipulation. Insight into the function of these cells is provided by the IPEX (immunodysregulation, polyendocrinopathy, enteropathy, X-linked) syndrome. This rare X-linked immunodeficiency is caused by defects in the Foxp3 transcription factor. The murine counterpart of

TABLE 36.1. Examples of emigration paradigms and involved molecules.

Cell	Selectin/R	Chemokine(1)/R	Integrin/R	Chemokine(2)/R	Tissue
Neutrophil	P-selectin/PSGL-1	IL-8/CXCR1,2	$\alpha_L\beta_2$/ICAM-1	?	Airway
	L-selectin/PSGL-1	Gro-α/CXCR1,2		?	
	E-selectin/PSGL-1	ENA78/CXCL5, GCP-2/CXC2		?	
Neutrophil	P-selectin/PSGL-1	IL-8/CXCR1,2	$\alpha_4\beta_1$/VCAM-1	?	Parenchyma
	L-selectin/PSGL-1		$\alpha_L\beta_2$/ICAM-1		
	E-selectin/PSGL-1		$\alpha_5\beta_1$		
Monocyte	?	CCL2/CCR1?	$\alpha_L\beta_2$/ICAM-1	?	Airway
		CX3CL1/CX3CR1			
Monocyte	?	?	$\alpha_L\beta_2$/ICAM-1	?	Parenchyma
T-Cell					
T_{cm}	L-selectin/PNAd	ELC (CCL19)/CCR7	$\alpha4\beta7$	?	Lymph node
T_{em}	?	Variable	?	?	Blood tissues
T_{ps}	?	CCL1/CCR8	?	?	
Th1	?	Mig/(CXCL9)/CCR3	?	?	
		MCP-2 (CCL8)/CCR5			Periphery
Th2	?	Eotaxin (CCL11)/CCR3	?	?	
Dendritic Cell	L-selectin/PNAd	ELC (CCL19)/CCR7	?	?	Lymph node
		SLC (CCL21)/CCR7			

Note: ELC, Epstein-Barr virus–induced-molecule ligand 1 chemokine; ENA78, epithelial neutrophil-activating protein 78; GCP-2, granulocyte chemotactic protein-2; Gro-α, growth-related oncogene-α; ICAM, intercellular cell adhesion molecule; IL, interleukin; VCAM, vesicular cell adhesion molecule; MCP-2, monocyte chemoattractant protein-2); Mig, monokine-induced by interferon-γ; PNad, peripheral node vascular adressin); PSGL-1, P-selectin glycoprotein ligand-1; SLC, secondary lymphoid organ chemokine); Tcm, memory T cell; Tem, effector memory T cell; Tps, peripheral immune surveillance T cell.

this disease is the *scurfy* mouse.[63] In both the human and mouse, this defect results in widespread autoimmune disease. However, it is now clear that the T_R cells also are essential for regulating the immune response to limit inflammatory damage. This activity extends to innate as well as adaptive immunity.[62] This activity is accomplished through the secretion of TGF-β and IL-10.

Tissue Distribution of Lymphocytes

As previously mentioned for neutrophils, emigration of other leukocytes from the circulation also follows a similar paradigm.[46] Lymphocytes and other leukocytes are recruited from the circulation into specific tissue locations through a coordinated series of events mediated by interaction of the circulating cells with endothelium to slow the velocity of the leukocytes so that firm adhesion, a prerequisite for eventual exit from the circulation, can take place. The slowing of the cells is accomplished through interactions of proteins known as *selectins*, with O-linked fucose-containing polysaccharide ligands containing many repeats of the oligosaccharide binding unit sialyl-Lewis X or sialyl-Lewis A. There are three known selectin molecules, L-selectin, P-selectin, and E-selectin. The mucin-like polysaccharide molecules that serve as ligands for the selectins include mucosal addressins and P-selectin glycoprotein ligand-1. Firm adhesion is pro-

vided by integrin molecules, which are $\alpha\beta$-heterodimers, and their ligands including vascular cell adhesion molecule-1 and intercellular adhesion molecule-1. The latter molecules belong to the immunoglobulin superfamily of proteins. For the above series of events to work, integrins on the endothelial surface must be activated (an obvious requirement to limit leukocyte emigration), and a mechanism for directed movement of the leukocytes must exist. The latter two requirements are served by chemokines and their receptors.

In the human, more than 50 chemokines are known with somewhat fewer receptors. Most chemokines have a signature motif of four cysteines that are in tandem (CC chemokines) or interrupted by a single amino acid flanked on either side by two cysteines (CXC chemokines). Exceptions to these variations are chemokines containing only one cysteine (XC chemokine, XCL1, 2) and a single example of a chemokine containing three uninterrupted cysteines (CX3CL1/fractalkine). These ligands interact with their receptors on leukocytes that belong to the seven-transmembrane spanning heterotrimeric G protein–coupled receptor family (Figure 36.4). Because these receptors are sensitive to pertussis toxin, they utilize one or more of the Gi proteins. On combination of these ligand–receptor pairs, the Gi subunit separates from the $\beta\gamma$ subunits after the complex binds guanosine triphosphate, triggering intracellular signaling

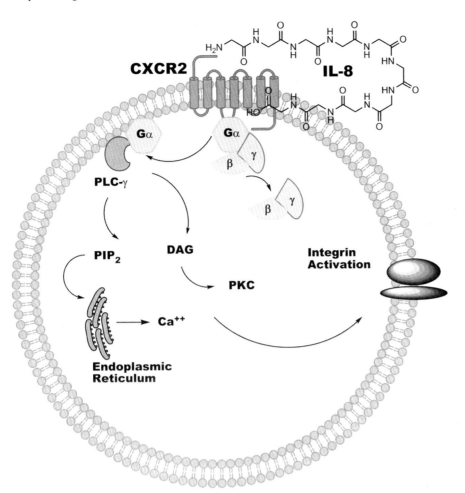

FIGURE 36.4. Simplified schematic drawing of signaling pathways for interleukin (IL)-8. Interleukin-8 is depicted interacting with one of its receptors, CXCR2. This seven-membrane spanning G protein–coupled receptor is activated by ligation of IL-8 with binding of guanosine triphosphate and uncoupling of the heterotrimer protein consisting of Gα-, β-, and γ-subunits. Phospholipase c-γ (PLC-γ) is activated with production of inositol triphosphate and diacylglycerol (DAG) from membrane lipids. Calcium ions are released from the endoplasmic reticulum with activation of calmodulin-sensitive protein kinases, and protein kinase C (PKC) is directly activated by DAG. These signaling events cause intermediary molecules between the cytoskeleton and membrane integrins to be assembled with the result that the membrane integrins are activated. PIP$_2$, phosphatidylinositol bisphosphate.

that results in activation of the integrin molecules (so-called inside-out signaling). The leukocytes follow a gradient of these chemokines, probably initially as a two-dimensional gradient (haptotaxis) of the molecules arranged on the endothelial surface. This last point requires initial binding of the chemokine to the endothelial surface through specific anchors. These anchors are matrix glycoproteins, including certain syndecans. After emigration from the vasculature, a three-dimensional gradient (chemotaxis) of chemokines may further localize the leukocytes. More than one chemokine may participate in the movement of a leukocyte from the vasculature. These processes appear to control different lymphocyte subpopulations' appearance in tissue locations, including the lung. The complexity of this system is illustrated by bronchial epithelial cells that can produce CCL5, a chemokine that binds CCR1, -3, and -5. This chemokine can activate not only lymphocytes but also macrophages and dendritic cells. Initial experiments with antibody against this chemokine appeared to decrease Th1 responses in mycobacterial infections in mice.[64] In contrast, CCL5 knockout mice had increased Th1 responses to *Leishmania donovani* compared with wild-type mice.[65] Furthermore, CCL5 appears to be important in the induction and maintenance of immunity against pneumococcal pneumonia.[66]

Natural Killer and Natural Killer T Cells

Unlike Th1/Tc1 or Th2/Tc2 cells that must interact with specific antigens on pathogen surfaces, both NK and NKT cells do not require such interactions, although NKT cells have a limited repertoire of αβ T-cell receptor origin. Both of these cell types have inhibitory receptors that either recognize the lack of class I MHC expression or activating receptors that detect the expression of the non-classic human leukocyte antigen (HLA) E molecule. In the case of decreased class I MHC expression, this is accomplished through polymorphic invariant receptors for HLA-A, -B, or -C antigens. For HLA-E, the CD95/NKG2A protein recognizes this molecule. These mechanisms are exquisitely sensitive, allowing these cells to recognize the loss of a single class of MHC. These mechanisms are of considerable importance in clearance of those infections that cause the loss of MHC expression. The mechanism of killing of these cells is similar to the same perforin and granzyme pathways described for CD8[+] cytolytic cells.

Dendritic Cells

Dendritic cells assume two different morphologies, plasmacytoid or myeloid. Although it was once thought that these two morphologically distinct cells types presented antigen to different T cell compartments, more recent work indicates that presentation by these cells overlap. They are professional antigen presenting cells and have regulatory functions for both innate and adaptive immunity. They express characteristic cell surface markers, including CD1a, Mac-1, HLA-DR, CD80, CD83, CD86, TLR2, and TLR4, that allow them to directly interact with bacterial products. In the lung these cells occupy a peripheral location and then migrate to the lymph nodes after contact with antigen. In comparison to alveolar macrophages, these cells probably provide the bulk of the antigen delivery to mediastinal lymph nodes utilizing the same CCR7 and CCR8 receptors to direct migration as do skin dendritic cells.[67] Remarkably, deletion of alveolar macrophages greatly increases traffic of lung dendritic cells to the mediastinal lymph nodes.[67] Thus the presence of alveolar macrophages may serve as a governor to inappropriate antigen delivery to mediastinal lymph nodes. As mentioned previously, neutrophils may interact with these cells with mutual signaling. It was originally thought that bronchial-associated lymphoid tissue was part of the gut-associated lymphoid system. This more recent information is most consistent with a distinct immunologic system for the lung.

These cells then play a fundamental role in the orientation and activation of the lymphocyte compartment of the lung. Because certain of these cells may retain antigen for long periods of time, initial contact with antigen and the state of the dendritic cells may determine the long-term polarization and function of immune system as it relates to the lung. Interestingly, Vitamin D3 appears to limit activation of T lymphocytes by dendritic cells.[68] These events are well illustrated by work with *Aspergillus* sp. in the mouse.[69]

Humoral Immunity (B Lymphocytes and Antibodies)

The importance of B cells and antibody to susceptibility of the lung to infection is well illustrated by the previously mentioned congenital immunodeficiency, Bruton's tyrosine kinase deficiency.[70] Defects in Bruton's tyrosine kinase results in arrest of B-cell maturation in the bone marrow at the pro-B-cell stage.[71] These cells do not develop a B-cell receptor and do not proliferate. Although some small amounts of antibodies are produced, they lack specificity. Individuals with this defect suffer from repeated sinopulmonary infections due to common respiratory bacterial pathogens. They have less difficulty with viruses with one notable exception, chronic echovirus infection. The latter virus may cause a disseminated infection that superficially resembles dermatomyositis.[72] However, chronic meningoencephalitis is the most devastating characteristic of this infection. If IgG is not replaced, bronchiectasis will develop early in life with eventual destruction of their lungs. Comparison of Bruton's tyrosine kinase deficiency with specific IgA deficiency, the most common of the known congenital immunodeficiencies (~1:700 incidence) provides further insight. Although secretory IgA would be expected to be the major humoral defense of the lung surfaces because of its secreted nature, many people with IgA deficiency are asymptomatic. This is a testament to the overlapping mechanisms of defense present in humans. It is sometimes suggested that secretory IgM in the lung is sufficient to account for this observation. However, patients with Bruton's tyrosine kinase deficiency have significant protection from sinopulmonary infections, although the replacement products contain only small amounts of IgA and IgM.

Part of the explanation for this behavior may be the hematogenous origin of many bacterial lung infections, a portal that would allow protection based on IgG. Both the antigen binding and constant, class determining regions of the immunoglobulin molecule are important in host defense. Binding and cross-linking the surface of bacteria by immunoglobulin to create aggregates of exposed Fc regions creates a powerful opsonin that directs phagocytosis and eventual killing of these organisms. Interaction of the Fc receptors (FcI, FcII, and FcIII) also result in extensive cell signaling on both neutrophils and monocytes that vary with the context of the cell at the time of receptor ligation.

Conclusion

Protection of the lung against invasion by bacteria, viruses, and fungi is multifaceted and complexly controlled. There is a carefully (or occasionally not so carefully) choreographed dance between pro- and antiinflammatory mechanisms. The control mechanisms are not unidirectional, but multidirectional, blurring the distinctions between innate and adaptive immunity. Another insight provided by this description of lung host defense is that even identical twins, depending on their antigenic exposure, might alter their immune systems as evidenced by subtle differences in T-cell polarization such that they respond differently to subsequent challenges.

Based on the CFTR knockout mice spontaneously demonstrating lung pathology in the absence of infection,[73] it is likely that small, genetically determined differences in expression of genes after infection or other insults play a significant role in determining the outcome of lung infection in the individual. These associations are already being realized as evidenced by association of TLR4 polymorphism Asp299Gly with less carotid artery atherogenesis but increased risk of severe bacterial infections[74] and by the effect of an IL-6-174 promoter polymorphism on clearance of *Strep. pneumonia* from the lung.[75] In addition, certain polymorphisms in IL-10[76] and the IL-1 receptor antagonist[77] predispose the host to infection. As genomics and proteomics methods continue to advance and mature in their scope and speed, there is the prospect that it may be possible eventually to predict the response of individuals to pathogen challenge.

References

1. Ochs M, Nyengaard JR, Jung A, et al. The number of alveoli in the human lung. Am J Respir Crit Care Med 2004; 169:120–124.
2. Marston BJ, Plouffe JF, File TM Jr, et al. Incidence of community-acquired pneumonia requiring hospitalization. Results of a population-based active surveillance Study in Ohio. The Community-Based Pneumonia Incidence Study Group. Arch Intern Med 1997;157:1709–1718.
3. Charan NB, Turk GM, Dhand R. Gross and subgross anatomy of bronchial circulation in sheep. J Appl Physiol 1984;57:658–664.
4. Doerschuk CM, Beyers N, Coxson HO, et al. Comparison of neutrophil and capillary diameters and their relation to neutrophil sequestration in the lung. J Appl Physiol 1993;74:3040–3045.
5. Hogg JC, Coxson HO, Brumwell ML, et al. Erythrocyte and polymorphonuclear cell transit time and concentration in human pulmonary capillaries. J Appl Physiol 1994;77:1795–1800.
6. Kubo H, Doyle NA, Graham L, et al. L- and P-selectin and CD11/CD18 in intracapillary neutrophil sequestration in rabbit lungs. Am J Respir Crit Care Med 1999;159:267–274.
7. Doerschuk CM. The role of CD18-mediated adhesion in neutrophil sequestration induced by infusion of activated plasma in rabbits. Am J Respir Cell Mol Biol 1992;7:140–148.
8. Stothert JC Jr, Ashley KD, Kramer GC, et al. Intrapulmonary distribution of bronchial blood flow after moderate smoke inhalation. J Appl Physiol 1990;69:1734–1739.
9. Sakurai H, Johnigan R, Kikuchi Y, et al. Effect of reduced bronchial circulation on lung fluid flux after smoke inhalation in sheep. J Appl Physiol 1998;84:980–986.
10. Widdicombe JH, Bastacky SJ, Wu DX, Lee CY. Regulation of depth and composition of airway surface liquid. Eur Respir J 1997;10:2892–2897.
11. Afzelius BA, Eliasson R, Johnsen O, Lindholmer C. Lack of dynein arms in immotile human spermatozoa. J Cell Biol 1975;66:225–232.
12. Zhan X, Li D, Johns RA. Expression of endothelial nitric oxide synthase in ciliated epithelia of rats. J Histochem Cytochem 2003;51:81–87.
13. Lindberg S, Cervin A, Runer T. Nitric oxide (NO) production in the upper airways is decreased in chronic sinusitis. Acta Otolaryngol 1997;117:113–117.
14. Widdicombe JG. Neurophysiology of the cough reflex. Eur Respir J 1995;8:1193–1202.
15. Addington WR, Stephens RE, Widdicombe JG, Rekab K. Effect of stroke location on the laryngeal cough reflex and pneumonia risk. Cough 2005;1:4.
16. Molina H, Holers VM, Li B, Fung Y, et al. Markedly impaired humoral immune response in mice deficient in complement receptors 1 and 2. Proc Natl Acad Sci USA 1996;93:3357–3361.
17. Kaya Z, Afanasyeva M, Wang Y, et al. Contribution of the innate immune system to autoimmune myocarditis: a role for complement. Nat Immunol 2001;2:739–745.
18. Kerr AR, Paterson GK, Riboldi-Tunnicliffe A, Mitchell TJ. Innate immune defense against pneumococcal pneumonia requires pulmonary complement component C3. Infect Immun 2005;73:4245–4252.
19. Knapp S, Leemans JC, Florquin S, et al. Alveolar macrophages have a protective antiinflammatory role during murine pneumococcal pneumonia. Am J Respir Crit Care Med 2003;167:171–179.
20. Geertsma MF, Nibbering PH, Haagsman HP, et al. Binding of surfactant protein A to C1q receptors mediates phagocytosis of *Staphylococcus aureus* by monocytes. Am J Physiol 1994;267:L578–L584.
21. van Iwaarden F, Welmers B, Verhoef J, et al. Pulmonary surfactant protein A enhances the host-defense mechanism of rat alveolar macrophages. Am J Respir Cell Mol Biol 1990;2:91–98.
22. Wu H, Kuzmenko A, Wan S, et al. Surfactant proteins A and D inhibit the growth of Gram-negative bacteria by increasing membrane permeability. J Clin Invest 2003;111:1589–1602.
23. Kuzmenko AI, Wu H, McCormack FX. Pulmonary collectins selectively permeabilize model bacterial membranes containing rough lipopolysaccharide. Biochemistry 2006;45:2679–2685.
24. Schagat TL, Wofford JA, Wright JR. Surfactant protein A enhances alveolar macrophage phagocytosis of apoptotic neutrophils. J Immunol 2001;166:2727–2733.

25. Noah TL, Murphy PC, Alink JJ, et al. Bronchoalveolar lavage fluid surfactant protein-A and surfactant protein-D are inversely related to inflammation in early cystic fibrosis. Am J Respir Crit Care Med 2003;168:685–691.

26. Linke MJ, Harris CE, Korfhagen TR, et al. Immunosuppressed surfactant protein A–deficient mice have increased susceptibility to *Pneumocystis carinii* infection. J Infect Dis 2001;183:943–952.

27. Message SD, Johnston SL. Host defense function of the airway epithelium in health and disease: clinical background. J Leukoc Biol 2004;75:5–17.

28. McAllister F, Henry A, Kreindler JL, et al. Role of IL-17A, IL-17F, and the IL-17 receptor in regulating growth-related oncogene-alpha and granulocyte colony-stimulating factor in bronchial epithelium: implications for airway inflammation in cystic fibrosis. J Immunol 2005;175:404–412.

29. Pier GB, Grout M, Zaidi TS, Goldberg JB. How mutant CFTR may contribute to *Pseudomonas aeruginosa* infection in cystic fibrosis. Am J Respir Crit Care Med 1996;154: S175–S182.

30. Pier GB, Grout M, Zaidi TS, et al. Role of mutant CFTR in hypersusceptibility of cystic fibrosis patients to lung infections. Science 1996;271:64–67.

31. Darling KE, Dewar A, Evans TJ. Role of the cystic fibrosis transmembrane conductance regulator in internalization of *Pseudomonas aeruginosa* by polarized respiratory epithelial cells. Cell Microbiol 2004;6:521–533.

32. Flaherty DM, Monick MM, Hinde SL. Human alveolar macrophages are deficient in PTEN. The role of endogenous oxidants. J Biol Chem 2006;281:5058–5064.

33. Tang TT, Dowbenko D, Jackson A, et al. The forkhead transcription factor AFX activates apoptosis by induction of the BCL-6 transcriptional repressor. J Biol Chem 2002;277: 14255–14265.

34. Platt N, Haworth R, Darley L, Gordon S. The many roles of the class A macrophage scavenger receptor. Int Rev Cytol 2002;212:1–40.

35. Pearson AM. Scavenger receptors in innate immunity. Curr Opin Immunol 1996;8:20–28.

36. Teder P, Vandivier RW, Jiang D, et al. Resolution of lung inflammation by CD44. Science 2002;296:155–158.

37. Reidy MF, Wright JR. Surfactant protein A enhances apoptotic cell uptake and TGF-beta1 release by inflammatory alveolar macrophages. Am J Physiol Lung Cell Mol Physiol 2003;285:L854–L861.

38. Huynh ML, Fadok VA, Henson PM. Phosphatidylserine-dependent ingestion of apoptotic cells promotes TGF-beta1 secretion and the resolution of inflammation. J Clin Invest 2002;109:41–50.

39. Fadok VA, Bratton DL, Konowal A, et al. Macrophages that have ingested apoptotic cells in vitro inhibit proinflammatory cytokine production through autocrine/paracrine mechanisms involving TGF-beta, PGE2, and PAF. J Clin Invest 1998;101:890–898.

40. Liu PT, Stenger S, Li H, et al. Toll-like receptor triggering of a vitamin D–mediated human antimicrobial response. Science 2006;311:1770–1773.

41. Hajjar AM, Harowicz H, Liggitt HD, et al. An essential role for non-bone marrow-derived cells in control of *Pseudomonas aeruginosa* pneumonia. Am J Respir Cell Mol Biol 2005;33:470–475.

42. Dockrell DH, Marriott HM, Prince LR, et al. Alveolar macrophage apoptosis contributes to pneumococcal clearance in a resolving model of pulmonary infection. J Immunol 2003;171:5380–5388.

43. Segal AW. How neutrophils kill microbes. Annu Rev Immunol 2005;23:197–223.

44. Chandra A, Katahira J, Schmalstieg FC, et al. P-selectin blockade fails to improve acute lung injury in sheep. Clin Sci (Lond) 2003;104:313–321.

45. Anderson DC, Miller LJ, Schmalstieg FC, et al. Contributions of the Mac-1 glycoprotein family to adherence-dependent granulocyte functions: structure-function assessments employing subunit-specific monoclonal antibodies. J Immunol 1986;137:15–27.

46. Springer TA. Traffic signals for lymphocyte recirculation and leukocyte emigration: the multistep paradigm. Cell 1994;76:301–314.

47. Mizgerd JP, Horwitz BH, Quillen HC, et al. Effects of CD18 deficiency on the emigration of murine neutrophils during pneumonia. J Immunol 1999;163:995–999.

48. Sabroe I, Prince LR, Jones EC, et al. Selective roles for Toll-like receptor (TLR)2 and TLR4 in the regulation of neutrophil activation and life span. J Immunol 2003;170: 5268–5275.

49. Madden JF, Burchette JL Jr, Hale LP. Pathology of parainfluenza virus infection in patients with congenital immunodeficiency syndromes. Hum Pathol 2004;35:594–603.

50. Schmalstieg FC, Goldman AS. Immune consequences of mutations in the human common gamma-chain gene. Mol Genet Metab 2002;76:163–171.

51. Schmalstieg FC, Palkowetz KH, Rudloff HE, Goldman AS. Blood gammadelta T cells and gammadelta TCR V gene specificities in a single missense mutation (L→Q271) in the common gamma chain gene. Scand J Immunol 2001;54: 592–598.

52. Goldman AS, Palkowetz KH, Rudloff HE, et al. Genesis of progressive T-cell deficiency owing to a single missense mutation in the common gamma chain gene. Scand J Immunol 2001;54:582–591.

53. Schmalstieg FC, Leonard WJ, Noguchi M, et al. Missense mutation in exon 7 of the common gamma chain gene causes a moderate form of X-linked combined immunodeficiency. J Clin Invest 1995;95:1169–1173.

54. Fieschi C, Casanova JL. The role of interleukin-12 in human infectious diseases: only a faint signature. Eur J Immunol 2003;33:1461–1464.

55. Fallarino F, Gajewski TF. Cutting edge: differentiation of antitumor CTL in vivo requires host expression of Stat1. J Immunol 1999;163:4109–4113.

56. Sun J, Walsh M, Villarino AV, et al. TLR ligands can activate dendritic cells to provide a MyD88-dependent negative signal for Th2 cell development. J Immunol 2005;174:742–751.

57. van Gisbergen KP, Sanchez-Hernandez M, Geijtenbeek TB, van Kooyk Y. Neutrophils mediate immune modulation of dendritic cells through glycosylation-dependent interactions between Mac-1 and DC-SIGN. J Exp Med 2005;201: 1281–1292.

58. van Gisbergen KP, Ludwig IS, Geijtenbeek TB, van Kooyk Y. Interactions of DC-SIGN with Mac-1 and CEACAM1 regulate contact between dendritic cells and neutrophils. FEBS Lett 2005;579:6159–6168.

59. Filippi C, Hugues S, Cazareth J, et al. CD4+ T cell polarization in mice is modulated by strain-specific major histocompatibility complex-independent differences within dendritic cells. J Exp Med 2003;198:201–209.

60. Moser B, Willimann K. Chemokines: role in inflammation and immune surveillance. Ann Rheum Dis 2004;63 Suppl 2: ii84–ii89.

61. Langenkamp A, Nagata K, Murphy K, et al. Kinetics and expression patterns of chemokine receptors in human CD4+ T lymphocytes primed by myeloid or plasmacytoid dendritic cells. Eur J Immunol 2003;33:474–482.

62. Gavin M, Rudensky A. Control of immune homeostasis by naturally arising regulatory CD4+ T cells. Curr Opin Immunol 2003;15:690–696.

63. Wildin RS, Freitas A. IPEX and FOXP3: clinical and research perspectives. J Autoimmun 2005;(Suppl 25):56–62.

64. Chensue SW, Warmington KS, Allenspach EJ, et al. Differential expression and cross-regulatory function of RANTES during mycobacterial (type 1) and schistosomal (type 2) antigen-elicited granulomatous inflammation. J Immunol 1999;163:165–173.

65. Sato N, Kuziel WA, Melby PC, et al. Defects in the generation of IFN-gamma are overcome to control infection with Leishmania donovani in CC chemokine receptor (CCR) 5-, macrophage inflammatory protein-1 alpha-, or CCR2-deficient mice. J Immunol 1999;163:5519–5525.

66. Palaniappan R, Singh S, Singh UP, et al. CCL5 modulates pneumococcal immunity and carriage. J Immunol 2006;176: 2346–2356.

67. Jakubzick C, Tacke F, Llodra J, et al. Modulation of dendritic cell trafficking to and from the airways. J Immunol 2006;176:3578–3584.

68. van Etten E, Mathieu C. Immunoregulation by 1,25-dihydroxyvitamin D3: basic concepts. J Steroid Biochem Mol Biol 2005;97:93–101.

69. Bozza S, Gaziano R, Spreca A, et al. Dendritic cells transport conidia and hyphae of Aspergillus fumigatus from the airways to the draining lymph nodes and initiate disparate Th responses to the fungus. J Immunol 2002;168:1362–1371.

70. Puck JM. Molecular and genetic basis of X-linked immunodeficiency disorders. J Clin Immunol 1994;14:81–89.

71. Nomura K, Kanegane H, Karasuyama H, et al. Genetic defect in human X-linked agammaglobulinemia impedes a maturational evolution of pro-B cells into a later stage of pre-B cells in the B-cell differentiation pathway. Blood 2000;96:610–617.

72. Weiner LS, Howell JT, Langford MP, et al. Effect of specific antibodies on chronic echovirus type 5 encephalitis in a patient with hypogammaglobulinemia. J Infect Dis 1979;140: 858–863.

73. Guilbault C, Novak JP, Martin P, et al. Distinct pattern of lung gene expression in the Cfr-KO mice developing spontaneous lung disease compared to their littermate controls. Physiol Genomics 2006;25:179–193.

74. Kiechl S, Lorenz E, Reindl M, et al. Toll-like receptor 4 polymorphisms and atherogenesis. N Engl J Med 2002; 347:185–192.

75. Schaaf B, Rupp J, Muller-Steinhardt M, et al. The interleukin-6-174 promoter polymorphism is associated with extrapulmonary bacterial dissemination in Streptococcus pneumoniae infection. Cytokine 2005;31:324–328.

76. Lowe PR, Galley HF, Abdel-Fattah A, Webster NR. Influence of interleukin-10 polymorphisms on interleukin-10 expression and survival in critically ill patients. Crit Care Med 2003;31:34–38.

77. Fang XM, Schroder S, Hoeft A, Stuber F. Comparison of two polymorphisms of the interleukin-1 gene family: interleukin-1 receptor antagonist polymorphism contributes to susceptibility to severe sepsis. Crit Care Med 1999;27:1330–1334.

37
Molecular Pathology of Viral Respiratory Diseases

Geoffrey A. Land

Introduction

Virology has long been the gold standard by which advances in molecular biology and methodology have been measured.[1] As new molecular tools have been developed, new viruses or variants of older, established taxons have been described. Recent advances in genetic sequencing and amplification technologies were pivotal in detecting and describing the two newest agents with a tropism for the respiratory system, severe acute respiratory syndrome (SARS) and avian influenza virus,[2-4] both of which have the potential to be pandemic agents with a high mortality and morbidity rate. The rapid development of specific molecular tests led to effective public health measures to be put in place to successfully quarantine these agents thus far. The identification of these two new agents underscores the fact that the major cause of nonbacterial epidemics in history has been viruses with a predilection for the respiratory system. The classic example is the global "Spanish flu" pandemic of 1918, attributed to causing the deaths of 20–40 million people within 1 year, a mortality rate greater than that recorded for World War I and the 4 worst years of the Black Plague (AD 1347–1351) combined.[4-7]

The recognition of viruses as entities and as potential agents of infection has occurred only within a little more than the past 115 years.[8,9] The Russian bacteriologist Dimitrii Ivanovsky presented evidence of small infective agents that could pass through unglazed porcelain filters that retained bacteria. Martinus Beijerinck, in 1898, hypothesized that these "filterable agents" could cause tobacco mosaic disease in a nondiseased plant. Similar filterable agents were described in 1901 by Walter Reed and James Carroll as the probable etiology of yellow fever, and soon thereafter there were descriptions of similar agents that caused malignancies in birds or that could eradicate bacteria.[8] The actual isolation and propagation of human viruses was a difficult process and languished behind the advances made in animal, plant, and bacterial viruses.[9] The major stumbling block in the development of animal virology was finding a satisfactory milieu or substrate for culturing human viruses. Initial success at growing viruses used animals or eggs, making human virology beyond the scope of everything but research laboratories. However, the development in the 1950s of eukaryotic cell culturing techniques and cell lines that sustained viral growth and propagation enabled the rapid development of diagnostic virology.[8]

The first human respiratory virus, influenza virus, was described in 1933 by Wilson Smith, Christopher Andrews, and Patrick Laidlaw.[4] Interest in human influenza research had become stimulated over the devastation left by the Spanish flu pandemic, but it was not until a suitable host was found that the virus could be studied in depth.[8] Studies to date have determined that this virus can undergo degrees of spontaneous mutation of some of the major proteins on its outer surface, the hemagglutinin (H) and neuraminidase (N) proteins, at a fairly regular rate.[10] Minor changes to these proteins (antigenic drift) lead to localized epidemics, whereby the antibodies stimulated in response to the previous strain are not as protective as they should be. There is, however, enough immunologic memory in the population that the virus cannot find a large group of unexposed individuals and cause a pandemic (worldwide epidemic). More profound changes in the composition of the H and N molecules can also occur (antigenic shift) in which the global immunologic memory of these antigens has been lost or never stimulated and a pandemic ensues.[11,12] The reason for the current concern over SARS and avian flu is based not only on the rate of change of the H and N molecules over the last 100 years in the case of influenza viruses[11] but also on the similarity both of these virus genomes have to their respective animal and avian counterparts[3,11,13] as well as recent evidence pointing to the human influenza flu virus family evolving from a crossover that occurred during the domestication of animals approximately 8,000 years ago.[14]

The intimate relationship of viral structure and extent and severity of influenza virus infections in humans has served as a benchmark for describing the relationship between the various macromolecules produced by other viruses and the course and pathology of their infections.[4,7,10,15–17] This chapter focuses on recent discoveries in the macromolecular structures of respiratory viruses and their contribution in establishing infection and concomitant pathology. This includes sections on viral structure, genomics, replication, the molecular events leading to respiratory tropism and pathology, and a brief description of the viruses involved.

General Principles

Structure and Invasion

Viruses are nonliving macromolecular complexes made up of proteins and either DNA or RNA that, upon gaining access to the host cell's energy and reproductive system, effectively redirect host cell metabolism and synthetic capabilities in order to replicate and transmit progeny virus (release).[9,18] Their general structure consists of an outer protein shell (capsid) composed of subunits, which are single folded polypeptides that link together as the basic structural unit (protomer).[8] These basic structural units may consist of one specific peptide type or multiple types, each with various functions relative to attaching and gaining entry into the cell as they condense to form the outer shell or, in the case of some viruses, that have condensed around a protein–genomic complex called the nucleocapsid.[19] In the case of enveloped viruses, these protomers may also become surface structures (capsomers, peplomers) such as spikes, projections, or knobs that give a virus its characteristic shape and appearance in electron micrographs. Finally, the tertiary folding of single polypeptides and their quaternary interaction and folding as they condense around the genome (packaging) impart a characteristic symmetry to the resulting macromolecular complex.[8] Viral symmetry is defined as either icosahedral or helical, and its geometry is directed by the steric interaction of folded structural units. In addition to their combined structure protecting the genome, the outer proteins function in binding the virus to specific receptors on the cell,[20,21] helping to prepare the virus for entry into the host cells by having protease and/or nuclease activities, interaction with the host cell membranes (budding) to develop the outer envelope,[8,22] or, in some cases, eventually inducing fusion with host cell membranes.[23–25]

Viruses enter host cells by (1) uptake through attachment to specific receptors or ligands (attachment) on the surface membrane of the target cells (receptor-mediated endocytosis)[8,23,26–28] or (2) by being absorbed into the cell by the cellular vesicular/endosome system (pinocytosis, fluid phase endocytosis, absorption).[20,29–31] Receptor–mediated or ligand entry is facilitated by the attachment of a specific epitope on the protein outer coat of the virus (capsid) with its corresponding receptor that gives a particular virus its characteristic tropism. For example, adenoviruses gain entry into respiratory epithelial cells by attachment of 1 of the 10 structural proteins with an integrin or immunoglobulin-like (Ig) receptor on the host cell surface, whereupon a second receptor (integrins $\alpha_v\beta_5$ and $\alpha_v\beta_5$) binds with the penton base of the virus with further molecular events introducing the capsid to the endosome system for transport.[10,32–34] The absorption form of viral entry is characterized by the presence of an outer envelope that is similar in structure to the host cell membrane, that is, coronavirus cold viruses (coronaviruses, SARS virus, rhinoviruses)[3,28,35] and the myxoviruses (influenza, measles, respiratory syncytial, human metapneumovirus, and parainfluenza viruses) with respiratory cells.[20,36,37] The similarity in lipoprotein structures of the two lead to fusion of the viral envelope with the cellular membrane/endosome system, and the virus is transported into the cell.

Once the virus gains access to the endosome system, a series of early molecular events (incubation period), some of which are still under the direction of the infective virion, uncoats the virus and releases the naked genome or nucleocapsid into the cell.[8,9] The uncoating process may be the result of changing internal pH-ionic concentration or some other internal aspect of the host cell environment (lipids, proteins), virion-directed enzymatic activity, or multiple mechanisms in concert stimulating the unfolding of structural proteins away from the genome. At the same time, another set of coordinated events modifies the reproductive and macromolecular synthetic capabilities of the host cell to become a factory for replicating the next generation of viruses (replication).[38–41] The way in which viruses store structural components in infected cells are released from infected cells or how their released components effect adjacent cells is what produces the characteristic changes in cells called cytopathic effects.[23,42]

Envelope

The envelope is not a structural component of all viruses, but its presence more than ensures the carrier virion's predilection for certain organs, tissues, or cells and adds protective layer(s) to the capsid. It is a lipid membrane derived from the host plasma membrane with the integration of glycosylated viral proteins.[8,9] These proteins carry covalently linked oligosaccharide (poly-sugar) chains that are added posttranslation as the peptides are being transported to the cell membrane assembly point. These glycoproteins span the lipid bilayer by one or more transmembrane segments, providing an anchor point for the molecule at the interior side and the characteristic knobs, projections, bonding sites, and so forth, of a specific viral group, for example, the HA, NA, and M2 proteins of the influenza A viruses.[12,13,43,44] Envelopes are developed by one of two mechanisms (1) they are assembled internally and sequentially with subsequent budding from the host cell at maturation, and (2) the progeny and envelope are synthesized and assembled at the same time.[9,45]

Type 1 envelope formation is a feature of influenza A viruses and is characterized by the replication and assembly of the ribonucleoprotein in the nucleus with subsequent M1 and NEP protein-dependent transport to the cytoplasm. At the same time, the viral glycoproteins (HA, NA) and the M2 membrane protein are synthesized and follow the cell secretory pathway and modify the outer host cell membrane.[4] The M1 protein aligns the nucleocapsid and the inner layer of the modified membrane, and assembly is completed. In type 2 envelope formation, a feature of retroviruses, the virus is assembled around the MA segment of the Gag polyprotein bound to the inner surface of the plasma membrane.[8] The Gag appears to direct the assembly process and the enfolding of the plasma membrane around the maturing viruses. Both pathways complete progeny development and prepare them for *release* to infect adjacent cells.[25]

Genome

One of the most unique features of viruses is that they may contain either a DNA or an RNA genome. Every other replicating organism has both DNA and RNA, but DNA is the single source of genetic information for its reproduction. Moreover, the way and degree of competency with which progeny genomes are reproduced often govern the virulence and pathology characteristic of specific viral groups.[8,9,40] Viral nucleic acids are defined as to whether or not they are single or double stranded, circular or linear, single or multiple copies, single or segmented, or ends are joined covalently or noncovalently. The *sense* of the viral polymerases is also considered an important characteristic of their respective genomes. *Sense* refers to the mechanism necessary for the genome to transcribe its genetic information to a functional messenger RNA (positive "+" strand mRNA). The complementing RNA and DNA strands would then be characterized as negative sense. This characteristic of strand complementarity relative to functional mRNA has been developed into a very effective schema for the molecular classification of viruses as shown below.[46]

Recombination

The fact that there are a number of genotypes of the same virus as well as the emergence of new human viruses that share some fraction of their genome with similar animal viruses (avian influenza virus), provides de facto evidence that recombinant types of events can occur during viral replication.[11,47–49] Some viruses exhibit rearrangements of nucleic acid sequences (genome copying errors, insertions, inversions, tandem repeats, reassortments), whereas others show that there has been recombination between two different genomes. Reassortment is common among segmented RNA viruses, such as the influenza virus, whereby two different segmented viruses infect the same cell and exchange RNA by exchanging segments during packaging. Because RNA viruses form many progeny with varying degrees of accurate template(s) replication, copying errors changing sequence information or exchanging of genetic information is not uncommon.[50]

DNA viruses exhibit two forms of recombination, homologous and site specific.[8,9,40] Site-specific recombination takes place along short DNA sequences flanked by codons recognized by catalytic recombination proteins and may occur with either or both nucleic acid strands. Homologous recombination occurs with all viral DNA, and it is an exchange between any pair of related sequences. These recombinant events are important in maintaining the virus in a changing environment, such as selection of a specific Influenza virus serotype or in perpetuating the virus without destroying the host as in the latent or persistent phase of the Herpetoviridae.[8,9,51,52]

One occasional result of recombination is the enhancement of virulence and/or lethality of an infection. In the case of SARS or avian influenza virus infections, a wild-type human virus has exchanged (gained) genetic information from an animal or avian counterpart.[3,11,47,53] The recombinant virus was different enough that the human immune memory repertoire did not completely recognize the new viral capsid epitopes and a de novo immune response was mounted against the virus. Because there was no herd immunity or "immune braking" to halt the spread of the virus, resultant infections in the local immune naive populations had a high morbidity and mortality with the potential for wide spread. The most studied group of respiratory viruses that undergo recombination-induced structural change is the influenza A viruses. The effects of such recombinant viral activity in human disease were discussed previously in the paragraphs on antigenic drift and antigenic shift.

Viral Pathogenesis

Once gaining entry into the host, the virus must invade the host immune defense to establish the infection. This is accomplished by ligand attachment, followed by replication within the initial cell, and spread to contiguous cells. Once local infection is established, many viruses are spread further by one or more general disseminations via the lymphatics, reticuloendothelial cells, and/or the bloodstream (viremia)[8] to other tissues or cells with receptors that bind to the capsid epitopes. Viruses are capable of causing acute infections (influenza, common colds),[2,3,54–57] persistent infections (cytomegalovirus, herpes simplex virus), or latent infections (Epstein-Barr virus, herpes simplex virus, varicella-zoster virus).[25,36,58–60] Acute infections are characterized by a short incubation period, with a sudden explosion of symptoms (replication and release) that rise to a nadir and then descend as the host develops an adaptive immune response to the infection.[4,8,61,62] Cellular damage is usually the result of a combination of release by cell lysis and the influx of host cytokines, antibodies, and immune-activated cells, which limit the spread of the virus and destroys infected cells. The cells and effectors of the adaptive immune response begin to remove the virus particles, and the attendant antibodies and memory cells produced during this process provide immunity to reinfection.[8] Persistent infections are chronic and have some intervals between periods of waxing and waning. After the initial infection and limited viral release (or steady low level viral release without host cell damage), the adaptive response limits the infection and it appears quiescent only to appear later with repeated wax and wane cycles.[51] Latent infections are the extreme end of the persistent infection spectrum—longer periods between overt signs of infection and adaptive control.

Adaptive immune clearance is accomplished by at least two mechanisms: (1) similarity of viral epitopes to host antigens and (2) genomic changes leading to changes in viral surface structure. In the first scenario, some viral epitopes are very similar to host cell surface epitopes, such that host immune clearance mechanisms do not recognize them as being non-self.[18,26,56,63,64] These are usually viruses that attach near or are similar to antigens/receptors of the major histocompatibility complex (*HLA*, *MHC*) such that their epitopes create a condition of tolerance by downregulating MHC expression, neutralizing host immune response. The second adaptive mechanism involves the mutation frequency of the genome, extent of copying errors in replication, or recombination frequency of the genome.[65] In the first scenario, small changes may occur in the structural peptides that do not interfere with the major mechanism of immune clearance, or small changes may occur in the viral structural peptides that slightly effect antibody or cytotoxic T-lymphocyte clearance, but there is some degree of protection (antigenic drift). These are usually due to random mutations and/or copy errors during replication. There are, however, instances when major changes occur in viral surface proteins, for example, when the capsid epitopes have changed so completely that the immune memory and clearance mechanisms directed against previous strains of the virus will not prevent infection (antigenic shift). These major changes in surface structure result from coinfection of two or more viral serotypes (same or different host origin) and subsequent recombination of their respective genomes.[7,11,21,66]

The classic example of such an abrupt change or shift in viral surface structure with devastating virulence is the 1918 Spanish flu.[9,11,44,67] The above-mentioned SARS and avian influenza strains are considered contemporary viruses with equal potential for similar lethal pandemics. It was only through a Herculean effort to isolate and quarantine infected humans, exposed family members and friends, exposed health care workers, and exposed and infected birds that the latter two viruses, for the present, have been localized to the Far East.[2–4]

Thus far, there have been six major Influenza A antigen shifts since 1889.[8,10,68] These long-term and discrete changes in antigenic structure teamed with the more common copying error–induced drift result in a diversity of immune memory within the population and serves to explain why some ethnic or age groups appear more or less protected by the current vaccine than others.[4]

In summary, the type of pathology induced by a specific virus is a combination of several factors, including but not limited to its mode of attachment, where it attaches (the predilection for a specific organ, tissue), ease of cell-to-cell spread, its mode of replication, frequency of genetic change (extent of mutation, copy errors during replication, recombination), whether or not it destroys the host cell upon release or buds off the plasma membrane slowly or quickly, the presence of a characteristic pattern of cell destruction (cytopathic effect), and the point at which some form of immunomodulation occurs. The acute infection may, with its intense protein load spread over several cells, stimulate the production of antibodies, release cytokines, and attract cells that process and present viral antigens specific to various components, leading eventually to lytic release as observed in hepatitis virus infections. In other instances, there may be a downregulation of the T-cell cytolytic response to cells presented viral antigens as observed in latent herpesvirus infections or slow and persistent infections such as measles.[18,26,56,69]

Finally, the virus may turn off some aspect of the immune system such as seen in the effect that human immunodeficiency virus has on T-helper cells at the time of attachment.[8] Once attached the T-helper response is downregulated, having a cumulative effect over a long period of time, and may only be suspected when the ratios of CD4[+] competent cells to CD8[+] cells becomes inverted and the patient begins to exhibit a variety of opportunistic infections.

Classification

Traditional viral classification was based on a variety of physicochemical parameters reflecting the character and the geometry of the capsid as well as its size, structure, composition, organization, presence of an envelope, and

TABLE 37.1. Classification of viruses.

Family and viruses	Gen (–)/BC; E; S*	Receptors†	Infection type‡				
			Common Cold	Pharyngitis	Laryngitis	Sinusitis	Pneumonia
Orthomyxoviridae	ssRNA (–)/V; E; H						
Influenza A virus		Cell surface sialyloligosaccharides	C	C	C		C
Influenza B virus		Cell surface sialyloligosaccharides	PU, AC	C	C		PU, AC
Avian influenza virus		α-2-6-Sialyloligosaccharides					AC
Paramyxoviridae	ssRNA (–)/V; E; H						
Parainfluenza virus types 1, 2, 3		Cell surface sialyloligosaccharides	C	C	C		PC, AU
Respiratory syncytial virus		Pattern recognition receptors: TLR4, CD14	C				PC, AU
Measles virus		CD46, signaling lymphocyte activation molecule (SLAM, CD121)	C			C	U
Metapneumovirus							
Metapneumovirus		Unclear (TLR4?)	U		C		U
Adenoviridae	dsDNA/I; E; IC						
Adenovirus types 1, 2, 3, 5		Coxsackie and adenovirus receptor (CAR)	C	C	C	U	U
Adenovirus types 4, 7 (military)		Major histocompatibility class II, CD46	AC	C	C	U	C
		Integrins $\alpha_v\beta_3$ and $\alpha_v\beta_5$					
Coronaviridae	ssRNA (+)/VI; E; H						
Common coronavirus		CEA glycoprotein family, aminopeptidase N, 9-O-acetylated sialic acid oligosaccharides	C	C	C		C
SARS virus							
SARS virus		Angiotensin-converting enzyme 2		AC			
Enteroviridae (Picornaviridae)	ssRNA (+)/VI; IC						
Coxsackievirus		Decay accelerating factor (DAF; CD55) CAR, $\alpha_v\beta_3$-integrin (vironectin)	U	U			U
Echovirus		DAF (CD55), $\alpha_2\beta_1$-integrin	U	C	U	U	U
Poliovirus		Poliovirus receptor		C	C	C	U
Rhinovirus		Intracellular adhesion molecule 1 Some—sialic acid	C	C	C	C	U
Bunyaviridae	ssRNA (–)/V; E; H						
Hantavirus§		β_3-integrin, upregulation RANTES	U	U	U	U	PU, AC
Herpesviridae	dsDNA/I; E; IC						
Herpes simplex virus		Heparan sulfate, herpesvirus entry mediator (HVEM/HveA), nectin 1 (PRR1/HveC), nectin 2 (PRR2/HveB)	U	C	U	U	U
Cytomegalovirus		Heparan sulfate, epidermal growth factor	PC, AU	U	C	U	U
Epstein-Barr virus		Complement receptor 2 (CD21)	C	C	C	U	U
Varicella-zoster virus		Insulin degrading enzyme, Fc receptor	PC, AU	PC, AU	U	U	U
Human herpesvirus 6		CD46	PC				AU

*Gen (–), strandedness and nucleic acid type of genome (polymerase sense: + or –)/I–VI, Baltimore classification); ss, single strand; ds, double strand; E, envelope present; S, symmetry: IC, icosahedral, or H, helical.
†CEA, carcinoembryonic antigen; SARS, severe acute respiratory syndrome; TLR4, Toll-like receptor 4.
‡P, pediatric; A, adult; C, common; U, uncommon.
§Hantavirus: adult respiratory disease syndrome.

nucleic acid content.[8,9] To take into account the unique aspects of replicating, transcribing, and translating viral genetic information, current classification schemes use a combination of viral physical characteristics and those of its genome (Table 37.1). The molecular approach, described by David Baltimore in 1971,[46] makes the assumption that all viruses have to replicate to the point of creating a positive (+) sense RNA (functional mRNA) in order for the message to be translated by cellular ribosomes into the proteins necessary for the production and packaging of progeny viruses. This divides the currently known viruses into six functional groups, with groups II and III not represented by agents causing respiratory infections.[8,9,46]

I. *Double-stranded DNA (dsDNA)*: DNA separates into positive and negative strands, with the negative strand being translated to mRNA (adenoviruses, herpesviruses).
II. *Single-stranded DNA (+ssDNA)*: A positive sense DNA strand replicates a −ssDNA intermediate that is then translated to mRNA.
III. *Double-stranded RNA (dsRNA)*: The two strands separate, and the positive strand becomes the functional mRNA and the negative strand is translated to a functional mRNA.
IV. *Single-stranded RNA (+ssRNA), pathway (1)*: The +ssRNA is translated to a −ssRNA replicative intermediate that is converted to a functional mRNA (picornaviruses/enteroviruses, togaviruses, coronaviruses).
V. *Single-stranded RNA (−ssRNA), pathway (2)*: The −ssRNA directly replicates the functional mRNA (bunyaviruses, orthomyxoviruses, paramyxoviruses).
VI. *Single-stranded RNA (−ssRNA), pathway 3*: The +ssRNA is translated to a −ssRNA replicative intermediate that is gives rise to mRNA. This method of replication appears an exclusive characteristic of the Retroviridae. None of the known retroviruses causes overt respiratory pathology, but they do suppress the immune system and permit those viruses capable of respiratory disease to gain a foothold.

Viral Respiratory Diseases

Orthomyxoviridae

The orthomyxoviruses are ubiquitous enveloped viruses, approximately 90–120 nm in diameter with helical symmetry and segmented, negative sense, ssRNA genome.[4] They are extremely stable in small droplet aerosols and are shed in large numbers, both characteristics adding in their efficient spread among immunologically naïve individuals and young schoolchildren.[8] The most important

member of the Orthomyxoviridae family is the influenza A virus, which reaches its peak infection rate in winter. Infections are described in terms of being local severe respiratory epidemic respiratory disease due to small changes in the peptide structure of the H and N peplomers on the envelope surface (antigenic drift) or severe pandemic respiratory disease due to major structural shifts in these same molecules (antigenic drift).[1,10,14,37] The salient points of their replication, structure, and antigen changes were described earlier in this chapter. Influenza viruses attach to mucosal surfaces, whereupon they replicate and spread in the respiratory tract leading to an acute, rapid-onset, febrile respiratory infection. There is a prodrome of fever, malaise, sore throat, and cough that progresses to croup, myositis, otitis media, abdominal pain, and vomiting or to viral pneumonia as the virus invades the central nervous system and muscles, as well as further damaging the lung parenchyma. The latter may be so severe as to cause hemorrhage, hyalination of the alveoli and alveolar ducts, and ulceration paving the way for secondary bacterial pneumonia.

Laboratory diagnosis is built around a number of quick serology tests based on the viral antigen and in latex agglutination, enzyme-linked immunosorbent assay (ELISA), or dipstick format.[4,70] These viruses can be cultured, and confirmatory polymerase chain reaction (PCR) tests have been developed.[49,66]

Paramyxoviridae

Paramyxoviruses are enveloped viruses with helical symmetry and are 150–300 nm in diameter with a nonsegmented negative sense ssRNA genome.[8,9] This viral group runs the gamut of respiratory symptoms from severe respiratory syncytial virus infections in infants (common), to the moderate to severe parainfluenza virus (common) and metapneumovirus (uncommon) infections, to the common measles (rubeola) virus with its mild respiratory prodrome and accompanying rash, its most identifying characteristic.

The parainfluenza viruses have four distinct HN fibers attached to their outer envelope, dividing the group into four distinct types.[15,62] Parainfluenza type 3 virus is the most common type isolated, especially in children ≤6 months of age, and endemic peak infectivity occurs in late spring.[8,62] Type 1 viruses are isolated about half as frequently as type 3 and type 2 about half as frequently type 1. Both types 1 and 2 appear seasonally, with their peak isolation period occurring in the autumn and alternate years. Infections range from mild upper respiratory infections (common cold-like syndromes) to severe infections of the large airways of the lower respiratory tract (croup, laryngotracheobronchitis).

The HN fibers serve as a ligand to sialylated molecules on the cell surface of ciliated respiratory epithelial cells.

Anchoring the virus to the cell surface activates the F (fusion) protein, which in turn is cleaved by cell surface serine proteases, and the virus enters the host cell.[8,62] Upon entry, the nucleocapsid complex that consists of the NP (nucleocapsid), L (polymerase), and P (phosphorylated nucleocapsid-associated protein) is released along with −ssRNA. These proteins and accompanying viral genome serve to direct mRNA synthesis. The mRNA replicates an antisense strand for progeny genomes and is also translated to form the necessary proteins for new virus production. Viral assembly occurs in the cytoplasm, with the new NP proteins condensing around the newly replicated genomes forming a helical structure that complex with the P and L proteins to form a complete nucleocapsid.

Envelope proteins have been simultaneously transported to the cell surface by the secretory endoplasmic reticulum, and the entire complex is assembled at the apical position of the host cell and released by budding.[62] This apical release is into the mucin layer, preventing infection of the deeper cell layers, and the presence of the fusion protein results in some syncytia formation. Laboratory diagnosis is most commonly by cell culture and antigen–antibody detection, with some successful molecular techniques having been reported.[8,62,71,72]

The most common cause of severe lower respiratory disease in children is respiratory syncytial virus.[73–75] These viruses are typical paramyxoviruses and are similar to the parainfluenza viruses in that they are ubiquitous, are 120–300 nm in diameter, and have a ssRNA, negative sense, nonsegmented genome with a fusion glycoprotein (F protein) on the envelope surface.[8,76] The envelope is highly pleomorphic and is circumscribed with glycoprotein projections that, in contrast to the parainfluenza viruses, consist of three transmembrane glycoproteins: the aforementioned F protein as well as the G and SH proteins.[8,76] Infection begins when the F protein fuses viral and cellular envelopes together with subsequent attachment to pattern recognition receptors such as Toll-like receptor 4 and CD14 via the G glycoprotein.[64,76] Upon progeny release, these surface glycoproteins also catalyze infection of other cells by fusing newly released viruses with the cell membranes of adjacent cells, giving rise to the characteristic syncytium formation of the infection.

Most individuals exhibit evidence of infection by the end of early childhood, with severe disease requiring hospitalization occurring in children ≤24 months, peaking in children <6 months old.[54,73–75] Infections are seasonal, with onset in winter to early spring. Severity of disease is age related, as adults exhibit mild cold-like symptoms with or without rhinitis, children exhibit mild disease to pneumonia (inversely proportional to age), and infants exhibit severe seasonal pneumonia, bronchiolitis, and tracheobronchitis.[54] The severe bronchial disease seen in infants is probably due to a combination of narrow airways and swelling tracheal and bronchial tissue due to viral-induced pathology and host immune response. The economic impact of this seasonal infection, because of the virus' highly contagious nature and virulence, has led to recommending administering prophylactic immune globulin to prevent epidemic infection in susceptible populations.[54,77,78]

These viruses grow in culture in HEp2 cells, HeLa cells, and cells adapted from a type II human alveolar epithelial lung carcinoma (A549). However, because of the extreme lability of the virus in clinical specimens, culture is not the most commonly used laboratory diagnostic procedure.[76] Routine laboratory diagnosis is made through a variety of rapid direct or indirect antigen and/or antibody tests in either the immunofluorescence or ELISA format.[76] Some recent reports have shown that molecular tests, especially reverse transcriptase PCR (RT-PCR) may also be effective in the rapid diagnosis of this infection.[71,72]

The rubeola virus (measles virus), also a paramyxovirus, is ubiquitous and highly contagious in an immune naïve population.[69] Infections are transmitted by inhalation of large droplet aerosols, with the peak infection period occurring from autumn to spring.[8] Their structure is typical of the family, consisting of an outer envelope (100–250 nm diameter) surrounding the helical NPL nucleocapsid complex. The outer envelope exhibits two types of peplomeric projections, a conical-shaped hemagglutinin (H glycoprotein) and a dumbbell-shaped fusion (F glycoprotein),[8,69] and a neuraminidase (NA) protein has also been described.[79] As with the other paramyxoviruses, these peplomers are involved with attachment and fusion of the virus with the host cell. Attachment and virus entry occurs via the F protein liganding with CD46 or a signaling lymphocyte activation molecule (SLAM, CD121/CDw150) on mucosal epithelial surfaces.[69,79,80] Once the virus enters the cell and the genome is uncoated, replication is typical for the nonsegmented paramyxovirus ssRNA genome.

Adjacent cells are infected through membrane release and syncytium formation, eventually giving rise to a primary viremia, and further spread is by blood-borne cells of the reticuloendothelial system.[8,69] Multiple organs become infected, more viruses are released, and a secondary viremia occurs, leading to the characteristic rash and Koplik's spots associated with the disease. The primary viremia also gives rise to the upper respiratory prodrome that is present prior to the rash's appearance, and symptoms range from mild to severe in nature and with or without a cough. In severe cases, respiratory symptoms may be augmented by the secondary viremia, which affects the entire respiratory mucosa, including denuding ciliated cells from the mucosal surfaces, and compromises the patient further through cough, croup, bronchiolitis, and pneumonia.

Diagnosis is primarily clinical, based on cough, coryza, rash, and Koplik's spots. The most common laboratory test is a fourfold specific antibody titer movement using a number of techniques, including complement fixation, ELISA, immunofluorescence, and, to a lesser extent, neutralization.[69] There are also several antigen detection tests available in a variety of formats for detecting rubeola antigen from serum, nasal discharge, and urinary sediments, and an RT-PCR test for measles RNA has been described.[69,81]

The recently described human metapneumovirus appears also to be a ubiquitous pathogen of children like respiratory syncytial virus and exhibits a close genetic association with avian pneumoviruses.[48,82] Whereas Respiratory syncytial virus tends to be severe in infants, with most children exhibiting seroevidence of infection by age 2 years, only 50% of children have metapneumovirus antibodies by 2 years, eventually reaching 100% seroprevalence by age 5.[83–85] They are typical paramyxoviruses with a negative sense, ssRNA, helical nucleocapsid, and a pleomorphic outer lipid envelope with peplomers projecting from the surface.[86] These surface projections are the F (fusion) protein, which permit viruses to enter host cells, release progeny, and infect adjacent cells, leading to characteristic syncytia. The actual receptor molecule is unclear but appears to be associated with Toll-like receptor 4.[8,86] Major symptoms include nasal congestion, cough, fever, and rhinorrhea, and the peak periods of infection appear to coincide with influenza and respiratory syncytial virus.[84,85] Diagnostic tests include serology (enzyme immunoassay, indirect fluorescent antibody), viral culture, and RT-PCR.[86–88]

Adenoviruses

Adenoviruses are nonenveloped, 70–90 nm diameter, icosahedral, double-stranded DNA viruses.[8,9,61] Their clinical importance resides in the ability to cause acute respiratory and conjunctival infections, diarrhea, central nervous system disease in humans, as well as latent or persistent infections in certain animals and cell lines.[8,9,32,61] They have been shown in two large epidemiologic studies to be the most commonly isolated virus in either clinical or subclinical infections.[61] Their typical cytopathic effect in susceptible cells consists of large rounded cells with fibrils or strands attaching them together.[42] They gained their name in the early 1950s as a result of their association with spontaneous degeneration of explanted adenoid tissue.[61] There are currently 52 serotypes as defined by their capsid proteins, and about half these serotypes are considered the etiologies of specific human diseases.[41] Group- and type-specific immunologic identities are conferred by hexon, penton, and fiber capsid proteins. Viruses enter the cell by attachment of knob-capped spikes or fibers projecting from the base of penton capsomeres

with the coxsackie adenovirus receptor and subsequent endocytosis.[19,21,32,33,89] This is facilitated by the association of the penton base with a cellular integrin and the partial uncoating of the virion. Upon entering the cell and further uncoating, the genome is transported to the nucleus; mRNAs are formed and then exported to the cytoplasm for transcription of progeny proteins.[8,38,61] Viruses are then assembled through a series of steps that neutralize host defense mechanisms, cleaving of precursor proteins, and release of cell. Infections may be lytic, persistent or chronic, or oncogenic depending on the host cell type or source (humans, animals, cell cultures).[89]

Respiratory-associated adenoviruses in children and adults consist of a few specific serotypes including members of subgenus B,[46,83] subgenus C,[18,34,51,70] and serotype 4, the only member of subgenus E.[8,61,90] These viruses have been shown to be latent in lymphoepithelial tissue, nasopharynx, and other tissues. Adenoviruses 1, 2, and 5 have been isolated from infants with pharyngitis and coryza or who have otherwise been asymptomatic, and children exhibit a wide variety of clinically apparent respiratory syndromes associated with tonsils and adenoids,[18,34,51,70] upper respiratory disease,[18,34,51,61,70] intussusception,[18,51,61,70] and pharyngoconjunctival fever.[46,83] Serotypes 3, 4, and 7 are common etiologies of acute viral respiratory disease in young adults, with serotype 4 often associated with epidemic infections in closed populations such as military recruits and types 5, 31, and 34 responsible for viral pneumonia with concomitant dissemination in immunocompromised patients.

Depending on the syndrome, adenoviruses may be cultured from pharynx, sputum, conjunctival scrapings, urine, and stool. However, two large and independent studies of symptomatic and asymptomatic individuals demonstrated that adenoviruses are more commonly isolated from stools than from respiratory or other clinical specimens.[61] They are readily cultured in human epithelial cells with characteristic cytopathic effects visible within 2–7 days.[42] They may also be visualized in purified preparations or in direct specimens by electron microscopy. Their DNA can be detected in cultures or clinical specimens by amplification or amplification probe methods with appropriate primers.[71] The standard method of laboratory diagnosis still remains the detection of a fourfold movement in antibody or antigen titer by a variety of serologic techniques, including complement fixation, neutralization, hemagglutination, immunofluorescence, and ELISA.[8,61]

Coronaviruses

Coronaviruses are highly pleomorphic viruses named for the "corona-like" array of club-shaped surface glycoproteins (S proteins) that project from their surface.[3,8] These viruses are ubiquitous and have been traditionally considered major pathogens of the upper respiratory tract in humans, causing approximately 15% of upper respiratory infections reported in temperate climates. They occasionally cause viral diarrhea and are also considered a major animal pathogen, likely composed of three distinct antigenic groups. Coronaviruses are enveloped, 80–160 nm diameter helical viruses with an infectious, single stranded, polyadenylated positive sense RNA genome.[8] The genome is the largest known viral RNA and forms a unique mRNA that has a 3′ polyadenylated cap that forces transcription to occur from the 5′ direction.

They gain entry by attachment of S-protein projections or rays to aminopeptidase M or 9-O-acetylated sialic acid containing oligosaccharides on the surface of nasal epithelial cells but do not produce characteristic cytopathic effects.[28,35] Once attached, viruses enter the cell by pinocytosis, and all progeny synthesis occurs in the cytoplasm. The positive sense genome is released to form a negative sense intermediate; the resultant positive mRNAs nest at their 3′ polyadenylated ends and translation occurs at the 5′ ends.[8,61] The mRNAs are translated into nonstructural proteins and a variety of structural and biosynthetic proteins, including RNA′-RNA polymerase, ATP-helicase, surface hemagglutinin-esterase (HE) protein (some coronaviruses), small envelope protein (E), membrane glycoprotein (M), and the nucleocapsid protein (N). Viruses are assembled in the cytoplasm and then bud into vesicles from the endoplasmic reticulum and are released from the cell membrane by reverse pinocytosis or by lysis, destroying the host cell. Changes in envelope or capsid antigenic structure, as described above, may result in immunologically different peptides being formed, making it difficult to develop consistent serodiagnostic reagents or vaccines for this group.[8,61,91] Because of the difficulty in growing coronavirus strains in culture, the benign and self-limiting nature of the disease (common cold), and the difficulty in obtaining definitive reagents for the laboratory, diagnosis is clinical and treatment is palliative.

Severe Adult Respiratory Distress Syndrome

The recently described SARS coronavirus (SARS-CoV), first identified in China's Guangdong Province, has been identified as the etiology of an acute, severe, and often fatal lower respiratory and systemic disease (SARS), characterized by a severe atypical pneumonia.[2,3] Although morphologically consistent with common coronaviruses, the SARS virus is genetically quite different from its human and animal counterparts, appearing to comprise a fourth antigenic group evolutionarily equidistant from the three major groups of coronaviruses.[3,8] This may reflect a closer relationship to the animal virus from which it was derived. The SARS virus lacks the HE protein and appears to attach to host cells by 9-O-acetylated sialic acid containing oligosaccharides, and it

may be cultured in VERO cell lines, where it may produce a syncytium. Its ease in culturing has permitted the development of some very sophisticated molecular approaches to strain identification, such as real-time PCR and sequence-based typing.[3]

Bunyaviridae (Hantaviruses)

The hantaviruses are ubiquitous and are associated with adult respiratory distress syndrome (Hantaan virus) and pulmonary syndrome, shock, and pulmonary edema (Sin Nombre virus).[92,93] Viruses are inhaled from aerosolized rodent urine with each virus species apparently adapted to its own specific rodent vector. These are enveloped RNA viruses about 90–110 nm in diameter with helical symmetry and contain three negative sense ssRNA segments. The genome is referred to as "ambisense" because not only can it be translated into a functional messenger but also the negative strand encodes information for six proteins, some nonstructural proteins, viral RNA′-RNA polymerase, and the G1 and G2 proteins. The latter are associated with cell fusion and hemagglutination and act as a receptor for neutralizing antibodies. The virus attaches to respiratory mucosal surface β_3-integrin molecules, and replication is cytoplasmic with subsequent release by budding via the Golgi/endoplasmic reticulum/vesicle pathway.[93,94] The Sin Nombre virus differs in that it is assembled at the cell cytoplasmic membrane and then is released by budding. Symptoms include acute onset fever and malaise, indicative of localized cellular damage and viremia leading to increased lung vascular permeability and shock.[55,95] A secondary viremia results in spread to target organs as well as increased vascular endothelial damage and invasion of macrophages.[95] Within 4–5 days, there are generalized respiratory symptoms (dyspnea, cough, hypotensive, malaise) that, if untreated, can abruptly accelerate to acute pulmonary failure, pulmonary edema, renal failure, and shock. The characteristic histopathologic picture is that of alveolar edema accompanied by nonnecrotic, interstitial T lymphocytic infiltrates and few to no visible polymorphonuclear leukocytes.[93,95] Laboratory diagnosis is by ELISA serology for the detection of specific IgM (acute disease) and/or IgG titers or antigen, RT-PCR of blood or other specimens, and cell culture.[93,96] The latter is discouraged in all but designated public health laboratories because of the extremely infectious nature of the virus.

Picornaviruses

The picornaviruses are a large heterogenous group of small (20–30 nm), nonenveloped, icosahedral viruses that include some of the enteroviruses: (1) coxsackie A with 24 antigen types, (2) echovirus with 33 types, (3) poliovirus with 3 types, and (4) rhinovirus with over 100 types.[8]

These are ubiquitous, positive sense ssRNA viruses and attach to host cells by a variety of receptors that give each virus species its characteristic tropism (see Table 37.1). Transmission is either by the fecal–oral route (enteroviruses) or by aerosol and contaminated hands (rhinoviruses).[8] Poliovirus has been nearly eradicated on a global basis and infection is sporadic, enteroviral infections are more common in summer, and rhinovirus infections appear in early autumn and late spring. The mucosal surface of the oropharynx serves as the primary portal of infection for picornaviruses, with enteroviruses also having the gastrointestinal tract as an additional port of entry. These cells have a variety of receptors that can accommodate the different capsid proteins of members of this group (see Table 37.1).[21,27,34,97] Rhinovirus infections are thought to be limited to the upper respiratory tract and are associated with common cold-like infections and exacerbations of asthma,[8] although there are some indications that they can cause lower respiratory infections.[57,98] as well. Enteroviruses exhibit a wide variety of secondary targets and host age depending on the species. For example, enterovirus infections are characterized by a serious central nervous system component (paralysis, encephalitis, meningitis); coxsackie A and B viruses and echoviruses are also associated with carditis, rash, and serious infections in newborns and neonates; whereas poliovirus infections occur more often in young children.[8] Laboratory diagnosis of picornaviruses is by serologic tests for antibody and antigen and by PCR.[8,72,99]

Herpetoviridae

The herpesviruses, in general, are minor viral respiratory pathogens. It is only when an infection occurs during the peak season of one of the more common respiratory pathogens do they have to be considered in a differential diagnosis.[8,100] The human Herpetoviridae are large (150–200 nm), enveloped, icosahedral dsDNA viruses that undergo recombination with the host cell genome to establish a latent (asymptomatic) relationship with the host. Infections may be primary only or progress to dissemination and, in either case, may result in a latent infection. Primary infections occur through exchange of saliva or other bodily fluids and subsequent viral attachment to mucosal surfaces via specific receptors for each member of the group,[16,25,29,31,58,96,101,102] and initial replication of the virus occurs through a double-stranded linear DNA that leads directly to a positive mRNA.[100] After progeny release, there is adjacent cell infection and eventual cell-to-cell spread from mucosal epithelium to target cells, organs, or tissues with a latent state set up in neurons or reticuloendothelial cells.[52,58–60,100,102] During the initial replication or during the viremic state, viruses may be transported via lymph nodes, macrophages, or B cells to various extramucosal tissues or organs. The respiratory compo-

nent of these infections consists of a viral prodrome of headache, fever, malaise, rhinitis, and/or pharyngitis due to the release of various cytokines.[103] The following are the major herpesviruses and their clinical manifestations:

1. Herpes simplex virus[16,17,30,31,39,100,101,104–106]: Virus attaches to the mucosal surface by nectin or heparin sulfate. After progeny release, there is adjacent cell infection and eventual cell-to-cell spread from mucosal epithelium to the sensory and autonomic ganglia of the peripheral nervous system, where a latent infection is established. Primary replicated virus may also be transported by the bloodstream to other organ systems and then establish latency in the sensory and autonomic ganglia. Reactivation of these latent peripheral nerve viruses or those from infected organs may also directly infect the brain and spinal cord. Diagnosis is made by antigen/antibody tests to respective types, a polyclonal test for both in fluorescence or EIA format, and molecular tests.[100,107,108]

2. Cytomegalovirus[18,58]: Viruses attach to the host mucosal cells by heparin sulfate or epidermal growth factor and then spreads to lymph nodes, where T cells and macrophages are infected. T-cell infection leads to a mononucleosis-type presentation, and macrophage infection leads to multiorgan dissemination and cytomegalic inclusion disease. Cytomegalovirus usually causes subclinical infections in immunocompetent individuals, with more devastating infections occurring among the immunosuppressed (e.g., hematology and oncology patients and allograft recipients). Diagnosis is made by antigen/antibody serology (fluorescence and ELISA) and molecular tests.[36,58,109–111]

3. Epstein-Barr virus[29,59]: Epstein-Barr virus infects the oral mucosa and B cells by attaching to complement receptor 2 (CD21). The B cells are transformed (immortalized) and transport the virus to the liver (hepatitis), tracheobronchial tree (pharyngitis), or spleen. In cases of mononucleosis, the spleen is highly enlarged and exhibits atypical lymphocytes. Epstein-Barr virus is also associated with lymphomas in the immunosuppressed, Burkitt's lymphoma, and nasopharyngeal carcinoma. Diagnosis is made by antigen/antibody serology (fluorescence and ELISA) and molecular tests.

4. Varicella-zoster virus[25,60]: Using the insulin-degrading enzyme or Fc receptor as a point of attachment, varicella-zoster virus infects epithelial cells and fibroblasts. Viruses spread from mucosa to lymph nodes with subsequent transport to liver, spleen, and respiratory systems. It then spreads by viremia to the skin, where it causes the characteristic skin lesions (chickenpox). The virus eventually establishes a latent infection in the sensory ganglia, with later reactivation possible (shingles). Other than the clinical presentation, serology is the

primary means of diagnosis; a few molecular alternatives have been described.[60]

5. Human herpesvirus type 6 (roseola)[102,112–114]: Formerly called human B-cell lymphotrophic virus, human herpesvirus type 6 is a ubiquitous and typical herpesvirus in structure and replicative mechanism. It infects most children before they reach 2 years of age, with specific antibodies found in 64%–83% of children within their first 13 months of life. Viruses attach to $CD4^+$ cells (T cells, monocytes, macrophages, etc.) by a CD46 ligand and, in fact, upregulate $CD4^+$ in $CD4^-$ cells. Primary infection appears to occur by droplet/body fluid aerosols reaching the oropharynx. From the oral mucosa, the virus spreads to the regional lymphatics and then to mononuclear cells. Lymphocytes are the main carrier during primary infection but the virus persists in monocytes and macrophages. The infection expresses itself with a high fever of moderate duration (3–5 days), with accompanying mild upper respiratory symptoms and cervical lymphadenopathy, and, as the fever resolves, a classic maculopapular rash appears (exanthem subitum, sixth disease). Laboratory diagnosis is by fourfold titer movement of specific antibody or by molecular techniques.[102,113,115,116]

Conclusion

We have seen that respiratory manifestations of viral infections may be only a minor harbinger of more serious systemic disease, or viral invasion, in and of itself, may have the potential for causing lethal pandemic respiratory infections.[11,106] Regardless of the degree of initial respiratory compromise, viral respiratory diseases are the cause of more human morbidity, mortality, and health care spending than all other infectious diseases. What makes controlling these viruses an almost insurmountable task is the frequency of mistakes in replication or in recombination that give rise to variants for which there is no immune memory in the population, and hence no immune protection, or to variants that are resistant to current antiviral therapies.[65] As the human population increases, the average age of the population increases with its parallel decrease in immune function and increase in the number of immunosuppressed individuals or well-maintained terminally ill individuals; therefore, the chance for one of these mutant viruses or one that has adapted to humans directly from a natural reservoir increases geometrically.[73,106,117]

Because of the proven devastating potential of viral respiratory infections, the one common thread has been the search for more rapid and more accurate means of diagnosing these infections and identifying their etiologic agents.[42] These lines of endeavor are mandatory for two primary reasons: (1) the lack of vaccines specific enough to protect against reinfection or against all variants within a virus taxon and (2) the very narrow window for effective antiviral therapy during early infection.[118] Understanding the molecular biology of the respiratory viruses has helped to address this "need for speed" by directing the development of rapid molecular diagnostic techniques such as the application of specific probes for virus identification in tissue slides or specimen smears (fluorescence in situ hybridization, PCR) or in fluids and cells (real-time PCR, RT-PCR, sequence-specific oligonucleotide probes, multiplex PCR techniques).[41,70–72,106,109,111,116,119,120] Molecular tests will enable pathology departments and laboratories to offer rapid identification of a specific infectious agent when several cause the same set of symptoms, permitting more accurate therapy to be more effectively administered and, ultimately, decreasing patient stays and health care costs.[78,118] To accomplish this, however, there must be a dramatic increase in funding for research into the genetics of these viruses, the development of recombinant polyvalent vaccines, the development of public health care strategies to control pandemics, and the development and bringing to market of rapid, accurate, and specific diagnostic tests.

References

1. Colman P, Ward C. Structure and diversity of influenza virus neuraminidase. Curr Top Microbiol Immunol 1985; 114:178–254.
2. Peiris J, Lai S, Poon L, et al. SARS study group. Coronavirus as a possible cause of severe acute respiratory syndrome. Lancet 2003;361:1319–1325.
3. McIntosh K, Anderson L. Coronavirus, including severe acute respiratory syndrome (SARS)–associated coronavirus. In Mandell G, Bennett J, Dolin R, eds. Principles and Practice of Infectious Diseases, 6th ed, vol 2. Philadelphia: Elsevier; 2005:1990–1987.
4. Treanor J. Influenza virus. In Mandell G, Bennett J, Dolin R, eds. Principles and Practice of Infectious Diseases, 6th ed, vol 2. Philadelphia: Elsevier; 2005:2060–2085.
5. Rogers G, Paulson J. Receptor determinants of human and animal influenza virus isolates: differences in receptor specificity of the H3 hemagglutinin based on species of origin. Virology 1983;127:361–373.
6. Laver G, Garman E. The origin and control of pandemic influenza. Science 2001;293:1776–1777.
7. Reid A, Janczewski T, Lourens R, et al. 1918 Influenza pandemic caused by highly conserved viruses with two receptor-binding variants. Emerg Infect Dis 2003;9: 1249–1253.
8. Flint S, Enquist L, Racaniello V, Skalka A. Principles of Virology, 2nd ed. Washington, DC: ASM; 2004:918.
9. Dermody T, Tyler K. Introduction to viruses and viral diseases. In Mandell G, Bennett J, Dolin R, eds. Principles and Practice of Infectious Diseases, 6th ed. Philadelphia: Elsevier; 2005:1729–1742.

10. Webster R, Laver W, Air G, et al. The mechanism of antigenic drift in influenza viruses: analysis of Hong Kong (H3N2) variants with monoclonal antibodies to the hemagglutinin molecule. Ann NY Acad Sci 1980;354:142–161.

11. Brownlee G, Fodor E. The predicted antigenicity of the haemagglutinin of the 1918 Spanish influenza pandemic suggests an avian origin. Philos Trans R Soc Lond Biol Sci 2001;356:1871–1876.

12. Hatta M, Gao P, Halfmann P, Kawaoka Y. Molecular basis for high virulence of Hong Kong H5N1 influenza A viruses. Science 2001;293:1840–1842.

13. Hay A, Gregory V, Douglas A, Lin Y. The evolution of human influenza viruses. Philos Trans R Soc Lond Biol Sci 2001;356:1861–1869.

14. Suzuki Y, Nei N. Origin and evolution of influenza virus hemagglutinin genes. Mol Biol Evol 2002;19:501–509.

15. Prince G, Ottolini M, Moscona A. Contribution of the human parainfluenza virus type 3 HN-receptor interactions to pathogenesis in vivo. J Virol 2001;75:2446–12451.

16. Shukla D, Spear P. Herpes virus and heparin sulfate: an intimate relationship in aid of viral entry. J Clin Invest 2001;108:503–510.

17. Spear P, Longenecker R. Herpes virus entry: and update. J Virol 2003;77:10179.

18. Beersma M, Bizlemaker M, Pleogh H. Human cytomegalovirus down regulates HLA class I expression by reducing the stability of class I H chains. J Immunol 1993;151:4455–4464.

19. Chiu C, Mathias P, Nemerow G, Stewart P. Structure of adenovirus complexed with its membrane receptor, $\alpha_v\beta_5$ integrin. J Virol 1999;73:6759–6768.

20. Connor R, Kawaoka Y, Webster R, Paulson J. Receptor specificity in human, avian, and equine H2 and H3 influenza virus isolates. Virology 1994;205:17–23.

21. Cohen CJ, Shieh JT, Pickles RJ, et al. The coxsackie and adenovirus receptor is a transmembrane component of the tight junction. Proc Natl Acad Sci USA 2001;98:15191–15196.

22. Condit R. Principles of virology. In Knipe D, Howley P, eds. Fields Virology, 4th ed. Philadelphia: Lippincott-Raven; 2001:19–51.

23. Horvath C, Paterson R, Shaughnessy M, et al. Biological activity of paramyxovirus fusion proteins: factors influencing formation of syncytia. J Virol 1992;66:4564–4569.

24. Lamb R. Paramyxovirus fusion: a hypothesis for changes. Virology 1993;197:1–11.

25. Li Q, Ali M, Cohen J. Insulin degrading enzyme is a cellular receptor mediating varicella-zoster virus infection and cell to cell spread. Cell 2006;127:305–331.

26. Burgert H, Maryanski J, Kvist S. E3/19K protein of adenovirus type 2 inhibits lysis of cytolytic T lymphocytes by blocking cell-surface expression of histocompatibility class I antigens. Proc Natl Acad Sci USA 1987;84:1356–1360.

27. Kolatkar P, Bella J, Olson N, et al. Structural studies of two rhinovirus serotypes complexed with fragments of their cellular receptor. EMBO J 1999;18:6249–6259.

28. Li W, Vasilieva N, et al. Angiotensin-converting enzyme 2 is a functional receptor for the SARS coronavirus. Nature 2003;426:450–454.

29. Frade R, Barel M, Ehlin-Henriksson B, et al. gp140, the C3d receptor of human B lymphocytes is also the Epstein-Barr virus receptor. Proc Natl Acad Sci USA 1985;82:1490–1493.

30. Shieh M, WuDunn D, Montgomery R, et al. Cell surface receptors for herpes simplex virus are heparin sulfate proteoglycans. J Cell Biol 1992;116:1273–1281.

31. Mauri D, Ebner R, Montgomery R, et al. LIGHT, a new member of the TNF superfamily and lymphotoxin α are ligands for herpesvirus entry mediator. Immunity 1998;8:21.

32. Varga M, Weibull C, Everitt E. Infectious entry pathway of adenovirus type 2. J Virol 1991;65:6061–6070.

33. Wickham T, Mathias P, Cheresh D, Nemerow G. Integrins $\alpha_v\beta_3$ and $\alpha_v\beta_5$ promote adenovirus internalization but not virus attachment Cell 1993;73:309–319.

34. Bergelson J, Cunningham J, Droguett G, et al. Isolation of a common receptor for Coxsackie B viruses and adenoviruses 2 and 5. Science 1997;275:1320–1323.

35. Yeager C, Ashmun R, Williams R, et al. Human aminopeptidase N is a receptor for human coronavirus 229E. Nature 1991;357:420–422.

36. Prince A, Szmuness W, Millian S, David D. A serologic study of cytomegalovirus infections associated with blood transfusions. N Engl J Med 1971;284:1125–1131.

37. Nobusawa E, Ishihara H, Morishita T, et al. Change in receptor-binding specificity of recent human influenza A viruses (H3N2): a single amino acid change in hemagglutinin altered its recognition of sialyloligosaccharides. Virology 2000;278:587–596.

38. Horwitz M. The adenoviridae and their replication. In Fields B, Knipe D, eds. Virology. Raven Press: New York; 1990:1679–1721.

39. Knopf C. Molecular mechanisms of replication of herpes simplex virus I. Acta Virol 2000;44:289–307.

40. DiMaio D, Coen D. Replication strategies in DNA viruses. In Knipe D, Howley P, eds. Fields Virology, 4th ed. Philadelphia: Lippincott-Raven; 2001:119–132.

41. Flexman J, Kay I, Fonte R, et al. Differences between the quantitative antigenemia assay and cobas amplicor monitor quantitative PCR for detecting CMV viraemia in bone marrow and solid organ transplants. J Med Virol 2001;64:275–282.

42. Wagner R. Cytopathic effect of viruses: a general survey. In Fraenkel-Conrat H, Wagner R, eds. Comprehensive Virology. New York: Plenum Press; 1984:1–63.

43. Ito T, Couceiro J, Kelm S, et al. Molecular basis for the generation in pigs of influenza A viruses with pandemic potential. J Virol 1998;72:7367–7373.

44. Glaser L, Stevens J, Zamarin D, et al. A single amino acid substitution in 1918 influenza virus hemagglutinin changes receptor binding specificity. J Virol 2005;79:11533–11536.

45. D'Halluin J. Virus assembly. Curr Top Microbiol Immunol 1995;99:47–66.

46. Baltimore D. Expression of animal virus genomes. Bacteriol Rev 1971;35:235–241.

47. Castrucci M, Donatelli I, Sidoli I, et al. Genetic reassortment between avian and human influenza A viruses in Italian pigs. Virology 1993;193:503–506.

48. Jacobs J, Njenga M, Alvarez R, et al. Subtype B avian metapneumoviruses resembles subtype A more closely than subtype C or human metapneumovirus with respect to the phosphoprotein, and second matrix and small hydrophobic proteins. Virus Res 2003;95:171–178.

49. Toquin D, de Boisseioson C, Beven V, et al. Subgroup C avian metapneumovirus (MPV) and the recently isolated human MPV exhibit a common organization but have extensive sequence divergence in their putative SH and G genes. J Gen Virol 2003;84:2169–2178.

50. Crotty S, Cameron C, Andino R. RNA virus error catastrophe: direct molecular test by using ribavirin. Proc Natl Acad Sci USA 2001;98:6895–6900.

51. de R, Morrison L, Knipe D. Viral Persistence. In Nathanson N, Ahmed R, Gonzalez-Scarano F, et al., eds. Viral Pathogenesis. Lippincott-Raven: New York; 1997: 181–205.

52. Corey L. Herpes simplex virus. In Mandell G, Bennett J, Dolin R, eds. Principles and Practice of Infectious Diseases, 6th ed. Philadelphia: Elsevier; 2005:1762–1780.

53. Milstone A, Brumble L, Barnes J, et al. A single-season prospective study of respiratory viral infections in lung transplant recipients. Eur Respir J 2006;28:131–137.

54. Brandt C, Kim H, Arrobio J, et al. Epidemiology of respiratory syncytial virus infection in Washington, DC: III. Composite analysis of eleven consecutive yearly epidemics. Am J Epidemiol 1973;98:355–364.

55. Ennis F, Cruz J, Spiropoulou C, et al. Hantavirus pulmonary syndrome: CD8$^+$ and CD4$^+$ cytotoxic T lymphocytes to epitopes on Sin Nombre virus nucleocapsid protein isolated during acute illness. Virology 1997;238:380–390.

56. Lin M, Tseng H, Trejaut J, et al. Association of HLA class I with severe acute respiratory syndrome coronavirus infection. BMC Med Genet 2003;4:1–7.

57. Papadopoulos N. Do rhinoviruses cause pneumonia in children? Paediatr Respir Rev 2005;5:s191–s195.

58. Crumpacker C, Wadhwa S. Cytomegalovirus. In Mandell G, Bennett J, Dolin R, eds. Principles and Practice of Infectious Diseases, 6th ed. Philadelphia: Elsevier; 2005: 1786–1801.

59. Johannsen E, Schooley R, Kaye K. Epstein-Barr virus. In Mandell G, Bennett J, Dolin R, eds. Principles and Practice of Infectious Diseases, 6th ed. Philadelphia: Elsevier; 2005:1801–1820.

60. Whitley R. Varicella-zoster virus. In Mandell G, Bennett J, Dolin R, eds. Principles and Practice of Infectious Diseases, 6th ed. Philadelphia: Elsevier; 2005:1780–1786.

61. Baum S. Adenoviruses. In Mandell G, Bennett J, Dolin R, eds. Principles and Practice of Infectious Diseases, 6th ed. Philadelphia: Elsevier; 2005:1835–1841.

62. Wright P. Parainfluenza viruses. In Mandell G, Bennett J, Dolin R, eds. Principles and Practice of Infectious Diseases, 6th ed. Philadelphia: Elsevier; 2005:1998–2002.

63. Wiertz E, Jones T, Sun L, et al. The human cytomegalovirus US11 gene product dislocates MHC class I heavy chains from the endoplasmic reticulum to the cytosol. Cell 1996;7:769–779.

64. Harcourt J, Alvarez R, Jones L, et al. Respiratory syncytial virus G protein CX3C motif adversely affects CX3CR1$^+$ T cell responses. J Immunol 2006;176:1600–1608.

65. Drake J, Holland J. Mutation rates among RNA viruses. Proc Natl Acad Sci USA 1999;96:13910–13913.

66. Taubenberger J, Reid A, Krafft A, et al. Initial genetic characterization of the 1918 "Spanish" influenza virus. Science 1997;275:1793–1796.

67. Gamblin S, Haire L, Russell R, et al. The structure and receptor binding properties of the 1918 influenza hemagglutinin. Science 2004;303:1838–1842.

68. Tumpey T, Garcia-Sastre A, Mikulasova A, et al. Existing antivirals are effective against influenza viruses with genes from the 1918 pandemic virus. Proc Natl Acad Sci USA 2002;99:13849–13854.

69. Gershon A. Measles virus (rubeola). In Mandell G, Bennett J, Dolin R, eds. Principles and Practice of Infectious Diseases, 6th ed. Philadelphia: Elsevier; 2005:2031–2038.

70. Allwinn R, Preiser W, Rabenau H, et al. Laboratory diagnosis of influenza—virology or serology? Med Microbiol Immunol 2002;191:157–160.

71. Freymouth F, Vabret A, Galateau-Salke F, et al. Detection of respiratory syncytial virus, parainfluenza 3, adenovirus, and rhinovirus sequences in respiratory tract of infants by polymerase chain reaction and hybridization. Clin Diagn Virol 1997;8:31–40.

72. Fan J, Henricksson K, Savatski L. Rapid simultaneous diagnosis of infections with respiratory syncytial viruses A and B, influenza viruses A and B, and human parainfluenza types 1, 2, and 3 by multiplex quantitation reverse transcriptase-polymerase chain reaction-enzyme hybridization assay (hexaplex). Clin Infect Dis 1998;s26:1397–1402.

73. Parrott R, Kim H, Arrobio J, et al. Epidemiology of respiratory syncytial virus infection in Washington, DC: II. Infection and disease with respect to age, immunologic status, race, and sex. Am J Epidemiol 1973;98:289–300.

74. Hall C, Hall W, Speers D. Clinical and physiologic manifestations of bronchiolitis and pneumonia: outcome of respiratory syncytial virus. Am J Dis Child 1979;133:798–802.

75. Glezen W, Taber L, Frank A, Kasel J. Risk of primary infection and reinfection with respiratory syncytial virus. Am J Dis Child 1986;140:543–546.

76. Hall C, McCarthy C. Respiratory syncytial virus. In Mandell G, Bennett J, Dolin R, eds. Principles and Practice of Infectious Diseases, 6th ed. Philadelphia: Elsevier; 2005:2008–2026.

77. Groothuis J, Simoes E, Levin M, et al. Prophylactic administration of respiratory syncytial virus immune globulin to high-risk infants and young children. N Engl J Med 1993;329:1524–1530.

78. Stang P, Brandenberg N, Carter B. The economic burden of respiratory syncytial virus associated bronchiolitis hospitalizations. Arch Pediatr Adolesc Med 2001;155:95–96.

79. Howe C, Schluederberg A. A neuraminidase associated with measles virus. Biochem Biophys Res Commun 1970;40:606.

80. Harcourt B, Rota P, Hummel K, et al. Induction of intercellular adhesion molecule 1 gene expression by measles virus in human umbilical vein endothelial cells. J Med Virol 1999;57:9–16.

81. Rota P, Liffick S, Jota J, et al. Molecular epidemiology of measles virus in the United States, 1997–2001. Emerg Infect Dis 2002;8:902–908.

82. Boivin G, Abed Y, Pelletier G, et al. Virological features and clinical manifestations associated with human metapneumovirus: a new paramyxovirus responsible for acute respiratory-tract infections in all age groups. J Infect Dis 2004;186:1330–1334.

83. Boivin G, De Serres G, Cote S, et al. Human metapneumovirus infections in young and elderly adults. Emerg Infect Dis 2003;9:634–640.

84. Williams J, Harris P, Tollefson S, et al. Human metapneumoviruses and lower respiratory tract disease in otherwise healthy infants and children. N Eng J Med 2004;350: 443–450.

85. Kahn J. Epidemiology of human metapneumoviruses. Clin Micro Rev 2006;19:546–557.

86. Falsey A. Human metapneumovirus. In Mandell G, Bennett J, Dolin R, eds. Principles and Practice of Infectious Diseases, 6th ed. Philadelphia: Elsevier; 2005:2026–2031.

87. Cole S, Abed Y, Boivin G. Comparative evaluation of real-time PCR assays for detection of the human metapneumoviruses. J Clin Microbiol 2003;41:3631–3635.

88. Mackay I, Jacob K, Woolhouse D, et al. Molecular assays for detection of human metapneumoviruses. J Clin Microbiol 2003;41:100–105.

89. Walters R, Freimuth P, Moninger TO, et al. Adenovirus fiber disrupts CAR-mediated intercellular adhesion allowing virus escape. Cell 2002;11:789–799.

90. Liu Q, Muruve D. Molecular basis of the inflammatory response to adenovirus vectors. Gene Ther 2003;10:935–940.

91. Zhou M, Xu D, Li X, et al. Screening and identification of severe acute respiratory syndrome-associated coronavirus-specific CTL epitopes. J Immunol 2006;177:2138–2145.

92. Zaki S, Greer P, Coffield L, et al. Hantavirus pulmonary syndrome. Pathogenesis of an emerging infectious disease. Am J Pathol 1995;146:552–579.

93. Peters C. California encephalitis, hantavirus pulmonary syndrome, and bunyavirid hemorrhagic fevers. In Mandell G, Bennett J, Dolin R, eds. Principles and Practice of Infectious Diseases, 6th ed. Philadelphia: Elsevier; 2005: 2086–2090.

94. Gavrilovskaya I, Shepley M, Shaw R, et al. β3 Integrins mediate the cellular entry of hantaviruses that cause respiratory failure. Proc Natl Acad Sci USA 1998;95: 7074–7079.

95. Sundstrom J, McMullan L, Spiropoulou C, et al. Hantavirus infection induces the expression of RANTES and IP-10 without causing increased permeability in human lung microvascular endothelial cells. J Virol 2001;75: 6070–6085.

96. Nichol S, Spiropoulou C, Morzunov S, et al. Genetic identification of a hantavirus associated with an outbreak of acute respiratory illness. Science 1993;262:914–917.

97. Rossman M, Arnold E, Erickson J, et al. Structure of a common cold virus and functional relationship to other picornaviruses. Nature 1985;317:145–153.

98. Hayden F. Rhinovirus and the lower respiratory tract. Rev Med Virol 2004;14:17–31.

99. Defferenz C, Wunderli W, Thomas Y, et al. Amplicon sequencing and improved detection of human rhinovirus in respiratory samples. J Clin Microbiol 2004;42:3212–3218.

100. Straus S. Introduction to Herpesvirinae. In Mandell G, Bennett J, Dolin R, eds. Principles and Practice of Infectious Diseases, 6th ed. Philadelphia: Elsevier; 2005:1757–1762.

101. Smith G, Gross S, Enquist L. Herpes use bidirectional fast-axonal transport to spread to sensory neurons. Proc Natl Acad Sci USA 2001;98:3466–3470.

102. Straus S. Human herpesvirus types 6 and 7. In Mandell G, Bennett J, Dolin R, eds. Principles and Practice of Infectious Diseases, 6th ed. Philadelphia: Elsevier; 2005: 1821–1825.

103. McMillan J, Weiner L, Higgins A, Lamparella V. Pharyngitis associated with herpes simplex virus in college students. Pediatr Infect Dis 1993;12:280.

104. Montgomery R, Warner M, Lum B, Spear P. Herpes simplex virus-1 entry into cells mediated by a novel TNF/TGF receptor family. Cell 1996;87:427–436.

105. Mettenleiter T. Herpesvirus assembly and egress. J Virol 2002;76:1537–1547.

106. Clark D, Griffiths P. Human herpesvirus relevance of infection in the immunocompromised host. Br J Haematol 2003;120:384–395.

107. Koelle D, Corey L. Recent progress in herpes virus immunobiology and vaccine research. Clin Microbiol Rev 2003;16:96–113.

108. Morrow R. Inaccuracy of certain commercial enzyme immunoassays in diagnosing genital infections with herpes simplex types 1 or 2. Am J Clin Pathol 2003;120: 829.

109. Masoka T, Hiroka A, Ohta K, et al. Evaluation of the amplicor CMV, cobas amplicor CMV monitor and antigenemia assay for cytomegalovirus disease. J Infect Dis 2001;54:12–16.

110. Caliendo A, St George K, Allega J, et al. Distinguishing cytomegalovirus (CMV) infection and disease with CMV nucleic acid assays. J Clin Microbiol 2002;40:1581–1586.

111. Piiparinen H, Hockerstedt K, Lappaleinen M, et al. Monitoring viral load by quantitative plasma PCR during active cytomegalovirus infection of individual liver transplant patients. J Clin Microbiol 2002;40:2945–2952.

112. Hall C, Long C, Schnabel K, et al. Human herpesvirus 6 infection in children: a prospective study of complications and reactivation. N Engl J Med 1994;33:432–438.

113. Gompels U, Nicholas J, Lawrence G, et al. The DNA sequence of human herpesvirus-6: structure, coding content, and genome evolution. Virology 1995;209:29–51.

114. Dockrell C. Human herpesvirus 6: molecular biology and clinical features. J Med Microbiol 2003;52:5–18.

115. Huang L, Lee C, Chen J, et al. Primary herpesvirus 6 infection in children: a prospective serologic study. J Infect Dis 1992;165:1163–1164.

116. Locatelli G, Santoro F, Veglia F, et al. Real-time quantitative PCR for human herpesvirus 6 DNA. J Clin Microbiol 2003;38:4042–4048.

117. Greenberg S. Respiratory viral infections in high-risk patients. Am J Respir Crit Care Med 2004;170:1142–1143.

118. Linde A. The importance of specific virus diagnosis and monitoring for antiviral treatment. Antiviral Res 2001;51:81–94.

119. Chan PK, Tam JS, Lam CW, et al. Human metapneumovirus detection in patients with severe acute respiratory syndrome. Emerg Infect Dis 2003;9:1058–1063.

120. Garbino J, Gerbase M, Wunderli W, et al. Lower respiratory viral illness: improved diagnosis by molecular methods and clinical impact. Am J Respir Crit Care Med 2004;170:1197–1203.

38
Molecular Pathology of Rickettsial Lung Infections

J. Stephen Dumler

Introduction

Rickettsial infections of humans comprise a diverse group of infections caused by pathogens that are obligate intracellular bacteria with a genetic relationship, including the genera *Rickettsia*, *Orientia*, *Ehrlichia*, and *Anaplasma*. The host cells of these pathogens largely belie the systemic clinical manifestations, because *Rickettsia* and *Orientia* infect endothelial cells, and *Ehrlichia* and *Anaplasma* infect circulating leukocytes (monocytes and neutrophils, respectively). Thus, the predominant manifestations (fever, headache, myalgia, with or without rash) do not usually focus attention on the respiratory system; however, the underlying pathogenesis of these infections involves degrees of vascular compromise either by direct injury and inflammation or by the action of vasoactive proinflammatory molecules such as cytokines, chemokines, and prostaglandins. Given that the lung possesses the largest vascular bed in the human body, it is not surprising that pulmonary involvement is periodically identified and, when severely affected, is considered a potentially life-threatening complication.[1,2]

The precise microbial molecular pathogenetic mechanisms and the relative contributions of molecular proinflammatory responses toward pulmonary infection with these pathogens are in general poorly understood. However, recent years have seen significant advances in understanding the principles of how these obligate intracellular pathogens interact with host cells to exert direct influence over cellular function and integrity and how the host immune system responds. The main purposes of this chapter are to briefly describe the histopathologic and pathophysiologic alterations observed with two major rickettsial infections that impact the lung, Rocky Mountain spotted fever (*Rickettsia rickettsii*) and human monocytic ehrlichiosis (*Ehrlichia chaffeensis*) and to describe the molecular basis of cellular alterations in the host and pathogen virulence mechanisms that belie the pulmonary pathology with these diseases.

Rickettsial Infections That Impact Lung Structure and Function

The order Rickettsiales is divided into two major families, Rickettsiaceae and Anaplasmataceae. The Rickettsiaceae family includes the genera *Rickettsia* and *Orientia*, obligate intracellular vasculotropic bacteria that live and propagate within the cytoplasmic compartments of endothelial cells in mammalian hosts. In contrast, genera within the family Anaplasmataceae include *Ehrlichia* and *Anaplasma*, which infect leukocytes, including those circulating in the bloodstream. Among these genera, important human infections that impact lung function and structure include the vasculotropic rickettsioses such as Rocky Mountain spotted fever (RMSF), epidemic typhus, and murine typhus, among other entities bearing geographic names. The major underlying theme of these is endothelial cell infection followed by vasculitis and increased vascular permeability.[3,4] Systemically, this leads to hypotension, organ ischemia and failure, and sometimes death. In the lung, this translates into potentially significant noncardiogenic pulmonary edema that can be life threatening.[3] Fundamental differences exist between spotted fever group rickettsiae, such as *R. rickettsii* that causes RMSF, and the typhus group rickettsiae, such as *Rickettsia prowazekii* and *Rickettsia typhi* that cause epidemic and murine typhus, respectively.[5] The molecular pathogenesis of typhus group infections is less well understood; thus, this chapter focuses in part on RMSF as an example of rickettsial pneumonitis.

In contrast, the Anaplasmataceae are known to infect predominantly circulating leukocytes in mammals, and, by virtue of this host cell niche, histopathologic vasculitis is not a significant component of *Ehrlichia* or *Anaplasma* infections in humans.[6] However, infections by *E. chaffeensis*, the cause of human monocytic ehrlichiosis, can present with a clinical picture similar to vasculitis, and this is now believed to be due to the local or systemic release of proinflammatory vasoactive cytokines that impair endothelial integrity and lead to increased vascular permeability as observed in vasculitis.[7,8] Of those Anaplasmataceae that are significant causes of human disease, *E. chaffeensis* is the most frequent cause of infection in which lung structure and function are impaired and thus is the other main topic of this chapter.

Rocky Mountain Spotted Fever

Clinical Disease and Pathophysiology

Rocky Mountain spotted fever is an acute febrile illness that results after transmission of *R. rickettsii* into a human or animal host after the bite of competent vector ticks. The infection is limited to the Western hemisphere, but infections by related spotted fever group rickettsiae are documented on every continent except Antarctica.[9] After tick bite, the rickettsiae usually disseminate within hours to days via the blood or lymphatics.[10] These obligate intracellular bacteria attach to host endothelial cells in which they become internalized, escape the endocytic vacuole, and propagate within the cytosol.[1] During this process, endothelial cell functions are altered, leading to proinflammatory and procoagulant conditions that favor leukocyte infiltration, focal thrombus formation and increase in vascular permeability.[11–13] Endothelial cells either release the rickettsiae into the bloodstream or the infected cell is lysed, also releasing bacteria for hematogenous spread into all organs and tissues, including the lung. In the extensive microvasculature of the lung, *R. rickettsii* infection may be widely spread.[3] Host inflammatory response, usually manifest as some combination of interstitial mononuclear cell pneumonitis and edema, is observed in histopathologic preparations, leading to the occasional interstitial infiltrative pattern observed with chest x-rays in RMSF.[14] The fact that pulmonary vasculature permeability increases at a time when multiorgan failure and hypotension are also observed sometimes leads to overly aggressive fluid therapy that can precipitate or aggravate pulmonary edema. Prompt treatment with doxycycline can arrest and reverse many clinical manifestations, indicating that much of the inflammatory process is initiated and maintained by the bacterium.

Early Events in the *Rickettsia*–Endothelial Cell Interaction

The molecular mechanisms by which infection of endothelial cells results in vasculitis and altered vascular permeability in the lung is an area of active study. Initially, bacteria that are inoculated into the host replicate locally and then disseminate into the lymphatics.[10] Thereafter, the rickettsiae enter the bloodstream and interact with endothelial cells in the microvasculature of many organs including the lung. The initial rickettsia–endothelial cell interface is a receptor–ligand mediated event, dependent on rickettsial expression of outer membrane proteins A and B (OmpA and OmpB).[15–17] The host cell ligand for OmpA, only found in the spotted fever group rickettsiae, is not known. However, for both the spotted fever group rickettsiae *Rickettsia japonica* and *Rickettsia conorii*, OmpB ligation occurs via binding to host cell Ku70 that is recruited to host membrane lipid microdomains.[15] After OmpB binding, Ku70 is ubiquitinated by the protein tyrosine kinase adaptor protein Cbl, an event linked to internalization of the rickettsia-containing endosome because its inhibition blocks *R. conorii* entry.

Similarly critical for internalization of rickettsiae is the recruitment of Arp2/3, c-Src, and p80/85 cortactin to binding sites that leads to localized actin cytoskeletal rearrangements in part mediated by Cdc42, phosphatidylinositol-3 kinase, and the Src family of kinases.[18] Spotted fever group rickettsiae also express RickA on one pole of the bacterium, a protein that mediates actin polymerization via Arp2/3 complex assembly, effectively creating an intracellular scaffold that allows propulsion through the host cell and occasionally through host membranes.[19]

On entry, the endosomal membrane that contains the rickettsiae is rapidly degraded, presumably by the action of rickettsial phospholipase D or membrane hemolysin TlyC that are actively expressed during this interval.[20,21] Rickettsial genomes encode an intact tricarboxylic acid cycle, but otherwise have only a limited capacity for energy generation, lacking genes for enzymes for carbohydrate, lipid, nucleotide, and amino acid metabolism.[5] These observations and the demonstration of active adenosine triphosphate/adenosine diphosphate translocases establish the concept of rickettsiae as energy parasites. The presence of an intact pathway for a type IV secretion mechanism underscores the potential importance of transporting rickettsial proteins into the host cytosol.[5]

Cellular and Tissue Injury

Rickettsia rickettsii infection of endothelial cells leads to membrane injury that can be antagonized by antioxidants, and this membrane injury leads to loss of cellular osmoregulation and eventually cell lysis, even in the absence of large organism loads.[22,23] The degree of membrane injury in typhus group infections is much less substantial, and cytolysis is generally believed to be mechanical owing to the accumulation of large bacterial quantities within infected cells.[1]

Endothelial cells infected by *R. rickettsii* undergo a number of transcriptional changes, including upregulation of proinflammatory cytokines and chemokines (interleukin [IL]-1α, IL-6, IL-8, monocyte chemoattractant protein 1), surface procoagulant activity and tissue factor expression, E-selectin upregulation, and release of von Willebrand factor multimers.[7,11,12,24,25] The net result of the intracellular infection is an increased proinflammatory and procoagulant endothelial cell phenotype. These changes are mediated in part by direct rickettsial activation and nuclear mobilization of nuclear factor (NF)-κB via a mechanism involving activation of inhibitory-κB kinase α and β and phosphorylation-proteolysis of the inhibitor protein IκBα.[26,27] This phenomenon is abrogated by the bacterial protein synthesis inhibitor doxycycline, implying a contribution of bacterial proteins toward NF-κB proinflammatory gene activation. The triggers for the transcriptional alterations are not completely defined but appear to involve interactions with protein kinase C isoforms, and are modulated in part by p38 mitogen-activated protein (MAP) kinase.[28,29] Interestingly, this process also inhibits apoptosis, prolonging survival of infected cells, an obvious advantage for the bacterium. Intracellular rickettsial infection also yields upregulated expression of heme oxygenase 1, a host defense against oxidative injury and a

critical regulator of the cyclooxygenases, including cyclooxygenase-2, that are upregulated with rickettsial infection and is a key enzyme that governs prostaglandin production, increased release of prostaglandins I_2 and E_2, and, indirectly, vascular tone and integrity.[13]

The upregulated presence of E-selectin and procoagulant molecules on infected endothelial cells promotes inflammation and focal thrombosis, features considered typical of rickettsial vasculitis.[11,12] Although large-vessel thrombosis is atypical for RMSF, fibrin clots are not infrequently detected as eccentrically localized lesions among vessels in which only focal infection is demonstrated (Figure 38.1). When rickettsial infection occurs within the confines of the pulmonary parenchyma, capillaries are the dominant vascular structure and support the heaviest burden of rickettsiae.[3] As a consequence of infection in these small-caliber vessels, interstitial inflammatory cell infiltration is the dominant feature and appears as widened, hypercellular alveolar septae, some of which may be edematous; capillaries that are dispersed within the alveolar septae are often surrounded by mononuclear cells, chiefly lymphocytes and macrophages (Figure 38.2).

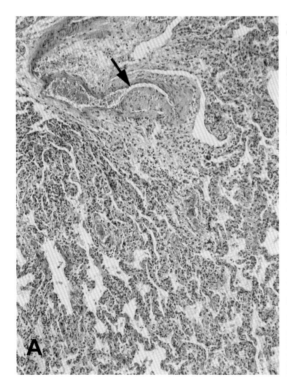 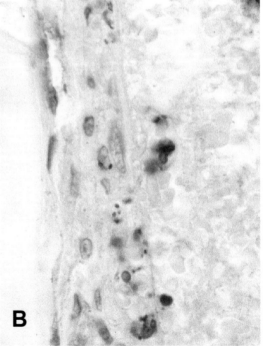

FIGURE 38.1. **(A)** *Rickettsia rickettsii* vasculitis with eccentric microthrombus (arrow) in pulmonary venule and diffuse interstitial pneumonitis. (Hematoxylin and eosin; original magnification, ×16.) **(B)** Note the intracellular distribution of infected endothelial cells along a venule as demonstrated by immunohistochemistry. (Anti-*Rickettsia rickettsii* with hematoxylin counterstain; original magnification, ×260.)

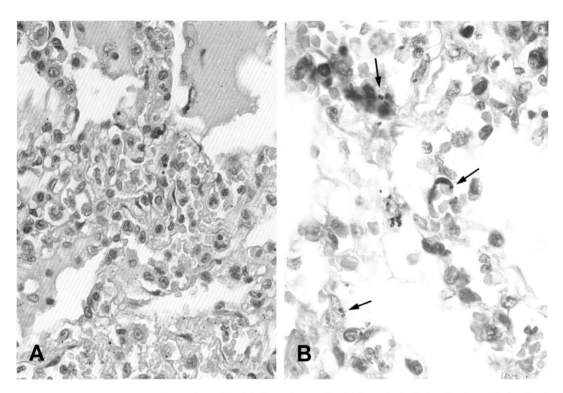

FIGURE 38.2. **(A)** Interstitial pneumonitis and capillaritis in Rocky Mountain spotted fever. (Hematoxylin and eosin; original magnification, ×160.) **(B)** Immunohistochemistry for *Rickettsia rickettsii* demonstrates the presence of small bacilli (arrows) within endothelial cells of capillaries in alveolar interstitial spaces. (Hematoxylin counterstain; original magnification, ×260.)

Host Innate and Adaptive Immune Responses to Infection

Host response to rickettsial infection is dominated by the infiltration of tissues and vessel walls by lymphocytes and macrophages. Immunophenotyping methods of rickettsial inflammatory lesions have identified a polymorphous mixture of CD4 and CD8 T lymphocytes, admixed with scattered B lymphocytes, macrophages, and occasional neutrophils.[1,30] Infection by rickettsiae leads to substantial chemokine production by endothelial cells, including IL-8, monocyte chemoattractant protein 1, and fractalkine (CX3CL1), and it is likely that these signals in part recruit and retain inflammatory cells and primed immune cells that participate in the localized tissue vasculitis.[30] As anticipated, effective antirickettsial immunity is predominantly dependent on cellular immunity, especially on expansion of adaptive immunity via CD4 and CD8 cells that produce interferon (IFN)-γ and mediate cytotoxic responses. However, recent investigations provide evidence that antibody plays a more important role than previously ascribed.[30]

The inflammatory and immune response to the presence of rickettsiae in cells is at first heralded by expansion of natural killer cell populations, and depletion of these cells allows greater rickettsial propagation and reduced production of suppressive IFN-γ. Depletion of both CD4 and CD8 T lymphocytes also adversely impacts survival in murine models, and the most dramatic effect implicates a role for major histocompatibility complex I–mediated, perforin-dependent adaptive immune responses.[1,30] The molecular mechanism of rickettsial restriction by immune cells appears to be dependent on the synergistic effects of IFN-γ, tumor necrosis factor (TNF)-α, IL-1β, and CCL5 produced from natural killer cells, CD8 T cells, and macrophages; critical effectors include both nitric oxide and hydrogen peroxide, accentuated by tryptophan starvation after enhanced host cell degradation of this amino acid essential for bacterial propagation. Interestingly, there appears to be a critical balance between beneficial and deleterious immune responses, because adoptive transfer of immune CD8 T cells into rickettsia-infected naïve animals accelerates death if introduced during early phases of infection.[1]

In the context of RMSF lung involvement, it is likely that many of the events are simultaneously occurring, with outcome dependent on degree of pulmonary microvascular infection and compromise and the degree to which a rapid and protective immune response is induced.[1,30] Fundamental studies have identified several novel targets for intervention at the level of the bacterium (inhibition of OmpB–Ku70 interaction, inhibition of type IV secretion system activity, inhibition of phospholipase D or hemolysin activity) and at the level of the host (inhibition of ubiquitination of Ku70, inhibition of induced actin cytoskeletal rearrangements or signaling via protein kinase C, p38 MAP kinase, cyclooxygenase-2, and NF-κB nuclear translocation).

Diagnosis

When involvement of the lung by RMSF becomes evident, it is usually during the course of increasing decompensation, hypotension, and multiorgan failure. Diagnosis of the infection at this interval is often too late to prevent significant morbidity, long-term sequelae, or death, prompting physicians to have a low threshold for empirical doxycycline therapy at earlier times. Rocky Mountain spotted fever is best diagnosed during the active phase of infection by skin biopsy of petechial lesions followed by immunohistochemical or in situ hybridization demonstration of R. rickettsii in the tissue.[31] Antibodies are infrequently present during active infection, but demonstration of seroconversion or a fourfold titer change in convalescence can retrospectively confirm a clinical diagnosis. Molecular diagnostic methods are less often used and generally focus on polymerase chain reaction (PCR) amplification of R. rickettsii nucleic acids from whole blood samples obtained during the active phase of infection, although this is not currently considered highly sensitive.[32] Additional data suggest that PCR on freshly obtained skin biopsies or other tissues may also work well because the rickettsiae live predominantly within tissue-bound endothelial cells.[33] Immunohistochemistry is often used to establish a postmortem diagnosis, and PCR methods should be excellent adjuncts to this approach.[34]

Human Monocytic Ehrlichiosis

Clinical Disease and Pathophysiology

Human monocytic ehrlichiosis (HME) is a febrile illness with many similarities to rickettsial infections such as RMSF.[35] Some authors have used the terminology "spotless" spotted fever to indicate the clinical and historical similarity of HME to RMSF. After tick bite, E. chaffeensis gains access to the blood and may be visualized in peripheral blood smears from some patients after an incubation period of 7–10 days. The infection has been well-characterized to occur only in North America, although increasing evidence suggests that the pathogen and infection may be worldwide in distribution.[35]

Unlike the situation for R. rickettsii, E. chaffeensis infects almost exclusively mononuclear phagocytes in both tissues and blood. It has been detected in blood, bone marrow, lymph node, liver, spleen, and many tissues and organs that possess mononuclear phagocyte populations or acquire these cells via inflammatory cell infiltration.[2,6] Presumably, E. chaffeensis infects mononuclear phagocytes at the site of tick bite or passes via lymphatics to draining lymph nodes where initial infection occurs. Once E. chaffeensis attaches to and enters the mononuclear phagocyte, it accumulates in an endosomal vacuole that is arrested in maturation at the early endosome stage.[36] The bacteria replicate within this vacuole to form an intracytoplasmic inclusion called a morula that is occasionally visualized in peripheral blood monocytes on Romanowsky-stained blood smears. The infected cells undergo substantial alterations in function that presumably diminish innate and adaptive immune recognition and response; however, cells that manage to ingest E. chaffeensis via opsonophagocytosis generate considerable proinflammatory cytokine responses that could drive the underlying inflammatory cell infiltration and tissue necrosis observed in some cases.[2,37] This response does not occur via typical lipopolysaccharide or peptidoglycan-mediated Toll-like receptor signaling because E. chaffeensis, like other Anaplasmataceae, lacks biosynthetic pathways for both of these bacterial components.[38] The majority of clinical infections present with fever and myalgias accompanied by thrombocytopenia, leukopenia, anemia, and evidence of mild to moderate hepatic injury supported by elevated liver transaminase activities in serum.[2,35]

Although E. chaffeensis has no known predilection for the respiratory system, when circulating mononuclear phagocytes become activated for proinflammatory function during passage through the pulmonary microvasculature, the result would be increased vascular permeability and inflammatory cell infiltration of the interstitial spaces—the typical interstitial pneumonitis observed with HME in severe cases.[6,39,40] Infection can precede diffuse alveolar damage (Figure 38.3), even in the absence of large numbers of bacteria and a vigorous inflammatory cell infiltrate. In advanced stages, lung involvement can appear as macrophage-rich intraalveolar infiltrates, again absent substantial quantities of bacteria (Figure 38.4).[6] The clinical and histopathologic sequelae of lung involvement can take days or weeks to resolve. This process often occurs in the context of systemic inflammatory response with fulminant E. chaffeensis infections in patients with preexisting immune compromise such as with human immunodeficiency virus and immune suppression for organ transplantation or for autoimmune diseases.[2,41,42] Very often the presentation is septic-like or toxic shock–like and includes a component of acute respiratory distress syndrome.[39,43,44] Despite clinical similarities to RMSF and vasculitis, histopathologic investigations do not provide any support for vasculitis as a component

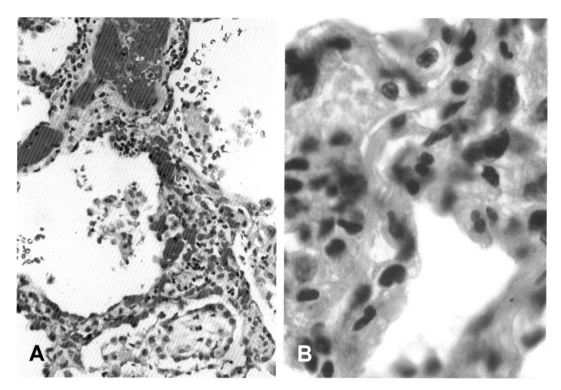

FIGURE 38.3. **(A)** *Ehrlichia chaffeensis*–induced interstitial pneumonitis accompanied by diffuse alveolar damage. (Hematoxylin and eosin; original magnification, ×80.) **(B)** Ordinarily, *E. chaffeensis* is infrequently found, except in patients with underlying immunocompromise. (*Ehrlichia chaffeensis* immunohistochemistry with hematoxylin counterstain; original magnification, ×400.)

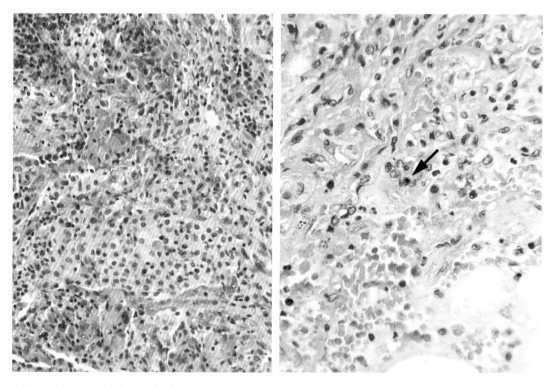

FIGURE 38.4. **(A)** *Ehrlichia chaffeensis*–induced macrophage-rich alveolar infiltrates and resolving diffuse alveolar damage in human monocytic ehrlichiosis. (Hematoxylin and eosin; original magnification, ×40.) **(B)** The tissue injury is usually greatly out of proportion to the bacterial load. (*Ehrlichia chaffeensis* immunohistochemistry with hematoxylin counterstain; original magnification, ×80.)

of HME.[6,41] Although a rapid clinical response is often demonstrated even after 1 to 2 days of doxycycline treatment, given the mononuclear phagocyte niche, it is difficult to explain pancytopenia and hepatic or pulmonary injury based on direct bacterial injury.[2] Most data now support a role for *E. chaffeensis* triggering of host proinflammatory response as a major pathogenetic feature in HME.[8,45]

Early Events in the *Ehrlichia*–Mononuclear Phagocyte Interaction

During the initial encounter with a mononuclear phagocyte, *E. chaffeensis* binds to E- and L-selectins probably via the bacterial membrane glycoprotein gp120.[46,47] Interestingly, there are two morphologic forms of *E. chaffeensis*, analogous to the situation with the Chlamydiae—a lower metabolic activity dense core form that expresses the gp120 adhesin and a more substantially metabolic reticulate form that expresses lower gp120 quantities and undergoes active binary fission.[47] The initial internalization leads to interactions via glycosylphosphatidylinositol-anchored proteins and caveolin in host cell membrane lipid rafts that is followed by intracellular calcium fluxes and changes in tyrosine phosphorylation, activation of phospholipase Cγ2, and inositol 1,4,5-triphophate production.[48] The emerging parasitophorous vacuoles accumulate only early endosomal markers, including an increasing amount of transferrin receptor, a characteristic of recycling endosomes diverted from the phagosome-lysosome fusion pathway.[36] Likewise, *E. chaffeensis*-infected THP-1 cells show downregulated transcription of *RAB5A*, *SNAP23*, and *STX16*, critical components of vesicular transport and fusogenic events.[49]

Intracellular entry also occurs in the absence of significant proinflammatory cell activation and triggering.[37] Although pretreatment of macrophages with IFN-γ leads to restriction of ehrlichial growth, infection is associated with inhibition of IFN-γ–inducing pathways such as JAK/STAT, and induction of important cytokines for maturation of Th1 and immune responses, such as IL-12, IL-15, IL-18, Toll-like receptors 2 and 3, and CD14.[48,49] The IFN-γ–mediated restriction occurs via its action in reducing expression of transferrin receptors, thereby reducing accessible free iron for bacterial growth, because *E. chaffeensis* lacks effective siderophores.[48] Similar to *R. rickettsii*, *E. chaffeensis* infection inhibits apoptosis of infected cells, presumably via its action on transcription of cell cycle proteins and inhibition of NF-κB activation.[48,49]

Cellular and Tissue Injury

Cytolysis of cells infected by *E. chaffeensis* in vitro is the usual outcome. However, most in vivo examinations demonstrate only meager quantities of bacteria, out of proportion to the degree of histopathologic injury, cytopenias, and hepatic injury in nonfulminant cases.[2] Because no good animal model of *E. chaffeensis* infection exists, data extrapolated from murine models of infection by related *Ehrlichia* species provides additional evidence that most tissue injury results from the induction of aberrant and dysfunctional immune responses.[8] Humans infected with *E. chaffeensis* have a marked expansion of CD8 T lymphocytes in lymph nodes and presumably other tissues, and this feature is associated with a high frequency of hemophagocytic macrophages, suggesting activation of macrophages as a component of the pathogenesis.[50] Similarly, a dose- and route-dependent induction of CD8 T lymphocyte overproduction of TNF-α has been implicated as a mechanism of severe tissue injury in murine models.[8,45] Infection of TNF receptor–deficient mice substantially abrogates manifestations of shock in murine models, yet depletion of TNF-α from mice does not alter shock manifestations.[51] In contrast, at least one severe infection in a human occurred while receiving the TNF-α inhibitor etanercept, seeming to contradict the murine model data.[52] Despite these advances, little investigation of the specific effectors of tissue injury, whether immunologic or not, has been conducted.

Host Innate and Adaptive Immune Responses to Infection

Ehrlichia chaffeensis subverts many innate immune responses via interactions with nonopsonophagocytic macrophage receptors (L-selectin or E-Selectin) and by its early downregulation of inflammation- and immune-inducing signals, receptors, and signaling pathways.[48,49] Classic cellular immune pathways appear important for restriction of *E. chaffeensis* infection.[53] In mice that ordinarily are not susceptible, infection persists when devoid of Toll-like receptor 4 and major histocompatibility complex II.[54,55] Murine models of monocytic ehrlichiosis generally employ the related species *Ehrlichia muris* or an *Ehrlichia* species isolated from *Ixodes ovatus* ticks.[8,56,57] In this model, infection and severity are decreased with low infectious doses and intradermal inoculation, and resistance to challenge depends on CD4 but not CD8 T lymphocytes and requires IL-12, IFN-γ, and TNF-α but not IL-4.[8,45,51,58] Likewise, intact adaptive immunity is critical because severe combined immunodeficiency mice cannot resist infection.[53,59] Despite the evidence that cellular immunity, chiefly Th1-polarized responses, are critical for control of *Ehrlichia* infections, a role for antibody has also been demonstrated with passive immunization using anti-*E. chaffeensis* or *Ehrlichia* monoclonal antibodies or with infection of animals devoid of Fc receptors or effector pathways such as phagocyte oxidase (gp91[phox] knockout mice).[53,57,60–62]

In the context of HME lung involvement, it is most likely that host immune response is a critical determinant of pathologic injury and outcome. The tissue injury that is disproportionate to bacterial load and the lack of any direct evidence of *Ehrlichia*-mediated cellular injury argue that the predominant pathologic force is an overly aggressive or misdirected host inflammatory or immune response triggered by active infection.[2,41,45,50] Why some infections are asymptomatic yet others are fatal is not understood, although studies with mouse models are yielding important clues regarding infectious load and genetic background.[8,53,58] If pathologic injury is driven primarily by host response, the most prudent approach as a supplement to antimicrobial treatment involves strategies to dampen overly aggressive production of proinflammatory cytokines or strategies that dampen vigorous Th1 responses culminating in excessive macrophage activation. That fulminant infection occurs with defects in T-cell immunity dictates that this approach must be carefully evaluated and implemented with great caution.[6,41,42,45,52] Molecular tools that could interfere with *Ehrlichia*-mediated host transcriptional changes or that interfere with *Ehrlichia*-initiated signal transduction events and apoptosis delay might provide adjunctive treatments, especially among immunocompromised patients with fulminant infections.[2,49]

Diagnosis

Approximately 20% of patients with HME demonstrate cough or other respiratory manifestations; however, significant respiratory disease is relatively infrequent, presenting as acute respiratory distress syndrome, and usually accompanied by other severe systemic manifestations such as multiorgan failure, a shock syndrome, and meningoencephalitis.[2,41] Even at this late stage, a diagnosis may prevent and reverse adverse outcomes by prompting doxycycline treatment. Although examination of peripheral blood smears will identify bacterial inclusion vacuoles in circulating monocytes in less than 10% of cases, and antibodies will be present in a small minority of infected persons, approximately 60% or more will have *E. chaffeensis* DNA demonstrable in peripheral blood by PCR.[2,52] Tissue examination by immunohistochemistry and in situ hybridization is useful in some cases, although these methods may lack sensitivity.[63,64] Polymerase chain reaction has also been applied as a diagnostic tool for *E. chaffeensis* on tissues including lung, although no careful evaluation of this approach has been conducted.

Conclusion

Many current advances in understanding the molecular pathogenesis of RMSF and HME have been facilitated by the availability and improved annotations of rickettsial genomes; however, these efforts continue to be undermined by the lack of effective gene ablation methods for these pathogens.[5,65–67] In time even this research bottleneck will be circumvented, and rickettsial organisms will release their unique secrets for the molecular and cellular perturbations that allow their intracellular survival and pathogenicity.

References

1. Walker DH, Valbuena GA, Olano JP. Pathogenic mechanisms of diseases caused by *Rickettsia*. Ann NY Acad Sci 2003;990:1–11.
2. Dumler JS. Anaplasma and ehrlichia infection. Ann NY Acad Sci 2005;1063:361–373.
3. Walker DH, Crawford CG, Cain BG. Rickettsial infection of the pulmonary microcirculation: the basis for interstitial pneumonitis in Rocky Mountain spotted fever. Hum Pathol 1980;11:263–272.
4. Walker DH, Mattern WD. Rickettsial vasculitis. Am Heart J 1980;100:896 906.
5. Walker DH, Yu XJ. Progress in rickettsial genome analysis from pioneering of *Rickettsia prowazekii* to the recent *Rickettsia typhi*. Ann NY Acad Sci 2005;1063:13–25.
6. Walker DH, Dumler JS. Human monocytic and granulocytic ehrlichioses. Discovery and diagnosis of emerging tick-borne infections and the critical role of the pathologist. Arch Pathol Lab Med 1997;121:785–791.
7. Sporn LA, Marder VJ. Interleukin-1 alpha production during *Rickettsia rickettsii* infection of cultured endothelial cells: potential role in autocrine cell stimulation. Infect Immun 1996;64:1609–1613.
8. Ismail N, Soong L, McBride JW, et al. Overproduction of TNF-alpha by CD8+ type 1 cells and down-regulation of IFN-gamma production by CD4+ Th1 cells contribute to toxic shock-like syndrome in an animal model of fatal monocytotropic ehrlichiosis. J Immunol 2004;172:1786–1800.
9. Walker DH. Rickettsioses of the spotted fever group around the world. J Dermatol 1989;16:169–177.
10. Murphy JR, Wisseman CL Jr, Fiset P. Mechanisms of immunity in typhus infection: some characteristics of *Rickettsia mooseri* infection of guinea pigs. Infect Immun 1978;21:417–424.
11. Shi RJ, Simpson-Haidaris PJ, Lerner NB, et al. Transcriptional regulation of endothelial cell tissue factor expression during *Rickettsia rickettsii* infection: involvement of the transcription factor NF-kappaB. Infect Immun 1998;66:1070–1075.
12. Sporn LA, Lawrence SO, Silverman DJ, Marder VJ. E-selectin-dependent neutrophil adhesion to *Rickettsia rickettsii*–infected endothelial cells. Blood 1993;81:2406–2412.
13. Sahni SK, Rydkina E, Sahni A, et al. Potential roles for regulatory oxygenases in rickettsial pathogenesis. Ann NY Acad Sci 2005;1063:207–214.
14. McCook TA, Briley C, Ravin CE. Roentgenographic abnormalities in Rocky Mountain spotted fever. South Med J 1982;75:156–157.
15. Martinez JJ, Seveau S, Veiga E, et al. Ku70, a component of DNA-dependent protein kinase, is a mammalian

receptor for *Rickettsia conorii*. Cell 2005;123:1013–1023.

16. Uchiyama T, Kawano H, Kusuhara Y. The major outer membrane protein rOmpB of spotted fever group rickettsiae functions in the rickettsial adherence to and invasion of Vero cells. Microbes Infect 2006;8:801–809.

17. Li H, Walker DH. rOmpA is a critical protein for the adhesion of *Rickettsia rickettsii* to host cells. Microb Pathog 1998;24:289–298.

18. Martinez JJ, Cossart P. Early signaling events involved in the entry of *Rickettsia conorii* into mammalian cells. J Cell Sci 2004;117:5097–5106.

19. Gouin E, Egile C, Dehoux P, et al. The RickA protein of *Rickettsia conorii* activates the Arp2/3 complex. Nature 2004;427:457–461.

20. Renesto P, Dehoux P, Gouin E, et al. Identification and characterization of a phospholipase D–superfamily gene in rickettsiae. J Infect Dis 2003;188:1276–1283.

21. Whitworth T, Popov VL, Yu XJ, et al. Expression of the *Rickettsia prowazekii pld* or *tlyC* gene in *Salmonella enterica* serovar *Typhimurium* mediates phagosomal escape. Infect Immun 2005;73:6668–6673.

22. Eremeeva ME, Silverman DJ. Effects of the antioxidant alpha-lipoic acid on human umbilical vein endothelial cells infected with *Rickettsia rickettsii*. Infect Immun 1998;66:2290–2299.

23. Silverman DJ, Santucci LA. Potential for free radical-induced lipid peroxidation as a cause of endothelial cell injury in Rocky Mountain spotted fever. Infect Immun 1988;56:3110–3115.

24. Clifton DR, Rydkina E, Huyck H, et al. Expression and secretion of chemotactic cytokines IL-8 and MCP-1 by human endothelial cells after *Rickettsia rickettsii* infection: regulation by nuclear transcription factor NF-kappaB. Int J Med Microbiol 2005;295:267–278.

25. Sporn LA, Shi RJ, Lawrence SO, et al. *Rickettsia rickettsii* infection of cultured endothelial cells induces release of large von Willebrand factor multimers from Weibel-Palade bodies. Blood 1991;78:2595–2602.

26. Clifton DR, Rydkina E, Freeman RS, Sahni SK. NF-kappaB activation during *Rickettsia rickettsii* infection of endothelial cells involves the activation of catalytic IkappaB kinases IKKalpha and IKKbeta and phosphorylation-proteolysis of the inhibitor protein IkappaBalpha. Infect Immun 2005;73:155–165.

27. Sporn LA, Sahni SK, Lerner NB, et al. *Rickettsia rickettsii* infection of cultured human endothelial cells induces NF-kappaB activation. Infect Immun 1997;65:2786–2791.

28. Rydkina E, Silverman DJ, Sahni SK. Activation of p38 stress-activated protein kinase during *Rickettsia rickettsii* infection of human endothelial cells: role in the induction of chemokine response. Cell Microbiol 2005;7:1519–1530.

29. Sahni SK, Turpin LC, Brown TL, Sporn LA. Involvement of protein kinase C in *Rickettsia rickettsii*–induced transcriptional activation of the host endothelial cell. Infect Immun 1999;67:6418–6423.

30. Valbuena G, Feng HM, Walker DH. Mechanisms of immunity against rickettsiae. New perspectives and opportunities offered by unusual intracellular parasites. Microbes Infect 2002;4:625–633.

31. Dumler JS, Walker DH. Rocky Mountain spotted fever—changing ecology and persisting virulence. N Engl J Med 2005;353:551–553.

32. Sexton DJ, Kanj SS, Wilson K, et al. The use of a polymerase chain reaction as a diagnostic test for Rocky Mountain spotted fever. Am J Trop Med Hyg 1994;50:59–63.

33. Demma LJ, Traeger MS, Nicholson WL, et al. Rocky Mountain spotted fever from an unexpected tick vector in Arizona. N Engl J Med 2005;353:587–594.

34. Paddock CD, Greer PW, Ferebee TL, et al. Hidden mortality attributable to Rocky Mountain spotted fever: immunohistochemical detection of fatal, serologically unconfirmed disease. J Infect Dis 1999;179:1469–1476.

35. Paddock CD, Childs JE. *Ehrlichia chaffeensis*: a prototypical emerging pathogen. Clin Microbiol Rev 2003;16:37–64.

36. Barnewall RE, Rikihisa Y, Lee EH. *Ehrlichia chaffeensis* inclusions are early endosomes which selectively accumulate transferrin receptor. Infect Immun 1997;65:1455–1461.

37. Lee EH, Rikihisa Y. Anti-*Ehrlichia chaffeensis* antibody complexed with *E. chaffeensis* induces potent proinflammatory cytokine mRNA expression in human monocytes through sustained reduction of IkappaB-alpha and activation of NF-kappaB. Infect Immun 1997;65:2890–2897.

38. Lin M, Rikihisa Y. *Ehrlichia chaffeensis* and *Anaplasma phagocytophilum* lack genes for lipid A biosynthesis and incorporate cholesterol for their survival. Infect Immun 2003;71:5324–5331.

39. Paparone PW, Ljubich P, Rosman GA, Nazha NT. Ehrlichiosis with pancytopenia and ARDS. NJ Med 1995;92:381–385.

40. Marty AM, Dumler JS, Imes G, et al. Ehrlichiosis mimicking thrombotic thrombocytopenic purpura. Case report and pathological correlation. Hum Pathol 1995;26:920–925.

41. Walker DH. Ehrlichia under our noses and no one notices. Arch Virol Suppl 2005:147–156.

42. Safdar N, Love RB, Maki DG. Severe *Ehrlichia chaffeensis* infection in a lung transplant recipient: a review of ehrlichiosis in the immunocompromised patient. Emerg Infect Dis 2002;8:320–323.

43. Patel RG, Byrd MA. Near fatal acute respiratory distress syndrome in a patient with human ehrlichiosis. South Med J 1999;92:333–335.

44. Smith Sehdev AE, Sehdev PS, Jacobs R, Dumler JS. Human monocytic ehrlichiosis presenting as acute appendicitis during pregnancy. Clin Infect Dis 2002;35:e99–e102.

45. Ismail N, Walker DH. Balancing protective immunity and immunopathology: a unifying model of monocytotropic ehrlichiosis. Ann NY Acad Sci 2005;1063:383–394.

46. Zhang JZ, McBride JW, Yu XJ. L-selectin and E-selectin expressed on monocytes mediating *Ehrlichia chaffeensis* attachment onto host cells. FEMS Microbiol Lett 2003;227:303–309.

47. Popov VL, Yu X, Walker DH. The 120 kDa outer membrane protein of *Ehrlichia chaffeensis*: preferential expression on dense-core cells and gene expression in *Escherichia coli* associated with attachment and entry. Microb Pathog 2000;28:71–80.

48. Rikihisa Y. *Ehrlichia* subversion of host innate responses. Curr Opin Microbiol 2006;9:95–101.

49. Zhang JZ, Sinha M, Luxon BA, Yu XJ. Survival strategy of obligately intracellular *Ehrlichia chaffeensis*: novel modulation of immune response and host cell cycles. Infect Immun 2004;72:498–507.

50. Dierberg KL, Dumler JS. Lymph node hemophagocytosis in rickettsial diseases: a pathogenetic role for CD8 T lymphocytes in human monocytic ehrlichiosis (HME)? BMC Infect Dis 2006;6:121.

51. Ismail N, Stevenson HL, Walker DH. Role of tumor necrosis factor alpha (TNF-alpha) and interleukin-10 in the pathogenesis of severe murine monocytotropic ehrlichiosis: increased resistance of TNF receptor p55- and p75-deficient mice to fatal ehrlichial infection. Infect Immun 2006;74: 1846–1856.

52. Stone JH, Dierberg K, Aram G, Dumler JS. Human monocytic ehrlichiosis. JAMA 2004;292:2263–2270.

53. Winslow GM, Bitsaktsis C, Yager E. Susceptibility and resistance to monocytic ehrlichiosis in the mouse. Ann NY Acad Sci 2005;1063:395–402.

54. Ganta RR, Cheng C, Wilkerson MJ, Chapes SK. Delayed clearance of *Ehrlichia chaffeensis* infection in CD4⁺ T-cell knockout mice. Infect Immun 2004;72:159–167.

55. Ganta RR, Wilkerson MJ, Cheng C, et al. Persistent *Ehrlichia chaffeensis* infection occurs in the absence of functional major histocompatibility complex class II genes. Infect Immun 2002;70:380–388.

56. Sotomayor EA, Popov VL, Feng HM, et al. Animal model of fatal human monocytotropic ehrlichiosis. Am J Pathol 2001;158:757–769.

57. Yager E, Bitsaktsis C, Nandi B, et al. Essential role for humoral immunity during *Ehrlichia* infection in immunocompetent mice. Infect Immun 2005;73:8009–8016.

58. Stevenson HL, Jordan JM, Peerwani Z, et al. An intradermal environment promotes a protective type-1 response against lethal systemic monocytotropic ehrlichial infection. Infect Immun 2006;74:4856–4864.

59. Winslow GM, Yager E, Shilo K, et al. Infection of the laboratory mouse with the intracellular pathogen *Ehrlichia chaffeensis*. Infect Immun 1998;66:3892–3899.

60. Li JS, Chu F, Reilly A, Winslow GM. Antibodies highly effective in SCID mice during infection by the intracellular bacterium *Ehrlichia chaffeensis* are of picomolar affinity and exhibit preferential epitope and isotype utilization. J Immunol 2002;169:1419–1425.

61. Winslow GM, Yager E, Li JS. Mechanisms of humoral immunity during *Ehrlichia chaffeensis* infection. Ann NY Acad Sci 2003;990:435–443.

62. Winslow GM, Yager E, Shilo K, et al. Antibody-mediated elimination of the obligate intracellular bacterial pathogen *Ehrlichia chaffeensis* during active infection. Infect Immun 2000;68:2187–2195.

63. Dumler JS, Dawson JE, Walker DH. Human ehrlichiosis: hematopathology and immunohistologic detection of *Ehrlichia chaffeensis*. Hum Pathol 1993;24:391–396.

64. Dawson JE, Paddock CD, Warner CK, et al. Tissue diagnosis of *Ehrlichia chaffeensis* in patients with fatal ehrlichiosis by use of immunohistochemistry, in situ hybridization, and polymerase chain reaction. Am J Trop Med Hyg 2001;65:603–609.

65. Dunning Hotopp JC, Lin M, Madupu R, et al. Comparative genomics of emerging human ehrlichiosis agents. PLoS Genet 2006;2:e21.

66. Long SW, Whitworth TJ, Walker DH, Yu XJ. Overcoming barriers to the transformation of the genus *Ehrlichia*. Ann NY Acad Sci 2005;1063:403–410.

67. Rachek LI, Hines A, Tucker AM, et al. Transformation of *Rickettsia prowazekii* to erythromycin resistance encoded by the *Escherichia coli ere*B gene. J Bacteriol 2000;182: 3289–3291.

39
Bacteria

Nabin K. Shrestha and Gary W. Procop

Introduction

This chapter begins with a general description of the etiology, pathogenesis, pathology, clinical features, and diagnosis of bacterial pneumonia. Specifics of pathogenesis, clinical features, antibiotic resistance, and diagnostic testing for the important bacterial causes of community-acquired pneumonia are then discussed.

Bacterial Causes of Pneumonia

Bacteria are the most common group of microorganisms that cause pneumonia. Pneumonia can be classified into several clinical subgroups, such as community-acquired pneumonia, health care–associated pneumonia, necrotizing pneumonia, and pneumonia in immunocompromised patients. The important bacterial causes of the different clinical syndromes of pneumonia are listed in Table 39.1.

Burkholderia pseudomallei is an important bacterial cause of pneumonia in southeast Asia.[1] Various occupational exposures lead to specific pneumonias. Exposure to cattle, sheep, or goats could lead to pneumonia caused by *Coxiella burnetii* (Q fever).[2] Exposure to birds may lead to psittacosis, caused by *Chlamydophila psittaci*. Many of the important potential bioterrorism agents could also cause pneumonia.[3]

Pathogenesis of Pneumonia

Pneumonia results when inhaled, aspirated, or hematogenously deposited microorganisms overcome the host's immune responses in the lung. The initial event in the pathogenesis of pneumonia is usually colonization of the upper nasopharyngeal or respiratory passages with the microorganism. In susceptible hosts, the bacteria then travel down the respiratory passages and establish lower respiratory tract infection. Conditions that impair local defenses or systemic immunity facilitate invasion by microorganisms and allow otherwise less virulent microorganisms to establish infection.

Conditions of impaired local defenses include loss of the cough reflex (due to coma, stroke or neuromuscular disorders, drugs, or chest pain), damage to the mucociliary escalator (due to smoking, toxic inhalation, viral infection, or the immotile cilia syndrome), pulmonary congestion and disturbance of pulmonary alveolar macrophage function (due to smoking, alcohol, hypoxia, congestion or diabetes mellitus), and local obstruction (due to secretions or mass effect). In some instances, damage to the respiratory epithelium by a viral infection such as influenza facilitates a secondary superadded bacterial infection. Systemic predisposing conditions include extremes of age, congenital or acquired immunodeficiency states, splenectomy or functional asplenia, and chronic diseases (chronic obstructive pulmonary disease [COPD], bronchiectasis, cystic fibrosis, heart failure, diabetes mellitus).[4]

Aspiration of gastric or oropharyngeal contents is a common precedent to the development of pneumonia in hospitalized or debilitated patients. This event introduces the flora colonizing the upper pharyngeal and respiratory epithelium into the lungs.

Pathology

Morphologically, bacterial pneumonia may lead to one of three gross anatomic patterns. Lobar pneumonia is a fibrinosuppurative consolidation of an entire lobe or of a large portion of the lobe of a lung. This is the typical pattern in pneumonia caused by *Streptococcus pneumoniae*. Bronchopneumonia is a patchy consolidation of multiple small areas of a lobe, many lobes, or both lungs. This is the pattern usually seen in pneumonia caused by *Haemophilus influenzae* or *Moraxella catarrhalis*. There

TABLE 39.1. Important bacterial causes of pneumonia.

Community-acquired pneumonia
  Streptococcus pneumonie
  Haemophilus influenzae
  Moraxella catarrhalis
  Mycoplasma pneumoniae
  Chlamydophila pneumoniae
  Legionella pneumophila
  Bordetella pertussis
  Staphylococcus aureus

Health care–associated pneumonia
  Staphylococcus aureus
  Enterobacteriaceae members *(Escherichia coli, Klebsiella
    pneumoniae, Serratia marcescens)*
  Pseudomonas aeruginosa
  Oropharyngeal anaerobic flora (in cases of aspiration)

Necrotizing pneumonia and lung abscess
  Anaerobic oral flora exclusively, or mixed with other bacteria
  Staphylococcus aureus
  Klebsiella pneumoniae
  Streptococcus pyogenes
  Streptococcus pneumoniae
  Nocardia spp.

Pneumonia in immunocompromised hosts
  Nocardia spp.
  Mycobacterium spp.
  Rhodococcus equi
  Bacteria that cause pneumonia in immunocompetent patients

are all ranges of overlap between these two anatomic forms, and the same bacterium may produce different morphologic patterns in different patients.

The third morphologic pattern is an interstitial pneumonia. The predominant finding is interstitial infiltration with inflammatory cells and widening of the alveolar septae. There may be scattered areas of bronchopneumonic consolidation. This is the usual pattern in patients who present with atypical pneumonia, which is often caused by *Mycoplasma pneumoniae* or *Chlamydophila pneumoniae*, and it is also the predominant pattern seen in patients with viral pneumonia.[4]

Clinical Features

Community-acquired pneumonia may present as an acute illness or as an atypical pneumonia. The typical symptoms of acute pneumonia are fever, pleuritic chest pain, cough, and expectoration of purulent sputum. Physical findings include splinting of the chest wall on the affected side along with signs of consolidation, which include increased vocal fremitus, dullness to percussion, and bronchial breath sounds with increased vocal resonance, aegophony, and whispering pectoriliquoy.[5] Crackles on the

affected side occur later. These classic symptoms and signs are usually seen in lobar pneumonia. Although the presentation of bronchopneumonia is also usually acute, physical findings are usually less prominent. In these patients, the predominant finding is scattered areas with bronchial breath sounds or crackles. Patients suffering from atypical pneumonia often are not very ill at the time of presentation. There may be very few physical findings. Because of the indolent presentation, this is also sometimes called *walking pneumonia*. In these patients chest radiographic findings are more dramatic than the physical findings.

Diagnosis

In patients without preexisting cardiac or pulmonary disease, making a clinical diagnosis of pneumonia is often straightforward and is based on clinical features and radiographic imaging. Unfortunately, there are no pathognomonic clinical or radiographic features that allow a definitive etiologic diagnosis to be made for pneumonia caused by any specific microorganism. Every patient with suspected pneumonia should have a chest radiographic study to confirm the clinical diagnosis of pneumonia, but additional tests are required to determine the etiology. Etiologic diagnosis requires laboratory confirmation.

The most rigorous studies have been successful in establishing an etiologic diagnosis of pneumonia only 50% of the time.[6] Laboratory diagnostic modalities include culture of sputum (or other respiratory samples) and blood, serology, antigen detection, and molecular diagnostic techniques such as detection using hybridization probes and nucleic acid amplification. Molecular diagnostic techniques are increasingly complementing traditional diagnostic modalities for the diagnosis of bacterial pneumonias and have revolutionized the diagnosis of infections for which culture was difficult and other modalities inadequate.

Molecular tests that look for all the significant pathogens causing pneumonia are of more clinical value than tests that specifically target a single microorganism. A multiplex polymerase chain reaction (PCR) assay that successfully detected the presence of *S. pneumoniae*, *H. influenzae*, *M. catarrhalis*, and *C. pneumoniae* has recently been described.[7] The use of real-time PCR for the diagnosis of pathogens causing lower respiratory tract infection increases the yield of pathogens identified but also increases cost; this, however, did not significantly change antibiotic prescribing in one study.[8] Furthermore, culture of microorganisms is also usually required for determination of antimicrobial susceptibility. Although in some instances genetic markers of resistance to antimicrobials have been described, the full spectrum of genetic markers that confer resistance is not known. Therefore, molecular testing for resistance, in its current state, cannot replace conventional antimicrobial susceptibility testing. Clearly, the optimum use of molecular diagnostic techniques will evolve with technologic advances and decreasing cost, and they can be expected to supplement current tests, not replace them entirely.

Streptococcus pneumoniae

Streptococcus pneumoniae is the most common cause of community-acquired pneumonia worldwide. It is restricted entirely to humans, there being no other known host or reservoir. It may be a commensal (i.e., part of the human normal microbiota) or a pathogen. Other serious infections that are commonly caused by this pathogen include sinusitis, otitis media, and meningitis.

Pathogenesis

Streptococcus pneumoniae is a part of the endogenous nasopharyngeal flora in 20% of healthy individuals. Some studies have shown carriage rates as high as 70% in children. Colonization is necessary for subsequent infection but does not always lead to infection.

For pneumonia to develop, bacteria travel down the respiratory passages, successfully avoid clearance by the mucociliary apparatus, and gain access to the alveolar epithelium and multiply in the alveolar spaces. Complement is activated, cytokine production is upregulated, and exudative fluid accumulates in the alveolar septae and the alveolar spaces. This can extend to uninvolved areas through the pores of Kohn. Filling of alveolar spaces by the inflammatory fluid constitutes consolidation and can be detected clinically and radiographically when it becomes more extensive.

Several virulence factors help the bacterium in successfully thwarting the host's immune defenses.[9] Attachment to nasopharyngeal cells is mediated by bacterial surface adhesins such as pneumococcal surface protein A, the major cell wall hydrolase, and choline binding protein A. The polysaccharide capsule protects the microorganism from phagocytosis by macrophages. Pneumococcal surface protein A is present in almost all pneumococci, and, in addition to mediating attachment, it also appears to protect the microorganism from the host complement system. Pneumolysin is present in all pneumococci, is released with bacterial lysis, and is cytotoxic to phagocytic and respiratory epithelial cells. It also induces inflammation by activating complement and inducing the production of inflammatory cytokines. Both of these actions contribute to tissue damage in pneumococcal pneumonia.

Clinical Features

Streptococcus pneumoniae is the most common cause of community-acquired pneumonia. Persons at the extremes of age, patients who have had a splenectomy or have functional asplenia, persons with primary or acquired hypogammaglobulinemia, and people with acquired immunodeficiency syndrome are at increased risk of invasive pneumococcal infection. Patients with *S. pneumoniae* pneumonia present with an acute febrile illness associated with chest pain and cough with expectoration. They may produce rust-colored or blood-tinged sputum. Physical findings of consolidation are often present. The typical chest radiographic finding is a lobar infiltrate, but patchy infiltrates may also be seen. Pleural effusion may also occur. Complications include development of empyema, pericarditis, and meningitis.

Antimicrobial Resistance

During the past three decades pneumococci have become increasingly more resistant to many antimicrobials to which they had previously been susceptible.[10] Resistance to fluoroquinolones and trimethoprim-sulfamethoxazole result from mutations within the bacterial genome, whereas resistance to other agents are usually from importation of foreign genetic material.[11] Resistance to β-lactam antibiotics is due to modification of genes encoding penicillin-binding proteins (PBPs), which are surface enzymes that are important for the synthesis of peptidoglycan. The products of these modified genes are altered PBPs that have decreased affinity for penicillin. Many of the altered PBPs that encode penicillin resistance also render the bacteria resistant to third-generation cephalosporins such as ceftriaxone and cefotaxime. The two major mechanisms of macrolide resistance are inhibition of binding and drug efflux. The *ermB* gene product causes methylation of a base in the 23S ribosomal subunit, which results in inhibition of macrolide binding and subsequent high-level resistance. The *mefA* and *mefE* genes, in contrast, encode for macrolide efflux pumps. Their presence results in a lower degree of resistance that might be overcome with higher concentrations of drug. Fluoroquinolone resistance is due to stepwise chromosomal mutations in the *parC* gene encoding DNA topoisomerase IV and in the *gyrA* gene encoding DNA gyrase.

Diagnostic Testing

The diagnosis of pneumonia caused by *S. pneumoniae* is most readily made by sputum Gram stain. The characteristic appearance on Gram stain is elongated Gram-positive cocci in pairs (lanceolate diplococci). However, the microorganism is detected by sputum Gram stain in the minority of patients. Sputum culture increases the sensitivity, but the specificity is limited because this bacterium normally colonizes the nasopharynx. Blood cultures may provide an etiologic diagnosis, but only one third of blood cultures taken during the first 4 days after onset of symptoms are positive for *S. pneumoniae*.[12] Urine antigen tests have sensitivities around 80% and specificities that range from 77% to 97%. Urine antigen tests cannot differentiate between infection and nasopharyngeal colonization and are particularly less useful for children because of the high rate of nasopharyngeal colonization.

Molecular tests based on nucleic acid amplification by PCR for detection of *S. pneumoniae* have been studied. Genes that have been targeted for detection include the DNA polymerase gene, the pneumolysin gene *(ply)*, the autolysin gene *(lytA)*, penicillin binding protein genes *pbp2a* and *pbp2b*, and the pneumococcal surface protein A gene *(pspA)*. Polymerase chain reaction is more sensitive than sputum culture for the detection of *S. pneumoniae*.[13] However, PCR does not differentiate between colonization and infection.

Haemophilus influenzae

Haemophilus influenzae is an important cause of pneumonia in adults. Humans are the only known host for *H. influenzae*. Other important illnesses caused by *H. influenzae* include meningitis, otitis media, sinusitis, epiglottitis, and facial cellulitis. With widespread *Haemophilus influenzae* type b vaccination, most disease seen in areas with adequate vaccination is not due to this strain.

Pathogenesis

Respiratory colonization with *H. influenzae* is very common. Infection is acquired through airborne droplets or direct contact with secretions. Several adhesins mediate attachment to the host epithelium.[14] After colonization, in susceptible hosts, bacteria travel to the lower respiratory passages to cause pneumonia. *Haemophilus influenzae* type b is able to gain access to the bloodstream and causes invasive disease, a virulence that is not seen with nonencapsulated *H. influenzae*. The capsular polysaccharide of encapsulated microorganisms protects the microorganisms from the host's defenses when they invade the body. The lower respiratory tract of patients with COPD is chronically colonized by nontypeable *H. influenzae*. Acquisition of new strains is an important cause of acute exacerbations of COPD.[15]

Clinical Features

The symptoms are indistinguishable from those caused by other bacteria causing acute pneumonia. Physical findings of consolidation are often not obvious at the time of presentation. Chest radiograph reveals a patchy or lobar distribution of infiltrates.

Antimicrobial Resistance

Up to one third or more of *H. influenzae* isolates are resistant to ampicillin.[16] These isolates are usually resistant to most other β-lactam antibiotics also. In the majority of cases resistance is due to production of plasmid-encoded β-lactamases.[17] Resistance can be overcome by the use of β-lactam/β-lactamase inhibitor combinations. Estimates of resistance to clarithromycin have ranged from 2% to 23% in large studies. Azithromycin is more active than clarithromycin. One large study found 14% of isolates to be resistant to trimethoprim-sulfamethoxazole.[18] Resistance is due to different mutations affecting enzymes of the folate biosynthesis system.[19]

Diagnostic Testing

Sputum (or other respiratory sample obtained more aggressively) and blood are the specimens most likely to yield a diagnosis. Sputum Gram stain may reveal the presence of small, pleomorphic Gram-negative coccobacilli. Because of their small size, *H. influenzae* may easily be missed on Gram-stained smears. Successful culture requires the use of media, (e.g., chocolate agar) that provide the growth factors hemin (factor X) and nicotinamide adenosine dinucleotide (factor V). A DNA probe based on recognition of specific 16S rRNA sequences for the identification of *H. influenzae* once the microorganism grows in culture is commercially available (Accuprobe, Gen-Probe Inc., San Diego, CA). This test is simple, rapid, and compares favorably with conventional tests of identification for the bacterium.[20] Polymerase chain reaction assays can also accurately detect the presence of *H. influenzae* in respiratory specimens, but the specificity of such assays suffers because disease cannot be readily differentiated from colonization.[21]

Moraxella catarrhalis

Moraxella catarrhalis is an important cause of upper and lower respiratory tract infections. Other important infections caused by this microorganism are otitis media and sinusitis.

Pathogenesis

About 1%–5% of healthy adults are colonized with *M. catarrhalis*. The rate of colonization is much higher in children than in adults. Adults with chronic lung diseases such as COPD and bronchiectasis have higher rates of colonization. For pneumonia to occur, the microorganism must spread to the lower respiratory tract. The mechanisms underlying this spread are not entirely clear. Virulence of the colonizing microorganism may be one factor, as studies suggest that some strains are more virulent than others.[22] Virulence factors include various outer membrane proteins that mediate attachment and protection from host bactericidal agents.[23]

Clinical Features

Moraxella catarrhalis is an important cause of pneumonia in elderly patients. Most of such patients have underlying chronic lung or heart conditions, especially COPD and congestive heart failure. It is also an important cause of acute exacerbations in patients with COPD.

Antimicrobial Resistance

Production of β-lactamases by *M. catarrhalis* was first described in 1976, and now more than 90% of strains produce β-lactamases.[24] These β-lactamases are chromosomally encoded. There are two major β-lactamases produced by *M. catarrhalis*. These have been designated BRO-1 and BRO-2.[25] These enzymes are unique to *M. catarrhalis*, and their origin is not clear. Strains producing these enzymes remain susceptible to ceftriaxone. About 10% of isolates are resistant to trimethoprim-sulfamethoxazole.[18] Resistance to trimethoprim-sulfamethoxazole is due to different mutations that affect different steps of the folate biosynthesis system.[19] *Moraxella catarrhalis* remains susceptible to the other commonly used antibiotics for treating respiratory tract infections, such as macrolides and respiratory quinolones.

Diagnostic Testing

Sputum (or other more aggressively obtained respiratory sample) is the best clinical sample for establishing an etiologic diagnosis of pneumonia caused by *M. catarrhalis*. Gram stain may reveal large numbers of extracellular Gram-negative diplococci. *Moraxella catarrhalis* grows well on blood and chocolate agars. Specific tests are necessary to distinguish the microorganism from *Neisseria* species, which may be part of the colonizing flora in the upper respiratory tract. *Moraxella catarrhalis* can also been detected by PCR with high sensitivity and specificity.[26]

Legionella pneumophila

Legionella pneumophila is the causative agent of Legionnaires' disease, a severe pneumonia, and Pontiac fever, a milder febrile illness. It is implicated in 0.5%–6% of cases of community-acquired pneumonia.[27] Legionellae are distributed worldwide in natural and artifical water systems.[28] They are intracellular parasites of freshwater protozoa, where they are able to obtain their nutritional requirements. Warm aquatic environments provide legionellae with a growth advantage over many other environmental bacteria. They also thrive in biofilms.[29]

Pathogenesis

Legionella pneumophila is ubiquitous in the environment. Some strains are virulent enough to produce disease in immunocompetent individuals. More than 70% of Legionnaires' disease cases are caused by serogroup 1. For infection to occur, virulent strains become aerosolized and enter the lungs of a susceptible host. The bacteria reach the lungs via inhalation of infective aerosols or microaspiration of bacteria. Infection with the microorganism may lead to a self-limiting influenza-like illness known as *Pontiac fever* or to pneumonia known as *Legionnaires' disease*.

Legionella pneumophila has several virulence factors that aid its survival within the host.[30] A lipid-modifying enzyme affords protection against cationic antimicrobial peptides, catalase peroxidase protects the bacterium from catalase, and the copper-zinc superoxide dismutase protects the bacterium from toxic superoxide anions. Attachment and entry into mammalian cells are mediated by type IV pili, flagella, and heat shock protein 60. The macrophage infectivity potentiator protein is important for initiation of intracellular infection. Intracellularly legionellae reside within unique phagosomes where they are protected from the host's immune system. The type IV secretion system of *L. pneumophila* inhibits phagosome–lysosome fusion. Proteins of the type II secretion system are important for intracellular growth of *L. pneumophila*.

Clinical Features

The incubation period for Legionnaires' disease is between 2 and 10 days. The clinical presentation is indistinguishable from that of pneumococcal pneumonia. Localizing symptoms may be preceded by a prodromal illness lasting several days. The majority of patients have fever, cough, and dyspnea at presentation. Some patients have severe headache. Physical examination usually reveals areas of scattered bronchial breath sounds or crackles, findings indicating patchy consolidation. Radiographically, segmental to lobar infiltrates are seen. These correspond to multiple areas of consolidation. In immunocompromised patients, pulmonary nodules may be seen. Cavitation may occur in about 10% of immunocompromised patients.

Antimicrobial Resistance

Legionella pneumophila is an intracellular organism. Hence it is intrinsically resistant to drugs that do not work in an intracellular environment, such as β-lactam antibiotics, aminoglycosides, and chloramphenicol. Azithromycin, the newer quinolones, and ketolides are more effective than erythromycin, clarithromycin, and doxycyline.[31]

Diagnostic Testing

Available methods for detection include culture, urinary antigen detection, serology, direct fluorescence antibody (DFA) staining, and PCR. The first two are the most easily available. The microorganism is fastidious and requires special culture conditions for growth. Culture on selective media requires 3–7 days for growth. The sensitivity of culture is 50%–60%.[32] Urinary antigen detection tests targeting *L. pneumophila* serogroup 1 have sensitivities ranging from 56% to 90% and specificities of 99%.[32]

Legionella pneumophila can also be detected by PCR of respiratory samples with high sensitivity and specificity.[33] Genetic targets for nucleic acid amplification assays have included the 5S rRNA gene, the *mip* gene, and the 16S rRNA gene.

Chlamydophila pneumoniae

Chlamydiae are obligate intracellular bacteria characterized by a biphasic life cycle consisting of an elementary body and a reticulate body. The elementary body is the infectious form and is adapted for survival outside the host cell. After internalization by receptor-mediated endocytosis, the elementary body differentiates into the reticulate body. The reticulate body divides by binary fission leading to the formation of a microcolony, which is visible by light microscopy and referred to as a *chlamydia inclusion body*. After growth and division, the products of the reticulate body condense to form infectious elementary bodies.

Chlamydophila (formerly *Chlamydia*) *pneumoniae* accounts for up to 10% of cases of patients hospitalized with pneumonia.[34] *Chlamydophila pneumoniae* is also an important cause of upper respiratory infections and bronchitis. *Chlamydophila pneumoniae* has also been associated with the development of adult-onset asthma. It is known to be one of the agents responsible for exacerbation of COPD. Infection with *C. pneumoniae* was shown to be associated with the occurrence of coronary artery disease in 1988. Since then, a large body of evidence has accumulated examining this association, with some studies supporting the association and others refuting it.

Pathogenesis

Asymptomatic carriage of *C. pneumoniae* occurs in about 5% of children.[35] In susceptible hosts, colonization is followed by infection. In animal studies infection with *C. pneumoniae* leads to patchy inflammatory infiltrates interspersed among areas of normal histology.[36]

Clinical Features

In symptomatic patients, the incubation period is about 21 days. It often causes an atypical pneumonia. Symptoms and signs of upper respiratory infection are nonspecific and include rhinitis, sore throat, and hoarseness. Patients who develop pneumonia often have a biphasic illness in which the upper respiratory symptoms subside and are followed days to weeks later with cough. Most patients with *C. pneumoniae* pneumonia are not very ill. Hoarseness of voice is a common accompanying condition. Symptoms usually develop gradually and tend to have a prolonged course despite appropriate treatment. Chest radiographs are nonspecific and may include segmental or subsegmental infiltrates, lobar or sublobar consolidation, interstitial infiltrates, multilobar infiltrates, hilar adenopathy, and pleural effusions.[37] Extrapulmonary syndromes that have been associated with *C. pneumoniae* include meningoencephalitis, Guillain-Barré syndrome, and endocarditis.

Antimicrobial Resistance

Chlamydophila pneumoniae is an intracellular pathogen. Thus β-lactam antibiotics and the sulfa drugs are not effective. Macrolides, quinolones, and doxycycline that achieve high concentrations intracellularly are all effective. No clinically significant acquired antimicrobial resistance has been recognized.

Diagnostic Testing

Cultures are not sensitive. Serologic tests are difficult to interpret; these have low sensitivity if only IgM is tested and require acute and convalescent sera tested together when IgG is tested. To make a diagnosis on the basis of serology either a fourfold rise in IgG titer or a single IgM titer ≥1:16 using a microimmunofluorescence test must be demonstrated.[38] Nucleic acid amplification tests are probably the most sensitive for the diagnosis of *C. pneumoniae*, but in the absence of a gold standard it is difficult to standardize these tests. Thus, the reported sensitivities have ranged from 33% to 76.5%.

Several PCR-based *C. pneumoniae* assays have been developed, but their sensitivities and specificities are largely unknown. In general, PCR is at least as sensitive as culture, but specificity is an issue because of the inability to differentiate between colonization and infection especially with upper respiratory samples.[13] An expert panel convened by the Centers for Disease Control and Prevention to address the interpretation of diagnostic test results for *C. pneumoniae* has provided recommendations that should help in improving diagnostic specificity.[38] *Chlamydophila pneumoniae* can also be readily detected in tissue specimens, when available, by immunofluorescence, in situ hybridization, and immunohistochemistry.

Mycoplasma pneumoniae

Mycoplasmas are the smallest organisms that are capable of a cell-free existence.[39] They are characterized by the permanent lack of a cell wall, thus distinguishing them from the L forms of bacteria that temporarily lack a cell wall under certain environmental conditions. Among the mycoplasmas, *Mycoplasma pneumoniae* is the only important cause of pneumonia.

Pathogenesis

Mycoplasma pneumoniae lives exclusively in close association with the respiratory mucosa of humans. The microorganism has a specialized attachment structure that facilitates the attachment of the microorganism to the host epithelial cell. The P1 adhesin is concentrated in the attachment tip and plays a major role in the interaction between the microorganism and the host cell.[40] Whether the microorganism invades the host cell and replicates intracellularly is not known at this time. *Mycoplasma pneumoniae* is not known to produce any exotoxin. It is able to produce hydrogen peroxide, and this molecule along with toxic oxygen radicals produced by the host inflammatory response lead to damage to the respiratory epithelium, including loss of cilia and ultimately exfoliation.[41] This exfoliation is responsible for the persistent, hacking cough that is associated with infection with this microorganism.

Mycoplasma pneumoniae can be detected in the airways of patients with chronic stable asthma more frequently than of controls. Acute pneumonia caused by *M. pneumoniae* has been shown to be followed by pulmonary function abnormalities for months. These findings suggest that *M. pneumoniae* may have a role in the pathogenesis of asthma. Infection with *M. pneumoniae* has also been associated with acute exacerbations in patients with COPD.

Some of the extrapulmonary manifestations of *M. pneumoniae* infection are thought to be autoimmune phenomena. However, the microorganism has been isolated from extrapulmonary lesions, suggesting a direct pathogenic effect.[42,43]

Clinical Features

Most *M. pneumoniae* infections lead to subclinical illness. When symptomatic, the incubation period is 2–3 weeks,[44] and the majority of those afflicted have a mild illness. Infection with *M. pneumoniae* may lead to tracheobronchitis, bronchiolitis, pharyngitis, croup, and pneumonia. *Mycoplasma pneumoniae* pneumonia occurs mostly in children and young adults. The typical symptoms of patients with pneumonia are fever, malaise, headache, and cough. Symptoms gradually worsen over 1–2 days but most illness appears to be mild in the majority of patients. Physical findings may be minimal, and chest radiographic findings are out of proportion to them. Some, especially the elderly, may develop severe illness.

Many extrapulmonary manifestations have been described with *M. pneumoniae* infection. These include Stevens-Johnson syndrome, meningoencephalitis, ascending paralysis, transverse myelitis, Guillain-Barré syndrome, pericarditis, and arthritis. After infection, the microorganism may persist for several months in the respiratory tract. In patients with hypogammaglobulinemia, the microorganism may persist in the respiratory tract for years.[45]

Antimicrobial Resistance

Mycoplasma pneumoniae is inhibited by tetracyclines, macrolides, fluoroquinolones, and ketolides.[46] Macrolides and tetracyclines are primarily bacteriostatic, but fluoroquinolones have been shown to be bactericidal. Because of the lack of a cell wall, cell wall–active antimicrobials such as β-lactam antibiotics are ineffective against *M. pneumoniae*. Sulfonamides, trimethoprim, and rifampin are also ineffective. Clinically significant antimicrobial resistance of *M. pneumoniae* to any drug class is not known, although tetracycline resistance has been well documented in *Mycoplasma hominis* and *Ureaplasma* species, mediated by the presence of the *tetM* determinant.[47]

Diagnostic Testing

Because of their lack of a cell wall, mycoplasmas are not stained by Gram stain. Culture for *Mycoplasma* is expensive, time consuming, and labor intensive. Because of their small size and the limited genetic material, mycoplasma need many exogenous nutrients to survive or grow in culture. Growth on special media takes 4 days to several weeks. It is far less sensitive than PCR.[48] Culture is thus not recommended for routine diagnosis. Until recently, serology was the most reliable way of making a diagnosis of *M. pneumoniae* infection. Most modern serology assays are ELISA based. These tests are more specific than the previous complement fixation tests and are able to detect IgM and IgG antibodies. A serologic diagnosis of *Mycoplasma* pneumonia requires either an elevated IgM level or a fourfold rise in IgG antibody titer. Rapid antigen detection tests are far simpler to perform but are limited by cross-reactivity with other mycoplasmas and lower sensitivity compared with PCR.[49]

DNA hybridization probes have about the same diagnostic sensitivity as antigen detection tests.[50] Nucleic acid amplification has emerged as the most sensitive method for the detection of *M. pneumoniae*.[13] Polymerase chain reaction has several advantages, including rapidity, need for only one specimen, becoming positive earlier than serology, and not requiring viable microorganisms.

Bordetella pertussis

Bordetella pertussis is a small coccobacillary microorganism. It is the cause of pertussis or whooping cough. It is a strict human pathogen, although it can experimentally be made to infect other animals. It causes illness in all persons who have not been previously infected or immunized. Pertussis was classically a disease of infants and children. Reported cases of pertussis have been increasing over the past decade, and a greater proportion of cases are now being reported in adolescents and adults.[51] Pertussis is very much underreported, because most illnesses are mild and do not come to clinical attention, illness is frequently not recognized because of the misconception that pertussis is a childhood disease, and lack of adequate diagnostic facilities preclude making a diagnosis even when considered by the clinician.

Pathogenesis

Pertussis is a contagious disease. Infection is spread person to person via infected droplets.[52] The microorganisms invade and destroy the ciliated epithelial cells lining the trachea, bronchi, and bronchioles. A lymphoid hyperplasia of the peribronchial and tracheobronchial lymph nodes occurs. Necrosis of the surface epithelial cells follows, and desquamation may occur. Numerous small areas of atelectasis occur, and most patients with fatal cases of pertussis have bronchopneumonia.[53]

Important virulence factors are adhesins and toxins.[54] Filamentous hemagglutinin is the major adhesion. This helps the microorganism bind to various cells and extracellular structures in the respiratory epithelium. Two important toxins are tracheal cytotoxin and pertussis toxin. Tracheal cytotoxin destroys ciliated epithelial cells. The pertussis toxin is a complex protein consisting of five subunits, S1–S5. It is responsible for inducing lymphocytosis, but its target tissue has not yet been recognized.

Clinical Features

The classic form of pertussis presents with a paroxysmal cough, posttussive vomiting, inspiratory whoop, and prolonged cough. This is a severe and potentially life-threatening disease. This form occurs in infants and is infrequently seen in places with adequate childhood vaccination. In adolescents and adults most cases of pertussis are mild illnesses.[55] Adults with prior immunization have mild illness and in some cases may be asymptomatic. When symptomatic, the important clinical feature is prolonged cough.

Antimicrobial Resistance

Erythromycin has been the mainstay of treatment for pertussis. The newer macrolides clarithromycin and azithromycin are also effective, as is trimethoprim-sulfamethoxazole. Reports of erythromycin resistance are very rare.[53]

Diagnostic Testing

Available diagnostic methods include culture, direct antigen detection (DFA testing), serology, and PCR. For culture, nasopharyngeal cultures must be obtained using calcium alginate or Dacron swabs because cotton and rayon contain fatty acids that are toxic to *B. pertussis*. The specimen must be transported in appropriate transport media and plated on appropriate enrichment media. From a practical standpoint, it may be difficult to have all these in place for the diagnosis of one type of microorganism.

The mainstay of serologic diagnosis now is ELISA using specific *B. pertussis* proteins as antigens. The biggest drawback to serologic diagnosis is that by the time the diagnosis is considered it is often already too late to obtain an acute phase sample. The serologic response will have already peaked, and no difference will be observed between the sample and a subsequent one. The DFA test, although easy to perform, lacks sensitivity because it does not involve amplification and lacks specificity because of cross-reactions with normal nasopharyngeal flora.[56] Polymerase chain reaction, which is more sensitive than culture and DFA, is now the gold standard for direct detection.[57]

Staphylococcus aureus

Staphylococcus aureus has been recognized to be an important cause of secondary bacterial pneumonia after an episode of viral pneumonia and has been thought to be responsible for significant morbidity and mortality during influenza pandemics. It is also an important cause of health care–associated pneumonia, and many of these infections are caused by methicillin-resistant *S. aureus* (MRSA). Until recently community-associated strains of *S. aureus* have usually been methicillin-susceptible. In recent years, community-associated methicillin-resistant *S. aureus* (CA-MRSA) has increasingly been recognized as a cause of severe community-acquired pneumonia and skin and skin structure infections.[58]

Pathogenesis

Staphylococcus aureus can reach the lungs by inhalation, aspiration, or hematogenous spread from a distant focus. Community-associated MRSA causes a necrotizing type of pneumonia with extensive tissue damage. Panton-Valentine leukocidin (PVL) appears to be an important virulence factor contributing to the pathogenesis of necrotizing *S. aureus* pneumonia.[59] Most strains of CA-MRSA that cause severe pneumonia produce PVL. Cases of severe pneumonia caused by PVL-producing strains of methicillin-susceptible *S. aureus* have also been reported, again suggesting that PVL is an important virulence factor.

Clinical Features

Pneumonia caused by CA-MRSA is rapidly progressive. It is often associated with high fever, purulent expectoration, hemoptysis, respiratory failure, and shock. Most people who develop pneumonia caused by CA-MRSA have been previously healthy.

Antimicrobial Resistance

Community-associated MRSA strains are by definition resistant to methicillin. In contrast to hospital-associated strains, these strains are usually susceptible to many other antibiotics to which the former are resistant.[60] The *mecA* gene is an acquired gene that is the major determinant of methicillin resistance. It is carried on a mobile genetic element, the staphylococcal chromosomal cassette *mec* (SCC*mec*). There are at least four different types of SCC*mec*. Community-associated MRSA carries SCC*mec* type IV, which is smaller and does not carry other resistance determinants that are found in the SCC*mec* types I–III that are present in hospital-associated strains.[61]

Diagnostic Testing

Staphylococcus aureus can be detected by Gram stain of respiratory samples. It grows readily in sputum and blood cultures, and routine laboratory testing allows easy recognition of methicillin resistance. Methicillin resistance can also be determined by PCR for the *mecA* gene, and this method is being increasingly used for detection of methicillin resistance. Rapid tests for identification of MRSA are also available. Identification as a CA-MRSA requires determination of the specific SCC*mec* type by PCR. Presence of PVL can also be determined by PCR.

Agents with Bioterrorism Potential

A new concern with respect to causative agents of pneumonia is bioterrorism. The agents that are considered likely to have the most devastating impact if used as agents for bioterrorist attacks have been classified as class A agents. The bacteria that are capable of causing pneumonia in this class are *Bacillus anthracis*, *Yersinia pestis*, and *Francisella tularensis*.[3] Other agents that have been identified as potential agents for bioterrorism have been classified as class B agents. The bacteria in this class that can cause pneumonia are *Coxiella burnetii*, *Brucella* spp., *Burkholderia mallei*, *Burkholderia pseudomallei*, *Rickettsia prowazekii*, and *Chlamydophila psittaci*.[3]

Pathogenesis

Inhalational anthrax almost always indicates bioterrorism. Pneumonia caused by the other agents may be natural or a result of bioterrorism. Pneumonia from these agents in the context of bioterrorism will result from the intentional release of the viable pathogenic agent in an aerosolized form. The bacteria will be released with the intent that they gain access to the respiratory tract via inhalation, overcome the host's immune response, and produce a respiratory tract infection. Infection with *Bacillus anthracis* leads to hemorrhagic mediastinal adenopathy, hemorrhagic pleural effusions, and bacteremia.[62] Infections with the other agents lead to multilobar pneumonia.[63]

Clinical Features

Being able to recognize an illness as inhalational anthrax rather than community-acquired pneumonia would promptly initiate an investigation, and the sooner this could be initiated, the more lives would be saved. Inhalational anthrax has a median incubation period of 4 days and begins with nonspecific symptoms referable to the respiratory and gastrointestinal tracts. A wide mediastinum on chest radiograph, hyperdense mediastinal nodes on chest computed tomography scan, and bloody pleural effusions are highly characteristic of inhalational anthrax.[62] Pneumonia caused by one of the other potential bioterrorism agents would not have any pathognomonic clinical features that would point toward the diagnosis. Such infections will likely be recognized early in the setting of a recognized outbreak but will otherwise only be likely to be recognized when microbiologic tests turn up the offending agent.

Antimicrobial Resistance

A valid concern with bioterrorism is the possibility that the agent used may be genetically engineered to be resistant to the drugs that would ordinarily be prescribed to treat the infection. It has been reported that genetically engineered antibiotic-resistant biologic agents had been developed in the former Soviet Union.[64] In the event of a bioterrorism event, it will be important to perform antibiotic susceptibility tests without delay.

Diagnostic Testing

Public health officials are acutely aware of the importance of rapid and accurate detection of agents of bioterrorism. Currently available tests are based on biochemical, immunologic, bioluminescence, and nucleic acid amplification procedures.[65] Other innovative technologies are being developed. No test or platform is going to be perfect, but the focus should be on developing those that are rapid, highly sensitive and specific, and able to simultaneously detect several different agents.

References

1. White NJ. Melioidosis. Lancet 2003;361(9370):1715–1722.
2. Parker NR, Barralet JH, Bell AM. Q fever. Lancet 2006;367(9511):679–888.
3. Rotz LD, Khan AS, Lillibridge SR, et al. Public health assessment of potential biological terrorism agents. Emerg Infect Dis 2002;8(2):225–230.
4. Husain AN, Kumar V. The Lung. In Kumar V, Abbas AK, Fausto N, eds. Robbins and Cotran Pathologic Basis of Disease, 7th ed. Philadelphia: Elsevier Saunders; 2005: 711–772.
5. Moore-Gillon J. The Respiratory System. In Swash M, ed. Hutchison's Clinical Methods, 21st ed. London: Elsevier Saunders; 2002:60–78.
6. Reimer LG, Carroll KC. Role of the microbiology laboratory in the diagnosis of lower respiratory tract infections. Clin Infect Dis 1998;26(3):742–748.
7. Stralin K, Tornqvist E, Kaltoft MS, et al. Etiologic diagnosis of adult bacterial pneumonia by culture and PCR applied to respiratory tract samples. J Clin Microbiol 2006;44(2):643–645.
8. Oosterheert JJ, van Loon AM, Schuurman R, et al. Impact of rapid detection of viral and atypical bacterial pathogens by real-time polymerase chain reaction for patients with lower respiratory tract infection. Clin Infect Dis 2005;41(10):1438–1444.
9. Jedrzejas MJ. Pneumococcal virulence factors: structure and function. Microbiol Mol Biol Rev 2001;65(2):187–207.
10. Doern GV, Pfaller MA, Kugler K, et al. Prevalence of antimicrobial resistance among respiratory tract isolates of Streptococcus pneumoniae in North America: 1997 results from the SENTRY antimicrobial surveillance program. Clin Infect Dis 1998;27(4):764–770.
11. Jacobs MR. Streptococcus pneumoniae: epidemiology and patterns of resistance. Am J Med 2004;117 Suppl 3A:3S–15S.
12. Kalin M, Lindberg AA. Diagnosis of pneumococcal pneumonia: a comparison between microscopic examination of expectorate, antigen detection and cultural procedures. Scand J Infect Dis 1983;15(3):247–255.
13. Murdoch DR. Molecular genetic methods in the diagnosis of lower respiratory tract infections. APMIS 2004;112(11–12):713–727.
14. Rao VK, Krasan GP, Hendrixson DR, et al. Molecular determinants of the pathogenesis of disease due to nontypable Haemophilus influenzae. FEMS Microbiol Rev 1999;23(2):99–129.
15. Sethi S, Murphy TF. Bacterial infection in chronic obstructive pulmonary disease in 2000: a state-of-the-art review. Clin Microbiol Rev 2001;14(2):336–363.
16. Hoban DJ, Doern GV, Fluit AC, et al. Worldwide prevalence of antimicrobial resistance in Streptococcus pneumoniae, Haemophilus influenzae, and Moraxella catarrhalis in the SENTRY Antimicrobial Surveillance Program, 1997–1999. Clin Infect Dis 2001;32 Suppl 2:S81–S93.
17. Williams JD, Moosdeen F. Antibiotic resistance in Haemophilus influenzae: epidemiology, mechanisms, and therapeutic possibilities. Rev Infect Dis 1986;8 Suppl 5:S555–S61.
18. Ehrhardt AF, Russo R. Clinical resistance encountered in the respiratory surveillance program (RESP) study: a review of the implications for the treatment of community-acquired respiratory tract infections. Am J Med 2001;111 Suppl 9A:30S–38S.
19. Then RL. Mechanisms of resistance to trimethoprim, the sulfonamides, and trimethoprim-sulfamethoxazole. Rev Infect Dis 1982;4(2):261–269.
20. Daly JA, Clifton NL, Seskin KC, Gooch WM 3rd. Use of rapid, nonradioactive DNA probes in culture confirmation tests to detect Streptococcus agalactiae, Haemophilus influenzae, and Enterococcus spp. from pediatric patients with significant infections. J Clin Microbiol 1991;29(1):80–82.
21. Marty A, Greiner O, Day PJ, et al. Detection of Haemophilus influenzae type b by real-time PCR. J Clin Microbiol 2004;42(8):3813–3815.
22. Bootsma HJ, van der Heide HG, van de Pas S, et al. Analysis of Moraxella catarrhalis by DNA typing: evidence for a distinct subpopulation associated with virulence traits. J Infect Dis 2000;181(4):1376–1387.
23. Karalus R, Campagnari A. Moraxella catarrhalis: a review of an important human mucosal pathogen. Microbes Infect 2000;2(5):547–559.
24. Felmingham D, Washington J. Trends in the antimicrobial susceptibility of bacterial respiratory tract pathogens—

findings of the Alexander Project 1992–1996. J Chemother 1999;11(Suppl 1):5–21.

25. Bootsma HJ, van Dijk H, Vauterin P, et al. Genesis of BRO beta-lactamase–producing *Moraxella catarrhalis*: evidence for transformation-mediated horizontal transfer. Mol Microbiol 2000;36(1):93–104.

26. Greiner O, Day PJ, Altwegg M, Nadal D. Quantitative detection of *Moraxella catarrhalis* in nasopharyngeal secretions by real-time PCR. J Clin Microbiol 2003;41(4): 1386–1390.

27. Mandell LA, Bartlett JG, Dowell SF, et al. Update of practice guidelines for the management of community-acquired pneumonia in immunocompetent adults. Clin Infect Dis 2003;37(11):1405–1433.

28. Fliermans CB, Cherry WB, Orrison LH, et al. Ecological distribution of *Legionella pneumophila*. Appl Environ Microbiol 1981;41(1):9–16.

29. Rogers J, Keevil CW. Immunogold and fluorescein immunolabelling of *Legionella pneumophila* within an aquatic biofilm visualized by using episcopic differential interference contrast microscopy. Appl Environ Microbiol 1992; 58(7):2326–2330.

30. Fields BS, Benson RF, Besser RE. *Legionella* and Legionnaires' disease: 25 years of investigation. Clin Microbiol Rev 2002;15(3):506–526.

31. Roig J, Rello J. Legionnaires' disease: a rational approach to therapy. J Antimicrob Chemother 2003;51(5):1119–1129.

32. Breiman RF, Butler JC. Legionnaires' disease: clinical, epidemiological, and public health perspectives. Semin Respir Infect 1998;13(2):84–89.

33. Hayden RT, Uhl JR, Qian X, et al. Direct detection of *Legionella* species from bronchoalveolar lavage and open lung biopsy specimens: comparison of LightCycler PCR, in situ hybridization, direct fluorescence antigen detection, and culture. J Clin Microbiol 2001;39(7):2618–2626.

34. Grayston JT, Diwan VK, Cooney M, Wang SP. Community- and hospital-acquired pneumonia associated with *Chlamydia* TWAR infection demonstrated serologically. Arch Intern Med 1989;149(1):169–173.

35. Schmidt SM, Muller CE, Mahner B, Wiersbitzky SK. Prevalence, rate of persistence and respiratory tract symptoms of *Chlamydia pneumoniae* infection in 1211 kindergarten and school age children. Pediatr Infect Dis J 2002;21(8): 758–762.

36. Hammerschlag MR. *Chlamydia pneumoniae* and the lung. Eur Respir J 2000;16(5):1001–1007.

37. McConnell CT Jr, Plouffe JF, File TM, et al. Radiographic appearance of *Chlamydia pneumoniae* (TWAR strain) respiratory infections. CBPIS Study Group. Community-Based Pneumonia Incidence Study. Radiology 1994; 192(3):819–24.

38. Dowell SF, Peeling RW, Boman J, et al. Standardizing *Chlamydia pneumoniae* assays: recommendations from the Centers for Disease Control and Prevention (USA) and the Laboratory Centre for Disease Control (Canada). Clin Infect Dis 2001;33(4):492–503.

39. Wilson MH, Collier AM. Ultrastructural study of *Mycoplasma pneumoniae* in organ culture. J Bacteriol 1976; 125(1):332–339.

40. Waites KB, Talkington DF. *Mycoplasma pneumoniae* and its role as a human pathogen. Clin Microbiol Rev 2004;17(4): 697–728.

41. Collier AM. Attachment by mycoplasmas and its role in disease. Rev Infect Dis 1983;5(Suppl 4):S685–S691.

42. Meseguer MA, Perez-Molina JA, Fernandez-Bustamante J, et al. *Mycoplasma pneumoniae* pericarditis and cardiac tamponade in a ten-year-old girl. Pediatr Infect Dis J 1996;15(9):829–831.

43. Abramovitz P, Schvartzman P, Harel D, et al. Direct invasion of the central nervous system by *Mycoplasma pneumoniae*: a report of two cases. J Infect Dis 1987;155(3): 482–487.

44. Foy HM, Grayston JT, Kenny GE, et al. Epidemiology of *Mycoplasma pneumoniae* infection in families. JAMA 1966;197(11):859–866.

45. Taylor-Robinson D, Webster AD, Furr PM, Asherson GL. Prolonged persistence of *Mycoplasma pneumoniae* in a patient with hypogammaglobulinaemia. J Infect 1980;2(2): 171–175.

46. Waites KB, Crabb DM, Duffy LB. Inhibitory and bactericidal activities of gemifloxacin and other antimicrobials against *Mycoplasma pneumoniae*. Int J Antimicrob Agents 2003;21(6):574–577.

47. Roberts MC, Koutsky LA, Holmes KK, et al. Tetracycline-resistant *Mycoplasma hominis* strains contain streptococcal *tetM* sequences. Antimicrob Agents Chemother 1985;28(1): 141–143.

48. Ieven M, Ursi D, Van Bever H, et al. Detection of *Mycoplasma pneumoniae* by two polymerase chain reactions and role of *M. pneumoniae* in acute respiratory tract infections in pediatric patients. J Infect Dis 1996;173(6):1445–1452.

49. Daxboeck F, Krause R, Wenisch C. Laboratory diagnosis of *Mycoplasma pneumoniae* infection. Clin Microbiol Infect 2003;9(4):263–273.

50. Razin S. DNA probes and PCR in diagnosis of mycoplasma infections. Mol Cell Probes 1994;8(6):497–511.

51. Guris D, Strebel PM, Bardenheier B, et al. Changing epidemiology of pertussis in the United States: increasing reported incidence among adolescents and adults, 1990–1996. Clin Infect Dis 1999;28(6):1230–1237.

52. Schellekens J, von Konig CH, Gardner P. Pertussis sources of infection and routes of transmission in the vaccination era. Pediatr Infect Dis J 2005;24(5 Suppl):S19–S24.

53. Mattoo S, Cherry JD. Molecular pathogenesis, epidemiology, and clinical manifestations of respiratory infections due to *Bordetella pertussis* and other *Bordetella* subspecies. Clin Microbiol Rev 2005;18(2):326–382.

54. Locht C, Antoine R, Jacob-Dubuisson F. *Bordetella pertussis*, molecular pathogenesis under multiple aspects. Curr Opin Microbiol 2001;4(1):82–89.

55. Jenkinson D. Natural course of 500 consecutive cases of whooping cough: a general practice population study. BMJ 1995;310(6975):299–302.

56. Ewanowich CA, Chui LW, Paranchych MG, et al. Major outbreak of pertussis in northern Alberta, Canada: analysis of discrepant direct fluorescent-antibody and culture results by using polymerase chain reaction methodology. J Clin Microbiol 1993;31(7):1715–1725.

57. Loeffelholz MJ, Thompson CJ, Long KS, Gilchrist MJ. Comparison of PCR, culture, and direct fluorescent-antibody testing for detection of *Bordetella pertussis*. J Clin Microbiol 1999;37(9):2872–2876.

58. Zetola N, Francis JS, Nuermberger EL, Bishai WR. Community-acquired methicillin-resistant *Staphylococcus aureus*: an emerging threat. Lancet Infect Dis 2005;5(5): 275–286.

59. Lina G, Piemont Y, Godail-Gamot F, et al. Involvement of Panton-Valentine leukocidin-producing *Staphylococcus aureus* in primary skin infections and pneumonia. Clin Infect Dis 1999;29(5):1128–1132.

60. Fey PD, Said-Salim B, Rupp ME, et al. Comparative molecular analysis of community- or hospital-acquired methicillin-resistant *Staphylococcus aureus*. Antimicrob Agents Chemother 2003;47(1):196–203.

61. Palavecino E. Community-acquired methicillin-resistant *Staphylococcus aureus* infections. Clin Lab Med 2004;24(2): 403–418.

62. Kuehnert MJ, Doyle TJ, Hill HA, et al. Clinical features that discriminate inhalational anthrax from other acute respiratory illnesses. Clin Infect Dis 2003;36(3):328–336.

63. Karwa M, Currie B, Kvetan V. Bioterrorism: preparing for the impossible or the improbable. Crit Care Med 2005;33(1 Suppl):S75–S95.

64. Greenfield RA, Bronze MS. Prevention and treatment of bacterial diseases caused by bacterial bioterrorism threat agents. Drug Discov Today 2003;8(19):881–888.

65. Lim DV, Simpson JM, Kearns EA, Kramer MF. Current and developing technologies for monitoring agents of bioterrorism and biowarfare. Clin Microbiol Rev 2005;18(4): 583–607.

40
Immunopathology of Tuberculosis

Jeffrey K. Actor, Robert L. Hunter, Jr., and Chinnaswamy Jagannath

Introduction: Magnitude of Disease

Tuberculosis remains one of the world's leading infectious causes of death. According to the World Health Organization, the disease is currently spreading at the rate of one person per second. Tuberculosis is a contagious bacterial disease primarily involving the lungs, which develops after inhalation of infected droplets released following a cough from someone infected with the *Mycobacterium tuberculosis* (M-TB) agent. One third of the world's population is infected with M-TB, resulting annually in approximately 9 million new tuberculosis cases and approximately 2 million tuberculosis deaths. The virulence of the combination of tuberculosis and human immunodeficiency virus and the rise of multidrug-resistant organisms are ominous developments. In response to the challenge of resurgent disease, numerous investigators are using the best tools of modern science to combat the disease. Nevertheless, there are surprising gaps in our knowledge of tuberculosis, especially secondary tuberculosis, the form that produces most clinical illness and nearly all transmissions of infection.

Mycobacterium tuberculosis is a facultative intracellular pathogen that replicates and survives inside mammalian macrophage hosts. It is an acid-fast, Gram-positive aerobe that contains a unique cell wall with dominant mycolic acid constituents. The genome of M-TB is approximately 4.41 Mb^2 and can code for roughly 4,000 proteins.[3] It has an extremely slow growth rate (a doubling time of 18 hr), perhaps contributed by a cell envelope that is rich in waxes and lipids, especially mycolic acids, which are covalently linked to arabinogalactans. Multiple clinical strains exist, distinguished primarily by genetic methods that identify copy numbers of unique insertion sequences (IS6110 chromosomal elements).[4]

Primary and Secondary Tuberculosis Pathology

The different human responses to clinical isolates manifest as a broad range of pathologic states in humans. Many people remain asymptomatic throughout life, harboring latent organisms, whereas others die of rapidly progressing disease. Latent organisms usually reactivate in the lung but may selectively attack kidney, bone, brain, or other organs, or they may disseminate widely in a miliary fashion.[5] Infections can be controlled, but seldom eradicated, by immunologic mechanisms requiring T lymphocytes.[6] The "cycle" of infection is outlined in Figure 40.1. *Mycobacterium tuberculosis* produces two major forms of disease (primary and secondary–postprimary manifestation) that arise via different pathologic processes.[7–9]

Primary infection initiates within the lungs following the first exposure to infection when M-TB are inhaled. The infection spreads via lymphatics and may involve multiple sites. In the majority of cases within immunocompetent hosts, infection is controlled and usually regresses, leaving behind little to no evidence of past encounter with organisms. Primary infection can produce progressive disease. Development of pathologic manifestations can occur in which organism load increases and immune mechanisms dictate development of protective sequestration of organisms. Patients with primary tuberculosis may be quite ill, but they almost never transmit infection to others, because the organisms remain deep within tissue. In this scenario, the organisms rapidly spread from the lung to lymph nodes and then hematogenously throughout the body. The infection is typically arrested and the lesions heal in 10–12 weeks with the development of effective cell-mediated immunity. Complications arise when immune function is impaired, or

419

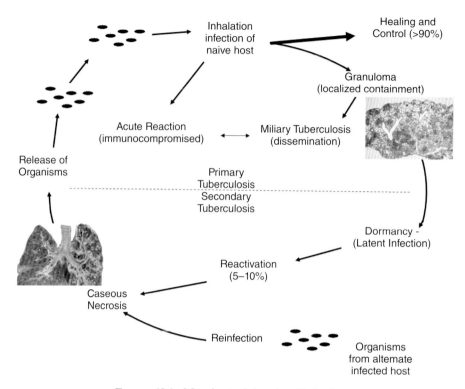

FIGURE 40.1. Mycobacterial cycle of infection.

responses are delayed, in which case syndrome may progress to meningitis or other disseminated disease. The lesions arise when proliferative (sometimes called *productive*) granulomas grow progressively in tissue to form discrete nodules or tubercles.[7] In the lung, these granulomas are located within alveolar septa and lung tissue. In primary tuberculosis, the alveolar spaces remain empty. The initial focal lesion is referred to as a *Ghon complex*, a subpleural lesion characterized by enlarged caseous lymph nodes stemming from draining pulmonary parenchyma. At this point, the patient is asymptomatic.

The granulomatous response is the characteristic histologic feature of M-TB infection essential for organism containment and control of organism growth (Figure 40.2). Both strong delayed type hypersensitivity response (DTH) and cell-mediated immunity are required for protection against active disease. Macrophages are continuously recruited to developing granulomas. However, the macrophages do not kill the bacteria until they are sufficiently activated by cell-mediated function, and the bacteria do not injure macrophages before the development of a different type of both cell-mediated immunity and DTH response involving lymphocytes.[10] If insufficiently activated to kill ingested organisms, the macrophages are destroyed by DTH and accumulate as slowly expanding caseating granulomas.[9,11] Caseation results from destruction of insufficiently activated macrophages with bacilli.[6] The lesions grow when intracellular multiplication and death of M-TB at the periphery of granulomas produce sufficient antigens to activate DTH, leading to overall increase in size of lesions.[10] High local concentrations of tuberculin-like products induce strong DTH reactions that cause necrosis.[10] Caseous centers enlarge progres-

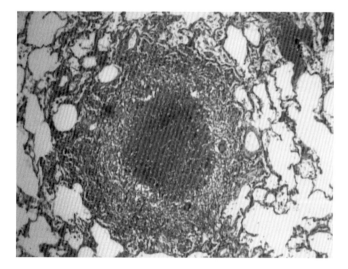

FIGURE 40.2. Primary infection with *Mycobacterium tuberculosis*. Alveolar macrophages that internalize *M. tuberculosis* are sequestered within granulomas during primary infection, allowing survival of the host and containment of organisms.

sively and destroy adjacent tissue because of ineffective macrophage activation.[6] These lesions typically heal within a few weeks in humans. The necrotic tissue is not absorbed but eventually calcifies and scars, leaving the characteristic Gohn complex. It is important to note that healing of primary tuberculosis does not kill all organisms. Some persist in the body for years to decades before they reactivate to produce secondary tuberculosis. In addition, a small proportion of patients fail to heal primary pulmonary lesions, in which case pathology may progress and regress many times over a period of years to decades.

In the absence of immune function defects, it is estimated that >90% of all contained infections will remain dormant, with a strong genetic component dictating outcome.[12] However, in the remaining minority of cases, reactivation occurs at a later time, representing secondary pulmonary tuberculosis. The secondary lesion is located at the apex of both lungs, thought to initiate when granulomatous inflammation is unable to eliminate organisms or control expansion. The lesion starts as a small, focal nidus of tissue destruction, followed by fibrous encapsulation of an emergent necrotizing granuloma. At this stage appearance of a core of degenerating epithelioid and multinucleated giant (Langhans) cells are histologically prominent (Figure 40.3).[5,9]

The largest portion of human disease and nearly all transmission of infection result from secondary tuberculosis in the lung in which caseating granulomas give rise to cavities (Figure 40.4).[13–15] Secondary tuberculosis differs from primary infection in several important respects. Most importantly, it occurs only in persons with a high degree of specific immunity resulting from previ-

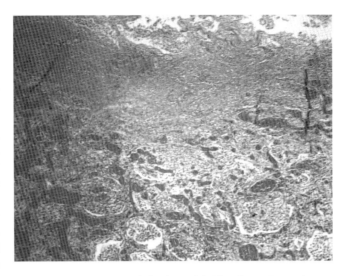

FIGURE 40.3. Secondary infection with *Mycobacterium tuberculosis*. Secondary tuberculosis, or reactivation tuberculosis, manifests as series of events culminating in necrotic damage. Depicted is a caseous pulmonary lesion with necrotic damage to bronchial walls **(top)**, with underlying acellular fibrosis **(middle)**. Immune responses are present, with evidence of pneumonitis and activated macrophages filling alveolar space **(bottom)**.

ous primary infection. In essence, its manifestation of pathology requires a strong competent immune response. Secondary tuberculosis may result from reactivation of dormant M-TB or, in some cases, reinfection with new organisms.[16,17] The infection does not spread via

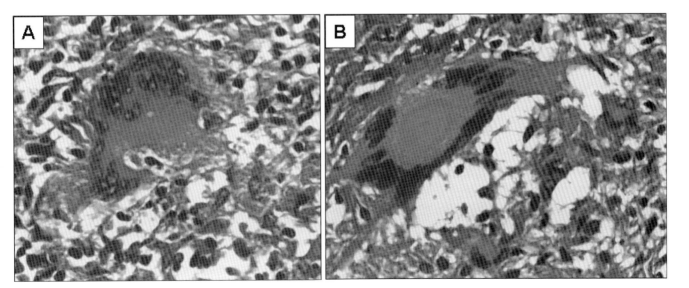

FIGURE 40.4. Multinucleated giant cells. Histologically prominent multinucleated giant cells are found during both primary **(A)** and secondary **(B)** manifestations of disease.

lymphatics and is typically confined to a small number of large foci usually in the lung.[12,13] It is characterized by nonhealing cavities in the lung that produce massive numbers of organisms that are coughed into the environment.[18]

Mycobacterium tuberculosis proliferate extracellularly within cavities and are coughed into the environment to infect new hosts. Secondary tuberculosis should not be confused with reactivation tuberculosis caused by immunosuppression, because immunosuppression reduces both caseating granulomas and cavities.[14,15] Rather, secondary tuberculosis is associated with strong immune responses that have been coopted by M-TB to produce caseating granulomas and cavities that facilitate extracellular proliferation of large numbers of organisms and their escape into the environment.[12,13,18]

Secondary human tuberculosis frequently begins abruptly as an exudative reaction of tuberculous pneumonia.[9,10] Whereas proliferative lesions are discrete granulomas, exudative lesions are inflammatory exudates that fill body spaces. They occur in adults primarily in the lung as tuberculous pneumonia.[13–15] Exudative pulmonary tuberculosis can be considered the inverse of proliferative tuberculosis in that the inflammation is confined to alveolar spaces with little or no disease in alveolar septa, whereas proliferative disease characteristically consists of granulomas within alveolar septa with little or no disease in alveolar spaces. Necrosis of exudative reactions produces caseating granulomas and cavities in human tuberculosis.[6,12,19] Caseating granulomas and secondary tuberculosis in humans develop through complex and prolonged processes subject to many controls and influences.

The term *caseation* is commonly used to embrace all forms of gross necrosis associated with tuberculosis.[20] Although there are several variations, caseation generally is a process of coagulation necrosis in which the cells, primarily macrophages, lose their outline, become irregular, no longer take stains and are finally converted into a homogeneous, structure-less substance composed largely of lipids.[5] The necrotic material forms a cheesy mass that may undergo softening, fibrous encapsulation, and calcification. During secondary infection, clinical presentations include classic symptoms of cough, weight loss, fatigue and fever, night sweats, and chills. Upon continued progression, the patient will experience anorexia, hemoptysis (coughing up blood), and pain with breathing or coughing due to pleurisy. At this time, clearly evident within tissue are small rounded tubercle nodules prominently attached to bone, mucous membrane, or skin. Miliary tuberculosis is characterized by a chronic, contagious bacterial infection caused by M-TB that has spread to other organs of the body by the blood or lymph system.

Tuberculosis generally affects the lungs but may cause infection in many other organs in the body, as exemplified by tuberculous meningitis in which M-TB is spread from other anatomic sites. The onset of symptoms is usually gradual. Risk factors include a history of pulmonary tuberculosis, excessive alcohol use, acquired immunodeficiency syndrom, and/or other disorders that compromise the immune system. Approximately 1% of people affected with tuberculosis will develop associated arthritis (tuberculous arthritis, granulomatous arthritis). The joints most frequently involved are the spine, hips, knees, wrists, and ankles. Most cases involve just one joint. Tuberculosis involving the spine is often referred to as *Pott's disease*. Indeed, secondary pulmonary tuberculosis develops preferentially in young immunocompetent adults aged 15–45 years.[7] In the aged, tuberculosis typically runs a slower course with pulmonary interstitial inflammation leading to pulmonary fibrosis rather than cavities.[13–15,18] Finally, secondary tuberculosis should not be confused with accelerated tuberculosis in immunocompromised states. People with acquired immunodeficiency syndrome are more likely to die of disseminated tuberculosis because they fail to develop cell-mediated immunity. However, they seldom develop pulmonary cavities and are less able to transmit infection to others than are fully immunocompetent people.[21,22] On clinical and epidemiologic grounds, secondary tuberculosis requires fully immunocompetent hosts to develop strong cell-mediated immune responses that can be subverted in the lung to produce cavities.

Immune Response to Tuberculosis

Many of the mechanisms leading to our understanding of the immunopathology have been identified through animal models. Research on tuberculosis is limited by available models. There are no models of secondary tuberculosis, the form of disease that is responsible for most disease in adults and nearly all transmissions of infection.[16,23,24] In addition, existing models in mice do not produce the most characteristic lesions of tuberculosis in humans, caseating granulomas.[16,23] However, it is clear that tissue damage in tuberculosis is not a direct result of bacterial toxicity but is largely an immunopathology associated with strong immune responses.

Protection against M-TB infection is highly dependent on the host's ability to launch an effective cell-mediated immune response.[25–27] A major hallmark of this response is the formation of granulomas, nodule-like masses of cells consisting primarily of activated macrophages and T lymphocytes.[28] T-cell–derived cytokines and macrophage products establish an environment for bacterial containment.[29–32] While the granulomas function to contain the infection and prevent dissemination, they also contribute to tissue damage within the host.[33,34] Antigen-specific T cells are essential in maintenance of the granuloma and secrete cytokines, which help to activate macrophages and increase bacterial killing [19,26]. Despite initiation of the host immune response, M-TB employs various mechanisms to avoid detection and destruction within the macrophage. The lipid-rich cell wall of M-TB contains several factors that contribute to its survival within the host.[20,35,36] Glycolipids, such as trehalose 6,6′-dimycolate (TDM), located in the mycobacterial cell wall are important components of this defense mechanism.[20,36,37]

The immune response to tuberculosis may be divided into phases encompassing initial reactivity to organisms and responses generated leading to either protection or active disease. The primary encounter of inhaled organisms leads to infection of alveolar cells, of which encounter with either dendritic cells or macrophages leads to a cascade of events that push the immune response toward generating a protective antiinfective response.[38] More than likely, initial interactions involve recognition by way of the Toll-like receptors (TLRs)[39] on the surface of the host cell, with response mediated through both myeloid differentiation factor 88[40,41] and Toll-like domain-containing adaptor protein pathways.[42,43] The interactions include lipids, lipoarabinomannans, and phosphatidylinositol mannosides ($PIM_{1,2}$, $PIM_{4,6}$) and mycobacterial DNA through TLR1, TLR2, TLR4, and TLR9.[40,44,45] Production of interleukin (IL)-12 occurs, leading to generation of natural killer, CD4+, and CD8+ cellular responses.[46] all of which are considered required for protection against mycobacteria.[47-49] A strong T-cell response involves both interferon-γ and tumor necrosis factor-α,[47,50-52] which assist in control of pathogen proliferation. CD4+ T helper cells assist in activation of macrophages to kill internalized organisms as well as provide assistance to CD8+ cells to kill via perforin and granulysin mechanisms.[53,54] What remains is a nidus of latently infected macrophages that are contained by T cells creating a granulomatous response that limits organism dissemination to other tissue and subdues active immunopathologic response.

The net result of granuloma formation is of benefit to both the host and the organism, allowing control of infection while providing a place for organisms to hide until time for expansion and subsequent transmission to other individuals.[33,34] The goal of the mycobacterium is to survive in the host long enough to be passed to other hosts. The organism has evolved perfect adaptation with the human host to circumvent immune function and allow survival within the professional phagocyte. Indeed, evasion mechanisms are multifaceted, benefiting persistence and long-term survival of organisms to allow later infection of hosts at sites far from the initial site of organism encounter. Table 40.1[55-70] lists some of the mechanisms used by M-TB toward achieving immune evasion.

Mycobacterium tuberculosis has the unique ability to survive within macrophages using diverse strategies,

TABLE 40.1. Mechanisms of immune evasion.

Mechanisms	References
Evasion of phagosome–lysosome fusion and phagosome maturation events	55–59
Differential entry mechanisms into phagocytes	60
Occupation of phagocytes that express low levels of presentation molecules; downregulation of class II/CD1 expression in infected cells	61, 62
Differential processing of mycobacterial antigens	63, 64
Regulation of cortisol and glucocorticoid response	65–67
Delay of CD4+ and CD8+ cellular responses	68
Regulation in trafficking and recruitment	69, 70

become dormant, and revive to cause reactivation. The pathogenesis of M-TB within macrophages is one of the most intensely studied topics and is mechanistically outlined in Figure 40.5. It should be noted that M-TB infects the alveolar macrophages when it comes in contact with the human host, and yet the plethora of studies performed to date have mostly been on macrophages derived from either human peripheral blood or mouse tissue such as bone marrow. Although some functional differences are likely to exist between the phenotype of alveolar macrophages and macrophages from other tissues such as lungs, spleens, lymph nodes and peripheral blood mononuclear cells, M-TB within macrophages shows some common themes of survival. Armstrong and Hart observed that M-TB phagosomes do not fuse with lysosomes in murine peritoneal macrophages, to avoid being killed by lysosomal hydrolases.[71] This observation has been repeatedly confirmed by over the years by other investigators using mouse as well as human macrophages.[72-75] Studies have also confirmed that surface TDM is critically involved in inhibition of trafficking of mycobacteria to acidic compartments.[55,76]

Our understanding of the phagosome–lysosome fusion phenomenon has been enhanced by advances in understanding endosomal sorting events within macrophages. Thus, "phagosome maturation" is an orderly process in which the phagocytosed bacteria are enclosed within a membrane sac termed *phagosome* that progressively fuses with various early and late endosomal compartments to culminate in the fusion with lysosomes. A distinct set of endosome traffic regulating proteins such as Rab and SNARE proteins regulate these endosomal sorting events. There is general agreement that the consequence of phagosome–lysosome fusion is the enzymatic breakdown of bacteria in the lysosomes through a variety of lipases and proteases. Interestingly, a series of studies have shown that M-TB does not fuse with the lysosomes, although it does fuse with early endosomes and certain late endosomal compartments. Thus, M-TB phagosomes can acquire membrane-derived glycosphingolipids as well as transferrin through docking with early

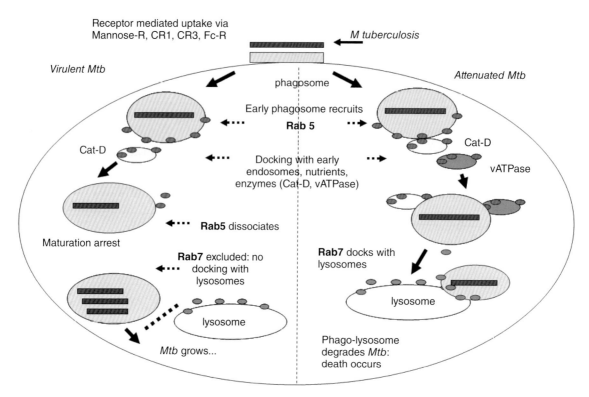

FIGURE 40.5. Survival with macrophages. Alveolar macrophages that internalize *Mycobacterium tuberculosis* (Mtb) are not capable of killing virulent organisms. Virulent organisms (e.g., H37Rv, Erdman) **(left)** are trafficked different from avirulent strains (e.g., H37Ra) **(right)**, which are eliminated. Virulent *M. tuberculosis* acquire Rab5 that enables fusion with early endosomes delivering nutrients but without acquisition of molecules allowing fusion with lysosomes. Thus, virulent organisms are not killed by lysosomal enzymes. In contrast, avirulent mycobacteria acquire enzymes (cathepsins [Cat-D], ATPase) that allow acidification of the phagosomes that will fuse with lysosomes and activate hydrolases to lower pH. Recent evidence suggests that virulent *M. tuberculosis* also excludes phagocyte oxidase and inducible nitric oxide synthase, that are normally involved in killing *M. tuberculosis* within the phagosomes.

endosomes.[77,78] It has been proposed that these events are necessary for the pathogen to receive nutrients from macrophages and grow. Consistent with these early fusion events, M-TB phagosomes label for early traffic-regulating proteins as such Rab5, but they do not label for Rab7, a marker of lysosomes.[72] *Mycobacterium tuberculosis* phagosomes also dock with endosomes originating from the trans-Golgi network that deliver cathepsin-D [79]. However, mycobacteria exclude the enzyme vacuolar proton adenosine triphosphatase that is essential for the acidification of the phagosome.[73] As a consequence, the cathepsin-D enzyme, that is dependent on an acidic pH-dependent autocatalysis, remains in an immature 46kDa form.

Recent studies have also obtained molecular evidence for the propensity of M-TB phagosomes to fuse with early endosomes and avoid phagosome–lysosome fusion. The mycobacterial phosphatidylinositol analog phosphatidylinositol mannoside has been found to stimulate early endosomal fusion.[80] In contrast, glycosylated phosphatidylinositol has been found to cause phagosome maturation arrest.[81]

A major mechanism of bactericidal activity of macrophages against M-TB is the production of nitric oxide by inducible nitric oxide synthase (iNOS).[82,83] Treatment of murine macrophages by the nitric oxide inhibitor N-monomethyl arginine enhances the survival of M-TB, and iNOS knockout mice are more susceptible to tuberculosis.[82] It should be noted here that the expression of iNOS in human macrophages has been disputed as is the role of iNOS against M-TB in human infections. *Mycobacterium tuberculosis* appears to be less susceptible to reactive oxygen species (ROS) produced by phagocyte oxidase, because it produces superoxide dismutase and catalase that inactivate ROS.[82] However, a *katG* mutant M-TB strain deficient in catalase grows better than the wild-type M-TB in ROS-deficient mice.[84] It has been proposed that ROS are indeed active within macrophages against M-TB and that they may synergize with nitric oxide to form peroxynitrite, which in turn can potentially kill M-TB.[82] Interestingly, mycobacteria exclude iNOS in murine macrophages, and M-TB has been proposed to avoid killing by iNOS by similarly excluding iNOS [85]. Recent evidence suggests that M-TB also excludes phagocyte oxidase in murine macrophages (C. Jagannath, personal communication, in press).

The foregoing studies indicate that M-TB is capable of modulating and maintaining the pathogenicity within macrophages by altering its trafficking behavior. It should be noted that only live virulent M-TB has the ability to maintain a dynamic M-TB phagosome that contains nutrients and membranes sufficient for survival of the pathogen. It appears to inactivate proteolytic host enzymes by excluding acid pumps and to avoid killing by oxidants by excluding iNOS and phagocyte oxidase. For these reasons, live virulent M-TB exhibit a "phagosome maturation arrest," and M-TB has been considered as the most elusive of all intracellular pathogens.

The immune signals for reactivation tuberculosis, and subsequent cavitary disease leading to spread of infection to new individuals, remains unclear. However, most observations and models of late-stage infection include aspects of immune mediation revolving around the pathogenic Koch phenomenon in which strong secondary responses are involved at the terminal stage of disease, leading to tissue damage and release of bacteria to spread to other individuals. Multiple factors come into play, many involving a depression in regulation of lymphocytic responses,[86,87] with a possible requirement for complement component C5 in granulomatous formation.[88] Recent evidence also suggests that lipids from the surface of organisms may be released, allowing interaction with natural lung lipids to form a toxic monolayer.[20] What is clear is that reactivation involves both local mediation, as well as systemic interplay, such as that identified by systemic dysregulation in active cortisol (11-hydroxy) relative to inactive (11-keto) glucocorticoid derivatives.[65,66,89–91]

Conclusion

The underlying pathology of tuberculosis is heavily dependent on host immune function. Indeed, a strong immune response is critical for development of the caseating granulomas, which are the characteristic lesion of active tuberculosis. The entire granulomatous process is one that benefits both the host and parasite in tuberculosis. Sequestration of organisms in a hostile environment allows survival, which eventually facilitates transmission to new hosts. Improved understanding of primary protection that leads to latency where bugs survive for long periods of time and of secondary response that initiates caseating granulomas critical for spread of disease is a high priority for researchers in the coming years.

References

1. World Health Organization. Global tuberculosis control. Surveillance, planning, financing. In The World Health Report 2006. Geneva: World Health Organization; 2006.
2. Garnier T, Eiglmeier K, Camus JC, et al. The complete genome sequence of *Mycobacterium bovis*. Proc Natl Acad Sci USA 2003;100(13):7877–7882.
3. Camus JC, Pryor MJ, Medigue C, Cole ST. Re-annotation of the genome sequence of *Mycobacterium tuberculosis* H37Rv. Microbiology 2002;148(Pt 10):2967–2973.
4. Mostrom P, Gordon M, Sola C, et al. Methods used in the molecular epidemiology of tuberculosis. Clin Microbiol Infect 2002;8(11):694–704.
5. Gunn FD. Tuberculosis. St Louis: Mosby; 1961.
6. Dannenberg AM Jr. Roles of cytotoxic delayed-type hypersensitivity and macrophage-activating cell-mediated immunity in the pathogenesis of tuberculosis. Immunobiology 1994;191(4–5):461–473.
7. Florey H. Tuberculosis. Philadelphia: WB Saunders; 1958.
8. Garay S. Pulmonary Tuberculosis. Boston: Little Brown & Co.; 1996.
9. Dannenberg AM Jr, Thoashefski JFJ. Pathogenesis of Pulmonary Tuberculosis. New York: McGraw Hill; 1988.
10. Dannenberg AM Jr, Collins FM. Progressive pulmonary tuberculosis is not due to increasing numbers of viable bacilli in rabbits, mice and guinea pigs, but is due to a continuous host response to mycobacterial products. Tuberculosis (Edinb) 2001;81(3):229–242.
11. Kumar V, Fausto N, Abbas A. Pathologic Basis of Disease, 7th ed. Philadelphia: WB Saunders; 2005.
12. Alcais A, Fieschi C, Abel L, Casanova JL. Tuberculosis in children and adults: two distinct genetic diseases. J Exp Med 2005;202(12):1617–1621.
13. Osler W. Tuberculosis. New York: D. Appleton and Co.; 1892.
14. Slavin RE. Late generalized tuberculosis: a clinical and pathologic analysis of a diagnostic puzzle and a changing pattern. Pathol Annu 1981;16(Pt 1):81–99.
15. Slavin RE, Walsh TJ, Pollack AD. Late generalized tuberculosis: a clinical pathologic analysis and comparison of 100 cases in the preantibiotic and antibiotic eras. Medicine (Baltimore) 1980;59(5):352–366.
16. North RJ, Jung YJ. Immunity to tuberculosis. Annu Rev Immunol 2004;22:599–623.
17. Smith I. *Mycobacterium tuberculosis* pathogenesis and molecular determinants of virulence. Clin Microbiol Rev 2003;16(3):463–496.
18. Levine ER. Classification of reinfection pulmonary tuberculosis. In E. Hayes E, ed. The Fundamentals of Pulmonary Tuberculosis and its Complications. Springfield, IL: Charles C. Thomas; 1949:97–113.
19. Ulrichs T, Kaufmann SH. New insights into the function of granulomas in human tuberculosis. J Pathol 2006;208(2): 261–269.
20. Hunter RL, Olsen M, Jagannath C, Actor JK. Trehalose 6,6′-dimycolate and lipid in the pathogenesis of caseating granulomas of tuberculosis in mice. Am J Pathol 2006; 168(4):1249–1261.

21. Aaron L, Saadoun D, Calatroni I, et al. Tuberculosis in HIV-infected patients: a comprehensive review. Clin Microbiol Infect 2004;10(5):388–398.

22. Ledru E, Ledru S, Zoubga A. Granuloma formation and tuberculosis transmission in HIV-infected patients. Immunol Today 1999;20(7):336–337.

23. McMurray DN, Collins FM, Dannenberg AM Jr, Smith DW. Pathogenesis of experimental tuberculosis in animal models. Curr Top Microbiol Immunol 1996;215:157–179.

24. Druilhe P, Hagan P, Rook GA. The importance of models of infection in the study of disease resistance. Trends Microbiol 2002;10(10 Suppl):S38–S46.

25. Kaufmann SH, Cole ST, Mizrahi V, et al. Mycobacterium tuberculosis and the host response. J Exp Med 2005;201(11): 1693–1697.

26. Kaufmann SH. Protection against tuberculosis: cytokines, T cells, and macrophages. Ann Rheum Dis 2002;61 (Suppl 2):ii54–ii58.

27. Rook GA, Zumla A. Advances in the immunopathogenesis of pulmonary tuberculosis. Curr Opin Pulm Med 2001;7(3): 116–123.

28. Maes HH, Causse JE, Maes RF. Tuberculosis I: a conceptual frame for the immunopathology of the disease. Med Hypotheses 1999;52(6):583–593.

29. Actor JK, Leonard CD, Watson VE, Wells A, et al. Cytokine mRNA expression and serum cortisol evaluation during murine lung inflammation induced by Mycobacterium tuberculosis. Comb Chem High Throughput Screen 2000;3(4):343–51.

30. Johnson CM, Cooper AM, Frank AA, Orme IM. Adequate expression of protective immunity in the absence of granuloma formation in Mycobacterium tuberculosis–infected mice with a disruption in the intracellular adhesion molecule 1 gene. Infect Immun 1998;66(4):1666–1670.

31. Orme IM, Andersen P, Boom WH. T cell response to Mycobacterium tuberculosis. J Infect Dis 1993;167(6):1481–1497.

32. Orme IM, Lee BY, Appelberg R, et al. T cell response in acquired protective immunity to Mycobacterium tuberculosis infection. Bull Int Union Tuberc Lung Dis 1991;66(1): 7–13.

33. Actor JK, Olsen M, Jagannath C, Hunter RL. Relationship of survival, organism containment, and granuloma formation in acute murine tuberculosis. J Interferon Cytokine Res 1999;19(10):1183–1193.

34. Flynn JL, Chan J. What's good for the host is good for the bug. Trends Microbiol 2005;13(3):98–102.

35. Karakousis PC, Bishai WR, Dorman SE. Mycobacterium tuberculosis cell envelope lipids and the host immune response. Cell Microbiol 2004;6(2):105–116.

36. Fenton MJ, Vermeulen MW. Immunopathology of tuberculosis: roles of macrophages and monocytes. Infect Immun 1996;64(3):683–690.

37. Perez RL, Roman J, Roser S, et al. Cytokine message and protein expression during lung granuloma formation and resolution induced by the mycobacterial cord factor trehalose-6,6'-dimycolate. J Interferon Cytokine Res 2000;20(9): 795–804.

38. Hickman SP, Chan J, Salgame P. Mycobacterium tuberculosis induces differential cytokine production from dendritic cells and macrophages with divergent effects on naive T cell polarization. J Immunol 2002;168(9):4636–4642.

39. Brightbill HD, Libraty DH, Krutzik SR, et al. Host defense mechanisms triggered by microbial lipoproteins through toll-like receptors. Science 1999;285(5428):732–736.

40. Scanga CA, Bafica A, Feng CG, et al. MyD88-deficient mice display a profound loss in resistance to Mycobacterium tuberculosis associated with partially impaired Th1 cytokine and nitric oxide synthase 2 expression. Infect Immun 2004;72(4):2400–2404.

41. Feng CG, Scanga CA, Collazo-Custodio CM, et al. Mice lacking myeloid differentiation factor 88 display profound defects in host resistance and immune responses to Mycobacterium avium infection not exhibited by Toll-like receptor 2 (TLR2)- and TLR4-deficient animals. J Immunol 2003;171(9):4758–4764.

42. Shi S, Blumenthal A, Hickey CM, et al. Expression of many immunologically important genes in Mycobacterium tuberculosis infected macrophages is independent of both TLR2 and TLR4 but dependent on IFN-alphabeta receptor and STAT1. J Immunol 2005;175(5):3318–3328.

43. Bulut Y, Michelsen KS, Hayrapetian L, et al. Mycobacterium tuberculosis heat shock proteins use diverse Toll-like receptor pathways to activate pro-inflammatory signals. J Biol Chem 2005;280(22):20961–20967.

44. Quesniaux V, Fremond C, Jacobs M, et al. Toll-like receptor pathways in the immune responses to mycobacteria. Microbes Infect 2004;6(10):946–959.

45. Bafica A, Scanga CA, Feng CG, et al. TLR9 regulates Th1 responses and cooperates with TLR2 in mediating optimal resistance to Mycobacterium tuberculosis. J Exp Med 2005; 202(12):1715–1724.

46. Trinchieri G, Gerosa F. Immunoregulation by interleukin-12. J Leuk Biol 1996;59(4):505–511.

47. Cooper AM, Flynn JL. The protective immune response to Mycobacterium tuberculosis. Curr Opin Immunol 1995;7(4): 512–516.

48. Cooper AM, Magram J, Ferrante J, Orme IM. Interleukin 12 (IL-12) is crucial to the development of protective immunity in mice intravenously infected with Mycobacterium tuberculosis. J Exp Med 1997;186(1):39–45.

49. Cooper AM, Roberts AD, Rhoades ER, et al. The role of interleukin-12 in acquired immunity to Mycobacterium tuberculosis infection. Immunology 1995;84(3):423–432.

50. Orme IM, Cooper AM. Cytokine/chemokine cascades in immunity to tuberculosis. Immunol Today 1999;20(7):307–312.

51. Saunders BM, Cooper AM. Restraining mycobacteria: role of granulomas in mycobacterial infections. Immunol Cell Biol 2000;78(4):334–341.

52. Mohan VP, Scanga CA, Yu K, et al. Effects of tumor necrosis factor alpha on host immune response in chronic persistent tuberculosis: possible role for limiting pathology. Infect Immun 2001;69(3):1847–1855.

53. Serbina NV, Liu CC, Scanga CA, Flynn JL. CD8+ CTL from lungs of Mycobacterium tuberculosis–infected mice

express perforin in vivo and lyse infected macrophages. J Immunol 2000;165(1):353–363.

54. Scanga CA, Mohan VP, Joseph H, et al. Reactivation of latent tuberculosis: variations on the Cornell murine model. Infect Immun 1999;67(9):4531–4538.

55. Indrigo J, Hunter RL Jr, Actor JK. Influence of trehalose 6,6′-dimycolate (TDM) during mycobacterial infection of bone marrow macrophages. Microbiology 2002;148(Pt 7):1991–1998.

56. Russell DG. Phagosomes, fatty acids and tuberculosis. Nat Cell Biol 2003;5(9):776–778.

57. Pieters J, Gatfield J. Hijacking the host: survival of pathogenic mycobacteria inside macrophages. Trends Microbiol 2002;10(3):142–146.

58. Vergne I, Chua J, Lee HH, et al. Mechanism of phagolysosome biogenesis block by viable *Mycobacterium tuberculosis*. Proc Natl Acad Sci USA 2005;102(11):4033–4038.

59. Deretic V, Singh S, Master S, et al. *Mycobacterium tuberculosis* inhibition of phagolysosome biogenesis and autophagy as a host defense mechanism. Cell Microbiol 2006;8(5):719–727.

60. Ernst JD. Macrophage receptors for *Mycobacterium tuberculosis*. Infect Immun 1998;66(4):1277–1281.

61. VanHeyningen TK, Collins HL, Russell DG. IL-6 produced by macrophages infected with *Mycobacterium* species suppresses T cell responses. J Immunol 1997;158(1):330–337.

62. Stenger S, Niazi KR, Modlin RL. Down-regulation of CD1 on antigen-presenting cells by infection with *Mycobacterium tuberculosis*. J Immunol 1998;161(7):3582–3588.

63. Ramachandra L, Smialek JL, Shank SS, et al. Phagosomal processing of *Mycobacterium tuberculosis* antigen 85B is modulated independently of mycobacterial viability and phagosome maturation. Infect Immun 2005;73(2):1097–1105.

64. Ramachandra L, Noss E, Boom WH, Harding CV. Processing of *Mycobacterium tuberculosis* antigen 85B involves intraphagosomal formation of peptide–major histocompatibility complex II complexes and is inhibited by live bacilli that decrease phagosome maturation. J Exp Med 2001;194(10):1421–1432.

65. Actor JK, Indrigo J, Beachdel CM, et al. A Mycobacterial glycolipid cord factor trehalose 6,6′-dimycolate causes a decrease in serum cortisol during the granulomatous response. Neuroimmunomodulation 2002;10(5):270–282.

66. Rook GA, Hernandez-Pando R. The pathogenesis of tuberculosis. Annu Rev Microbiol 1996;50:259–284.

67. Dheda K, Booth H, Huggett JF, et al. Lung remodeling in pulmonary tuberculosis. J Infect Dis 2005;192(7):1201–1209.

68. Feng CG, Bean AG, Hooi H, et al. Increase in gamma interferon-secreting CD8(+), as well as CD4(+), T cells in lungs following aerosol infection with *Mycobacterium tuberculosis*. Infect Immun 1999;67(7):3242–3247.

69. Peters W, Ernst JD. Mechanisms of cell recruitment in the immune response to *Mycobacterium tuberculosis*. Microbes Infect 2003;5(2):151–158.

70. Actor JK, Breij E, Wetsel RA, et al. A role for complement C5 in organism containment and granulomatous response during murine tuberculosis. Scand J Immunol 2001;53(5):464–474.

71. Armstrong JA, Hart PD. Phagosome–lysosome interactions in cultured macrophages infected with virulent tubercle bacilli. Reversal of the usual nonfusion pattern and observations on bacterial survival. J Exp Med 1975;142(1):1–16.

72. Via LE, Deretic D, Ulmer RJ, et al. Arrest of mycobacterial phagosome maturation is caused by a block in vesicle fusion between stages controlled by rab5 and rab7. J Biol Chem 1997;272(20):13326–13331.

73. Sturgill-Koszycki S, Schlesinger PH, Chakraborty P, et al. Lack of acidification in *Mycobacterium* phagosomes produced by exclusion of the vesicular proton-ATPase. Science 1994;263(5147):678–681.

74. Kusner DJ, Barton JA. ATP stimulates human macrophages to kill intracellular virulent *Mycobacterium tuberculosis* via calcium-dependent phagosome–lysosome fusion. J Immunol 2001;167(6):3308–3315.

75. Clemens DL, Lee BY, Horwitz MA. The *Mycobacterium tuberculosis* phagosome in human macrophages is isolated from the host cell cytoplasm. Infect Immun 2002;70(10):5800–5807.

76. Indrigo J, Hunter RL Jr, Actor JK. Cord factor trehalose 6,6′-dimycolate (TDM) mediates trafficking events during mycobacterial infection of murine macrophages. Microbiology 2003;149(Pt 8):2049–2059.

77. Clemens DL, Horwitz MA. The *Mycobacterium tuberculosis* phagosome interacts with early endosomes and is accessible to exogenously administered transferrin. J Exp Med 1996;184(4):1349–1355.

78. Sturgill-Koszycki S, Schaible UE, Russell DG. *Mycobacterium*-containing phagosomes are accessible to early endosomes and reflect a transitional state in normal phagosome biogenesis. EMBO J 1996;15(24):6960–6968.

79. Ullrich HJ, Beatty WL, Russell DG. Direct delivery of procathepsin D to phagosomes: implications for phagosome biogenesis and parasitism by *Mycobacterium*. Eur J Cell Biol 1999;78(10):739–748.

80. Vergne I, Fratti RA, Hill PJ, et al. *Mycobacterium tuberculosis* phagosome maturation arrest: mycobacterial phosphatidylinositol analog phosphatidylinositol mannoside stimulates early endosomal fusion. Mol Biol Cell 2004;15(2):751–760.

81. Fratti RA, Chua J, Vergne I, Deretic V. *Mycobacterium tuberculosis* glycosylated phosphatidylinositol causes phagosome maturation arrest. Proc Natl Acad Sci USA 2003;100(9):5437–5442.

82. Nathan C, Shiloh MU. Reactive oxygen and nitrogen intermediates in the relationship between mammalian hosts and microbial pathogens. Proc Natl Acad Sci USA 2000;97(16):8841–8848.

83. Jagannath C, Actor JK, Hunter RL Jr. Induction of nitric oxide in human monocytes and monocyte cell lines by *Mycobacterium tuberculosis*. Nitric Oxide 1998;2(3):174–186.

84. Ng VH, Cox JS, Sousa AO, et al. Role of KatG catalase-peroxidase in mycobacterial pathogenesis: countering the

phagocyte oxidative burst. Mol Microbiol 2004;52(5):1291–1302.

85. Miller BH, Fratti RA, Poschet JF, et al. Mycobacteria inhibit nitric oxide synthase recruitment to phagosomes during macrophage infection. Infect Immun 2004;72(5): 2872–2878.

86. Scanga CA, Mohan VP, Yu K, et al. Depletion of CD4(+) T cells causes reactivation of murine persistent tuberculosis despite continued expression of interferon gamma and nitric oxide synthase 2. J Exp Med 2000;192(3):347–358.

87. Chan J, Flynn J. The immunological aspects of latency in tuberculosis. Clin Immunol 2004;110(1):2–12.

88. Jagannath C, Hoffmann H, Sepulveda E, et al. Hypersusceptibility of A/J mice to tuberculosis is in part due to a deficiency of the fifth complement component (C5). Scand J Immunol 2000;52(4):369–379.

89. Rook GA, al Attiyah R. Cytokines and the Koch phenomenon. Tubercle 1991;72(1):13–20.

90. Rook GA, Stanford JL. The Koch phenomenon and the immunopathology of tuberculosis. Curr Top Microbiol Immunol 1996;215:239–262.

91. Rook GA, al Attiyah R, Filley E. New insights into the immunopathology of tuberculosis. Pathobiology 1991; 59(3):148–52.

41
Molecular Pathology of Fungal Lung Infection

Michael R. McGinnis, Michael B. Smith, and Abida K. Haque

Introduction

Fungi are eukaryotic, unicellular or multicellular organisms that are larger and genomically more complex than bacteria. The fungal cell wall is complex and has polysaccharides, proteins, sugars, and glycoproteins. Plasma membranes of fungi contain ergosterol, which is the primary target for antifungal drugs such as amphotericin B. Although more than 1.3 million fungal species exist in the environment, only about 150 are pathogenic to humans.[1] The virulence factors of fungi resemble those of bacteria, such as possession of a capsule, adhesion molecules, toxins, free radicals, and so forth. Thus, fungi can elicit acute exudative, necrotizing, and granulomatous reactions in tissues. Although some generalizations are possible, the diverse structural and antigenic properties of individual fungi produce unique patterns of infection in individual hosts.[2,5]

Fungi have emerged as a major cause of infection within the past two decades. Although natural and acquired host defense systems are in place to prevent fungal infections, compromise of these mechanisms can result in serious progressive fungal infection. The principal defense mechanisms against fungal infections are innate and adaptive immunity. Both of these are interdependent, and effective host response requires a coordinated innate and adaptive immune response.

Innate Immunity

Innate immunity consists of protective mechanisms that were developed and maintained through evolution and exert a direct antifungal effect. Innate immunity plays a predominant role in clearance of inhaled fungal spores.[6] It also has an instructive role regarding adaptive immunity through antigen uptake and presentation and production of chemokines and cytokines. Initial mechanisms of innate immunity include the mechanical barrier of mucosa, microbial antagonism by normal flora, and peptides such as defensins and collectins involved in the uptake and phagocytosis of microorganisms by effector cells.[7,8] The second defense mechanism includes cells with innate phagocytic and antigen-presenting capability, including macrophages, monocytes, neutrophils, and dendritic cells. A third group that is involved to a variable extent includes natural killer (NK) cells, $\gamma\delta$T cells, and epithelial and endothelial cells.

Within the respiratory tract, mucociliary clearing is an essential first line of defense, forming a physical, chemical, and biologic barrier. The mucus contains secretory immunoglobulin A (sIgA), lysozyme, surfactant, and peroxidases, as well as phagocytic cells. Any spores that escape the mucociliary mechanism are ingested and killed by the phagocytic cells. The phagocytic cell surface receptors can recognize the surface structure of fungal mannan, allowing recognition and phagocytosis of fungal spores even in the absence of complement or specific antibodies. After binding and phagocytosis, the macrophages secrete proinflammatory cytokines such as interleukin (IL)-1, IL-6, interferon (IFN)-γ, and tumor necrosis factor (TNF)-α that activate other cells and augment the phagocytic and killing capacity of other phagocytes through oxidative mechanisms. The cytokines further activate the respiratory epithelial cells to induce a second wave of phagocytic cells to eliminate the fungal organisms.

Cellular Component of Immunity

Cells involved in innate immunity recognize fungal organisms mainly through components of the fungal cell wall acting as pathogen-associated molecular patterns (PAMPS). The PAMPS are recognized by pattern-recognizing receptors on the surface of the host cells, including Toll-like receptors (TLRs). Recognition leads to activation of phagocytic functions and induction of adaptive T-helper (Th) cell responses by dendritic cells.[9,10]

The antifungal phagocytic functions involve production of reactive oxygen molecules through oxidative enzymes such as nicotinamide adenine dinucleotide phosphate oxidase and nitric oxide synthase. The nonoxidative functions include degranulation and release of defensins, neutrophil cationic peptides, and other effector molecules.[8,11] Antifungal host response also includes production and activation of phagocytic cells from hematopoietic progenitor cells by granulocyte colony-stimulating factor, granulocyte–macrophage colony-stimulating factor, and macrophage colony-stimulating factor.[12,13]

Complement Component

Complement activation and deposition on the surface of the fungi enhance their phagocytosis and killing. The C3 component activation is particularly effective in respiratory defense. The sIgA is a specific adaptive immune response, because binding of the sIgA to the fungal surface prevents the binding of spores to the epithelium, thus facilitating clearance.

Phagocytic cells, an essential part of the innate defense mechanism against inhaled fungal spores, include macrophages, monocytes, and neutrophils. Spores that escape the first line of defense may germinate and grow as hyphae. Neutrophils are the most effective protection against the fungal hyphae, because they are too large for effective phagocytosis. Neutrophils attach to the hyphae and release toxic oxygen radicals and cationic peptides to induce damage.[14] Neutropenia is thus the most significant predisposing factor for invasive candidiasis and aspergillosis. That oxygen radicals are critical for defense against fungal hyphae is supported by the finding of increased risk of fungal infections in chronic septic granulomatosis, a hereditary disease with defect in oxygen radical formation. Immune defenses also include cell-mediated immunity, activation of the complement system, and generation of antibody response.

Adaptive Immunity

Cell-Mediated Immunity and Cytokines

Cell-mediated immunity includes the different Th lymphocyte subsets and is considered an adaptive immunity to fungal infections. The phagocytosis of fungal particles and antigens by the antigen-presenting cells activates specific T cells and cytokines, which in turn induce production of antibodies by B cells.[15] The innate resistance and adaptive immunity are interdependent, with crosstalk occurring between these two mechanisms that are essential for protection against fungal infections.[16] Depending on the host immunologic status, an equilibrated cytokine response, or a predominantly Th1- or

Th2-like cytokine response develops. The adaptive Th cell responses may be "protective" type 1 (Th1) or "nonprotective" type 2 (Th2). In the type 1 response, there is production of Th1 cytokines, such as IFN-γ and interleukins (IL-2, IL-12, IL-18), that stimulate macrophage activation, generate cytotoxic CD4+ T cells, and produce opsonizing antibodies and delayed-type hypersensitivity response. In the type 2 response, there is production of Th2 cytokines, such as IL-4, IL-5, and IL-13, that elicit production of nonopsonizing antibodies and allergic reactions and downregulate the inflammatory response produced by Th1 cytokines.[17] Cytokines IL-4 and IL-12 induce the production of Th2 cells that favor allergic responses and humoral immunity, whereas IL-2 and IFN-γ induce Th1 cells that favor cell-mediated immune responses and production of opsonizing antibodies.[6] Several other cytokines are also involved in the antifungal immune response, such as IL-1, IL-6, IL-8, IL-10, IL-15, TNF-α, and transforming growth factor (TGF)-β. Interleukin-10 and IL-12 play an important role in regulating the development of Th cells.[8,9] A role for regulatory T cells (T_{reg}) has been recently shown in fungal immune response.[18] The T_{reg} cells decreased inflammation, attenuated Th1 response, induced tolerance, and mediated resistance to reinfection.

Impairment of cell-mediated immunity predisposes patients to fungal infections. Patients with primary or acquired cell-mediated immune deficiency and taking drugs that suppress cell-mediated immunity are highly susceptible to fungal infections. Experimental evidence suggests that Th2 cells rather than Th1 cells are protective against fungi.[6] Resistance to *Candida* infection is shown to correlate with cell-mediated immunity in vivo as well as Th1 cytokine secretion in vitro.[19] There is some clinical evidence to support the activation of Th2 cells by *Candida*.

Dendritic Cells

Dendritic cells are essential in linking the innate and adaptive immune responses to the fungi.[20,21] The interaction of dendritic cells with fungi is important for the type of adaptive T-cell response.[22] This interaction is determined by the ligation of conidia or hyphae of different fungi to distinct pattern-recognizing receptors and the mechanism of their phagocytosis (coiling or zipper-type phagocytosis) by dendritic cells.[11,23] The *Aspergillus conidia* stimulate both TLR2 and TLR4 to induce a Th1 response, whereas *Aspergillus* hyphae lose the TLR4 response, resulting in IL-10 production and impaired host response to invasive disease [24,25]. *Candida albicans* similarly stimulate the TLR2 pathway to attenuate the host response. Modulation of the TLR pathways may thus provide immune intervention for treatment of invasive fungal infections. Differentiation of CD4+ T lymphocytes to Th1 or Th2 types is an essential determinant of the host's susceptibility or resistance to infection. Development of the Th1 cell response is mediated through cytokines IFN-γ, IL-6, IL-12, and TNF-α in the relative absence of Th2 cytokines. The predominance of Th1 cytokines is protective against fungal infection.[22,26] Interferon-γ produced by T and NK cells is a key cytokine in the immune response to invasive fungal infections and stimulates migration, adherence, and antifungal activities of neutrophils and macrophages. Interferon-γ also regulates the Th1 antifungal adaptive response through IL-1.[27]

Humoral Immunity

The role of humoral immunity in fungal infections is not completely understood. Data support the presence of protective antibodies in *Candida* and *Cryptococcus* infections.[28] These antibodies may protect the host by inhibition of adhesion to respiratory cells, inhibition of germ-tube formation, opsonization, and neutralization of virulence enzymes.[29,30] Fungal infections are also associated with various allergic disorders characterized by high serum IgE levels.[31] Serum IgE levels against *Aspergillus* are elevated in allergic bronchopulmonary aspergillosis. T cells from these patients express a typical Th2-type cytokine pattern, with high IL-4 and little or no IFN-γ.[32] Additionally, specific IgE antibody production against distinct allergens specific for allergic bronchopulmonary aspergillosis have been shown.[33]

Pathology and Pathogenesis of Fungal Infections

Fungi that cause invasive pulmonary infection can be divided in two groups: (1) primary or true pathogens and (2) opportunistic pathogens. The primary or true pathogenic fungi infect healthy, immunologically competent individuals.[34,35] In immunocompromised patients, however, these fungi can be very aggressive and produce severe, disseminated, and fatal infections. While endemic fungi such as *Histoplasma capsulatum* and *Coccidioides immitis* are the most common, *Penicillium marneffei*, *Fusarium* species, *Scedosporium* species, and *Malassezia* species are increasing in incidence as opportunistic infections in immunocompromised hosts, especially in those with acquired immunodeficiency syndrome (AIDS).[36,37] Each of these fungi can cause systemic life-threatening infections. The opportunistic fungi cause infections in critically ill or immunosuppressed patients. Almost all opportunistic fungi gain entry through the lungs, except endogenous *Candida* species. The most common opportunistic fungi include *Candida*, *Aspergillus*, *Cryptococcus*, zygomycetes, *Pseudallescheria*, *Fusarium*, and *Trichosporon*.

The dramatic increase in opportunistic fungal infection in recent years is related to several factors,[36,38,39] including immunosuppression of transplant recipients, chemotherapy for malignancies, broad-spectrum therapy for bacterial infections, the long-term placements of catheters for various therapies, and last, but not the least, AIDS.[37,40] Host factors responsible for increased susceptibility to fungal infections include a decrease in the number or functional impairment of mature granulocytes and mononuclear phagocytes, depressed B-lymphocyte (humoral) immunity resulting in decreased production of immunoglobulins and impaired opsonization, depressed T-lymphocyte (cell-mediated) immunity, abnormal host immune regulation,[39–42] and neutropenia. Other factors include disruption of mucosal and skin barriers, disorders of complement system, and hereditary immune dysfunctions.[42,43]

Fungal infections in severely immunocompromised patients present with clinical features that are often different from those of immunocompetent patients. The tissue response is also different, because there may be little or no inflammatory response or granulomas with even massive infection. Special stains or immunostains for fungi and other organisms should be routinely used for demonstrating fungi in severely immunocompromised patients.

In general, fungal infections are associated with a higher mortality than either bacterial or viral infections in this patient population. This is because of the limited number of available therapies, dose-limiting toxicities of the antifungal drugs, fewer symptoms due to lack of inflammatory response, and lack of sensitive tests to aid in the diagnosis of invasive fungal infections.[44] A recent study of patients with fungal infections admitted to a university-affiliated hospital indicated that community-acquired infections are becoming a serious problem; 67% of the 140 patients had community-acquired fungal pneumonia.[45] There is also an increase in nosocomial fungal infections.[46]

Three pathogenic fungi, species of *Aspergillus*, *Coccidioides*, and *Histoplasma*, are excellent models that illustrate the gamut of host–pathogen interactions that vary from fungi growing through tissue as invasive hyphae, developing spherules with endospores, to survival, growth, replication within phagocytic cells.

Aspergillus

Invasive aspergillosis is caused by several species of *Aspergillus*, *A. fumigatus* being the most commonly encountered species causing invasive aspergillosis in the lungs. With the exception of *A. terreus*, which can produce lateral aleurioconidia in the vegetative hyphae and, *A. niger*, which can form calcium oxalate crystals in tissue near its hyphae, the vegetative hyphae of *Aspergillus* species look alike. Under some conditions, *Aspergillus* species may produce fruiting structures consisting of conidiophores, phialides, and phialoconidia in lung cavities that are like those seen in culture. These fruiting structures can be used to achieve a tentative species level of identification if the phialides and their arrangement are clearly evident.

Within the diagnostic laboratory, some isolates that would have been traditionally identified as *A. fumigatus* using morphologic criteria are now being identified with molecular-based data as *A. lentulus*, a species that has a decreased in vitro susceptibility to amphotericin B, itraconazole, voriconazole, and caspofungin,[47] *A. viridinutans*,[48,49] *A. thermomutatus*,[50] and *A. fischeri*.[51] It has been suggested that *A. fumigatus* consists of two different phylogenetic species that are morphologically identical.[52] Hong et al. have proposed the names *A. fungatiaffinis* and *A. novofumigatus* for two species they worked with that were originally identified as members of the *A. fumigatus* group.[53]

Coccidioides

Coccidioidomycosis is believed by some to be caused by two species of *Coccidioides*, *C. immitis* and *C. posadasii*.[54] These two species are morphologically identical both in vivo and in vitro, being distinguished from one another by DNA polymorphisms, different growth rates on high salt concentration media, and different biogeographic distributions. There are no known differences in their infectivity, and both species are classified as biosafety level 3 agents and are regulated by the laws governing bioterrorism.

Histoplasma

Even though separate species names for the six clades of *Histoplasma capsulatum* have not been proposed, the distinct genetic populations have been clearly defined.[55] Different clinical presentations and geographic distribution patterns for the six clades are recognized. Currently, the three varieties *H. capsulatum* var. *capsulatum*, *H. capsulatum* var. *duboisii*, and *H. capsulatum* var. *farciminosum* are named, the latter not being associated with human infection. Additional studies of *Histoplasma* isolates lead Komori et al. to distinguish nine different populations.[56] For the discussion in this chapter, *H. capsulatum* will reflect all of the varieties and phylogenetic species described to date.

Molecular Basis of Pathogenesis

Molecular strain typing has demonstrated that there is apparently no difference between environmental and patient isolates of *A. fumigatus*. Thus, in an immunocompromised patient, any *A. fumigatus* isolate from anywhere in the world (Figure 41.1) has the potential to cause infection in an immunocompromised patient. Aspergilli are actively involved with the decomposition of organic material such as vegetation and other cellulose-containing material. Nosocomial infections occur when *Aspergillus* grows on cellulytic substrates in the hospital environment and produce conidia that are inhaled by immunocompromised patients. With the exception of the rare case of *Aspergillus* being transferred from one patient to another during trachea–lung transplantation, an infection follows the inhalation of inoculum from the environment. Like *Aspergillus*, *Coccidioides* has been transmitted in organs being transplanted into another patient. In the case of coccidioidomycosis, arthroconidia formed in specialized soil-based ecologic niches become airborne, often in dust, and are subsequently inhaled. When *Coccidioides* and *Histoplasma* are isolated in the diagnostic laboratory, they are always considered pathogens. This is not the situation with the isolation of *Aspergillus* because of its ubiquitous nature and common occurrence in air samples. It is not known for sure what the inoculum for histoplasmosis is. It is thought that microconidia or hyphal fragments formed by the fungus growing in soil enriched with bird or bat fecal material become aerosolized and are then inhaled. It is highly unlikely that a yeast form of this dimorphic fungus is the primary inoculum originating from nature.

Following the inhalation of *A. fumigatus* conidia, the rodAp protein (16 kDa) in the rodlets on the conidial outer cell wall provides resistance to conidia being killed by mouse alveolar macrophages.[57] Apparently, the macrophage reactive oxidants are not able to effectively pass through the hydrophobic protein barrier surrounding the conidia. A second hydrophobin called rodBp (14 kDa) has been found, and it participates only in cell wall development. This protein does not provide protection to the conidia. Both rodAp and rodBp are found only in the rodlets of the outer cell walls of conidia and do not occur on the cell wall surface of hyphae. Even though hydrophobins have not been reported for *Coccidioides* and *Histoplasma* conidia, these proteins may be present as they are in other fungi that have airborne dispersal of conidia.

Aspergillus fumigatus synthesizes a bluish green conidial pigment using the 1,8-dihydroxynaphthalene pathway (DHN-melanin) that is deposited in the outer conidial wall near the rodlets. The DHN-melanin pathway protects the conidia by quenching reactive oxygen species formed by alveolar macrophages and polymorphonuclear neutrophils. Following phagocytosis, phagocytes primarily kill fungi using oxidative mechanisms. These host defense reactive oxygen species can be neutralized by fungal oxidoreductases and other metabolites. In addi-

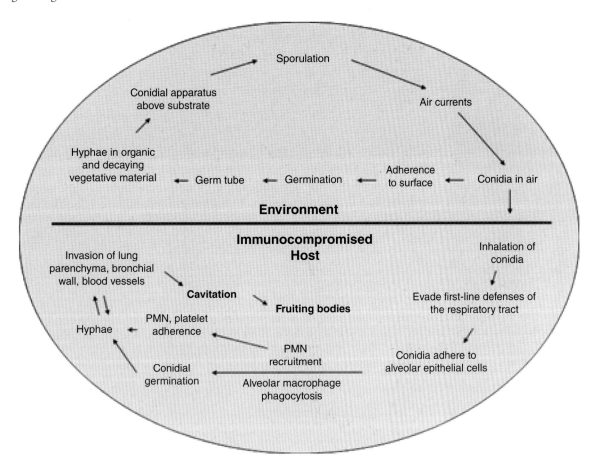

FIGURE 41.1. *Aspergillus* is present in the environment as conidia in the air that can germinate and transform to hyphae. Inhalation of the conidia by an immunocompromised host results in germination and formation of hyphae within the lung and invasive aspergillosis. Fruiting bodies may be seen in cavitary lesions. PMN, polymorphonuclear leukocytes.

tion, there are mycotoxins in the conidial wall that can prevent phagocytosis and interfere with T-lymphocyte function. The histologic Fontana-Masson stain for melanin does not demonstrate the presence of melanin in the tissue form of *A. fumigatus, C. immitis,* or *H. capsulatum.*[58] Conidia of *C. immitis* and *H. capsulatum* are also negative when stained by the Fontana-Masson method. Recent studies have clearly shown that melanin does exist on the yeast cells of *H. capsulatum* in vivo and conidia grown in vitro. The melanin on the cell walls of the yeast cells can bind amphotericin B and caspofungin as a protective devise by the fungus.[59] Unlike *A. fumigatus* and *H. capsulatum* melanin formed by the DHN-melanin pathway, the yeast cells of *H. capsulatum* form melanin by the L-3,4-dihydroxyphenylalanine pathway during infection in mammalian tissue.[60] Melanin is also important because of its antigenic antiinflammatory properties.

Following germination of conidia, germ tubes are formed that develop into hyphae. Neutrophils attach to the hyphae and cause hyphal damage and death by using a respiratory burst, secretion of reactive oxygen interme-diates, and degranulation. Toxic components of the immune system can be eliminated by the fungus through the use of efflux pumps. Efflux pumps are resistance mechanisms used by some fungi to remove antifungal agents from the fungus.

All fungi require iron for growth. Even though serum transferrin is fungistatic to many fungi, *A. fumigatus* possesses siderophores belonging to the hydroxamate family of compounds (fericrocin and triacetylfusarinine) that can remove iron from the transferrin molecule. This not only protects the hyphae against host attack but also provides needed iron for fungal growth. *Aspergillus* commonly invades blood vessels as it causes invasive infection. The intracellular yeast cells of *H. capsulatum* modify the microenvironment inside of the macrophage by regulating its pH toward acidity. This allows the release of iron from the internal transferrin molecule that compromises its killing ability while providing the yeast with iron for growth.[61]

Aspergillus hyphae invade lung parenchyma, the bronchial wall, and blood vessels. Hyphae release extracellular elastinolytic and collagenolytic enzymes that break down the elastin and collagen lung matrix. Similar functional proteases are formed by *Coccidioides* and *Histoplasma*. In addition to obtaining nutrients needed for fungal growth, fungal proteases such as alkaline serine protease, metalloprotease, and aspartic protease interfere with the immune response. *Aspergillus* hyphae may produce the mycotoxin gliotoxin[62] while growing in host tissue. Gliotoxin suppresses mast cell activation (degranulation, leukotriene C_4 secretion, TNF-α, and IL-13 production), induces apoptosis of monocytes, lymphocytes, and neutrophils, and suppresses T-cell activation by inhibiting antigen presentation. In vitro studies have shown that amphotericin B enhances gliotoxin synthesis and release.[63] Mycotoxins have not been reported in *Coccidioides* and *Histoplasma*.

Coccidioides arthroconidia inhaled from the environment do not form germ tubes in lung tissue; they swell and develop directly into spherules containing numerous endospores (Figure 41.2). An exception to this rule occurs when endospores germinate and form germ tubes that

develop into hyphae within pulmonary cavities. The hyphae in cavities form arthroconidia that are converted into spherules containing endospores. Arthroconidia of *C. immitis* that are inhaled release a chemotactic component that attracts polymorphonuclear leukocytes (PMNs). Following their ingestion, a respiratory burst occurs, after which only approximately 20% of the arthroconidia are killed. It has been suggested that PMNs may promote the development of spherules from arthroconidia. Owing in part to their size and to an extracellular fibrillar matrix, spherules are resistant to phagocytosis and killing by PMNs. Following the rupture of the spherule wall and subsequent endospore release, additional PMNs are summoned. Newly released endospores are covered with an extracellular fibrillar matrix. The respiratory burst associated with endospores is less intense than that caused by arthroconidia. Inhibition of phagosome–lysosome fusion may be used by *C. immitis* to survive phagocytosis by macrophages. In addition to neutrophils, macrophages, and monocytes, NK lymphocytes are an important component of innate immunity.[64]

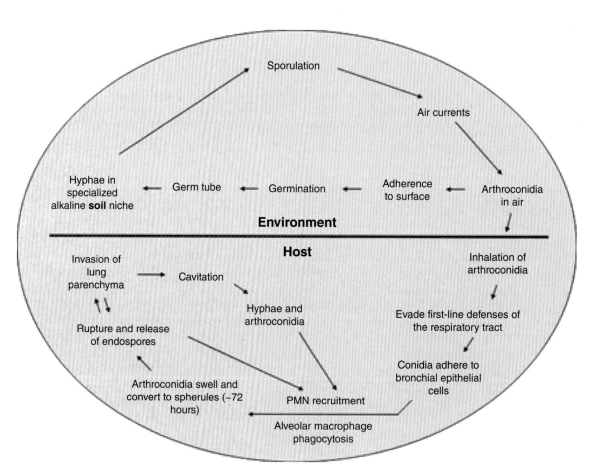

FIGURE 41.2. *Coccidioides* is present in air as arthroconidia that can form germ tubes and hyphae in soil. Inhalation of arthroconidia results in conversion to spherules with rupture and release of endospores, invasion of lung parenchyma, and infection. PMN, polymorphonuclear leukocytes.

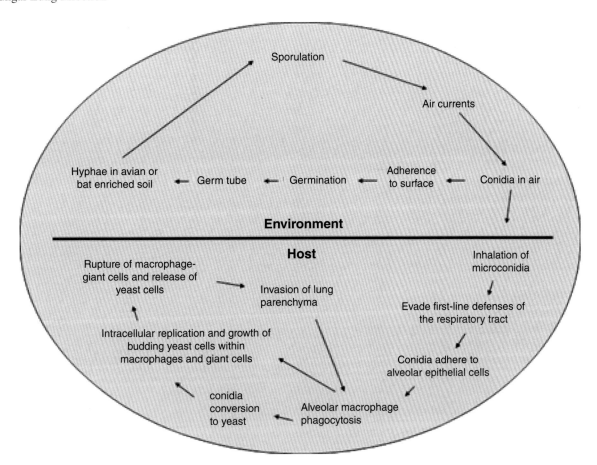

FIGURE 41.3. Histoplasma exist in air as conidia and germinate with formation of hyphae in avian-enriched soil. Inhalation of microconidia results in development of yeast forms, growth and replication of yeast in macrophages, and lung invasion following the release of yeast with rupture of these macrophages.

Following the inhalation of *H. capsulatum*, the microconidia, hyphal fragments, or both are recognized, bound to alveolar macrophages, and then ingested (Figure 41.3). Within the macrophage, the *H. capsulatum* converts to yeast cells that reproduce by budding. In addition, cell-mediated immunity is activated where *H. capsulatum* antigens are processed and presented to T cells, followed by cytokine activation, after which the macrophages contain and kill the yeast. The macrophage is stimulated to express a respiratory burst of toxic oxygen species and the fusion of lysosomes with the phagocytic vacuole. The yeast cells, which reside within a membrane-bound vacuole, are not destroyed by the toxic oxygen radicals (hydrogen peroxide, superoxide anion, hydroxyl radical) and reactive nitrogen intermediates such as nitric oxide released by the respiratory burst. Within the phagocytic cell, the yeast controls the intraphagosomal environment by maintaining a pH of approximately 6–6.5. At this pH, lysosome acid hydolases are inactivated, and transferrin gives up iron that is then used by the fungus. The loss of iron from transferrin inactivates the fungistatic activity of the transferrin.[61,62]

Pathology

Tissue histology for the diagnosis of fungal lung disease is important because the signs and symptoms and radiographic findings are not specific for any particular fungal infection. Ideally, histology, fungal serology, molecular detection of fungal components, epidemiologic information, and culture should be used to make a diagnosis of a fungal infection. When there is a question regarding the role of an isolated fungus such as *Aspergillus* species, histology becomes especially important in distinguishing between invasion, environmental contamination, or colonization. In addition, the tissue reaction can be used to distinguish between allergic disease and invasion.

Hematoxylin and eosin staining provides valuable information regarding the host response, especially the Splendore-Hoeppli phenomenon. Hematoxylin and eosin allows for the detection of fungal melanin in the fungal cell wall and the detection of fungal nuclei, which may be important in distinguishing the multinucleated yeast cells of *Blastomyces dermatitidis* from the uninucleate yeast cells of *H. capsulatum*. Unfortunately, fungi often do not stain well by the hematoxylin and eosin method, which may cause fungi to be overlooked. Gomori's methenamine silver is a good special stain for the detection and evaluation of fungal structures in lung. Because silver precipitates onto the fungus, the dematiaceous nature of some fungi can be masked. If the staining procedure is not done properly, fungal structures may be overstained, making an accurate evaluation of the fungal structures questionable. An advantage of overstaining occurs when looking for *H. capsulatum* in the central portion of old calcified pulmonary granulomata where the fungal cells have deteriorated following their death.

Aspergillus species may cause a broad spectrum of diseases depending on the immune status of the host. These include allergic disease, colonization of preexisting cavities in immunocompetent patients, noninvasive to superficial invasive necrotizing tracheobronchitis, chronic to destructive infection in mildly compromised patients, and rapidly progressive, invasive aspergillosis in severely immunocompromised patients. Dissemination occurs in 25%–33% of seriously immunocompromised patients. *Aspergillus* is not a dimorphic fungus, because, regardless of the growth temperature, the fungus vegetatively forms only hyphae. In tissue, *Aspergillus* grows as hyaline, septate, dichotomously branching, 3–6μm hyphae with a propensity for vascular invasion and occlusion and the development of wedge-shaped, pleural-based nodular pulmonary infarcts. When physical space (cavitation) with adequate aeration is available, fungal fruiting bodies may be formed.

The tissue response in invasive aspergillosis is a mixed purulent and necrotizing inflammatory reaction. Necrosis may be caused by gliotoxins and vascular obstruction. Initially, hyphae develop small to large radiating aggregates that spread in a radial manner. The peripheral hyphae are usually surrounded by neutrophils. Chronic lesions are usually focal, granulomatous, and contain giant cells, neutrophils, and eosinophils. Lesions become walled off by a granulomatous tissue reaction that contains Langerhans giant cells. A cavity may form when the central area of the granuloma becomes necrotic and caseous and liquefies. In this instance, cavity formation occurs as a result of the disease process and is not a preexisting entity. If the cavity is associated with a bronchiole, hyphae may be coughed up in sputum. Hematogenous dissemination of *Aspergillus* to other organs occurs rapidly owing to its propensity to invade blood vessels. Interestingly, blood cultures are typically negative, yet thrombosis leading to hemorrhage, infarction, and death are well documented.

Coccidioidomycosis may occur in either immunocompetent or immunocompromised hosts. As with other pulmonary fungal pathogens, infection in the immunocompromised patient is more severe. *Coccidioides immitis* is a dimorphic fungus because it grows into entirely different vegetative forms depending on the incubation temperature. In tissue, *C. immitis* vegetatively develops spherules that form endospores. At the edges of pulmonary cavities, *C. immitis* may form hyphae in approximately 10%–30% of coccidioidal cavities. The hyphae are similar to those that grow in culture and may subsequently develop into arthroconidia. Depending on the environmental conditions in the pulmonary cavity, the morphology of the fungus can be extremely variable in form, shape, and size.

A mixed granulomatous and purulent tissue reaction occurs in pulmonary, disseminated, or cutaneous coccidioidomycosis. When endospores are released by the rupture of the spherule wall, a severe local purulent reaction occurs. As the endospores (2–5μm) mature and become spherules (20–200μm), neutrophils are gradually replaced by lymphocytes, plasma cells, epithelioid cells, and Langerhans or foreign body-type giant cells. The mature spherule is surrounded by epithelioid cells and multinucleated giant cells. Because of the rapid rate of *Coccidioides* growth, a spectrum of spherule development is usually present within a single area. Fibrosis, scarring, and occasional calcification follow granuloma formation if the patient's immunity is good. If the immunity is poor, a purulent reaction predominates. Thus, primary coccidioidomycosis tends to be granulomatous, whereas secondary disseminated disease is purulent.

All three varieties of *H. capsulatum* are dimorphic fungi that form intracellular yeast cells in tissue and vegetative hyphae in culture. *Histoplasma capsulatum* var. *duboisii* differs in tissue from the other two varieties by forming larger yeast cells in tissue and being distributed within Africa. Hyphae are not formed in tissue, but occasionally several budded cells may remain attached to each other to form primitive or rudimentary pseudohyphae.

Like coccidioidomycosis, the majority (90%–95%) of *Histoplasma* infections are asymptomatic. Patients with acute pulmonary infection often have nodular densities on x-ray study that result from the inhalation of the fungus from environmental sources such as disturbed soil containing bird or bat fecal material. The primary lesion begins as a patchy bronchopneumonia with yeast-laden macrophages and giant cells in the alveolar spaces. As the disease progresses, granulomata, with or without central caseation, develop. Larger granulomata commonly become fibrocaseous nodules that frequently calcify.

Diagnosis

Historically, the use of fluorescein-labeled antibody reagents designed to attach to specific fungal antigenic sites, and then be detected by fluorescence, provided a sensitive and specific method for identifying fungi in pulmonary tissue. Owing to the scarcity and absence of many fluorescein-labeled antibody reagents, such testing is no longer readily available. Instead, DNA-based technology has been introduced to meet the needs of tissue identification of pulmonary pathogens.[66,67] There are two fundamental approaches, the use of specific probes to detect known fungal gene sequences associated with specific pathogens[68] and the use of species specific DNA sequence data from databases to identify an unknown fungus after sequencing of its DNA. The latter approach has greater applicability because there are many fungi for which probes do not exist. Even though both techniques can result in fungal identifications, they are not widely used at present because of either an absence of standardized probes and methodologies or the limited availability of space, trained personnel, cost effectiveness, and equipment. Both fluorescein-labeled antibody and DNA probes can be used not only on tissue sections but also on nearly any clinical specimen.

Currently available laboratory methods for diagnosing invasive fungal infections include (1) isolation of fungi in the laboratory, (2) histologic evidence of invasion, and (3) molecular diagnostic techniques. A combination of these approaches is recommended but is not always possible.[69]

Molecular Diagnostic Techniques

Several molecular diagnostic techniques are now available for identification and confirmation of fungi.[70,71]

Serologic Diagnosis

Diagnosis by serology is limited for immunocompromised patients, because they do not mount a good antibody response during infection. Therefore, most of the research has been focused on identifying antigens or metabolites that can be detected in the blood or urine during invasive fungal infection. Some of the recent markers developed for the diagnosis of invasive infections include $(1\rightarrow3)$-β-D-glucan, a cell wall component of yeast and filamentous fungi detectable in the blood during invasive fungal infection. The reported sensitivity and specificity of the assay has been good, ranging from 78% to 100% and 88% to 100%, respectively.[72,73] This assay can detect invasive *Aspergillus, Candida, Fusarium, Trichosporon, Saccharomyces,* and *Acremonium* but not *Cryptococcus*. In addition, for the diagnosis of invasive candidiasis, antigens or metabolites thus far investigated include cell wall mannoprotein (mannan), heat-labile antigen, D-arabinose, and enolase. β-Glucan mannan is available for identification of candida antigen.[74] Unfortunately, none of the assays has sensitive enough predictive value to be used routinely. Several assays have been developed for the detection of galactomannan, a polysaccharide antigen component of *Aspergillus* cell wall, in the serum and urine of patients with invasive aspergillosis. An enzyme-linked immunosorbent assay (ELISA) for detection of galactomannan has shown a sensitivity of 65%–100% and specificity of 81%–100%.[75,76] Although the results for therapeutic monitoring using these tests are encouraging, there is an 8% false-positive rate.

Polymerase Chain Reaction

Polymerase chain reaction (PCR) assays for the diagnosis of invasive fungal infections have used a highly conserved area in the 18S ribosomal DNA gene as a target.[77] This gene has allowed the design of primers that are specific for a wide variety of medically important fungi. The PCR-based assays are very sensitive, with detection limits down to 1 cfu/mL. A sensitivity of 100% and specificity of 65% was found in prospective trials. Specific oligonucleotide probes have been developed to identify fungi that display yeast-like morphology in vivo.[78] Universal fungal primers ITS1 and ITS4, directed to the conserved regions of rDNA, were used to amplify DNA from *H. capsulatum, B. dermatitidis, C. immitis, Paracoccidioides brasiliensis, P. marneffei, S. schenckii, C. neoformans,* five *Candida* species, and *Pneumocystis carinii*. With the exception of minor cross-reactivity, all probes were found to be highly specific. There is, however, a possibility of high false-positive results with this high degree of sensitivity. In a recent study, PCR for *Aspergillus* on whole blood samples was found to be highly sensitive for the detection and prediction of invasive pulmonary aspergillosis.[79] In addition, a PCR assay using the LightCycler technology is now available, reducing the risk of contamination and thus false-positive results. The real-time LightCycler PCR assay used with automated DNA extraction from serum provides better reliability and safety than the standard PCR test. Specific probes using oligonucleotide primers from the nuclear rDNA for PCR identification and sero-diagnosis using galactomannan are now available.[80]

Traditionally, fungi have been identified using morphology. For fungi such as *C. immitis* and *H. capsulatum* that have morphologically similar-appearing molds, additional testing is obviously required. Animal studies, temperature-dependent tissue form-to-laboratory form conversion testing for dimorphic fungi, and exoantigen testing are no longer used. These methods have been replaced with species-specific DNA probes. For isolates that exhibit unusual morphologic variation, they are unfortunately force fitted into a traditional genus and species or sent to an extramural laboratory for additional testing. At this level of identification, specific gene regions such as the *ITS* or *D1–D2* portion of the 26S ribosomal gene can be sequenced from which the fungus is identified.[81] From a practical perspective, this type of identification is rarely required.

The detection of metabolites or fungal genetic material is an ideal approach for the diagnosis of mycoses. Because the hyphae of *A. fumigatus* and several other species of *Aspergillus* produce the mycotoxin gliotoxin when the fungus grows in tissue, it is of potential diagnostic value. Gliotoxin production is independent of the host's immune status or underlying disease state. Unfortunately, not all isolates of *A. fumigatus* produce gliotoxin in tissue.[62]

For the diagnosis of coccidioidomycosis, the tube precipitin-reacting test (TP) for IgM antibodies and complement fixing antibody test (CF) for IgG antibodies are the most useful test procedures.[82] Both of these tests use antigen to look for specific types of antibody produced in response to *C. immitis*. The IgM TP antibodies appear first and disappear before IgM CF antibodies. The CF antibodies are important because they remain for longer periods of time and have prognostic importance. As with other systemic mycoses, antigen detection has been shown to be potentially useful.

Antibody is not always detected in aspergillosis using precipitin tests, immunodiffusion test, or CF because of the low sensitivity of the tests. Testing for metabolites and cell wall components such as D-mannitol and β-(1,3)-glucan using methods such as latex agglutination or immunoblotting have been helpful. Detection of serum galactomannan by ELISA has shown that up to 93% of patients with infection can be positive (with a specificity of 95%). More importantly, in up to two-thirds of patients, the ELISA test results were positive prior to the first clinical or radiologic features of infection. Combined with the appropriate predisposing host factors, and signs and symptoms, two consecutive positive galactomannan assay tests can be equated with probable invasive aspergillosis.[69]

Antibody to *H. capsulatum* arises in 2–6 weeks. It may be absent in immunocompromised patients and, if present, may be from a previous exposure to the fungus. The immunodiffusion test and CF are used to measure antibody production in histoplasmosis. The immunodiffusion test measures the presence of H and M precipitin bands and is less sensitive than the CF test. There is no titer cut-off point for CF testing. Cross-reactivity has been observed in patients having aspergillosis, blastomycosis, candidiasis, coccidioidomycosis, and paracoccidioidomycosis.[83] In immunocompromised patients, the detection of *H. capsulatum* antigen is more useful because it does not rely on the ability to form antibody or on previous infection [84]. Antigen was detected in the urine of 95% of AIDS patients and in 85% of their serum samples. Skin test reagents for histoplasmosis skin testing are no longer used.

Molecular Basis of Therapy

Reconstitution of the immune system is ideal but is not typically attainable in many of the immunocompromised patient populations. The use of colony-stimulating factor, granulocyte transfusions, and IFN-γ to augment the immune system has been successfully used in patients with aspergillosis.[69] Prevention through the use of vaccines is being explored for several mycoses.[85,86] Unfortunately, there are no vaccines available for aspergillosis,[87,88] coccidioidomycosis, or histoplasmosis.[89]

The primary antifungal agents used to treat invasive infection include amphotericin B, usually as a lipid formulation, azoles, echinocandins, or these classes of antifungals used together as combined therapy. The polyenes such as amphotericin B attach to ergosterol in the fungal plasma membrane and cause leakage of ions and small molecules from the fungal cell. To reduce toxicity, amphotericin B is often used as a liposomal formulation. The most commonly used azoles are the triazoles fluconazole, itraconazole, posaconazole, ravuconazole, and voriconazole, all of which inhibit 14-α-demethylation (cytochrome P450-erg 11p) of lanosterol in the fungal ergosterol biosynthetic pathway. Echinocandins such as anidulafungin, caspofungin, and micafungin inhibit fungal β-glucan biosynthesis. 5-Fluorocytosine, which acts as an antimetabolite after it is converted to 5-fluorouracil within the fungal cell, is given with a second antifungal agent to avoid its use as a monotherapeutic agent, potentially for treatment of aspergillosis, candidiasis, and cryptococcosis.

Voriconazole is more effective than amphotericin B for initial therapy of invasive aspergillosis. Recent clinical data indicate that posaconazole is at least as effective as voriconazole for treating aspergillosis caused by *A. terreus*. Caspofungin has a favorable response in salvage aspergillosis cases, that is, when other antifungal drugs have failed. It appears that caspofungin used with either amphotericin B or voriconazole has favorable benefit. For some patients who were refractory to voriconazole, posaconazole has been effective.[69] Treatment of coccidioidomycosis with amphotericin B, fluconazole, and itraconazole frequently results in failure and relapse. Posaconazole in a small number of patients can be effective. Amphotericin B, itraconazole, and fluconazole are the primary antifungals used to treat histoplasmosis. Of these, fluconazole is less effective than voriconazole.[90] Posaconazole has also been successfully used to treat histoplasmosis.[91]

Conclusion

Major advances have been made recently in understanding the innate and adaptive immunity to fungal infections. The regulatory role of cellular immunity, including the T lymphocytes, macrophages, neutrophils, and dendritic cells, are being studied in humans and experimental animals. The role of many cytokines is complex, pleiotropic, and sometimes opposing, depending on the timing of their participation in the immune process. Some of the cytokines that were originally believed to play a role in innate immunity are recently shown to be involved in adaptive immunity also. The data on the clinical use of cytokines are still in preliminary stages and being evaluated. Future therapies for fungal infections may also utilize agents that augment the activity of various effector cells involved in the immune response and manipulate the cell signaling cascade.

References

1. Speth C, Rambach G, Lass-Florl C, et al. The role of complement in invasive fungal infections. Mycoses 2004;47:93–103.
2. Waldorf AR. Pulmonary defense mechanisms against opportunistic fungal pathogens. Immunol Ser 1989;47:243–271.
3. Deepe GS, Bullock WE. Immunologic aspects of fungal pathogenesis. Eur J Clin Microbiol Dis 1990;9:567–579.
4. Shoham S, Levitz SM. The immune response to fungal infections. Br J Haematol 2005;129:569–582.
5. Levitz SM. Overview of host defenses in fungal infections. Clin Infect Dis 1992;14(Suppl 1):S37–S42.
6. Crameri R, Blaser K. Allergy and immunity to fungal infections and colonization. Eur Respir J 2002;19:151–157.
7. McCormack FX, Gibbons R, Ward SR, et al. Macrophage-independent fungicidal action of the pulmonary collectins. J Biol Chem 2003;278:36250–36256.
8. Romani L. Immunity to fungal infections. Nat Rev Immunol 2004;4:1–23.
9. Huffnagle GB, Deepe GS. Innate and adaptive determinants of host susceptibility to medically important fungi. Curr Opin Microbiol 2003;6:344–350.
10. Mambula SS, Sau K, Henneke P, et al. Toll-like receptor (TLR) signaling in response to Aspergillus fumigatus. J Biol Chem 2002;277:39320–39326.
11. Mansour MK, Levitz SM. Interactions of fungi with phagocytes. Curr Opin Microbiol 2002;5:359–365.
12. Roilides E, Dignani MC, Anaissie EJ, Rex JH. The role of immunoreconstitution in the management of refractory opportunistic infections. Med Mycol 1998a;36(Suppl 1):12–25.
13. Lohmeyer J. Role of hematopoietic growth factors and cytokines in host defense against fungal infections. Mycoses 1997;40(Suppl 2):37–39.
14. Schaffner A, Douglas H, Braude A. Selective protection against conidia by mononuclear and mycelia by polymorphonuclear phagocytes in resistance to Aspergillus. J Clin Invest 1982;69:617–631.
15. Romani L. The T cell response against fungal infections. Curr Opin Immunol 1997;9:484–490.
16. Trinchieri G, Kubin M, Bellone G, Cassatella MC. Cytokine cross-talk between phagocytic cells and lymphocytes: relevance for differentiation/activation of phagocytic cells and regulation of adaptive immunity. J Cell Biochem 1993;53:301–308.
17. Antachopoulos C, Roilides E. Cytokines and fungal infections. Br J Hematol 2005;129:583–596.
18. Montagnoli C, Bacci A, Bozza S, et al. B7/CD28-dependent CD4+CD25+ regulatory T cells are essential components of the memory-protective immunity to Candida albicans. J Immunol 2002;169:6298–6308.
19. Ausiello CM, Urbani F, Gessani S, et al. Cytokine gene expression in human peripheral blood mononuclear cells stimulated by mannoprotein constituents from Candida albicans. Infect Immun 1993;61:4105–4111.
20. Bauman SK, Nicholas KL, Murphy JW. Dendritic cells in the induction of protective and nonprotective anticryptococcal cell-mediated immune response. J Immunol 1998;165:158–167.
21. Braedel S, Radsak M, Einsele H, et al. Aspergillus fumigatus antigens activate innate immune cells via toll-like receptors 2 and 4. Br J Hematol 2004;125:392–399.
22. Huang Q, Liu D, Majewski P, et al. The plasticity of dendritic cell responses to pathogens and their components. Science 2001;294:870–875.
23. Romani L, Bistoni F, Puccetti P. Fungi, dendritic cells and receptors: a host perspective of fungal virulence. Trends Microbiol 2002;10:508–514.
24. Netea MG, Warris A, Van der Meer JW, et al. Aspergillus fumigatus evades immune recognition during germination through loss of toll-like receptor-4–mediated signal transduction. J Infect Dis 2003;188:320–326.
25. Netea MG, Van Der Graaf CA, Vonk AG, et al. The role of toll-like receptors (TLR) 2 and TLR4 in the host defense against disseminated candidiasis. J Infect Dis 2002;185:1483–1489.
26. Roilides E, Tsaparidou S, Kadiltsoglou I, et al. Interleukin-12 enhances antifungal activity of human mononuclear phagocytes against Aspergillus fumigatus: implications for a gamma interferon-independent pathway. Infect Immun 1999;67:3047–3050.
27. Cenci E, Mencacci A, Del Sero G, et al. IFN-gamma is required for IL-12 responsiveness in mice with Candida albicans infection. J Immunol 1998a;161:3543–3550.
28. Cassone A, Conti S, De Bernardis F, Polonelli L. Antibodies, killer toxins and antifungal immunoprotection: a lesson from nature?. Immunol Today 1997;18:164–169.
29. Nosanchuck JD. Protective antibodies and endemic dimorphic fungi. Curr Mol Med 2005;5:435–442.
30. Magliani W, Conti S, Arseni S, et al. Antibody-mediated protective immunity in fungal infections. New Microbiol 2005;28:299–309.
31. Horner SE, Helbling A, Salvaggio JE, Lehrer SB. Fungal allergens. Clin Microbiol Rev 1995;8:161–179.
32. Knutsen AP, Mueller KR, Levine AD, et al. Asp f 1 CD4+ TH2-like T-cell lines in allergic bronchopulmonary aspergillosis. J Allergy Clin Immunol 1994;94:215–221.
33. Hemmann S, Menz G, Ismail C, et al. Skin test reactivity to 2 recombinant Aspergillus fumigatus allergens in A. fumigatus–sensitized asthmatic subjects allows diagnostic separation of allergic bronchopulmonary aspergillosis from fungal sensitization. J Allergy Clin Immunol 1999;104:601–607.
34. Haque AK. Pathology of common pulmonary fungal infections. J Thorac Imaging 1992;7(4):1–11.
35. Saubolle MA. Fungal pneumonias. Semin Respir Infect 2000;15(2):162–177.

36. Walsh TJ, Hiemenz JW, Siebel NL, et al. Amphotericin B lipid complex for invasive fungal infections: analysis on safety and efficacy in 556 cases. Clin Infect Dis 1998;26: 1383–1396.

37. American Thoracic Society statement. Fungal infections in HIV infected persons. Am J Respir Crit Care Med 1995;152:816.

38. Walsh TJ, Groll A, Hiemenz J, et al. Infections due to emerging and uncommon medically important fungal pathogens. Clin Microbiol Infect 2004;10(Suppl 1):48–66.

39. Hawkins C, Armstrong D. Fungal infections in the immunocompromised host. Clin Hematol 1984;13:599–630.

40. Murray, JF, Mills J. Pulmonary infectious complications of human immunodeficiency virus infection. Part II. Am Rev Respir Dis 1990;141:1582.

41. Crum NF, Lederman ER, Stafford CM, et al. Coccidioidomycosis: a descriptive survey of a reemerging disease. Clinical characteristics and current controversies. Medicine (Baltimore) 2004;83(3):149–175.

42. Grieco MH. Humoral and cellular responses to infection. In Grieco MH, ed. Infections in the Abnormal Host. New York: Yorke Medical; 1980:131–304.

43. Elliott K, Whelan J, eds. Enzyme Defects and Immune Dysfunction. Ciba Foundation Symposium No. 68. Amsterdam: Excerpta Medica; 1979.

44. Alexander BD. Diagnosis of fungal infection: new technologies for the mycology laboratory. Transpl Infect Dis 2002;4(Suppl 3):32–37.

45. Chen KY, Ko SC, Hsueh PR, et al. Pulmonary fungal infection: emphasis on microbiological spectrum, patient outcome, and prognostic factors. Chest 2001;120:177–184.

46. Liu ZY, Sheng RY, Li XL, et al. Nosocomial fungal infections, analysis of 149 cases. Zhonghua Yi Xue Za Zhi 2003;83(5):399–402.

47. Balajee SA, Gribskov JL, Hanley E, et al. *Aspergillus lentulus* sp. nov., a new sibling species of *A. fumigatus*. Eukaryot Cell 2005;4(3):625–632.

48. Varga J, Vida Z, Toth B, et al. Phylogenetic analysis of newly described *Neosartorya* species. Antonie van Leeuwenhoek 2000;77:235–239.

49. Katz ME, Dougall AM, Weeks K, Cheetham BF. Multiple genetically distinct groups revealed among clinical isolates identified as atypical *Aspergillus fumigatus*. J Clin Microbiol 2005;43(2):551–555.

50. Balajee SA, Gribskov J, Brandt M, et al. Mistaken identity: *Neosartorya pseudofischeri* and its anamorph masquerading as *Aspergillus fumigatus*. J Clin Microbiol 2005;43(12): 5996–5999.

51. Nierman WC, Pain A, Anderson MJ, et al. Genomic sequence of the pathogenic and allergenic filamentous fungus *Aspergillus fumigatus*. Nature 2005;438(7071):1151–1156.

52. Pringle A, Baker DM, Platt JL, et al. Cryptic speciation in the cosmopolitan and clonal human pathogenic fungus *Aspergillus fumigatus*. Evol Int J Org Evol 2005;59(9): 1886–1899.

53. Hong SB, Shin HD, Frisvad JC, Samson RA. Polyphasic taxonomy of *Aspergillus fumigatus* and related species. Mycologia 2005;97(6):1316–1329.

54. Fischer MG, Koenig GL, White TJ, Taylor JW. Molecular and phenotypic description of *Coccidioides posadasii* sp.

nov., previously recognized as the non-California population of *Coccidioides immitis*. Mycologia 2002;94(1):73–84.

55. Kasuga T, Taylor JW, White TJ. Phylogenetic relationships of varieties and geographical groups of the human pathogenic fungus *Histoplasma capsulatum* Darling. J Clin Microbiol 1999;37(3):653–663.

56. Komori T, Sano A, Yarita K, et al. Phylogenetic analysis of *Histoplasma capsulatum* based on partial sequence of the D1/D2 region of the 28S rRNA gene. Nippon Ishinkin Gakkai Zasshi 2005;46(4):291–295.

57. Paris S, Debeaupuis JP, Crameri R, et al. Conidial hydrophobins of *Aspergillus fumigatus*. Appl Environ Microbiol 2003;69(3):1581–1588.

58. Kwon-Chung KJ, Hill WB, Bennett JE. New, special stain for histopathological diagnosis of cryptococcosis. J Clin Microbiol 1981;13(2):383–387.

59. Gomez BL, Nosanchuk JD. Melanin and fungi. Curr Opin Infect Dis 2003;16(2):91–96.

60. Nosanchuk JD, Gomez BL, Youngchim S, et al. *Histoplasma capsulatum* synthesizes melanin-like pigments in vitro and during mammalian infection. Infect Immun 2002; 70(9):5124–5131.

61. Newman SL, Gootee L, Hilty J, Morris RE. Human macrophages do not require phagosome acidification to mediate fungistatic/fungicidal activity against *Histoplasma capsulatum*. J Immunol 2006;176(3):1806–1813.

62. Lewis RE, Wiederhold NP, Lionakis MS, et al. Frequency and species distribution of gliotoxin-producing *Aspergillus* isolates recovered from patients at a tertiary-care cancer center. J Clin Microbiol 2005;43(12):6120–6122.

63. Reeves EP, Murphy T, Daly P, Kavanagh K. Amphotericin B enhances the synthesis and release of the immunosuppressive agent gliotoxin from the pulmonary pathogen *Aspergillus fumigatus*. J Med Microbiol 2004;53(Pt 8):719–725.

64. Cox RA, Magee DM. Coccidioidomycosis: host response and vaccine development. Clin Microbiol Rev 2004;17(4): 804–803.

65. Woods JP, Heinecke EL, Luecke JW, et al. Pathogenesis of *Histoplasma capsulatum*. Semin Respir Infect 2001;16(2): 91–101.

66. Bialek R, Konrad F, Kern J, et al. PCR based identification and discrimination of agents of mucormycosis and aspergillosis in paraffin wax embedded tissue. J Clin Pathol 2005;58(11):1180–1184.

67. Rickerts V, Just-Nubling G, Konrad F, et al. Diagnosis of invasive aspergillosis and mucormycosis in immunocompromised patients by seminested PCR assay of tissue samples. Eur J Clin Microbiol Infect Dis 2006;25(1):8–13.

68. Playford EG, Kong F, Sun Y, et al. Simultaneous detection and identification of *Candida*, *Aspergillus*, and *Cryptococcus* species by reverse line blot hybridization. J Clin Microbiol 2006;44(3):876–880.

69. Segal BH, Walsh TJ. Current approaches to diagnosis and treatment of invasive aspergillosis. Am J Respir Crit Care Med 2006;173(7):707–717.

70. Naber PS. Molecular pathology—diagnosis of infectious disease. N Engl J Med 1994;331:1212–1215.

71. Symposium: Molecular techniques in diagnostic pathology. Hum Pathol 1994;25:555–614.

72. Obayashi T, Yoshida M, Mori T, et al. Plasma (1→3)-beta-D-glycan measurement in diagnosis of invasive deep mycosis and fungal febrile episodes. Lancet 1995;345:17–20.

73. Mori T, Ikemoto H, Matsumura M, et al. Evaluation of plasma (1→3)-beta-D-glucan measurement by the kinetic turbidimetric Limulus test, for the clinical diagnosis of mycotic infections. Eur J Clin Chem Clin Biochem 1997;35: 553–560.

74. Pfaller MA, Cabezudo I, Buschelman B, et al. Value of the Hybritech ICON *Candida* assay in the diagnosis of invasive candidiasis in high-risk patients. Diagn Microbiol Infect Dis 1993;16:53–60.

75. Lindsley MD, Hurst SF, Iqbal NJ, et al. Rapid identification of dimorphic and yeast-like fungal pathogens using specific DNA probes. J Clin Microbiol 2001;39(10):3505–3511.

76. Raad I, Hanna H, Sumoza D, Albitar M. Polymerase chain reaction on blood for the diagnosis of invasive pulmonary aspergillosis in cancer patients. Cancer 2002;94:1032–1036.

77. Costa C, Costa JM, Desterke C, et al. Real-time PCR coupled with automated DNA extraction and detection of galactomannan antigen in serum by enzyme-linked immunosorbent assay for diagnosis of invasive aspergillosis. J Clin Microbiol 2002;40(6):2224–2227.

78. Kraus PR, Boily MJ, Giles SS, et al. Identification of *Cryptococcus neoformans* temperature-regulating genes with a genomic-DNA microarray. Eukaryot Cell 2004;3:1249–1260.

79. Raad I, Hanna H, Sumoza D, Albitar M. Polymerase chain reaction on blood for the diagnosis of invasive pulmonary aspergillosis in cancer patients. Cancer 2002;94:1032–1036.

80. Maertens J, Van Eldere J, Verhaegen J, et al. Use of circulating galactomannan screening for early diagnosis of invasive aspergillosis in allergenic stem cell transplant recipients. J Infect Dis 2002;186:1297–306.

81. Hinrikson HP, Hurst SF, Lott TJ, et al. Assessment of ribosomal large-subunit D1–D2, internal transcribed spacer 1, and internal transcribed spacer 2 regions as targets for molecular identification of medically important *Aspergillus* species. J Clin Microbiol 2005;43(5):2092–2103.

82. Chiller TM, Galgiani JN, Stevens DA. Coccidioidomycosis. Infect Dis Clin North Am 2003;7(1):41–45.

83. Wheat LJ. Current diagnosis of histoplasmosis. Trends Microbiol 2003;11(10):488–494.

84. Wheat LJ, Garringer T, Brizendine E, Connolly P. Diagnosis of histoplasmosis by antigen detection based upon experience at the histoplasmosis reference laboratory. Diagn Microbiol Infect Dis 2002;43(1):29–37.

85. Polonelli L, Casadevall A, Han Y, et al. The efficacy of acquired humoral and cellular immunity in the prevention and therapy of experimental fungal infections. Med Mycol 2000;38:281–292.

86. Dan JM, Levitz SM. Prospects for development of vaccines against fungal diseases. Drug Resist Update 2006;9(3): 105–110.

87. Casadevall A, Pirofski LA. Polysaccharide-containing conjugate vaccines for fungal diseases. Trends Mol Med 2006;12(1):6–9.

88. Stevens DA. Vaccinate against aspergillosis! A call to arms of the immune system. Clin Infect Dis 2004;38(8):1131–1136.

89. Deepe GS Jr, Wuthrich M, Klein BS. Progress in vaccination for histoplasmosis and blastomycosis: coping with cellular immunity. Med Mycol 2005;43(5):381–389.

90. Adderson E. Histoplasmosis. Pediatr Infect Dis J 2006;25(1): 73–74.

91. Keating GM. Posaconazole. Drugs 2005;65(11):1553–67; 1568–1569.

42
Parasites

Juan P. Olano

Introduction

In this chapter, I explore the advances made in understanding the molecular pathogenesis and basic immunologic principles of the most common protozoan and metazoan organisms that affect the lungs. These eukaryotic organisms are far more complex genetically than their bacterial and viral counterparts. Genome sizes range from 7,000 to 20,000 protein-encoding genes.[1] This level of complexity is needed in order to survive through multiple stages of development that occur in intermediate and definitive hosts. As a rule, most parasitic diseases lead to chronicity, suggesting that the host–parasite relationship enters a level of "tolerance" that we are beginning to understand at the molecular level through a complex interaction between parasite-derived immunomodulatory products and the host immune response.

Principles of Parasitic Molecular Pathogenesis

The term pathogenesis encompasses several steps including transmission, entry, initial spread from point of entry to other organs, contact with target cell/organ, survival within the host (immune evasion and adaptation to the host environment), and extension of the niche (multiplication, survival, and modulation of host biology). Mechanisms of transmission and entry of pulmonary parasites are as diverse as the parasites capable of causing pulmonary disease (see discussions of mode of transmission under each pathogen heading). Most of the discussion in this section will focus on the interaction between the parasite and the host, with special emphasis on the immune response as a pathogenetic mechanism in some of these infections.

Human parasitic infections range from asymptomatic carriers to lethal infections. This variability is determined by several factors, including host response, virulence factors, and infectious dose. From the immunologic point of view, responses to parasites follow the usual T-helper type 1 (Th1) and type 2 (Th2) types.[2] The Th1 responses are associated with the activation of cells by interferon (IFN)-γ and interleukin (IL)-2, induction of cytolytic CD8+ T cells, and production of complement fixing antibodies. The Th1 responses are very useful when the host is battling an intracellular infectious agent.[3] The Th2 responses are driven by IL-4, IL-5, IL-10, and IL-13 and are characterized by high levels of neutralizing antibodies and cell-bound antibodies, activation of mast cells, and eosinophils. The Th2 responses are most useful for extracellular organisms. Both responses can become detrimental to the host if unchecked because of side effects produced by their effectors such as nitric oxide, reactive oxygen species, and tumor necrosis factor (TNF)-α in Th1 responses and formation of immune complexes, complement activation, and hypersensitivity reactions in strong Th2 responses. As a rule, the host tries to strike a balance between these two responses. Inhibitors of the Th1 response include IL-10, transforming growth factor (TGF)-β and IL-4, whereas the Th2 response is mostly controlled by IFN-γ, IL-12, and IL-10. Experimental rodent models have shown that IL-10–deficient mice have increased mortality with normally avirulent *Toxoplasma gondii* (an intracellular protozoan) due mostly to overproduction of IFN-γ, TNF-α, and IL-12.[4–6] At the same time, *T. gondii* levels in these animals were lower than in their control counterparts. On the other hand, Th2 responses can also be beneficial and detrimental. It has been widely believed that *Schistosoma* species cause disease because of the granulomatous response to egg deposition in tissues, especially in the mesenteric circulation and liver, leading to scarring and subsequent portal hypertension. In these cases, the host develops a strong Th2 response driven mostly by IL-4 leading to granuloma formation around the eggs. However, in animal models where the IL-4 response is nonexistent, and therefore granuloma formation is markedly impaired, the host succumbs to acute infection rapidly, for the most part because of the deleterious effects of a sustained proinflammatory cytokine response.[7,8] Even though these animal models illustrate the protective role of the Th2 response during the early phases of the infection, the sequelae in the liver during chronic infections, namely, hepatic fibrosis, seems to be driven by IL-13, a potent fibrogenic Th2 cytokine.[9] It appears then that in these animal models, polarized Th1 and Th2 responses are detrimental to the host, whereas a balanced Th1, Th2 response is necessary for the control of egg-induced immunopathology.[10]

Innate Immunity to Parasitic Infections

The traditional view of innate immunity playing a small role in parasitic infections has changed in recent years. Innate immunity plays a very important role in determining the class of the adaptive immune response, be it Th1 or Th2 dominated. Innate immunity operates through both humoral and cellular mechanisms. One of the best-studied humoral mechanisms is the activation of the complement cascade through the alternative pathway (parasite membrane components) or lectins present on the parasite surface. Activation of the classic pathway requires parasite antigen–antibody complexes and therefore occurs when adaptive immunity is already active and production of antibodies is underway. Parasites have developed different strategies present at certain developmental stages that prevent killing by the activated complement cascade and include expression of parasite-derived regulatory proteins (gp160 or gp63) or acquisition of regulatory proteins from the host on the parasite surface such as decay accelerating factor (DAF) and factors H and I, which inhibit formation of the membrane attack complex by acting on C3b.[11] The glycoprotein gp160 present in trypomastigotes of *Trypanosoma cruzi* is homologous to DAF and therefore bind to C3b or C4b, inhibiting the downstream members of the cascade. On the other hand, gp63 present on *Leishmania* species can cleave C3b to its inactive from, iC3b, and prevent deposition of the C5b–C9 attack complex.[11] Other examples include the cleavage of C3 by a cysteine proteinase from *Entamoeba histolytica* that leads to complement activation via the alternative pathway, but it also inactivates C3a and C5a, preventing immunoregulatory and chemotactic functions of these two molecules.[12] Amoebas and certain helminths such as *Echinococcus granulosus* can also acquire host regulatory proteins on their surface.[12,13] Larvae and adults of *Schistosoma mansoni* can also express DAF on their tegumental surface.[13]

Examples of evasion of innate cellular mechanisms include the ability of *Leishmania* species to survive in the macrophage after phagocytosis because of internalization via complement receptors CR1 and CR3, which fails to trigger the respiratory burst.[14] *Trypanosoma cruzi* escapes the phagosome by expressing a C9 homolog that disrupts the phagosomal membrane.[15] *Toxoplasma gondii* prevents acidification of the parasitophorous vacuole.[16] The host at the same time responds to intracellular pathogens by producing IL-12, which activates natural killer cells and macrophages to control the intracellular pathogen. Interleukin-12 is produced by several cells, including macrophages, dendritic cells, and neutrophils. The most studied molecule in protozoans that is thought to be responsible for the production of proinflammatory cytokines is the lipid molecule known as glycosylphosphatidylinositol.[17,18] On the other hand, lipophosphoglycans and glycosylinositolphospholipids of *Leishmania* species have been shown to downregulate production of IL-12 and TNF receptor, therefore favoring the parasite in its initial interaction with the host.[19,20]

Natural killer cells seem to play a very important role in the initial response to parasitic infections. The early production of IFN-γ by these cells seems to prevent the parasite from rapid proliferation in the host.[21] Ultimately, adaptive immunity takes over, and T cells are the main players in controlling intracellular protozoan infections.

Regarding helminths, innate humoral mechanisms are associated with resistance to such infections. T-cell–dependent mast cell responses play a role in infections caused by nematodes. Eosinophils are also important in resistance to helminthic infections during their larval stages, which requires IL-5 production by T cells and opsonization (antibody production). Other components of the innate immune response that have been shown to play a role in protection against parasites include B1 cells (B cells that express the CD5 molecule and are mostly present in body cavities) and γδ-T cells, which seem to play an important role in epithelial mucosal barriers.[21]

Adaptive Immune Response

The ultimate effector mechanisms that control parasitic infections depend largely, as with any other infectious agents, on location within the host (organ and intracellular vs. extracellular), life cycle stages within the host, and evasion strategies of the parasite. Interleukin-12 plays a critical role in starting protective immune responses against intracellular parasites. Interleukin-12 upregulates production of IFN-γ and therefore favors Th1 responses.[22] The main sources of IL-12 are macrophages and dendritic cells, which secrete IL-12 after ingestion of whole parasites or parasite products. Other sources include T cells through ligation of CD40 by CD40 ligand and ligation of CCR5 on dendritic cells by macrophage inflammatory proteins 1a and 1b ligands.[3,23,24] Killing of parasites present in macrophages is achieved mostly through activation of these cells by IFN-γ and TNF-α. Activated macrophages then produce both reactive oxygen intermediates and reactive nitrogen intermediates. In protozoan infections that target other cells different from macrophages, the immune system has to eliminate the parasites from non-phagocytic cells. CD8$^+$ T cells seem to play a critical role in this situation because they recognize antigen in the context of major histocompatibility complex class I molecules, which are expressed by all cells in the body. In these cases, CD8$^+$ T cells aid macrophages by producing IFN-γ.[3] Humoral immunity also has the potential of playing a role in infections produced by intracellular parasites. Antibodies act in different ways by lysing the pathogen directly, playing a role in opsonization, promoting antibody-dependent cell-mediated cytotoxicity, and blocking invasion.[3]

The Th2 responses are important in infections produced by intestinal nematodes. Studies rely on animal models, especially rodents, and have revealed that the two most important cytokines are IL-4 and IL-13 in the process of expulsion of intestinal nematodes from the host.[25] Recently, IL-9 has been implicated and also seems to play an important role in the expulsion process.[25] However, the effector mechanisms responsible for the parasite clearance are not clear. The role of eosinophils and antibodies seems nil or absent. In some animal models of helminth infection mast cells present in the intestinal mucosa may play an important effector role in clearance of intestinal nematodes by production of specific proteases.[26] Other studies have suggested the role of subtle chemical changes in goblet cells in the intestinal mucosa making the microenvironment for worm survival less amenable.[26] Another important observation is the effect of type 1 responses. Both IL-12 and IL-18 suppress or downregulate the type 2 response, leading to delayed expulsion of intestinal nematodes. Most certainly, other factors are in play also, such as host nutrition. Gut nematodes can also produce immunomodulatory molecules that would tip the balance toward a type 1 response by an IFN-γ mimic in *Trichuris muris* infections.[27] Other observations have implicated the size of the initial inoculum as an important determinant of susceptibility or resistance. When the host is infected by a low-level inoculum, susceptibility develops, whereas a large inoculum is associated with a very strong type 2 response followed by expulsion from the host.[3]

After successful entry into a host, bacterial and viral infections are usually followed by rapid replication that leads to tissue damage and therefore disease. The outcome is either recovery if the immune system is able to control the infectious burden or the host's demise if the bacterial/viral burden is overwhelming. In some cases, chronic infections arise in which the host tolerates a certain amount of infectious burden. For parasitic infections, most of these principles apply to protozoan pathogens. In humans, many protozoan infections are followed by a

rapid expansion of the infectious agent within the host followed by chronic infection. Chronicity is due to either antigenic variation or the parasite becoming quiescent or dormant. In helminthic infections, expansion of the initial infectious burden is much more complex because of the life cycle of most helminths. For most helminths, adults mate and try to produce eggs or larvae capable of infecting new hosts. In most cases of human infection, these stages are the ones responsible for the pathology observed in human hosts.

Parasitic Proteases and Their Role in Pathogenesis

A common theme in protozoan and helminthic infections is the presence of proteases that play an important role in virulence and pathogenesis (Tables 42.1 and 42.2). Their roles have been described in establishing, maintaining, and expanding or exacerbating infections. Larval stages of several helminth nematodes directly invade the human host through the skin (*Schistosoma, Strongyloides,* and *Ancylostoma*).[28] The third stage of larval maturation is the invasive one, and several serine and

TABLE 42.1. Summary of representative parasitic proteases and protease inhibitors identified in protozoan pulmonary pathogens.

Protease	Parasite	Mechanism(s) of action
EhCP1	*Entamoeba histolytica*	Inflammatory dysregulation
EhCP2	*E. histolytica*	Cytotoxic; disruption of intestinal epithelium
		Enhancement of chemokine activity (CXCL8)
EhCP5	*E. histolytica*	Enhancement of cytokine activity (IL-1β)inactivation of IL-18
		Caspase-3 activator (apoptotic signal)
Toxopain 1	*Toxoplasma gondii*	Cysteine protease; rhoptry biogenesis; protein processing
Tg SUB1	*T. gondii*	Serine protease; host cell invasion
Microneme processing proteases (Tg MPP1-3)	*T. gondii*	Host cell invasion
Toxamepsin II	*T. gondii*	Aspartyl protease; host cell invasion
CAD98424	*Cryptosporidium parvum*	Aspartyl protease; host cell invasion

TABLE 42.2. Summary of representative parasitic proteases and protease inhibitors identified in helminthic pulmonary pathogens.

Protease	Parasite	Mechanism(s) of action
Elastase-like serine proteases	*Schistosoma mansoni*	Immunoglobulin degradation
Onchocystatin	*Onchocerca volvulus*	Inhibition of host cysteine proteases
		Decreased antigen presentation by antigen-presenting cells and T-cell hyperreactivity
		Cuticle molting
Bm-CPI-1	*Brugia malayi*	Inhibition of host cysteine proteases; unknown
Bm-CPI-2	*B. malayi*	Inhibition of host cysteine proteases (cathepsins L, S, AM)
		T-cell hyporeactivity via altered major histocompatibility complex antigen presentation
Bm-SPN-1	*B. malayi*	Inhibition of host serine proteases; regulation of proteolysis
Bm-SPN-2	*B. malayi*	Unknown
SMpi56	*S. mansoni*	Inhibition of host serine proteases
		Possible inhibition of coagulation cascade and complement
		Activation; inhibition of host neutrophil elastase
SHSPI	*Schistosoma haematobium*	Inhibition of host serine proteases
		Same as SMpi56
Excreted–secreted proteins	*Paragonimus* spp.	Cysteine proteases; tissue degradation
Strongylastacin	*Strongyloides stercolaris*	Metalloproteinase; skin invasion

metalloproteases have been found to be expressed during this stage of development. Likewise, *Onchocerca* migrates extensively within the body once the infection is established after a vector bite.[29] Tissue migration is indeed mediated by proteases expressed in the mature microfilaria. Trematodes such as *Fasciola* species, *Paragonimus* species, and *Clonorchis* species also produce several proteolytic enzymes during the tissue invasive stage of the life cycle in order to form a niche in their target organs.[30,31] In addition, proteases can also play a role in the immunomodulatory process by degrading immunoglobulins or altering cytokine production, especially IL-8.[32] As a general rule, proteases produced during the larval stage play an important role in tissue invasion or immune evasion, whereas proteases produced during the adult stage primarily degrade gut proteins (those who use the bowel as niche for adult stages) and have roles in anticoagulation and immune evasion.

The best-studied proteases are the ones produced by schistosomes and have been described in several stages of development.[33] They can be present in the parasite gut and excreted or present on the surface of the parasite where they can coat it and play a role in anticoagulation or degradation of immunoglobulins. Some of the proteases are also potent immunogens and could be used as vaccine candidates.[34]

Other kinds of proteins produced by helminths are protease inhibitors that play an important role in perpetuating these infections for the entire life span of the host. Molecules released from filarial parasites such as phosphorylcholine can interfere with activation and proliferation of T and B cells and favor Th responses toward the Th2 type. Inhibitors of cysteine and serine proteases, known as cystatins and serpins, respectively, can also have a role in immunomodulation.[34]

The best-known cystatin is the one found in *Onchocerca volvulus* (onchocystatin) and is responsible for inhibition of protease activity in antigen-presenting cells, leading to low T-cell responses.[35] Other cystatins have been described in *Brugia malayi*, which inhibit host cathepsins leading to altered digestion of antigens necessary for presentation of antigen-derived peptides to immune cells via major histocompatibility complex molecules.[36] Serpins have been described in *Schistosoma* species and are possibly responsible for anticoagulation. *Ascaris* and *Ancylostoma* species secrete protease inhibitors that might be responsible for inhibition of host enzymes, such as trypsin and chymotrypsin in the gut lumen, and key coagulation factors.[37]

Protozoans also produce potent proteases that play an important role in pathogenesis and immune response. For example the genome of *E. histolytica* is thought to contain up to 20 proteases, three of which are very well studied, and they all belong to the family of cysteine proteases: EhCP1, EhCP2, and EhCP5. Two of them, 1 and 5, are actually absent in other nonpathogenic amebas.[38] They are cytolytic and therefore contribute to intestinal layer degradation and trigger strong inflammatory responses via enhanced activity of chemokines such as CXCL8. Other protozoan proteases have been described in *T. gondii* and their role elucidated during entrance and exit from parasitized cells. Examples include cell surface proteins such as Tg MIC (*Toxoplasma* microneme protein) and Tg AMA1 (*T. gondii* apical membrane antigen); proteins present in the rhoptries, such as Tg toxopain I and Tg SUB1 and SUB2, important in processing and targeting rhoptry proteins ROP2, ROP3, and ROP4; and proteins of the aspartyl protease group such as toxamepsin II are also important for invasion.[34]

Molecular Pathogenesis of Pulmonary Protozoan Pathogens

Toxoplasmosis

Toxoplasmosis is a systemic disease due to an obligate intracellular coccidian named *Toxoplasma gondii,* which is a very homogeneous species with only three strains worldwide, responsible for more than 95% of infections. Its distribution is worldwide, and the range of animal species that can be affected by it is broad.[39] The life cycle involves a wide range of mammalian intermediate hosts.[39] *Toxoplasma gondii* is found in three forms in nature, namely, tachyzoites (asexual forms), tissue cysts enclosing bradyzoites (found mostly in brain and muscle), and oocysts containing sporozoites (sexual forms). The invasive form in humans and other hosts is the tachyzoite and is also the form responsible for cellular and tissue damage. Tissue cysts containing bradyzoites serve as reservoirs for tachyzoites and therefore play an important role in disease transmission (ingestion of contaminated meat) and latent infection. Oocysts with sporozoites are found only in the definitive hosts, the wild and domestic Felidae, where they are produced in the intestinal epithelium and then shed in the stool. After sporulation, the cysts are infectious and can then be ingested/inhaled by humans. Other routes of transmission include ingestion of raw or undercooked infected meats, perinatal exposure from infected mothers, transfusion of infected blood products, and transplantation of infected organs.

Regardless of the route of infection, tissue cysts or oocysts are digested in the gastrointestinal tract, and bradyzoites (tissue cysts) or sporozoites (oocysts) are released in the intestine where they invade neighboring cells and become tachyzoites. Invasion of the eukaryotic host cell is an active process mediated completely by the parasite's cytoskeleton.[40] The host cell cytoskeleton does not play any role nor does phosphorylation of any proteins upon attachment of the parasite to the host cell via glycosaminoglycans and sialic acid.[41] The ubiquity of the receptor explains the wide distribution of the parasite in human infections. The parasite adhesins also play an important role in entry. They are not displayed continuously on the surface, as opposed to bacterial and viral adhesins. Instead, the adhesins are contained in cytoplasmic structures called *micronemes* that discharge their contents upon contact mediated by a controlled release of calcium from the parasite.[41] A "baseline" secretion of the adhesion is sufficient for the initial interaction followed by a dramatic increase in microneme secretion. Such secretion is only apical facilitating interaction in a polarized way that is necessary for entry.

The best-characterized of the microneme proteins is MIC2, which belongs to the TRAP (thrombospondin anonymous repeat protein) family of proteins.[41,42] Type A domains (or von Willebrand factor–like domains) interact with heparin-like molecules and glycosaminoglycans and therefore are important as adhesins. After apical secretion, MIC2 is transported to the posterior pole of the parasite via the actin cytoskeleton, where it is cleaved and released from the cell surface. Microneme protein 2 in turn is tightly related to an accessory protein (M2AP) that is also necessary for upregulation of MIC2 secretion from the micronemes. The cytoplasmic domain of MIC2 in turn binds aldolase in the host cell, and this complex is able to recruit actin monomers.[41] The actual protein responsible for the gliding motility in *T. gondii* is a class XIV myosin, Tg MyoA, that is present beneath the plasma membrane.[43] This protein is anchored to the inner membrane complex by accessory proteins, and myosin filaments can propel actin filaments recruited by the aldolase–MIC2 complex and induce motility. Entry also depends on a calcium-regulated secretion of the parasite.[44] However, calcium signals in the host cell do not play a role in entry either. Because entry relies completely on active motility of the parasite, research into this area has been active and has elucidated some molecular mechanisms responsible for the unique "gliding" motility seen in all apicomplexans. *Toxoplasma gondii* motility is highly predictable and consists of circular gliding (counterclockwise) and helical gliding (clockwise). Once inside the cell, *T. gondii* resides in a modified vacuole that does not fuse with any of the endocytic or exocytic vesicles. Most of the vacuolar membranes come from apical organelles called *rhoptries,* which secrete their contents after entry. The main component identified so far is the transmembrane protein ROP2, which mediates interactions between the vacuolar membrane and the host cell's mitochondria and endoplasmic reticulum.[45] Another component of the vacuolar membrane is the host's glycosylphosphatidylinositol-anchored proteins.

The damage during the acute infection is due to cell death of parasitized cells and a vigorous inflammatory reaction that initially is neutrophilic in nature and turns lymphocytic when acquired immunity sets in. Most human hosts control the disease in the acute phase, and critical determinants are IL-12 and IFN-γ followed by CD8+ T cells.[46,47] Antibodies are also capable of neutralizing or killing circulating tachyzoites.[48] Tissue cysts containing bradyzoites are then formed, and tissue integrity is usually restored completely. In some cases, infection persists in the lymph nodes, leading to chronic lymphadenopathy, usually in the cervical region accompanied by mild constitutional symptoms. The spectrum of disease ranges from asymptomatic infections (the most common form) to severe disseminated disease seen mostly in immunocompromised patients. In the lungs, the main presentation is that of a diffuse confluent bronchopneumonia that appears secondary to hematogenous and lymphatic dissemination, followed by shock. In acquired immunodeficiency syndrome, pulmonary toxoplasmosis is seen in up to 3% of cases, and CD4+ T cells are usually below 100 cells/μL.

Amebiasis

Pulmonary amebiasis is due to *E. histolytica*, a protozoan primarily responsible for colonic infections in humans. Pulmonary infections are the result of complications seen in cases of intestinal amebiasis in which *E. histolytica* becomes systemic after invasion of the colonic mucosa, spreading to the liver, lungs, and other organs. Most of these infections occur in the tropics in developing countries. The life cycle of *E. histolytica* comprises an infective cyst and an invasive trophozoite. Cyst formation appears to be mediated by quorum sensing triggered by a lectin (Gal/GalNAc) on the parasite's surface.[49] Excystation occurs in the intestine, and eight trophozoites are produced from each cyst that then invade the colonic mucosa, leading to ulcer formation. Killing of host cells occurs only after contact of trophozoites with the host cell, and adhesion is mediated by an amebic adhesin, the Gal/GalNAc lectin, referred to earlier. The lectin recognizes N- and O-linked oligosaccharides on the cell surface. This lectin also appears to be cytotoxic, because monoclonal antibodies directed against certain epitopes block cytotoxicity in vitro, although adhesion is conserved.[49] Invasion and hematogenous spread activates the immune system, and in cases of amebiasis both the alternate and classic complement pathways are activated. However, trophozoites are resistant to the C5b–C9 attack complex, which is inhibited by the above-mentioned lectin.[50] Mechanisms of cell killing by *E. histolytica* are under intense scrutiny and may include dramatic rises in cytoplasmic calcium upon contact leading to cell blebbing and death, apoptosis, and a pore-forming protein isolated from amoeba.[51] Amoebic cytoplasm also contains collagenases and cysteine proteases that play a role in pathogenesis by degrading extracellular matrix and producing cell detachment, respectively.[34]

Immunity to amebic infections is usually both humoral (secretory IgA antibodies directed against the surface lectin) and cell mediated in the form of cytokine activation of macrophages and neutrophils that become amebicidal after stimulation by IFN-γ, IL-12, and TNF-α.[52–54] Most infections are acquired via the fecal–oral route, but cases can also be acquired via the anal route in homosexual men. Pleuropulmonary complications of amebiasis are seen in cases of hepatic amebiasis (up to 20%) or invasive colonic amebiasis (up to 3%). Multiple forms have been described, including a pleuritis that results from the inflammatory reaction in the liver "traveling" via the right dome of the diaphragm, empyema or pulmonary amebic complications (pneumonitis, abscess or fistulas) secondary to rupture of a hepatic abscess, and hematogenous spread.

Microsporidiosis

Phylum Microsporidia are spore-forming, obligate intracellular protozoans that reside in the intestine, liver, kidneys, brain, and other tissues of wild and domesticated mammals and several other animal species. Eight genera out of more than 144 (containing more than 1,000 species) have been documented as human pathogens, namely, *Encephalitozoon, Enterocytozoon, Pleistophora, Brachiola, Nosema, Trachipleistophora, Vittaforma,* and *Microsporidium*.[55] Of these, *Encephalitozoon hellem, Encephalitozoon cuniculi,* and *Enterocytozoon bieneusi* have been documented as the main culprits in pulmonary microsporidiosis. Microsporidia in general are rare diseases in humans that have received attention because of the increased incidence of infections present in patients with acquired immunodeficiency syndrome. In cases of pulmonary microsporidiosis, there usually is intestinal involvement and in many cases systemic involvement.

Histologically, the microsporidia are seen as faintly basophilic intracellular round structures in the apical portion of the cell measuring 1–1.5 μm in diameter inside the cells lining the bronchial and bronchiolar epithelium. Microsporidia are eukaryotes with Golgi apparatus, mitochondrial remnants, a double-layered spore structure (exo- and endospore layers), and a typical extrusion apparatus anchored to the anterior end of the spore by a disc.[55] Upon invasion of the host cell, the sporoplasm is extruded through the polar tube, which pierces the phagocytic vacuole, into the cytoplasm of the host cell.[56] Spores gain access to humans via ingestion or inhalation. Once they germinate in the host, the sporoplasm undergoes merogony, in which proliferation occurs (meronts), followed by sporogony, in which the membranes thicken again and from sporoblasts that turn into mature spores and are released from the distended cell and into the environment to complete the cycle.

Characterization of the process of extrusion of the sporoplasm is lacking. Early events in the process include rupture of the anterior attachment complex upon host cell attachment and cell penetration. Thus far three polar proteins have been identified—protein-tyrosine phosphatase (PTP) 1, PTP2, and PTP3.[56] Protein-tyrosine phosphatase 1 is O-mannosylated, a posttranslational modification that seems to be necessary for its function.[57] Protein-tyrosine phosphatase 1 represents at least 70% of the polar tube mass. Furthermore, it has been demonstrated in humans that PTP1 is one of the immunodominant proteins that triggers formation of neutralizing antibodies of the IgG type in humans.[58] The major epitope is indeed the posttranslational carbohydrate modification, namely, O-mannosylation. Protein-tyrosine phosphatase 2 is also immunodominant, and PTP3 seems to be involved in sporoblast-to-spore polar tube biogenesis.[59] Protein-tyrosine phosphatase 1 and PTP2 contribute to the high tensile strength of the polar tube via extensive disulfide linkages.[59] Another mechanism of infection is phagocytosis upon attachment of the microsporidia to the host cell. In these cases, penetration of the host cell by the polar apparatus and extrusion of the spore contents does not occur on the cell surface. Instead, the spore is phagocytosed, and some of them extrude their contents using the polar tube, thus escaping the endosomes.[60] The spores that remain in the endosomes at some point fuse with lysosomes and disappear after 72 hr. The phagocytosis route is 10 times more effective than the attachment followed by extrusion in an in vitro model using *Enc. cuniculi*. Adhesion mechanisms have also been studied with *Encephalitozoon intestinalis*, and host cell glycosaminoglycans seem to play an important role in the adhesion process. Another interesting pathogenetic mechanism is manipulation of the host cell cycle. In models using *Encephalitozoon*, it has been shown that levels of cyclin D1 are decreased and cyclin B1 are elevated, suggesting that host cells can go into arrest to ensure optimal growth of the parasitophorous vacuole in a nondividing cell.[61]

Cryptosporidiosis

Cryptosporidium was first diagnosed as a human pathogen in 1976 in two immunocompromised patients in whom persistent diarrhea developed. The largest outbreak occurred in Milwaukee in 1984 and involved 400,000 people most of whom recovered completely.[62] However, in immunocompromised patients, the diarrhea persists for weeks or months and is debilitating. Currently the main risk factor is the presence of human immunodeficiency virus infection/acquired immunodeficiency syndrome. Cryptosporidiosis is endemic in developing countries and is responsible for childhood diarrhea. Respiratory cryptosporidiosis results in cough, dyspnea, fever, and chest pain and is always associated with gastrointestinal symptoms. Histologically, there is tracheitis, bronchitis, and bronchiolitis with mild to moderate mononuclear inflammatory infiltrate in the mucosa and submucosa. The organisms are usually seen in the epithelial surface and rarely in submucosal glands.

Cryptosporidium belongs to the phylum Apicomplexa (some other members of the phylum include *Toxoplasma*, *Plasmodia*, and *Babesia*) and is a monoxenous genus (complete developmental cycle occurs in one host).[63] Oocysts are ingested by the host and release in the small bowel lumen four sporozoites (infective form). Upon attachment, sporozoites form an intracellular/extracytoplasmic parasitophorous vacuole in which they evolve

into trophozoites and then into meronts (schizonts). Schizonts undergo three nuclear divisions and become type I merozoites that invade neighboring cells and develop into type II merozoites or into trophozoites. The merozoites can infect other cells and restart the asexual part of the cycle. Type II meronts can also undergo two nuclear divisions and release four type II merozoites that invade other cells and become macro- and microgametocytes, which can then form a zygote (sexual reproduction). The zygote ultimately becomes either a thin-walled oocyst (autoinfectious) or a thick-walled cyst shed in feces. There are several species within the genus *Cryptosporidium*, and the ones known to infect humans include *C. parvum* (humans and bovines), *C. hominis* (humans), *C. meleagridis* (turkeys and humans), and *C. felis* (cats and humans).[63] Infectious doses are very low. As few as 10 oocysts are capable of starting an infection in humans. In addition, cysts are extremely resistant to chlorination treatments and pass through filters relatively easily. Forms of the disease include endemic childhood diarrhea in developing countries, traveler's diarrhea in visitors to endemic countries, chronic diarrhea in immunosuppressed patients, and diarrhea outbreaks in developed countries.

The pathogenesis of these infections is virtually unknown. Several mechanisms have been proposed, such as malabsorption produced by villous inflammation and blunting, prostaglandin secretion at the local levels, cellular damage secondary to IL-8 and TNF-α secretion, and substance P release in the microenvironment.[64–68] Entry into the unique compartment (intracellular/extracytoplasmic) requires protein kinase C activation and actin rearrangements in vitro.[69] In cultured biliary epithelial cells, *C. parvum* has been shown to induce apoptosis via Fas/FasL interactions.[69] In fact, *C. parvum* is responsible for cases of ascending cholangitis in immunocompromised patients. The full genomic sequence of *C. parvum* "type II" isolate was finalized in 2004 and revealed 9.1 Mbp in eight chromosomes, coding for approximately 3,807 proteins.[70] Cryptosporidia lack mitochondria and apicoplasts, unlike *Plasmodia* and *Toxoplasma*, making the genomes simpler and smaller. Its metabolic pathways are very efficient and rely mostly on glycolysis as a source of adenosine triphosphate due to absence of mitochondrial genes. Because of its unique intracellular but extracytoplasmic location, several genes are present for transport of sugars and amino acids into the parasitophorous vacuole. Motility and adhesion seems to be mediated by a family of proteins known as thrombospondin-related-adhesive proteins (TRAPs). In the adhesion process, an apical complex glycoprotein (CSL) has been shown to play an important role, and its receptor is an 85-kDa protein in intestinal epithelial cells.

Cell-mediated immunity is important in controlling infections, and the most important cytokine seems to be

IFN-γ.[71] Humoral response appears to be irrelevant. Elevated levels of IL-15 in the intestinal mucosa seem to correlate with no fecal shedding in human volunteers infected with Cryptosporidia.[72] Other cytokines found elevated in Haitian children include IL-8, IL-13, and TNF-α.[64]

Molecular Pathogenesis of Pulmonary Helminthic Pathogens

Nematodes

Filariasis

Filariasis infections can be divided into lymphatic filariasis and zoonotic filariasis. The first type is caused by *Wuchereria bancrofti*, *Brugia malayi*, and *B. timori*. The latter is caused by filarial parasites that usually infect other animal hosts, and humans become accidental hosts.

Lymphatic filariasis is the cause of recurrent lymphadenitis leading to sequelae such as elephantiasis and hydrocele due to lymphatic obstruction. In some individuals infected with *W. bancrofti* or *B. malayi*, a distinct asthma-like syndrome develops, known as *tropical pulmonary eosinophilia*, in which there is paroxysmal cough and wheezing (typically at night due to nocturnal filarial periodicity), low-grade fever, and weight loss. Typically, the blood reveals severe eosinophilia (>3,000/μL) and elevated IgE levels in serum.[73] If not treated, the condition can develop into restrictive pulmonary disease with interstitial fibrosis.

The life cycle[73] of lymphatic filariae is very long and starts with the mosquito biting a patient with circulating microfilariae. Once in the mosquito, the filariae develop into first through third stage larvae in the thoracic muscles, which then introduce infective third stage larvae into the human circulation. Larvae migrate to lymphatics where they mature and differentiate into adult females and males, which then mate and start releasing microfilariae after 5–10 years. Up to 10,000 parasites can be released per day from pregnant female worms.

Initial immune responses to the third and fourth larval stages (early in human infection) are both proinflammatory Th1 and Th2 responses.[74] By the time microfilariae appear in the blood, several years later, there are markedly diminished antigen-specific T-cell responses, especially IFN-γ and IL-4.[75] Mechanisms of immune tolerance are multiple and poorly studied but include genetic predisposition, suppressor T cells, increased expression of downregulatory molecules such as cytotoxic T-lymphocyte–associated protein 4, and high levels of regulatory cytokines such as IL-10 and TGF-β.[76,77] Another potentially important pathogenetic mechanism is the presence of large numbers of the endosymbiont *Wolbachia pipientis* in filarial parasites that probably modulate the parasite's life cycle. Dying parasites probably release large numbers of *Wolbachia* cellular products, triggering an inflammatory reaction.[78–80]

The best known zoonotic filariasis is the one caused by *Dirofilaria immitis*.[81] These are all transmitted to humans by an infected arthropod and lead to solitary (sometimes multiple) "coin lesions" in the lungs that are easily confused with neoplastic processes on chest x-rays. Patients are usually asymptomatic, and the diagnosis is made when the lesion is taken out for histologic examination. Peripheral eosinophilia can be seen in blood smears. Pathogenetically, the lesion appears as a reaction around a dead or dying worm. *Dirofilaria immitis* is mainly a dog pathogen, although it can infect other mammals such as cats. This nematode has a similar life cycle as described for the lymphatic filariasis. However, *D. immitis* is mostly a vascular pathogen.[82] In humans, who are resistant to chronic infections, the microfilariae lodge in pulmonary vessels and subcutaneous vessels and the immune system destroys the parasite, at which time the histopathology appears.

Strongyloidiasis

Strongyloidiasis is caused by *Strongyloides stercolaris*. The genus contains more than 40 named species, and only one is capable of completing its cycle in humans.[83] The disease is mostly tropical, but endemic foci can be seen in temperate areas. The infection is acquired at the time filariform larvae enter the human body via the skin (usually the lower extremities) and gain access to vascular or lymphatic channels that take them to the lungs where they rupture the capillaries and gain access to alveolar spaces. Location of an adequate host depends on detection of thermal and chemical signals by the larvae using specialized amphidial neurons located in the amphidial channel.[84] A metalloproteinase expressed in the third larval stage, named *strongylastacin*, is possibly responsible for skin penetration. This protein belongs to the metzincin superfamily of zinc metalloendopeptidases.[85] From the lungs, they migrate up to the bronchi, trachea, and upper aerodigestive tract where they are swallowed and develop into hermaphroditic adults in the small bowel mucosa. The adults then penetrate the mucosa and release eggs that hatch into rhabditiform larvae. At this point of the cycle, two possible scenarios come into play: (1) larvae are shed in the stool and develop into free-living male and female adults that mate and release eggs into the soil, followed by hatching of rhabditiform larvae that then develop into filariform larvae (indirect or heterogonic development); and (2) larvae shed in stool develop directly into filariform larvae (direct development). In addition, a third possible scenario is that of autoinfection in which rhabditiform larvae in the bowel lumen mature into filariform larvae that then can invade the body through bowel mucosa or perianal skin. The latter scenario is the one responsible for the so-called pruritic larva currens syndrome and hyperinfection leading to systemic disease (pneumonitis, colitis, polymicrobial sepsis, and meningitis).[83]

Chronic infections with *S. stercolaris* are as a rule asymptomatic. However, in cases of hyperinfection, dissemination is marked, and in the lungs it can lead to diffuse bronchopneumonia, often with intraalveolar hemorrhage or abscess formation. These infections are usually mixed with intestinal bacteria carried by the parasites in their cuticles. Rhabditiform and filariform larvae, and even eggs can be seen in tissue sections. The mortality rates for hyperinfected patients approach 90% and are usually associated with administration of exogenous steroids for conditions such as asthma and chronic obstructive pulmonary disease. Steroids seem to upregulate metabolism of ecdysteroids (molting hormones) in the parasite via receptor-mediated uptake of the corticosteroid by the parasites.[86,87] Eggs and rhabditiform larvae receive molting signals, and the number of filariform larvae increases dramatically. Intestinal populations in these cases approach 100,000 adults, and, even if steroids are discontinued and molting rates are low, the burden of adult worms is so high that population growth cannot be arrested. The described developmental processes might be regulated by a family of transcription factors that control genes in response to fat-soluble hormones such as steroids. A gene homolog of *daf-12* present in *Caenorhabditis elegans* has been described in *S. stercolaris*.[88] Such genes play an important role in the development of *C. elegans*.

Other risk factors include human T-cell lymphoma/leukemia virus (HTLV) 1 infections, autoimmune diseases, hematologic malignancies, and solid organ allografts.[83] However, the common denominator in many of these conditions seems to be steroid administration. In HTLV-1 infections, it has been demonstrated that the cytokine profile in humans infected with this retrovirus favors the parasite by way of high levels of IFN-γ and TGF-β, leading to decreased levels of IL-4, IL-5, IgE, and IL-13.[89] Interestingly, *S. stercolaris* has also been shown to decrease the period of time to develop acute T-cell lymphoma/leukemia (ATLL) in patients infected with HTLV-1. In such cases, *S. stercolaris* induces a significant expansion of restricted T-cell clones infected with HTLV-1.[90] On average, the incubation period of acute T-cell lymphoma/leukemia is decreased by 30 years in patients infected with *S. stercolaris*.

Other Nematodes (Ascaris lumbricoides), Hookworms (Ancylostoma duodenale, Necator americanus), Toxocara canis *(Visceral larva migrans), and* Trichinella *Species*

Ascaris lumbricoides and hookworms are acquired through the mouth, and, once eggs hatch in the intestines, larva migrate throughout the body, including the lungs, where they cross from capillaries to airways and migrate up to the upper airways to be ingested and mature into adults in the intestine. The larval stage is capable of producing mechanical damage to tissues in the lungs and hypersensitivity reactions elicited by larval antigens leading to pulmonary and bronchial lesions rich in neutrophils, eosinophils, and macrophages (eosinophilic pneumonitis). Pulmonary signs and symptoms are known clinically as Loeffler's syndrome, which tends to be more severe in cases of ascaridiasis. *Toxocara* infections tend to be as severe as ascaridiasis and can also lead to acute or chronic eosinophilic pneumonitis whose severity also depends on the larval burden. *Trichinella* is also a nematode that can affect several organ systems including the lungs, and its presentation is similar to the described syndromes.

Trematodes

Paragonomiasis

The best known pathogen in the genus *Paragonimus* is *P. westermani*, although seven more species have been described as human pathogens: *P. westermani* is mostly found in the Far East (from India to Japan and the Philippines); *P. heterotremus* in China and southeast Asia; *P. skrjabini* and *P. hueitungensis* from China; *P. miyazakii* from Japan; *P. uterobilateralis* and *P. africanis* from central and western Africa; *P. mexicanus* from Central and South America; and *P. kellicotti* from North America.[91]

The life cycles are very similar but the best-studied one is *P. westermani*. The cycle[92] starts with ingestion of metacercariae in uncooked crab or crayfish. The metacercariae are then excysted in the stomach and small bowel and migrate through the bowel wall, mesenteric fat, and diaphragm until they reach the pleural cavity and lungs where they mature into hermaphroditic flukes that cross-fertilize. The body surrounds the parasites with a capsule that then cavitates, causing hemoptysis and cough. Adults lay eggs after fertilization, which are found in sputum and feces if swallowed. The eggs then embryonate in water, and miracidia are released that then penetrate *Thiara* or *Semisulcospira* snails. Once in this intermediate host, miracidia turn into sporocysts, rediae and then short-tailed cercaria. The infected snails are then ingested by crabs or crayfish, and cercariae encyst as metacercariae in gills and muscles of these crustaceans.

The spectrum of disease ranges from pleuropulmonary infections due to *P. westermani*, *P. heterotremus*, *P. africanis*, and *P. uterobilateralis* to mostly cutaneous manifestations due to *P. skrjabini*. Adults can live up to 5–10 years in human tissues and acute disease manifestations can occur any time during this period, but usually acute symptoms occur days after ingestion. They include diarrhea and abdominal pain followed days later by fever, chest pain, fatigue, urticaria, and cough that can turn productive with rusty-colored sputum.[92] Pathologically, the lesions consist of cavitary lesions when adult flukes appear. Excised lesions reveal adult worms with fibrous cysts and egg-induced granulomas. Bronchiectasis, vasculitic lesions, and consolidation can also occur. Other organs affected include skin, brain, liver, spleen, and peritoneum.

Paragonimus species secrete several biologically active molecules called *excretory–secretory products* (ESPs), and several of them are cysteine proteases whose role is probably host tissue degradation.[92,93] In addition, they might play a role in immune modulation. In vitro, microglial cells exposed to low levels of EPSs secrete nitric oxide, whereas at high levels microglial cells die.[94] Likewise, coincubation of eosinophils with ESPs induces rapid degranulation and elevated levels of granule products such as eosinophil-derived neurotoxin.[95] In addition, ESPs can also induce apoptosis in eosinophils via caspase-3 activation, facilitating survival of parasitic larvae early in the infectious process.[96] Another important mechanism of survival is production of a copper/zinc-containing superoxide dismutase at various stages of development, including the adult stage.[97]

Cytokines and chemokines found elevated in human serum or pleural effusions of humans infected with *Paragonimus* species included thymus and activated-regulated chemokine, eotaxin, RANTES, and IL-8.[98] The immune response in general is that of a Th2-dominated response with an IgG4 subclass.

Schistosomiasis

Schistosomiasis is one the main human helminthiasis around the world with an estimated prevalence of 200 million people infected worldwide. The main human pathogens are *Schistosoma mansoni*, *S. japonicum*, and *S. haematobium*. Two other species, *S. intercalatum* and *S. mekongi*, have also been described in humans, although their geographic distribution is more limited.[99]

The life cycle[100] starts with penetration of the host's skin by forked tail cercaria after which they shed their tail and become schistosomulae. At the site of penetration, they induce an inflammatory response called *swimmers' itch*. The schistosomulae then migrate to the portal circulation in liver where they become adults that start to mate for the life of the parasite (3–30 years). Mating adults of *S. mansoni* and *S. japonicum* migrate to the mesenteric venules of bowel and rectum where females start laying eggs that reach the liver and eventually the stools. *Schistosoma haematobium* adults migrate to the venous plexus of the bladder where females lay eggs, leading to bacterial infections in the bladder, hematuria, and later in the disease process scarring and calcification of the venules. Eggs are shed in the urine. In cases with heavy parasitism, eggs can embolize to other parts of the body, including brain and lungs. Once eggs are shed in stools or urine, they hatch in the outside environment and release miracidia that then penetrate the different snails (*Bulinis*, *Biomphalaria*, and *Oncomelania*) in which they develop as two generations of sporocysts. When mature, the snails release the forked tail cercaria to restart the cycle.

The disease itself is divided into the acute and chronic phases. During the acute phase the patient develops dermatitis, and the circulation of schistosomulae through the hepatic and pulmonary vascular beds followed by maturation and initial oviposition induces a systemic response that includes fever, chills, sweats, cough, and headaches (seen only in *S. japonicum* or *S. mansoni* exposure).[101] Lymphadenopathy and hepatosplenomegaly can also be seen. The chronic phase is characterized by a granulomatous response to eggs deposited in the intestinal, portal, or urinary tract veins. Pulmonary schistosomiasis is the result of egg deposition in the pulmonary vascular bed resulting in granuloma formation and fibrosis.[101] If a large area of the pulmonary circulation is involved, secondary pulmonary hypertension can ensue. Eggs reach the pulmonary circulation via urinary veins draining into the inferior vena cava or bypassing the liver through portosystemic collaterals in cases of *S. mansoni* and *S. japonicum* infection in which liver damage has led to portal hypertension.[102]

One of the main driving forces in mouse models of *S. mansoni* behind the formation of liver granulomas once eggs are deposited in the hepatic microcirculation is IL-13 and the IL-13 receptor complex.[9] Liver fibrogenesis is greatly decreased in animals deficient in IL-13 or treated with IL-13 antagonists. It has been shown that IL-13 promotes expression of arginase in myofibroblasts, a step necessary to increase collagen production. Other less important mediators include IL-4/IL-4Rα and STAT6.[103] In fact, granulomas evolve in two phases: during the early stages, a short-lived type 1 cytokine response predominates, whereas in later stages a type 2 response takes over and is longlived.[10] The immune response to the eggs is necessary to neutralize an uncontrolled inflammatory response to egg antigens, leading even to death in the early stages of the disease. The most important cell at this stage is the CD4+ Th2 cell. From the parasite's point of view, several molecules have been described as important in skewing the immune response toward the Th2 phenotype. An area of intense research is now focused on the role of several schistosomal glycans, including Lewis X and lacto-N-fucopentose III conjugates. These molecules act via Toll-like receptor 4 and possibly C-type lectins.[104]

With regard to the acute phase of the disease called *snail fever*, *Katayama fever*, or *acute toxemic schistosomiasis*, it is widely accepted that the signs and symptoms are due to large amounts of circulating immune complexes, elevated levels of proinflammatory cytokines, and low type 2 responses.[105] In fatal animal models an overwhelming type 1 response is usually seen that can be controlled by IL-4 and IL-10. Interleukin-4 in vitro is necessary for development of CD4+ Th2 cells.

Cestodes: Echinococcosis

Echinococcosis is caused by cestodes belonging to the genus *Echinococcus* to which more than five species have been described, namely, *E. granulosus*, *E. multilocularis*, *E. oligarthrus*, *E. vogeli*, and *E. shiquicus*.[106] The first four are well known as human pathogens but the newly described *E. shiquicus* is of unknown human pathogenicity. *Echinococcus granulosus* contains several strains (G1–G10) based on their definitive host isolation.[106] The classic form of the disease (cystic echinococcosis) is due to *E. granulosus*. Another form of the disease, known as *alveolar echinococcosis*, is a highly lethal and infiltrative disease in humans caused by *E. multilocularis*. Infections by *E. vogeli* and *E. oligarthrus* lead to polycystic echinococcosis. The latter three are far less frequent in humans because their host specificity is limited to wild animals as opposed to *E. granulosus*.

The life cycles of all of them involve two mammalian hosts. Definitive hosts are carnivores in which adult worms live in their intestines. The eggs from adult worms are shed in the environment and, when ingested by intermediate hosts (such as humans), hatch and liberate embryos that migrate to extraintestinal tissues (liver, lungs, brain, etc.) and turn into metacestode or larval forms. It is these larval forms that are known as *hydatid cysts* that take different morphologies when causing disease (polycystic, alveolar, or cystic).[107] In nature, the passage from intermediate host (except for humans) to definitive host is the result of predator–prey interactions between those two hosts.

Echinococcus granulosus, as mentioned earlier, is the most common in humans because dogs are one of the definitive hosts. Infected dogs can harbor up to 40,000 tapeworms, which in turn can release up to 1,000 eggs each per day. Fecal–oral transmission is therefore relatively easy during close contact with the dog. Indirect transmission via arthropods, fomites, soil, water, and vegetables is also possible. Other hosts besides dogs include sheep, cattle, camels, pigs, and cervids.

Signs and symptoms are extremely variable and depend on the localization of the cyst (lungs, brain, liver, etc.), size of the cyst, and condition of the cyst (intact vs. ruptured). Conversely, in the brain and eyes, signs and symptoms appear more quickly. Cyst rupture can cause a variety of complications, including mild to severe allergic reactions, chest pain, cough, dyspnea, and hemoptysis. The immune response is usually biphasic. The first phase is directed against the oncosphere or egg hatching in the intestine and penetrating the gut wall. This response is far more effective in controlling the infection, because the metacestode in the extraintestinal tissues has more means of evading the immune response.

Conclusion

The classic triad of infectious agent, host, and environment plays a key role in parasitic as well as in any other infectious agents. The geographic distribution seen with some of the parasitic diseases, especially the ones due to helminths, is in large part because of the complex life cycles that most of the helminthic parasites need to survive in nature. The interplay between host and parasite is also a very complex system in which virulence factors, developmental cycles, parasite nutrition, host immune response, and immune modulation by the parasite interact in a complicated network that we are beginning to elucidate at the molecular level. The availability of small animal models has provided great insights into the pathogenesis of these diseases. Likewise, with the use of powerful molecular techniques, both in vivo and in vitro experiments can now be designed to elucidate the host–parasite relationship and move the research to a new level.

References

1. Pearce EJ, Tarleton RL. Overview of Parasitic Pathogens. In Kaufmann SHE, Sher A, Ahmed R, eds. Immunology of Infectious Diseases. Washington, DC: ASM Press; 2002: 39–52.
2. Mosmann TR, Cherwinski H, Bond MW, et al. Two types of murine helper T cell clone. I. Definition according to profiles of lymphokine activities and secreted proteins. J Immunol 1986;136:2348–2357.
3. Scott P, Grencis RK. Adaptive immune effector mechanisms against intracellular protozoa and gut-dwelling nematodes. In Kaufmann SHE, Sher A, Ahmed R, eds. Immunology of Infectious Diseases. Washington, DC: ASM Press; 2002:235–246.
4. Gazzinelli RT, Wysocka M, Hieny S, et al. In the absence of endogenous IL-10, mice acutely infected with *Toxoplasma gondii* succumb to a lethal immune response dependent on CD4+ T cells and accompanied by overproduction of IL-12, IFN-gamma and TNF-alpha. J Immunol 1996;157:798–805.

5. Bessieres MH, Swierczynski B, Cassaing S, et al. Role of IFN-gamma, TNF-alpha, IL4 and IL10 in the regulation of experimental *Toxoplasma gondii* infection. J Eukaryot Microbiol 1997;44:87S.

6. Butcher BA, Kim L, Panopoulos AD, Watowich SS, Murray PJ, Denkers EY. IL-10–independent STAT3 activation by *Toxoplasma gondii* mediates suppression of IL-12 and TNF-alpha in host macrophages. J Immunol 2005;174:3148–3152.

7. Dunne DW, Pearce EJ. Immunology of hepatosplenic schistosomiasis mansoni: a human perspective. Microbes Infect 1999;1:553–560.

8. Cheever AW, Yap GS. Immunologic basis of disease and disease regulation in schistosomiasis. Chem Immunol 1997;66:159–176.

9. Chiaramonte MG, Schopf LR, Neben TY, et al. IL-13 is a key regulatory cytokine for Th2 cell-mediated pulmonary granuloma formation and IgE responses induced by *Schistosoma mansoni* eggs. J Immunol 1999;162:920–930.

10. Wynn TA, Thompson RW, Cheever AW, Mentink-Kane MM. Immunopathogenesis of schistosomiasis. Immunol Rev 2004;201:156–167.

11. Norris KA, Schrimpf JE. Biochemical analysis of the membrane and soluble forms of the complement regulatory protein of *Trypanosoma cruzi*. Infect Immun 1994;62:236–243.

12. Reed SL, Ember JA, Herdman DS, et al. The extracellular neutral cysteine proteinase of *Entamoeba histolytica* degrades anaphylatoxins C3a and C5a. J Immunol 1995;155:266–274.

13. Pearce EJ, Hall BF, Sher A. Host-specific evasion of the alternative complement pathway by schistosomes correlates with the presence of a phospholipase C-sensitive surface molecule resembling human decay accelerating factor. J Immunol 1990;144:2751–2756.

14. Da Silva RP, Hall BF, Joiner KA, Sacks DL. CR1, the C3b receptor, mediates binding of infective *Leishmania* major metacyclic promastigotes to human macrophages. J Immunol 1989;143:617–622.

15. Andrews NW, Abrams CK, Slatin SL, Griffiths G. A *T. cruzi*–secreted protein immunologically related to the complement component C9: evidence for membrane pore-forming activity at low pH. Cell 1990;61:1277–1287.

16. Sibley LD, Weidner E, Krahenbuhl JL. Phagosome acidification blocked by intracellular *Toxoplasma gondii*. Nature 1985;315:416–419.

17. Nebl T, De Veer MJ, Schofield L. Stimulation of innate immune responses by malarial glycosylphosphatidylinositol via pattern recognition receptors. Parasitology 2005;130(Suppl):S45–S62.

18. Ropert C, Ferreira LR, Campos MA, et al. Macrophage signaling by glycosylphosphatidylinositol-anchored mucin-like glycoproteins derived from *Trypanosoma cruzi* trypomastigotes. Microbes Infect 2002;4:1015–1025.

19. Proudfoot L, O'Donnell CA, Liew FY. Glycoinositolphospholipids of *Leishmania major* inhibit nitric oxide synthesis and reduce leishmanicidal activity in murine macrophages. Eur J Immunol 1995;25:745–750.

20. Carrera L, Gazzinelli RT, Badolato R, et al. *Leishmania* promastigotes selectively inhibit interleukin 12 induction in bone marrow-derived macrophages from susceptible and resistant mice. J Exp Med 1996;183:515–526.

21. Hunter CA, Sher A. Innate immunity to parasitic infections. In Kaufmann SHE, Sher A, Ahmed R, eds. Immunology of Infectious Diseases. Washington, DC: ASM Press; 2002:111–127.

22. Trinchieri G. Interleukin-12: a cytokine at the interface of inflammation and immunity. Adv Immunol 1998;70:83–243.

23. Aliberti J, Reis e Sousa C, Schito M, et al. CCR5 provides a signal for microbial induced production of IL-12 by CD8 alpha+ dendritic cells. Nat Immunol 2000;1:83–87.

24. Soong L, Xu JC, Grewal IS, et al. Disruption of CD40–CD40 ligand interactions results in an enhanced susceptibility to *Leishmania amazonensis* infection. Immunity 1996;4:263–273.

25. Finkelman FD, Shea-Donohue T, Goldhill J, et al. Cytokine regulation of host defense against parasitic gastrointestinal nematodes: lessons from studies with rodent models. Annu Rev Immunol 1997;15:505–533.

26. Donaldson LE, Schmitt E, Huntley JF, Newlands GF, Grencis RK. A critical role for stem cell factor and c-kit in host protective immunity to an intestinal helminth. Int Immunol 1996;8:559–567.

27. Grencis RK, Entwistle GM. Production of an interferon-gamma homologue by an intestinal nematode: functionally significant or interesting artefact? Parasitology 1997;115(Suppl):S101–S106.

28. Tort J, Brindley PJ, Knox D, et al. Proteinases and associated genes of parasitic helminths. Adv Parasitol 1999;43:161–266.

29. Lackey A, James ER, Sakanari JA, et al. Extracellular proteases of *Onchocerca*. Exp Parasitol 1989;68:176–185.

30. Park H, Kim SI, Hong KM, et al. Characterization and classification of five cysteine proteinases expressed by *Paragonimus westermani* adult worm. Exp Parasitol 2002;102:143–149.

31. Na BK, Lee HJ, Cho SH, et al. Expression of cysteine proteinase of *Clonorchis sinensis* and its use in serodiagnosis of clonorchiasis. J Parasitol 2002;88:1000–1006.

32. Shin MH, Lee SY. Proteolytic activity of cysteine protease in excretory-secretory product of *Paragonimus westermani* newly excysted metacercariae pivotally regulates IL-8 production of human eosinophils. Parasite Immunol 2000;22:529–533.

33. Curwen RS, Wilson RA. Invasion of skin by schistosome cercariae: some neglected facts. Trends Parasitol 2003;19:63–68.

34. McKerrow JH, Caffrey C, Kelly B, Loke P, Sajid M. Proteases in parasitic diseases. Annul Rev Pathol Mech Dis 2006:497–536.

35. Hartmann S, Lucius R. Modulation of host immune responses by nematode cystatins. Int J Parasitol 2003;33:1291–1302.

36. Manoury B, Gregory WF, Maizels RM, Watts C. Bm-CPI-2, a cystatin homolog secreted by the filarial parasite *Brugia malayi*, inhibits class II MHC-restricted antigen processing. Curr Biol 2001;11:447–451.

37. Silverman GA, Bird PI, Carrell RW, et al. The serpins are an expanding superfamily of structurally similar but

functionally diverse proteins. Evolution, mechanism of inhibition, novel functions, and a revised nomenclature. J Biol Chem 2001;276:33293–33296.

38. Bruchhaus I, Jacobs T, Leippe M, Tannich E. *Entamoeba histolytica* and *Entamoeba dispar*: differences in numbers and expression of cysteine proteinase genes. Mol Microbiol 1996;22:255–263.

39. Hill DE, Chirukandoth S, Dubey JP. Biology and epidemiology of *Toxoplasma gondii* in man and animals. Anim Health Res Rev 2005;6:41–61.

40. Dobrowolski JM, Sibley LD. Toxoplasma invasion of mammalian cells is powered by the actin cytoskeleton of the parasite. Cell 1996;84:933–939.

41. Sibley LD. Intracellular parasite invasion strategies. Science 2004;304:248–253.

42. Dowse T, Soldati D. Host cell invasion by the apicomplexans: the significance of microneme protein proteolysis. Curr Opin Microbiol 2004;7:388–396.

43. Meissner M, Schluter D, Soldati D. Role of *Toxoplasma gondii* myosin A in powering parasite gliding and host cell invasion. Science 2002;298:837–840.

44. Lovett JL, Marchesini N, Moreno SN, Sibley LD. *Toxoplasma gondii* microneme secretion involves intracellular Ca(2+) release from inositol 1,4,5-triphosphate (IP[3])/ryanodine-sensitive stores. J Biol Chem 2002;277:25870–25876.

45. Sinai AP, Joiner KA. The *Toxoplasma gondii* protein ROP2 mediates host organelle association with the parasitophorous vacuole membrane. J Cell Biol 2001;154:95–108.

46. Aliberti J, Jankovic D, Sher A. Turning it on and off: regulation of dendritic cell function in *Toxoplasma gondii* infection. Immunol Rev 2004;201:26–34.

47. Sher A, Collazzo C, Scanga C, et al. Induction and regulation of IL-12–dependent host resistance to *Toxoplasma gondii*. Immunol Res 2003;27:521–528.

48. Fadul CE, Channon JY, Kasper LH. Survival of immunoglobulin G–opsonized *Toxoplasma gondii* in nonadherent human monocytes. Infect Immun 1995;63:4290–4294.

49. Eichinger D. A role for a galactose lectin and its ligands during encystment of *Entamoeba*. J Eukaryot Microbiol 2001;48:17–21.

50. Reed SL, Gigli I. Lysis of complement-sensitive *Entamoeba histolytica* by activated terminal complement components. Initiation of complement activation by an extracellular neutral cysteine proteinase. J Clin Invest 1990;86:1815–1822.

51. Ravdin JI, Moreau F, Sullivan JA, et al. Relationship of free intracellular calcium to the cytolytic activity of *Entamoeba histolytica*. Infect Immun 1988;56:1505–1512.

52. Haque R, Ali IM, Sack RB, Farr BM, Ramakrishnan G, Petri WA, Jr. Amebiasis and mucosal IgA antibody against the *Entamoeba histolytica* adherence lectin in Bangladeshi children. J Infect Dis 2001;183:1787–1793.

53. Salata RA, Martinez-Palomo A, Murray HW, et al. Patients treated for amebic liver abscess develop cell-mediated immune responses effective in vitro against *Entamoeba histolytica*. J Immunol 1986;136:2633–2639.

54. Denis M, Chadee K. Human neutrophils activated by interferon-gamma and tumour necrosis factor-alpha kill *Entamoeba histolytica* trophozoites in vitro. J Leuk Biol 1989;46:270–274.

55. Weiss LM, Schwartz DA. Microsporidiosis. In Guerrant RL, Walker DH, Weller PF, eds. Tropical Infectious Diseases: Principles, Pathogens and Practice, vol 2. Philadelphia: Churchill Livingstone; 2006:1126–1140.

56. Xu Y, Weiss LM. The microsporidian polar tube: a highly specialised invasion organelle. Int J Parasitol 2005;35:941–953.

57. Xu Y, Takvorian PM, Cali A, et al. Glycosylation of the major polar tube protein of *Encephalitozoon hellem*, a microsporidian parasite that infects humans. Infect Immun 2004;72:6341–6350.

58. Peek R, Delbac F, Speijer D, et al. Carbohydrate moieties of microsporidian polar tube proteins are targeted by immunoglobulin G in immunocompetent individuals. Infect Immun 2005;73:7906–7913.

59. Peuvel I, Peyret P, Metenier G, et al. The microsporidian polar tube: evidence for a third polar tube protein (PTP3) in *Encephalitozoon cuniculi*. Mol Biochem Parasitol 2002;122:69–80.

60. Franzen C, Muller A, Hartmann P, Salzberger B. Cell invasion and intracellular fate of *Encephalitozoon cuniculi* (Microsporidia). Parasitology 2005;130:285–292.

61. Scanlon M, Shaw AP, Zhou CJ, et al. Infection by microsporidia disrupts the host cell cycle. J Eukaryot Microbiol 2000;47:525–531.

62. MacKenzie WR, Hoxie NJ, Proctor ME, et al. A massive outbreak in Milwaukee of *Cryptosporidium* infection transmitted through the public water supply. N Engl J Med 1994;331:161–167.

63. Bushen OY, Lima AAM, Guerrant RL. Cryptosporidiosis. In Guerrant RL, Walker DH, Weller PF, eds. Tropical Infectious Diseases: Principles, Pathogens and Practice, vol 2. Philadelphia: Churchill Livingstone; 2006:1003–1014.

64. Kirkpatrick BD, Daniels MM, Jean SS, et al. Cryptosporidiosis stimulates an inflammatory intestinal response in malnourished Haitian children. J Infect Dis 2002;186:94–101.

65. Argenzio RA, Rhoads JM, Armstrong M, Gomez G. Glutamine stimulates prostaglandin-sensitive Na(+)–H+ exchange in experimental porcine cryptosporidiosis. Gastroenterology 1994;106:1418–1428.

66. Kandil HM, Berschneider HM, Argenzio RA. Tumour necrosis factor alpha changes porcine intestinal ion transport through a paracrine mechanism involving prostaglandins. Gut 1994;35:934–940.

67. Seydel KB, Zhang T, Champion GA, et al. *Cryptosporidium parvum* infection of human intestinal xenografts in SCID mice induces production of human tumor necrosis factor alpha and interleukin-8. Infect Immun 1998;66:2379–2382.

68. Robinson P, Okhuysen PC, Chappell CL, et al. Substance P expression correlates with severity of diarrhea in cryptosporidiosis. J Infect Dis 2003;188:290–296.

69. Hashim A, Mulcahy G, Bourke B, Clyne M. Interaction of *Cryptosporidium hominis* and *Cryptosporidium parvum* with primary human and bovine intestinal cells. Infect Immun 2006;74:99–107.

70. Abrahamsen MS, Templeton TJ, Enomoto S, et al. Complete genome sequence of the apicomplexan, *Cryptosporidium parvum*. Science 2004;304:441–445.

71. White AC, Robinson P, Okhuysen PC, et al. Interferon-gamma expression in jejunal biopsies in experimental human cryptosporidiosis correlates with prior sensitization and control of oocyst excretion. J Infect Dis 2000; 181:701–709.

72. Robinson P, Okhuysen PC, Chappell CL, et al. Expression of IL-15 and IL-4 in IFN-gamma-independent control of experimental human *Cryptosporidium parvum* infection. Cytokine 2001;15:39–46.

73. Nutman TB, Kazura JW. Filariasis. In Guerrant RL, Walker DH, Weller PF, eds. Tropical Infectious Diseases: Principles, Pathogens and Practice, vol 2. Philadelphia: Churchill Livingstone; 2006:1152–1162.

74. Babu S, Nutman TB. Proinflammatory cytokines dominate the early immune response to filarial parasites. J Immunol 2003;171:6723–6732.

75. Graham SP, Trees AJ, Collins RA, et al. Down-regulated lymphoproliferation coincides with parasite maturation and with the collapse of both gamma interferon and interleukin-4 responses in a bovine model of onchocerciasis. Infect Immun 2001;69:4313–4319.

76. Steel C, Nutman TB. CTLA-4 in filarial infections: implications for a role in diminished T cell reactivity. J Immunol 2003;170:1930–1938.

77. King CL, Mahanty S, Kumaraswami V, et al. Cytokine control of parasite-specific anergy in human lymphatic filariasis. Preferential induction of a regulatory T helper type 2 lymphocyte subset. J Clin Invest 1993;92:1667–1673.

78. Hise AG, Gillette-Ferguson I, Pearlman E. The role of endosymbiotic *Wolbachia* bacteria in filarial disease. Cell Microbiol 2004;6:97–104.

79. Taylor MJ. A new insight into the pathogenesis of filarial disease. Curr Mol Med 2002;2:299–302.

80. Taylor MJ, Cross HF, Bilo K. Inflammatory responses induced by the filarial nematode *Brugia malayi* are mediated by lipopolysaccharide-like activity from endosymbiotic *Wolbachia* bacteria. J Exp Med 2000;191: 1429–1436.

81. Eberhard ML. Zoonotic Filariasis. In Guerrant RL, Walker DH, Weller PF, eds. Tropical Infectious Diseases: Principles, Pathogens and Practice, vol 2. Philadelphia: Churchill Livingstone; 2006:1189–1203.

82. Theis JH. Public health aspects of dirofilariasis in the United States. Vet Parasitol 2005;133:157–180.

83. Siddiqui AA, Genta RM, Berk LB. Strongyloidiasis. In Guerrant RL, Walker DH, Weller PF, eds. Tropical Infectious Diseases: Principles, Pathogens and Practice, vol 2. Philadelphia: Churchill Livingstone; 2006:1274–1285.

84. Ashton FT, Li J, Schad GA. Chemo- and thermosensory neurons: structure and function in animal parasitic nematodes. Vet Parasitol 1999;84:297–316.

85. Gomez Gallego S, Loukas A, Slade RW, et al. Identification of an astacin-like metallo-proteinase transcript from the infective larvae of *Strongyloides stercoralis*. Parasitol Int 2005;54:123–133.

86. Genta RM. Dysregulation of strongyloidiasis: a new hypothesis. Clin Microbiol Rev 1992;5:345–355.

87. Escobedo G, Roberts CW, Carrero JC, Morales-Montor J. Parasite regulation by host hormones: an old mechanism of host exploitation? Trends Parasitol 2005;21: 588–593.

88. Siddiqui AA, Stanley CS, Berk SL. A cDNA encoding the highly immunodominant antigen of *Strongyloides stercoralis*: gamma-subunit of isocitrate dehydrogenase (NAD+). Parasitol Res 2000;86:279–283.

89. Carvalho EM, Da Fonseca Porto A. Epidemiological and clinical interaction between HTLV-1 and *Strongyloides stercoralis*. Parasite Immunol 2004;26:487–497.

90. Gabet AS, Mortreux F, Talarmin A, et al. High circulating proviral load with oligoclonal expansion of HTLV-1 bearing T cells in HTLV-1 carriers with strongyloidiasis. Oncogene 2000;19:4954–460.

91. Velez ID, Ortega JE, Velasquez LE. Paragonimiasis: a view from Colombia. Clin Chest Med 2002;23:421–431.

92. Maclean JD, Cross J, Mahanty S. Liver, Lung, and Intestinal Fluke Infections. In Guerrant RL, Walker DH, Weller PF, eds. Tropical Infectious Diseases: Principles, Pathogens and Practice, vol 2. Philadelphia: Churchill Livingstone; 2006:1349–1369.

93. Lee EG, Na BK, Bae YA, et al. Identification of immunodominant excretory–secretory cysteine proteases of adult *Paragonimus westermani* by proteome analysis. Proteomics 2006;6:1290–1300.

94. Jin Y, Lee JC, Choi IY, et al. Excretory–secretory products produced by *Paragonimus westermani* differentially regulate the nitric oxide production and viability of microglial cells. Int Arch Allergy Immunol 2006;139: 16–24.

95. Shin MH, Chung YB, Kita H. Degranulation of human eosinophils induced by *Paragonimus westermani*–secreted protease. Korean J Parasitol 2005;43:33–37.

96. Min DY, Lee YA, Ryu JS, et al. Caspase-3–mediated apoptosis of human eosinophils by the tissue-invading helminth *Paragonimus westermani*. Int Arch Allergy Immunol 2004;133:357–364.

97. Li AH, Na BK, Kong Y, et al. Molecular cloning and characterization of copper/zinc-superoxide dismutase of *Paragonimus westermani*. J Parasitol 2005;91:293–299.

98. Matsumoto N, Mukae H, Nakamura-Uchiyama F, et al. Elevated levels of thymus and activation-regulated chemokine (TARC) in pleural effusion samples from patients infested with *Paragonimus westermani*. Clin Exp Immunol 2002;130:314–318.

99. Ross AG, Bartley PB, Sleigh AC, et al. Schistosomiasis. N Eng J Med 2002;346:1212–1220.

100. King CH. Schistosomiasis. In Guerrant RL, Walker DH, Weller PF, eds. Tropical Infectious Diseases: Principles, Pathogens and Practice, vol 2. Philadelphia: Churchill Livingstone; 2006:1341–1348.

101. King CH. Acute and chronic schistosomiasis. Hosp Pract (Off Ed) 1991;26:117–130.

102. Cheever AW. Schistosomiasis. Infection versus disease and hypersensitivity versus immunity. Am J Pathol 1993; 142:699–702.

103. Jankovic D, Kullberg MC, Noben-Trauth N, et al. Schistosome-infected IL-4 receptor knockout (KO) mice, in contrast to IL-4 KO mice, fail to develop granulomatous

pathology while maintaining the same lymphokine expression profile. J Immunol 1999;163:337–342.

104. Hokke CH, Yazdanbakhsh M. Schistosome glycans and innate immunity. Parasite Immunol 2005;27:257–264.

105. Stadecker MJ, Asahi H, Finger E, et al. The immunobiology of Th1 polarization in high-pathology schistosomiasis. Immunol Rev 2004;201:168–179.

106. Thompson RC, McManus DP. Towards a taxonomic revision of the genus *Echinococcus*. Trends Parasitol 2002; 18:452–457.

107. Schantz PM, Kern P, Brunett E. Echinococcosis. In Guerrant RL, Walker DH, Weller PF, eds. Tropical Infectious Diseases: Principles, Pathogens and Practice, vol 2. Philadelphia: Churchill Livingstone; 2006:1304–1326.

Section 6
Molecular Pathology of Other Nonneoplastic Pulmonary Diseases: General Principles

43
Inflammation

Armando E. Fraire

The Inflammatory Response

In the lung, as in other anatomic sites, inflammation can be regarded as a complex, generally salutary response of the body to injurious agents. This bodily response derives from a series of interconnected cellular and molecular events acting in concert with an equally complex array of neurogenic[1,2] and vasogenic factors.[3–5] Principal cellular actors playing a role in the inflammatory process include polymorphonuclear leukocytes, lymphocytes, plasma cells, eosinophils, mast cells, monocytes, and macrophages. Leading molecular compounds regulating cellular responses are chemical mediators such as vasoactive amines, prostaglandins, and leukotrienes, as well as members of the kinin and complement activation system (Table 43.1).[6] This chapter discusses the major forms of the inflammatory response, namely, acute and chronic inflammation, and addresses granulomatous inflammation. In addition, it covers mechanisms of response selection, innate immunity (Toll receptors), and specific cellular constituents, in particular, pulmonary alveolar macrophages and dendritic cells and their roles in antigen presentation and human leukocyte antigen (HLA)–linked diseases.

As aptly stated by Muller, inflammation can be thought of as an attempt to restore homeostasis.[7] In the early story of humans, when life spans were short and people were more likely to die young from infection or trauma, the ability to fight pathogens and heal wounds was much more critical for the survival of the species.[7] However, now that we live longer, we have come to realize that inflammation can paradoxically act as a "double-edged sword" with potentially harmful as well as beneficial effects.[7] Harmful effects of inflammation, stemming from excessive or defective inflammation, have been succinctly summarized by Kumar et al. and are discussed further below.[8]

A considerable amount of particulates and other environmental pollutants contaminate the air entering the airways. To these, virus- and bacteria-containing droplets can be added when respiratory secretions are released from others' airways by coughing or sneezing. The respiratory system must recognize and eliminate these unwanted elements in inspired air.[9] This is accomplished by a complex and multifaceted line of defenses designed to protect the integrity of the respiratory tract.[9] Along with the cough reflex, mucociliary clearance, and humoral immunity, inflammation ranks among the most clinically and physiologically important defense mechanisms of the respiratory tract.[9]

Like the genitourinary tract, the skin, and the gut, the lung is one of the interfaces of the sterile body sanctuary with the environment.[10] As noted, the lung is equipped with defense mechanisms involving cellular and humoral immunity. In the complex processes of cellular defense, two cells of hematopoietic origin, the lymphocyte and the pulmonary macrophage, play key roles in the inflammatory response. In many ways, they represent two very different sides of this inflammatory response. The macrophage, as a phagocytic cell, is of ancient phylogenetic lineage, is not antigen specific, and may be triggered by many inflammatory stimuli. The lymphocyte is present only in vertebrates and represents a significant refinement in the inflammatory response: it displays antigen specificity and participates in discrimination of self and nonself.[10]

Recognized since antiquity and recorded in ancient texts, inflammation is characterized by the well-known cardinal signs of *tumor, rubor, calor,* and *dolor* (swelling, redness, heat, and pain). The overall purpose of the inflammatory response is to respond to an injury and its attendant damage. Two forms of inflammation are classically recognized: acute and chronic. By definition, acute inflammation takes place over a short period of time: hours or days. Chronic inflammation, on the other hand, refers to inflammation of prolonged duration. The time frame for chronic inflammation is quite variable, ranging from weeks to months or years. Some authors, perhaps

459

TABLE 43.1. Inflammatory mediators.

Polypeptides	Lipids
Cytokines	Thromboxane
Complement activation products	Leukotrienes
Clotting cascade products	Prostaglandins
Reactive oxygen intermediates	Vasoactive amines
Superoxide	Histamine
Hydrogen peroxide	Serotonin
Metabolites of arginine	Nucleotides
Nitric oxide	
Adenosine diphosphate	

Source: From Kunkel et al.,[6] with permission.

arbitrarily, define chronic inflammation as inflammation lasting longer than 4 weeks. Regardless of its duration, however, chronic inflammation usually has an antecedent stage of acute inflammation, with the acute process evolving into a chronic one. In some situations, however, chronic inflammation begins de novo without a preceding acute phase. Furthermore, acute and chronic inflammations may coexist in a superimposed state.

What causes chronicity? For an inflammatory process to become chronic, the stimulus, most often injury or infection, must persist. Chronic inflammation differs considerably from acute inflammation and is characterized by three components: active inflammation, tissue destruction, and attempts at repair. The component of active inflammation is characterized primarily by cellular recruitment of macrophages. This recruitment evolves from continued recruitment of monocytes through activated endothelium. In addition, macrophages are stimulated to proliferate at sites of inflammation. Thus, both recruitment and proliferation contribute to the mononuclear infiltrates. Tissue destruction takes place in necrotizing diseases such as in lung abscesses secondary to bacterial infection. Repair is dominated by fibroblastic proliferation and collagen deposition.

Harmful Effects of Inflammation

Excessive inflammation is the basis of many categories of human disease. This is particularly true for disorders of the immune system.[8] Recent studies, however, point to an important role of inflammation in a wide variety of human diseases that are not primarily disorders of the immune system. These include cancer, atherosclerosis, and ischemic heart disease as well as some neurodegenerative diseases such as Alzheimer's disease.[8]

Defective inflammation typically results in increased susceptibility to infections, delayed healing of wounds, and tissue damage.[8] The susceptibility to infections

reflects the fundamental role of the inflammatory response in host defense and is the reason why this response is a central component of the defense mechanisms that are called *innate immunity*.[8] Delayed repair occurs because the inflammatory response is essential for clearing damaged tissue and debris and provides the necessary stimulus to get the repair process started.[8]

Innate Immunity: Toll-Like Receptors

The mammalian immune system is an intricate system that can discriminate between self and nonself, affording protection from a wide variety of pathogenic insults. This system can be viewed as consisting of two parts or subsystems, one dealing with innate immunity and the other with adaptive immunity. In general, innate immunity is a nonspecific inducible response to pathogens.[11] It is present at birth, does not show specificity, and does not become more efficient upon subsequent exposure to pathogens. Components of the innate immune response include mechanical barriers (skin, mucosal surfaces), physiologic defenses (soluble factors such as lysozyme, interferon, complement), phagocytic cells in concert with some families of antimicrobial proteins (defensins), compounds such as resolvins that reduce chronic inflammation by inhibiting the production and transportation of inflammatory cells and chemical mediators to the site of inflammation, and Toll-like receptors (TLRs) that serve to recognize complex molecular patterns known as *pathogen-associated molecular patterns* (PAMPs).[12] To this list of components of the innate immune system, natural killer (NK) cells can be added on account of their nonspecific cytotoxicity against some viruses and tumor cells.[12] This chapter, however, focuses primarily on the important roles of the *toll* gene and TLRs in the innate immunity subsystem and their relationship to some selected inflammatory conditions affecting the lung.

Deriving its name from the German, and literally meaning "mad, wild, or terrific,"[13] the *toll* gene has generated an excitement in the scientific community that seems to match its name. First identified in the fruit fly (*Drosophila melanogaster*), the *toll* gene is important not only in the fly's embryogenesis (helping to establish the dorsal–vertical axis) but also in contributing to its protection against fungal infections.[14-16] Following their recognition in *Drosophila* in 1988, TLRs were identified in mammals in 1997 and later in humans. As noted, TLRs serve to recognize PAMPs and are part of the innate immune host defenses in a great variety of infectious and noninfectious inflammatory conditions of the lung.[17] Generally, TLR proteins serve a protective role in infectious diseases, particularly in tuberculosis. The progression of chronic inflammatory lung disease can be influenced by TLR-dependent responses.[18] In higher vertebrates, TLRs play a pivotal role in innate immune responses by enabling the host to recognize a wide range of PAMPs such as bacterial lipo-saccharides, viral RNA, and flagellin.[18] The engagement of TLR proteins leads to upregulation of costimulatory and proinflammatory cytokines, as well as nitrogen and oxygen products. The role of TLR proteins in lung diseases such as allergic asthma, airway hyperreactivity, and tuberculosis is currently the subject of much research. As the identification of new receptors continues to expand our understanding of the evolving family of TLRs and their ligands (PAMPs) and activation factors has grown exponentially, now including 13 numerically designated TLRs. Among these, TLR2 and TLR4 have been the subject of considerable attention, particularly in connection with chronic obstructive pulmonary disease, bacterial pneumonias, fungal infections of the lung, and some allergic disorders.

Pons and associates investigated the role of TLRs in the induction of the inflammatory response in patients with chronic obstructive pulmonary disease (COPD).[19] These authors used flow cytometry to analyze the expressions of TLR2, TLR4, and CD14 in monocytes. To study the functional responses of these receptors, monocytes were stimulated with peptidoglycan or lipo-saccharide and levels of tumor necrosis factor (TNF)-α and interleukin (IL)-6 were quantitated. In this model, the expression of TLR2 was upregulated in the peripheral blood of patients with COPD as compared with never-smokers or smokers with normal lung function.[19]

Toll-like receptors recognize highly conserved microbial molecular patterns, such as those found in endotoxin.[20] Using a murine model, Velasco et al. tested whether TLR4 and TLR2 stimulation in vivo would modulate subsequent adaptive (allergic) immune responses.[20] The authors analyzed the effects of pulmonary administration of a TLR4 agonist, lipid A, and two TLR2 agonists, peptidoglycan and pan-cys, in their murine model of allergic inflammation. In their experiment, Velasco et al. showed that both types of TLR agonists decreased the allergen-induced recruitment of eosinophils when administered at sensitization or challenge. The authors concluded that both TLR4 and TLR2 agonists decrease allergen responses, supporting the concept that exposure to bacterial components under defined conditions may protect against allergic disease.[20]

Toll-like receptor 4 is considered by some to be critical for inducing host innate immunity against many Gram-negative bacteria, including some respiratory pathogens.[21] *Francisella tularensis*, the causative agent of tularemia, is a Gram-negative facultative intracellular bacterium. To determine the role of TLR4 in host defense against airborne *F. tularensis*, Chen et al. challenged TLR4-deficient and wild-type mice with low doses of aerosolized type A

F. tularensis.[21] Host responses were compared at 2 and 4 days postinoculation (dpi). At dpi 2, bacterial burdens were similar between the two strains of mice, but TLR4-deficient mice harbored approximately 10-fold fewer bacteria in their spleens and livers. At dpi 4, the bacterial burdens were indistinguishable between the two groups. These data, along with the lack of differences in survival and cytokine levels, prompted these authors to conclude that TLR4 does not contribute to resistance of mice to airborne type A *F. tularensis*.[21]

Acinetobacter baumannii is a Gram-negative bacterial pathogen increasingly associated with bacterial pneumonia in humans.[22] To gain insight into the role of CD14, TLR4, and TLR2 in the host response to *A. baumannii*, Knapp et al. used gene-deficient mice that had been intranasally infected with *A. baumannii* and challenged with *A. baumannii*–derived lipopolysaccharide.[22] Bacterial counts were increased in CD14 and TLR4 gene-deficient mice, and only these animals developed bacteremia. The pulmonary cytokine–chemokine response was impaired in TLR4 knockout mice, and the onset of lung inflammation was delayed. In contrast, TLR2-deficient animals displayed an earlier cellular influx into their lungs, combined with increased macrophage inflammatory protein 2 and monocyte chemoattractant protein 1 concentrations, that was associated with accelerated elimination of bacteria from the pulmonary compartment. Neither CD14 nor TLR4 gene-deficient mice responded to intranasal administration of lipopolysaccharide, whereas TLR2 knockout mice were indistinguishable from wild-type animals.[22] Knapp and associates concluded that CD14 and TLR4 play a key role in the innate detection of *A. baumannii* via the lipopolysaccharide moiety, resulting in effective elimination of the bacteria from the lung, whereas TLR2 signaling seems to counteract the robustness of innate responses during acute *A. baumannii* pneumonia.[22]

Acquired Immunity: Macrophages, Dendritic Cells and Antigen Presentation

Macrophages are ubiquitous phagocytic cells of monocytic lineage that reside within various tissue compartments in a variety of organs.[10] They are particularly prominent in the lung where they serve multiple functions, including augmenting particle removal on the muco-ciliary escalator, transporting particles to regional lymph nodes, and promoting the generation of B and T cells.[10] Several types of macrophages and antigen-presenting cells are found in the lung: blood monocytes, alveolar macrophages, dendritic cells, epithelioid histiocytes, and Langerhans cells. This section focuses on alveolar macrophages, dendritic cells, and epithelioid histiocytes occurring within granulomas.

Macrophages play an important part in the inflammatory response, producing TNF, interleukin (IL)-1, and IL-6. In addition, more than 100 other substances are known to be secreted by pulmonary macrophages. Macrophages are important in lymphocyte activation, where they act as important antigen-presenting cells for T lymphocytes. They take up antigen, from which they cleave immunogenic fragments. Binding and display of these fragments on either class I or class II HLA antigens stimulates T cells. Macrophages are commonly seen at sites of infection, a prime example being tuberculosis.[23] The macrophages are first attracted to an infected area by both bacterial and neutrophil fragments as well as by endotoxins, complement, immune complexes, and collagen fragments. Macrophages remain at a focus of infection because of a migration-inhibition factor generated by T lymphocytes.[23] Besides killing organisms, macrophages play an important role in lysis of tumor cells by releasing substances such as TNF, complement components, and proteases. Macrophages are present in wounds immediately after injury, where they synthesize collagenase and elastase, which clean the wound. They also release factors regulating the physiologic activity of bronchial epithelial cells. Pulmonary macrophages not only have a phagocytic role, keeping the lung sterile, but are also secretory and regulatory cells.[23] For example, alveolar macrophages and epithelial cells may act in concert in the clearance process of removing inhaled particulate matter. Fujii et al. have shown that human alveolar macrophages and bronchial epithelial cells produce cytokines when macrophages phagocytize atmospheric particles.[24] This cell-to-cell interaction results in production of cytokines growth factors such as granulocyte-macrophage colony-stimulating factor, add TNF-α, IL-7β, and IL-6.[24] Histologically, macrophages are particularly prominent in smoking-related lung diseases such as desquamative interstitial pneumonia and respiratory bronchiolitis.

Abbas et al. proposed a maturation scheme for mononuclear phagocytes that is shown in Table 43.2.[25] Although, the most commonly held view is that lung macrophages originate from blood monocytes, alveolar proliferation has also been demonstrated. However, interstitial macrophages, as compared with alveolar ones, have an increased ability to replicate and synthesize DNA.

The alveolar macrophage varies in size from 12 to 40μm in diameter and has a lobulated and sometimes kidney-shaped nucleus, numerous mitochondria, and electron-dense secondary lysosomes in its cytoplasm. Increased numbers of macrophages are found in smokers. In smokers, they are larger (up to 50μm) and contain pigmented intracytoplasmic inclusions. Alveolar macrophages have been separated into different subpopulations. Membrane receptor expression and functions, such as phagocytosis and mediator release, vary among these different cell populations. Apart from circulating monocytes and interstitial macrophages, a third and morphologically distinct population of pulmonary macrophages have been described in humans. Although most attention has been given to parenchymal (alveolar) macrophages, it has been shown that if the lung is fixed by submersion, intravascular fixation, or vapor fixation, many macrophages can be seen in the bronchial tree. Airway fixation displaces most airway macrophages. Some of these cells are present in the mucociliary escalator system, but others are adherent to the bronchial epithelium.[23]

Originally identified by Steinman and colleagues, dendritic cells represent the pacemakers of the immune response.[26–28] They are crucial for the presentation of antigenic peptides to T lymphocytes and are widely recognized as the key antigen-presenting cells. Dendritic cells are distributed throughout the respiratory tract, from the nasal mucosa to the lung and pleura.[29] The most prominent populations of dendritic cells are located within the epithelium of conducting airways. In the airways, dendritic cells form a rich cellular network comparable to that of Langerhans cells in the epidermis. Within the lung parenchyma, dendritic cells lie near or at interseptal junctions between adjacent alveolar units.[29]

TABLE 43.2. Maturation of mononuclear phagocytes.

Bone marrow	Peripheral blood		Tissues
Stem cell → Monoblast	→ Monocyte →	Macrophage	Activated macrophages / Activation / Differentiation / Microglia (brain) / Kupffer cells (liver) / Alveolar macrophages (lung) / Osteoclasts (bone)

Source: From Abbas et al.,[25] with permission.

Monocytes continuously exit the bloodstream and enter body tissues, where many differentiate to macrophages.[30] Because there is no net accumulation of macrophages in tissues during the steady state, monocyte entry into tissues may be just sufficient to replace dying macrophages, or monocytes may only transiently traverse tissues.[30] During resolution of inflammation, at least some monocytes leave tissues by migrating to draining lymph nodes. However, the state of differentiation of monocyte-derived cells that arrive in lymph nodes has not been well characterized.[30]

Randolph et al. investigated the differentiation and trafficking of inflammatory monocytes that phagocytosed subcutaneously injected fluorescent latex microspheres.[30] As expected, most of the monocytes became microsphere-containing macrophages, which remained in subcutaneous tissue. However, about 25% of latex-containing cells migrated to the T-cell area of draining lymph nodes, where they expressed dendritic cell–restricted markers and high levels of costimulatory molecules.[30] Microsphere-transporting cells were distinct from resident skin dendritic cells, and this transport was reduced by more than 85% in monocyte-deficient osteopetrotic mice. Thus, the authors concluded that a substantial minority of inflammatory monocytes carry phagocytosed particles to lymph nodes and differentiate into dendritic cells.[30]

Holt and others have implicated populations of dendritic cells in lung parenchyma and tissue from the airways as key regulators of qualitative and quantitative aspects of T-cell responses to antigenic challenge.[29] Under steady-state conditions, dendritic cells are specialized for antigen uptake but require maturation signals for full expression of their T-cell–stimulating activity. The functional phenotype of dendritic cells appears to be controlled via a complex series of regulatory interactions with bone marrow–derived cells, mesenchymal cells, and possibly neuroendocrine cells.[29] Failure in one or more of these regulatory interactions may be an important etiopathogenetic factor in a variety of respiratory immunoinflammatory diseases.[29] For instance, a growing body of evidence suggests that upregulation of the dendritic cell population in the respiratory tract may be an etiologic factor in allergic respiratory disease. Holt and others have called attention to such upregulation of dendritic cells in the nasal mucosal of patients with rhinitis, after deliberate or environmental allergen challenge, and also in bronchial mucosa of subjects with atopic asthma.[31–33]

Variants of Inflammation

Granulomatous Inflammation

Chronic inflammation can take a variety of morphologic forms. It may present as a chronic abscess or granulation tissue or as an ulcer or granuloma. Currently, two major

types of granulomas are recognized. The first is the foreign-body type of granuloma, which is usually secondary to agents such as suture material, glass particles, or crystals. The immune (hypersensitivity) type of granulomas represent the second largest category of granulomas.[34] The causes of granulomas are many (Table 43.3), and some are idiopathic.[35]

What is a granuloma? The answer to this question may be approached by attempting to provide a definition. Briefly, one may say that a granuloma is a granule-like microstructure with a central collection of epithelioid macrophages surrounded by a rim of peripheral lymphocytes. Epithelioid cells are essentially modified macrophages bearing some resemblance to epithelial cells, hence the term *epithelioid*. Epithelioid cells have large, usually oval, but sometimes elongated, pale, vesicular nuclei with visible nuclear membranes and a small nucleolus. Multinucleated giant cells often accompany the epithelioid cells; these cells are histiocytic cells with two or

TABLE 43.3. Some common causes of pulmonary granulomas.

Infection	Bacteria	*Brucella abortus*
		Francisella tularensis
		Yersinia pestis
	Mycobacteria	*Mycobacterium tuberculosis*
		M. kansasii
		M. leprae
		M. marinum
	Spirochetes	*Treponema pallidum*
		T. carateum
	Metazoa	*Schistosoma* sp.
		Toxocara canis
	Fungi	*Coccidioides immitis*
		Histoplasma capsulatum
	Protozoa	*Toxoplasma gondii*
		Leishmania sp.
Hypersensitivity pneumonitis		Farmer's lung
		Parakeet lung
		Suberosis, bagassosis
		Mushroom picker's lung
		Pigeon breeder's lung
Drugs/medications		Dilantin
		Methotrexate
		Bacille Calmette-Guerin
		Mineral oil
		Talc
Chemicals		Beryllium
		Zirconium
		Hard metals
		Silica
Neoplastic diseases		Lymphoma
		Carcinoma
Idiopathic		Sarcoidosis
		Wegener's granulomatosis
		Lymphomatoid granulomatosis
		Vasculitides

Source: From Sharma,[35] with permission.

more nuclei and similar histologic characteristics to epithelioid cells. Epithelioid histiocytes react strongly with CD68 and are cytokeratin negative; these features help to distinguish them from epithelial cells. A hypersensitivity type of granuloma with epithelioid histiocytes and a multinucleated giant cell in a case of hot-tub lung (believed secondary to nontuberculous mycobacteria) is shown in Figure 43.1.

How do granulomas form? In an organ that is chronically inflamed, the cellular infiltrate usually spreads more or less evenly throughout the tissue, or it can gather into tiny, separate, more or less rounded clusters of macrophages with a sprinkling of other cell types such as lymphocytes, eosinophils, and plasma cells.[34] The actual evolutionary mechanism leading to the formation of a granuloma, starting with an inflicted injury, going through a mid phase of macrophage accumulation, and culminating in a well-formed granuloma is shown in Table 43.4.[36]

As stated by Kumar et al., macrophages are the *prima donnas* of chronic inflammation and more so in the case of granulomatous inflammation, such as that seen in sarcoidosis and tuberculosis of the lung.[8] What is the function or mission of a granuloma? Paraphrasing Majno and Joris, we may think of a granuloma as a "specialized device for focusing and concentrating the cellular counter attack."[34] When bacteria are the offending agents, the granuloma per se does not act as a bacterial defense but rather as a manufacturing site for the production and release of chemical mediators, chiefly cytokines. Immune granulomas may undergo necrosis, particularly in granulomas associated with tuberculosis, syphilis, and rheuma-

TABLE 43.4. Mechanism of evolution of a granuloma.

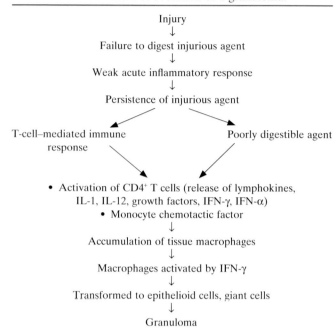

Source: From Mohan,[36] with permission.

toid arthritis. The necrosis is of the coagulative type and develops in the centers of the granulomas. The cause of the necrosis is not entirely clear. Prime causative agents, according to Majno and Joris, are macrophage-derived cytokines such as TNF.[34] The pathogenesis of tuberculous granulomas is discussed more extensively in Chapter 40.

Interstitial Inflammation

Broadly characterized, the interstitium of the lung is its connective tissue framework.[23] It can also be thought of as that part of the interalveolar septal wall that lies between the alveolar epithelial and capillary endothelial basement membranes.[37] The interstitium is abundant around the airways and arteries in the centers of the lobules, and around the veins. The interstitium consists of collagen and elastin fibers, among which are fibroblasts, myofibroblasts, histiocytes, and mast cells with scanty nerves and nerve terminals.[23] The myofibroblasts are closely related to the capillaries, and it is suggested that they control perfusion of the alveoli. Other interstitial cells include mast cells and a form of histiocyte intermediate between a blood monocyte and an alveolar macrophage. Lymphoid elements, Langerhans cells, and dendritic reticular cells are also contained within the interstitium.[23]

The interstitium is the target of a rather long list of disorders known collectively as *interstitial lung diseases.* To date, more than 100 such disorders have been identi-

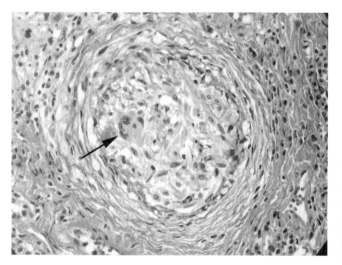

FIGURE 43.1. Nonnecrotizing granuloma found in a patient with hot-tub lung. Note the arrangement of centrally located epithelioid macrophages with a multinucleated giant cell (arrow). (Hematoxylin and eosin; ×200.)

fied. The term is often used somewhat imprecisely to refer to a group of disorders associated with physiologic restrictive changes and a histologic abnormality—usually inflammation—of the lung interstitium, leading to slow accumulation of collagen (fibrosis) in the interstitium. However, the accumulation of other substances or cells, such as neoplastic cells or amyloid, may also result in "interstitial lung disease."[38–40]

What prompts the development of interstitial inflammation? The location of the stimulating antigen(s) in the alveolar septum is believed to be an important factor. Antigens bound to or expressed by alveolar lining cells can be recognized by CD4- or CD8-expressing T cells, depending on whether there is class 1 or class 2 antigen presentation. Disorders associated with interstitial inflammation of the lung classically include viral interstitial pneumonias, hypersensitivity pneumonia, and autoimmune processes such as rheumatoid arthritis, systemic lupus erythematosus, and scleroderma. The predominant inflammatory cells in interstitial lung diseases may be lymphocytic, as in nonspecific interstitial pneumonia, or neutrophilic, as in usual interstitial pneumonia (UIP). Nonspecific interstitial pneumonia has been identified as a distinct entity with a more favorable prognosis and better response to immunosuppressive therapies than UIP. However, an increasing number of cases are being reported with mixed features of nonspecific interstitial pneumonia and UIP, suggesting that at least in some cases these disorders share a common pathogenesis.

For several decades, UIP, also known to pulmonologists and radiologists as *idiopathic pulmonary fibrosis* (IPF), has largely been regarded as an inflammatory interstitial process.[41] This belief was based to a large extent on the observation that bronchoalveolar lavage fluid from patients with UIP/IPF had increased numbers of inflammatory cells (mostly neutrophils) as compared with normal controls.[41,42] This concept pervaded the literature, suggesting that UIP/IPF resulted from an unremitting inflammatory response to an exogenous insult, culminating in progressive fibrosis and honeycombing. The belief had profound clinical and therapeutic implications[41] by targeting therapies toward interfering with the inflammatory response. The basic tenet was that the fibrosis could be limited and/or prevented with appropriate use of antiinflammatory agents such as corticosteroids. More recently, however, structural abnormalities in lung architecture (traction bronchiectasis) have been recognized to play an important role in the pathogenesis of UIP/IPF, and the observed changes in inflammatory cell trafficking have been suggested to follow from the fibrotic changes.[41] Although the role of inflammation in the pathology of UIP/IPF remains controversial, it is difficult to ignore the lack of efficacy of corticosteroids.[41]

Inflammation and a fibrogenic response can be seen concurrently. An example of this occurrence is observed

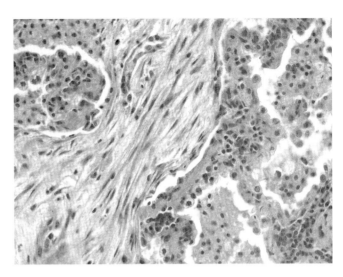

FIGURE 43.2. Organizing pneumonia. A plug of young fibroblastic tissue fills an alveolar duct. The chronic inflammatory response in the surrounding alveolar walls is rather mild. (Hematoxylin and eosin; ×200.)

in organizing pneumonia. In this condition, an infiltrate of mononuclear inflammatory cells (lymphocytes and macrophages) is seen in the pulmonary interstitium, while the alveolar ducts and sacs are filled by organizing plugs of young fibroblastic tissue (Figure 43.2). In contrast to UIP/IPF, organizing pneumonia is corticosteroid responsive in a significant majority of cases.

Human Leukocyte Antigen–Linked Lung Disease

The HLA system plays a major role in the immunoregulation of inflammatory processes in the human lung and is the correlate of the major histocompatibility complex (MHC) system in mice. A variety of pulmonary disorders such as hypersensitivity pneumonitis, transfusion reactions, nosocomial pneumonias, bronchiolitis obliterans, and diffuse panbronchiolitis are immunomodulated by the HLA system. Class I HLA receptors are widely expressed, whereas class II receptors are constitutively expressed only by professional antigen-presenting cells, particularly dendritic cells and B cells.[43] During inflammatory responses, expression can be upregulated by other cells, such as endothelial cells. There are three class I genes, *HLA-A, HLA-B,* and *HLA-C,* and at least six class II genes, although only three (*DR, DQ,* and *DP*) are particularly important in antigen presentation. For each gene, there exist many different alleles recognized originally through serotypes and more recently by sequencing so that at a nucleotide level individuals are relatively unique in their HLA structures.[43]

T cells in the periphery (as opposed to the thymus) will not respond to free antigen but only to antigen properly presented by HLA receptors. This represents an important biologic control mechanism that limits reactivity to self-antigens. The interaction between the T-cell receptor and the HLA molecule is exquisitely specific, with alterations in single amino acids in either the peptide, the HLA receptor, or the T-cell receptor profoundly altering the response. Certain peptides will bind only to certain HLA alleles, which probably explains the association between particular HLA phenotypes and certain autoimmune diseases. Ankylosing spondylitis, in which over 90% of sufferers have the *HLA-B27* allele compared with less than 10% of the general population, is an example.[43]

Superantigens are microbial toxins that can activate up to one third of T cells. Such activation is accomplished through simultaneous binding to the V_B domain of the T-cell receptor and to the complementary chain of the class II HLA molecule. This common mechanism of microbial virulence causes a number of clinical syndromes, including toxic shock syndrome, tissue necrosis, and food poisoning.[44-46] Some HLA class II molecules are better at binding and presenting a specific superantigen.[44,45,47] This leads to an HLA class II association of superantigen action, with its clinical effects resulting from high T-cell cytokine responses. Microorganisms that produce superantigens include *Staphylococcus, Streptococcus, Mycoplasma, Yersinia,* and certain retroviruses, including endogenous retroviruses. Superantigens have an important role in atopic dermatitis and, possibly, chronic severe asthma, type I diabetes, multiple sclerosis, rheumatoid arthritis, Kawasaki's disease, and psoriasis.[44,48,49]

Antigen presentation by macrophages is regulated by HLA-DR[47]–activated macrophages characterized by specific alterations of the expression of their surface markers under certain pathologic conditions, such as pneumonia. In particular, myeloid-related proteins MRP8/MRP14 are involved in the regulation of macrophage migration and adhesion.[50] Myeloid-related proteins are proteins of the S100 family of proteins that are regarded as having antimicrobial, chemotactic, and cytostatic properties.[50] Bühling et al. studied the cytofluorometric expression of MRP8/MRP14 and HLD-DR in patients with pneumonia, COPD, interstitial lung disease, and controls with no known lung disease.[51] These investigators correlated phenotypic characteristics with levels of transforming growth factor (TGF)-β1 and IL-8 in bronchoalveolar lavage fluid from the above-cited patients and controls and then analyzed the influence of TGF-β1 and IL-8 on the expression of MRP8/MRP14 and HLA-DR in cultured monocytes. Significantly, more MRP8/MRP14-positive macrophages and less HLA-DR–positive macrophages were found in pneumonia patients but not in COPD or interstitial lung disease patients, suggesting that in pneumonia, but not in COPD or interstitial lung

disease, alveolar macrophages are characterized by increased (salutarious) expression of myeloid-related proteins and a concurrent decrease in HLA-DR expression. The authors suggested that characterization of subpopulations of macrophages such as cited earlier may be a useful tool for the monitoring of disease progression.[51]

Anti-HLA and antineutrophil antibodies have been implicated in some cases of transfusion-related acute lung injury, which is a potentially lethal pulmonary complication of transfusion.[52] Nishimura et al. postulate that anti-HLA and antineutrophil antibodies activate leukocytes in recipients of blood transfusion, resulting in the release of soluble factors such as reactive oxygen species and detrimental cytokines and chemokines (such as TNF-α, interferon-γ, and IL-18), derived from said activated leukocytes.[52] The harmful effects of these factors on lung tissues are strongly suspected to be profoundly involved in the pathogenesis of transfusion-related acute lung injury reactions.[52]

A serious condition of small airways, obliterative bronchiolitis is characterized by fibrous obstruction of bronchiolar lumina. Obliterative bronchiolitis developing after lung transplantation is considered to be the end result of multiple airway insults inflicted by immunologic and microbiologic processes that vary for individual patients and are influenced in their outcomes by genetic and environmental factors. Schulman et al. analyzed risk factors for obliterative bronchiolitis in 152 lung transplant recipients and determined that mismatching at the *HLA-A* locus was a significant risk factor for obliterative bronchiolitis and a determinant of its severity.[53,54]

A number of studies have revealed relationships between HLA antigen expression and the development of pulmonary infections. Specifically, low levels of HLA-DR expression on peripheral blood monocytes have been demonstrated to correlate with the risk of infection in pediatric lung transplant recipients as well as in trauma patients.[55-57] Furthermore, antigens of the HLA system are known to modulate resistance or susceptibility to a variety of viruses and members of the mycoplasma family. Human leukocyte antigen B40, for example, appears to be associated with resistance to influenza A, whereas B18 and B21 appear to be associated with resistance to parainfluenza. In addition, B15 and B35 appear to be associated with resistance to *Mycoplasma pneumoniae.*[58]

As noted earlier, the HLA system plays a significant role in hypersensitivity pneumonitis. In experimental models of hypersensitivity pneumonitis, there is increasing evidence that a high level of antigen-specific suppressor cell activity contributes to either completely inhibiting or modulating the degree of pulmonary inflammation.[59] There is also evidence that a genetic predisposition linked to the HLA system determines the occurrence of hypersensitivity pneumonitis. For example, in the animal model of hypersensitivity pneumonitis developed by Wilson et al., pigeon feces extracts were given to two different strains of mice.[60] One (high responder) mouse strain developed intense and diffuse interstitial inflammation of the lung along with delayed hyperreactivity to avian antigens. The other (low responder) strain showed only mild perivascular inflammation and did not demonstrate delayed reactivity.[59,60] Several studies looking at links between HLA and hypersensitivity pneumonitis have shown a statistically significant predisposition to hypersensitivity pneumonitis in individuals with certain alleles such as *HLA-DR3* and *HLA-DQw3*.[59,61,62]

Asthma is known to be associated with eosinophilic inflammation of the airways, bronchial hyperresponsiveness, increased production of IgE, and increased levels of cytokines IL-4, IL-5, and IL-13. Development of inflammation within the asthmatic lung depends to some extent on HLA class II–restricted antigen presentation leading to stimulation of CD4[+] T cells with cytokine generation.[57]

Diffuse panbronchiolitis, a disorder of unknown etiology, is characterized by accumulation of foamy histiocytes in respiratory bronchioles and alveoli. More common in the Far East, particularly in Japan, diffuse panbronchiolitis has shown a strong association with HLA class I alleles, supporting the view that diffuse panbronchiolitis is an immune-mediated disease. In Japanese patients, there is a strong association between the *HLA-Bw54* locus and the disease.[63] In one study, 37% of patients possessed the *HLA-B5401* allele, which is conserved predominantly in East Asians, as compared with 15% of healthy controls.[63,64] In Koreans, an association with the HLA class I serotype was also seen, although in this group it was with *HLA-A11* (53% vs. 18% of controls) and *HLA-B55* (17% vs. 3.5%).[63,64]

Conclusion

The subject of inflammation is vast and complex. A recent access to a PubMed yielded 57,860 citations for inflammation of the lung alone and 183,184 citations for the subject of inflammation at large. Such a level of knowledge has taken centuries to accumulate. The past two to three decades, however, have seen an accelerated level of accrued new data.

This brief review of the inflammatory process in the lung does not pretend to be comprehensive. Rather, it is an attempt to present the reader with recent developments, namely, the tissue response to immunoinflammatory agents, how granulomas form, mechanisms of response selection, and an introduction to the TLR–PAMP story. In addition, this chapter discussed the role of dendritic cells in antigen presentation and the influence of the HLA system in a variety of inflammatory lung disorders.

Acknowledgments. The author is grateful to Dr. Bruce Woda for his critical review of the manuscript and to Ms. Karen Balcius for her expert secretarial assistance and typing of the manuscript.

References

1. Tracey KJ. The inflammatory reflex. Nature 2002;420:853–859.
2. Richardson JD, Vasko MR. Cellular mechanisms of neurogenic inflammation. Pharmacol Exp Ther 2002;302:839–845.
3. Majno G, Palade GE. Studies on inflammation. I. The effect of histamine and serotonin on vascular permeability: an electron microscopic study. J Biophys Biochem Cytol 1961;11:571–596.
4. Majno G, Palade GE, Schoefl GI. Studies on inflammation. II. The site of action of histamine and serotonin along the vascular tree: a topographic study. J Biophys Biochem Cytol 1961;11:607–626.
5. Majno G. Commentary. Chronic inflammation: links with angiogenesis and wound healing. Am J Pathol 1998;153:1035–1039.
6. Kunkel SL, Strieter RM. Cytokines and chemokines in lung inflammation and injury. In Fishman AP, ed. Fishman's Pulmonary Diseases and Disorders, 3rd ed, vol 1. New York: McGraw-Hill; 1998:315–324.
7. Muller WA. Leukocyte–endothelial cell interactions in the inflammatory response. Lab Invest 2002;82:521–534.
8. Kumar V, Abbas AK, Fausto N, ed. Robbins and Cotran Pathologic Basis of Disease, 7th ed. Philadelphia: Elsevier, 2005:47–86.
9. Reynolds HY, Elias JA. Pulmonary defense mechanisms against infections. In Fishman AP, ed. Pulmonary Diseases and Disorders, 3rd ed, vol 1. New York: McGraw-Hill; 1998:265–274.
10. Berman JS, Center DM. Lymphocyte- and macrophage-mediated inflammation in the lung. In Fishman AP, ed. Pulmonary Diseases and Disorders, 3rd ed, vol 1. New York: McGraw-Hill; 1998:275–287.
11. Inlay M. A response to Chapter 6 of Darwin's Black Box. Minlay@biomail.UCSD.edu, June 2002.
12. Goldsby RA, Kindt TJ, Osborne BA, et al. Immunology, 5th ed. New York: W.H. Freeman; 2003:69.
13. Collins German Concise Dictionary, 3rd ed. Glasgow, Scotland: Harper Collins, 2006:333.
14. Goldstein DR. Toll like receptors and other links between innate and acquired alloimmunity. Curr Opin Immunol 2004;16:538–544.
15. Luke AJ, O'Neill LA. Immunity's early-warning system. Sci Am 2005;292:38–45.
16. Dunne A, O'Neill LA. The interleukin-1 receptor/Toll like receptor superfamily: signal transduction during inflammation and host defense. Sci STKE 2003;171:R-3.
17. Lazarus R, Ruby BA, Louge C, et al. Toll-like receptor 10 genetic variation is associated with asthma in two independent samples. Am J Respir Crit Care Med 2004;170:594–600.

18. Basu S, Fenton MJ. Toll-like receptors: function and roles in lung disease. Am J Physiol Lung Cell Mol Physiol 2004;286:L887–L892.

19. Pons J, Sauleda J, Regueriro V, et al. Expression of toll-like receptor 2 is up-regulated in monocytes from patients with chronic obstructive pulmonary disease. Respir Res 2006;7:64A.

20. Velasco G, Campo M, Manrique OJ, et al. Toll-like receptor 4 or 2 agonists decrease allergic inflammation. Am J Respir Cell Mol Biol 2005;32:218–224.

21. Chen W, Kuo Lee R, Shen H, et al. Toll-like receptor 4 (TLR 4) does not confer a resistance advantage on mice against low-dose aerosol infection with virulent type A Francisella tularensis. Microb Pathog 2004;37:185–191.

22. Knapp S, Wieland CW, Florquin S, et al. Differential roles of CD14 and Toll-like receptors 4 and 2 in murine Acinetobacter pneumoniae. Am J Respir Crit Care Med 2006;173:122–129.

23. Corrin B, Nicholson AG. Pathology of the Lungs, 2nd ed. Philadelphia: Churchill Livingstone; 2006:1–34.

24. Fujii T, Hayashi S, Hogg JC, et al. Interaction of alveolar macrophages and airway epithelial cells following exposure to particulate matter produces mediators that stimulate the bone marrow. Am J Respir Cell Mol Biol 2002;27:34–41.

25. Abbas AK, Lichtman AH, Pober JS. Cellular and Molecular Immunology, 4th ed. Philadelphia: W.B. Saunders; 2000:22–24.

26. Steinman R, Cohn Z. Identification of a novel cell type in peripheral lymphoid organs of mice. J Exp Med 1973;137:1142–1162.

27. Satthaporn S, Eremin O. Dendritic cells (1): Biological functions. J R Coll Surg Edinb 2001;46:9–20.

28. Banchereau J, Steinman RM. Dendritic cells and the control of immunity. Nature 1998;392:245–252.

29. Holt PG. Antigen presentation in the lung. Am J Respir Crit Care Med 2000;162:S151–S156.

30. Randolph GJ, Beaulieu S, Lebecque S, et al. Differentiation of monocytes into dendritic cells in a model of transendothelial trafficking. Science 1998;282:480–483.

31. Godthelp T, Fokkens WJ, Kleinjan A, et al. Antigen presenting cells in the nasal mucosa of patients with allergic rhinitis during allergen provocation. Clin Exp Allergy 1996;26:677–688.

32. Fokkens WJ, Vroom M, Rijntjes E, et al. Fluctuation of the number of CD-1 (T6)-positive dendritic cells, presumably Langerhans cells, in the nasal mucosa of patients with an isolated grass-pollen allergy before, during, and after the grass-pollen season. J Allergy Clin Immunol 1989;84:39–43.

33. Tunon-de-Lara JM, Redington P, Bradding MK, et al. Dendritic cells in normal and asthmatic airways: expression of the α subunit of the high affinity immunoglobulin E receptor (Fcε RI-α). Clin Exp Allergy 1996;26:648–655.

34. Majno G, Joris I. Cells, Tissues and Disease. Principles of General Pathology, 2nd ed. New York: Oxford University Press; 2004:442–476.

35. Sharma OP. Clinical diagnosis and types of granulomas. In: Cagle PT, ed. Diagnostic Pulmonary Pathology. New York: Marcel-Dekker; 2000:331–347.

36. Mohan H, ed. Textbook of Pathology, 5th ed. New Delhi: Jaypee Brothers, 2005:153–154.

37. Hasleton PS, ed. Spencer's Pathology of the Lung, 5th Ed. New York: McGraw-Hill; 1996:1–44.

38. Laga AC, Allen T, Cagle PT. Usual interstitial pneumonia. In: Cagle PT, ed. Color Atlas and Text of Pulmonary Pathology. Philadelphia: Lippincott Williams & Wilkins; 2005:427–429.

39. Laga A, Allen T, Cagle PT. Non specific interstitial pneumonia. In: Cagle PT, ed. Color Atlas and Text of Pulmonary Pathology. Philadelphia: Lippincott Williams & Wilkins, 2005:431–432.

40. Laga A, Allen T, Cagle PT. Cryptogenic organizing pneumonia (idiopathic bronchiolitis obliterans organizing pneumonia). In Cagle PT, ed. Color Atlas and Text of Pulmonary Pathology. Philadelphia: Lippincott Williams & Wilkins; 2005:433–434.

41. Noble PN. Idiopathic pulmonary fibrosis: new insight into classification and pathogenesis usher in a new era in therapeutic approaches. Am J Respir Cell Mol Biol 2003;29:S27–S31.

42. Merrill WW, Reynolds HY. Bronchial lavage in inflammatory lung disease. Clin Chest Med 1983;4:71–84.

43. Wardlaw A. Immunologic basis of lung disease. In Wardlaw AJ, Hamid Q, eds. Textbook of Respiratory Cell and Molecular Biology. London: Martin Dunitz LTD; 2002:47–71.

44. Schubert MS. A superantigen hypothesis for the pathogenesis of chronic hypertrophic rhinosinusitis, allergic fungal sinusitis and related disorders. Ann Allergy Asthma Immunol 2001;87:181–188.

45. Kappler, J, Kotzin, B, Herron L, et al. Vβ-specific stimulation of human T cells by staphylococcal toxins. Science 1989:244;811–813.

46. Kotb M, Norrby-Teglund A, McGeer A, et al. An immunogenetic and molecular basis for differences in outcomes of invasive group A streptococcal infections. Nat Med 2002;8:1398–1404.

47. Krakauer T. Immune response to staphylococcal superantigens. Immunol Res 1999;20:163–173.

48. Paliard X, West SG, Lafferty JA, et al. Evidence for the effects of a super antigen in rheumatoid arthritis. Science 1991;253:325–329.

49. Hauk PJ, Wenzel SE, Trumble AE, et al. Increased T-cell receptor Vβ8+T cells in bronchoalveolar lavage fluid of subjects with poorly controlled asthma: a potential role for microbial superantigens. J Allergy Clin Immunol 1999;103:37–45.

50. Rammes A, Roth J, Goebeler M, et al. Myeloid-related protein (MRP) 8 and MRP14 calcium-binding proteins of the S100 family, are secreted by activated monocytes via a novel, tubulin-dependent pathway. J Biol Chem 1997;272:9496–9502.

51. Bühling F, Ittenson A, Kaiser D, et al. MRP8 / MRP14, CD11b and HLA-DR expression of alveolar macrophages in pneumonia. Immunol Lett 2000;71:185–190.

52. Nishimura M, Mitsunaga S, Ishikawa Y, et al. Possible mechanisms underlying development of transfusion related acute lung injury: roles of anti-major histocompatibility

complex class II DR antibodies. Transfusion Med 2003;13:141–147.

53. Schulman LL, Weinberg AD, McGregor CC, et al. Influence of donor and recipient HLA locus mismatching on development of obliterative bronchiolitis after lung transplantation. Am J Respir Crit Care Med 2001;163:437–442.

54. Chalermskulrat W, Neuringer IP, Schmitz JL, et al. Human leukocyte antigen mismatches predispose to the severity of bronchiolitis obliterans syndrome after lung transplantation. Chest 2003;123:1825–1831.

55. Hoffman JA, Weinberg RI, Azen CG, et al. Human leukocyte antigen-DR expression on peripheral blood monocytes and the risk of pneumonia in pediatric lung transplant recipients. Transplant Infect Dis 2004;6:147–155.

56. Muehlstedt SO, Lyte M, Rodriguez JL. Increased IL-10 production and HLA-DR suppression in the lungs of injured patients precede the development of nosocomial pneumonia. Shock 2002;17:443–450.

57. Ye Q, Finn PW, Sweeney R, et al. MCH class II–associated invariant chain isoforms regulate pulmonary immune responses. J Immunol 2003;170:1473–1480.

58. Tsybalova LM, Popova TL, Karpukhin GI. HLA system antigens in persons with differing susceptibilities to the causative agents of acute respiratory diseases. Zh Mikrobiol Epidemiol Immunobiol 1989;10:64–68.

59. Selman LM, Chapela R, Salas J, et al. Hypersensitivity pneumonitis: clinical approach and an integral concept about its pathogenesis. A Mexican point of view. In Selman-Lama M, Barrios R, eds. Interstitial Pulmonary Diseases: Selected Topics. Boston: CRC Press; 1991:171–195.

60. Wilson BD, Sternick JL, Yoshizawa Y, et al. Experimental murine hypersensitivity pneumonitis: multigenic control and influence by genes within the I-B subregion of the H-2 complex. J Immunol 1982;129:2160–2163.

61. Rittner G, Sennenkamp J, Mollenhauer E, et al. Pigeons breeder's lung association with HLA-DR3. Tissue Antigens 1983;21:374–379.

62. Ando M, Hirayama K, Soda K, et al. HLA-DQw3 in Japanese summer-type hypersensitivity pneumonitis induced by *Trichosporon cutaneum*. Am Rev Respir Dis 1989;140:948–950.

63. Park MH, Kim YW, Yoon HI, et al. Association of HLA class I antigens with diffuse panbronchiolitis. 1999;159:526–529.

64. Keicho N, Tokunaga K, Nakata K, et al. Contribution of HLA genes to genetic predisposition in diffuse panbronchiolitis. Am J Respir Crit Care Med 1998;158:846–850.

44
Oxidants and Antioxidants

Hanzhong Liu and Gary A. Visner

Introduction

Oxidants are an important source of injury to cells and tissues. The lung is exposed to significantly more oxidants than are most other organs. The lung is unique because of its large epithelial surface area that is directly exposed to high levels of oxygen tension, that is, oxygen pressure in inhaled air is 20kPa (150mmHg). Ambient air contains additional oxidants, including cigarette smoke, asbestos fibers, mineral dust, and environmental carcinogens. A common component in most lung disease is activation of the inflammatory response, which leads to the generation of a relatively large quantity of oxidants. Even some therapeutic interventions, such as ventilation and oxygen therapy in the treatment of prematurely born neonates and acute respiratory distress syndrome, or chemotherapeutic agents, including bleomycin, carmustine, and anthracyclines, enhance oxidant burden to lung tissue.[1] Thus, the lung represents a unique tissue exposed not only directly to external environmental oxidants under normal conditions but also to inflammation- and therapy-associated oxidants in disease state.

To maintain normal lung homeostasis and function, lung tissue is endowed with a well-established defense system against oxidant-mediated damage through non-enzymatic and enzymatic antioxidants. Under certain circumstance, however, oxidative stress, resulting from disequilibrium between oxidant burden and antioxidant reserve, can occur and consequently lead to a series of pathophysiologic events that include activation of inflammation, widespread tissue damage, and eventually pulmonary dysfunction. In this chapter, the generation of oxidants and antioxidants in lung tissue and their regulatory role in expression of transcription factors involved in the molecular mechanisms of most lung diseases are discussed.

Oxidants in the Lung

Reactive Oxygen Species

Oxidation of organic compounds during aerobic metabolism is an essential process by which mammalian cells generate sufficient energy to maintain their growth and function. However, the resulting reactive oxygen species (ROS), which mainly include superoxide (O_2^-), hydrogen peroxide (H_2O_2), and hydroxyl radicals ($\cdot OH$), are potentially toxic to almost every biologic molecule in living cells. Indeed, oxidants are capable of damaging cell membranes, especially those rich in polyunsaturated fatty acids, resulting in lipid peroxidation.[2] This not only damages the integrity of cell membranes but also produces additional products, peroxides and aldehydes, that are cytotoxic.[3] Reactive oxygen species also modify proteins, resulting in functional impairment or marking them for early destruction. In addition, DNA is a sensitive target to oxidative injury, resulting in base modification, base-free sites, deletions, frame shifts, and strand breaks.[4]

During normal aerobic metabolism, intracellular O_2^- is continually produced by a reaction catalyzed by cytochrome oxidase in the mitochondrial respiratory chain. It has been estimated that each living cell is exposed to approximately 10^{10} molecules of O_2^- per 24 hr. A much higher level of O_2^- can be generated by the NADPH oxidase enzymatic system in "professional" phagocytes, that is, neutrophils and macrophages, at the site of inflammation.[5] O_2^- is a free radical, that is, it contains an unpaired electron that can be transferred to nonradical H_2O_2 by a nonenzymatic or superoxide dismutase (SOD)–catalyzed reaction ($O_2^- + O_2^- + 2H^+ \rightarrow H_2O_2 + O_2$). Unlike O_2^-, H_2O_2 is not charged and can diffuse freely through cell membranes. Both O_2^- and H_2O_2 can be used as a source for producing $\cdot OH$. For example, H_2O_2 can be oxidized by eosinophil-specific peroxidase and neutrophil-specific peroxidase using Br or Cl as a cosubstrate to form hypobromous acids (HOBr) and hypochlorous acid (HOCl), respectively. These hypohalous acids can further react with $O_2^-\cdot$ to produce $\cdot OH$ (HOBr + $O_2^-\cdot \rightarrow$ $\cdot OH$ + O_2 + Br$^-$ or HOCl + $O_2^-\cdot \rightarrow \cdot OH$ + O_2 + Cl$^-$). Another example for $\cdot OH$ generation from $O_2^-\cdot$ and H_2O_2 is the combination of the iron-catalyzed Haber-Weiss reaction ($Fe^{3+} + O_2^-\cdot \rightarrow Fe^{2+} + O_2$) and the Fenton reaction ($Fe^{2+} + H_2O_2 \rightarrow Fe^{3+} + OH^- + \cdot OH$). These reactions are important, as most of the damage done by $O_2^-\cdot$ and H_2O_2 in vivo is due to their production of $\cdot OH$, a very reactive oxygen species that plays a major role in tissue damage associated with acute and chronic lung inflammation.[6]

Reactive Nitrogen Species

Nitric oxide (NO) is widely present in environmental pollutants and cigarette smoke.[7] In addition, this gas is continuously being generated throughout the body and plays important physiologic functions such as the regulation of blood pressure. Nitric oxide is formed from the semiessential amino acid L-arginine by the action of nitric oxide synthase (NOS). There are three isoforms of NOS. The constitutive forms, which include neuronal NOS (nNOS) and endothelial NOS (eNOS), are Ca^{2+}–calmodulin dependent and release low levels of NO in response to receptor and physical stimulation. The inducible form of NOS (iNOS) is Ca^{2+}–calmodulin independent and usually produces large amounts of NO in response to pathologic stimuli. Nitric oxide is highly reactive, as the paramagnetic molecule contains an odd number of electrons. In addition, it also serves as a source for generation of other reactive nitrogen species (RNS).

Two major pathways have been identified in the formation of RNS from NO in vivo. First, autooxidation of NO with O_2 results in the formation of nitrite (NO_2^-), which can be further oxidized by hemeperoxidases such as neutrophil-specific peroxidase and eosinophil-specific peroxidase to generate nitrogen dioxide radical ($NO_2\cdot$) or related molecules, which are capable of nitrating reactions. Another pathway is the reaction of NO with free radicals (radical–radical reaction). Nitric oxide can react quickly with $O_2\cdot$ to form peroxynitrite ($ONOO^-$), which can be protonated to give peroxynitrous acid (ONOOH). Like $NO_2\cdot$, ONOOH is highly reactive and can cause nitration of protein, lipids, and DNA bases and consequently damage cellular functions.[8] It should be noted that, compared with other amino acids, tyrosine is particularly prone to nitration, and thus formation of its nitrated product, 3-nitrotyrosine, has be used as a biomarker for the generation of RNS in lung tissue in vivo.[9]

Antioxidants in the Lung

As mentioned, both ROS and RNS are continuously generated in lung tissue even during normal metabolism. Therefore, lung cells have developed a highly effective defense system that is crucial for ensuring the proper balance between oxidant and antioxidant molecules and maintaining normal pulmonary function.

Nonenzymatic Antioxidants

Lung extracellular fluids including epithelial lining fluid (ELF) act as an interface between ambient air and the epithelium and constitute the first line of defense against inhaled oxidants. Epithelial lining fluid contains large amounts of free radical scavengers, which represent a group of compounds that can react directly with oxidizing agents and inactivate them. Several vitamins contained in ELF can act as scavengers under certain conditions. Vitamin E (α-tocopherol) is a membrane-bound agent that can scavenge lipid peroxides, thereby terminating lipid peroxidation. Vitamin C is capable of scavenging $O_2^-\cdot$ and $\cdot OH$; however, it can also convert Fe^{3+} to Fe^{2+}, which can then react with H_2O_2 producing $\cdot OH$.[6] A typical feature in the antioxidant defense of the human lung is that its ELF is rich in glutathione (approximately 140 times higher than in the circulating blood).[10] Additional antioxidant species contained in ELF include iron-binding proteins (ceruloplasmin, transferrin, ferritin, lactoferrin, etc.), proteins with free radical scavenging capacity such as albumin, and low-molecular-weight substances such as bilirubin and uric acid.[11] Moreover, some proteins expressed in lung cells, such as surfactant protein D in type II cells, also have an antioxidant function.[1]

Enzymatic Antioxidants

A variety of antioxidant enzymes, mainly glutathione peroxidases (GPs), SODs, and catalase, constitute the main protective mechanism of lung tissue against ROS-mediated injury. The selenoprotein GPs are the central mechanism for reducing H_2O_2 and lipid peroxides in lung tissue. Four isoforms of GPs encoding different genes have been identified: two are cytosolic enzymes, another one is a membrane-associated GP, and the last one is an extracellular GP, which is highly expressed in ELF.[12] The GP-mediated reaction uses glutathione (GSH) as the electron donor and produces glutathione disulfide (GSSG) (ROOH + 2GSH$\rightarrow$ ROH + GSSG + H_2O or $ONOO^-$ + 2GSH$\rightarrow$ ONO^- + GSSG + H_2O). The GSSG formed in the course of the reaction can be transferred back to the reduced form of GSH through the action of glutathione reductase, which uses NADPH generated from the hexose monophosphate shunt system as an electron donor.[13] The concentration of GSH in a living cell ranges from 1 to 10 mM, and the GSH/GSSG ratio has been widely used as an indicator of the cell's oxidative state. Glutamylcysteine ligase is the rate-limiting enzyme catalyzing the conversion of the amino acid cysteine to GSH. This enzyme is a heterodimer composed of a 73-KDa catalytic heavy subunit and a 30-KDa regulatory light subunit.[14] Like other enzyme-mediated reactions, glutamylcysteine ligase can be inhibited by high levels of GSH through a feedback mechanism.[13,14]

Superoxide dismutases are the only enzymatic antioxidant catalyzing the dismutation of superoxide to H_2O_2 and are believed to play an important protective role against oxidant-related lung injury. There are three different forms of SOD. Two are intracellular, the cytoplasmic copper/zinc (Cu/ZnSOD) and the mitochondrial manganese SOD (MnSOD), and the third is extracellular SOD normally found on the outside of the plasma membrane (ECSOD).[1] Superoxide dismutase expression has been observed in all types of lung cells, but individual isoforms show significant variability in distribution. For example, it has been reported that ELF contains a much higher level of ECSOD than MnSOD and Cu/ZnSOD.[6] In contrast, alveolar type II cells have higher expression of CuZnSOD and MnSOD compared with ECSOD.[15]

Catalase, a tetrameric hemoprotein generally found only in peroxisomes, catalyzes the very rapid dismutation of H_2O_2 into water. Thus, there may be a functional overlap between catalase and GPs. However, catalase is most effective in the presence of high levels of H_2O_2, whereas the GPs system is able to reduce H_2O_2 at very low levels. In addition, unlike GPs, catalase cannot reduce large molecular peroxides such as lipid hydroperoxide, products of lipid peroxidation, or peroxynitrites.[6,13]

In addition to the above-mentioned "classic" antioxidant enzymes, increasing evidence indicates that lung tissue from both human and animals expresses indoleamine 2,3-dioxygenase (IDO), a cytosolic enzyme catalyzing the oxidative cleavage of the indole ring of L-tryptophan to N-formyl-kynurenine that decomposes spontaneously to formate and L-kynurenine then to the terminal metabolites picolinic and quinolinic acid.[16] This enzyme is unique in that it utilizes $O_2^-\cdot$ as a substrate and a cofactor in its catalytic process. Upon consumption of $O_2^-\cdot$, the dioxygenase initiates the formation of tryptophan metabolites including 3-hydroxyanthranilic acid and 3-hydroxykynurenine that are potent radical scavengers. The capability of transferring a prooxidant ($O_2^-\cdot$) into antioxidants makes IDO a powerful antioxidant enzyme.[17] Indeed, induction of this enzyme has been proposed as a local antioxidant defense aimed at preventing inflammation-mediated injury.[18] In supporting the idea that IDO modulates the lung's oxidative state, we obtained evidence showing that IDO-overexpressed lung cells were resistant to oxidant-induced necrosis and apoptosis by limiting intracellular ROS formation[16]. However,

the physiologic role of IDO in lung tissue is still not fully understood.

Redox-Sensitive Transcription Factors

Oxidants and antioxidants have been shown to regulate gene expression by altering the activity of specific redox-sensitive transcription factors. The transcription factors about which there is the most information regarding lung inflammation and antioxidant responses are nuclear factor-κB (NF-κB) and activator protein-1 (AP-1). The binding sites for these two transcription factors are located in the promoter region of a variety of proinflammatory genes associated with different lung diseases. In this section the mechanisms involved in the oxidative regulation of these transcription factors are briefly reviewed.

Nuclear factor-κB controls expression of many genes involved in inflammation/oxidative stress–associated lung injury. For example, activation of NF-κB leads to gene expression of a variety of adhesion molecules, including intercellular adhesion molecule-1, vascular cell adhesion molecule-1, and E-selectin, which play key roles in recruiting inflammatory cells such as neutrophils, eosinophils, and T lymphocytes from the circulation to the site of inflammation.[19] This transcription factor is a member of the Rel family of proteins, which share sequence homology over a 300-amino acid region termed the *NF-κB/Rel domain*.[20] Nuclear factor-κB is a dimer, with the most abundant form being a heterodimer of a 50-kDa (p50) and a 65-kDa (p65) polypeptide subunit. In resting cells, NF-κB resides in the cytoplasm, and its subunits are bound to the inhibitor protein inhibitory κB (IκB), which masks the nuclear translocation signals and thus prevents translocation of NF-κB to the nucleus. Upon activation of the cell, IκB is phosphorylated by IκB kinase, leading to the release of NF-κB (p65/p50) from IκB. The free IκB is degraded by proteasomes, whereas the active p65/p50 translocates to the nucleus and binds to specific motifs in the promoter regions of target genes. The NF-κB/DNA binding activates transcription of mRNA for producing various mediators, including chemokines, cytokines, and growth factors.[20]

There is mounting evidence that NF-κB can be regulated by oxidants and antioxidants. Rahman et al. demonstrated that depletion of GSH with buthionine sulfoximine led to activation of NF-κB and consequently enhanced H_2O_2-induced lung epithelial cell injury.[21] It was also found that $O_2^-\cdot$ accumulation caused by cigarette smoke increased the DNA-binding activity of NF-κB and interleukin (IL)-8 mRNA expression in the airways of guinea pigs.[22] Lipid peroxidation products were shown to induce rapid phosphorylation and degradation of IκB and consequently activate NF-κB.[23] In supporting the view that oxidants enhance NF-κB expression/activity, other studies using antioxidants reported opposite effects. In vitro study demonstrated that treatment of airway epithelial cells with N-acetyl-cysteine or GSH prevented translocation of the NF-κB p65 unit from the cytoplasm to the nucleus and subsequent *IL-8* gene expression in response to tumor necrosis factor (TNF)-α.[24] Similarly, it has been shown that a natural antioxidant pomegranate wine could act as a potent inhibitor of NF-κB activation in bovine artery endothelial cells by preventing its migration into the nucleus and DNA binding activity.[25]

Activator protein-1 is a leucine-zipper transcription factor composed of homo- or heterodimers of the Jun (e.g., JunB and JunD) and the Fos (FosB, Fra-1, and Fra-2) protein families. These proteins control the transcription of several genes involved in cell proliferation, apoptosis, and tumor promotion. Specifically, AP-1 can bind to the 12-O-tetradecanoylphorbol 13-acetate–responsive element (5′-TGAG/CTCA-3′) in the promoter region of a number of genes involved in pulmonary inflammation such as transforming growth factor (TGF)-β.[19,26] Whereas the Jun family of proteins is capable of forming homo- and heterodimers, Fos proteins, which cannot be bound to each other, are capable of associating with any member of the Jun family to produce stable heterodimers with enhanced DNA binding activity. It should be noted that the individual Jun and Fos proteins have significantly different transactivation potentials. In general, Jun, Fos, and FosB exhibit higher transactivation potential than JunB, JunD, Fra-1, and Fra-2 proteins.[26]

Activator protein-1 activation is achieved by the Jun N-terminal kinases (JNK) cascade. The JNKs are members of the mitogen-activated protein kinase superfamily and comprise three isoforms: JNK1, JNK2, and JNK3.[27] The activated JNKs in the nucleus can phosphorylate the N-terminal transactivation domain (residues Ser63 and Ser73) of Jun protein as well as Fos protein, which dimerize to produce active AP-1.[27] Evidence suggests direct involvement of ROS in activation of AP-1 and its downstream target gene expression. In bleomycin-induced lung fibrosis, Jun and Fos protein were found to be overexpressed in alveolar macrophages and type II pneumocytes.[28] Clinical studies provided similar results. For example, it has been shown that free radicals in cigarette smoke increased DNA binding of AP-1 in human type II alveolar epithelial cells.[29] Moreover, cigarette smoke led to overexpression of AP-1 and its subunits Jun and Fos in human airways.[30] On the other hand, it has been shown that the antioxidant N-acetyl-cysteine was able to inhibit AP-1 activation and prevent the induction of Jun and Fos mRNA expression in mesothelial cells in vitro.[19]

It is important to note that the two oxidant-sensitive transcription factors AP-1 and NF-κB can physically and functionally interact. For example, the *IL-2* gene contains DNA binding sites for both AP-1 and NF-κB.[31] Moreover, it has been shown that the NF-κB p65 unit can directly cross-couple with AP-1 subunits and synergistically promote their biologic function.[32]

Oxidative Stress-Associated Lung Disease/Injury

There is good evidence that oxidative stress plays a major role in the development of chronic obstructive pulmonary disease (COPD), a progressively disabling condition characterized by airflow limitation resulting from pathologic changes of chronic bronchitis/bronchiolitis in the airways and destruction of alveolar walls. Cigarette smoke contains a large amount of free radicals and has been identified as a major etiologic factor for this disease. Indeed, a high level of H_2O_2 in breath condensate, which is a direct measurement of oxidant burden in lung tissue, has been found in patients with COPD.[33] Furthermore, lipid peroxidation products are significantly increased in urine, plasma, and bronchoalveolar lavage fluid of smokers and patients with COPD compared with healthy controls.[34,35] Increased levels of NO in exhaled breath, a marker of nitrosative stress, was also found in patients with stable COPD.[36] In addition to the direct evidence showing enhanced oxidant burden, infiltration of neutrophils occurs in lung tissue from patients with COPD.[37] Activated neutrophils have a high capacity to produce ROS and have been used as a reliable marker for inflammation-associated oxidative stress in lung tissue.[38]

Free radicals also participate in the pathogenesis of lung disease with evidence of chronic inflammation, possibly through activating TGF-β and inflammatory cells. Heme oxygenase-1 is a sensitive marker of oxidative stress, and we found that the development of cystic fibrosis is closely associated with induction of heme oxygenase-1 in the airway.[39] Occupational exposure to crystalline silica has been linked to pulmonary fibrosis (i.e., chronic silicosis). The production of ROS and NO caused by silica is believed to be an important part of the pathogenesis of the resulting fibrotic lung disease through activation of NF-κB and AP-1 pathways.[40] In addition, the role of ROS/RNS in other lung diseases, including asthma,[41] idiopathic pulmonary fibrosis,[42] and primary pulmonary hypertension,[43] has also been documented.

Allogeneic lung transplantation has become a common life-saving therapy for many patients with end-stage lung disease. However, lung allografts are especially prone to ischemia/reperfusion injury and acute rejection, which, in addition to infiltrating lymphocytes, are accompanied by neutrophil infiltration and neutrophil-associated oxidative stress.[44] The inflammation-associated oxidative stress contributes importantly to the lung allograft injury, as demonstrated by our findings that treatment with the anti-TNF-α drug pirfenidone[38] and genetic upregulation

of the antioxidant enzyme IDO in donor lungs[16] significantly attenuated neutrophil-related oxidative stress and
consequently showed therapeutic effects. Thus, oxidative
stress is involved not only in the pathogenesis of lung
diseases but also in lung injury caused by therapeutic
interventions. At the present time, however, few effective
antioxidant therapies are available for treating oxidant-
related human lung disease/injury, indicating that the
molecular mechanisms of oxidative stress effects on lung
cells and integrated function remain a subject for further
study.

References

1. Kinnula V, Crapo J. Superoxide dismutases in the lung and
   human lung diseases. Am J Respir Crit Care Med 2003;167:
   1600–1619.
2. Gutteridge J. Lipid peroxidation and antioxidants as biomarkers of tissue damage. Clin Chem 1995;41:1819–1828.
3. Esterbauer H, Zollner H. Methods for determination of
   aldehydic lipid peroxidation products. Free Radic Biol Med
   1989;7:197–203.
4. Valko M, Izakovic M, Mazur M, et al. Role of oxygen radicals in DNA damage and cancer incidence. Mol Cell
   Biochem 2004;266:37–56.
5. Babior B. NADPH oxidase. Curr Opin Immunol 2004;16:
   42–47.
6. Comhair S, Erzurum S. Antioxidant responses to oxidant-
   mediated lung diseases. Am J Physiol Lung Cell Mol Physiol
   2002;283:L246–L255.
7. Langen R, Korn S, Wouters E. ROS in the local and systemic pathogenesis of COPD. Free Radic Biol Med 2003;35:
   226–235.
8. Dedon P, Tannenbaum S. Reactive nitrogen species in the
   chemical biology of inflammation. Arch Biochem Biophys
   2004;423:12–22.
9. van der Vliet A, Eiserich J, Shigenaga M, et al. Reactive
   nitrogen species and tyrosine nitration in the respiratory
   tract: epiphenomena or a pathobiologic mechanism of
   disease? Am J Respir Crit Care Med 1999;160:1–9.
10. Cantin A, North S, Hubbard R, et al. Normal alveolar epi-
    thelial lining fluid contains high levels of glutathione. J
    Appl Physiol 1987;63:152–157.
11. MacNee W. Oxidants/antioxidants and COPD. Chest
    2000;117:303S–317S.
12. Ren B, Huang W, Akesson B, et al. The crystal structure
    of seleno-glutathione peroxidase from human plasma at 2.9
    A resolution. J Mol Biol 1997;268:869–885.
13. Rahman I, Biswas S, Jimenez L, et al. Glutathione, stress
    responses, and redox signaling in lung inflammation. Anti-
    oxid Redox Signal 2005;7:42–59.
14. Krzywanski D, Dickinson D, Iles K, et al. Variable regula-
    tion of glutamate cysteine ligase subunit proteins affects
    glutathione biosynthesis in response to oxidative stress.
    Arch Biochem Biophys 2004;423:116–125.
15. Gutteridge J, Halliwell B. Free radicals and antioxidants in
    the year 2000. A historical look to the future. Ann NY Acad
    Sci 2000;899:136–147.
16. Liu H, Liu L, Fletcher B, et al. Novel action of indoleamine
    2,3-dioxygenase attenuating acute lung allograft injury. Am
    J Respir Crit Care Med 2006;173:566–572.
17. Thomas S, Stocker R. Redox reactions related to indole-
    amine 2,3-dioxygenase and tryptophan metabolism
    along the kynurenine pathway. Redox Rep 1999;4:199–
    220.
18. Christen S, Peterhans E, Stocker R. Antioxidant activities
    of some tryptophan metabolites: possible implication for
    inflammatory diseases. Proc Natl Acad Sci USA 1990;87:
    2506–2510.
19. Rahman I, MacNee W. Role of transcription factors in
    inflammatory lung diseases. Thorax 1998;53:601–612.
20. Chen F, Castranova V, Shi X, et al. New insights into the
    role of nuclear factor-kappaB, a ubiquitous transcription
    factor in the initiation of diseases. Clin Chem 1999;45:7–
    17.
21. Rahman I, Mulier B, Gilmour P, et al. Oxidant-mediated
    lung epithelial cell tolerance: the role of intracellular gluta-
    thione and nuclear factor-kappaB. Biochem Pharmacol
    2001;62:787–794.
22. Nishikawa M, Kakemizu N, Ito T, et al. Superoxide medi-
    ates cigarette smoke-induced infiltration of neutrophils into
    the airways through nuclear factor-kappaB activation and
    IL-8 mRNA expression in guinea pigs in vivo. Am J Respir
    Cell Mol Biol 1999;20:189–198.
23. Bowie A, O'Neill L. Oxidative stress and nuclear factor-
    kappaB activation: a reassessment of the evidence in the
    light of recent discoveries. Biochem Pharmacol 2000;59:
    13–23.
24. Harper R, Wu K, Chang M, et al. Activation of nuclear
    factor-kappa b transcriptional activity in airway epithelial
    cells by thioredoxin but not by N-acetyl-cysteine and gluta-
    thione. Am J Respir Cell Mol Biol 2001;25:178–185.
25. Schubert S, Neeman I, Resnick N. A novel mechanism for
    the inhibition of NF-kappaB activation in vascular endothe-
    lial cells by natural antioxidants. FASEB J 2002;16:1931–
    1933.
26. Hess J, Angel P, Schorpp-Kistner M. AP-1 subunits: quarrel
    and harmony among siblings. J Cell Sci 2004;117:5965–
    5973.
27. Davis R. Signal transduction by the JNK group of MAP
    kinases. Cell 2000;103:239–252.
28. Haase M, Koslowski R, Lengnick A, et al. Cellular distribu-
    tion of c-Jun and c-Fos in rat lung before and after bleomy-
    cin induced injury. Virchows Arch 1997;431:441–448.
29. Rahman I, Smith C, Lawson M, et al. Induction of gamma-
    glutamylcysteine synthetase by cigarette smoke is associ-
    ated with AP-1 in human alveolar epithelial cells. FEBS
    Lett 1996;396:21–25.
30. Wodrich W, Volm M. Overexpression of oncoproteins in
    non-small cell lung carcinomas of smokers. Carcinogenesis
    1993;14:1121–1124.
31. Paliogianni F, Raptis A, Ahuja S, et al. Negative transcrip-
    tional regulation of human interleukin 2 (IL-2) gene by
    glucocorticoids through interference with nuclear transcrip-
    tion factors AP-1 and NF-AT. J Clin Invest 1993;91:1481–
    1489.
32. Stein B, Baldwin A Jr, Ballard D, et al. Cross-coupling of
    the NF-kappa B p65 and Fos/Jun transcription factors pro-

duces potentiated biological function. EMBO J 1993;12: 3879–3891.

33. Nowak D, Antczak A, Krol M, et al. Increased content of hydrogen peroxide in the expired breath of cigarette smokers. Eur Respir J 1996;9:652–657.

34. Morrison D, Rahman I, Lannan S, et al. Epithelial permeability, inflammation, and oxidant stress in the air spaces of smokers. Am J Respir Crit Care Med 1999;159: 473–479.

35. Pratico D, Basili S, Vieri M, et al. Chronic obstructive pulmonary disease is associated with an increase in urinary levels of isoprostane F2alpha-III, an index of oxidant stress. Am J Respir Crit Care Med 1998;158:1709–1714.

36. Corradi M, Majori M, Cacciani G, et al. Increased exhaled nitric oxide in patients with stable chronic obstructive pulmonary disease. Thorax 1999;54:572–575.

37. Shapiro S, Ingenito E. The pathogenesis of chronic obstructive pulmonary disease: advances in the past 100 years. Am J Respir Cell Mol Biol 2005;32:367–372.

38. Liu H, Drew P, Cheng Y, et al. Pirfenidone inhibits inflammatory responses and ameliorates allograft injury in a rat lung transplant model. J Thorac Cardiovasc Surg 2005;130: 852–858.

39. Zhou H, Lu F, Latham C, et al. Heme oxygenase-1 expression in human lungs with cystic fibrosis and cytoprotective effects against *Pseudomonas aeruginosa* in vitro. Am J Respir Crit Care Med 2004;170:633–640.

40. Castranova V. Signaling pathways controlling the production of inflammatory mediators in response to crystalline silica exposure: role of reactive oxygen/nitrogen species. Free Radic Biol Med 2004;37:916–925.

41. Hanazawa T, Kharitonov S, Barnes P. Increased nitrotyrosine in exhaled breath condensate of patients with asthma. Am J Respir Crit Care Med 2000;162:1273–1276.

42. Gross T, Hunninghake G. Idiopathic pulmonary fibrosis. N Engl J Med 2001;345:517–525.

43. Archer S, Rich S. Primary pulmonary hypertension: a vascular biology and translational research "work in progress." Circulation 2000;102:2781–2791.

44. Wilkes D, Egan T, Reynolds H. Lung transplantation: opportunities for research and clinical advancement. Am J Respir Crit Care Med 2005;172:944–955.

45
Epithelial Repair and Regeneration

Steven L. Brody and Jeffrey J. Atkinson

Introduction

Contact with the environment positions the respiratory epithelium at risk for acute and chronic injury from infectious pathogens, noxious agents, and inflammatory processes. Thus, to protect gas transfer within the lung the epithelium is programmed for routine maintenance and repair. Programs for repair are directed by epithelial, mesenchymal, and inflammatory signals that collectively constitute highly regulated networks. Principal components of the repair network are developmental morphogens, integrin and growth factor signaling molecules, and transcription factors. The epithelium responds to these signals with a remarkable plasticity and is bulwarked by a population of lung progenitor cells to ensure maintenance and repair for fluid balance and host defense functions.

Insight into mechanisms of injury response and epithelial cell repair comes from observations of human disease that have been tested using in vivo and in vitro models. Epithelial cell responses have been studied by numerous methods, initially based on morphologic image analysis, cell radiolabeling, and more recently by immunolabeling of molecular markers, receptors, ligands, and genetic tags for lineage analysis. Together, these data have been integrated with a classic injury-wound healing paradigm to create a multistage model (Figure 45.1). Although specific injury/repair responses initiate programs, the resulting steps of epithelial differentiation for repair recapitulate embryonic patterns. In the pathologic state, repair programs are perturbed, leading to states characterized by fibrosis, metaplasia, or carcinogenesis.

Repair mechanisms discussed in this chapter encompass mainly the airway and alveolar epithelium of the lung. The proximal airway epithelium lines the trachea and bronchi and forms the attendant bronchial glands. The distal airway includes bronchiolar epithelium that extends to the junction of the alveolar ducts. Major epithelial types of the airway include ciliated, secretory (Clara), mucous (goblet), and basal cells. Neuroendocrine cells are also found in the epithelial layer. The alveolar epithelium covers the surfaces of the alveolar ducts and alveoli and is composed of primarily the type I and type II pneumocytes. Differences in cell populations and gene expression dictate some differences in repair mechanisms between these regions.

Steady-State Kinetics of Lung Epithelial Cells

Studies of pulmonary cell kinetics in rodents have demonstrated that the epithelial compartment in the adult lung is mitotically inactive, based on ^{3}H-thymidine labeling indices.[1] This overall low proliferation rate and the diverse number of cell types in the lung have made determination of steady-state kinetics difficult. Following postnatal growth, the mitotic index in the rodent lung was calculated to be less than 0.4% per day.[2] In tracheal epithelial cells, 4-week-old rats had a turnover of about 1 month, whereas very low mitotic activity has been identified in the epithelial cells of the postgrowth trachea and terminal bronchiolar epithelium.[3] Prolonged studies achieved by the addition of radiolabeled thymidine to drinking water have demonstrated that alveolar epithelial cells can survive for 125 days in young animals.[4] These observations were obscured by the prolonged period of postnatal alveolar growth that occurs in animals and humans. When labeling of alveolar wall cells was considered relative to age, cell turnover in the alveolar epithelium was noted to decrease even further.[5] Thus, in the absence of injury, the epithelial cells of all lung compartments are mitotically quiescent.

Steps in Injury and Repair

Classic wound healing has been investigated in great detail in the skin where a paradigm for repair that is similar to the lung has been established.[6] This regenera-

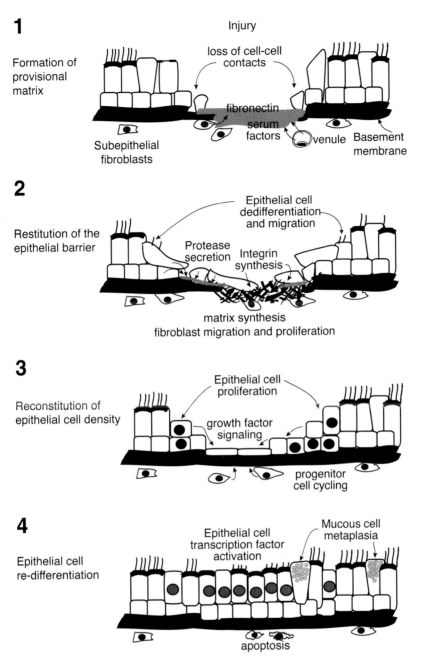

FIGURE 45.1. Steps in repair of airway epithelial cell injury. Conceptual stages of repair of the airway epithelium. See text and Table 45.1 for details of each step. Mitotic or label-retaining cells are indicated by dark nuclei.

tive response was observed over 50 years ago following direct wound injury of the tracheas of rats[7] and subsequently in large numbers of in vivo and in vitro models utilizing mechanical injury in airway and alveolar cell models.[8-15] A similar pattern of behavior is often observed in respiratory epithelial cells injured by chemical or infectious agents, suggesting a stereotypical repair program.[16-18] Although not a simple linear process, the programmed response to injury and repair can be condensed into a model, shown in Figure 45.1 and Table 45.1.

Although shown for an airway epithelial cell model, concepts are similar during alveolar epithelial cell repair.[15] Each of these stages involves participation of multiple factors that are directed by the mesenchymal and epithelial cells. For the purpose of this section, we discuss repair after classic wounding that includes loss of the epithelial cell barrier and, critically, disruption of the basement membrane and underlying interstitial matrix. However, injured epithelial cells may also be selectively removed without disruption of the basement membrane.

TABLE 45.1. Stages and components of repair after epithelial cell injury.

1. Formation of provisional matrix
   Loss of epithelial cells during injury
   Loss of normal basement membrane matrix
   Vascular-derived factors for fibrin clot production
2. Restitution of the epithelial barrier
   Epithelial cell dedifferentiation, spreading, and migration
   Integrin-dependent epithelial cell signaling
   Proteolytic degradation of intracellular adhesions
   Subepithelial fibroblast migration and proliferation
3. Reconstitution of epithelial cell density
   Growth factor–mediated epithelial cell proliferation
   Progenitor and stem cell cycling
4. Epithelial cell redifferentiation
   Growth/transcription factor–mediated epithelial cell differentiation
   Metaplasia and hyperplasia of epithelial cell populations
   Compensatory apoptosis of cell populations

Formation of A Provisional Matrix

Loss of Normal Basement Membrane

In the steady state, the basement membrane is composed of two parallel sheets of laminin and collagen. The uppermost layer (adjacent to the epithelial cells) is composed primarily of laminin-5 and laminin-10, while the lower layer is collagen IV.[19] The layers are connected by entactin/nidogen and multiple, highly charged, heparan sulfate proteoglycans (HSPGs) that are distributed throughout the basement membrane.[19,20] The underlying interstitial matrix contains fibroblasts in a fibrillar collagen (types I and III) matrix with additional HSPGs. Following disruption of the epithelial cell layer and basement membrane, a provisional matrix is formed predominantly by passive leakage of serum factors from local vasculature into the disrupted epithelial basement membrane and into the exposed airspace.[6,21] Cellular components including red blood cells (passively) and neutrophils (actively) move into the wound. The serum components form a fibrin clot that is present for up to 4 days.[7] In acute alveolar injury, the "hyaline membranes" seen in acute respiratory distress syndrome (ARDS) are an example of exuberant provisional matrix after breach of epithelial and endothelial barriers.[22] Inhibitors of fibrinolysis, such as serine protease inhibitors, are present at this point to stabilize the provisional matrix.[23] The passive provisional matrix formation is accompanied by active production of fibronectin by fibroblasts and epithelial cells.[24] Although many molecules compose the provisional matrix, the major factors are fibrin (most prominently), fibronectin, and vitronectin.

Functions of the Provisional Matrix

The provisional matrix provides a temporary barrier and contains multiple molecules to signal subsequent steps in repair. At the defect, a fibrin plug acts as a scaffold for fibronectin and vitronectin molecules but must be removed during reepithelialization.[25] The fibronectin and vitronectin contain multiple arginineglycine-aspartic acid (RGD) epitopes that are not present within the steady-state matrix. This peptide sequence provides sites for interaction of epithelial and fibroblast cell surface receptors (predominantly integrins) during cell migration and barrier restitution.[26–28] In addition to RGD epitopes, proinflammatory neoepitopes and exposed cryptic sites are present that function in growth factor signaling and immune cell recruitment.[29] Furthermore, alterations in matrix-associated HSPGs result in liberation of sequestered growth factors and cytokines.[30] Also, inflammatory and epithelial cells secrete platelet-derived growth factor that acts as both a mitogen and motogen (stimulating cell motility) for fibroblasts[31] that subsequently restore normal matrix components. Once established, the provisional matrix provides a rich source of matrix epitopes and sequestered growth factors that function as a scaffold and signaling unit for future reepithelialization.

Restitution of the Epithelial Barrier

Processes to return basement membrane to a fully established barrier covered with a layer of epithelial cells are initiated almost immediately following injury by several simultaneous processes. First, as discussed earlier, a change in basement membrane composition as mediated by epithelial and mesenchymal cell secretion occurs rapidly to provide barrier protection and matrix-dependent signals for epithelial cells and fibroblasts.[32] Second, epithelial cells, in response to matrix and growth factors, dedifferentiate, stretch, and migrate to cover the basement membrane for reestablishment of functional epithelial cells for barrier, host defense, and fluid equilibrium. Third, proteolytic cleavage of the provisional matrix returns the steady-state composition.[33] Using morphologic methods, these changes are observed to occur within hours following mechanical injury.[8,11]

Epithelial Cell Dedifferentiation

Soon after injury (1–2 hr), the epithelial cells at the edge of the wound undergo dynamic cytoskeletal rearrangement resulting in changes in morphology, featuring formation of lamellipodia.[14] This is the result of the loss of components of cell–matrix and cell–cell junctions leading to dissolution of focal adhesions, adherens junctions, and hemidesmosomes, untethering of intermediate filaments, and thus reorganization of the actin cytoskeleton. The change in morphology is accompanied by loss of features of differentiation (e.g. microvilli) as cells spread over the newly formed surface of provisional matrix. Following mechanical or naphthalene (selectively toxic for Clara cells) injury, the ciliated cells assume a squamous cell-like form and lose cilia.[7,8,16] Molecular marker studies indicate that following naphthalene injury virtually all of the cells participating in the squamous cell-like barrier are from endodermally derived epithelial cells that were present at the time of injury.[34,35]

Signals for Dedifferentiation

Regulation of cell dedifferentiation is thought to result from alterations in matrix–integrin binding, growth factor secretion, and loss of cell–cell junctions. The Wingless (Wnt)/β-catenin pathway is intimately related to cell–cell junction complexes and epithelial cell differentiation.[36] Following injury, the disassembly of E-cadherin at cell junctions releases β-catenin to the cytoplasm where it can be translocated to the nucleus in a Wnt-dependent process.[37] Nuclear β-catenin activates signaling via the transcription factor lymphoid enhancer factor-1/T-cell factor. Consistent with this, after naphthalene-induced injury, β-catenin is diffusely upregulated in the cytoplasm of epithelial cells that are dedifferentiating to cover the provisional matix.[38]

Epithelial Cell Migration

In large wounds, both cell extension and migration occur. The rate of cell migration based on a moving front of cells has been determined to be 1–3 μm/min over the first 8 hr of mechanical injury.[8] Migration is dependent on growth factor activation, matrix–epithelial integrin binding, and matrix metalloprotease expression. Migration can be activated by growth factors such as epidermal growth factor (EGF) and trefoil factor in airway cell models; however, it is likely that other growth factors in serum also potentiate cell movement.[39,40] The predominant cell that migrates varies with the injury model, the cell type targeted, and the animal species studied.[17,35,41] In all cases, the matrix integrins play a critical role in directing epithelial adhesion and fibroblast movement into the wound. Simultaneously, proteases from epithelial and mesenchymal sources release cell–cell and cell–matrix contacts for epithelial cell cytoskeletal reorganization and migration.

Matrix–Epithelial Cell Interactions During Migration

Migrating cells must alter surface receptors for adhesion and traction across the provisional matrix. Integrins are heterodimeric proteins that adhere to many matrix substrates[27] but also transmit signals after ligation of substrate.[42] Alveolar and bronchiolar epithelial cells demonstrate directional migration (both chemotactic and haptotactic) toward many matrix proteins. Fibronectin is the most potent promigratory substance for these cells.[12,28] There is a switch in the expression of integrin receptors on epithelial cells during injury that facilitates migration over the provisional matrix. During steady state, the matrix-associated receptors in lung epithelial cells are predominantly collagen and laminin binding integrins (α2β1, α3β1, and α6β4) but α5 and αv are not present.[43] With injury, integrins α5 and αv are expressed on epithelial cells at the wound edge.[43] These integrins are specific receptors for RGD epitopes in fibronectin and vitronectin and are required for migration.[12,28] Fibroblasts also express α5 to facilitate migration on fibronectin. In addition to integrins, cell surface proteoglycan adhesion molecules such as syndecan and CD44 are also increased on migrating fibroblasts to bind components of provision matrix.[44,45]

Protease Functions in Epithelial Cell Migration

Two major categories of proteases are involved in cellular spreading and migration, matrix metalloproteases (MMPs) and serine. These proteases function by releasing epithelial cell–cell junctions and primordial contacts with the matrix. Of the MMPs, both MMP-7 and MMP-9 are required for normal airway epithelial cell migration.[46,47] Migrating epithelial cells secrete MMP-7 (matrilysin) in a basolateral direction to degrade the extracellular domain of E-cadherin,[46] contributing to cell detachment and spreading at the wound edge. Gelatinase B (MMP-9) releases lamellipodia of migrating cells from the matrix surface to allow extension.[47,48] Tissue inhibitor of matrix metalloproteinase (TIMP)-1 present in early wounding inhibits all secreted MMPs (including MMP-7 and MMP-9). A deficiency of this antiprotease accelerates wound closure.[49] Serum-derived serine protease plasminogen within the wound is activated to plasmin by uroplasminogen activator secreted by bronchial epithelial cells.[50] The primary role of plasmin is fibrinolysis of the provisional fibrin plug. Plasmin also promotes MMP synthesis and activation.[48] Plasmin activator inhibitor-1 is also present and blocks migration by binding to and obscuring vitronectin epitopes.[51] Fibroblasts also require proteases for migration, and membrane type 1 MMP (MT1-MMP, MMP-14) may be crucial for migration through fibrillar collagen and fibrin.[52] Additionally, inflammatory cells present in the wound can alter the activation of these proteases and alter the epitopes present in the provisional matrix.[53]

Reestablishment of the Normal Basement Membrane

Epithelial cells synthesize and remodel basement membrane components during migration. Migrating epithelial cells grown on glass slides secrete a trail of synthesized basement membrane composed of fibronectin, laminin, collagen IV, and factors that newly arriving cells can use as a path for repairing a wound.[54] Other matrix components such as HSPGs, entactin/nidogen, and fibrillar collagens are supplied by the underlying fibroblasts. Restitution of basement membrane also requires removal of the provisional matrix. Failure to do so may result in prolonged signaling, recruitment of fibroblasts, and scar formation.[55] Furthermore, reestablishment of stable cell–matrix adhesions is not passive, and some proteases must continue to be expressed for proteolytic modification of the basement membrane.[54,56] For instance, laminin-5, the major matrix component of hemidesmosomes, requires proteolytic cleavage by serine proteases for enucleation of the hemidesmosomes.[56] Once the basement membrane and extracellular matrix are in the mature, stable confirmation, promigratory signals are quenched.

Reconstitution of Epithelial Cell Density

Epithelial Cell Proliferation

Following epithelial cell stretch and migration to cover a reestablished basement membrane, the epithelium must replace the cells lost during injury. A major mediator of proliferation during this stage is EGF and related family members; however, other growth factors, including fibroblast growth factor (FGF)-7 and hepatocyte growth factor (HGF), contribute to this function (Table 45.2) and are discussed later.[57–59] Epithelial cell proliferation has been noted to occur within 24–48 hr of mechanical and inhalation injury (e.g., ozone, nitrogen dioxide).[7,8,13,18] After injury, 20%–30% of undifferentiated epithelial cells covering the wound contain proliferation markers at 24–48 hr, followed by a marked decrease by 72 hr.[8,13,41,60] After nitrogen dioxide injury, an increase from 1% to 24% labeling index (proportion of labeled cells) of Clara cells and type II cells is observed at 24 hr.[41] The appearance of differentiated epithelial cells follows the peak of mitotic activity (the final stage in the repair model).[10]

Lung Progenitor and Lung Epithelial Stem Cells Roles

Observations many decades ago, based on thymidine labeling during development and after injury, suggested that the basal cell was the progenitor cell of the tracheal epithelium, the Clara cell provided this function in the distal airway,[61,62] and type II cells proliferated and gave rise to type I pneumocytes in the alveoli.[18,63] Recent injury–repair models and genetic approaches have confirmed many of these observations. Lineage tagging by conditional recombination in mice engineered with airway and alveolar epithelial cell specific promoters that drive cell markers has identified a single pool of progenitor epithelial cells present during early lung development.[64] Within fully formed adult lung, injury models reveal regional niches (proximal airway, distal airway, alveolar) for progenitor cells.[34,64–66] These lung cells are considered to be slow cycling but can give rise to progenitor cells that are capable of further cell division (transit amplifying cells). In the proximal airway, a niche of label-retaining cells has been localized within the submucosal glands and basal cells of the mouse trachea.[65,67] The expression of cell cycle protein Ki-67 in basal cells of cystic fibrosis bronchi identifies a similar proliferating population in human disease.[68]

In the distal airways, naphthalene injury models suggest that pulmonary neuroendocrine cells provide a protective niche for label-retaining Clara-like cells that are capable of epithelial reconstitution.[35] Similar studies identified injury-resistant cells expressing Clara cell secretory protein (CCSP) at the bronchoalveolar duct junction that are reparative.[34] Consistent with this, in the terminal airways of humans, 20%–40% of the proliferating cells express CCSP.[69] Cells expressing ciliated cell markers (e.g., transcription factor Foxj1) were not observed to proliferate in naphthalene or virus injury models.[17,38] Progenitor cells that repair the alveolar epithelium are less well defined. During alveolar injury, labeling studies show that type II but not type I cells proliferate and that type II can generate type I cells after lung injury.[70] Subpopulations of type II alveolar epithelial

TABLE 45.2. Growth factors in epithelial cell repair.

Ligand	Major sources	Key targets	Proliferation	Migration	Differentiation	Reference
EGF family	Epi	Epi	+	+	+	57
TGF-β	Epi, Fib, Mφ	Epi, Fib	−	−	+	58
FGF-7 (KGF)	Fib, SM	Epi	+	+	+	59
HGF	Fib, En, Epi, Mφ	Epi	+	+	−	59
PDGF	Mφ, Epi	Fib	+	+	−	31

Note: EGF, epidermal growth factor; En, endothelial; Epi, epithelial; FGF, fibroblast growth factor; Fib, fibroblast; HGF, hepatocyte growth factor; KGF, keratinocyte growth factor; Mφ, macrophage; PDGF, platelet-derived growth factor; SM, smooth muscle; TGF, transforming growth factor.

cells resistant to injury and capable of proliferation have been identified in vitro,[71] but compelling data suggests that a bronchoalveolar duct cell may function as a progenitor for both alveolar type II pneumocytes and Clara cells.[72]

Bone Marrow Stem Cells in Repair

New information is evolving concerning the reparative role of bone marrow–derived cells in lung injury repair (see Chapter 47). Some evidence suggests that adult stem cells can function to reconstitute at least a small percentage of the airway and alveolar epithelium of an injured lung.[66]

Growth Factor Functions in Epithelial Cell Reconstitution

Signaling between cells of endodermal and mesenchymal origin is a fundamental process in development that is shared with repair and is predominantly mediated by growth factors (see Table 45.2 and later discussion).[73,74] Growth factors that play key roles in epithelial cell repair include EGF, transforming growth factor (TGF)-β, FGF-7, platelet-derived growth factor, and HGF family members. Other growth factors are known to be critical in lung development, but specific roles in repair are not described.[73,74] Growth factors function during epithelial cell repair and reconstitution by motogenic, mitogenic, and prodifferentiation effects.

Epithelial Cell Redifferentiation

Differentiating epithelial cells within a repairing wound arise primarily from three different populations: dedifferentiated cells, proliferating cells, and multipotent stem or progenitor cells. In turn, differentiation is regulated by three major groups of molecules: secreted growth factors and other developmental signaling molecules, transcription factors, and extracellular matrix proteins (discussed earlier). In addition, multiple cofactors play important roles in differentiation, including retinoic acid[75] and those known to be critical for in vitro differentiation of primary epithelial cells such as insulin, epinephrine, thyroid hormone, and corticosteroids.[70,76] Epithelial cell differentiation during repair relies on programs similar to those used during lung development.[17,38,73]

Epithelial Cell Redifferentiation and Transdifferentiation

Morphologic evidence of redifferentiation commences at 3–10 days in vivo depending on wound model.[7,8,11] Multi-

ple epithelial cell populations contribute to the redifferentiating airway epithelia within the repairing wound.[34,38,62,67,77] First, a large number of the redifferentiated cells arise from previously differentiated cells that have dedifferentiated to cover the provisional matrix. It has been observed that, following naphthalene injury, former ciliated cells that squamate to cover a wound continue to express the Foxj1 transcription factor for subsequent ciliated cell redifferentiation.[38] Second, proliferating cells also become differentiated cells. As noted earlier, these are either of Clara cell or basal cell origin in the airway or of type II cell origin in the alveolar compartment.[78,79] Third, it is likely that there is a multipotent or progenitor cell that can contribute to lung-specific lineages that is capable of resupplying all epithelial cell types. Here, genetic tagging and clonogenic studies have indicated that niches of specialized cells can generate multiple differentiated cell types.[65,67,72]

Developmental Signaling Pathways Mediating Differentiation

Developmental signaling proteins that are members of the Wnt, Sonic hedgehog (Shh), and bone morphogenic protein (BMP) pathways play essential roles in differentiation.[73,74] Each pathway contains multiple members and receptors that are functionally interdependent. Although these families have been studied in detail during lung development (specifically in branching morphogenesis), their roles in repair are not as well defined.

Wnt signaling regulates cell proliferation, migration, and differentiation.[36,80] The canonical Wnt/β-catenin pathway involves the binding of Wnt ligands to the receptor complex and regulation of β-catenin. Noncanonical Wnt signaling, such as utilized by Wnt5, is required for normal alveolar differentiation and alters expression of Shh and BMP4.[80] Sonic hedgehog is expressed in developing lung epithelium where it signals through its receptor Patch to activate the transcription factor Gli. Gli1 and Gli2 are expressed in developing lung mesenchymal cells budding from the foregut and instruct the tracheal epithelial cells during branching morphogenesis.[81] However, Shh and Gli are also highly expressed in the epithelium following naphthalene injury and are upregulated in small cell lung cancer.[82] Overactivation of the Shh pathway results in proliferation and perturbation of differentiation, notably in epithelial neuroendocrine cells of the lung, but the role in normal lung epithelial cells is unclear.[82] BMP4 is expressed in the lung epithelium, regulates proximal–distal patterning, and is required for normal alveolar epithelial cell differentiation.[83] This pathway may be interrupted in inflammatory states where activation of transcription factor NF-κB has been shown to alter epithelial–mesenchymal signaling through interruption of BMP4 in a chick lung model.[84]

Transcription Factors Mediating Differentiation Following Injury

Transcription factor expression in epithelial cells during injury and repair also recapitulates developmental sequences.[17,38] Transcription factors with central roles in lung epithelial cell differentiation are homeodomain thyroid transcription factor 1 (TITFI or TTF-1; Nkx2.1), forkhead family members (Foxa1, Foxa2, Foxj1), and GATA-6.[85] Lung morphogenesis requires both Gli and TITF-1.[86,87] Molecular analysis of mice deficient in TITF-1 showed a requirement for this factor in differentiation of epithelial cells of the distal airways and alveoli.[86] Thyroid transcription factor 1 and Foxa2 are expressed in epithelium in early development, persist in the adult, and activate epithelial cell-specific genes such as surfactant proteins and CCSP, suggesting major roles in epithelial differentiation.[85] Persistent Foxa2 and TITF-1 expression during injury in airway and alveolar (type II) epithelial cells may be due to a relative resistance of some cell populations and indicates that early programs of epithelial cell differentiation remain intact.[17,38,78] Selective cytotoxic injury of alveolar epithelial cells markedly increased transient expression of Foxn1 in airway and alveolar proliferating cells; however, a specific role for this factor in differentiation has not been described. Foxj1 is expressed later in repair when it is required for ciliogenesis.[17,38,88] Similarly, GATA-6 is required for differentiation of alveolar epithelial cells and the transition of type II to type I cells.[89]

Metaplasia and Compensatory Apoptosis of Epithelial Cell Populations

Mucous cell metaplasia commonly occurs during abnormal airway repair. Injury-associated inflammatory cells secrete proteases (neutrophil elastase) and cytokines (e.g., IL-13 and IL-9) to induce mucous cell metaplasia in animal models and human disease.[90–93] Metaplasia may be persistent or be remedied through apoptosis.[94] In normal repair of alveolar epithelium, type II cell hyperplasia after lung injury is followed by compensatory apoptosis.[95,96]

Roles for Growth Factors in Epithelial Cell Repair

Growth factor–mediated signaling between cells is a constant feature of repair and does not exist as a discrete stage of repair; however, specific growth factors may dominate at one point. Several growth factors with roles

in injury an repair are noted in Table 45.2 and discussed in this section.

Epidermal Growth Factor Family

Epidermal growth factor is the prototypic member of the EGF family of ligands.[57] Epidermal growth ligands are key factors in airway and alveolar epithelial repair through their activation of epithelial cell migration, proliferation, and differentiation.[15,39,40,92] The EGF receptor Her1 (EGFR, ErbB1) and other family members (Her2-4) are receptor tyrosine kinases with affinity for multiple EGF ligands, including TGF-α, heparin binding EGF, amphiregulin, epiregulin, and neuregulin. Signaling occurs after homo- or heterodimerization of receptor family members. At steady state, EGF receptors are localized predominantly on the basolateral surface of epithelial cells, providing ligand–receptor exclusion. Following injury, there is redistribution of receptors to apical cell surfaces, enhancing ligand receptor interaction and subsequent repair.[79,92,97] Epidermal growth factor, TGF-α, and other ligands are elevated in human disease (e.g., cystic fibrosis, asthma) and cell and animal models of airway and alveolar epithelial cell injury.[68,97–99]

Transforming Growth Factor-β Family

Transforming growth factor-β functions in both epithelial maintenance and injury–repair.[21,58] The three TGF-β forms all signal through the same receptor but have unique functions.[100] Abundant latent TGF-β is stored within the extracellular matrix at steady state and is activated after injury through proteolytic and nonproteolytic mechanisms.[58] Transforming growth factor-β activation results in increased synthesis of matrix factors by epithelial cells and fibroblasts, differentiation of epithelial cells, enhanced survival and proliferation of fibroblasts, inhibition and apoptosis of inflammatory cells, and maturation of certain inflammatory cell subsets. Failure to activate TGF-β in the lung matrix results in excessive inflammation and lung destruction.[101] Excessive or prolonged TGF-β activation leads to fibrosis (see Chapter 46). It also prevents normal epithelial cell differentiation due to TGF-β signaling via Smad that inhibits TITF-1 to subsequently reduce surfactant protein gene expression.[102] Additionally, TGF-β promotes epithelial-to-mesenchymal transdifferentiation.[103]

Fibroblast Growth Factor

Fibroblast growth factor-7 (keratinocyte growth factor [KGF]) functions as a potent mitogen for both Clara and type II cells.[104,105] In lung injury, FGF-7 is produced by fibroblasts and vascular smooth muscle cells and has high affinity for only the FGFR2-IIIb splice variant that is expressed on airway and alveolar epithelia.[59] Proinflammatory cytokines stimulate fibroblast production of FGF-7 in vitro.[106] Fibroblast growth factor-7 enhances epithelial cell spreading and motility[107] by increasing MMP-9 and uroplasminogen activator secretion from wounded epithelial cells.[108] It also enhances differentiation and surfactant synthesis by alveolar type II cells.[109] Fibroblast growth factor-7 is elevated in human ARDS bronchoalveolar lavage fluid and in models of acute lung injury.[59] Exogenous intratracheal or systemic delivery prior to lung injury ameliorates damage in animal models.[59]

Hepatocyte Growth Factor

Hepatocyte growth factor is a mitogen and motogen for alveolar type II cells.[59] Hepatocyte growth factor is synthesized by fibroblasts, bronchial epithelial cells, endothelial cells, and alveolar macrophages as a precursor that is proteolytically processed.[110] The HGF receptor c-Met is a receptor tyrosine kinase that is present on epithelial cells, fibroblasts, endothelial cells, and hematopoietic cells. Hepatocyte growth factor is increased in human and animal models of lung injury, in part through proinflammatory cytokines (e.g., IL-1 and IL-6) that stimulate HGF secretion from fibroblasts.[59] Following alveolar epithelial cell injury, HGF secretion precedes FGF-7[111] and is temporally related to type II cell DNA synthesis during the cell proliferation phase, suggesting that HGF is a prominent mitogen in ARDS.[59]

Epithelial Cell Repair Following Prototypic Injuries

Human diseases characterized by respiratory epithelial cell injury provide insight into normal and abnormal repair mechanisms. Epithelial injury and repair occur commonly after respiratory viral and bacterial infections but may also occur with acid aspiration or toxic gas or steam inhalation. In contrast, chronic injury associated with cigarette smoking, asthma, and chronic bronchitis results in an interruption of normal repair. Normal and pathogenic mechanisms that follow acute respiratory epithelial injury in human disease demonstrate the importance of each stage of the injury–repair model described earlier (see Figure 45.1). Below, events occurring during repair of the airway after respiratory virus infection (Figure 45.2) and of the alveolar epithelium in ARDS demonstrate the relevance of the repair model.

Airway Epithelial Cell Repair Following Respiratory Virus Infection

Reestablishment of epithelium following viral injury mirrors the stages of the classic wound injury–repair model (compare Figures 45.1 and 45.2). Information regarding airway epithelial injury induced by respiratory viruses has been derived from natural human infections, but especially from studies of experimental infections in animals with paramyxovirus (e.g., parainfluenza and respiratory syncytial virus) and influenza virus. These infections result in loss of cilia and ciliated cells (based on virus-specific receptor targeting) and metaplasia of epithelial cells during repair.[17,112-115]

Morphologic Events Following Respiratory Virus Infection

Morphologic events of injury and repair following respiratory virus infection, as observed by electron and light microscopy studies, are similar across several animal infection models (see Figure 45.2A). A common initial event is sloughing of epithelial cells, resulting in denuded basement membrane in airways and alveoli.[17,112] This is followed by cell dedifferentiation, marked particularly by cell elongation covering the provisional basement membrane and by ciliary shorting and loss.[17,112,113] Concomitant are subepithelial cell inflammatory infiltrates and/or alveolar pneumonitis.[113] Virus clearance is coupled with regeneration of the epithelium, typically at days 5–8 postinoculation. In contrast to mechanical injury, experimental virus infection in animals showed that airway and alveolar epithelial cell proliferation occurred at 5 days after inoculation.[17,113] In the Sendai virus–infected mouse, bromodeoxyuridine labeling peaked at day 12 and was absent by day 21.[17] Airway and alveolar epithelial cell differentiation normalizes within 3–4 weeks postinoculation.[17,112,113] Functionally, injury is marked by decreased bacterial clearance and secondary bacterial infections, and repair tracks with measured mucociliary clearance.[17,113]

Molecular Correlates of Morphologic Events

Molecular markers of epithelial cell differentiation characterized in the developing lung have been assessed in postinfection repair (see Figure 45.2B).[17,85] As in naphthalene injury, throughout virus injury and repair Foxa2 and TITF-1 remain expressed.[38] Depressed expression of ciliated cell marker Foxj1 and Clara cell marker CCSP during injury and early repair reflects a relatively undifferentiated state of the epithelium as has been observed following human respiratory syncytial virus infection.[17] A relative absence of CCSP in epithelial cells postinjury suggests it is unlikely that mature Clara cells are functioning as a reservoir for new differentiated cells. Foxj1 expression was not detected in proliferating cells identified by bromodeoxyuridine labeling,[17] suggesting mature ciliated cells are nonmitotic. Instead, it is more probable that Foxj1 is important for late-stage ciliogenesis.[88] The

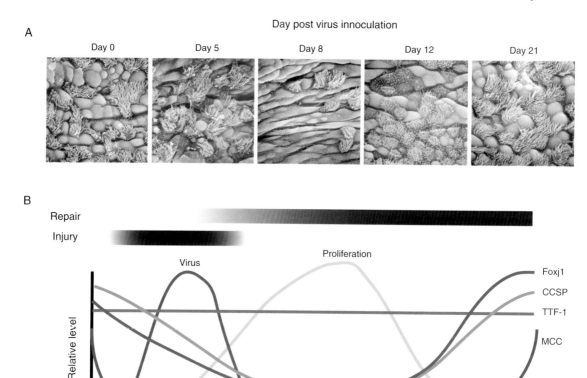

FIGURE 45.2. Airway epithelial cell repair following respiratory viral injury. **(A)** Scanning electron micrographs of mouse trachea following in vivo infection with Sendai paramyxovirus. (Reprinted from Am J Pathol 2001;159:2055–2069, with permission of the American Society for Investigative Pathology.) **(B)** Molecular and functional events following the respiratory virus infection shown in A. Relative changes in expression of airway epithelial cell markers and transcription factors. CCSP, Clara cell secretory protein; Foxj1, transcription factor; MCC, mucociliary clearance; TITF-1 (also known as TITF1, Nkx2.1), thyroid transcription factor 1.

sequence of differentiation during the repair phase, including the lag of CCSP expression relative to the appearance of cilia markers, is similar to that seen in the developing lung, supporting the idea that repair recapitulates development.[85]

Mucous Cell Metaplasia Following Respiratory Virus Infection

Mucous cell (goblet cell) metaplasia is a feature of chronic airway diseases including asthma and COPD. These diseases have been linked to preceding respiratory virus infections and have implicated several factors including aberrant EGF receptor and IL-13 signaling.[92] Mouse models of respiratory virus infection show mucous cell metaplasia in the late repair phase that persists despite virus clearance, suggesting that the virus

reprograms epithelial cell responses through persistent immune responses.[92,93,116,117]

Alveolar Epithelial Cell Repair Following Acute Respiratory Distress Syndrome

Acute lung injury and the clinical manifestation ARDS are a classic example of alveolar injury and repair. Diffuse alveolar damage, the histologic correlate of acute lung injury/ARDS has been subdivided into three phases that parallel the wound–repair model.[22] The early exudative phase (days 1–7) is characterized by necrosis of pneumocytes and endothelial cells and by interstitial and alveolar edema with hemorrhage and hyaline membranes. The ensuing proliferative phase (days 7–21) is marked by type II cell hyperplasia, fibroblast migration into organizing areas of luminal fibrosis, and inflammation. The fibrotic phase entails fibrosis with variable degrees of architectural remodeling.

Establishment of a Provisional Matrix in Acute Respiratory Distress Syndrome

The hallmark of the early exudative phase is the leakage of serum proteins, including serum albumin, β_2-microglobulin, ceruloplasmin and fibrinogen, into the alveolar space for provisional matrix formation.[22,118] An influx of platelets and inflammatory cells also occurs by passive and active mechanisms. Antiprotease production in this phase favors stabilization of the provisional matrix by inhibition of fibrinolytic activity.[23] Gene profiling of animals in this phase of acute lung injury suggests that three major cellular processes occur: (1) loss of the functional activity of differentiated type II cells, (2) production of inhibitors of the serine and matrix metalloproteinase family, and (3) production of cytokines and growth factors.[23] The loss of differentiated alveolar epithelial cells (type II cells) is likely due to injury and dedifferentiation to replace necrotic type I cells and is marked by decreased ion channel and surfactant-associated gene production.[23] Transforming growth factor-β_1-induced genes are rapidly upregulated within 72 hr after alveolar epithelial damage.[23,119] Blockade of TGF-β signaling in the exudative phase prevents alveolar edema, suggesting that TGF-β activation inhibits alveolar epithelial repair during this stage.[120]

Restitution and Reconstitution of the Epithelial Cell Barrier

The proliferative phase is characterized by migration of alveolar epithelial cells over the provisional matrix and type II cell proliferation. These processes are responsive to growth factors EGF and KGF as well as to matrix RGD epitopes.[28] Also during this phase, fibroblasts and myofibroblasts migrate toward the fibronectin cross-linked within the fibrin of the provisional matrix.[25] Failure of repair, associated with inability to reconstitute the epithelial barrier, results in fibroblast/myofibroblast production of collagen and fibronectin, contraction, and fibrosis.

Summary: Epithelial Cell Repair Following Injury

Repair of the epithelium can be conceptualized as a stage-dependent process, but lines of division of biologic activities are not discrete. Instead, an orchestration of mesenchymal and epithelial interactions directed by matrix and epithelial signaling in response to fundamental development, growth, and matrix factors results in the

repair process. Models of repair after respiratory viral infection and acute lung injury provide useful information for understanding the molecular basis of repair in human lung diseases.

References

1. Kauffman SL. Cell proliferation in the mammalian lung. Int Rev Exp Pathol 1980;22:131–191.
2. Enesco M, Leblond CP. Increase in cell number as a factor in the growth of the young male rat. J Embryol Exp Morphol 1962;10:530–562.
3. Kauffman SL. Alteration in cell proliferation in mouse lung following urethane exposure. II. Effects of chronic exposure on terminal bronchiolar epithelium. Am J Pathol 1971;64(3):531–538.
4. Cameron IL. Cell renewal in the organs and tissues of the nongrowing adult mouse. Tex Rep Biol Med 1970; 28(3):203–248.
5. Simnett JD, Heppleston AG. Cell renewal in the mouse lung. The influence of sex, strain, and age. Lab Invest 1966; 15(11):1793–1801.
6. Clark RAF. The Molecular and Cellular Biology of Wound Repair, 2nd ed. New York: Plenum Press; 1996.
7. Wilhelm DL. Regeneration of tracheal epithelium. J Pathol Bacteriol 1953;65(2):543–550.
8. Erjefalt JS, Erjefalt I, Sundler F, Persson CG. In vivo restitution of airway epithelium. Cell Tissue Res 1995;281 (2):305–316.
9. Keenan KP, Combs JW, McDowell EM. Regeneration of hamster tracheal epithelium after mechanical injury. I. Focal lesions: quantitative morphologic study of cell proliferation. Virchows Arch B Cell Pathol Incl Mol Pathol 1982;41(3):193–214.
10. Lane BP, Gordon R. Regeneration of rat tracheal epithelium after mechanical injury. I. The relationship between mitotic activity and cellular differentiation. Proc Soc Exp Biol Med 1974;145(4):1139–1144.
11. Gordon RE, Lane BP. Regeneration of rat tracheal epithelium after mechanical injury. II. Restoration of surface integrity during the early hours after injury. Am Rev Respir Dis 1976;113(6):799–807.
12. Rickard KA, Taylor J, Rennard SI, Spurzem JR. Migration of bovine bronchial epithelial cells to extracellular matrix components. Am J Respir Cell Mol Biol 1993;8(1): 63–68.
13. Shimizu T, Nishihara M, Kawaguchi S, Sakakura Y. Expression of phenotypic markers during regeneration of rat tracheal epithelium following mechanical injury. Am J Respir Cell Mol Biol 1994;11(1):85–94.
14. Zahm JM, Chevillard M, Puchelle E. Wound repair of human surface respiratory epithelium. Am J Respir Cell Mol Biol 1991;5(3):242–248.
15. Kheradmand F, Folkesson HG, Shum L, et al. Transforming growth factor-alpha enhances alveolar epithelial cell repair in a new in vitro model. Am J Physiol 1994;267(6 Pt 1):L728–L738.
16. Lawson GW, Van Winkle LS, Toskala E, et al. Mouse strain modulates the role of the ciliated cell in acute tra-

cheobronchial airway injury—distal airways. Am J Pathol 2002;160(1):315–327.

17. Look DC, Walter MJ, Williamson MR, et al. Effects of paramyxoviral infection on airway epithelial cell Foxj1 expression, ciliogenesis, and mucociliary function. Am J Pathol 2001;159(6):2055–2069.

18. Adamson IY, Bowden DH. The type 2 cell as progenitor of alveolar epithelial regeneration. A cytodynamic study in mice after exposure to oxygen. Lab Invest 1974; 30(1):35–42.

19. Sannes PL, Burch KK, Khosla J, et al. Immunohistochemical localization of chondroitin sulfate, chondroitin sulfate proteoglycan, heparan sulfate proteoglycan, entactin, and laminin in basement membranes of postnatal developing and adult rat lungs. Am J Respir Cell Mol Biol 1993; 8(3):245–251.

20. Yurchenco PD, Amenta PS, Patton BL. Basement membrane assembly, stability and activities observed through a developmental lens. Matrix Biol 2004;22(7):521–538.

21. McGowan SE. Extracellular matrix and the regulation of lung development and repair. FASEB J 1992;6(11):2895–2904.

22. Tomashefski JF Jr. Pulmonary pathology of acute respiratory distress syndrome. Clin Chest Med 2000;21(3):435–466.

23. Wesselkamper SC, Case LM, Henning LN, et al. Gene expression changes during the development of acute lung injury: role of transforming growth factor beta. Am J Respir Crit Care Med 2005;172(11):1399–1411.

24. Rosi E, Beckmann JD, Pladsen P, et al. Modulation of human bronchial epithelial cell IIICS fibronectin mRNA in vitro. Eur Respir J 1996;9(3):549–555.

25. Greiling D, Clark RA. Fibronectin provides a conduit for fibroblast transmigration from collagenous stroma into fibrin clot provisional matrix. J Cell Sci 1997;110(Pt 7):861–870.

26. Hocking DC, Chang CH. Fibronectin matrix polymerization regulates small airway epithelial cell migration. Am J Physiol Lung Cell Mol Physiol 2003;285(1):L169–L179.

27. Sheppard D. Functions of pulmonary epithelial integrins: from development to disease. Physiol Rev 2003;83(3):673–686.

28. Kim HJ, Henke CA, Savik SK, Ingbar DH. Integrin mediation of alveolar epithelial cell migration on fibronectin and type I collagen. Am J Physiol 1997;273(1 Pt 1):L134–L41.

29. Laskin DL, Kimura T, Sakakibara S, et al. Chemotactic activity of collagen-like polypeptides for human peripheral blood neutrophils. J Leuk Biol 1986;39(3):255–266.

30. Li Q, Park PW, Wilson CL, Parks WC. Matrilysin shedding of syndecan-1 regulates chemokine mobilization and transepithelial efflux of neutrophils in acute lung injury. Cell 2002;111(5):635–646.

31. Bonner JC. Regulation of PDGF and its receptors in fibrotic diseases. Cytokine Growth Factor Rev 2004;15(4):255–273.

32. Clark RA. Fibrin is a many splendored thing. J Invest Dermatol 2003;121(5):XXI–XXII.

33. Van Leer C, Stutz M, Haeberli A, Geiser T. Urokinase plasminogen activator released by alveolar epithelial cells modulates alveolar epithelial repair in vitro. Thromb Haemost 2005;94(6):1257–1264.

34. Giangreco A, Reynolds SD, Stripp BR. Terminal bronchioles harbor a unique airway stem cell population that localizes to the bronchoalveolar duct junction. Am J Pathol 2002;161(1):173–182.

35. Hong Ku, Reynolds SD, Giangreco A, et al. Clara cell secretory protein-expressing cells of the airway neuroepithelial body microenvironment include a label-retaining subset and are critical for epithelial renewal after progenitor cell depletion. Am J Respir Cell Mol Biol 2001;24(6):671–681.

36. Seto ES, Bellen HJ. The ins and outs of Wingless signaling. Trends Cell Biol 2004;14(1):45–53.

37. Orsulic S, Huber O, Aberle H, et al. E-cadherin binding prevents beta-catenin nuclear localization and beta-catenin/LEF-1–mediated transactivation. J Cell Sci 1999; 112(Pt 8):1237–1245.

38. Park KS, Wells JM, Zorn AM, et al. Transdifferentiation of ciliated cells during repair of the respiratory epithelium. Am J Respir Cell Mol Biol 2006;34(2):151–157.

39. Oertel M, Graness A, Thim L, et al. Trefoil factor family-peptides promote migration of human bronchial epithelial cells: synergistic effect with epidermal growth factor. Am J Respir Cell Mol Biol 2001;25(4):418–424.

40. Kim JS, McKinnis VS, Nawrocki A, White SR. Stimulation of migration and wound repair of guinea-pig airway epithelial cells in response to epidermal growth factor. Am J Respir Cell Mol Biol 1998;18(1):66–74.

41. Evans MJ, Stephens RJ, Freeman G. Effects of nitrogen dioxide on cell renewal in the rat lung. Arch Intern Med 1971;128(1):57–60.

42. Akiyama SK. Integrins in cell adhesion and signaling. Hum Cell 1996;9(3):181–186.

43. Pilewski JM, Latoche JD, Arcasoy SM, Albelda SM. Expression of integrin cell adhesion receptors during human airway epithelial repair in vivo. Am J Physiol 1997;273(1 Pt 1):L256–L263.

44. Clark RA, Lin F, Greiling D, et al. Fibroblast invasive migration into fibronectin/fibrin gels requires a previously uncharacterized dermatan sulfate-CD44 proteoglycan. J Invest Dermatol 2004;122(2):266–277.

45. Lin F, Ren XD, Doris G, Clark RA. Three-dimensional migration of human adult dermal fibroblasts from collagen lattices into fibrin/fibronectin gels requires syndecan-4 proteoglycan. J Invest Dermatol 2005;124(5):906–913.

46. McGuire JK, Li Q, Parks WC. Matrilysin (matrix metalloproteinase-7) mediates E-cadherin ectodomain shedding in injured lung epithelium. Am J Pathol 2003;162(6):1831–1843.

47. Legrand C, Gilles C, Zahm JM, et al. Airway epithelial cell migration dynamics. MMP-9 role in cell–extracellular matrix remodeling. J Cell Biol 1999;146(2):517–529.

48. Legrand C, Polette M, Tournier JM, et al. UPA/plasmin system–mediated MMP-9 activation is implicated in bronchial epithelial cell migration. Exp Cell Res 2001;264(2):326–36.

49. Chen P, Farivar AS, Mulligan MS, Madtes DK. tissue inhibitor of metalloproteinase-1 deficiency abrogates obliterative airway disease after heterotopic tracheal

transplantation. Am J Respir Cell Mol Biol 2006;34(4):
464–472.

50. Chu EK, Cheng J, Foley JS, et al. Induction of the plasminogen activator system by mechanical stimulation of
human bronchial epithelial cells. Am J Respir Cell Mol
Biol 2006;35(6):628–638.

51. Lazar MH, Christensen PJ, Du M, et al. Plasminogen
activator inhibitor-1 impairs alveolar epithelial repair by
binding to vitronectin. Am J Respir Cell Mol Biol 2004;
31(6):672–678.

52. Hotary KB, Yana I, Sabeh F, et al. Matrix metalloproteinases (MMPs) regulate fibrin-invasive activity via MT1-
MMP-dependent and -independent processes. J Exp Med
2002;195(3):295–308.

53. Parks WC, Shapiro SD. Matrix metalloproteinases in lung
biology. Respir Res 2001;2(1):10–19.

54. Hintermann E, Quaranta V. Epithelial cell motility on
laminin-5: regulation by matrix assembly, proteolysis, integrins and ErbB receptors. Matrix Biol 2004;23(2):75–
85.

55. De Giorgio-Miller A, Bottoms S, Laurent G, et al. Fibrin-
induced skin fibrosis in mice deficient in tissue plasminogen activator. Am J Pathol 2005;167(3):721–732.

56. Baker SE, Hopkinson SB, Fitchmun M, et al. Laminin-5
and hemidesmosomes: role of the alpha 3 chain subunit in
hemidesmosome stability and assembly. J Cell Sci 1996;109
(Pt 10):2509–2520.

57. Citri A, Yarden Y. EGF-ErbB Signalling: towards the
systems level. Nat Rev Mol Cell Biol 2006;7(7):505–516.

58. Sheppard D. Transforming growth factor-beta: a central
modulator of pulmonary and airway inflammation and
fibrosis. Proc Am Thorac Soc 2006;3(5):413–417.

59. Ware LB, Matthay MA. Keratinocyte and hepatocyte
growth factors in the lung: roles in lung development,
inflammation, and repair. Am J Physiol Lung Cell Mol
Physiol 2002;282(5):L924–L40.

60. Evans MJ, Johnson LV, Stephens RJ, Freeman G. Cell
renewal in the lungs of rats exposed to low levels of ozone.
Exp Mol Pathol 1976;24(1):70–83.

61. Bindreiter M, Schuppler J, Stockinger L. Cell proliferation
and differentiation in the tracheal epithelium of the rat.
Exp Cell Res 1968;50(2):377–382.

62. Evans MJ, Cabral-Anderson LJ, Freeman G. Role of the
Clara cell in renewal of the bronchiolar epithelium. Lab
Invest 1978;38(6):648–653.

63. Evans MJ, Cabral LJ, Stephens RJ, Freeman G. Transformation of alveolar type 2 cells to type 1 cells following
exposure to NO$_2$. Exp Mol Pathol 1975;22(1):142–150.

64. Perl AK, Wert SE, Loudy DE, et al. Conditional recombination reveals distinct subsets of epithelial cells in
trachea, bronchi, and alveoli. Am J Respir Cell Mol Biol
2005;33(5):455–462.

65. Hong Ku, Reynolds SD, Watkins S, et al. Basal cells are a
multipotent progenitor capable of renewing the bronchial
epithelium. Am J Pathol 2004;164(2):577–588.

66. Neuringer IP, Randell SH. Stem cells and repair of lung
injuries. Respir Res 2004;5(1):6.

67. Borthwick DW, Shahbazian M, Krantz QT, et al. Evidence
for stem-cell niches in the tracheal epithelium. Am J
Respir Cell Mol Biol 2001;24(6):662–670.

68. Voynow JA, Fischer BM, Roberts BC, Proia AD. Basal-
like cells constitute the proliferating cell population in
cystic fibrosis airways. Am J Respir Crit Care Med
2005;172(8):1013–1018.

69. Boers JE, Ambergen AW, Thunnissen FB. Number
and proliferation of Clara cells in normal human airway
epithelium. Am J Respir Crit Care Med 1999;159(5 Pt 1):
1585–1591.

70. Danto SI, Shannon JM, Borok Z, et al. Reversible transdifferentiation of alveolar epithelial cells. Am J Respir
Cell Mol Biol 1995;12(5):497–502.

71. Reddy R, Buckley S, Doerken M, et al. Isolation of a putative progenitor subpopulation of alveolar epithelial type 2
cells. Am J Physiol Lung Cell Mol Physiol 2004;286(4):
L658–L667.

72. Kim CF, Jackson EL, Woolfenden AE, et al. Identification
of bronchioalveolar stem cells in normal lung and lung
cancer. Cell 2005;121(6):823–835.

73. Demayo F, Minoo P, Plopper CG, et al. Mesenchymal–
epithelial interactions in lung development and repair: are
modeling and remodeling the same process? Am J Physiol
Lung Cell Mol Physiol 2002;283(3):L510–L517.

74. Shannon JM, Hyatt BA. Epithelial–mesenchymal interactions in the developing lung. Annu Rev Physiol 2004;66:
625–645.

75. Cardoso WV, Williams MC, Mitsialis SA, et al. Retinoic
acid induces changes in the pattern of airway branching
and alters epithelial cell differentiation in the developing
lung in vitro. Am J Respir Cell Mol Biol 1995;12(5):464–
476.

76. Lechner JF, Haugen A, Autrup H, et al. Clonal growth of
epithelial cells from normal adult human bronchus. Cancer
Res 1981;41(6):2294–2304.

77. Reynolds SD, Hong KU, Giangreco A, et al. Conditional
Clara cell ablation reveals a self-renewing progenitor func-
tion of pulmonary neuroendocrine cells. Am J Physiol
Lung Cell Mol Physiol 2000;278(6):L1256–L1263.

78. Kalinichenko VV, Lim L, Shin B, Costa RH. Differential
expression of forkhead box transcription factors following
butylated hydroxytoluene lung injury. Am J Physiol Lung
Cell Mol Physiol 2001;280(4):L695–L704.

79. Casalino-Matsuda SM, Monzon ME, Forteza RM. Epidermal growth factor receptor activation by epidermal growth
factor mediates oxidant-induced goblet cell metaplasia in
human airway epithelium. Am J Respir Cell Mol Biol
2006;34(5):581–591.

80. Li C, Xiao J, Hormi K, et al. Wnt5a participates in distal
lung morphogenesis. Dev Biol 2002;248(1):68–81.

81. Motoyama J, Liu J, Mo R, et al. Essential function of Gli2
and Gli3 in the formation of lung, trachea and oesophagus.
Nat Genet 1998;20(1):54–57.

82. Watkins DN, Berman DM, Burkholder SG, et al. Hedgehog signalling within airway epithelial progenitors and in
small-cell lung cancer. Nature 2003;422(6929):313–337.

83. Weaver M, Yingling JM, Dunn NR, et al. BMP signaling
regulates proximal–distal differentiation of endoderm in
mouse lung development. Development 1999;126(18):
4005–4015.

84. Muraoka RS, Bushdid PB, Brantley DM, et al. Mesenchymal expression of nuclear factor-kappaB inhibits epithelial

growth and branching in the embryonic chick lung. Dev Biol 2000;225(2):322–338.

85. Costa RH, Kalinichenko VV, Lim L. Transcription factors in mouse lung development and function. Am J Physiol Lung Cell Mol Physiol 2001;280(5):L823–L838.

86. Minoo P, Su G, Drum H, et al. Defects in tracheoesophageal and lung morphogenesis in Nkx2.1(−/−) mouse embryos. Dev Biol 1999;209(1):60–71.

87. Pepicelli CV, Lewis PM, McMahon AP. Sonic hedgehog regulates branching morphogenesis in the mammalian lung. Curr Biol 1998;8(19):1083–1086.

88. Brody SL, Yan XH, Wuerffel MK, et al. Ciliogenesis and left-right axis defects in forkhead factor Hfh-4-null mice. Am J Respir Cell Mol Biol 2000;23(1):45–51.

89. Yang H, Lu MM, Zhang L, et al. GATA6 regulates differentiation of distal lung epithelium. Development 2002; 129(9):2233–2246.

90. Fischer BM, Voynow JA. Neutrophil elastase induces MUC5AC gene expression in airway epithelium via a pathway involving reactive oxygen species. Am J Respir Cell Mol Biol 2002;26(4):447–452.

91. Longphre M, Li D, Gallup M, et al. Allergen-induced IL-9 directly stimulates mucin transcription in respiratory epithelial cells. J Clin Invest 1999;104(10):1375–1382.

92. Tyner JW, Kim EY, Ide K, et al. Blocking airway mucous cell metaplasia by inhibiting EGFR antiapoptosis and IL-13 transdifferentiation signals. J Clin Invest 2006;116(2): 309–321.

93. Walter MJ, Morton JD, Kajiwara N, et al. viral induction of a chronic asthma phenotype and genetic segregation from the acute response. J Clin Invest 2002;110(2):165–175.

94. Tesfaigzi Y. Roles of apoptosis in airway epithelia. Am J Respir Cell Mol Biol 2006;34(5):537–547.

95. Bardales RH, Xie SS, Schaefer RF, Hsu SM. Apoptosis is a major pathway responsible for the resolution of type II pneumocytes in acute lung injury. Am J Pathol 1996; 149(3):845–852.

96. Fehrenbach H, Kasper M, Koslowski R, et al. Alveolar epithelial type II cell apoptosis in vivo during resolution of keratinocyte growth factor–induced hyperplasia in the rat. Histochem Cell Biol 2000;114(1):49–61.

97. Vermeer PD, Einwalter LA, Moninger TO, et al. Segregation of receptor and ligand regulates activation of epithelial growth factor receptor. Nature 2003;422(6929): 322–326.

98. Madtes DK, Busby HK, Strandjord TP, Clark JG. Expression of transforming growth factor-alpha and epidermal growth factor receptor is increased following bleomycin-induced lung injury in rats. Am J Respir Cell Mol Biol 1994;11(5):540–551.

99. Amishima M, Munakata M, Nasuhara Y, et al. Expression of epidermal growth factor and epidermal growth factor receptor immunoreactivity in the asthmatic human airway. Am J Respir Crit Care Med 1998;157(6 Pt 1):1907–1912.

100. Bandyopadhyay B, Fan J, Guan S, et al. A "traffic control" role for TGFbeta3: orchestrating dermal and epidermal cell motility during wound healing. J Cell Biol 2006; 172(7):1093–1105.

101. Morris DG, Huang X, Kaminski N, et al. Loss of integrin alpha(V)beta6-mediated TGF-beta activation causes MMP12-dependent emphysema. Nature 2003;422(6928): 169–173.

102. Kumar AS, Gonzales LW, Ballard PL. Transforming growth factor-beta(1) regulation of surfactant protein B gene expression is mediated by protein kinase-dependent intracellular translocation of thyroid transcription factor-1 and hepatocyte nuclear factor 3. Biochim Biophys Acta 2000;1492(1):45–55.

103. Willis BC, Liebler JM, Luby-Phelps K, et al. Induction of epithelial–mesenchymal transition in alveolar epithelial cells by transforming growth factor-beta1: potential role in idiopathic pulmonary fibrosis. Am J Pathol 2005;166(5): 1321–1332.

104. Fehrenbach H, Fehrenbach A, Pan T, et al. Keratinocyte growth factor–induced proliferation of rat airway epithelium is restricted to Clara cells in vivo. Eur Respir J 2002;20(5):1185–1197.

105. Yano T, Mason RJ, Pan T, et al. KGF regulates pulmonary epithelial proliferation and surfactant protein gene expression in adult rat lung. Am J Physiol Lung Cell Mol Physiol 2000;279(6):L1146–L1158.

106. Chedid M, Rubin JS, Csaky KG, Aaronson SA. Regulation of keratinocyte growth factor gene expression by interleukin 1. J Biol Chem 1994;269(14):10753–10757.

107. Waters CM, Savla U. Keratinocyte growth factor accelerates wound closure in airway epithelium during cyclic mechanical strain. J Cell Physiol 1999;181(3): 424–432.

108. Putnins EE, Firth JD, Uitto VJ. Keratinocyte growth factor stimulation of gelatinase (matrix metalloproteinase-9) and plasminogen activator in histiotypic epithelial cell culture. J Invest Dermatol 1995;104(6):989–994.

109. Chelly N, Henrion A, Pinteur C, et al. Role of keratinocyte growth factor in the control of surfactant synthesis by fetal lung mesenchyme. Endocrinology 2001;142(5):1814–1819.

110. Miyazawa K, Shimomura T, Naka D, Kitamura N. Proteolytic activation of hepatocyte growth factor in response to tissue injury. J Biol Chem 1994;269(12):8966–8970.

111. Sakai T, Satoh K, Matsushima K, et al. Hepatocyte growth factor in bronchoalveolar lavage fluids and cells in patients with inflammatory chest diseases of the lower respiratory tract: detection by RIA and in situ hybridization. Am J Respir Cell Mol Biol 1997;16(4):388–397.

112. Bryson Dg, McNulty MS, McCracken RM, Cush PF. Ultrastructural features of experimental parainfluenza type 3 virus pneumonia in calves. J Comp Pathol 1983; 93(3):397–414.

113. Castleman WL, Chandler SK, Slauson DO. Experimental bovine respiratory syncytial virus infection in conventional calves: ultrastructural respiratory lesions. Am J Vet Res 1985;46(3):554–560.

114. Ibricevic A, Pekosz A, Walter MJ, et al. Influenza virus receptor specificity and cell tropism in mouse and human airway epithelial cells. J Virol 2006;80(15):7469–7480.

115. Aherne W, Bird T, Court SD, et al. Pathological changes in virus infections of the lower respiratory tract in children. J Clin Pathol 1970;23(1):7–18.

116. Park JW, Taube C, Yang ES, et al. Respiratory syncytial virus–induced airway hyperresponsiveness is independent of IL-13 compared with that induced by allergen. J Allergy Clin Immunol 2003;112(6):1078–1087.

117. Hashimoto K, Graham BS, Ho SB, et al. Respiratory syncytial virus in allergic lung inflammation increases MUC5AC and GOB-5. Am J Respir Crit Care Med 2004; 170(3):306–312.

118. Schnapp LM, Donohoe S, Chen J, et al. Mining the acute respiratory distress syndrome proteome: identification of the insulin-like growth factor (IGF)/IGF-binding protein-3 pathway in acute lung injury. Am J Pathol 2006;169(1): 86–95.

119. Kaminski N, Allard JD, Pittet JF, et al. Global analysis of gene expression in pulmonary fibrosis reveals distinct programs regulating lung inflammation and fibrosis. Proc Natl Acad Sci USA 2000;97(4):1778–1783.

120. Pittet JF, Griffiths MJ, Geiser T, et al. TGF-beta is a critical mediator of acute lung injury. J Clin Invest 2001;107(12): 1537–1544.

46
Fibrogenesis

John S. Munger and William N. Rom

Introduction

Pulmonary fibrosis can be idiopathic or secondary to inflammatory states or injuries (Table 46.1). The tempo ranges from insidious to rapid, and the location of the fibrous tissue can be centered around or in the airways (bronchiolitis obliterans) or in the alveolar compartment (idiopathic pulmonary fibrosis [IPF]). In this chapter, we focus on IPF, the paradigmatic fibrosing lung disorder.

Early attempts to explain IPF emphasized inflammation ("alveolitis") and the effects of inflammatory and profibrotic cytokines.[1] The current consensus proposes instead that an initial epithelial injury provokes a wound repair response (Figure 46.1). Instead of restoring normal tissue architecture, in some cases the repair process goes awry, and persistent matrix deposition ensues; in turn, these events may produce signals that further damage epithelium.[2] Experimental models have allowed us insight into many cellular processes and molecular mediators that are triggered by injury and lead to fibrosis in susceptible animals. What remains elusive is the nature of the inciting injury in IPF and the host and environmental factors that determine whether the response to injury is adaptive or maladaptive.

Experimental Models of Lung Fibrosis

Animal models are valuable for testing the roles of specific molecules by using genetically altered mice or administering a specific factor or inhibitor; testing potential therapeutic compounds; distinguishing between the roles of resident lung cells and marrow-derived cells; and assessing the genetic factors through comparative genetics studies (e.g., linkage analysis using intercrosses of fibrosis-prone and fibrosis-resistant strains of mice).

Bleomycin, given either intratracheally or systemically, is the most commonly used model. Bleomycin interacts

with oxygen and a transition metal to form an activated complex, which binds and cleaves DNA. Activated bleomycin can also damage proteins and lipids, in part by release of hydroxyl radicals. Bleomycin toxicity is most prominent in the lung; vascular injury, cell death, and inflammation occur acutely, followed by collagen deposition. The pathology is more similar to the acute respiratory distress syndrome (ARDS) than it is to IPF. Other fibrosis models utilize radiation exposure; intratracheal silica, asbestos, or fluorescein isothiocyanate; and adenoviral or transgenic expression of transforming growth factor (TGF)-β or interleukin (IL)-13.

Most experimental models consist of two components: an injury and a fibrotic response. In most models the injury is severe, associated with inflammation, and produces fibrosis rapidly. Hence, these are poor models of the postulated initial injury in IPF, which is so subtle that it has not yet been identified. Only one model has been reported that reproduces many of the histologic features of UIP/IPF: interferon-γ receptor knockout mice (which preferentially develop a Th2 cytokine response) chronically infected with murine γ-herpesvirus 68 (MHV68).[3] Using these models, in particular the murine bleomycin model, investigators have identified many factors involved in fibrosis. For example, around 40 different knockout mice have an altered fibrotic response in the bleomycin model (Table 46.2).

Fibroblastic Foci and the Fibroblast Phenotype

Ultimately, IPF is a disease of fibroblasts and the connective tissue they deposit. In seminal studies, Kuhn, McDonald, and colleagues used antibodies against procollagen I that stain cells actively synthesizing collagen.[4] These antibodies preferentially react with small clusters of fibroblasts in IPF lungs. These clusters, called *fibroblastic foci*, are one of the pathologic hallmarks of UIP/IPF. The

TABLE 46.1. Disorders associated with pulmonary fibrosis.

Usual interstitial pneumonia/idiopathic pulmonary fibrosis and other
   idiopathic pneumonias
Acute respiratory distress syndrome
Collagen vascular diseases
Bronchiolitis obliterans
Cryptogenic organizing pneumonia
Sarcoidosis
Langerhans cell histiocytosis
Dust exposures
Radiation injury
Asthma (subepithelial fibrosis)

TABLE 46.2. Gene products involved in bleomycin-induced fibrosis, revealed by use of knockout mice.

Profibrotic	Antifibrotic
Chemokines	
CCL11, CCR2	CXCR3, CXCL10
Cytokine and other signaling pathways	
IL-4, Smad3, IFN-γ, TGF-β, TNF receptors, angiotensin 1a receptor	Stat1, GM-CSF, IL12p40, CD73
Coagulation	
TAFI, PAR-1, PAI-1	
ROS	
p47phox, iNOS	Nrf2
Lipid mediators	
Leukotriene C(4) synthase, cytosolic phospholipase A_2, 5-lipoxygenase	CysLT2 receptor
Leukocyte function	
L-selectin, ICAM-1, perforin, CD28	
Proteases	
Matrix metalloproteinase-7	Cathepsin K
Apoptosis	
Bid, Fas, Fas ligand	
Other	
β6-Integrin (activates TGF-β1), C5, γ-glutamyl transpeptidase	SP-C, SPARC, Thy-1

Note: C5, complement factor 5; CysLT2, cysteinyl leukotriene 2; GM-CSF, granulocyte-macrophage colony-stimulating factor; ICAM, intercellular adhesion molecule; IFN, interferon; IL, interleukin; iNOS, inducible nitric oxide synthase; Nrf2, nuclear factor E2 p45-related factor 2; PAI-1, plasminogen activator inhibitor-1; PAR-1, protease-activated receptor-1; SPARC, secreted protein, acidic and rich in cysteine; SP-C, surfactant protein C; TAFI, thrombin-activatable fibrinolysis inhibitor; TGF, transforming growth factor; TNF, tumor necrosis factor.

extent of fibroblastic foci in IPF lung biopsy material predicts mortality (the extent of fibrosis and inflammation, in contrast, do not).[2]

Fibroblastic foci are relatively small collections of fibroblasts (as few as 3, up to 30 or more) located just below the alveolar gas–tissue interface (Figure 46.2). Inflammatory cells are rarely present. The fibroblasts are arranged parallel to the alveolar surface and are often hypertrophied. The fibroblasts stain for procollagen I and for cellular fibronectin, indicative of active matrix protein synthesis. The fibroblasts also express α-smooth muscle actin, indicating that they are contractile myofibroblasts. The remnants of a basement membrane, identifiable by collagen IV staining, are typically present *below* the fibroblastic focus, indicating that the fibroblasts have migrated into the alveolar space. If basement membrane can be

identified at the epithelial layer rather than buried within the focus, it is frequently interrupted and distorted. Occasionally, two or three layers of basement membrane are detectable within a focus, suggesting repeated episodes of fibroblast invasion and epithelial repair. Fibrin is often present, indicating leakage of plasma.

The epithelium overlying fibroblastic foci is abnormal. The epithelial cells are cuboidal and hyperplastic. A basement membrane is often lacking, placing epithelial cells in direct contact with fibroblasts. Perhaps as a result, the epithelial cells are poorly adherent. In addition, by morphologic criteria and in situ end labeling, many epithelial cells are apoptotic or necrotic; dead or dying epithelial cells are preferentially located at fibroblastic foci.[5] Paradoxically, the underlying myofibroblasts are not apoptotic.

These observations suggest that an initial epithelial injury leads to a disruption of the normal barrier of the alveolus, with formation of a fibrin-rich exudate that is

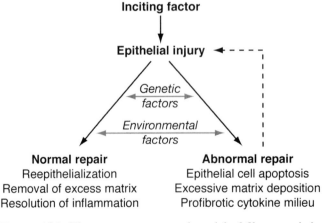

FIGURE 46.1. The current conceptual model of fibrogenesis in idiopathic pulmonary fibrosis. An inciting factor causes epithelial injury. Depending on the nature and repetitiveness of the injury, as well as genetic and environmental factors, the injury undergoes either normal repair or an abnormal repair process with associated fibrosis. Signals related to the abnormal repair process (e.g., oxidative stress or angiotensin II) may cause further epithelial injury.

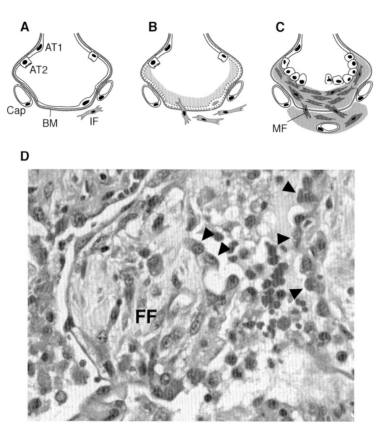

FIGURE 46.2. The fibroblastic focus. **(A)** A normal alveolus with alveolar type 1 (AT1) and type 2 (AT2) cells, capillaries (Cap), and an interstitial fibroblast (IF). BM, basement membrane. **(B)** Epithelial injury is followed by formation of a fibrin-rich provisional matrix on the alveolar surface. Fibroblasts are activated, and an inflammatory response may occur (not shown).

(C) A fibroblastic focus with numerous myofibroblasts (MF) forms. The alveolar epithelium is hyperplastic and poorly adherent. A collagen-rich matrix is formed, and neovascularization occurs. **(D)** Photomicrograph of a fibroblastic focus (FF). Hyperplastic epithelial cells are indicated by arrowheads. (Courtesy of Herman Yee, PhD, MD.)

then invaded by activated, contractile fibroblasts (see Figure 46.2). The perpetuation of fibroblast activation, matrix synthesis and contraction, accompanied by epithelial cell death, defines the pathobiology of IPF.

Many laboratory investigators have compared IPF and normal lung fibroblasts. These studies consistently find that IPF fibroblasts behave differently in culture—but not always in the same way. For example, IPF fibroblast growth rates have been reported as increased and decreased compared with normal fibroblasts.[2] Several proteins are selectively expressed by IPF fibroblasts, including discoidin domain receptor 1 (a receptor tyrosine kinase that binds collagen),[6] fibroblast activation protein α (a membrane protease),[7] and Thy-1.

Thy-1 is a glycosylphosphatidylinositol-anchored cell surface protein expressed on many cells, including some fibroblasts.[8] It is a ligand for several integrins, interacts with signaling molecules such as the Src family kinase c-fyn, and localizes to lipid rafts. Cross-linking Thy-1 with antibodies triggers apoptosis. The activated fibroblasts in fibroblastic foci are Thy-1 negative, whereas most fibro-

blasts in normal human lung are Thy-1 positive. Thy-1 knockout mice are generally healthy; however, upon challenge with bleomycin, Thy-1 knockout mice develop increased fibrosis. In addition, absence of Thy-1 expression in lung fibroblasts correlates with higher TGF-β expression, the ability to activate latent TGF-β in response to fibrogenic stimuli, increased expression of the platelet-derived growth factor-α receptor, enhanced migration, and increased α-smooth muscle actin expression.[8]

Sources of Fibroblasts

Three sources of the increased number of fibroblasts in interstitial lung disease have been proposed: proliferation of existing interstitial fibroblasts, transdifferentiation of epithelial cells into fibroblasts (epithelial–mesenchymal transition), and bone marrow–derived precursor cells referred to as *circulating fibrocytes*. The relative contribution of each source is not known for lung fibrosis models, but in a model of kidney fibrosis (unilateral ureteral obstruction) it was estimated that approximately one third of interstitial fibroblasts derived from epithelial–mesenchymal transition and one sixth originated from bone marrow.[9]

Circulating fibrocytes constitute <1% of circulating leukocytes and express a distinctive set of proteins, including collagens I and III, vimentin, CD34, CD45, CXCR4, CXCR7, major histocompatibility complex class II, and CD86.[10,11] When cultured, fibrocytes adopt a spindle shape, continue to express extracellular matrix proteins, and become α-smooth muscle actin positive; TGF-β enhances these changes. The fibrocytes undergo chemotaxis in response to the chemokines CCL21 and CXCL12 and are recruited from the circulation to sites of tissue injury, including the lung.

In two models, the degree of lung fibrosis correlated with the extent of fibrocyte recruitment. Phillips et al. showed that fibrocytes are recruited to lung in the bleomycin model, that the kinetics of recruitment parallel collagen deposition, and that blocking recruitment of fibrocytes with anti-CXCL12 antibody reduces fibrosis.[12] Similarly, Moore and colleagues found, in the fluorescein isothiocyanate–induced lung fibrosis model, that fibrocytes are recruited to the lung in a CCL12- and CCR2-dependent manner and that CCR2 knockout mice have reduced lung fibrosis.[13]

Epithelial–mesenchymal transition may also be a source of fibroblasts in lung fibrosis. The fact that TGF-β, a key mediator of fibrosis, induces epithelial–mesenchymal transition in a variety of epithelial cells in cell culture, including alveolar type 2 (AT2) cells,[14,15] lends appeal to this idea. Willis and colleagues have presented evidence that epithelial–mesenchymal transition occurs in human IPF lung based on the identification, by three-dimensional deconvolution microscopy, of cells that coexpress epithelial and mesenchymal markers.[14]

Mechanisms of Fibrosis

Oxidative Stress

Lung cells must deal with a significant oxidant load derived from high oxygen tension, inhaled substances (e.g., tobacco smoke, ozone, and particulates), and activated leukocytes.[16] Endogenously generated oxidants include superoxide (O_2^-), hydrogen peroxide (H_2O_2), hypochlorous acid (HOCl), and hydroxyl radical (OH·). Oxidants modify biologic macromolecules, potentially leading to cellular dysfunction and death. In addition, the redox state can alter gene expression via effects on redox-sensitive transcription factors such as nuclear factor-κB and activator protein-1. Defenses against oxidants include superoxide dismutases, which convert O_2^- to H_2O_2; catalase and other enzymes that decompose H_2O_2; and antioxidants such as glutathione, a tripeptide derived from

glutamate, cysteine, and glycine. Glutathione concentrations in epithelial lining fluid (≈400 μM) are approximately two orders of magnitude higher than in nonlung extracellular fluids and plasma, and within cells glutathione constitutes ≈90% of the nonprotein thiol groups.[16]

Circumstantial evidence suggests that alterations in redox balance promote fibrosis. Many agents that induce fibrosis (e.g., asbestos, silica, bleomycin, ionizing radiation) produce reactive oxygen species (ROS) directly. Inflammatory cells from IPF lungs produce higher concentrations of oxidants than normal cells, and lavage fluid from IPF patients contains a high level of 8-isoprostane, a product of lipid peroxidation widely used as a marker of oxidative stress. Epithelial lining fluid from IPF patients has a reduced glutathione concentration (≈25% of normal).[17]

There are compelling links between redox biology and the fibrotic process. Transforming growth factor-β, a key profibrotic cytokine, causes reduced expression of γ-glutamyl cysteine synthetase, the rate-limiting enzyme for glutathione production, and induces the production of ROS by myofibroblasts isolated from IPF lung.[18] In addition, the latent form of TGF-β is activated by ROS.[19] Mice deficient in the redox-regulated transcription factor Nrf2, which is involved in the expression of several antioxidant enzyme systems, have increased fibrosis after bleomycin injury.[20] Reactive oxygen species can increase proliferation of fibroblasts and cause epithelial cell death.

There is also evidence that enhancing lung antioxidant functions reduces fibrosis. Administration of superoxide dismutase, or small molecules with superoxide dismutase activity, reduces fibrosis in several models. Because the availability of cysteine is rate limiting for glutathione synthesis, N-acetyl cysteine, which is converted to cysteine, has been used to augment glutathione levels. N-acetyl cysteine attenuates bleomycin-induced lung inflammation and subsequent fibrosis in mice and stabilizes lung function in IPF patients.[21]

Apoptosis

Apoptosis is a form of programmed cell death characterized by activation of a set of cysteine proteases (caspases), packaging of the cell remnants into membrane-bound vesicles that are taken up by surrounding cells, and lack of an inflammatory response.[22] Apoptosis is conceptually distinct from another form of programmed cell death (autophagy) and from nonprogrammed cell death (necrosis), although in practice these forms of cell death are often not clearly distinguishable. Triggers of apoptosis involve extrinsic signals that trigger tumor necrosis factor receptor superfamily members with a death domain (e.g., the Fas receptor) and/or intrinsic signals such as DNA damage that cause release of mitochondrial cytochrome c and subsequent activation of a caspase cascade. Apoptosis can be induced by interruption of normal cell adhesion to the extracellular matrix, a process referred to as *anoikis*.

Increased numbers of apoptotic epithelial cells are present in IPF lungs, particularly adjacent to fibroblastic foci, but also in relatively normal areas of lung.[5,22] In animal models, apoptosis is causally related to fibrosis. Inhibition of apoptosis with the broad-spectrum caspase inhibitor zVADfmk inhibits fibrosis in the bleomycin model. The role of apoptosis has also been studied in mice with an inducible *TGF-β* transgene expressed in lung epithelium; *TGF-β* expression in these mice causes a wave of apoptosis, followed by fibrosis, both of which are blocked by zVADfmk.[23,24] Finally, intratracheal administration of an activating anti-Fas antibody, which binds to Fas expressed on epithelial cells, leads to lung epithelial cell apoptosis and fibrosis.[22]

There are several possible causes for increased numbers of apoptotic epithelial cells in IPF. Epithelial cells overlying a fibroblastic focus may undergo anoikis. Li and colleagues showed that IPF myofibroblasts release angiotensin II, which triggers epithelial cell apoptosis, and captopril prevents fibrosis in several rodent models.[25] Oxidant stress and TGF-β signaling may also contribute to epithelial apoptosis. In patients with mutations in the gene encoding surfactant protein-C (SP-C), cellular dysfunction and the endoplasmic reticulum stress response may cause apoptosis of AT2 cells, and one can speculate that protein misfolding or trafficking abnormalities in AT2 cells might occur in IPF due to environmental and/or genetic factor(s). Vandivier and colleagues suggest that impaired apoptotic cell removal may also be a factor.[26]

How epithelial cell apoptosis leads to fibrosis is not known. A simple explanation is that loss of epithelial barrier function leads to formation of a fibrinous exudate followed by an abnormal fibroblast response. Also, apoptotic cells or the cells that engulf them can release the profibrotic cytokine TGF-β,[26] triggering other cellular and biochemical changes that promote development of fibrosis.

Transforming Growth Factor-β

Transforming growth factor-β is a multifunctional cytokine involved in development, the immune system, matrix production, angiogenesis, and control of proliferation. Essentially all cells express TGF-β and have TGF-β receptors. Overwhelming evidence implicates TGF-β as a major factor in fibrosis.[27] Transforming growth factor-β levels are increased in IPF lung. In animal studies, overexpression of TGF-β in lung causes fibrosis,[24,28] and interruption of TGF-β signaling prevents fibrosis in lung,[29,30] kidney, skin, and liver models. There are three isoforms

of TGF-β; TGF-β1 is the main isoform involved in the pathogenesis of fibrosis.

The activated TGF-β receptor complex has serine/threonine kinase activity, and its major substrates are the receptor Smad (R-Smad) proteins Smad2 and Smad3. Phosphorylated R-Smads combine with a Co-Smad (Smad4), translocate to the nucleus, and, in conjunction with cell- and context-specific coactivators and corepressors, alter transcription of target genes.[31] Smad3 knockout mice have impaired fibrosis and wound healing responses.

Transforming growth factor-β is secreted in a latent form that results from noncovalent interaction between TGF-β and its propeptide (latency-associated peptide [LAP]). Latency-associated peptide also forms a disulfide linkage with proteins of the latent TGF-β binding protein (LTBP) family. Latent TGF-β binding proteins, in turn, are covalently attached to extracellular matrix proteins.[32]

Latent TGF-β must be released from LAP before it can bind to its receptors. This process, called *latent TGF-β activation*, is highly regulated and can be accomplished in several ways.[32] Proteases (plasmin and several matrix metalloproteinases) can degrade LAP and release TCFβ-1. Reactive oxygen species activate latent TGF-β1 by denaturing LAP. Thrombospondin-1 binds to LAP, triggering a conformational change that releases active TGF-β. Finally, the integrins αvβ6 and αvβ8 activate TGF-β1 by binding to an integrin binding motif (arginine-glycine-aspartic acid) near the C terminus of LAP.

Sime et al. demonstrated the critical importance TGF-β activation in lung fibrosis.[28] Using an adenoviral system, they expressed either wild-type TGF-β1 or a mutated form bearing mutations in the LAP domain that eliminate the inhibitory function of LAP. Only the constitutively active form of TGF-β1 produced fibrosis, despite the presence of high lung levels of total TGF-β1 protein in both cases. This result indicates that TGF-β activating capacity, rather than the amount of substrate (latent TGF-β), can be the limiting factor in TGF-β–mediated fibrotic lung reactions.

αvβ6-mediated TGF-β activation appears to be a particularly important activation mechanism in the lung. Integrins are heterodimeric cell surface receptors, each composed of an α- and a β-subunit. αvβ6 is one of 24 mammalian integrins, 8 of which bind arginine-glycine-aspartic acid sequences. αvβ6 is mainly expressed in epithelial cells. Activation of TGF-β1 by αvβ6 requires an intact actin cytoskeleton and tethering of latent TGF-β1 to the extracellular matrix by LTBP1.[33] Protease-activated receptor-1 signaling enhances actin contractility and αvβ6-mediated TGF-β1 activation.[34]

In the lung, αvβ6 normally is expressed at a low level but is sharply upregulated by inflammatory stimuli. β6-

integrin knockout mice develop lung inflammation and ultimately emphysema, are protected from acute lung injury, and are resistant to fibrosis.[35,36] All these effects are due to, or at least consistent with, reduced TGF-β signaling. Bleomycin-treated β6 knockout mice have more lung inflammation than wild-type controls, indicating that inflammation and fibrosis can be dissociated. Other mechanisms of TGF-β activation in the lung may also come into play; for example, IL-13–dependent lung fibrosis is dependent on TGF-β signaling, and proteases (plasmin and matrix metalloproteinases) appear to be the activators.[29,30] Also, bleomycin-stimulated alveolar macrophages activate TGF-β using plasmin and thrombospondin-1.[37]

Once activated, TGF-β sets in motion a wide range of profibrotic processes (Figure 46.3). In addition to its direct effects, TGF-β upregulates other profibrotic molecules such as platelet-derived growth factor, ROS, and connective tissue growth factor. Connective tissue growth factor, a member of the CCN family of matricellular proteins, is a downstream mediator of TGF-β effects. Its signaling function is not well understood but may derive in part from its ability to enhance binding of TGF-β to TGF-β receptors.[38] Transforming growth factor-β signaling causes autoinduction of the *TGFβ-1* gene and upregulation of TGF-β activators (αvβ6 and ROS), suggesting the possibility of a positive feedback loop in TGF-β signaling. Endogenous negative regulators of TGF-β signaling include an inhibitory Smad (Smad7), which is induced by TGF-β, and extracellular molecules such as decorin and α2-macroglobulin. Impaired Smad7 expression may contribute to scarring in scleroderma.[39]

Viral Infection

Accumulating evidence supports the intriguing hypothesis that chronic viral infection of alveolar epithelial cells triggers fibrosis in susceptible hosts.[40] Tang et al.[41] found that 97% of IPF biopsy specimens were positive for one or more of four herpesviruses tested compared with only 36% of controls, and others have reported the presence of actively replicating Epstein-Barr virus (EBV) in IPF lung.[42] Although EBV DNA can be detected in the blood of most people, it is less commonly detected in the lung; EBV can be detected in lungs of IPF patients about four times more frequently than in controls. Furthermore, a specific form of EBV (the Wzhet rearrangement) that favors active replication was found to occur much more frequently in IPF patients (59%) than in controls (2%).[42]

Causality cannot be proved in such studies but can be assessed in animal models. The murine γ-herpesvirus 68 (MHV68), analogous to EBV, has been used in several studies.[40] BALB/c mice, normally fibrosis resistant, develop fibrosis if infected with MHV68 prior to bleomycin injury. Also, MHV68 infection of interferon receptor knockout mice results in lung fibrosis with many of the pathologic features of human UIP/IPF.

Angiogenesis

Idiopathic pulmonary fibrosis lungs have abnormal anastomoses between the systemic and pulmonary circulations, and neovascularization also occurs in animal models. In addition, extracts of fibrotic lungs have angiogenic activity when tested in the corneal pocket assay. Strieter and colleagues showed that the abnormal angiogenic activity of fibrotic lung is due to an imbalance between angiogenic CXC chemokines (e.g., CXCL5 and CXCL8, which signal through the receptor CXCR2) and interferon-inducible angiostatic CXC chemokines (CXCL9, CXCL10, and CXCL11, which signal through CXCR3).[43,44] Increasing angiostatic activity (e.g., by administration of recombinant CXCL10 or CXCL11) or reducing angiogenic activity (e.g., in CXCR2 knockout mice) reduces fibrosis in the bleomycin model, supporting the concept that neovascularization may be causally connected to the fibrotic process.

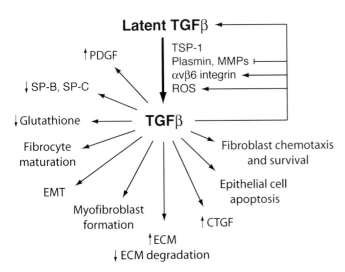

FIGURE 46.3. The central role of transforming growth factor-β (TGF-β) in lung fibrosis. Latent TGF-β is converted to active TGF-β by thrombospondin-1 (TSP-1), αvβ6 integrin, proteases, or reactive oxygen species (ROS). Transforming growth factor-β may positively regulate its own signaling by upregulating two activation mechanisms (ROS and αvβ6 expression) and autoinducing transcription of the TGF-β1 gene. Transforming growth factor-β signaling also positively regulates multiple fibrogenic factors and processes. CTGF, connective tissue growth factor; ECM, extracellular matrix; EMT, epithelial-mesenchymal transition; MMPs, matrix metalloproteinases; PDGF, platelet-derived growth factor; SP, surfactant protein.

Inherited Forms of Interstitial Lung Disease

Surfactant Protein C Mutations

Surfactant protein C (SP-C) mutations are the best-characterized genetic cause of IPF-like lung disease. Surfactant protein C is produced by AT2 cells and contributes to the surface tension–reducing properties of surfactant and to innate immune defense. Because of its hydrophobicity and tendency to form insoluble aggregates, including amyloid fibrils in aqueous solution, SP-C poses a processing challenge to the AT2 cell. The 3.7-kDa mature protein is generated from a 21-kDa precursor (Figure 46.4). Surfactant protein C processing involves translocation of the proprotein to the endoplasmic reticulum,

folding, and addition of two palmitic acid residues, a total of four proteolytic cleavages of the N- and C-terminal propeptide domains to generate mature SP-C, release of SP-C into the lumen of the lamellar body where it associates with surfactant phospholipids and proteins, and secretion into the alveolar space.[45]

Surfactant protein C mutations in patients with interstitial lung disease occur in several locations and act in an autosomal dominant fashion. Almost all mutations occur in the luminal part of the proprotein, and most are within the ≈100 amino acid C-terminal region (Phe94–Ile197) that forms a so-called BRICHOS domain. The BRICHOS domain affects targeting, processing, and folding of proteins that contain them.

The clinical manifestations of these mutations are varied. Some patients present within weeks of birth, whereas others manifest disease as adults. Pathologic findings range from UIP and nonspecific interstitial pneumonia to pulmonary alveolar proteinosis.

The molecular basis of the lung disease appears to be loss of normal SP-C levels in surfactant and/or toxic effects of misfolded mutant SP-C within the AT2 cell. The toxic "gain-of-function" effects of mutant proteins have been studied by expressing mutant SP-C in epithelial cells. Depending on the mutation and level of expression, mutant protein accumulates in the endoplasmic reticulum, in perinuclear collections termed *aggresomes* or in endosomal vesicles. Misfolded protein can induce the endoplasmic reticulum stress response, leading to apoptosis or increased expression of inflammatory mediators.[46] Also, accumulations of mutant protein may be directly toxic to the cell, as postulated for other proteins that form amyloid.

Mutant SP-C acts in a dominant-negative fashion to block release of wild-type, mature SP-C. This effect appears to be restricted to SP-C mutations within the BRICHOS domain; patients with these mutations fail to secrete mature SP-C. Amin and colleagues described a patient with interstitial lung disease who had no detectable mature SP-C within the lung despite the absence of mutations within the SP-C gene coding regions, suggesting that absence of SP-C may cause lung disease.[47] However, patients with SP-C mutations outside the BRICHOS domain produce mature SP-C, suggesting that toxic gain-of-function effects may be the dominant mechanism leading to lung disease.

Mice lacking SP-C or overexpressing mutant SP-C have lung abnormalities but do not recapitulate the findings found in humans. Surfactant protein C knockout mice are viable and develop lung inflammation and emphysema; when exposed to bleomycin they have an exaggerated fibrotic response.[48] Mice overexpressing a mutant *SFTPC* transgene lacking much of the BRICHOS domain have a lethal disruption of branching morphogenesis.[49]

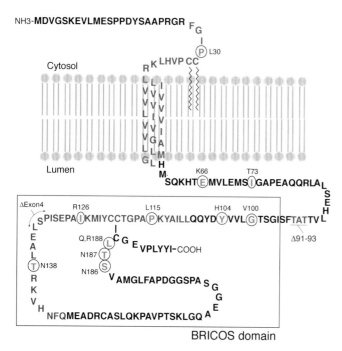

FIGURE 46.4. Schematic diagram of prosurfactant protein C and mutations that cause interstitial lung disease. Mature surfactant protein C (SP-C) is shown in blue. Pro-SP-C associates with the cell membrane via a transmembrane domain and two palmitic acid residues before it is translocated into the lumen of the lamellar body. After removal of the N- and C-terminal prodomains, mature SP-C is translocated to the lumen of the lamellar body where it associates with the other constituents of surfactant. Lamellar bodies are lysosome-related organelles unique to AT2 cells. Amino acid substitutions causing interstitial lung disease are shown in green. Two deletions causing interstitial lung disease are shown in red. The mutations interfere with normal processing, causing protein aggregation and in some cases impaired secretion of mature SP-C.

Hermansky-Pudlak Syndrome

Hermansky-Pudlak syndrome (HPS) is another inherited disorder leading to interstitial lung disease, and, interestingly, the defect also targets AT2 cells. Hermansky-Pudlak syndrome is due to mutations in one of eight genes in humans *(HPS1–8)*[50–52]; corresponding mutations occur in mice (Table 46.3). Patients manifest reduced skin and eye pigmentation, a bleeding diathesis due to platelet dysfunction, and, in some cases, progressive lung fibrosis in middle age. The defect underlying these abnormalities is impaired genesis or function of lysosome-related organelles.[51] These organelles are variants of lysosomes that perform specialized functions. The affected organelles are melanosomes in melanocytes, cytotoxic granules in lymphocytes, platelet dense granules, and lamellar bodies in AT2 cells. Biopsy specimens reveal proliferative, enlarged AT2 cells containing giant lamellar bodies packed with surfactant. The AT2 cells appear degenerative and often desquamated. There is inflammation centered on respiratory bronchioles and fibrosis with honeycombing.

The disorder is autosomal recessive and involves two classes of genes. One group encodes proteins with known roles in protein trafficking (e.g., adaptor protein-3). The second group encodes proteins that are subunits of protein complexes called BLOCs (biogenesis of lysosome-related organelles complex). The BLOCs are ubiquitously expressed, but the cellular localization and precise function of these multiprotein complexes have not been defined.

While the mouse strains with HPS mutations have pigmentation and platelet defects that mimic HPS, the lung pathology is quite different.[52] The HPS-like strains in general have reduced life spans and develop emphysema. Lyerla and colleagues generated a double homozygous mutant (*HPS1* and *HPS2* genes); the AT2 cells in these mice are enlarged and contain enlarged lamellar bodies engorged with surfactant, as well as significant inflammation, as seen in humans with HPS lung disease.[53]

The mechanism connecting the genetic defects and lung fibrosis in humans is not known. Toxicity to AT2 cells and/or reductions in surfactant components may be involved. Toxicity to AT2 cells is readily apparent in biopsy tissues of patients. Alterations in surfactant secretion in patients have not been defined. In *HPS1/HPS2* double mutant mice, total lung phospholipid, SP-B, and SP-C levels are increased (and SP-C is processed to the 3.7-kDa form), but alveolar levels of these components are reduced and isolated AT2 cells from these mice have reduced basal and stimulated phospholipid secretion.[52,53]

Genetic Studies of Sporadic and Familial Interstitial Lung Disease

Case–control studies have been carried out to test the association of polymorphic variants of candidate genes with the risk for IPF. Positive results have been reported for genes encoding angiotensin-converting enzyme, complement receptor-1, IL-1 receptor antagonist, TNF-α, and SP-A and SP-B.[54] Interestingly, the SP-A1 variant (6A^4) encodes a protein with an altered amino acid (tryptophan rather than arginine) that appears to affect aggregation.[55]

Sometimes interstitial lung disease cases cluster within families. Inheritance is autosomal dominant with reduced penetrance. In about half the families the disease is uniformly UIP/IPF, and in the others there are various presentations (as occurs in families with SP-C mutations).

TABLE 46.3. Hermansky-Pudlak syndrome (HPS) genes in humans and mice.

Mouse	Human	Product	Lung fibrosis
Pale ear	*HPS1*	BLOC-3 subunit	Yes
Pearl	*HPS2*	AP-3 β3A subunit	
Cocoa	*HPS3*	BLOC-2 subunit	
Light ear	*HPS4*	BLOC-3 subunit	Yes
Ruby eye-2	*HPS5*	BLOC-2 subunit	
Ruby eye	*HPS6*	BLOC-2 subunit	
Sandy	*HPS7*	BLOC-1 subunit	
Reduced pigmentation	*HPS8*	BLOC-1 subunit	
Pallid		BLOC-1 subunit	
Muted		BLOC-1 subunit	
Cappuccino		BLOC-1 subunit	
Buff		Vps33A	
Mocha		δ-Subunit of AP-3	
Gunmetal		Rab geranylgeranyl transferase α-subunit	

Note: AP, adaptor protein; BLOC, biogenesis of lysosome-related organelles complex.

References

1. Noble PW, Homer RJ. Back to the future: historical perspective on the pathogenesis of idiopathic pulmonary fibrosis. Am J Respir Cell Mol Biol 2005;33(2):113–120.
2. Selman M, Pardo A. Idiopathic pulmonary fibrosis: an epithelial/fibroblastic cross-talk disorder. Respir Res 2002; 3(1):3.
3. Mora AL, Woods CR, Garcia A, et al. Lung infection with gamma-herpesvirus induces progressive pulmonary fibrosis in Th2-biased mice. Am J Physiol Lung Cell Mol Physiol 2005;289(5):L711–L721.
4. Kuhn C 3rd, Boldt J, King TE Jr, Crouch E, Vartio T, McDonald JA. An immunohistochemical study of architectural remodeling and connective tissue synthesis in pulmonary fibrosis. Am Rev Respir Dis 1989;140(6):1693–1703.
5. Uhal BD, Joshi I, Hughes WF, Ramos C, Pardo A, Selman M. Alveolar epithelial cell death adjacent to underlying myofibroblasts in advanced fibrotic human lung. Am J Physiol 1998;275(6 Pt 1):L1192–L1199.

6. Matsuyama W, Watanabe M, Shirahama Y, et al. Discoidin domain receptor 1 contributes to the survival of lung fibroblast in idiopathic pulmonary fibrosis. Am J Pathol 2006; 168(3):866–877.

7. Acharya PS, Zukas A, Chandan V, Katzenstein AL, Pure E. Fibroblast activation protein: a serine protease expressed at the remodeling interface in idiopathic pulmonary fibrosis. Hum Pathol 2006;37(3):352–360.

8. Rege TA, Hagood JS. Thy-1 as a regulator of cell–cell and cell–matrix interactions in axon regeneration, apoptosis, adhesion, migration, cancer, and fibrosis. FASEB J 2006; 20(8):1045–1054.

9. Iwano M, Plieth D, Danoff TM, Xue C, Okada H, Neilson EG. Evidence that fibroblasts derive from epithelium during tissue fibrosis. J Clin Invest 2002;110(3):341–350.

10. Abe R, Donnelly SC, Peng T, Bucala R, Metz CN. Peripheral blood fibrocytes: differentiation pathway and migration to wound sites. J Immunol 2001;166(12):7556–7562.

11. Bucala R, Spiegel LA, Chesney J, Hogan M, Cerami A. Circulating fibrocytes define a new leukocyte subpopulation that mediates tissue repair. Mol Med 1994;1(1):71–81.

12. Phillips RJ, Burdick MD, Hong K, et al. Circulating fibrocytes traffic to the lungs in response to CXCL12 and mediate fibrosis. J Clin Invest 2004;114(3):438–446.

13. Moore BB, Murray L, Das A, Wilke CA, Herrygers AB, Toews GB. The Role of CCL12 in the recruitment of fibrocytes and lung fibrosis. Am J Respir Cell Mol Biol 2006;35(2):175–181.

14. Willis BC, Liebler JM, Luby-Phelps K, et al. Induction of epithelial–mesenchymal transition in alveolar epithelial cells by transforming growth factor-β1: potential role in idiopathic pulmonary fibrosis. Am J Pathol 2005;166(5): 1321–1332.

15. Yao HW, Xie QM, Chen JQ, Deng YM, Tang HF. TGF-β1 induces alveolar epithelial to mesenchymal transition in vitro. Life Sci 2004;76(1):29–37.

16. Rahman I, MacNee W. Oxidative stress and regulation of glutathione in lung inflammation. Eur Respir J 2000;16(3): 534–554.

17. Cantin AM, Hubbard RC, Crystal RG. Glutathione deficiency in the epithelial lining fluid of the lower respiratory tract in idiopathic pulmonary fibrosis. Am Rev Respir Dis 1989;139(2):370–372.

18. Waghray M, Cui Z, Horowitz JC, et al. Hydrogen peroxide is a diffusible paracrine signal for the induction of epithelial cell death by activated myofibroblasts. FASEB J 2005;19(7): 854–856.

19. Barcellos-Hoff MH, Dix TA. Redox-mediated activation of latent transforming growth factor-β1. Mol Endocrinol 1996;10(9):1077–1083.

20. Cho HY, Reddy SP, Kleeberger SR. Nrf2 defends the lung from oxidative stress. Antioxid Redox Signal 2006;8(1–2): 76–87.

21. Demedts M, Behr J, Buhl R, et al. High-dose acetylcysteine in idiopathic pulmonary fibrosis. N Engl J Med 2005;353(21): 2229–2242.

22. Thannickal VJ, Horowitz JC. Evolving concepts of apoptosis in idiopathic pulmonary fibrosis. Proc Am Thorac Soc 2006;3(4):350–356.

23. Lee CG, Kang HR, Homer RJ, Chupp G, Elias JA. Transgenic Modeling of Transforming Growth Factor-β1: Role of Apoptosis in Fibrosis and Alveolar Remodeling. Proc Am Thorac Soc 2006;3(5):418–423.

24. Lee CG, Cho SJ, Kang MJ, et al. Early growth response gene 1–mediated apoptosis is essential for transforming growth factor β1–induced pulmonary fibrosis. J Exp Med 2004;200(3):377–389.

25. Li X, Shu R, Filippatos G, Uhal BD. Apoptosis in lung injury and remodeling. J Appl Physiol 2004;97(4):1535–1542.

26. Vandivier RW, Henson PM, Douglas IS. Burying the dead: the impact of failed apoptotic cell removal (efferocytosis) on chronic inflammatory lung disease. Chest 2006;129(6): 1673–1682.

27. Branton MH, Kopp JB. TGF-β and fibrosis. Microbes Infect 1999;1(15):1349–1365.

28. Sime PJ, Xing Z, Graham FL, Csaky KG, Gauldie J. Adenovector-mediated gene transfer of active transforming growth factor-β1 induces prolonged severe fibrosis in rat lung. J Clin Invest 1997;100(4):768–776.

29. Kolb M, Margetts PJ, Galt T, et al. Transient transgene expression of decorin in the lung reduces the fibrotic response to bleomycin. Am J Respir Crit Care Med 2001;163 (3 Pt 1):770–777.

30. Lee CG, Homer RJ, Zhu Z, et al. Interleukin-13 induces tissue fibrosis by selectively stimulating and activating transforming growth factor β. J Exp Med 2001;194(6): 809–821.

31. Shi Y, Massague J. Mechanisms of TGF-β signaling from cell membrane to the nucleus. Cell 2003;113(6):685–700.

32. Annes JP, Munger JS, Rifkin DB. Making sense of latent TGFβ activation. J Cell Sci 2003;116(Pt 2):217–224.

33. Annes JP, Chen Y, Munger JS, Rifkin DB. Integrin αvβ6-mediated activation of latent TGF-β requires the latent TGF-β binding protein-1. J Cell Biol 2004;165(5):723–734.

34. Jenkins RG, Su X, Su G, et al. Ligation of protease-activated receptor 1 enhances αvβ6 integrin-dependent TGF-β activation and promotes acute lung injury. J Clin Invest 2006;116(6):1606–1614.

35. Munger JS, Huang X, Kawakatsu H, et al. The integrin αvβ6 binds and activates latent TGFβ1: a mechanism for regulating pulmonary inflammation and fibrosis. Cell 1999;96(3):319–328.

36. Morris DG, Huang X, Kaminski N, et al. Loss of integrin αvβ6-mediated TGF-β activation causes MMP12-dependent emphysema. Nature 2003;422(6928):169–173.

37. Yehualaeshet T, O'Connor R, Green-Johnson J, et al. Activation of rat alveolar macrophage-derived latent transforming growth factor β1 by plasmin requires interaction with thrombospondin-1 and its cell surface receptor, CD36. Am J Pathol 1999;155(3):841–851.

38. Abreu JG, Ketpura NI, Reversade B, De Robertis EM. Connective-tissue growth factor (CTGF) modulates cell signalling by BMP and TGF-β. Nat Cell Biol 2002;4(8): 599–604.

39. Dong C, Zhu S, Wang T, et al. Deficient Smad7 expression: a putative molecular defect in scleroderma. Proc Natl Acad Sci USA 2002;99(6):3908–3913.

40. Doran P, Egan JJ. Herpesviruses: a cofactor in the pathogenesis of idiopathic pulmonary fibrosis? Am J Physiol Lung Cell Mol Physiol 2005;289(5):L709–L710.

41. Tang YW, Johnson JE, Browning PJ, et al. Herpesvirus DNA is consistently detected in lungs of patients with idiopathic pulmonary fibrosis. J Clin Microbiol 2003;41(6): 2633–2640.

42. Kelly BG, Lok SS, Hasleton PS, et al. A rearranged form of Epstein-Barr virus DNA is associated with idiopathic pulmonary fibrosis. Am J Respir Crit Care Med 2002;166(4): 510–513.

43. Strieter RM, Belperio JA, Keane MP. CXC chemokines in angiogenesis related to pulmonary fibrosis. Chest 2002; 122(6 Suppl):298S–301S.

44. Burdick MD, Murray LA, Keane MP, et al. CXCL11 attenuates bleomycin-induced pulmonary fibrosis via inhibition of vascular remodeling. Am J Respir Crit Care Med 2005; 171(3):261–268.

45. Beers MF, Mulugeta S. Surfactant protein C biosynthesis and its emerging role in conformational lung disease. Annu Rev Physiol 2005;67:663–696.

46. Mulugeta S, Nguyen V, Russo SJ, Muniswamy M, Beers MF. A surfactant protein C precursor protein BRICHOS domain mutation causes endoplasmic reticulum stress, proteasome dysfunction, and caspase 3 activation. Am J Respir Cell Mol Biol 2005;32(6):521–530.

47. Amin RS, Wert SE, Baughman RP, et al. Surfactant protein deficiency in familial interstitial lung disease. J Pediatr 2001;139(1):85–92.

48. Lawson WE, Polosukhin VV, Stathopoulos GT, et al. Increased and prolonged pulmonary fibrosis in surfactant protein C–deficient mice following intratracheal bleomycin. Am J Pathol 2005;167(5):1267–1277.

49. Bridges JP, Wert SE, Nogee LM, Weaver TE. Expression of a human surfactant protein C mutation associated with interstitial lung disease disrupts lung development in transgenic mice. J Biol Chem 2003;278(52):52739–5246.

50. Morgan NV, Pasha S, Johnson CA, et al. A germline mutation in BLOC1S3/reduced pigmentation causes a novel variant of Hermansky-Pudlak syndrome (HPS8). Am J Hum Genet 2006;78(1):160–166.

51. Bonifacino JS. Insights into the biogenesis of lysosome-related organelles from the study of the Hermansky-Pudlak syndrome. Ann NY Acad Sci 2004;1038:103–114.

52. Li W, Rusiniak ME, Chintala S, Gautam R, Novak EK, Swank RT. Murine Hermansky-Pudlak syndrome genes: regulators of lysosome-related organelles. Bioessays 2004; 26(6):616–628.

53. Lyerla TA, Rusiniak ME, Borchers M, et al. Aberrant lung structure, composition, and function in a murine model of Hermansky-Pudlak syndrome. Am J Physiol Lung Cell Mol Physiol 2003;285(3):L643–L653.

54. Grutters JC, du Bois RM. Genetics of fibrosing lung diseases. Eur Respir J 2005;25(5):915–927.

55. Selman M, Lin HM, Montano M, et al. Surfactant protein A and B genetic variants predispose to idiopathic pulmonary fibrosis. Hum Genet 2003;113(6):542–550.

47
Stem Cells in Nonneoplastic Lung Disorders

Dani S. Zander

Introduction

Over the past decade, our knowledge regarding pulmonary stem cells has undergone dramatic expansion. Research has focused on (1) identifying and characterizing populations of resident pulmonary stem cells and (2) determining whether, and to what extent, bone marrow–derived stem cells contribute to pulmonary repair. It is hoped that the regenerative properties of stem cells can be harnessed to provide a new approach to treatment of diffuse lung diseases that are poorly responsive to current therapies. Acute respiratory distress syndrome is a prime example. Acute respiratory distress syndrome is associated with a mortality rate as high as 60% and leads to pulmonary disability in the majority of survivors. Whether stem cells could be utilized to promote recovery has been a topic of intense interest. Chronic obstructive pulmonary disease and usual interstitial pneumonia produce chronic lung dysfunction and, in their advanced forms, represent common indications for lung transplantation. Given the lack of curative therapies for these disorders, stem cell–based approaches have been viewed as a potential avenue for development. Gene therapy administered via stem cells represents another focus of investigation because of its potential applications to the treatment of inherited genetic disorders such as cystic fibrosis.[1-4] The roles of stem cells in pulmonary carcinogenesis represent another topic of current investigation.

Criteria for defining stem cells vary, but, at minimum, stem cells are viewed as having the properties of self-renewal and differentiation. Organs that undergo continuous regeneration throughout postnatal life, such as the gastrointestinal tract, blood, and hair follicles, contain "dedicated" adult stem cells that undergo long-term self-renewal, have a relatively low proliferation rate, and live

in localized regions know as *stem cell niches* that regulate their behavior.[5-8] The stem cell niche is the microenvironment that supplies the external signals that control stem cell behavior. Secreted factors, cell–cell interactions mediated by membrane proteins, and interactions with extracellular matrix proteins via adhesion molecules are important elements of the stem cell niche. Transit-amplifying (TA) cells arising from these dedicated stem cells demonstrate a high rate of proliferation, short-term self-renewal capability, and the ability to produce one or more differentiated cell types characteristic of the particular organ.[5]

Although the classic stem cell hierarchy presented in Figure 47.1 is generally well established, it is not unalterable.[9] Under appropriate environmental conditions, some TA cells may be induced to acquire properties of stem cells.[9-11] Transdifferentiation, that is, transformation of one differentiated cell type into another, may occur via TA cells that are given particular signals.[5,12] The concept of the "facultative" stem cell has also been put forth to explain how organs without functional undifferentiated stem cell populations can regenerate themselves in the face of injury, probably through the acquisition of capabilities for self-renewal and differentiation by a differentiated cell type.[13,14]

In human and animal lungs, several populations of resident cells with properties of self-renewal and differentiation have been defined. Recently, also, the phenomenon of repopulation of the postnatal lung by progeny of bone marrow–derived cells has been a topic of active investigation. Evidence for both circulating mesenchymal and epithelial progenitor cells that traffic to the lungs has been increasingly published over the past few years. Nonetheless, our understanding of these phenomena is incomplete, and effective therapeutic strategies remain to be developed.

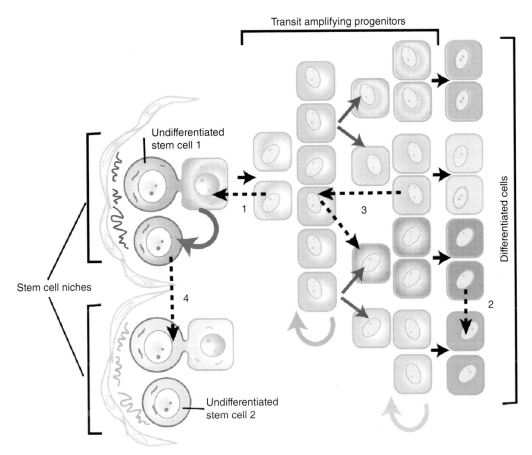

FIGURE 47.1. Classic stem cell hierarchy. Model of the "classic" hierarchy of undifferentiated epithelial stem cells, transit-amplifying (TA) progenitor cells, and mature postmitotic differentiated cells. Cell fate choices are indicated by red arrows. In this model, the stem cell in its "niche" and different TA cell subclasses can self-renew (curved arrows). Stem cells self-renew infrequently and TA cells more rapidly. Early TA cells may be able to replace stem cells if the niche is depleted (dashed arrow 1). The niche probably consists of several cell types and associated molecules, including blood vessels and nerves. "Transdif-ferentiation" of one well-defined differentiated cell type into another could occur directly, without cell division (dashed arrow 2) or might also involve reversion or dedifferentiation between distinct TA progenitor populations (dashed arrows 3). Rarely, stem cells switch from one tissue-specific lineage to another (dashed arrow 4) in a process called *metaplasia* or *transdetermination*. (Adapted from Watt and Hogan,[8] with permission. Modified and reprinted from Rawlins and Hogan,[5] with permission of the Company of Biologists.)

Pulmonary Repopulation by Bone Marrow–Derived Adult Stem Cells

A large number of studies have sought to determine whether bone marrow–derived adult stem cells can repopulate the lung and participate in pulmonary repair. Although most data support the existence of this phenomenon, with subsequent differentiation into epithelial, endothelial, and mesenchymal cells, a significant minority of published studies have yielded negative results. The concept of adult stem cell plasticity remains controversial.[9,15–18]

Epithelial Cells

Most reports of adult stem cell plasticity show low frequencies of marrow-derived nonhematopoietic cells in target organs, usually 1 in 1,000 to 1 in 10,000 epithelial cells, frequencies that are likely to be insufficient to achieve therapeutic results.[15] Mechanisms accounting for the ability of bone marrow–derived cells to take on nonhematopoietic phenotypes have not yet been clarified, but possibilities include cell-to-cell fusion,[19,20] direct differentiation of a nonhematopoietic precursor cell from the bone marrow, and transdifferentiation of a bone marrow cell that had previously been committed to a different phenotype.[15] Existing data support the first two possibilities but are lacking to support the third process.[15]

Investigation is ongoing to identify mechanisms for increasing levels of engraftment and to explain how bone marrow–derived cells develop into mature-appearing epithelial cells.

Animal models used to study this process employ donor bone marrow that expresses a marker, such as the Y chromosome, green fluorescent protein (GFP), lacZ, or β-galactosidase, that distinguishes cells that are derived from the donor from those derived from the recipient. Similarly, human lung transplant and bone marrow transplant recipients with gender-mismatched donors have been frequent choices of experimental subjects for these studies. A landmark investigation published by Krause and colleagues tested whether a single bone marrow–derived cell could engraft into a lethally irradiated recipient mouse and generate epithelial cells of donor phenotype.[21] Examination of the mice 11 months after transplantation showed engraftment of cytokeratin-positive, CD45-negative cells in the lung (columnar respiratory epithelial cells and pneumocytes), gastrointestinal tract, liver, and skin.[21] Theise and colleagues treated mice with lethal irradiation and then subjected them to cross-gender bone marrow transplantation.[22] They discovered that up to 14% of the type II pneumocytes in the injured lung possessed the donor karyotype and that the kinetics of bone marrow engraftment as type II pneumocytes coincided with the development of severe radiation pneumonitis.[22] Grove et al. took wild-type bone marrow–derived cells from male mice that had been transfected with a lentivirus encoding the *GFP* transgene expressed on the constitutively active long terminal repeat promoter and transplanted these cells into irradiated female mice.[4] Between 1% and 7% of cytokeratin-positive cells expressed *GFP*, and these cells had characteristics of type II and type I pneumocytes, indicating maintenance of transgene expression after differentiation of the bone marrow–derived cells to epithelial cells. These last results suggest that marrow-derived cells can be used as a vehicle for targeted transgene expression in epithelial cells of the lungs, an approach that could be important for diseases caused by single gene mutations, such as surfactant deficiencies or cystic fibrosis.

Bone marrow–transplanted mice subjected to lipopolysaccharide-induced airway injury were observed to demonstrate alveolar repopulation by donor-derived epithelial and endothelial cells.[23] Likewise, bone marrow–derived progenitor cells were shown to differentiate into alveolar epithelial cells and endothelial cells after treatment of elastase-induced emphysema with all-trans retinoic acid or granulocyte colony stimulating factor,[24] and administration of adrenomedullin was found to enhance this phenomenon.[25] Abe and colleagues employed a parabiotic mouse model and radiation and/or elastase to create lung injury.[26] They observed that cells with characteristics of interstitial monocytes/macrophages, subepi-

thelial fibroblast-like interstitial cells, and type I alveolar epithelial cells in one mouse appeared to be derived from the other mouse, ostensibly via circulating cells.[26] Another study showed that freshly isolated side population cells derived from ROSA26 adult bone marrow contributed to reconstitution of injured tracheal epithelium in vivo, and the donor-derived epithelial cells accounted for 0.83% of epithelial cells.[27] Bone marrow–derived mesenchymal cells administered systemically to mice also appeared to generate donor-derived respiratory bronchiolar cells.[28] Finally, Gomperts and colleagues identified a CK5-positive, CD45-positive, CXCR4-positive cell in the bone marrow and blood of mice and showed that these circulating cells were capable of contributing to large airway epithelial repair in a murine model of gender-mismatched tracheal transplantation.[29] Repopulation appeared to be dependent on the CXCR4/CXCL12 chemokine biologic axis.

In contrast, however, hematopoietic stem cell differentiation in the lung was not identified in transplantation and parabiotic models by Wagers and colleagues.[30] Kotton and colleagues also did not find evidence of reconstitution of pulmonary epithelial cells by bone marrow–derived stem cells in studies employing transplantation of GFP-expressing unfractionated bone marrow, bone marrow side population cells, or a single bone marrow side population cell into mice treated with lethal irradiation and then bleomycin to induce lung injury.[31] Although transplantation of GFP- or lacZ-labeled bone marrow into lethally irradiated wild-type mice revealed what appeared to be labeled bone marrow–derived cells with prosurfactant protein C expression and features of type II pneumocytes, deconvolution microscopy and flow cytometry did not demonstrate distal airway engraftment of bone marrow–derived cells as type II pneumocytes, and the original interpretation was thought to stem from artifact.[32]

Evaluations of gender-mismatched human lung allografts have also yielded conflicting results. Earlier in situ hybridization studies of lung allografts from female donors, which were transplanted into male recipients, revealed Y chromosome–expressing cells with phenotypic characteristics of leukocytes, but not epithelial cells, in the allografts.[33,34] Kleeberger et al., however, reported different results than the two earlier studies.[35] Using methods that included laser microdissection followed by short tandem repeat analysis of a polymorphic marker, these investigators studied lung allografts and reported significant numbers of recipient-derived epithelial cells, including 6%–26% of the bronchial epithelial cells, 9%–20% of the type II pneumocytes, and 9%–24% of the seromucinous glandular epithelial cells. These investigators associated higher percentages of recipient karyotype cells with histologic evidence of chronic injury. Tissue samples from gender-mismatched lung and bone marrow transplant specimens were studied by Albera and colleagues who reported finding evidence of repopulation with differentiation into type II pneumocytes and endothelial cells, but assessment of the percentages of donor-derived cells could not be performed because of technical factors.[36] No evidence of polyploidy was observed, suggesting that fusion was not responsible for the findings. Zander and colleagues likewise evaluated lung biopsy specimens from seven male recipients of transplanted lungs from female donors and performed sequential immunohistochemistry and fluorescent in situ hybridization to assess for Y chromosome–containing type II pneumocytes.[37] They found that Y chromosome–containing type II pneumocytes were present in approximately one-third of the biopsy specimens from five of the seven transplant recipients and accounted for 0%–0.553% of the type II pneumocytes. Furthermore, no evidence of polyploidy was identified to suggest cell–cell fusion, and, like the results of Kleeberger and colleagues, the number of type II pneumocytes of recipient origin appeared to correlate with lung injury. Fusion was also not observed in the lungs by Harris and colleagues, who used a Cre-Lox system together with β-galactosidase and enhanced GFP expression in transgenic mice to evaluate whether fusion plays a role in the development of marrow-derived epithelial cells.[38]

Hematopoietic cell transplant patients are vulnerable to many types of lung injury and represent a natural patient group to study. Diffuse alveolar damage is relatively common in this group of patients because of the administration of high-dose chemotherapeutic agents and radiation and the frequent development of opportunistic infections or graft versus host disease. Like the animal studies, investigations of tissues from human hematopoietic cell transplant recipients have produced a spectrum of results regarding the existence of pulmonary epithelial chimerism. Suratt and colleagues evaluated lung tissues from three female cross-gender hematopoietic cell transplant recipients and reported 2.5% and 8.0% epithelial chimerism in two of the patients' lungs, as well as very high degrees (35.7% and 42.3%) of endothelial chimerism.[39] The locations of the epithelial cells were described as alveolar and occasionally bronchiolar. Similar results were reported by Mattsson and colleagues in two female cross-gender hematopoietic cell transplant recipients.[40] On the other hand, the study by Kleeberger described no epithelial chimerism in bronchial tissues derived from three bone marrow transplant recipients, but pneumocytes were not evaluated in this work.[35] Finally, a recent study by Zander and colleagues evaluated the lungs of four cross-gender hematopoietic cell transplant recipients using sequential immunohistochemistry and fluorescent in situ hybridization to assess for Y chromosome–containing type II pneumocytes and found only a single Y chromosome–containing type II pneumocyte (Figure 47.2) in one lung biopsy specimen from one transplant recipient, accounting for 1.75% of all type II pneumocytes in the biopsy section.[41]

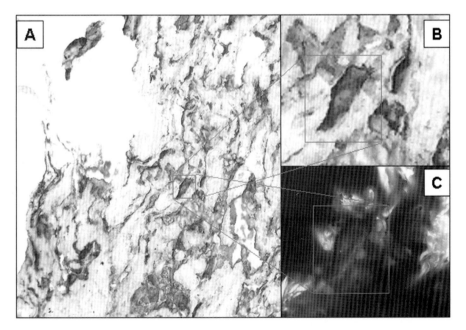

FIGURE 47.2. Hematopoietic cell transplant patient (female recipient of bone marrow from male donor). **(A,B)** A large reactive type II pneumocyte is stained for prosurfactant protein B (DAB, brown) and epithelial membrane antigen (Vector Blue, blue). (Original magnifications, A. ×200; B, ×1,000.) **(C)** The cell, viewed under fluorescence microscopy, has a Y chromosome (green) in the nucleus. (Original magnification ×1,000. Reprinted from Zander et al.,[41] with permission.)

The sources of the discrepancies among these reports have been addressed by many authors, who cite a number of variations in experimental methods. Regarding the animal studies performed by Wagers et al.,[30] explanations put forth by Theise et al.[42] to account for the lack of demonstration of engraftment included older donor and recipient pairs, shorter time periods of study after bone marrow transplantation, reliance of stem cell isolation protocols that may have selected for a less plastic cell than was used in other studies, and use of a GFP donor with expression of this protein as the sole marker of donor origin. Regarding the studies of human lung transplant recipients by Yousem et al.[33] and Bittman et al.,[34] which did not show the presence of recipient-derived type II pneumocytes, Zander and colleagues[37] noted that the pepsin digestion step used in the study published by Yousem et al.[33] was substantially shorter than the step used by their group, and may not have been long enough to allow for probe uptake by the type II pneumocyte nuclei, and that Bittman and colleagues[34] evaluated only 100 interphase pneumocyte nuclei, which may not have been sufficient to detect very low levels of microchimerism. Others have suggested that immunofluorescence microscopy cannot reliably detect rare engrafted cells in lung tissues and that artifact introduced by overlapping nuclei may account for many of the positive results reported.[31]

Finally, if bone marrow–derived stem cell repopulation of adult lungs occurs, can gene therapy be applied to progenitor cell populations in order to correct a genetic defect? There are undoubtedly many steps involved in the process of answering this question and devising a protocol that will provide safe, long-term restitution of gene function, but some progress has been made. Grove et al. transplanted male marrow that had been transduced with retrovirus encoding GFP into irradiated female mice and found transgene-expressing lung epithelial cells in all recipients analyzed at 2, 5, or 11 months after transplantation.[4] Wang and colleagues followed this work by showing that human bone marrow stromal stem cells have the potential to differentiate into airway epithelial cells; that MSCs from patients with cystic fibrosis can be isolated, expanded, and gene corrected ex vivo; and that these gene-corrected MSCs can contribute to apical chloride secretion in response to cyclic adenosine monophosphate stimulation, which is critical for successful therapy for cystic fibrosis.[1]

Endothelial Cells

As discussed above, Yamada et al.[23] and Ishizawa et al.[24] reported endothelial repopulation by donor-derived cells in bone marrow–transplanted mice subjected to lipopolysaccharide-induced airway injury and treatment of elastase-induced emphysema with all-trans retinoic acid or granulocyte colony-stimulating factor, respectively. Suratt and colleagues reported a high degree (37.5%–42.3%) of endothelial cell chimerism in lung biopsy specimens from female allogeneic hematopoietic stem cell transplant recipients who received stem cells from male donors,[39] but this result has not been confirmed by others. Nonetheless, others have shown in mice that adult bone marrow–derived, phenotypically defined hematopoietic stem cells (c-Kit positive, stem cell antigen-1 [Sca-1] positive, lineage negative) can give rise to functional endothelial cells that express CD31, produce von Willebrand factor, take up low-density lipoprotein, and are not the products of cell fusion.[43] Whether the number of circulating endothelial progenitor cells correlates with outcome in acute lung injury and acute respiratory distress syndrome was recently studied.[44] Endothelial progenitor cell colony numbers generated from buffy coat samples were significantly higher in patients with acute lung injury compared with healthy control subjects, and, in the patients with acute lung injury, a higher colony count correlated with improved survival.

That tumors may recruit CD34-positive progenitor cells to build their vascular networks was suggested by work done using the Lewis lung carcinoma (LLC) model.[45] In vitro studies showed that LLC cells could chemoattract CD34-positive cells predominantly through tumor production of vascular endothelial growth factor and that LLC-conditioned medium containing angiopoietin-1 could promote differentiation of CD34-positive cells toward endothelial cells expressing CD31 and CD144. Additional in vivo studies showed that infusion of lacZ-positive, CD34-positive cells from the bone marrow of transgenic mice into wild-type mice bearing LLC tumors resulted in the accumulation of lacZ-positive cells within the tumor mass, particularly at the tumor's periphery, and that these infused CD34-positive progenitor cells acquired the endothelial cell markers CD31 or CD144 within the tumor tissue. However, in a subsequent study, development of functional tumor vasculature from recruited lineage-negative, c-Kit-positive, Sca-1–positive cells was not observed.[46]

Fibrocytes

The peripheral blood includes small numbers (0.1%–0.5% of nucleated cells) of circulating collagen-, vimentin-, and CD34-positive cells with fibroblastic properties, termed *fibrocytes*, that participate in scar formation.[47] In culture, these cells express α-smooth muscle actin (αSMA), and exposure to transforming growth factor-β (TGF-β) or endothelin-1 increases their expression of αSMA while promoting acquisition of the morphologic features of myofibroblasts.[48,49] A loss of CD45 and CD34 expression accompanies increasing development of myofibroblast-like features,[49–52] suggesting a loss of stem cell marker expression with increased degrees of differentiation. Fibrocytes express CXCR4, migrate in response to CXCL12 under specific in vitro conditions, and traffic to the lungs, as shown in a murine model of bleomycin-induced pulmonary fibrosis.[50] Maximal intrapulmonary recruitment of these fibrocytes correlated with increased pulmonary collagen deposition, and treatment of the bleomycin-exposed mice with neutralizing antibodies to CXCL12 inhibited both fibrocyte recruitment and pulmonary fibrosis. Analysis of the lungs from bleomycin-treated wild-type mice previously transplanted with GFP-labeled bone marrow–derived cells showed that >80% of collagen I–expressing cells also demonstrated GFP expression, indicating an origin from circulating bone marrow–derived cells.[53] Another group induced radiation pneumonitis in mice transplanted with whole bone marrow or a clonal bone marrow stromal cell line and demonstrated repopulation by fibroblastic cells of bone marrow origin.[54] Furthermore, the numbers of donor-derived fibroblastic cells in the lungs could be reduced by prior administration of manganese superoxide dismutase–plasmid/liposome intratracheal injection, which inhibits development of radiation pneumonitis. Schmidt and colleagues studied the role of circulating fibrocytes in the genesis of subepithelial fibrosis, a feature of the remodeling process associated with asthma.[49] These investigators found that allergen exposure induced the accumulation of CD34-, collagen I-, and αSMA-positive fibrocyte-like cells in the subepithelial bronchial mucosa of patients with allergic asthma. Additionally, by tracking labeled circulating fibrocytes in a mouse model of allergic asthma, they demonstrated recruitment of fibrocytes into bronchi following allergen exposure, with a decrease in the expression of CD34 and an increase in collagen I and αSMA expression (greater myofibroblastic differentiation) in the cells in the airway tissues as compared with cells recovered from the peripheral blood.

Resident Pulmonary Stem Cells

A rich and voluminous literature has developed over several decades regarding pulmonary epithelial cell populations possessing the stem cell-like properties of self-renewal and differentiation. These cells are believed to give rise to the spectrum of histologically differentiated cell types that we recognize today, cell types that, for the most part, are believed to have little or no capacity to self-renew. Currently, these cell groups are believed to include undifferentiated basal cells residing in the epithelium of the large airways and populations of cells found at the bronchoalveolar duct junctions and in neuroepithelial bodies. Some or all type II pneumocytes may also be included in this category. The mechanisms controlling progenitor cell functionalities are not well understood,

but it is likely that future research will shed more light on the signaling pathways involved in these processes and provide insight into methods that can be used to enhance pulmonary repair.

Large Airways

Multiple studies suggest that undifferentiated (basal) cells in the bronchi and trachea represent a population of stem cells.[55–67] Basal cells appear to proliferate in association with injury and express the proliferation marker MIB1 to a higher degree than more differentiated cells.[68] Studies using heterotopically implanted tracheal grafts have shown that deepithelialized grafts that were inoculated with basal cell–rich cell suspension fractions or mixed tracheal cell fractions were eventually reepithelialized with an epithelium containing basal cells, goblet cells, other secretory cells, and ciliated cells.[60,69,70] Nettesheim and colleagues also demonstrated that vitamin A–depleted basal cell cultures can undergo squamous differentiation, analogous to the common process of squamous differentiation that occurs with airway epithelial injury.[60] Interesting studies performed by Borthwick and colleagues evaluated the localization of bromodeoxyuridine (BrdU) label-retaining cells (LRCs) in mice receiving weekly epithelial damage by intratracheal detergent or SO$_2$ inhalation.[71] At 3 and 6 days after injury, basal and lumenal BrdU-positive epithelial cells were distributed along the entire trachea. At 20 and 95 days after injury, LRCs were localized to gland ducts in the upper trachea and to systematically arrayed foci in the lower trachea, typically near the cartilage–intercartilage junction, suggesting that these areas represent stem cell niches in the tracheal epithelium. Furthermore, heterotopic tracheal grafts that were denuded of surface epithelium demonstrated epithelial reconstitution from gland remnants. A bronchial xenograft model of the human airway was also used by Engelhardt and colleagues to identify submucosal gland progenitor cells within the surface airway epithelium.[72] Replication-defective recombinant retroviruses were used to study the development of submucosal glands and led to the identification of a pluripotent progenitor cell in the airway epithelium that retains a capacity for glandular development. Other studies using tracheal grafts suggest that nonbasal (secretory or ciliated) cell populations can also restore the tracheal epithelium,[67,73,74] raising the question of "facultative" stem cell capabilities in the nonbasal cell populations studied.

Small Airways

A number of studies have supported the capacity of Clara cells to reproduce themselves and differentiate into ciliated cells in bronchioles.[75–79] Using a heterotopic tracheal xenograft model, Hook and colleagues observed repopulation of the denuded tracheas by Clara cell–rich isolates from the lungs of rabbits, with production of an epithelium resembling bronchiolar epithelium composed of ciliated cells and Clara-like cells.[80] Naphthalene has been used in animal models to destroy Clara cells and examine mechanisms of airway epithelial repair. Naphthalene is an aromatic hydrocarbon that selectively kills cells that express cytochrome P450–2F2, which is converted to toxic epoxides in such cells. Within a few hours of exposure, most of the Clara cells die, except for the few that do not express cytochrome P450–2F2. A small population of resistant Clara cell secretory protein (CCSP)-expressing Clara cells (variant CCSP-expressing cells) that survive naphthalene injury appear to proliferate and renew the Clara cell population, and these cells are found in the neuroepithelial bodies (NEBs).[81,82] Localization of proliferating Clara cells at bronchiolar bifurcations was also noted by Stripp and colleagues after induction of naphthalene airway injury.[83]

A similar population of pollutant-resistant CCSP-expressing cells that localized to the bronchoalveolar duct junction and contributed to epithelial renewal in Clara cell–depleted terminal bronchioles with few NEBs was described by Giangreco et al.[84] Immunohistochemical colocalization studies involving CCSP and the NEB-specific marker calcitonin gene-related peptide showed that these bronchoalveolar duct junction–associated CCSP-expressing stem cells function independently of NEBs. Kim and colleagues[85] reported isolation of a CD34-positive cell population localized to the murine bronchioalveolar duct junction that they termed *bronchioalveolar stem cells* (BASCs), that may be the same cell population studied by Giangreco et al.[84] These cells exhibit self-renewal, are multipotent in clonal assays, are resistant to bronchiolar and alveolar damage, and coexpress the Clara cell–specific marker CCA (identical to CCSP) and prosurfactant protein C, a major product of type II pneumocytes. In culture, these cells gave rise to progeny expressing markers for either Clara cells or type I or type II pneumocytes. Further experiments showed that BASCs were increased in murine lung adenocarcinomas and precursor lesions and that cultured BASCs expanded in response to oncogenic K-ras, suggesting that these cells may represent candidate cells of origin for pulmonary adenocarcinomas.

Regarding pulmonary neuroendocrine stem cells, a transgenic mouse model was used to define the contribution of NEB-associated CCSP-expressing progenitor cells to pulmonary neuroendocrine cell hyperplasia after Clara cell ablation.[86] After selective ablation of CCSP-expressing cells, proliferation and hyperplasia of pulmonary neuroendocrine cells occurred without detectable proliferation among other residual airway epithelial cell populations, indicating that pulmonary neuroendocrine cells function as a self-renewing progenitor population.

The Sonic hedgehog pathway may play a role in neuroendocrine cell renewal; naphthalene-induced Clara cell depletion was followed by marked expression of both Sonic hedgehog ligand and Gli1, a transcriptional target of hedgehog signaling.[87] This pattern of signaling was also noted in airway development during normal differentiation of pulmonary neuroendocrine precursor cells, as well as in a subset of small cell lung cancers.

Type II pneumocytes may represent another population of resident cells manifesting the properties of self-renewal and differentiation into type I pneumocytes.[88–92] Whether the type II cells possessing stem cell properties reside at the bronchoalveolar duct junction and represent the same population identified by Kim and colleagues[85] as the "bronchioalveolar stem cell" is unclear. The identification of subsets of type II cells differing in expression of telomerase and E-cadherin suggest the existence of multiple populations of type 2 alveolar epithelial cells.[93] Telomerase expression, which is considered to be a characteristic of stem or progenitor cells, was increased in a subpopulation of type 2 alveolar epithelial cells with exposure to hyperoxia and showed a strong correlation with proliferating cell nuclear antigen expression.[94] Other in vitro studies have shown conversion of type I pneumocytes to type II pneumocytes with changes in culture conditions[95] or treatment with keratinocyte growth factor,[96] raising the question of whether type 1 pneumocytes may represent another potential pool of progenitor cells or exist in a dynamic continuum with type II cells under varying conditions in vivo.

Side Population Cells

Side population (SP) cells constitute a rare cell population that is enriched for stem cell activity and is identified by the cells' ability to efflux the vital dye Hoechst 33342.[97,98] In the murine lung, SP cells are found in proximal and distal lung regions and comprise 0.03%–0.07% of total lung cells.[99] These cells express hepatocyte nuclear factor-3β but not thyroid transcription factor-1 and demonstrate cell surface expression of Sca-1 and breast cancer resistance protein 1 (BCRP1), as well as variable expression of CD45.[99] Experiments using bone marrow transplantation revealed that both CD45-positive and CD45-negative lung SP cells are derived from the bone marrow.[100] CD45-positive lung and bone marrow SP cells showed similar morphologic features (small, round cells with scant cytoplasm), while CD45-negative lung SP cells were larger and contained abundant granular cytoplasm.[100] Gene expression patterns for hematopoietic transcription factors GATA-1, GATA-2, and PU.1, and for αSMA and cytokeratin, differed between bone marrow and lung SP subtypes, and considerable heterogeneity existed within each population of SP cells.[100] In another study, CD45-negative lung SP cells were found to express Sca-1 reactivity and molecular markers indicating either airway epithelial (CCSP) or mesenchymal (vimentin) characteristics.[101] A lack of cytochrome P450–2F2 RNA was found in the CD45-negative SP cell population, a property that is consistent with the molecular phenotype of a cell population residing in the NEB, a location previously found to harbor stem cells.

Conclusion

Multiple progenitor cell populations reside in the lung and contribute to recovery from lung injury. Identification and characterization of these cell populations continues to advance, fostered by use of modern technologies to create models of pulmonary injury and measure the responses of individual cell types to these environmental changes. Contributions of adult stem cells to pulmonary regeneration continue to be investigated, and the possibility of combining gene therapy with stem cell approaches represents another intriguing avenue of research. There is a need for additional mechanistic research to determine the molecular events responsible for stem cell behavior. The influences of neighboring cells and secreted substances must be defined. As a consequence, delineation of these events may lead to new therapeutic approaches that harness the regenerative capacities of stem cells to enhance the native processes involved in pulmonary repair.

References

1. Wang G, Bunnell BA, Painter RG, et al. Adult stem cells from bone marrow stroma differentiate into airway epithelial cells: potential therapy for cystic fibrosis. Proc Natl Acad Sci USA 2005;102:186–191.
2. Lee TW, Matthews DA, Blair GE. Novel molecular approaches to cystic fibrosis gene therapy. Biochem J 2005;387:1–15.
3. Copreni E, Penzo M, Carrabino S, et al. Lentivirus-mediated gene transfer to the respiratory epithelium: a promising approach to gene therapy of cystic fibrosis. Gene Ther 2004;11(Suppl 1):S67–S75.
4. Grove JE, Lutzko C, Priller J, et al. Marrow-derived cells as vehicles for delivery of gene therapy to pulmonary epithelium. Am J Respir Cell Mol Biol 2002;27:645–651.
5. Rawlins EL, Hogan BL. Epithelial stem cells of the lung: privileged few or opportunities for many? Development 2006;133:2455–2465.
6. Fuchs E, Tumbar T, Guasch G. Socializing with the neighbors: stem cells and their niche. Cell 2004;116:769–778.
7. Lanza R. Essentials of Stem Cell Biology. Burlington, MA: Elsevier Academic Press; 2006.
8. Watt FM, Hogan BL. Out of Eden: stem cells and their niches. Science 2000;287:1427–1430.
9. Raff M. Adult stem cell plasticity: fact or artifact? Annu Rev Cell Dev Biol 2003;19:1–22.
10. Kai T, Spradling A. Differentiating germ cells can revert into functional stem cells in Drosophila melanogaster ovaries. Nature 2004;428:564–569.
11. Pearton DJ, Ferraris C, Dhouailly D. Transdifferentiation of corneal epithelium: evidence for a linkage between the segregation of epidermal stem cells and the induction of hair follicles during embryogenesis. Int J Dev Biol 2004;48:197–201.
12. Pearton DJ, Yang Y, Dhouailly D. Transdifferentiation of corneal epithelium into epidermis occurs by means of a multistep process triggered by dermal developmental signals. Proc Natl Acad Sci USA 2005;102:3714–3719.
13. Dor Y, Brown J, Martinez OI, et al. Adult pancreatic beta-cells are formed by self-duplication rather than stem-cell differentiation. Nature 2004;429:41–46.
14. Alison MR, Vig P, Russo F, et al. Hepatic stem cells: from inside and outside the liver? Cell Prolif 2004;37:1–21.
15. Krause DS. Engraftment of bone marrow–derived epithelial cells. Ann NY Acad Sci 2005;1044:117–124.
16. Quesenberry PJ, Dooner G, Colvin G, et al. Stem cell biology and the plasticity polemic. Exp Hematol 2005;33:389–394.
17. Theise ND. Perspective: stem cells react! Cell lineages as complex adaptive systems. Exp Hematol 2004;32:25–27.
18. Wagers AJ, Weissman IL. Plasticity of adult stem cells. Cell 2004;116:639–648.
19. Terada N, Hamazaki T, Oka M, et al. Bone marrow cells adopt the phenotype of other cells by spontaneous cell fusion. Nature 2002;416:542–545.
20. Ying QL, Nichols J, Evans EP, et al. Changing potency by spontaneous fusion. Nature 2002;416:545–548.
21. Krause DS, Theise ND, Collector MI, et al. Multi-organ, multi-lineage engraftment by a single bone marrow–derived stem cell. Cell 2001;105:369–377.
22. Theise ND, Henegariu O, Grove J, et al. Radiation pneumonitis in mice: a severe injury model for pneumocyte engraftment from bone marrow. Exp Hematol 2002;30:1333–1338.
23. Yamada M, Kubo H, Kobayashi S, et al. Bone marrow–derived progenitor cells are important for lung repair after lipopolysaccharide-induced lung injury. J Immunol 2004;172:1266–1272.
24. Ishizawa K, Kubo H, Yamada M, et al. Bone marrow–derived cells contribute to lung regeneration after elastase-induced pulmonary emphysema. FEBS Lett 2004;556:249–252.
25. Murakami S, Nagaya N, Itoh T, et al. Adrenomedullin regenerates alveoli and vasculature in elastase-induced pulmonary emphysema in mice. Am J Respir Crit Care Med 2005;172:581–589.
26. Abe S, Boyer C, Liu X, et al. Cells derived from the circulation contribute to the repair of lung injury. Am J Respir Crit Care Med 2004;170:1158–1163.
27. MacPherson H, Keir P, Webb S, et al. Bone marrow–derived SP cells can contribute to the respiratory tract of mice in vivo. J Cell Sci 2005;118:2441–2450.

28. Anjos-Afonso F, Siapati EK, Bonnet D. In vivo contribution of murine mesenchymal stem cells into multiple cell-types under minimal damage conditions. J Cell Sci 2004; 117:5655–5664.

29. Gomperts BN, Belperio JA, Rao PN, et al. Circulating progenitor epithelial cells traffic via CXCR4/CXCL12 in response to airway injury. J Immunol 2006;176:1916–1927.

30. Wagers AJ, Sherwood RI, Christensen JL, et al. Little evidence for developmental plasticity of adult hematopoietic stem cells. Science 2002;297:2256–2259.

31. Kotton DN, Fabian AJ, Mulligan RC. Failure of bone marrow to reconstitute lung epithelium. Am J Respir Cell Mol Biol 2005;33:328–334.

32. Chang JC, Summer R, Sun X, et al. Evidence that bone marrow cells do not contribute to the alveolar epithelium. Am J Respir Cell Mol Biol 2005;33:335–342.

33. Yousem SA, Sonmez-Alpan E. Use of a biotinylated DNA probe specific for the human Y chromosome in the evaluation of the allograft lung. Chest 1991;99:275–279.

34. Bittmann I, Dose T, Baretton GB, et al. Cellular chimerism of the lung after transplantation. An interphase cytogenetic study. Am J Clin Pathol 2001;115:525–533.

35. Kleeberger W, Versmold A, Rothamel T, et al. Increased chimerism of bronchial and alveolar epithelium in human lung allografts undergoing chronic injury. Am J Pathol 2003;162:1487–1494.

36. Albera C, Polak JM, Janes S, et al. Repopulation of human pulmonary epithelium by bone marrow cells: a potential means to promote repair. Tissue Eng 2005;11:1115–1121.

37. Zander DS, Baz MA, Cogle CR, et al. Bone marrow–derived stem cell repopulation contributes minimally to the type II pneumocyte pool in transplanted human lungs. Transplantation 2005;80:206–212.

38. Harris RG, Herzog EL, Bruscia EM, et al. Lack of a fusion requirement for development of bone marrow–derived epithelia. Science 2004;305:90–93.

39. Suratt BT, Cool CD, Serls AE, et al. Human pulmonary chimerism after hematopoietic stem cell transplantation. Am J Respir Crit Care Med 2003;168:318–322.

40. Mattsson J, Jansson M, Wernerson A, et al. Lung epithelial cells and type II pneumocytes of donor origin after allogeneic hematopoietic stem cell transplantation. Transplantation 2004;78:154–157.

41. Zander DS, Cogle CR, Theise ND, et al. Donor-derived type II pneumocytes are rare in the lungs of allogeneic hematopoietic cell transplant recipients. Ann Clin Lab Sci 2006;36:47–52.

42. Theise ND, Krause DS, Sharkis S. Comment on "Little evidence for developmental plasticity of adult hematopoietic stem cells." Science 2003;299:1317.

43. Bailey AS, Jiang S, Afentoulis M, et al. Transplanted adult hematopoietic stems cells differentiate into functional endothelial cells. Blood 2004;103:13–19.

44. Burnham EL, Taylor WR, Quyyumi AA, et al. Increased circulating endothelial progenitor cells are associated with survival in acute lung injury. Am J Respir Crit Care Med 2005;172:854–860.

45. Young MR. Tumor skewing of CD34⁺ progenitor cell differentiation into endothelial cells. Int J Cancer 2004;109: 516–524.

46. Shinde Patil VR, Friedrich EB, Wolley AE, et al. Bone marrow-derived lin(−)c-kit(+)Sca-1+ stem cells do not contribute to vasculogenesis in Lewis lung carcinoma. Neoplasia 2005;7:234–240.

47. Bucala R, Spiegel LA, Chesney J, et al. Circulating fibrocytes define a new leukocyte subpopulation that mediates tissue repair. Mol Med 1994;1:71–81.

48. Abe R, Donnelly SC, Peng T, et al. Peripheral blood fibrocytes: differentiation pathway and migration to wound sites. J Immunol 2001;166:7556–7562.

49. Schmidt M, Sun G, Stacey MA, et al. Identification of circulating fibrocytes as precursors of bronchial myofibroblasts in asthma. J Immunol 2003;171:380–389.

50. Phillips RJ, Burdick MD, Hong K, et al. Circulating fibrocytes traffic to the lungs in response to CXCL12 and mediate fibrosis. J Clin Invest 2004;114:438–446.

51. Quan TE, Cowper S, Wu SP, et al. Circulating fibrocytes: collagen-secreting cells of the peripheral blood. Int J Biochem Cell Biol 2004;36:598–606.

52. Gomperts BN, Strieter RM. Stem cells and chronic lung disease. Annu Rev Med 2007;58:285–298.

53. Hashimoto N, Jin H, Liu T, et al. Bone marrow–derived progenitor cells in pulmonary fibrosis. J Clin Invest 2004; 113:243–252.

54. Epperly MW, Guo H, Gretton JE, et al. Bone marrow origin of myofibroblasts in irradiation pulmonary fibrosis. Am J Respir Cell Mol Biol 2003;29:213–224.

55. Breeze RG, Wheeldon EB. The cells of the pulmonary airways. Am Rev Respir Dis 1977;116:705–777.

56. Hackett NA. Proliferation of lung and airway cells induced by nitrogen dioxide. J Toxicol Environ Health 1979;5: 917–928.

57. Kauffman SL. Cell proliferation in the mammalian lung. Int Rev Exp Pathol 1980;22:131–191.

58. Donnelly GM, Haack DG, Heird CS. Tracheal epithelium: cell kinetics and differentiation in normal rat tissue. Cell Tissue Kinet 1982;15:119–130.

59. Breuer R, Zajicek G, Christensen TG, et al. Cell kinetics of normal adult hamster bronchial epithelium in the steady state. Am J Respir Cell Mol Biol 1990;2:51–58.

60. Nettesheim P, Jetten AM, Inayama Y, et al. Pathways of differentiation of airway epithelial cells. Environ Health Perspect 1990;85:317–329.

61. Evans MJ, Van Winkle LS, Fanucchi MV, et al. Cellular and molecular characteristics of basal cells in airway epithelium. Exp Lung Res 2001;27:401–415.

62. Bishop AE. Pulmonary epithelial stem cells. Cell Prolif 2004;37:89–96.

63. Hong KU, Reynolds SD, Watkins S, et al. Basal cells are a multipotent progenitor capable of renewing the bronchial epithelium. Am J Pathol 2004;164:577–588.

64. Hong KU, Reynolds SD, Watkins S, et al. In vivo differentiation potential of tracheal basal cells: evidence for multipotent and unipotent subpopulations. Am J Physiol Lung Cell Mol Physiol 2004;286:L643–L649.

65. Liu X, Driskell RR, Engelhardt JF. Airway glandular development and stem cells. Curr Top Dev Biol 2004;64:33–56.

66. Schoch KG, Lori A, Burns KA, et al. A subset of mouse tracheal epithelial basal cells generates large colonies in vitro. Am J Physiol Lung Cell Mol Physiol 2004;286: L631–42.

67. Avril-Delplanque A, Casal I, Castillon N, et al. Aquaporin-3 expression in human fetal airway epithelial progenitor cells. Stem Cells 2005;23:992–1001.

68. Boers JE, Ambergen AW, Thunnissen FB. Number and proliferation of basal and parabasal cells in normal human airway epithelium. Am J Respir Crit Care Med 1998; 157:2000–2006.

69. Inayama Y, Hook GE, Brody AR, et al. The differentiation potential of tracheal basal cells. Lab Invest 1988;58: 706–717.

70. Inayama Y, Hook GE, Brody AR, et al. In vitro and in vivo growth and differentiation of clones of tracheal basal cells. Am J Pathol 1989;134:539–549.

71. Borthwick DW, Shahbazian M, Krantz QT, et al. Evidence for stem-cell niches in the tracheal epithelium. Am J Respir Cell Mol Biol 2001;24:662–670.

72. Engelhardt JF, Schlossberg H, Yankaskas JR, et al. Progenitor cells of the adult human airway involved in submucosal gland development. Development 1995;121:2031–2046.

73. Johnson NF, Hubbs AF. Epithelial progenitor cells in the rat trachea. Am J Respir Cell Mol Biol 1990;3:579–585.

74. Liu JY, Nettesheim P, Randell SH. Growth and differentiation of tracheal epithelial progenitor cells. Am J Physiol 1994;266:L296–L307.

75. Evans MJ, Johnson LV, Stephens RJ, et al. Renewal of the terminal bronchiolar epithelium in the rat following exposure to NO₂ or O3. Lab Invest 1976;35:246–257.

76. Evans MJ, Cabral-Anderson LJ, Freeman G. Role of the Clara cell in renewal of the bronchiolar epithelium. Lab Invest 1978;38:648–653.

77. Boers JE, Ambergen AW, Thunnissen FB. Number and proliferation of Clara cells in normal human airway epithelium. Am J Respir Crit Care Med 1999;159:1585–1591.

78. Plopper CG, Nishio SJ, Alley JL, et al. The role of the nonciliated bronchiolar epithelial (Clara) cell as the progenitor cell during bronchiolar epithelial differentiation in the perinatal rabbit lung. Am J Respir Cell Mol Biol 1992;7:606–613.

79. Barth PJ, Muller B. Effects of nitrogen dioxide exposure on Clara cell proliferation and morphology. Pathol Res Pract 1999;195:487–493.

80. Hook GE, Brody AR, Cameron GS, et al. Repopulation of denuded tracheas by Clara cells isolated from the lungs of rabbits. Exp Lung Res 1987;12:311–329.

81. Reynolds SD, Giangreco A, Power JH, et al. Neuroepithelial bodies of pulmonary airways serve as a reservoir of progenitor cells capable of epithelial regeneration. Am J Pathol 2000;156:269–278.

82. Hong KU, Reynolds SD, Giangreco A, et al. Clara cell secretory protein–expressing cells of the airway neuroepithelial body microenvironment include a label-retaining subset and are critical for epithelial renewal after progenitor cell depletion. Am J Respir Cell Mol Biol 2001;24: 671–681.

83. Stripp BR, Maxson K, Mera R, et al. Plasticity of airway cell proliferation and gene expression after acute naphthalene injury. Am J Physiol 1995;269:L791–L799.

84. Giangreco A, Reynolds SD, Stripp BR. Terminal bronchioles harbor a unique airway stem cell population that localizes to the bronchoalveolar duct junction. Am J Pathol 2002;161:173–182.

85. Kim CF, Jackson EL, Woolfenden AE, et al. Identification of bronchioalveolar stem cells in normal lung and lung cancer. Cell 2005;121:823–835.

86. Reynolds SD, Hong KU, Giangreco A, et al. Conditional Clara cell ablation reveals a self-renewing progenitor function of pulmonary neuroendocrine cells. Am J Physiol Lung Cell Mol Physiol 2000;278:L1256–L1263.

87. Watkins DN, Berman DM, Burkholder SG, et al. Hedgehog signalling within airway epithelial progenitors and in small-cell lung cancer. Nature 2003;422:313–317.

88. Adamson IY, Bowden DH. The type 2 cell as progenitor of alveolar epithelial regeneration. A cytodynamic study in mice after exposure to oxygen. Lab Invest 1974;30: 35–42.

89. Adamson IY, Bowden DH. Derivation of type 1 epithelium from type 2 cells in the developing rat lung. Lab Invest 1975;32:736–745.

90. Evans MJ, Cabral LJ, Stephens RJ, et al. Transformation of alveolar type 2 cells to type 1 cells following exposure to NO₂. Exp Mol Pathol 1975;22:142–150.

91. Evans MJ, Dekker NP, Cabral-Anderson LJ, et al. Quantitation of damage to the alveolar epithelium by means of type 2 cell proliferation. Am Rev Respir Dis 1978;118: 787–790.

92. Kapanci Y, Weibel ER, Kaplan HP, et al. Pathogenesis and reversibility of the pulmonary lesions of oxygen toxicity in monkeys. II. Ultrastructural and morphometric studies. Lab Invest 1969;20:101–118.

93. Reddy R, Buckley S, Doerken M, et al. Isolation of a putative progenitor subpopulation of alveolar epithelial type 2 cells. Am J Physiol Lung Cell Mol Physiol 2004;286: L658–L667.

94. Driscoll B, Buckley S, Bui KC, et al. Telomerase in alveolar epithelial development and repair. Am J Physiol Lung Cell Mol Physiol 2000;279:L1191–L1198.

95. Danto SI, Shannon JM, Borok Z, et al. Reversible transdifferentiation of alveolar epithelial cells. Am J Respir Cell Mol Biol 1995;12:497–502.

96. Borok Z, Lubman RL, Danto SI, et al. Keratinocyte growth factor modulates alveolar epithelial cell phenotype in vitro: expression of aquaporin 5. Am J Respir Cell Mol Biol 1998;18:554–561.

97. Goodell MA, Brose K, Paradis G, et al. Isolation and functional properties of murine hematopoietic stem cells that are replicating in vivo. J Exp Med 1996;183:1797–1806.

98. Asakura A, Rudnicki MA. Side population cells from diverse adult tissues are capable of in vitro hematopoietic differentiation. Exp Hematol 2002;30:1339–1345.

99. Summer R, Kotton DN, Sun X, et al. Side population cells and Bcrp1 expression in lung. Am J Physiol Lung Cell Mol Physiol 2003;285:L97–L104.

100. Summer R, Kotton DN, Sun X, et al. The origin and phenotype of lung side population cells. Am J Physiol Lung Cell Mol Physiol 2004;287:L477–L483.

101. Giangreco A, Shen H, Reynolds SD, et al. Molecular phenotype of airway side population cells. Am J Physiol Lung Cell Mol Physiol 2004;286:L624–L630.

48
Gene Therapy in Nonneoplastic Lung Disease

Timothy Craig Allen and Philip T. Cagle

Introduction

The genetic basis of some nonneoplastic lung diseases and the accessibility of the pulmonary airways for administration of aerosol therapy make the concept of gene therapy for these diseases one worthy of the intense examination that it has been given.[1] Cystic fibrosis (CF) and α_1-antitrypsin deficiency (AATD), two common and incurable lung diseases that are caused by mutations in a single gene, have been closely investigated for potential treatment with gene therapy.[1]

Gene Therapy in the Lung

As a hollow organ, the respiratory tract is well-suited for topically administered therapies, and presently a variety of conventional therapies are delivered to airways via inhalers and nebulizers.[1] Other therapies, such as antibiotics, are typically delivered systemically. Both routes have been investigated for administration of gene therapy, and the one chosen depends on the nature of the disease being treated, the cellular site requiring gene expression, and the limitations of the gene transfer agents and delivery systems.[1]

Administration

Direct administration onto the airway surface is an appropriate method for delivering therapeutic epithelial membrane-bound proteins such as the cystic fibrosis transmembrane conductance regulator (CFTR) protein—mutated in CF—as well as for AATD, a disease characterized by protein secretion into the airway.[1] Widespread delivery is most likely to occur by inhalation or nebulization of the therapeutic agent.[1] Nebulization has been used widely for nongene-based drug delivery to airways and has been investigated for gene therapy delivery; however, nebulizer systems that are currently available generally destroy DNA because of the physical forces exerted on it during its passage through the equipment.[1,2] Newer nebulization systems, with single passage of DNA through a porous membrane, may allow for better results.[1] Bronchoscopic techniques such as injection or instillation are appropriate for single application localized gene therapy delivery, such as for treatment of endobronchial tumors; however, such a delivery system is not practical for diseases such as CF that require repeated deliveries to a widespread area.[1]

The inefficiency of current aerosol delivery systems has led to the development of more efficient systems such as soft mist inhalers.[2] Microspraying technology has been shown to be substantially superior to oral nebulization in animal studies but has the disadvantage of requiring bronchoscopy and administration through an endotracheal tube.[2] One challenge of any aerosol delivery system is overcoming the effect of airway obstruction on aerosol deposition in the lungs of adult CF patients with significant airways disease.[2] With respect to systemic therapy, several barriers exist, including crossing the bronchial and pulmonary circulatory systems, that limit that route's efficacy.[1]

Barriers to Gene Transfer

Several significant barriers hinder gene transfer to the lungs and airways.[3-5] Because of the need to protect itself from the environment, the lung has developed efficient mechanisms to exclude exogenous substances, including gene transfer agents.[1,3,4] Investigators, attempting to overcome these protective mechanisms, have used viral and nonviral vectors to achieve efficient, persistent, and sustained gene transfer to airway epithelial cells in vivo; however, that goal has been difficult to achieve despite high transduction levels and phenotypic correction demonstrated in vitro with a variety of vectors.[3,5-22]

A major reason for this difficulty arises from the role of the natural airway defenses to pathogens, which

510

provide a strong barrier to gene therapy delivery at the airway surface—including mucus and mucociliary clearance, the epithelial cell glycocalyx, and, for most viruses, the basolateral cellular localization of their cognate receptors.[3,23–29] Ciliated and mucous-secreting epithelial cells line the conducting airways and function in rapidly removing inhaled material via mucociliary clearance.[1,30] This mucous barrier prevents direct contact between inhaled particles and the cell surface and reduces the epithelial inflammatory response to pathogens.[1] In normal persons, the mucociliary clearance mechanism is a significant barrier to topical gene therapy delivery.[1]

As discussed in more detail later, CF patients have an even greater barrier to delivery because their sputum, abnormal in both volume and composition, inhibits gene transfer by both viral and nonviral vectors.[5,27,31–34] As these multiple barriers efficiently protect lung epithelium from infectious organisms and particulates, chemical modification of these barriers will almost certainly be necessary to achieve efficient and sustainable gene transfer to the airway epithelium.[3] Therapies that reduce mucus viscosity have been studied preclinically and have the potential of being clinically applicable.[1,35,36] Surfactant, other low surface tension liquids, and thixotropic agents (gels that become fluid when stirred or shaken and return to the semisolid state upon standing), as well as other gelling agents, have been investigated to facilitate the spread of gene transfer vectors throughout the respiratory tract and increase vector contact time; however, these agents could probably be clinically applicable only for targeting of distal airways and alveoli because they increase distal airway and alveolar expression of therapeutic genes at the expense of more proximal airway expression.[1,3,37–40]

The divalent cation chelator ethylene glycol-bis(2-aminoethylether)-N,N,N′N′-tetraacetic acid (EGTA), as well as sodium caprate and sodium laurate, were each shown by Johnson et al. to enhance gene delivery in vivo to tracheal epithelium with an adenoviral vector.[3,41] EGTA functions by disrupting epithelial cell tight junctions. Tight junction disruption might provide more efficient targeting of epithelial stem cells, because adult stem cells and progenitor cells reside in airways behind tight junctions.[3,42] Cystic fibrosis gene therapy involving stem cells and progenitor cells is discussed in greater detail later.

The detergents polidocanol and α-L-lysophosphatidylcholine have been investigated for their potential to enhance gene transfer by disrupting epithelial cell tight junctions.[3] Parsons et al. found that murine nasal airway treatment with polidocanol 1 hour before instillation with an adenoviral vector enhanced gene transduction in vivo and caused little histologically-identifiable airway damage.[43] Polidocanol has also been shown to enhance gene transfer with a lentiviral vector, which is discussed in detail below.[3,44] α-L-lysophosphatidylcholine was found

to provide sustainable (3 months) gene expression with no diminution in transduced cell number when used with a lentiviral vector carrying the *CFTR* gene.[45,46] Because α-L-lysophosphatidylcholine is found in low concentrations naturally in airways, it may be converted rapidly to the nontoxic dipalmitoylphosphatidylcholine, ubiquitous in biologic membranes, an additional benefit.[3,45] Perfluorocarbons have also been studied to enhance delivery of gene vectors.[3]

Cell Entry and Nuclear Entry

If a gene transfer agent can overcome the mucociliary clearance mechanisms and come into direct contact with a target cell, cell entry by the agent must be managed in a manner that protects the agent from destruction.[1] Cell surface glycocalyx is resistant to gene transfer agent entry, but investigators have studied methods, such as enzymatic removal of the agents' sialic acid moieties, to assist in overcoming that resistance.[1,23] Although their safety to the patient has not been determined, agents that break intercellular tight junctions permit basolateral cell surface access to gene therapy agents and increase viral and synthetic vector cell uptake.[4–49] Because some viral vectors can use specific cell surface receptors to enter a cell, ligands for specific cell surface receptors have been attached to synthetic vectors in an attempt to mimic the process, including the successful targeting of serpin–enzyme complex receptor (sec-R).[1] Ziady and Davis found that sec-R–targeted CFTR led to some chloride ion transport correction in the CF mouse nose, whereas nontargeted complexes did not.[31] Integrins, cell adhesion molecules located on the apical membrane of respiratory epithelium, were targeted by Scott et al. and showed increased uptake of plasmid coupled to an integrin-binding motif by receptor-mediated endocytosis.[50] The clinical effectiveness of targeting cell surface receptors for gene therapy agent cell entry has yet to be demonstrated.

Systemic delivery of gene therapy agents has been evaluated as a potential method of introducing therapy intracellularly while avoiding the hindering mucosal surface barriers.[1] The basolateral membrane of airway epithelial cells, having a higher rate of endocytosis and increased receptor density, can potentially be accessed with intravenous administration.[1] Unfortunately, studies to date have shown that systemic circulation-driven administration has resulted in little airway epithelial cell transfection, with primarily pulmonary endothelial cells and alveolar epithelial cells being transfected.[51–53] This phenomenon is considered to be related to the barriers to cell entry, including reticuloendothelial system clearance, serum protein inhibition, vascular compartment escape, the interstitium, and the epithelial cell basement membrane.[1,54,55]

After the gene therapy agent enters a cell, it must cross the cytoplasm to enter the nucleus while avoiding cytoplasmic DNase destruction.[56] Various methods to promote such avoidance have been investigated, including coupling the agent with peptides similar to those used by viruses to avoid escape, the use of proton sponges with intrinsic endosomolytic activity, the introduction of pH-responsive histidine-based systems, conjugation of nonviral vectors with specific sugar moieties, and the addition of peptides to facilitate cytoskeletal transport.[57–59] Normally, molecules required within the nucleus enter it through the nuclear pore complex, assisted by the possession of specific nuclear localizing sequences (NLS).[1] The nuclear envelope prevents entry of foreign material into the nucleus, and in nondividing cells it is a major barrier to gene transfer.[1] Incorporation of specific NLS peptide sequences, such as those from human immunodeficiency virus TAT protein, and the identification of novel NLS have been attempted to overcome the barrier.[1,60,61] Brisson et al. have attempted to avoid the nuclear envelope barrier by using cytoplasmic expression systems such as those incorporating the T7 promoter and RNA polymerase.[62]

Physical Methods of Overcoming Gene Transfer Barriers

Strategies to overcome airway gene transfer difficulties have resulted in the investigation of a variety of methods, including electroporation, ultrasound, and magnetism.[1] Electroporation is the application of an electronic pulse across tissue in an attempt to improve gene transfer agent uptake, probably by either cell membrane permeabilization or DNA electrophoresis, depending on the pulse administered.[1,63] Little tissue damage has been identified in animal models by the use of this method, with relatively successful attempts using skeletal muscle, various tumors, blood vessels, skin, and neural tissue.[1,64] Dean et al. showed a dose-dependent transfer of naked DNA by electroporation through the chest wall in mice.[65] Gene transfer was identified in both alveolar and airway cells, with no macroscopic or microscopic damage identified with the doses employed.[65] Pringle et al. showed reporter gene expression in mice lungs after thoracotomy and direct placement of electrodes on the lung surface.[66] Machado-Aranda et al. noted that the electroporation-mediated transfer of naked NDA encoding the Na^+-K^+/ATPase led to enhanced fluid clearance in rat lung.[67] The use of this technique in the larger chests of human beings and in isolated areas are challenges that the development of bronchoscopic techniques might address in the future.[1]

Ultrasound, via a mechanism of action that may include heating and cavitation, has been investigated in both preclinical and clinical studies to increase percutaneous absorption of drugs such as insulin, local anesthetics, and nonsteroidal antiinflammatory agents, with some studies demonstrating increased drug uptake.[1,68,69] Studies to date have been performed on tumors, joints, and blood vessels but not lung tissue or airways.[1,70–72] It may be suitable for pulmonary purposes, as studies have shown that low-frequency (<100 MHz) ultrasound can traverse air-filled spaces.[1]

Magnetofection, the application of a magnetic field to an organ or animal administration of gene transfer agent-linked magnetic nanoparticles, has been attempted in order to increase contact time between host cells and DNA, increasing uptake likelihood.[1] In vitro studies have shown vector particle binding to up to 100% of cells within a few minutes via mangetofection.[1] Scherer et al. found that coxsackie adenovirus receptor–deficient cells, resistant to adenoviral gene transfer, were transfectable by magnetofection, probably because of increased contact time and enhanced uptake.[73] Gersting et al., studying a porcine airway model, found significantly increased reporter gene expression in a short time with magnetofection partly because of reduced mucociliary escalator clearance.[74]

Gene Transfer Efficacy

Various mechanisms limit transgene expression duration. Gene transfer agents utilizing viral promoters often yield high, early peak expression levels, with rapid decline due to inflammatory cytokine-mediated transcriptional silencing.[1] Human promoters such as polyubiquitin C has extended expression of naked DNA from 2 weeks to 6 months in murine lung, and such prolonged expression might provide a major clinical benefit.[1,75] Transfected-cell death, from usual cell turnover or from host recognition response, is another reason for shortened transgene expression duration.[1] Terminally differentiated conducting airway cells live several months, but once one dies, the transgene is lost, and additional, repeated dosages are required.[5,76] Selective transfection of progenitor or stem cells has been considered as a method of overcoming this barrier, with the potential to effect long-term CFTR expression in progeny cells.[1,5] Clara cells, basal cells, neuroepithelial cells, and type II pneumocytes in the airways have been considered as potential target cells for such transfection.[1] Use of viral vectors could give rise to generations of corrected progeny cells, a benefit not apparent with the use of nonviral vectors here.[1] Insertion of DNA directly into the host genome, the transposon system, may also help extend transgene expression duration, but concerns over insertional mutagenesis, as with viral vector systems, would have to be addressed.[77,78]

Gene transfer efficiency and duration may be limited by innate and adaptive host immune responses regardless of administration route.[1] In the lung, alveolar macrophages rapidly clear topically applied gene transfer vectors.[1,79] Reticuloendothelial system macrophages can similarly clear systemically applied vectors.[1,80] Also adaptive immune responses, both humoral and cell mediated, can impair gene transfer and expression of viral and nonviral vectors.[1] Clinical trials have shown major toxicity with viral vectors in this capacity.[1] Transduced cells may be killed by initiation of a cytotoxic T lymphocyte response, thereby limiting transgene expression duration.[1] Antibody production to previously unencountered transgene-derived proteins is a potential risk.[1] Viral and non viral vectors in the context of CF are discussed in more detail.

Cystic Fibrosis

Cystic fibrosis occurs in about 1 in 2,500 live births and is one of the most common life-threatening monogenic disorders in Caucasian populations of Northern European ancestry.[3] Cystic fibrosis is caused by a variety of mutations in the gene encoding the CFTR protein, a cAMP-regulated chloride channel in the apical surface of epithelial cells.[5,81,82] Cystic fibrosis transmembrane conductance regulator protein is active in several organs, including the intestine, pancreas, lung, sweat glands, eyes, and kidneys.[3] Besides functioning as a cyclic adenosine monophosphate–regulated chlorine ion channel, the CFTR gene product regulates fluid secretion from various epithelial membranes, regulates the epithelial sodium channel, controls the efflux of glutathione, is involved in bicarbonate transport, and as such controls airway surface liquid and submucosal gland secretion; it also possibly plays a role in lipid metabolism.[3,83–90]

Cystic fibrosis manifests itself clinically in epithelial tissues of various organs, including the intestine, pancreas, respiratory tract, sweat glands, liver, and reproductive organs.[3] Lung disease, the cause of death in over 90% of patients, occurs because of impaired hydration and impaired mucociliary clearance caused by abnormal epithelial ion transport, chronic bacterial infection, and severe inflammation.[31,91] Treatment today at best slows the unrelenting progression of lung disease, and median survival is about 30 years.[1,3,5] Lung disease involves the proximal and distal airways and is characterized by severe and sustained neutrophil-mediated inflammation, purulent mucus, recurrent infections, chronic inflammation, epithelial cell necrosis, and progressive lung damage with functional deterioration.[3,5] Lung pathology is attributable to insufficient or absent CFTR in airway epithelial cells, with a resultant decrease in airway surface liquid volume and associated decreased mucus hydration, increased mucus viscosity, and poor mucociliary clearance, combining to produce mucus stasis and progressive microbial colonization and infection of airways.[92,93] New

therapeutic approaches, including curative therapies, are needed.

Cystic Fibrosis Transmembrane Conductance Regulator Protein and Gene Therapy

Since the CFTR gene was isolated in 1989, researchers have considered gene therapy as a promising treatment for CF lung disease.[3,94] The goal of CFTR gene therapy in CF patients is to deliver the CFTR gene in sufficient quantity specifically to affected cells for a period of time that allows for therapeutic benefit.[31] Different levels of CFTR gene expression may be required to restore the various CFTR functions, and studies have varied in determining how many cells require transfection.[1,5] Some authors have suggested that normal CFTR function in 20% of epithelial cells may correct or prevent the CF phenotype; whereas others believe over 80% of epithelial cells will require transfection in order to correct the CF phenotype.[3,31,95–97] Some researchers consider that as few as 10% of normal levels of CFTR are enough to prevent lung disease, suggesting that, as the number of transcripts per cell is usually low, the number of cells transduced, rather than the level of CFTR expression, will ultimately determine whether CFTR gene therapy succeeds.[5,31,98,99] It is unknown whether CFTR expression in other cell types such as the gland ducts will be required for successful treatment or whether ectopic expression in cells normally free of CFTR will yield any untoward side effects.[3,100]

Although organs other than the lung are affected in CF patients, the lung is the primary site of pathology. As such airways have been the target for the majority of CF gene therapy clinical trials, and trials with topical gene delivery to airway epithelium—inserting a normal copy of the CFTR gene into the cell, most often the nucleus—have aimed to normalize CFTR function, including its ion transport function.[1,5] Studies investigating the location of normal CFTR expression in the lung have found high levels of CFTR in serous cells of submucosal glands and much lower levels in the surface epithelium in distal small airways where clinically detectable CF begins.[3,5,101–103] Brochiero et al., in a recent study using improved reagents and techniques, found that CFTR expression diminishes from proximal to distal areas of the lung, and, although CFTR expression occurs in the terminal bronchioles and alveoli, it does so minimally.[104] Brochiero et al. identified no goblet cell, basal cell, or Clara cell CFTR expression, in contrast to previous studies, supporting the hypothesis that effective CF gene therapy will require ongoing CFTR expression in some proportion of ciliated airway epithelial cells.[104] It is presently unknown whether induction of CFTR expression in ciliated cells within gland ducts will be necessary in order to normalize mucus composition.[3]

Stem Cells and Progenitor Cells

In rodents, terminally differentiated airway epithelial cells have been found to have a life span of approximately 3 months, and other mammals, including human beings, likely have similar cell longevity.[3,105] Effective CF gene therapy therefore will require targeting of stem cells and other progenitor cells in order to produce prolonged, sustainable benefit.[3] Identification of populations of stem and progenitor cells in proximal and distal airways has been an active focus of investigation and is discussed in another chapter. Along with investigation of other potential pulmonary stem cells, researchers are examining the potential for hematopoietic cell stem cell engraftment in the lung as another potential stem cell approach to CF gene therapy.[106–113] Future studies will be required to develop delivery methods, target appropriate stem cell populations, and assess the affects of these interventions on patient safety.

Cystic Fibrosis Transmembrane Conductance Regulator Protein Function and Safety

Different levels of gene therapy may be required to restore CFTR functions.[1] Lower numbers of transfected cells would probably be required to restore chloride transport, and higher levels would be needed to normalize sodium absorption.[21] It is not known which CFTR functions would require correction to prevent CF progression or disease initiation; however, 5%–10% of wild-type CFTR levels might be enough to produce a disease-free phenotype.[114] Organs differ in their various epithelial sensitivities to low CFTR levels, with the male reproductive system being very sensitive, airways appearing of intermediate sensitivity, and pancreas exhibiting low sensitivity.[115] As such, although airways are the major targets for gene therapy, the levels of gene expression necessary for normal function will probably differ.[1] In addition, although mRNA or CFTR protein detection is evidence of gene expression, their presence is not necessarily indicative of functional correction.[1]

Ion transport, the first CFTR function identified, is considered to be critical in CF pathophysiology and is the function most commonly assessed in gene-based and pharmacologic clinical trials.[1,5] The measurement of transepithelial potential difference at baseline and in response to various drugs that block the sodium channel or that stimulate chloride secretion is the means most readily used to assess ion transport in vivo and is obtainable within the airway by bronchoscope and from nasal epithelium.[116–118] Ex vivo techniques such as epifluorescence microscopy have been helpful in some investigations, and alternative protein functions, such as those concerning bacterial adherence, have been used by some researchers to assess CFTR function.[116,119]

After clinical trials involving liposome-mediated *CFTR* gene transfer to nasal epithelium safely demonstrated functional correction, clinical trials of liposome-mediated *CFTR* gene therapy to the lower airways of CF patients were conducted.[22,116,120–124] Cystic fibrosis patients have tolerated inhalation treatments relatively well, with mild influenza-like symptoms generally thought to relate to the CF patients' lung inflammation.[125,126] In a trial examining the efficacy of gene therapy in the lower airway by measuring lower airway transepithelial potential difference, Alton et al. noted no change in sodium absorption parameters in patients given placebo, but found a significant response of about 25% of non-CF values to perfusion with low chloride and isoprenaline.[116] Hyde et al. found repeated nasal administration to be well tolerated and effective, unlike other studies identifying problems with readministration of adenoviral-mediated gene transfer.[127] Konstan et al. confirmed the safety and noted partial chloride transport correction in some CF patients by using nanoparticles composed of a single plasmid DNA molecule and polyethylene glycol–substituted polylysine.[128]

Vectors

As discussed earlier, sustained, effective gene therapy to airway epithelium has been a very difficult task, and in CF patients, thickened mucus is an additional barrier to gene delivery, as is the inflammation accompanying ongoing infections that impede gene delivery with various viral and nonviral vectors.[3,34,129–134]

Because of the low transfection levels achieved with naked DNA, most CF gene therapy research has involved viral vectors as facilitators of cell and nuclear DNA uptake.[5,31,135–139] Vectors for treating CF airway disease include both virus-derived and nonviral or synthetic vectors.[5] The majority of studies concerning CF gene therapy vectors have involved viruses that have a propensity for airway infection, specifically adenovirus and adeno-associated virus (AAV).[3,140] More recently, other respiratory viruses have been investigated for CF gene therapy, including Sendai virus, respiratory syncytial virus, polyomavirus, and human parainfluenza virus.[31,94,141–146] Unfortunately, sustained and efficient gene transfer to airway epithelium has not resulted from investigations of most vectors, even when *in vivo* studies have shown limited airway cell gene transduction.[3] As an efficient vector will be required for airway gene therapy, investigators have studied other potential vectors. Mitotically stable episomal plasmid vectors are being developed in an attempt to overcome the barrier of lack of persistence in airway epithelial cells.[3,147–149] These vectors also seem to provide more efficient delivery because of compacted DNA.[3,149] Adenoviral vectors using modified, replication-deficient adenoviruses have been by far the most widely studied viral vectors; however, nonintegrating viral vectors may be unusable as CF gene therapy vectors because of the patients' life-long requirement for repeated treatments and the patients' immune recognition of these vectors.[3,5] Development of neutralizing antibodies to viral proteins may significantly reduce the efficacy of treatment over time.[5] Clinical trials have borne this out.[3,33]

Adeno-associated virus and retroviral vectors, more recently investigated, have potential as CF gene therapy vectors.[6,27] Adeno-associated virus has the ability to transduce both dividing and nondividing cells, opening an avenue for stem cell transduction.[3,150] Adeno-associated virus vectors are therefore being intensely studied for CF gene therapy.[6,31,133,134,151] Adeno-associated viruses are non-enveloped viruses that have a protein capsid and a single strand of DNA encoding for two genes, *rep*, encoding replication proteins, and *cap*, encoding capsid proteins.[3] Adeno-associated viruses in human beings are nonpathogenic and are located in the respiratory and gastrointestinal systems.[3] Adeno-associated virus is capable of integrating into host cell chromosomes as tandem arrays.[3] McCarty et al., using recombinant AAV (rAAV) vectors, and Schnepp et al., using wild-type AAV vectors, have shown genomic persistence for relatively long time periods as episomes.[3,150,152] Adeno-associated virus vectors have several benefits, including their potential ability to integrate into host chromosomes, relatively high infectivity, and viral noninfectivity.[3,133] The primary disadvantage to AAV vectors is their relatively small size (4.7kb) that may be problematic given the relatively large size of the CFTR coding sequence (4.5kb).[3] Several researchers have constructed *CFTR* minigenes, used minimal promoter elements, and used split genome systems, including recombination and trans-splicing, in attempts to overcome the genomic capacity barrier.[3,153–155] Adeno-associated virus capsid immunogenicity is also a potential concern were readministration of CF gene therapy required.[3] A variety of studies have shown that AAV vector genomes remain stable, even after several months.[3,28,150]

Various serotypes of AAV vectors have been investigated for CF gene therapy.[3] Unfortunately, clinical studies with AAV vectors have been disappointing, possibly because most have used the AAV-2 serotype, which does not infect the apical surface of airway epithelial cells efficiently.[3,31] Newer AAV serotypes that target the apical surface might show improved transduction of lung airway epithelium.[3] As well as their potential improved transduction efficiency, other AAV serotypes, unlike AAV-2, are not naturally found in human beings, so concerns regarding preexisting immunity are not as great.[3,156,157] Adeno-associated virus-5, for example, has been found to bind strongly to apical surfaces of cells and result in a 50-fold more efficient gene transfer to ciliated human airway epithelial cells in vitro, with significantly higher

transduction efficiency in mouse lung airway epithelium in vivo.[3,156,158] Various agents, discussed earlier, including gelling agents and perfluorocarbons, have been shown to enhance airway gene delivery by several AAV serotypes.[40,159,160] Future studies using various AAV serotypes may produce efficient, sustainable gene transduction in CF patients.

Recombinant AAV vectors examined in preclinical studies have shown that they are capable of long-term gene transfer and expression in bronchial epithelium of animal models and importantly have shown that rAAV vectors did not increase inflammatory cells or proinflammatory cytokines.[32,161–165] Phase I and phase II clinical trials using rAAV vectors have been performed and showed evidence of dose-related DNA transfer and gene expression.[8,161,166–168] Neutralizing antibodies were also identified however, and repeated doses did not show evidence of repeated efficient gene transfer.[8,161,166–168] These studies have disclosed some key limitations in rAAV vector use, including the relative paucity of AAV receptors and coreceptors in airway cell luminal surfaces, inactivation of rAAV within the airway, rapid turnover of airway epithelium in CF patients, limiting the persistence of rAAV episomes, and development of neutralizing anti-AAV antibodies, limiting the efficiency of repeated dosing.[161] Presently, rAAV research is ongoing, with newer generations of rAAV vectors being developed in order to attempt to overcome these barriers, and additional technologies being applied to rAAV, for example, spliceosome-mediated RNA trans-splicing.[133,157,161,169,170]

Lentivirus, a retrovirus, is the only retroviral vector able to transduce nondividing cells.[3,171] Lentiviral vectors, relatively recently developed from lentiviruses such as human immunodeficiency virus, feline immunodeficiency virus, and equine infectious anemia virus, are promising vectors for CF gene therapy because of their ability to integrate in nondividing cells and, as retroviruses, integrate into the host cell chromosome.[31,94,171–173] Their chromosomal integration ability makes them especially attractive as potential stem cell–targeted vectors.[3,174] Lentivirus vectors may also be pseudotyped with various viral envelopes so that they can target the apical surface, the basolateral surface, or both surfaces of the epithelial cells.[40,175,176] More research is necessary with lentivirus vectors to further assess their potential benefits, as well as to assess safety concerns and whether their benefits can translate into CF patient benefit clinically.[3,177]

To circumvent the safety concerns of viral vectors, synthetic vectors are being investigated for use in CF gene therapy, and cationic liposomes or other synthetic polymers have undergone clinical trials.[5,178,179] DNA complexed to lipids (lipoplexes) and molecular conjugates (polyplexes) are less efficient in vivo than viruses, and much of the DNA fails to reach the nucleus with these vectors.[5,31] A major potential benefit of these nonviral vectors is their relative lack of toxicity or immunogenicity; however, lipoplexes have elicited a host cytotoxic response associated with bacterial unmethylated cytosine-pyrimidine-guanine sequences present in plasmid DNA.[5,31,180] Nanoparticles, short pieces of DNA that are compact and small in diameter—facilitating their transport through the nuclear pore—with the addition of a receptor to mediate cellular uptake, such as the sec-R, have shown promising results in animal models.[5] Research in nanomedicine for CF is ongoing.[181] Electroporation has enhanced transfer efficacy.[5] Both liposome-mediated and recombinant viral approaches have shown advantages, with generally well-tolerated administration; however, sodium absorption parameters have not been shown to change.[5] Some researchers believe that the unwanted and disabling immune reaction that reduces the ability to administer the vector subsequently presently eliminates current nonviral vectors as usable vectors for CF gene therapy.[3,6,33,94,136,179,182,183] At best, unique issues remain to be addressed for nonviral gene therapy to become a clinically viable treatment. Removal of damaging DNA sequences has reduced the risks inherent in lipoplexes, but lipoplexes may remain clinically unhelpful.[31] PEGylation might stabilize lipoplexes and reduce cytotoxicity.[31,184] PEGylation stabilizes DNA nanoparticles for relatively long time periods, allowing for aerosolization.[31,139] Polyplexes formed with polyK are nontoxic and have no vector-associated inflammation in human beings, allowing for readministration for long-term expression.[31,185] They can also be modified to target-specific cells, making them a vector with some reasonable potential for success in CF patients.[31]

Endpoint Assays

For clinical application of CF gene therapy research, dependable endpoint assays, both preclinical and clinical, must exist.[186,187] Reporter genes encoding for chloramphenicol acetyl transferase, firefly luciferase, or β-galactosidase have been used to identify and characterize viral and synthetic gene transfer agents.[52,75,143,186] Preclinical endpoints for *CFTR* gene airway epithelial cell transfer include the use of reporter genes in lung or nasal turbinate homogenate, immunohistochemical examination for reporter gene expression, and quantification of recombinant CFTR mRNA, protein, or chloride channel function, among other assays.[186] Clinical endpoints include direct assays to quantify CFTR mRNA, protein, and chloride channel activity, as well as a variety of invasive and noninvasive indirect assays for CFTR, including evaluating the reduction in attachment of *Pseudomonas aeruginosa* to ciliated epithelial cells, analysis of inflammatory markers in sputum and bronchoalveolar lavage fluid, analysis of inflammatory markers in exhaled breath condensate, and bacterial colonization, as assessed by the

number of exacerbations of infection or the requirement for intravenous antibiotics over a certain time period.[186]

Future Directions

Research in nonviral vectors is ongoing. Waterhouse et al. has developed a synthetic nonviral vector platform known as liposome:mu:DNA in an attempt to successfully address the relatively inefficient nucleic acid delivery associated with nonviral vectors.[188] There has been progress in CF gene therapy research with the advancement of AAV, stem cell, and progenitor cell targeting with integrating lentiviral vectors, new synthetic vectors, and the addition of physical energy such as magnetofection to enhance gene transfer.[101,135] Concerns remain regarding barriers to gene transfer and repeat administration, among other barriers.[101,135]

α₁-Antitrypsin Deficiency

Deficiency of α_1-antitrypsin, the principal endogenous antiprotease, causes pulmonary emphysema in adults and liver disease that may occur as early as infancy.[1,189] α_1-Antitrypsin deficiency is an autosomal recessive disease caused by various mutations in the corresponding gene, leading to absent or significantly reduced levels of circulating AAT protein, and is found in approximately 4% of human beings, a percentage similar to CF.[1,161,190] α_1-Antitrypsin deficiency is more homogeneous than CF, the so-called Z allele accounting for over 95% of mutant alleles and causing a defect in secretion of the antiprotease from hepatocytes into the circulation.[161] The protein's main action in the lung is to counter the adverse effects of proteases such as neutrophil elastase on the distal conducting airways and alveoli.[1] Reduced AAT activity causes long-term loss of pulmonary interstitial elastin because of the unopposed action of neutrophil elastase and other neutrophil products and leads to clinical chronic obstructive pulmonary disease that is usually diagnosed in adults.[161] Studies have shown that there is a greatly reduced risk of lung disease if plasma AAT levels are above $11\,\mu M$ (57–80 mg/dL).[161,191] The goal of gene therapy for these patients is therefore to bring AAT levels into range.[161] Presently, therapy consists of symptomatic therapy and avoiding environmental triggers such as cigarette smoke.[1] Plasma-derived AAT is suitable for intravenous administration but is expensive, has a risk of viral transmission, and suffers from a short half-life, requiring frequent dosages.[192] As such, gene therapy has been investigated as an alternative and potentially curative therapy for AATD.

Unlike CF, AATD is characterized by a deficiency in activity of a secreted protein so that exogenous gene transfer at another site is possible.[1] The natural site of

AAT synthesis, the liver, is a logical choice for transfection; however, protein produced at the local site of action, the distal lung, might allow for disease treatment at lower levels of transfection.[1] Preclinical trials have been performed with animals using viral vectors.[189,193] Canonico et al., studying aerosolized cationic liposome-mediated *AAT* gene transfer to rabbit lung, showed protein in airway and alveolar cells, and, based on those results, Brigham et al. conducted a clinical trial of *AAT* gene transfer.[194,195] In the investigation by Brigham et al., AATD patients receiving a single dose of cationic liposome-AAT in one nostril were found to exhibit protein in their nasal lavage fluid, with protein levels peaking at about day 5.[195] Levels of proinflammatory cytokine interleukin-8 were decreased in the treated nostril in these patients, a feature not found in patients intravenously administered purified AAT protein, leading the authors to suggest that different routes of administration might lead to variable responses at different sites of expression.[195] Recombinant AAV has been studied in animal models for AATD gene therapy with some success, and future research may lead to improved biologic efficacy and safe, effective, and sustainable rAAV-mediated gene transfer methods.[161,196–199]

Other Conditions

Besides CF and AATD, airway gene therapy has been considered for a variety of other reactive lung diseases, including acute respiratory distress syndrome, asthma, and fibrotic lung disease.[1] Acute respiratory distress syndrome is a condition of various etiologies for which no specific treatment exists, prognosis is poor, and therapy is generally supportive.[200] Investigators have attempted to reduce pulmonary inflammation by both antagonizing proinflammatory cytokines and increasing antiinflammatory cytokine levels utilizing conventional gene transfer techniques, predominantly employing viral vectors, and with antisense oligonucleotides that reduce protein translation by specific mRNA binding.[1,189] Conary et al., using a rabbit model of endotoxin-induced acute lung injury, administered a gene encoding the prostaglandin synthase gene complexed to cationic lipid and noted decreased pulmonary edema, a recognized feature of acute lung injury, and thromboxane B_2 release.[201] Stern et al. noted significantly reduced pulmonary edema in a mouse model of acute lung injury after using cationic liposomes to overexpress Na^+/K^+ ATPase, a protein that clears alveolar liquid in healthy individuals.[202]

Asthma, a common disorder characterized by type 2 T helper lymphocyte-mediated inflammation and airway hyperreactivity, is generally treated with bronchodilators and antiinflammatory agents.[203,204] A subgroup of asthma patients fails to respond to the use of these agents for treating their cough, wheezing, and breathlessness, and

for these patients benefit has been shown with a variety of cytokine genes.[1] Lee et al. used nonviral vectors to transfer an IL-12 variant to the airways of mice exhibiting dust mite–induced inflammation and demonstrated marked reduction in airway hyperresponsiveness, IL-5, and local eosinophils after treatment.[205] del Pozo et al., using a rat model of asthma, intratracheally administered plasmid DNA containing galectin-3, a molecule that selectively downregulates IL-5, and demonstrated a normalization of eosinophil counts and T-cell counts in bronchoalveolar lavage fluid.[206] Although these approaches have potential benefit for asthma patients, they will probably be appropriate only for the small subset of patients who do not benefit from standard asthma therapies.[1]

Several growth factors, including transforming growth factor-β, are thought to be critical for the progression of fibrotic lung diseases of various etiologies.[207,208] Epperly et al. demonstrated prevention of radiation-induced lung fibrosis and improved survival using liposome-mediated manganese superoxide dismutase.[209] Ziesche et al. noted that interferon-γ1b protein therapy, along with prednisolone, improved pulmonary function and oxygen saturation, suggesting that Fas-mediated alveolar cell apoptosis might be of potential benefit for the development of future gene therapy regimens for pulmonary fibrosis.[210,211]

References

1. Davies JC, Alton E. Airway gene therapy. Adv Genet 2005;54:291–314.
2. Laube BL. The expanding role of aerosols in systemic drug delivery, gene therapy, and vaccination. Respir Care 2005;50:1161–1174.
3. Anson DS, Smith GJ, Parsons DW. Gene therapy for cystic fibrosis airway disease. Is clinical success imminent? Curr Gene Ther 2006;6:161–179.
4. Zabner J, Fasbender AJ, Moninger T, et al. Cellular and molecular barriers to gene transfer by a cationic lipid. J Biol Chem 1995;270:18997–19007.
5. Davies JC. Gene and cell therapy for cystic fibrosis. Paediatr Respir Rev 2006;7S:S163–S165.
6. Lee TWR, Matthews DA, Blair GE. Novel molecular approaches to cystic fibrosis gene therapy. Biochem J 2005;387:1–15.
7. Drumm ML, Pope HA, Cliff WH, et al. Correction of the cystic fibrosis defect in vitro by retrovirus-mediated gene transfer. Cell 1990;1227–1233.
8. Flotte TR, Zeitlin PL, Reynolds TC, et al. Phase I trail of intranasal and endobronchial administration of a recombinant adeno-associated virus serotype 2 (rAAV2)–CFTR vector in adult cystic fibrosis patients: a two-part clinical study. Hum Gene Ther 2003; 14:1079–1088.
9. Goddard CA, Ratcliff R, Anderson JR, et al. A second dose of a CFTR cDNA-liposome complex is as effective as the first dose in restoring cAMP-dependent chloride secretion to null CF mice trachea. Gene Ther 1997;4:1231–1236.

10. Rich DP, Anderson MP, Gregory JR, et al. Expression of cystic fibrosis transmembrane conductance regulator corrects defective chloride channel regulation in cystic fibrosis airway epithelial cells. Nature 1990;347:358–363.

11. Zabner J, Ramscy BW, Meeker DP, et al. Repeat administration of an adenovirus vector encoding cystic fibrosis transmembrane conductance regulator to the nasal epithelium of patients with cystic fibrosis. J Clin Invest 1996;97: 1504–1511.

12. Rich DP, Couture LA, Cardoza LM, et al. Development and analysis of recombinant adenoviruses for gene therapy of cystic fibrosis. Hum Gene Ther 1993;4:461–476.

13. Grubb BR, Pickles RJ, Ye H, et al. Inefficient gene transfer by adenovirus vector to cystic fibrosis airway epithelia of mice and humans. Nature 1994;371:8026.

14. Lei DC, Kunzelmann K, Koslowsky T, et al. Episomal expression of wild-type CFTR corrects cAMP-dependent chloride transport in respiratory epithelial cells. Gene Ther 1996;3:27–36.

15. Halbert CL, Standaert TA, Aitken ML, et al. Transduction by adeno-associated virus vectors in rabbit airway: efficiency, persistence, and readministration. J Virol 1997;71:5932–5941.

16. Goldman MJ, Lee PS, Yang JS, et al. Lentiviral vectors for gene therapy of cystic fibrosis. Hum Gene Ther 1997; 8:2261–2268.

17. Wagner JA, Messner AH, Moran ML, et al. Safety and biological efficacy of an adeno- associated virus vector-cystic fibrosis transmembrane regulator (AAV–CFTR) in the cystic fibrosis maxillary sinus. Laryngoscope 1999; 109:266–274.

18. Jiang C, O'Connor SP, Armentano D, et al. Ability of adenovirus vectors containing different CFTR transcriptional cassettes to correct ion transport defects in CF cells. Am J Physiol 1996;271:L527–L537.

19. Harvey BG, Leopold PL, Hackett NR, et al. Airway epithelial CFTR mRNA expression in cystic fibrosis patients after repetitive administration of a recombinant adenovirus. J Clin Invest 1999;104:1245–1255.

20. Olsen JC, Johnson LG, Stutts MJ, et al. Correction of the apical membrane chloride permeability defect in polarized cystic fibrosis airway epithelia following retroviral-mediated gene transfer. Hum Gene Ther 1992;3:253–266.

21. Johnson LG, Boyles SE, Wilson J, et al. Normalization of raised sodium absorption and raised calcium mediated chloride secretion by adenovirus-mediated expression of cystic fibrosis transmembrane conductance regulator in primary human cystic fibrosis airway epithelial cells. J Clin Invest 1995;95:1377–1382.

22. Noone PG, Hohneker KW, Zhou Z, et al. Safety and biological efficacy of a lipid–CFTR complex for gene transfer in the nasal epithelium of adult patients with cystic fibrosis. Mol Ther 2000;1:105–111.

23. Pickles RJ, Fahrner JA, Petrella JM, et al. Retargeting the coxsackievirus and adenovirus receptor to the apical surface of polarized epithelial cells reveals the glycocalyx as a barrier to adenovirus-mediated gene transfer. J Virol 2000;74:6050–6057.

24. Ferrari S, Geddes DM, Alton EW. Barriers to and new approaches for gene therapy and gene delivery in cystic fibrosis. Adv Drug Deliv Rev 2002;54:1373–1393.

25. Stonebreaker JR, Wagner D, Lefensty RW, et al. Glycocalyx restricts adenoviral vector access to apical receptors expressed on respiratory epithelium in vitro and in vivo: role for tethered mucins as barriers to luminal infection. J Virol 2004;78:13755–13768.

26. Greber UF, Willetts M, Webster P, et al. Stepwise dismantling of adenovirus 2 during entry into cells. Cell 1993;75: 477–486.

27. Pickles RJ. Physical and biological barriers to viral vector-mediated delivery of genes to the airway epithelium. Proc Am Thorac Soc 2004;1:302–308.

28. Duan D, Yue Y, Yan Z, et al. Polarity influences the efficiency of recombinant adeno-associated virus infection in differentiated airway epithelia. Hum Gene Ther 1998; 9:2761–2776.

29. Summerford C, Samulski RJ. Membrane-associated heparin sulfate proteoglycan is a receptor for adeno-associated virus type 2 virions. J Virol 1998;72:1438–1445.

30. Houtmmeyers E, Gosselink R, Gayan-Ramirez G, et al. Regulation of mucociliary clearance in health and disease. Eur Respir J 1999;13:1177–1188.

31. Ziady AG, Davis PB. Current prospects for gene therapy of cystic fibrosis. Curr Opin Pharmacol 2006;6:1–7.

32. Driskell RA, Engelhardt JF. Current status of gene therapy for inherited lung diseases. Annu Rev Physiol 2003;65: 585–612.

33. Weiss DJ, Pilewski JM. The status of gene therapy of cystic fibrosis. Semin Respir Crit Care Med 2003;24:749–770.

34. Parsons DW. Airway gene therapy and cystic fibrosis. J Paediatr Child Health 2004;41:94–96.

35. Ferrari S, Kitson C, Farley R, et al. Mucus altering agents as adjuncts to non-viral gene transfer to airway epithelium. Gene Ther 2001;8:1380–1386.

36. Stern M, Caplen NJ, Browning JE, et al. The effects of mucolytic agents on gene transfer across a CF sputum barrier in vitro. Gene Ther 1998;5:91–98.

37. Raczka E, Kukowsak-Latallo JF, Rymaszewski M, et al. The effect of synthetic surfactant Exosurf on gene transfer in mouse lung in vivo. Gene Ther 1998;5:1333–1339.

38. Weiss DJ, Strandjord TP, Liggitt D, et al. Perflubron enhances adenovirus-mediated gene expression in lungs of transgenic mice with chronic alveolar filling. Hum Gene Ther 1999;10:2287–2293.

39. Seiler MP, Luner P, Moninger TO, et al. Thixotropic solutions enhance viral-mediated gene transfer to airway epithelia. Am J Respir Cell Mol Biol. 2002;27:133–140.

40. Sinn PL, Shah AJ, Donovan MD, et al. Viscoelastic gel formulations enhance airway epithelial gene transfer with viral vectors. Am J Respir Cell Mol Biol 2005;32:404–410.

41. Johnson LG, Vanhook MK, Coyne CB, et al. Safety and efficiency of modulating paracellular permeability to enhance airway epithelial gene transfer in vivo. Hum Gene Ther 2003;14:729–747.

42. Bishop AE. Pulmonary epithelial stem cells. Cell Prolif 2004;37:89–96.

43. Parsons DW, Grubb BR, Johnson LG, et al. Enhanced in vivo airway gene transfer via transient modification of host barrier properties with a surface-active agent. Hum Gene Ther 1998;9:2661–2672.

44. Limberis M, Anson DS, Fuller M, et al. Recovery of airway cystic fibrosis transmembrane conductance regulator function in mice with cystic fibrosis after single-dose lentivirus-mediated gene transfer. Hum Gene Ther 2002;13:1961–1970.

45. Koehler Dr, Frndova H, Leung K, et al. Aerosol delivery of an enhanced helper-dependent adenovirus formulation to rabbit lung using an intratracheal catheter. J Gene Med 2005;7:1409–1420.

46. Seidner SR, Jobe AH, Ikegami M, et al. Lysophosphatidylcholine uptake and metabolism in the adult rabbit lung. Biochim Biophys Acta 1988;961:3228–3236.

47. Croyle MA, Cheng X, Sandhu A, et al. Development of novel formulations that enhance adenoviral-mediated gene expression in the lung in vitro and in vivo. Mol Ther 2001;4:22–28.

48. Das A, Niven R. Use of perfluorocarbon (Fluorinert) to enhance reporter gene expression following intratracheal instillation into the lungs of Balb/c mice: implications for nebulized delivery of plasmids. J Pharm Sci 2001;90:1336–1344.

49. Meng ZH, Robinson D, Jenkins RG, et al. Efficient transfection of non-proliferating human airway epithelial cells with a synthetic vector system. J Gene Med 2004;6:210–221.

50. Scott ES, Wiseman JW, Evans MJ, et al. Enhanced gene delivery to human airway epithelial cells using an integrin-targeting lipoplex. J Gene Med 2001;3125–3134.

51. Zhu N, Liggitt D, Liu Y, et al. Systemic gene expression after intravenous DNA delivery into adult mice. Science 1993;261:209–211.

52. Griesenbach U, Chonn A, Cassady R, et al. Comparison between intratracheal and intravenous administration intravenous administration of liposome–DNA complexes for cystic fibrosis lung gene therapy. Gene Ther 1998;5:181–188.

53. Koehler Dr, Hannam V, Belcastro R, et al. Targeting transgene expression for cystic fibrosis gene therapy. Mol Ther 2001;4:58–65.

54. Fenske DB, MacLachlan I, Cullis PR. Long-circulating vectors for the systemic delivery of genes. Curr Opin Mol Ther 2001;3:153–158.

55. Niidome T, Huang L. Gene therapy progress and prospects: non-viral vectors. Gene Ther 2002;9:1647–1652.

56. Lechardeur D, Sohn KJ, Haardt M, et al. Metabolic instability of plasmid DNA in the cytosol: a potential barrier to gene transfer. Gene Ther 1999;6:482–497.

57. Grosse S, Tremeau-Bravard A, Aron Y, et al. Intracellular rate-limiting steps of gene transfer using glycosylated polylysines in cystic fibrosis airway epithelial cells. Gene Ther 2002;9:1000–1007.

58. Kitson C, Angel B, Judd D, et al. The extra- and intracellular barriers to lipid and adenovirus-mediated pulmonary gene transfer in native sheep airway epithelium. Gene Ther 1999;6:534–546.

59. Cho YW, Kim JD, Park K. Polycation gene delivery systems: escape from endosomes to cytosol. J Pharm Pharmacol 2003;55:721–734.

60. Snyder EL, Dowdy SF. Protein/peptide transduction domains: potential to delivery large DNA molecules into cells. Curr Opin Mol Ther 2001;3:147–152.

61. Munkonge FM, Hillery E, Griesenbach U, et al. Isolation of a putative nuclear import DNA shuttle protein. Mol Biol Cell 1998;9:187a.

62. Brisson M, He Y, Li S, et al. A novel T7 RNA polymerase autogene for efficient cytoplasmic expression of target genes. Gene Ther 1999;6:263–270.

63. Satkauskas S, Bureau MF, Puc M, et al. Mechanisms of in vivo DNA electrotransfer: respective contributions of cell electropermeabilization and DNA electrophoresis. Mol Ther 2002;5:133–140.

64. Bigey P, Bureau MF, Scherman D. In vivo plasmid DNA electrotransfer. Curr Opin Biotechnol 2002;13:443–447.

65. Dean DA, Machado-Aranda D, Blair-Parks K, et al. Electroporation as a method for high-level non-viral gene transfer to the lung. Gene Ther 2003;10:1608–1615.

66. Pringle IA, Davies LA, McLachlan G, et al. Duration of reporter gene expression from naked DNA in the mouse lung following direct electroporation and development of wire electrodes for sheep lung electroporation studies. Mol Ther 2004;9:S1–S56.

67. Machado-Aranda D, Adir Y, Young JL, et al. Gene transfer of the Na⁺, K⁺-ATPase β1 subunit using electroporation increases lung liquid clearance. Am J Respir Crit Care Med 2005;171:204–211.

68. Machet L, Boucaud A. Phonophoresis: efficiency, mechanisms and skin tolerance. Int J Pharm 2002;243:1–115.

69. Miller DL, Pislaru SV, Greenleaf JE. Sonoporation: mechanical DNA delivery by ultrasonic cavitation. Somat Cell Mol Genet 2002;27:115–134.

70. Kim HJ, Greenleaf JF, Kinnick R, et al. Ultrasound-mediated transfection of mammalian cells. Hum Gene Ther 1996;7:1339–1346.

71. Manome Y, Nakamura M, Ohno T, et al. Ultrasound facilitates transduction of naked plasmid DNA into colon carcinoma cells in vitro and in vivo. Hum Gene Ther 2000;11:1521–1528.

72. Amabile PG, Waugh JM, Lewis TN, et al. High-efficiency endovascular gene delivery via therapeutic ultrasound. J Am Coll Cardiol 2001;37:1975–1980.

73. Scherer F, Anton M, Schillinger U, et al. Magnetofection: enhancing and targeting gene delivery by magnetic force in vitro and in vivo. Gene Ther 2002;9:102–109.

74. Gersting SW, Schillinger U, Lausier J, et al. Gene delivery to respiratory epithelial cells by magnetofection. J Gene Med 2004;6:913–922.

75. Gill DR, Smyth SE, Goddard CA, et al. Increased persistence of lung gene expression using plasmids containing the ubiquitin C or elongation factor 1alpha promoter. Gene Ther 2001;8:1539–1546.

76. Warburton D, Wuenschell C, Flores-Delgado G, et al. Commitment and differentiation of lung cell lineages. Biochem Cell Biol 1998;76:971–995.

77. Yant SR, Meuse L, chu W, et al. Somatic integration and long-term transgene expression in normal and haemophilic mice using a DNA transposon system. Nature Genet 2000; 25:35–41.

78. Hacien-Bey-Abiina S, von Kalle C, Schmidt M, et al. A serious adverse event after successful gene therapy for X-linked severe combined immunodeficiency. N Engl J Med 2003;348:255–256.

79. Worgall S, Leopold PL, Wolff G, et al. role of alveolar macrophages in rapid elimination of adenovirus vectors administered to the epithelial surface of the respiratory tract. Hum Gene Ther 1997;8:175–184.

80. Plank C, Mechtler K, Szoka FC Jr, et al. Activation of the complement system by synthetic DNA complexes: a potential barrier for intravenous gene delivery. Hum Gene Ther 1996;7:1437–1446.

81. Welsh MJ, Smith AE. Molecular mechanisms of CFTR chloride channel dysfunction in cystic fibrosis. Cell 1993;73:1251–1254.

82. Rommens JM, Iannuzzi MC, Kerem B, et al. Identification of the cystic fibrosis gene: chromosome walking and jumping. Science 989;245:1059–1065.

83. Hyde SC, Emsley P, Hartshorn MJ, et al. Structural model of ATP-binding proteins associated with cystic fibrosis, multidrug resistance and bacterial transport. Nature 1990;346:362–365.

84. Akabas MH. Cystic fibrosis transmembrane conductance regulator. Structure and function of an epithelial chloride channel. J Biol Chem 2000;275:3729–3732.

85. Stutts MJ, Canessa CM, Olsen JC, et al. CFTR as a cAMP dependent regulator of sodium channels. Science 1995;269:847–850.

86. Metha A. CFTR: more than just a chloride channel. Pediatr Pulmonol 2005;39:292–298.

87. Kogan I, Ramjeesingh M, Li C, et al. CFTR directly mediates nucleotide-regulated glutathione flux. EMBO J 2004;1981–1989.

88. Hudson VM. New insights into the pathogenesis of cystic fibrosis: pivotal role of glutathione system dysfunction and implications for therapy. Treat Respir Med 2004;3:353–363.

89. Coakley RD, Grubb BR, Paradiso AM, et al. Abnormal surface liquid pH regulation by cultured cystic fibrosis bronchial epithelium. Proc Natl Acad Sci USA 2003;100:16083–16088.

90. Song Y, Salinas D, Nielson DW, et al. Hyperacidity of secreted fluid from submucosal glands in early cystic fibrosis. Am J Physiol Cell Physiol 2006;290:C741–C749.

91. Armstrong DS, Grimwood K, Carzino R, et al. Lower respiratory infection and inflammation in infants with newly diagnosed cystic fibrosis. BMJ 1995;310:1571–1572.

92. Kreda SM, Mall M, Mengos A, et al. Characterization of wild-type and deltaF508 cystic fibrosis transmembrane regulator in human respiratory epithelia. Mol Biol Cell 2005;16:2154–2167.

93. Tarran R, Grubb BR, Parsons D, et al. The CF salt controversy: in vivo observations and therapeutic approaches. Mol Cell 2001;8:149–158.

94. Klink D, Schindelhauer D, Laner A, et al. Gene delivery systems—gene therapy vectors for cystic fibrosis. J Cystic Fibrosis 2004;3:203–212.

95. Johnson LG, Olsen JC, Sarkadi B, et al. Efficiency of gene transfer for restoration of normal airway epithelial function in cystic fibrosis. Nat Genet 1992;2:21–25.

96. Farmen SL, Karp PH, Ng P, et al. Gene transfer of CFTR to airway epithelia: low levels of expression are sufficient to correct Cl- transport and overexpression can generate basolateral CFTR. Am J Physiol Lung Cell Mol Physiol 2005;289:L1123–L1130.

97. Boucher RC. Status of gene therapy for cystic fibrosis lung disease. J Clin Invest 1999;103:441–445.

98. Chu CS, Trapnell BC, Curristin SM, et al. Extensive posttranscriptional deletion of the coding sequences for part of nucleotide-binding fold 1 in respiratory epithelial mRNA transcripts of the cystic fibrosis transmembrane conductance regulator gene is not associated with the clinical manifestations of cystic fibrosis. J Clin Invest 1992;90:785–790.

99. Trapnell BC, Chu CS, Paakko PK, et al. Expression of the cystic fibrosis transmembrane conductance regulator gene in the respiratory tract of normal individuals and individuals with cystic fibrosis. Proc Natl Acad Sci USA 1991;88:6565–6569.

100. O'Dea S, Harrison DJ. CFTR gene transfer to lung epithelium—on the trail of a target cell. Curr Gene Ther 2002;2:173–181.

101. Griesenbach U, Geddes DM, Alton EWFW. Advances in cystic fibrosis gene therapy. Curr Opin Pulm Med 2004;10:542–546.

102. Engelhardt JF, Yankaskas JR, Ernst SA, et al. Submucosal glands are the predominant site of CFTR expression in the human bronchus. Nature Genet 1992;2:240–248.

103. Engelhardt JF, Zepeda M, Cohn JA, et al. Expression of the cystic fibrosis gene in adult human lung. J Clin Invest 1994;93:737–749.

104. Brochiero E, Dagenais A, Prive A, et al. Evidence of a functional CFTR Cl(−) channel in adult alveolar epithelial cells. Am J Physiol Lung Cell Mol Physiol 2004;287:L382–L392.

105. Borthwick DW, Shahbazian M, Krantz QT, et al. Evidence for stem-cell niches in the tracheal epithelium. Am J Respir Cell Mol Biol 2001;24:662–670.

106. Hong KU, Reynolds SD, Giangreco A, et al. Clara cell secretory protein-expressing cells of the airway neuroepithelial body microenvironment include a label-retaining subset and are critical for epithelial renewal after progenitor cell depletion. Am J Respir Cell Mol Biol 2001;24:671–681.

107. Hong KU, Reynolds SD, Watkins S, et al. Basal cells are a multipotent progenitor capable of renewing the bronchial epithelium. Am J Pathol 2004;164:577–588.

108. Giangreco A, Reynolds SD, Stripp Br. Terminal bronchioles harbor a unique airway stem cell population that localizes to the bronchoalveolar duct junction. Am J Pathol 2002;161:173–182.

109. Reddy R, Buckley S, Doerken M, et al. Isolation of a putative progenitor subpopulation of alveolar epithelial type 2 cells. Am J Physiol Lung Cell Mol Physiol 2004;286:L658–L667.

110. Wang G, Bunnell BA, Painter RG, et al. Adult stem cells from bone marrow stroma differentiate into airway epithelial cells: potential therapy for cystic fibrosis. Proc Natl Acad Sci USA 2005;102:186–191.

111. Kotton DN, Ma BY, Cardoso WV, et al. Bone marrow-derived cells as progenitors of lung alveolar epithelium. Development 2001;1128:5181–5188.

112. Krause DS, Theise ND, Collector MI, et al. Multi-organ, multi-lineage engraftment by a single bone marrow-derived stem cell. Cell 2001;105:369–377.

113. Kleeberger W, Versmold A, Rothamel T, et al. Increased chimerism of bronchial and alveolar epithelium in human lung allografts undergoing chronic injury. Am J Pathol 2003;162:1487–1494.

114. Gan KH, Veeze HJ, van den Ouweland AM, et al. A cystic fibrosis mutation associated with mild lung disease. N Engl J Med 1995;333:95–99.

115. Cutting GR. What we have learned from correlating genotype to phenotype. Pediatr Pulmonol 2004;S27:94.

116. Alton EWFW, Stern M, Farley R, et al. Cationic lipid-mediated CFTR gene transfer to the lungs and nose of patients with cystic fibrosis: a double-blind placebo-controlled trial. Lancet 1999;353:947–954.

117. Middleton PG, Geddes DM, Alton EWFW. Protocols for in vivo measurement of the ion transport defects in cystic fibrosis nasal epithelium. Eur Respir J 1994;7:2050–2056.

118. Knowles M, Gatzy J, Boucher R. Increased bioelectric potential difference across respiratory epithelia in cystic fibrosis. N Engl J Med 1981;305:1489–1495.

119. Stern M, Munkonge FM, Caplen NJ, et al. Quantitative fluorescence measurements of chloride secretion in native airway epithelium from CF and non-CF subjects. Gene Ther 1995;2:766–774.

120. Caplen NJ, Alton EW, Middleton PG, et al. Liposome-mediated CFTR gene transfer to the nasal epithelium of patients with cystic fibrosis. Nature Med 1995;1:39–46.

121. Gill DR, Southern DW, Mofford KA, et al. A placebo-controlled study of liposome-mediated gene transfer to the nasal epithelium of patients with cystic fibrosis. Gene Ther 1997;4:199–209.

122. Knowles MR, Noone PG, Hohneker K, et al. A double-blind, placebo controlled, dose ranging study to evaluate the safety and biological efficacy of the lipid–DNA complex GR213487B in the nasal epithelium of adult patients with cystic fibrosis. Hum Gene Ther 1998;9:249–269.

123. Porteous DJ, Dorin JR, McLachlan GK, et al. Evidence for safety and efficacy of DOTAP cationic liposome mediated CFTR gene transfer to the nasal epithelium of patients with cystic fibrosis. Gene Ther 1997;4:210–218.

124. Sorscher EJ, Logan JJ, Frizzell RA, et al. Gene therapy for cystic fibrosis using cationic liposome mediated gene transfer: a phase I trail of safety and efficacy in the nasal airway. Hum Gene Ther 1994;5:1259–1277.

125. Chadwick SL, Kingston HD, Stern M, et al. Safety of a single aerosol administration of escalating doses of the cationic lipid GL-67/DOPE/DMPE-PEG$_{5000}$ formulation to the lungs of normal volunteers. Gene Ther 1997;4:937–942.

126. Ruiz FE, Clancy JP, Perricone MA, et al. A clinical inflammatory syndrome attributable to aerosolized lipid-DNA administration in cystic fibrosis. Hum Gene Ther 2001;12:751–761.

127. Hyde SC, Southern KW, Gileadi U, et al. Repeat administration of DNA/liposomes to the nasal epithelium of patients with cystic fibrosis. Gene Ther 2000;7:1156–1165.

128. Konstan MW, Wagener JS, Hilliard KA, et al. Single dose escalation study to evaluate safety of nasal administration of CFTR001 gene transfer vector to subjects with cystic fibrosis. 2003;7:S386.

129. Perricone MA, Recs DD, Sacks CR, et al. Inhibitory effect of cystic fibrosis sputum on adenovirus-mediated gene transfer in cultured epithelial cells. Hum Gene Ther 2000;11:1997–2008.

130. Sanders NN, De Smedt SC, Van Rompaey E, et al. Cystic fibrosis sputum: a barrier to the transport of nanospheres. Am J Respir Crit Care Med 2000;162:1905–1911.

131. Virella-Lowell I, Poirer A, Chesnut KA, et al. Inhibition of recombinant adeno-associated virus (rAAV) transduction by bronchial secretions from cystic fibrosis patients. Gene Ther 2000;7:1783–1789.

132. Van Heeckeren A, Ferkol T, Tosi M. Effects of bronchopulmonary inflammation induced by pseudomonas aeruginosa on adenovirus-mediated gene transfer to airway epithelial cells in mice. Gene Ther 1998;5:345–351.

133. Flotte TR, Schwiebert EM, Zeitlin PL, et al. Correlation between DNA transfer and cystic fibrosis airway epithelial cell correction after recombinant adeno-associated virus serotype 2 gene therapy. Hum Gene Ther 2005;16:921–928.

134. Flotte TR. Recent developments in recombinant AAV-mediated gene therapy for lung diseases. Curr Gene Ther 2005;5:361–366.

135. Griesenbach U, Geddes DM, Alton EW. Update on gene therapy for cystic fibrosis. Curr Opin Mol Ther 2003;5:489–494.

136. Ziady AG, Davis PB, Konstan MW. Non-viral gene transfer therapy for cystic fibrosis. Exp Opin Biol Ther 2003;3:449–458.

137. Zabner J, Cheng SH, Meeker D, et al. Comparison of DNA–lipid complexes and DNA alone for gene transfer to cystic fibrosis airway epithelial in vivo. J Clin Invest 1997;100:1529–1537.

138. Glasspool-Malone J, Steenland PR, McDonald RJ, et al. DNA transfection of macaque and murine respiratory tissue is greatly enhanced by use of a nuclease inhibitor. J Gene Med 2002;4:323–332.

139. Ziady AG, Gedeon Cr, Miller T, et al. Transfection of airway epithelium by stable PEGylated poly-L-lysine DNA nanoparticles in vivo. Mol Ther 2003;8:936–947.

140. Flotte TR, Laube BL. Gene therapy in cystic fibrosis. Chest 2001;120:124S–131S.

141. Ferrari S, Griesenbach U, Shiraki-Iida T, et al. A defective nontransmissible recombinant Sendai virus mediates efficient gene transfer to airway epithelium in vivo. Gene Ther 2004;11:1659–1664.

142. Zhang L, Peeples ME, Boucher RC, et al. Respiratory syncytial virus infection of human airway epithelial cells is polarized, specific to ciliated cells, and without obvious cytopathology. J Virol 2002;76:5654–666.

143. Yonemitsu Y, Kitson C, Ferrari S, et al. Efficient gene transfer to airway epithelium using recombinant Sendai virus. Nat Biotechnol 2000;18:970–973.

144. Zhang L, Bukreyev A, Thompson CI, et al. Infection of ciliated cells by human parainfluenza virus type 3 in an

in vitro model of human airway epithelium. J Virol 2005;
79:1113–1124.

145. Griesenbach U, Boyton RJ, Somerton L, et al. Effect of
tolerance induction to immunodominant T-cell epitopes
of Sendai virus on gene expression following repeat administration to lung. Gene Ther 2006;13:449–456.

146. Wiseman JW, Scott ES, Shaw PA, et al. Enhancement of
gene delivery to human airway epithelial cells in vitro
using a peptide from the polyoma virus protein VP_1.
J Gene Med 2005;7:759–770.

147. Jenke AC, Stehle IM, Herrmann F, et al. Nuclear scaf-
fold/matrix attached region modules linked to a transcription unit are sufficient for replication and maintenance of
a mammalian episome. Proc Natl Acad Sci USA 2004;101:
11322–11327.

148. Glover DH, Lipps HJ, Jans DA. Towards safe, non-viral
therapeutic gene expression in humans. Nat Rev Genet
2005;6:299–310.

149. Konstan MW, Davis PB, Wagener JS, et al. Compacted
DNA nanoparticles administered to the nasal mucosa of
cystic fibrosis subjects are safe and demonstrate partial to
complete cystic fibrosis transmembrane regulator reconstitution. Hum Gene Ther 2004;15:1255–1269.

150. McCarty DM, Young SM Jr, Samulski RJ. Integration of
adeno-associated virus (AAV) and recombinant AAV
vectors. Annu Rev Genet 2004;38:819–845.

151. Flotte TR. Gene therapy progress and prospects: recombinant adeno-associated virus (rAAV) vectors. Gene Ther
2004;11:805–810.

152. Schnepp BC, Jensen RL, Chen CL, et al. Characterization
of adeno-associated virus genomes isolated from human
tissues. J Virol 2005;79:14793–14803.

153. Zhang L, Wang D, Fischer H, et al. Efficient expression
of CFTR function with adeno-associated virus vectors that
carry shortened CFTR genes. Proc Natl Acad Sci USA
1998;95:10158–10163.

154. Sirninger J, Muller C, Braag S, et al. Functional characterization of a recombinant adeno-associated virus 5-pseudo-
typed cystic fibrosis transmembrane conductance regulator
vector. Hum Gene Ther 2004;15:832–841.

155. Ostedgaard LS, Rokhlina T, Karp PH, et al. A shortened
adeno-associated virus expression cassette for CFTR gene
transfer to cystic fibrosis airway epithelia. Proc NatlAcad
Sci USA 2005;102:2952–2957.

156. Zabner J, Seiler M, Walters R, et al. Adeno-associated
virus type 5 (AAV5) but not AAV2 binds to the apical
surfaces of airway epithelia and facilitates gene transfer. J
Virol 2000;74:3852–3858.

157. Virella-Lowell I, Zusman B, Foust K, et al. Enhancing
rAAV vector expression in the lung. J Gene Med 2005;7:
842–850.

158. Walters RW, Yi SM, Keshavjee S, et al. Binding of adeno-
associated virus type 5 to 2,3- linked sialic acid is required
for gene transfer. J Biol Chem 2001;276:20610–20616.

159. Weiss DJ, Bonneau L, Allen JM, et al. Perfluorochemical
liquid enhances adeno-associated virus–mediated transgene expression in lungs. Mol Ther 2000;2:624–630.

160. Duan D, Yue Y, Yan Z, et al. Endosomal processing limits
gene transfer to polarized airway epithelia by adeno-
associated virus. J Clin Invest 2000;105:1573–1587.

161. Flotte TR. Adeno-associated virus-based gene therapy for
inherited disorders. Pediatr Res 2005;58:1143–1147.

162. Conrad CK, Allen SS, Afione SA, et al. Safety of single-
dose administration of an adeno-associated virus (AAV)–
CFTR vector in the primate lung. Gene Ther 1996;3:
658–668.

163. Afione SA, Conrad CK, Kearns WG, et al. In vivo model
of adeno-associated virus vector persistence and rescue.
J Virol 1996;70:3235–3241.

164. Flotte TR, Afione SA, Zeitlin PL. Adeno-associated virus
vector gene expression occurs in nondividing cells in the
absence of vector DNA integration. Am J Respir Cell Mol
Biol 1994;11:517–521.

165. Flotte TR, Afione SAS, Conrad C, et al. Stable in vivo
expression of the cystic fibrosis transmembrane conductance regulator with an adeno-associated virus vector.
Proc Natl Acad Sci USA 1993;90:10613–10617.

166. Wagner JA, Nepomuseno IB, Messner AH, et al. A phase
II, double-blind, randomized, placebo-controlled clinical
trial of tgAAVCF using maxillary sinus delivery in patients
with cystic fibrosis with antrostomies. Hum Gene Ther
2002;13:1349–1359.

167. Flotte TR, Brantly ML, Spencer LT, et al. Phase I trial of
intramuscular injection of a recombinant adeno-
associated virus alpha 1-antitrypsin (rAAV2-CB-hAAT)
gene vector to AAT-deficient adults. Hum Gene Ther
2002;13:1349–1359.

168. Moss RB, Rodman D, Spencer LT, et al. Repeated adeno-
associated virus serotype 2 aerosol-mediated cystic fibrosis
transmembrane regulator gene transfer to the lungs of
patients with cystic fibrosis: a multicenter, double-blind,
placebo-controlled trial. Chest 2004;125:509–521.

169. Liu X, Luo M, Zhang LN, et al. Spliceosome-mediated
RNA trans–splicing with recombinant adeno-associated
virus partially restores cystic fibrosis transmembrane
conductance regulator function to polarized human cystic
fibrosis airway epithelial cells. Hum Gene Ther 2005;16:
1116–1123.

170. Halbert CL, Miller AD, McNamera S, et al. Prevalence of
neutralizing antibodies against adeno-associated virus
(AAV) types 2, 5, and 6 in cystic fibrosis and normal populations: implications for gene therapy using AAV vectors.
Hum Gene Ther 2006;17:440–447.

171. Naldini L, Blomer U, Gallay P, et al. In vivo gene delivery
and stable transduction of nondividing cells by a lentiviral
vector. Science 1996;272:263–267.

172. Olsen JC. Gene transfer vectors derived from equine
infectious anemia virus. Gene Ther 1998;5:1481–1487.

173. Poeschla EM, Wong-Staal F, Looney DJ. Efficient transduction of nondividing human cells by feline immunodeficiency virus lentiviral vectors. Nat Med 1998;4:354–
357.

174. Copreni E, Penzo M, Carrabinio S, et al. Lentivirus-
mediated gene transfer to the respiratory epithelium: a
promising approach to gene therapy of cystic fibrosis.
Gene Ther 2004;11:S67–S75.

175. Kobayashi M, Iida A, Ueda Y, et al. Pseudotyped lentivi-
rus vectors derived from simian immunodeficiency virus
SIVagm with envelope glycoproteins from paramyxovirus.
J Virol 2003;77:2607–2614.

176. Kobinger GP, Weiner DJ, Yu QC, et al. Filovirus-pseudo-typed lentiviral vector can efficiently and stably transducer airway epithelia in vivo. Nat Biotechnol 2001;19:225–230.

177. Anson DS. The use of retroviral vectors for gene therapy-what are the risks? A review of retroviral pathogenesis and its relevance to retroviral vector–mediated gene delivery. Genet Vaccines Ther 2004;2:9.

178. Alton EWFW. Use of nonviral vectors for cystic fibrosis gene therapy. Proc Am Thorac Soc 2004;1:296–301.

179. Montier T, Delepine P, Pichon C, et al. Non-viral vectors in cystic fibrosis gene therapy: progress and challenges. Trends Biotechnol 2004;22:586–592.

180. Yew NS, Wang KX, Przybylska M, et al. Contribution of plasmid DNA to inflammation in the lung after administration of cationic lipid:pDNA complexes. Hum Gene Ther 1999;10:223–234.

181. Pison U, Welte T, Giersig M, et al. Nanomedicine for respiratory diseases. Eur J Pharmacol 2006;533:341–350.

182. Weiss DJ. Delivery of DNA to lung airway epithelium. Methods Mol Biol 2004;246:53–68.

183. Kinsey BM, Densmore CL, Orson FM. Non-viral gene delivery to the lungs. Curr Gene Ther 2005;5:181–194.

184. Sanders NN, De Smedt SC, Cheng SH, et al. PEGylated GL67 lipoplexes retain their gene transfection activity after exposure to components of CF mucus. Gene Ther 2002;9:363–371.

185. Ziady AG, Gedeon Cr, Muhammad O, et al. Minimal toxicity of stabilized compacted DNA in the murine lung. Mol Ther 2003;8:948–956.

186. Griesenbach U, Boyd AC. Pre-clinical endpoint assays for cystic fibrosis gene therapy. J Cystic Fibrosis 2005;4:89–100.

187. Amaral MD, Clarke LA, Ramalho AS, et al. Quantitative methods for the analysis of CFTR transcripts/splicing variants. J Cystic Fibrosis 2004;3:17–23.

188. Waterhouse JE, Harbottle RP, Keller M, et al. Synthesis and application of integrin targeting lipopeptides in targeted gene delivery. Chem Biochem 2005;6:1212–1223.

189. Stecenko AA, Brigham KL. Gene therapy progress and prospects: alpha-1-antitrypsin. Gene Ther 2003;10:95–99.

190. Coakley RJ, Taggart C, O'Neil S, et al. Alpha-1-antitrypsin deficiency: biological answers to clinical questions. Am J Med Sci 2001;321:33–41.

191. Crystal RG. The alpha 1-antitrypsin gene and its deficiency states. Trends Genet 1989;5:411–417.

192. Pierce JA. Alpha 1-antitrypsin augmentation therapy. Chest 1997;112:872–874.

193. Rosenfeld MA, Siegfried W, Yoshimura K, et al. Adenovirus-mediated transfer of a recombinant alpha1-antitrypsin gene to the lung epithelium in vivo. Science 1991;252:431–434.

194. Canonico AE, Corary JT, Meyrick BO, et al. Aerosol and intravenous transfection of human alpha 1-antigrypsin gene to lungs of rabbits. Am J Respir Cell Mol Biol 1994;10:24–29.

195. Brigham KL, Lane KB, Meyrick B, et al. Transfection of nasal mucosa with a normal alpha 1-antitrypsin gene in alpha 1-antitrypsin deficient subjects: comparison with protein therapy. Hum Gene Ther 2000;11:1023–1032.

196. Chao H, Liu Y, Rabinowitz J, et al. Several log increase in therapeutic transgene deliver by distinct adeno-associated viral serotype vectors. Mol Ther 2000;2:619–623.

197. Poirier A, Campbell-Thompson M, Tang Q, et al. Toxicology and biodistribution studies of a recombinant adeno-associated virus 2-alpha-1 antitrypsin vector. Preclinica 2004;2:43–51.

198. Song S, Lu Y, Choi YK, et al. DNA-dependent PK inhibits adeno-associated virus DNA integration. Proc Natl Acad Sci USA 2004;101:2112–2116.

199. Song S, Laipis PJ, Berns KI, et al. Effect of DNA-dependent protein kinase on the molecular fate of the rAAV2 genome in skeletal muscle. Proc Natl Acad Sci USA 2001;98:4084–4088.

200. Weinacker AB, Vaszar LT. Acute respiratory distress syndrome: physiology and new management strategies. Ann Rev Med 2001;52:221–237.

201. Conary JT, Parker RE, Christman BW, et al. Protection of rabbit lungs from endotoxin injury by in vivo hyper-expression of the prostaglandin G/H synthase gene. J Clin Invest 1994;93:1834–1840.

202. Stern M, Ulrich K, Robinson C, et al. Pretreatment with cationic lipid-mediated transfer of the Na+K+-TPase pump in a mouse model in vivo augments resolution of high permeability pulmonary oedema. Gene Ther 2000;7:960–966.

203. Lee NA, Gelfand EW, Lee JJ. Pulmonary T cells and eosinophils: co-conspirators or independent triggers of allergic respiratory pathology? J Allergy Clin Immunol 2001;107:945–957.

204. Suissa S, Ernst P. Inhaled corticosteroids: impact on asthma morbidity and mortality. J Allergy Clin Immunol 2001;107:937–944.

205. Lee YL, Ye L, Yu CI, et al. Construction of single-chain interleukin-12 DNA plasmid to treat airway hyperresponsiveness in an animal model of asthma. Hum Gene Ther 2001;12:2065–2079.

206. del Pozo V, Rojo M, Rubio ML, et al. Gene therapy with galectin-3 inhibits bronchial obstruction and inflammation in antigen-challenged rats through interleukin-5 gene down regulation. Am J Respir Crit Care Med 2002;166:732–737.

207. Fonseca C, Abraham D, Black CM. Lung fibrosis. Spring Semin Immunopathol 1999;21:453–474.

208. Sime PJ, O'Reilly KM. Fibrosis of the lung and other tissues: new concepts in pathogenesis and treatments. Clin Immunol 2001;99:308–319.

209. Epperly WM, Silora CA, DeFilippi SJ, et al. Pulmonary irradiation-induced expression of VCAM-1 and ICAM-1 is decreased by manganese superoxide dismutase- plasmid/liposome (MnSOD-PL) gene therapy. Biol Blood Marrow Transplant 2002;8:175–187.

210. Ziesche R, Hofbauer E, Wittmann K, et al. A preliminary study of long-term treatment with interferon gamma-1b and low-dose prednisolone in patients with idiopathic pulmonary fibrosis. N Engl J Med 1999;341:1264–1269.

211. Kuwano K, Hagimoto N, Kawasaki M, et al. Essential roles of the Fas-Fas ligand pathway in the development of pulmonary fibrosis. J Clin Invest 1999;104:13–19.

Section 7
Molecular Pathology of Other Nonneoplastic Pulmonary Diseases: Specific Entities

49
Smoking-Related Lung Diseases

Manuel G. Cosio and Helmut H. Popper

Effects of Tobacco Smoke on the Respiratory Tract

Tobacco smoking results in inhalation of various amounts of toxins, which can induce a wide variety of effects on different cell systems in the respiratory tract. The toxins are acidic as well as basic; heat additionally harms the respiratory tract. However, there is also a protective system working, which can reduce the effects of this toxic inhalation. We discuss the toxic effects of tobacco substances, briefly review the protective system, and finally focus on nontumorous tobacco smoke–induced lung diseases.

Most reports mainly focus on the oncogenic effects of tobacco smoke products. It is generally not mentioned that prior to an oncogenic effect there is usually a toxic effect with cell death, inflammation, and repair. Activation of proliferation and angiogenesis also affect normal cells and as such exert changes in the lung structure and cellular constituents and might affect matrix proteins long before the development of precancerous lesions starts.

Effects of Toxins

Among the more than 5,000 compounds in tobacco smoke are carcinogens such as nitrosamines, irritants such as phenolic compounds, volatiles such as carbon monoxide, different metal oxides in part depending on the location and the nutrition of the tobacco plants, and of course nicotine. Nicotine itself has quite complex actions, mediated in part by nicotinic cholinergic receptors that may have extraneuronal as well as neuronal distribution. Nicotine is a potent angiogenic agent. Nicotine hijacks an endogenous nicotinic cholinergic pathway present in endothelial cells that is involved in physiologic as well as pathologic angiogenesis.[1] Zhu and coworkers demonstrated that environmental tobacco smoke results in tumor angiogenesis and provide evidence that the responsible factor in environmental tobacco smoke is nicotine.[2] Although a weak carcinogen, nicotine promotes carcinogenesis by a number of different mechanisms.[2]

The most toxic substances are within the vapor phase of tobacco sidestream smoke and cause respiratory epithelium damage.[3] Many tobacco smoke constituents are potent inducers of oxygen radicals, thus causing DNA strand breaks, DNA adducts, oxidative DNA damage, chromosome aberrations, and micronuclei formation.[4] They can also affect the mitotic spindle apparatus and influence the methylation of promoter regions of tumor suppressor genes.[5-8] Multiple different compounds have been identified in tobacco main- and sidestream smoke, including tar (in filterless cigarettes), polycyclic aromatic hydrocarbons (PAHs), N-nitrosamines, many different N-nitroso compounds such as butanones and anatabines, and volatile N-nitrosamines. Just within PAHs, 150 different substances have been identified.[9] In addition, many metal oxides are generated during tobacco burning, such as chromium, cadmium, and arsenic oxides. Many of these can either generate oxygen radicals themselves or act as catalyzing agents in concert with nitroso compounds in generating radicals. Depending on environmental contamination, many other unusual metals can occur (e.g., lead contaminating tobacco plants grown close to highways).[10-12] Zaridze et al.[13] and Stabbert et al.[14] provide comprehensive lists of tobacco constituents; others can be found on the website of the International Agency for Cancer Research at http://www-cie.iarc.fr/monoeval/grlist.html. For some of these components, the mechanisms of their toxic and carcinogenic action have been elucidated.

Nitrosamine 4-(methylnitrosamino)-1-(3-pyridyl)-1-butanone (NNK) is formed by nitrosation of nicotine, and NNK simultaneously stimulates Bcl-2 and c-Myc phosphorylation through activation of both ERK1/2 and protein kinase Cα, which is required for NNK-induced survival and proliferation. Phosphorylation of Bcl-2 promotes a direct interaction between Bcl-2 and c-Myc in the nucleus and on the outer mitochondrial membrane that significantly enhances the half-life of the c-Myc protein. Thus, NNK induce a functional cooperation of Bcl-2 and c-Myc in promoting cell survival and proliferation.[15]

Nicotine and NNK activate the Akt pathway and increase cell proliferation and survival. Nicotinic activation of Akt increases phosphorylation of multiple downstream substrates of Akt in a time-dependent manner, including GSK-3, FKHR, tuberin, mTOR and p70S6K1. Nicotine or NNK binds to cell surface nicotinic acetylcholine receptors. Only nicotine decreased apoptosis. Protection conferred by nicotine was nuclear factor-κB (NF-κB) dependent. Collectively, these results identify tobacco component–induced, Akt-dependent proliferation and NF-κB–dependent survival of cancer cells.[16]

Carcinogenic Effects

In 1950, the first large-scale epidemiologic studies demonstrated that lung cancer is causatively associated with cigarette smoking. Although cigarette consumption has gradually decreased in most industrialized countries, death from lung cancer has reached a high among males and females. In the younger cohorts, the lung cancer death rate is decreasing in both men and women. On the contrary, a steeper increase in lung adenocarcinoma incidence is seen in recent decades. Contributors to this change in the histologic types of lung cancer are a decrease in average nicotine and tar delivery of cigarettes from about 2.7 and 38 mg, respectively, in 1955 to 1.0 and 13.5 mg in 1993. Other major factors relate to changes in the composition of the cigarette tobacco blend and to general acceptance of cigarettes with filter tips. Smokers compensate for the lowered nicotine content by inhaling the smoke more deeply and by smoking more intensely. Under these conditions, the peripheral lung is exposed to increased amounts of smoke carcinogens that are suspected to lead to lung adenocarcinoma. Importantly, because of the efficacy of the filters, particulate matter with bound carcinogens are withheld in the filters, but vaporized toxins and carcinogens are enriched in the tobacco smoke and delivered to the alveolar periphery. Among the important changes in the composition of the tobacco blend is a significant increase in nitrate content (from 0.5% to 1.2%–1.5%), which raises the yields of nitrogen oxides and N-nitrosamines in the smoke. Furthermore, the more intense smoking by the consumers of low-yield cigarettes increases N-nitrosamines in the smoke two- to threefold. Among the N-nitrosamines is NNK (see earlier), a powerful lung carcinogen in animals that is exclusively formed from nicotine. This organ-specific tobacco-specific nitrosamine induces adenocarcinoma of the lung.[17]

The effect of using filters has been evaluated in animal experiments. Mice were exposed to either full tobacco smoke or to filtered tobacco smoke devoid of particulate matter. Analysis of the filtered smoke showed reduced concentrations of PAHs and tobacco smoke–specific nitrosamines below 18%. Aldehydes and other volatile organic compounds such as 1,3-butadiene, benzene, and acrolein were not as much reduced (about 50%–90%). Some potentially carcinogenic metals reached levels in filtered smoke ranging from 77% to less than 1%. However, mice exposed to the filtered smoke atmosphere had practically identical lung tumor multiplicities and incidences as did the animals exposed to full smoke. The authors concluded that 1,3-butadiene might be an important contributor to lung tumorigenesis in this mouse model of tobacco smoke carcinogenesis.[18]

Temperature

Inhaled tobacco smoke is usually hot, with the temperature ranging between 400° and 800°C at the tip of the cigarette. When tobacco smoke aerosols are generated at 250° to 550°C, there are no mutagenic components below the generator temperature of 400°C, but mutagens are found above this temperature. This underlines the importance of the pyrolysis temperature.[19] The pyrolysis of tobacco depends on different conditions, including temperature and pH of the substances, such as hydrogen cyanide, benzo[a]pyrene, aldehydes, volatile organic compounds, phenolics, and aromatic amines. A few compounds are significantly affected by the pH.[20] The temperature of the inhaled smoke condensate on reaching the distal airways is still over 60°C.

Tobacco smoke, especially sidestream smoke, contains a high amount of fine dust. Particles below the PM10 type (fine dust, respirable size <5 μm) are thought to impact on genotoxicity as well as on cell proliferation via their ability to generate oxidants such as reactive oxygen species (ROS) and reactive nitrogen species (RNS). For mechanistic purposes, one should discriminate between (1) the oxidant-generating properties of the particles themselves (i.e., acellular), which are mostly determined by the physicochemical characteristics of the particle surface, and (2) the ability of particles to stimulate cellular oxidant generation. Because particles can induce an inflammatory response, a further subdivision needs to be made between primary (i.e., particle driven) and secondary (i.e., inflammation driven) formation of oxidants. Particles may also affect genotoxicity by their ability to carry surface-adsorbed carcinogenic components into the lung. Each of these pathways can impact on genotoxicity and proliferation, as well as on feedback mechanisms involving DNA repair or apoptosis.[21] It should be remembered that toxins and carcinogens such as NNK bound to the surface of PM2.5 not only reach the alveolar periphery but also, because of the surface activity and the low degrading rate, can act much longer on the epithelial cells.

From studies of mutations of the *TP53* gene, which usually precede the development of dysplasia as well as carcinomas but can be found in normal-appearing epithelial cells, it has become clear that many of the different tobacco carcinogens leave behind their specific "fingerprint" by interacting specifically with some genes within the cell cycle.[22]

Other Factors Relevant for the Action of Toxic and Carcinogenic Substances/Particles

The architecture of the human bronchial system is another site of modification caused by inhaled substances, especially tobacco smoke, as well as the composition of the epithelial lining system. In human as in primates, the branching of the bronchial tree is asymmetric. A bronchus divides into a main branch with a diameter of two thirds and a smaller one with one third of the diameter. This gives rise to air flow turbulences at the bifurcations, causing a deposition of particulate matter, according to their respective sizes: the larger the particles, the more they will be deposited at larger bronchial bifurcations. The particle phase in tobacco smoke is composed of ash, but it also contains incomplete combusted particles from tobacco plants, such as nitrosamines and PAHs, and metal oxides. Coal and incompletely combusted plant particles have the tendency to bind PAHs and nitrosylated hydrocarbons either chemically or physically and thus prolong the time of contact of the harmful chemicals with the respiratory epithelium. This has resulted in a toxin- and carcinogen-rich particle fraction acting at larger bifurcations in the era of the filterless cigarette.

The Repair Program and Its Impact on the Reaction of the Epithelium Toward Inhaled Toxins

After the acute inflammatory reaction normally the epithelium is restored to its full function. However, when the inhalation of toxic substances persists, adaptive changes will take place. This is dependent on the location of the lesion. Whereas columnar cell hyperplasia followed by goblet cell hyperplasia and finally transitional and squamous cell metaplasia are the main steps of repair and protection in the large bronchi,[23] proliferation of Clara cells, secretory and goblet cell hyperplasia, and type II pneumocytes resulting in the so-called cuboidal transformation of the epithelium can be found in the bronchoalveolar region. In the large bronchi this can result in squamous and transitional cell dysplasia.[23] Another type of dysplasia, however, is seen in bronchioles (bronchiolar

columnar cell dysplasia[24]) and alveoli (atypical adenomatous hyperplasia[25]). Rarely squamous cell metaplasia can be encountered in the peripheral lung, most often associated with the effects of cytotoxic drugs.

Neuroendocrine cell hyperplasia is another reactive lesion found especially in patients with obstructive lung disease, such as chronic obstructive pulmonary dysplasia (COPD), bronchiectasis, and emphysema.[26–28] Neuroendocrine cells, normally found as scattered single cells along bronchi and bronchioles,[29] start to proliferate upon chronic stimulation by disturbed air flow. It is supposed that this proliferation aims to restore normal lung architecture and thus function. However, neuroendocrine hyperplasia itself causes thickening of bronchial/bronchiolar walls and thus stenosis.[30,31]

The Defence System

Mucociliary Escalator and Clearance

One of the oldest defence systems is the mucociliary escalator system. The cilia are constantly beating to move the mucus produced by the bronchial glands, the goblet cells, and the secretory columnar cells toward the larynx. This mucus overlays the epithelium as a thin layer and protects the epithelium against toxic substances. Because of the constant movement, the time of contact and thus the action of toxins is reduced to a few seconds. Coughing and/or ingestion of the mucus together with substances dissolved in it quickly remove most of the harmful inhaled material from the bronchial system.

The Phagocytic System

In the alveolar periphery another old protection system is effective, the phagocytic cell system. Alveolar macrophages constantly enter the alveoli, patrol along the surface, phagocytose all inhaled material, and either vanish into the mucus, if irreversibly damaged by the ingested material, or enter the lymphatics and reach the draining lymph nodes, presenting the processed foreign material to dendritic cells and lymphocytes for a probable immune reaction.

The Enzymes

The action of enzymes with respect to tobacco toxins and carcinogens is not as simple as it looks at a first glance: Different substances are inhaled within the tobacco smoke: some of them are primarily toxic and carcinogenic, whereas others need activation. Cytochrome P450 2A13 (CYP2A13), an enzyme expressed predominantly in the human respiratory tract, exhibits high efficiency in the metabolic activation of tobacco carcinogen NNK. A-C to T transition in the *CYP2A13* gene causes Arg257Cys amino acid substitution and thus results in a significantly reduced activity toward NNK and other substrates. By genotyping patients with lung cancer and controls for the variant *CYP2A13* genotype, a substantially reduced risk for lung adenocarcinoma was found. This reduced risk of lung adenocarcinoma was associated with the genotype as well as with light smokers but not with other types of lung cancer.[32]

Phase II enzymes are implicated in the detoxication of many carcinogens and ROS, thereby protecting cells against DNA damage and subsequent malignant transformation. Although the induction of phase II enzymes is usually considered beneficial, in some cases these enzymes also bioactivate several hazardous chemicals. Furthermore, from the study of the protective actions of certain enzymes found in vegetables (e.g., isothiocyanate sulforaphane in broccoli), it should not be overlooked that these enzymes can also have adverse effects on phase I enzymes, which subsequently can bioactivate a variety of other carcinogens. For example, the bioprecursor of sulforaphane slightly induced phase II detoxifying enzymes, but powerfully induced phase I carcinogen-activating enzymes. Concomitantly it also generated ROS.[33]

The phase I enzyme microsomal epoxide hydrolase 1a plays an important role in both the activation and detoxification of tobacco-derived carcinogens. The low-activity variant genotype of microsomal epoxide hydrolase 1 polymorphism at exon 3 is associated with decreased risk of lung cancer. In contrast, the high-activity variant genotype (polymorphism at exon 4) was associated with a modest increase in risk of lung cancer.[34]

The cytochrome P450 family of enzymes is responsible for many of the initial metabolic conversions of procarcinogenic compounds in tobacco smoke to reactive metabolites. However, other enzyme-based systems such as myeloperoxidase may also be involved. Myeloperoxidase is a phase I metabolic enzyme that has a polymorphic region upstream of the gene that appears to reduce transcriptional activity. The polymorphic G to A shift is associated with a reduction in lung cancer risk in men, younger individuals, and current smokers but not in former smokers and those who have never smoked.[35]

In a lung cancer risk assessment study, the effects of different phase I and phase II enzymes were studied. By analyzing the activities of aryl hydrocarbon hydroxylase, ethoxycoumarin O-deethylase, epoxide hydrolase, UDP-glucuronosyltransferase, and glutathione S-transferase, a pronounced effect of tobacco smoke on pulmonary metabolism of xenobiotics and prooxidant were found, and the existence of a metabolic phenotype conferring higher risk for tobacco-associated lung cancer was documented.[36]

Polymorphisms of genes coding for some of these toxifying and detoxifying enzymes is of special importance as shown in the review by Norppa.[22] The lack of glutathione S-transferase M1 (GSTM1$^{-/-}$) is associated with increased sensitivity to the genotoxicity of tobacco smoke, and GSTM1$^{-/-}$ smokers also show an increased frequency of chromosomal aberrations and sister chromatid exchanges. N-Acetyltransferase slow acetylation genotype and glutathione S-transferase T1 (GSTT1$^{-/-}$) null genotype seem to elevate the baseline level of chromosomal aberrations and sister chromatid exchanges, respectively, possibly because of reduced capacity to detoxify some widespread or endogenous genotoxins. Some evidence exists for polymorphisms of x-ray cross-complementation group 1 (XRCC1) codon 280 and xeroderma pigmentosum group D codon 23 on baseline aberrations, for XRCC1 codon 399 on sister chromatid exchange, and for methylene tetrahydrofolate reductase codon 677 and methionine synthase reductase on spontaneous micronucleus formation.[22]

The effects of tobacco smoke on the DNA repair system have been investigated in recent years;, however, these studies focused on lung cancer.[37–39] An effect can also be anticipated for nontumorous lung diseases. Another important mechanism especially investigated in lung cancer is gene silencing by methylation. Promoter methylation of several tumor suppressor genes is an early event in tobacco-induced carcinogenesis and occurs long before dysplastic changes of the epithelium take place and thus might also influence the development of inflammatory diseases of the lung and remodeling of the architecture.[6,8,40–43]

Chronic Obstructive Pulmonary Disease

The Global Initiative on Obstructive Lung Disease defines COPD as a "disease state characterized by not fully reversible airflow limitation that is usually progressive and associated with abnormal inflammatory response of the lungs to noxious particles or gases."[44] Much of the recent research on COPD has focused on the nature of the inflammatory response and the cellular and molecular mechanisms involved. However, this knowledge is still at an early stage compared with the knowledge of asthma. This chapter reviews the present knowledge of these mechanisms, which are probably responsible for the pathologic abnormalities characteristic of COPD.

Anatomic Basis

The progressive airflow limitation in COPD is due to two major pathologic processes: remodeling and narrowing of small airways and destruction of the lung parenchyma with consequent destruction of the alveolar attachments of these airways as a result of emphysema (Figure 49.1). This results in higher resistance to flow, diminished lung recoil, gas trapping, difficulty breathing, and eventually ventilatory failure.

Both the small airway remodeling and narrowing and the emphysema are due to chronic inflammation and its byproducts, and this inflammation increases as the disease progresses.[45] The pattern of inflammation in airways and lung parenchyma comprises cells of the innate and adaptive immunity, such as macrophages, T lymphocytes, with predominantly CD8+ (cytotoxic) T cells, and in more severe disease B lymphocytes and increased numbers of neutrophils in the airway lumen.[45,46]

Multiple inflammatory mediators are increased in COPD and are derived from inflammatory and structural cells of the lungs.[47] Cigarette smoke may activate surface macrophages and airway epithelial cells to release chemotactic factors among which chemokines predominate and therefore play a key role in orchestrating the chronic inflammation in COPD. These might be the initial inflammatory events occurring in all smokers. However, in smokers who develop COPD, this inflammation progresses into a more complicated inflammatory pattern of innate and adaptive immunity involving dendritic cells as well as T and B lymphocytes along with a complicated interacting array of cytokines and other mediators. The molecular basis of this amplification of inflammation is not yet understood but may be, at least in part, genetically determined.

Cells and Mediators

Epithelial Cells

Epithelial cells function as a first line of defense and are capable of releasing inflammatory mediators, including tumor necrosis factor (TNF)-α, interleukin (IL)-1β, granulocyte–macrophage colony-stimulating factor, CXCL8 (IL-8), and leukotriene B4 upon stimulation or damage.[48] The epithelium is thus likely responsible for the initiation and maintenance of the innate inflammation seen in smokers. Epithelial cells also release C-C chemokines, including RANTES, monocyte chemoattractant protein 1, and eotaxin with activity in macrophages and dendritic cells.[48]

Inflammation and injury of the epithelium likely contributes to airway remodeling in several ways. Epithelial growth factor receptors (EGFR) and proliferation in basal airway epithelial cells, measured by proliferating cell nuclear antigen, are markedly increased in patients with chronic bronchitis and may contribute to basal cell proliferation, squamous metaplasia, and an increased risk of bronchial carcinoma.[49] Furthermore, activation of EGFR along with TNF-α and neutrophil elastase are responsible for mucin production and hypersecretion in airways probably mediated by protein kinase C.[48]

Epithelial cells can also modulate the extracellular matrix by directly producing matrix proteins, such as fibronectin and collagen mediated by transforming growth factor-β[50] and fibroblast activity, and recruitment and proliferation probably through the production of fibroblast growth factors (types 1 and 2; see Figure 49.1).[51] Matrix metalloproteinase (MMP)-9 expression is increased in the epithelium and may play a role in airway remodeling.

The alveolar epithelial response to injury resembles that of the airway epithelium in many respects. Of special interest is the increased expression of vascular epithelial growth factor (VEGF), a major regulator of vascular growth, in pulmonary vascular smooth muscle of patients with mild and moderate COPD but paradoxically a reduction in expression in severe COPD with emphysema where it is associated with apoptosis of endothelial cells.[49] In addition, VEGF is also an important proinflammatory cytokine produced by epithelial and endothelial cells, macrophages, and activated T cells that acts by increasing endothelial cell permeability by inducing expression of endothelial adhesion molecules via its ability to act as a monocyte chemoattractant. It also stimulates dendritic cells. Thus, VEGF is likely a intermediary between cell-mediated immune inflammation and the associated angiogenesis reaction.[49]

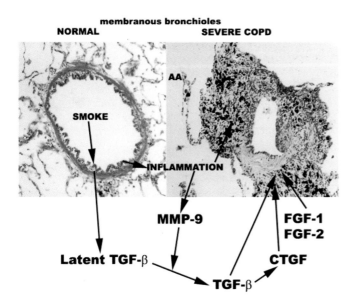

FIGURE 49.1. Membranous bronchioles (approximately 0.7 mm in diameter) in lungs of a nonsmoker and a patient with severe chronic obstructive pulmonary disease. The possible pathways for the remodeling of the airway fibrosis are indicated. AA, alveolar attachments; CTGF, connective tissue growth factor; FGF, fibroblast growth factor; MMP, matrix metalloproteinase; TGF, transforming growth factor.

Neutrophils

Activated neutrophils are found in sputum and bronchoalveolar lavage (BAL) fluid of patients with COPD[52] and to a lesser extent in the airways or lung parenchyma.[46] The role of neutrophils in COPD is not yet clear; however, they are correlated with the rate of decline in lung function.[53] There are several chemotactic signals derived from alveolar macrophages, T cells and epithelial cells that have the potential for neutrophil recruitment in COPD, including leukotriene B4, CXCL8, and related CXC chemokines CXCL1 (GRO-α) and CXCL5 (ENA-78), which are increased in COPD airways.[54]

Neutrophils have the capacity to induce tissue damage and emphysema through the release of serine proteases, including neutrophil elastase (NE), cathepsin G, proteinase-3, MMP-8, and MMP-9, and superoxide anion generation. It is likely that airway neutrophilia and their proteases are linked to mucous hypersecretion in COPD.[55]

Macrophages

There is a marked increase (5- to 10-fold) in the numbers of macrophages in all lung compartments in COPD. Furthermore, macrophages are localized to sites of alveolar wall destruction in patients with emphysema,[46] and there is a correlation between macrophage numbers in the lung and the severity of emphysema[46] and COPD.[53] Alveolar macrophages from patients with COPD secrete more inflammatory proteins and have a greater elastolytic activity than those from normal smokers.[56] Activated by cigarette smoke, alveolar macrophages release inflammatory mediators, including TNF-α, IL-1β, IL-6, IL-12, IL-18, CXCL8 and other CXC chemokines, CCL2 (monocyte chemoattractant protein 1), leukotriene B4, and reactive oxygen species, providing a cellular mechanism that links smoking with inflammation in COPD.[57,58] Alveolar macrophages also secrete elastolytic enzymes, including predominantly MMP-9 but also MMP-2, MMP-12, cathepsins K, L, and S, and neutrophil elastase taken up from neutrophils. Most of the inflammatory proteins produced by COPD macrophages are regulated by the transcription factor NF-κB, which is activated in the alveolar macrophages of COPD patients, particularly during exacerbations.[59]

There may be an increased recruitment of monocytes from the circulation in smokers in response to monocyte-selective chemokines, such as CCL2, that is increased in sputum, BAL, and alveolar macrophages of patients with COPD.[60] Macrophages may have a prolonged survival in smokers and patients with COPD,[61] very likely mediated by the T-cell production of interferon(IFN)-γ and the expression of CD40 ligand.

In vitro the release of CXCL8, TNF-α, and MMP-9 in macrophages of normal subjects and normal smokers are inhibited by corticosteroids, but not in macrophages from patients with COPD,[62] and this may be secondary to the marked reduction in activity of histone deacetylase (HDAC), which is recruited to activated inflammatory genes by glucocorticoid receptors to switch off inflammatory genes (see later discussion of oxidative stress).[63]

Eosinophils

Although eosinophils are the predominant leukocyte in asthma, their role in COPD is much less certain. The presence of eosinophils in patients with COPD predicts a response to corticosteroids and may indicate coexisting asthma.[64]

Dendritic Cells

The airways and parenchyma contain a rich network of dendritic cells that are localized near the surface, and cigarette smoking is associated with an expansion in the dendritic cell population in the lower respiratory tract with a marked increase in the number of mature cells in the airways and alveolar walls.[65] This is an indication that the lung response to cigarette smoke exposure follows the established immune response design, including innate immunity and readiness for a dendritic cell–modulated adaptive immune response, if necessary, which would promote a lymphocytic inflammation.

T Lymphocytes

There is an increase in the total numbers of T lymphocytes in lung parenchyma and peripheral and central airways of patients with COPD, with the greater increase in CD8+ than in CD4+ cells.[46,65-68] The majority of T cells in the lung in COPD are of the Tc1 and Th1 subtypes.[69,70]

The mechanisms by which T cells accumulate in the airways and parenchyma of patients with COPD must depend on some initial activation by presentation of antigenic products by dendritic cells and then adhesion and selective chemotaxis in the lung. CD4+ and CD8+ T cells in the lung in COPD show increased expression of CXCR3, a receptor activated by the chemokines CXCL9, CXCL10, and CXCL11. There is increased expression of CXCL10 by bronchiolar epithelial cells, and this could contribute to the accumulation of CD4+ and CD8+ T cells, which preferentially express CXCR3.[70] The T cells in COPD do not express any of the chemokine receptors described in asthma (CCR4 and CCR8), indicating that the infiltrating T cells in COPD are activated, Th1 committed and utilize Th1-type chemokines and receptors to home to the lung. These results are a strong indication that the T cells in COPD, which express phosphorylated signal transducers and activators of transcription (STAT) protein 4 and IFN-γ, are effector cells likely activated by antigenic peptides from the lung in the local lymphoid tissue and homing back to the lung, the source of the antigens, guided by Th1-selective chemokines.[71]

Activated T cells have the potential to produce extensive damage in the lung. CD8+ cells have the capacity to cause cytolysis and apoptosis, and there is an association between CD8+ cells and apoptosis of alveolar cells in emphysema.[67] In addition, CD8+ T cells also produce a number of cytokines of the Tc-1 phenotype, including TNF-α, lymphotoxin (TNF-β) and IFN-γ, which CD8+ T cells express in COPD.[58] The effector functions of the CD4+ T cell are mainly mediated by Th1 cytokines, which stimulate much greater inflammatory cell migration, the so-called immune inflammation.

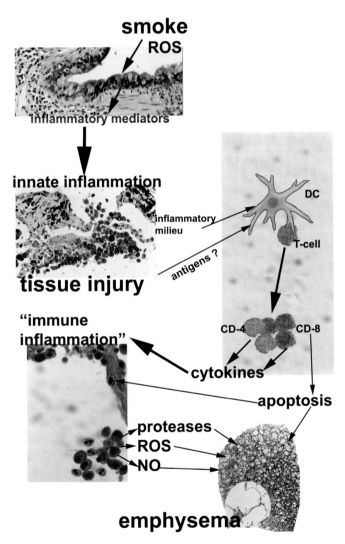

FIGURE 49.2. Possible mechanistic pathways in the pathogenesis of chronic obstructive pulmonary disease and emphysema. DC, dendritic cell; NO, nitric oxide; ROS, reactive oxygen species.

It is now apparent that the inflammatory process leading to disease in COPD results from a complex inflammatory and immune process, most likely orchestrated by the T cells (Figure 49.2). Consequently, it has been suggested that COPD could be considered an autoimmune disease triggered by antigens derived from the lung injury produced by smoking.[67,72,73]

Oxidative Stress

There is increasing evidence that oxidative stress is an important feature in COPD.[74] Besides cigarette smoke itself,[75] activated inflammatory and structural cells in the lungs of smokers, including, neutrophils, eosinophils, macrophages, and epithelial cells, produce ROS. Superoxide anions (O_2^-) are generated by NADPH oxidase and are converted to hydrogen peroxide (H_2O_2) by superoxide dismutases, which could also form the highly reactive hydroxyl radical (OH). Nitric oxide (NO) is generated in COPD from the inducible enzyme NO synthase (iNOS), which is expressed in macrophages and lung parenchyma in COPD.[76] Nitric oxide combines with ROS to form peroxynitrite, which can also generate ·OH.[77]

The normal production of oxidants is counteracted by several antioxidant mechanisms in the human respiratory tract, mainly catalase, superoxide dismutase, and glutathione.[78] There is a high concentration of reduced glutathione in lung epithelial lining fluid,[78] and concentrations are increased in cigarette smokers.

There is considerable evidence of increased oxidative stress in COPD,[79] and markers of oxidative stress, as well as oxidants such as H_2O_2, 8-isoprostane, and ethane, can be detected in exhaled air or breath condensates in smokers.[80] Furthermore, a specific marker of lipid peroxidation, 4-hydoxy-2-nonenal, can be detected by immunocytochemistry in airway of patients with COPD.[81]

Reactive oxygen species have several effects on the airways and parenchyma that increase the inflammatory response mediated either directly, by the actions of ROS on target cells in the airways and alveoli, or indirectly via activation of signal transduction pathways and transcription factors. Reactive oxygen species activate NF-κB and activator protein-1, which switch on multiple inflammatory genes resulting in amplification of the inflammatory response.[82] Nuclear factor-κB is activated in airways and alveolar macrophages of patients with COPD and is further activated during exacerbations,[59] likely by oxidative stress. This activation will induce a neutrophilic inflammation via increased expression of CXCL8 (IL-8) and other CXC chemokines, TNF-α, and MMP-9. Oxidants also activate mitogen-activated protein kinase pathways that regulate the expression of many inflammatory genes, their survival in certain cells, and many aspects of macrophage function.[83] Oxidative stress may also impair the function of antiproteases such as α_1-antitrypsin and secretory leukocyte protease inhibitor and thereby accelerates the breakdown of elastin in lung parenchyma.[84]

Reactive oxygen species and NO can affect different cellular functions, produce mitochondrial damage, DNA strand breaks, and structural/functional modification of proteins; and result in cell death.[85] Oxidative modification of proteins can render proteins antigenic and elicit an autoimmune T-cell response.[86] This might be a mechanism for the adaptive immune response seen in COPD.

Oxidative stress may play a key role in the inflammatory process by its role in the nuclear histones. The acetylation of histones plays an essential role in the nucleosome remodeling that permits access to the promoter sites of inflammatory and other genes; levels of histone acetylation (HAT) have been directly related to the levels of gene transcription. Deacetylation of histones by the recruitment of ston deacetylase (HDACs), either spontaneously or by corticosteroids, reverses the acetylation of histones and terminates gene transcription, thus terminating the inflammatory cascade. Cigarette smoke, probably through the induction of oxidative stress, plays an important role in the increased levels of HAT activity and decreased levels of HDAC found in epithelial cells, macrophages, and neutrophils in smokers.[63] Both acetylation of histones and inhibition of HDAC are associated with enhanced activation of activator protein-1 and NF-κB essential inflammatory genes, which will promote and maintain inflammation.[63]

Proteases

The paradigm of the pathogenesis of emphysema is an imbalance between proteases induced by cigarette smoke exposure and endogenous antiproteases. Several proteases are implicated in the pathogenesis of COPD and emphysema. *Neutrophil elastase* has a potent elastolytic effect, can produce emphysema in animals,[87] and has been shown by immunochemistry to localize on lung elastic fibers in human emphysema.[88] Neutrophil elastase is also a potent mucous secretagogue of submucosal glands and goblet cells and induces the expression of some cytokines, including IL-8, in airway epithelial cells. *Cysteine proteases (cathepsins)* are increased in BAL fluid in patients with emphysema,[89] but their role in COPD is uncertain. *Matrix metalloproteinases* with elastolytic and collagenolytic activities have been implicated in COPD. Matrix metalloproteinase-9 (elastase) and MMP-1 (collagenase) can be localized in macrophage alveolar II cells and are increased in BAL fluid in COPD.[90] Besides their proteolytic function, MMPs generate chemotactic peptides that promote macrophages, recruitment to the airways and parenchyma, and MMP-9 also plays an important role in the activation of the latent form of TGF-β to its active form, thereby regulating inflammation.[91]

The excess of proteases is counteracted by *endogenous antiproteases*; serine protease inhibitors include α_1-antitrypsin and to a lesser extent α_1-antichemotrypsin, elafin, and secretory leukocyte protease inhibitor, the major serine proteinase inhibitor in the airways. All these proteases can be inactivated by oxidative stress and cleavage by other proteinases such as MMP-9 and cathepsins L and S.[84,90] The tissue inhibitors 1–4 of MMPs counteract these proteases,[92] but their production by macrophages in COPD seems to be blunted.[56]

Other Tobacco Smoking-Induced Lung Diseases

Habits and changes in the fabrication of cigarettes have changed smoking habits and by this also the spectrum of lung diseases. Respiratory bronchiolitis was originally described in 1974.[93] In the 1980s respiratory bronchiolitis was rarely seen, but an increase in cases was seen by one of us since 1994. During the 1970s, filter cigarettes became more popular, and, in the 1980s, "light" cigarettes were invented. This has changed the composition of tobacco smoke carcinogens as well as the distribution within the airways (see the earlier explanations).

When discussing tobacco–induced lung diseases other than COPD, we have to deal with cigarette smoking–induced lung diseases, because cigar and pipe smoking usually causes diseases of the oral cavity and the larynx. Rarely this kind of tobacco smoke is inhaled. Cigarette smoking diseases can be classified into the following:

Pulmonary histiocytosis X (HX) or Langerhans cell histiocytosis (LCH)
Respiratory bronchiolitis–combined interstitial lung disease (RB-ILD)
Combined HX + RB-ILD
Desquamative interstitial pneumonia (DIP)

Pulmonary Histiocytosis X

Histiocytosis X (HX), presently called *Langerhans cell histiocytosis*, is a granulomatous inflammatory disease caused by a proliferation of Langerhans cells involving the bronchial tree from middle-sized bronchi down to bronchioles and the centroacinar portion of the lung lobules. An infiltration by eosinophils is present, which is the main cause of bronchiolar destruction (Figure 49.3). In the early lesion abundant eosinophilic granulocytes are found in the mucosa, and degranulation of eosinophils can be proven by immunohistochemistry for basic proteins or simply by a Congo red stain. In later lesions the granuloma undergoes fibrosis and scarring, and eosinophils are vanishing. In these late stages the lesions

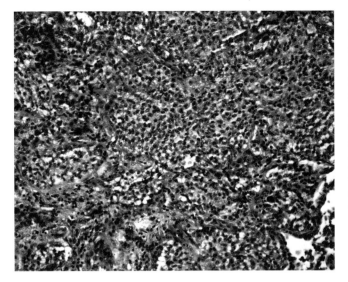

FIGURE 49.3. Florid Langerhans cell histiocytosis completely destroying a bronchiolus. In this early lesion eosinophils cause necrosis by a release of toxic basic proteins from their granules. (Hematoxylin and eosin; ×250.)

acquire a star-like shape, which can also quite characteristically be seen on high-resolution computed tomography scans.

Langerhans cells are part of the antigen-presenting dendritic cell system and are characterized by their expression of CD1a on the cell surface and by Birbeck granules demonstrated by electron microscopy.[94] Langerhans cells are also positive for S100 protein, similar to some alveolar macrophages. Langerhans cells can easily be differentiated from macrophages by their larger ovoid nuclei, their finely dispersed chromatin, and their invisible cell borders. In addition, Langerhans cells are negative for CD68, which is a classic macrophage marker.

The reason for this proliferation of Langerhans cells is not entirely clear; however, an excess of inhaled plant antigens, derived from incomplete combustion of tobacco plant proteins, is one of the underlying causes.[95] The disease usually affects young individuals, male as well as female, who all can be characterized as excessive cigarette smokers. Because many more individuals smoke excessively than get diseased, other underlying factors are likely.

Many cytokines have been proven in HX, released from alveolar macrophages and Langerhans cells, predominantly inducing a Th2 reaction with increased levels of IL-4 and IL-5.[96] These might be responsible for the eosinophilic infiltration. Eosinophils themselves contain a vast amount of basic proteins, such as major basic protein, which are cytotoxic for the respiratory epithelium.

Besides pulmonary LCH, a tumor-like "classic" LCH can be found confined to, for example, the skin, but also can involve different organs, such as bone and lung. This type of LCH usually occurs in preadolescents and is not related to smoking, whereas the pulmonary LCH is associated with smoking. In addition, dendritic cell tumors and sarcomas do exist at the malignant end of the spectrum.[97] Whereas the differential diagnosis of dendritic cell tumors and sarcomas can easily be made, the morphologic differentiation among diffuse versus tumor-like and tumorous Langerhans cell proliferations is still not solved. Multiorgan involvement, the absence of cigarette smoke exposure, and preadolescent age are the most reliable indicators.

Respiratory Bronchiolitis–Combined Interstitial Lung Disease

Similar to HX, RB-ILD is caused by excessive inhalation of cigarette smoke. In contrast to HX, there is usually no reaction and/or proliferation of antigen-presenting cells but a massive accumulation of alveolar macrophages. Similar to HX, the etiology and pathogenesis of RB-ILD is incompletely understood. It is supposed that the disease is caused by an excessive inhalation of cigarette smoke, causing an accumulation of waste products with which the alveolar macrophages cannot cope. This induces an influx of monocytic cells, which differentiate into macrophages. These cells accumulate within the terminal respiratory bronchioles, the alveolar ducts, and the adjacent centroacinar portion of the lobules (Figure 49.4). The airflow is reduced by this macrophage accumulation functionally similar to bronchiolar obstruction, and reduced airflow in the alveolar region causes decreased gas exchange. Therefore, clinically the disease shows

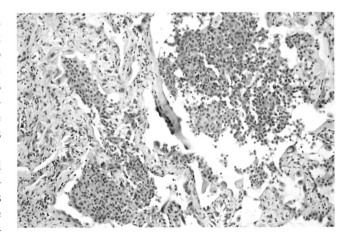

FIGURE 49.4. Respiratory bronchiolitis–combined interstitial lung disease. Alveolar macrophages functionally causing bronchiolar obstruction. (Hematoxylin and eosin; ×250.)

combined obstructive and restrictive ventilation disturbances.

In later stages destruction of lung parenchyma occurs, and emphysema can result. Most probably macrophages that have phagocytosed the waste products of cigarette smoke cause their own death by rupture of phagolysosomes and thus release their toxic enzymes into the surrounding lung.[98] A similar phenomenon was described in the 1950s and 1960s in experimental inhalation experiments. Titanium oxide was used as a control dust in animal inhalation studies, because it is inert and does not cause disease. However, if the amount of inhaled titanium oxide dust was increased excessively above the threshold that can be removed by the mucous escalator system and the phagocytic capacity of the macrophages, an accumulation of dust-laden macrophages occurred, macrophages died by release of their enzymes, and a secondary histiocytic and macrophage, sometimes granulomatous, inflammation started.[99] This reaction was called an *overload phenomenon*, and histologically it resembled RB-ILD.

It should be remembered that RB-ILD is not a common disease; it is less prevalent in contrast to the millions of heavy smokers in Europe. However, RB-ILD is underestimated clinically; in adjacent lung tissue in patients suffering from lung cancer, it is a quite common finding. Thus, the etiology is still not well understood.

Combined Respiratory Bronchiolitis–Combined Interstitial Lung Disease and Histiocytosis X

A combination of HX and RB-ILD in different parts of the lung is seen with increasing frequency. In biopsy specimens obtained during diagnostic video-assisted thoracic surgery, HX granulomas are seen in one subsegment, whereas accumulations of macrophages in respiratory bronchioles and centrolobular areas are observed in another one (Figure 49.5). This is not surprising, because patients are usually heavy smokers.

Desquamative Interstitial Pneumonia

Desquamative interstitial pneumonia is characterized by an accumulation of alveolar macrophages within the alveolar periphery. Respiratory bronchioles are not involved. Desquamative interstitial pneumonia can mimic a peripheral carcinoma radiologically, because the cellular accumulation is similarly dense, and the cells completely fill the alveoli. The etiology again is cigarette smoking in most cases.[101–102] However, it should be noted that cases have been reported that point to inhalation of toxic substances, such as aluminium welding fumes and nylon flock dust.[103–107]

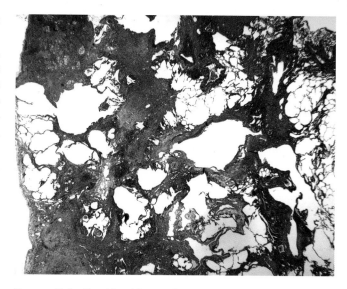

FIGURE 49.5. Combined Langerhans cell histiocytosis and respiratory bronchiolitis–interstitial lung disease in one patient. Foci of Langerhans cell proliferations can be seen occluding bronchioles. In addition, accumulation of alveolar macrophages is seen, occluding terminally bronchioles. (Hematoxylin and eosin; ×25.)

Desquamative interstitial pneumonia, in contrast to RB-ILD, is rare. In fact, there is no transition between both diseases. It is not imaginable where and why accumulation of macrophages should vanish and only concentrate in the alveolar periphery or how macrophage accumulation should extend to respiratory bronchioles. In reality, a transition between both diseases has never been reported. In contrast to RB-ILD, DIP will usually induce a restrictive pattern on functional tests.

Conclusion

Cigarette smoke exposure induces a florid inflammatory response in the lung involving structural and inflammatory cells and a large array of inflammatory mediators. The interactions among these complex steps eventually leads to tissue injury and abnormal repair, with airway remodeling and obstruction and lung destruction with emphysema, albeit in only 20% of chronic smokers. Of interest, the main difference between smokers who develop COPD and the ones who do not seems to be the presence of an adaptive immune response with CD8[+], CD4[+], and B cells that express obvious signs of being activated effector cells. It is likely that genetic and epigenetic factors are involved in determining the progression of the inflammatory cascade, as this is supported by animal models looking at strains of different susceptibilities for the development of smoke-induced emphysema.[108]

Which of the cells or inflammatory mediators described are responsible for the disease and its progression in smokers? Probably all are, acting together as redundant and obligatory players in a complex innate and adaptive immune response. Progress in understanding COPD would surely lie in the knowledge of which genes or gene master switches are orchestrating the progression, or even more likely the lack of progression, of inflammation toward the full disease.

References

1. Cooke JP, Bitterman H. Nicotine and angiogenesis: a new paradigm for tobacco-related diseases. Ann Med 2004; 36(1):33–40.

2. Zhu BQ, Heeschen C, Sievers RE, et al. Second hand smoke stimulates tumor angiogenesis and growth. Cancer Cell 2003;4:191–196.

3. Schick S, Glantz S. Philip Morris toxicological experiments with fresh sidestream smoke: more toxic than mainstream smoke. Tob Control 2005;14(6):396–404.

4. Husgafvel-Pursiainen K. Genotoxicity of environmental tobacco smoke: a review. Mutat Res 2004;567(2–3):427–445.

5. Dopp E, Saedler J, Stopper H, et al. Mitotic disturbances and micronucleus induction in Syrian hamster embryo fibroblast cells caused by asbestos fibers. Environ Health Perspect 1995;103(3):268–271.

6. Harden SV, Tokumaru Y, Westra WH, et al. Gene promoter hypermethylation in tumors and lymph nodes of stage I lung cancer patients. Clin Cancer Res 2003;9(4):1370–1375.

7. Lu C, Soria JC, Tang X, et al. Prognostic factors in resected stage I non–small-cell lung cancer: a multivariate analysis of six molecular markers. J Clin Oncol 2004;22(22):4575–4583.

8. Toyooka S, Maruyama R, Toyooka KO, et al. Smoke exposure, histologic type and geography-related differences in the methylation profiles of non-small cell lung cancer. Int J Cancer 2003;103(2):153–160.

9. Harke HP, Schuller D, Klimisch JH, Meissner K. [Investigations of polycyclic aromatic hydrocarbons in cigarette smoke.] Z Lebensm Unters Forsch 1976;162(3):291–297.

10. Andrew AS, Warren AJ, Barchowsky A, et al. Genomic and proteomic profiling of responses to toxic metals in human lung cells. Environ Health Perspect 2003;111(6):825–835.

11. Bachelet M, Pinot F, Polla RI, et al. Toxicity of cadmium in tobacco smoke: protection by antioxidants and chelating resins. Free Radic Res 2002;36(1):99–106.

12. Waalkes MP. Cadmium carcinogenesis. Mutat Res 2003; 533(1–2):107–120.

13. Zaridze DG, Safaev RD, Belitsky GA, et al. Carcinogenic substances in Soviet tobacco products. IARC Sci Publ 1991(105):485–488.

14. Stabbert R, Voncken P, Rustemeier K, et al. Toxicological evaluation of an electrically heated cigarette. Part 2:

15. Jin Z, Gao F, Flagg T, et al. Tobacco-specific nitrosamine NNK promotes functional cooperation of Bcl2 and c-Myc through phosphorylation in regulating cell survival and proliferation. J Biol Chem 2004;279(38):40209–40219.

16. Tsurutani J, Castillo SS, Brognard J, et al. Tobacco components stimulate Akt-dependent proliferation and NFkappaB-dependent survival in lung cancer cells. Carcinogenesis 2005;26(7):1182–1195.

17. Wynder EL, Muscat JE. The changing epidemiology of smoking and lung cancer histology. Environ Health Perspect 1995;103 Suppl 8:143–148.

18. Witschi H. Carcinogenic activity of cigarette smoke gas phase and its modulation by beta-carotene and N-acetylcysteine. Toxicol Sci 2005;84(1):81–87.

19. White JL, Conner BT, Perfetti TA, et al. Effect of pyrolysis temperature on the mutagenicity of tobacco smoke condensate. Food Chem Toxicol 2001;39(5):499–505.

20. Torikai K, Yoshida S, Takahashi H. Effects of temperature, atmosphere and pH on the generation of smoke compounds during tobacco pyrolysis. Food Chem Toxicol 2004;42(9):1409–1417.

21. Knaapen AM, Borm PJ, Albrecht C, et al. Inhaled particles and lung cancer. Part A: mechanisms. Int J Cancer 2004;109(6):799–809.

22. Norppa H. Cytogenetic biomarkers and genetic polymorphisms. Toxicol Lett 2004;149(1–3):309–334.

23. Wang GF, Lai MD, Yang RR, et al. Histological types and significance of bronchial epithelial dysplasia. Mod Pathol 2006;19(3):429–437.

24. Ullmann R, Bongiovanni M, Halbwedl I, et al. Bronchiolar columnar cell dysplasia—genetic analysis of a novel preneoplastic lesion of peripheral lung. Virchows Arch 2003;442(5):429–436.

25. Mori M, Rao SK, Popper HH, et al. Atypical adenomatous hyperplasia of the lung: a probable forerunner in the development of adenocarcinoma of the lung. Mod Pathol 2001;14(2):72–84.

26. Pilmane M, Luts A, Sundler F. Changes in neuroendocrine elements in bronchial mucosa in chronic lung disease in adults. Thorax 1995;50(5):551–554.

27. Shenberger JS, Shew RL, Johnson DE. Hyperoxia-induced airway remodeling and pulmonary neuroendocrine cell hyperplasia in the weanling rat. Pediatr Res 1997;42(4):539–544.

28. Stevens TP, McBride JT, Peake JL, et al. Cell proliferation contributes to PNEC hyperplasia after acute airway injury. Am J Physiol 1997;272(3 Pt 1):L486–L493.

29. Boers JE, den Brok JL, Koudstaal J, et al. Number and proliferation of neuroendocrine cells in normal human airway epithelium. Am J Respir Crit Care Med 1996;154(3 Pt 1):758–763.

30. Brown MJ, English J, Muller NL. Bronchiolitis obliterans due to neuroendocrine hyperplasia: high-resolution CT–pathologic correlation. AJR Am J Roentgenol 1997; 168(6):1561–1562.

31. Miller RR, Muller NL. Neuroendocrine cell hyperplasia and obliterative bronchiolitis in patients with peripheral

carinoid tumors. Am J Surg Pathol 1995;19(6):653–658.

32. Wang H, Tan W, Hao B, et al. Substantial reduction in risk of lung adenocarcinoma associated with genetic polymorphism in CYP2A13, the most active cytochrome P450 for the metabolic activation of tobacco-specific carcinogen NNK. Cancer Res 2003;63(22):8057–8061.

33. Paolini M, Perocco P, Canistro D, et al. Induction of cytochrome P450, generation of oxidative stress and in vitro cell-transforming and DNA-damaging activities by glucoraphanin, the bioprecursor of the chemopreventive agent sulforaphane found in broccoli. Carcinogenesis 2004;25(1):61–67.

34. Kiyohara C, Yoshimasu K, Takayama K, et al. EPHX1 polymorphisms and the risk of lung cancer: a HuGE review. Epidemiology 2006;17(1):89–99.

35. Schabath MB, Spitz MR, Zhang X, et al. Genetic variants of myeloperoxidase and lung cancer risk. Carcinogenesis 2000;21(6):1163–1166.

36. Bartsch H, Petruzzelli S, De Flora S, et al. Carcinogen metabolism in human lung tissues and the effect of tobacco smoking: results from a case–control multicenter study on lung cancer patients. Environ Health Perspect 1992;98:119–124.

37. Hu Z, Ma H, Lu D, et al. A promoter polymorphism (-77T>C) of DNA repair gene XRCC1 is associated with risk of lung cancer in relation to tobacco smoking. Pharmacogenet Genomics 2005;15(7):457–463.

38. Matullo G, Dunning AM, Guarrera S, et al. DNA repair polymorphisms and cancer risk in non-smokers in a cohort study. Carcinogenesis 2006;27(5):997–1007.

39. Zienolddiny S, Campa D, Lind H, et al. Polymorphisms of DNA repair genes and risk of non–small cell lung cancer. Carcinogenesis 2006;27(3):560–567.

40. Forgacs E, Zochbauer-Muller S, Olah E, et al. Molecular genetic abnormalities in the pathogenesis of human lung cancer. Pathol Oncol Res 2001;7(1):6–13.

41. He B, You L, Uematsu K, et al. SOCS-3 is frequently silenced by hypermethylation and suppresses cell growth in human lung cancer. Proc Natl Acad Sci USA 2003;100(24):14133–14138.

42. Lamy A, Sesboue R, Bourguignon J, et al. Aberrant methylation of the CDKN2a/p16INK4a gene promoter region in preinvasive bronchial lesions: a prospective study in high-risk patients without invasive cancer. Int J Cancer 2002;100(2):189–193.

43. Li QL, Kim HR, Kim WJ, et al. Transcriptional silencing of the RUNX3 gene by CpG hypermethylation is associated with lung cancer. Biochem Biophys Res Commun 2004;314(1):223–228.

44. GOLD. Global Initiative for Chronic Obstructive Lung Disease (GOLD): global strategy for the diagnosis mocopd. NHLBI/WHO Workshop Report. 2003.

45. Hogg JC. Pathophysiology of airflow limitation in chronic obstructive pulmonary disease. Lancet 2004;364:709–721.

46. Finkelstein R, Fraser RS, Ghezzo H, et al. Alveolar inflammation and its relation to emphysema in smokers. Am J Respir Crit Care Med 1995;152:1666–1672.

47. Barnes PJ. Mediators of chronic obstructive pulmonary disease. Pharmacol Rev 2004;56:515–548.

48. Spurzen JR, Renard IR. Epithelial cells. In Barnes PJ, ed. Chronic Obstructive Pulmonary Disease: Cellular and Molecular Mechanisms. New York: Taylor & Francis; 2005.

49. Barnes PJ, Cosio MG. Cells and mediators of COPD. European Respiratory Monograph: Management of COPD. 2006 (in press).

50. Takizawa H, Tanaka M, Takami K, et al. Increased expression of transforming growth factor-beta1 in small airway epithelium from tobacco smokers and patients with chronic obstructive pulmonary disease (COPD). Am J Respir Crit Care Med 2001;163:1476–1483.

51. Kranenburg AR, Willems-Widyastuti A, Mooi WJ, et al. Chronic obstructive pulmonary disease is associated with enhanced bronchial expression of FGF-1, FGF-2, and FGFR-1. J Pathol 2005;206:28–38.

52. Lacoste JY, Bousquet J, Chanez P, et al. Eosinophilic and neutrophilic inflammation in asthma, chronic bronchitis, and chronic obstructive pulmonary disease. J Allergy Clin Immunol 1993;92:537–548.

53. Di Stefano A, Capelli A, Lusuardi M, et al. Severity of airflow limitation is associated with severity of airway inflammation in smokers. Am J Respir Crit Care Med 1998;158:1277–1285.

54. Traves SL, Culpitt SV, Russell RE, et al. Increased levels of the chemokines GROalpha and MCP-1 in sputum samples from patients with COPD. Thorax 2002;57:590–595.

55. Sommerhoff CP, Nadel JA, Basbaum CB, et al. Neutrophil elastase and cathepsin G stimulate secretion from cultured bovine airway gland serous cells. J Clin Invest 1990;85:682–689.

56. Russell RE, Culpitt SV, DeMatos C, et al. Release and activity of matrix metalloproteinase-9 and tissue inhibitor of metalloproteinase-1 by alveolar macrophages from patients with chronic obstructive pulmonary disease. Am J Respir Cell Mol Biol 2002;26:602–609.

57. Barnes PJ. Macrophages as orchestrators of COPD. J COPD 2004;1:59–70.

58. Cosio MG. T-lymphocytes. In: Barnes PJ, ed. Chronic Obstructive Pulmonary Disease: Cellular and Molecular Mechanisms. New York: Taylor & Francis Group; 2005:321–325.

59. Caramori G, Romagnoli M, Casolari P, et al. Nuclear localisation of p65 in sputum macrophages but not in sputum neutrophils during COPD exacerbations. Thorax 2003;58:348–351.

60. de Boer WI, Sont JK, van Schadewijk A, et al. Monocyte chemoattractant protein 1, interleukin 8, and chronic airways inflammation in COPD. J Pathol 2000;190:619–626.

61. Tomita K, Caramori G, Lim S, et al. Increased p21(CIP1/WAF1) and B cell lymphoma leukemia-x(L) expression and reduced apoptosis in alveolar macrophages from smokers. Am J Respir Crit Care Med 2002;166:724–731.

62. Culpitt SV, Rogers DF, Shah P, et al. Impaired inhibition by dexamethasone of cytokine release by alveolar macro-

phages from patients with chronic obstructive pulmonary disease. Am J Respir Crit Care Med 2003;167: 24–31.

63. Barnes PJ, Adcock IM, Ito K. Histone acetylation and deacetylation: importance in inflammatory lung diseases. Eur Respir J 2005;25:552–563.

64. Papi A, Romagnoli M, Baraldo S, et al. Partial reversibility of airflow limitation and increased exhaled NO and sputum eosinophilia in chronic obstructive pulmonary disease. Am J Respir Crit Care Med 2000;162:1773–1777.

65. Soler P, Moreau A, Basset F, et al. Cigarette smoking-induced changes in the number and differentiated state of pulmonary dendritic cells/Langerhans cells. Am Rev Respir Dis 1989;139:1112–1117.

66. Hogg JC, Chu F, Utokaparch S, et al. The nature of small-airway obstruction in chronic obstructive pulmonary disease. N Engl J Med 2004;350:2645–2653.

67. Majo J, Ghezzo H, Cosio MG. Lymphocyte population and apoptosis in the lungs of smokers and their relation to emphysema. Eur Respir J 2001;17:946–953.

68. Saetta M, Baraldo S, Corbino L, et al. CD8+ve cells in the lungs of smokers with chronic obstructive pulmonary disease. Am J Respir Crit Care Med 1999;160:711–717.

69. Grumelli S, Corry DB, Song LZ, et al. An immune basis for lung parenchymal destruction in chronic obstructive pulmonary disease and emphysema. PLoS Med 2004;1: e8.

70. Saetta M, Mariani M, Panina-Bordignon P, et al. Increased expression of the chemokine receptor CXCR3 and its ligand CXCL10 in peripheral airways of smokers with chronic obstructive pulmonary disease. Am J Respir Crit Care Med 2002;165:1404–1409.

71. Di Stefano A, Caramori G, Capelli A, et al. STAT4 activation in smokers and patients with chronic obstructive pulmonary disease. Eur Respir J 2004;24:78–85.

72. Cosio MG, Majo J, Cosio MG. Inflammation of the airways and lung parenchyma in COPD: role of T cells. Chest 2002;121:160S–165S.

73. Cosio MG. Autoimmunity, T-cells and STAT-4 in the pathogenesis of chronic obstructive pulmonary disease. Eur Respir J 2004;24:3–5.

74. Bowler RP, Barnes PJ, Crapo JD. The role of oxidative stress in chronic obstructive pulmonary disease. J COPD 2004;2:255–277.

75. Pryor WA, Stone K. Oxidants in cigarette smoke. Radicals, hydrogen peroxide, peroxynitrate, and peroxynitrite. Ann NY Acad Sci 1993;686:12–27.

76. Maestrelli P, Paska C, Saetta M, et al. Decreased haem oxygenase-1 and increased inducible nitric oxide synthase in the lung of severe COPD patients. Eur Respir J 2003;21:971–976.

77. Beckman JS, Koppenol WH. Nitric oxide, superoxide, and peroxynitrite: the good, the bad, and ugly. Am J Physiol 1996;271:C1424–C1437.

78. Cantin AM, Fells GA, Hubbard RC, et al. Antioxidant macromolecules in the epithelial lining fluid of the normal human lower respiratory tract. J Clin Invest 1990;86:962–971.

79. Bowler RP, Crapo JD. Oxidative stress in airways: is there a role for extracellular superoxide dismutase? Am J Respir Crit Care Med 2002;166:S38–S43.

80. Paredi P, Kharitonov SA, Barnes PJ. Analysis of expired air for oxidation products. Am J Respir Crit Care Med 2002;166:S31–S37.

81. Rahman I, van Schadewijk AA, Crowther AJ, et al. 4-Hydroxy-2-nonenal, a specific lipid peroxidation product, is elevated in lungs of patients with chronic obstructive pulmonary disease. Am J Respir Crit Care Med 2002;166: 490–495.

82. Janssen-Heininger YM, Poynter ME, Baeuerle PA. Recent advances towards understanding redox mechanisms in the activation of nuclear factor kappaB. Free Radic Biol Med 2000;28:1317–1327.

83. Ogura M, Kitamura M. Oxidant stress incites spreading of macrophages via extracellular signal–regulated kinases and p38 mitogen-activated protein kinase. J Immunol 1998;161:3569–3574.

84. Carp H, Janoff A. Possible mechanisms of emphysema in smokers. In vitro suppression of serum elastase-inhibitory capacity by fresh cigarette smoke and its prevention by antioxidants. Am Rev Respir Dis 1978;118: 617–621.

85. Rao T, Richardson B. Environmentally induced autoimmune diseases: potential mechanisms. Environ Health Perspect 1999;107(Suppl 5):737–742.

86. Rose N, Afanasyeva M. Autoimmunity: busting the atherosclerotic plaque. Nat Med 2003;9:641–642.

87. Senior RM, Tegner H, Kuhn C, et al. The induction of pulmonary emphysema with human leukocyte elastase. Am Rev Respir Dis 1977;116:469–475.

88. Damiano VV, Tsang A, Kucich U, et al. Immunolocalization of elastase in human emphysematous lungs. J Clin Invest 1986;78:482–493.

89. Takeyabu K, Betsuyaku T, Nishimura M, et al. Cysteine proteinases and cystatin C in bronchoalveolar lavage fluid from subjects with subclinical emphysema. Eur Respir J 1998;12:1033–1039.

90. Shapiro SD, Senior RM. Matrix metalloproteinases. Matrix degradation and more. Am J Respir Cell Mol Biol 1999;20:1100–1102.

91. Dallas SL, Rosser JL, Mundy GR, et al. Proteolysis of latent transforming growth factor-beta (TGF-beta)-binding protein-1 by osteoclasts. A cellular mechanism for release of TGF-beta from bone matrix. J Biol Chem 2002;277:21352–21360.

92. Cawston T, Carrere S, Catterall J, et al. Matrix metalloproteinases and TIMPs: properties and implications for the treatment of chronic obstructive pulmonary disease. Novartis Found Symp 2001;234:205–218.

93. Niewöhner D KJ, Rice D. Pathologic changes in peripheral airways of young cigarette smokers. N Engl J Med 1974;291:755–758.

94. Nezelof C, Basset F. Langerhans cell histiocytosis research. Past, present, and future. Hematol Oncol Clin North Am 1998;12(2):385–406.

95. Youkeles LH, Grizzanti JN, Liao Z, et al. Decreased tobacco-glycoprotein-induced lymphocyte proliferation in

vitro in pulmonary eosinophilic granuloma. Am J Respir Crit Care Med 1995;151(1):145–150.

96. Egeler RM, Favara BE, van Meurs M, et al. Differential In situ cytokine profiles of Langerhans-like cells and T cells in Langerhans cell histiocytosis: abundant expression of cytokines relevant to disease and treatment. Blood 1999;94(12):4195–4201.

97. Pileri SA, Grogan TM, Harris NL, et al. Tumours of histiocytes and accessory dendritic cells: an immunohistochemical approach to classification from the International Lymphoma Study Group based on 61 cases. Histopathology 2002;41(1):1–29.

98. Stachura I, Singh G, Whiteside TL. Mechanisms of tissue injury in desquamative interstitial pneumonitis. Am J Med 1980;68(5):733–740.

99. Oberdorster G. Toxicokinetics and effects of fibrous and nonfibrous particles. Inhal Toxicol 2002;14(1):29–56.

100. Carrington CB, Gaensler EA, Coutu RE, et al. Natural history and treated course of usual and desquamative interstitial pneumonia. N Engl J Med 1978;298(15):801–809.

101. Liebow AA, Steer A, Billingsley JG. Desquamative interstitial pneumonia. Am J Med 1965;39:369–404.

102. Ryu JH, Colby TV, Hartman TE, et al. Smoking-related interstitial lung diseases: a concise review. Eur Respir J 2001;17(1):122–132.

103. Abraham JL, Hertzberg MA. Inorganic particulates associated with desquamative interstitial pneumonia. Chest 1981;80(1 Suppl):67–70.

104. Freed JA, Miller A, Gordon RE, et al. Desquamative interstitial pneumonia associated with chrysotile asbestos fibres. Br J Ind Med 1991;48(5):332–337.

105. Hammar SP, Hallman KO. Localized inflammatory pulmonary disease in subjects occupationally exposed to asbestos. Chest 1993;103(6):1792–1799.

106. Herbert A, Sterling G, Abraham J, et al. Desquamative interstitial pneumonia in an aluminum welder. Hum Pathol 1982;13(8):694–699.

107. Kern DG, Kuhn C, Ely EW, et al. Flock worker's lung: broadening the spectrum of clinicopathology, narrowing the spectrum of suspected etiologies. Chest 2000;117(1):251–259.

108. Hoshino Y, Radzioch D, Ghezzo H, et al. Smoke-induced and inherent differences at the level of gene expression in mice with different susceptibility to emphysema. Eur Respir J 2003;22(Suppl 45):195s.

50
Heritable α₁-Antitrypsin Deficiency

Richard N. Sifers

Introduction

A heritable deficiency of circulating α₁-antitrypsin (AAT) can lead to the development of pulmonary emphysema in response to the elastolytic destruction of lung connective tissue. Inappropriate accumulation of the molecule in hepatocytes, the primary site of biosynthesis, is an etiologic agent of liver injury. The deficiency results from inappropriate structural maturation of the newly synthesized molecule, whereas defective folding and incomplete clearance lead to intrahepatic accumulation. A small ensemble of processing enzymes modify the asparagine-linked oligosaccharides to generate fate determinants that promote the molecule's entrance into either pathway. The interconnection of these systems, thought to represent the decentralized surveillance of eukaryotic genome expression, is suspected to contain potential modifiers of both diseases. For this reason, the chapter focuses on the elucidation of cellular strategies used by cells to handle mutant forms of AAT.

Heritable α₁-Antitrypsin Deficiency

α₁-Antitrypsin is the archetypal member of the serine proteinase inhibitor (serpin) superfamily of proteins. Additional members include antithrombin, C1-inhibitor, α-antichymotrypsin, plasminogen activator inhibitor-1, neuroserpin, and heparin cofactor II.[1] All share common structure[2] but inhibit particular proteinases to different extents.[1] Severe deficiency of circulating proteinase inhibitor is one of the most common genetic disorders to affect the Caucasian population. Over 100 allelic variants of the *AAT* gene have been identified, but homozygosity for the *Z* allele (Glu342Lys) is most commonly associated with the severe deficiency phenotype. One in 25 individuals inherit a single *Z* allele, and approximately 1 in 2,000 are homozygotes for the allele at the *AAT* gene locus.[3,4]

Associated Disorders

The heritable phenomenon of severe AAT deficiency can lead to clinically relevant consequences. As the most abundant proteinase inhibitor in human plasma, a primary physiologic role for AAT is to protect lung elastin fibers from excessive degradation by neutrophil elastase.[5] In many individuals, a severe deficiency (10%–15% of normal) of the circulating proteinase inhibitor is an underlying cause for excessive proteolytic destruction of lung elastic tissues, resulting from the unopposed hydrolytic action of elastase released from activated neutrophils.[5,6] Early-onset panlobular emphysema has been designated as a primary loss-of-function phenotype.[5] The situation is exacerbated because the available *Z* variant is less effective than the wild-type molecule (fivefold diminished association rate between the *Z* variant and neutrophil elastase).[7] The problem is further intensified by the inappropriate structural conversion caused by the amino acid substitution (see later) that converts AAT to a chemoattractant for human neutrophils.[8]

The detection of periodic acid–Schiff positive inclusion bodies in hepatocytes corresponds to distended regions of the hepatocyte endoplasmic reticulum (ER), resulting from the inappropriately accumulated *Z* variant.[9] The observation, which is now a hallmark for the disorder, also led to the identification of the liver as the primary source for AAT biosynthesis.[4] Transgenic animal models have confirmed that the inclusion bodies contribute to chronic liver injury as a primary gain-of-toxic-function phenotype.[10] In some individuals the disorder can progress to hepatitis, cirrhosis, and/or hepatocellular carcinoma,[11,12] the latter of which has also been detected in some, but not all, transgenic mouse models.

Structural and Cellular Abnormalities

Experimental investigation of the accumulated Z variant eventually led to several significant discoveries. First, the Glu342Lys amino acid substitution is responsible for the molecule's inappropriate conformational transition into polymers following biosynthesis.[13] The perturbation generates a kinetically unstable late folding intermediate that can undergo spontaneous noncovalent polymerization in vitro and in the hepatocyte ER.[14] In the generally accepted "loop-sheet polymerization" model, sequential insertion of the reactive center loop into β-sheet A of another molecule generates noncovalent Z polymers.[15]

Intermolecular polymerization also underlies the severe deficiency associated with the rare *Siiyama* (Ser-53Phe) and *Mmalton* (deletion of residue 52) deficiency variants of AAT, plus the milder deficiency variants designated *S* (Glu264Val) and *I* (Arg39Cys).[16] That the structural anomaly is pathogenic is suggested by the fact that mutations suspected to most favor polymerization also coincide with the greatest risk of liver injury and most severe plasma deficiency.[7] Moreover, several members of the serpin family exhibit mutations that result in their spontaneous polymerization, intrahepatic retention, and plasma deficiency. Identification of the common molecular mechanism has allowed for the different disorders to be designated a new class of disorders called the *serpinopathies*.[16]

Polymerization not only limits the secretion of AAT, eventually affecting lung function, but also might directly contribute to the destruction of lung elastin. The recent use of a monoclonal antibody led to the detection of Z polymers in emphysematous tissue that colocalized with neutrophils in the lung alveoli.[17] The proinflammatory nature of the material was further substantiated by the influx of neutrophils into the lungs of mice instilled with polymers. Based on these observations, one must now consider whether the chemoattractant nature of AATZ polymers might promote the progression of severe lung damage. Finally, metabolic pulse-chase radiolabeling studies have convincingly demonstrated that the rate in which the Z variant is subject to intracellular transport is greatly hindered as compared with correctly folded monomers.[18–20]

A Case For Disease Modifiers

Importantly, not every individual who exhibits severe plasma AAT deficiency (AATD) will necessarily develop lung emphysema, again suggesting that modifiers likely exist for this disorder. Cigarette smoke, because of its capacity to reduce the activity of AAT, has been designated as a major environmental modifier of the lung disease.[6] The identification of genetic modifiers is in progress.

Importantly, only a small subset (10%–15%) of patients who accumulate Z polymers in the hepatocyte ER actually develop any demonstrable liver damage,[11,21] suggesting that additional genetic or environmental factors are likely required to induce a clinically relevant phenotype and especially end-stage liver disease. Because patients fall into two broad age categories in terms of the time of disease onset,[22] a genetic modifier might control the rate at which the disease is manifested. Notably, a delay in the degradation of the Z variant has been observed in transduced cells from patients who eventually underwent liver transplantation,[23] implying that the degradation process might contribute to disease pathogenesis. One suggestion is that the liver injury results from a greater burden[24] of accumulated molecules in response to their impaired intracellular clearance.

In recent years, several groups[25,26] have attempted to unravel the mechanisms by which glycoprotein folding and degradation alter the circulating AAT concentration and/or its accumulation within hepatocytes. Elucidation of the rules by which these systems are governed is expected to aid in the discovery of new disease biomarkers and novel sites to treat both the lung and liver diseases.

Glycoprotein Biosynthetic Quality Control

The transcription of a gene into mRNA does not constitute gene expression but merely represents one of the many steps that culminate in translation of an encoded polypeptide. Subsequent acquisition of native structure directly transforms the inherited information into biologic activity. The interconnected nature by which correct maturation is linked to subsequent protein deployment is, perhaps, best exemplified by the secretory pathway.[27] The system, consisting of large membranous organelles interconnected by transport vesicles, coevolved with the nuclear envelope in eukaryotes, implying its role in monitoring late stages in the eukaryote genome expression program.[28]

Biosynthetic quality control[29,30] refers to a system that assists the conformational maturation of all newly synthesized proteins in living cells. For our purposes, the phrase is used as an operational definition that refers to a complex system of requisite events[31] that work in concert to facilitate the productive transformation of genetic information into biologic activity.[28]

Glycoprotein Structural Maturation

Facilitated folding represents the initial stage of protein biosynthetic quality control.[31] Nascent secretory and membrane proteins begin their existence in the cytoplasm as nascent peptide still bound to the ribosomal translation machinery. A hydrophobic signal sequence located in the polypeptide backbone allows for binding by the large signal recognition particle. In turn, the complex docks with a designated ER protein translocation channel of which the primary component is Sec61p. During translocation, physical engagement of the polypeptide with one or more molecular chaperones facilitates the acquisition of native structure by preventing off-pathway events that can lead to nonspecific aggregation. The same interactions underlie the capacity by which newly synthesized proteins are able to acquire native structure within a biologically relevant time scale.[32] Adoption of native structure is coupled to productive transport through a series of subsequent membranous compartments (Figure 50.1).

Involvement of Asparagine-Linked Oligosaccharides

An important finding was that covalent modification of the asparagine-linked oligosaccharides plays a central role to assist the folding of newly synthesized AAT in the ER.[33–35] Asparagine-linked glycosylation assists the folding of attached polypeptides. The branched 14-unit oligosaccharide represents a common covalent modification attached to the Asn–X–Ser/Thr consensus sequence in nascent polypeptides during translocation into the ER lumen.[36] The appendage provides a scaffold onto which oligosaccharide processing enzymes can transmit information about the underlying protein structure (Figure 50.2).[37]

The Current Model

In a widely accepted model,[27] cotranslational hydrolysis of the two outermost glucose units by glucosidase I and glucosidase II generates a monoglucosylated oligosaccharide (see Figure 50.2). The processing intermediate functions as a ligand capable of promoting physical engagement[38] with two lectin-like members of the glycoprotein folding machinery designated *calnexin* and *calreticulin*[39,40] Disengagement coincides with removal of the remaining glucose unit by glucosidase II.[41] Post-translational reassembly with the folding machinery is driven by UDP-glucose:glycoprotein glucosyltransferase (UGGT),[38,42] which can catalyze the transfer of a single glucose unit back to the appendage upon recognition of

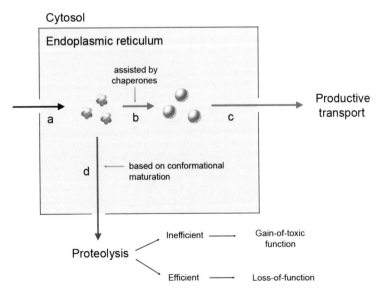

FIGURE 50.1. Schematic representation of the differential fates that await newly synthesized proteins in the endoplasmic reticulum. Following biosynthesis (step a), polypeptides can fold into their native conformation (step b) and undergo productive export from the endoplasmic reticulum (step c). In contrast, those unable to achieve this milestone are retained in the early secretory pathway and dislocated into the cytosol (step d) for proteolysis. Productive and nonproductive fates are designated by green and red arrows, respectively. How the efficiency of proteolysis can contribute to disease pathogenesis is designated at the bottom.

Fate determinants

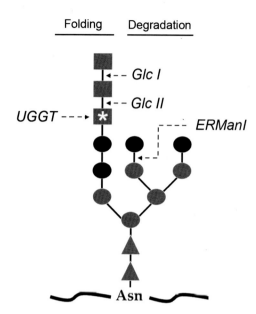

FIGURE 50.2. Generation of glycoprotein fate determinants. Shown is the 14-unit oligosaccharide cotranslationally attached to asparagine (Asn) units located in specific consensus sequences in the polypeptide backbone. The appendage consists of glucose (squares), mannose (ovals), and N-acetylglucosamine (triangles). The sites of hydrolysis by glucosidase I (Glc I), glucosidase II (Glc II), and endoplasmic reticulum mannosidase I (ERManI) are shown. The asterisk designates the specific glucose unit transferred by UDP-glucosidase:glycoprotein glucosyltransferase (UGGT). All $\alpha_{-1,2}$-linked mannose units that can be hydrolyzed by ERManI are shown (black ovals), as is the prominent glycosidic linkage (dashed arrow).

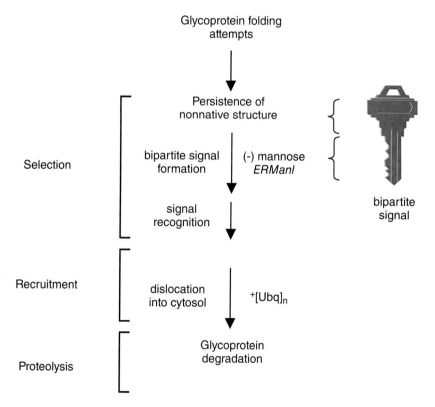

FIGURE 50.3. A triad of requisite events orchestrate the preferential degradation of nonnative glycoproteins on the basis of their inefficient conformational maturation. In the event that repeated folding attempts fail, the molecule's prolonged retention in the early secretory pathway leads to the opportunistic cleavage of mannose (via endoplasmic reticulum mannosidase I [ERManI]) from asparagine-linked oligosaccharides. The cleaved glycans and nonnative structure serve as the central components of a proximal degradation signal and are schematically represented as the shaft and handle of a key, respectively. Signal recognition is speculated to initiate the glycoprotein's recruitment to a proposed retrograde translocon. Polyubiquitination ($[Ubq]_n$) both facilitates dislocation of the protein into the cytosol and triggers proteolysis by 26S proteasomes.

residual nonnative protein structure. The resultant arrangement has been termed the *calnexin cycle*.[27] In the absence of further recognition by UGGT, biologically active glycoproteins are deployed to their sites of operation.

Orchestration of Glycoprotein Degradation

In the second stage of quality control, terminally misfolded glycoproteins are subject to selective clearance from the early secretory pathway by a conformation-based disposal system[43] designated ER-associated degradation (ERAD; Figure 50.3). Persistent engagement of AAT with one or more molecular chaperones[44] is generally diagnostic of a protein folding defect, preventing productive transport beyond the early secretory pathway (see Figure 50.1). The combination of nonnative protein structure and asparagine-linked oligosaccharides opportunistically cleaved by ER mannosidase I in response to prolonged retention has been proposed to generate a luminal bipartite signal that initiates the partitioning of terminally misfolded glycoproteins into glycoprotein ERAD (GERAD; see Figure 50.3).[28] In a recently proposed model, nonnative structure is incapable of initiating entrance into GERAD. Rather, the single determinant is held suspect until acquisition of the oligosaccharide cleavage by ER mannosidase I provides corroborative evidence for inefficient conformational maturation.[45]

Precision of Substrate Selection

Endoplasmic reticulum mannosidase I exists at a remarkably low intracellular concentration,[45] especially when compared with molecular chaperones that are generally plentiful. The stochastic basis by which substrates are selected for GERAD was recently supported by the accelerated degradation of misfolded glycoproteins in response to an experimentally elevated intracellular concentration of recombinant human ER mannosidase I.[45] In contrast to the stochastic model, Lederkremer and Glickman [46] recently suggested that vesicle recycling[47] rather than strict ER retention might contribute to the "timed" degradation of secretion-incompetent glycoproteins. In that model, ER mannosidase I is localized to a downstream compartment,[47] and the recycling of the substrate provides a window of opportunity for cleavage of the asparagine-linked appendages. Regardless of the model, the impaired progression of damaged gene products (i.e., encoded proteins) through the exocytic pathway is broadly reminiscent of the capacity by which damaged DNA impedes cell cycle progression.

Substrate Recruitment and Proteolysis

The trajectory toward proteasomal degradation is suspected to result from downstream machinery predicted to recognize the emergent bipartite signal anatomy (see Figure 50.3). Their role in recruiting the protease-destined molecules to a putative ER channel through which retrotranslocation into the cytosol takes place. The machinery has been discussed elsewhere, and several possible components have been tentatively identified.[28] Subsequent retrotranslocation into cytosol and destruction by cytosolic 26S proteasomes are both mediated by polyubiquitination of the eventual proteasomal substrates. The efficiency, or lack thereof, by which the proposed triad of requisite events operates and their chain of operation conspicuously contribute to the pathogenesis of both the lung and liver diseases (see Figure 50.1).

Potential Therapeutic Approaches

α₁-Antitrypsin deficiency represents one of many conformational diseases. There is currently no specific therapy for the aforementioned end-stage diseases apart from organ transplantation. Rather than attempting to replace the abnormal gene, or add a normal gene by homologous recombination, many have begun to consider pharmacologic intervention. In fact, this idea might very well work because misfolded proteins are degraded by multistep processes (Figure 50.4). For AATD, therapeutic intervention will be attempted for the purpose of enhancing variant Z secretion without affecting the folding or degradation of other molecules. For this reason, it is particularly advantageous that at least three different forms of the Z variant can simultaneously exist in cells (Figure 50.5), and three different degradation systems capable of eliminating AATZ have been identified.[48,49] Also, degradation of the Z variant has been shown to act in a cell type-specific manner, implying that certain conformations of the Z variant might predominate in one cell line over another (see Figure 50.5).

A reasonable, therapeutic strategy is to somehow hinder AAT polymerization in vivo. The idea is to develop small molecules that will block the structural anomaly in the hepatocyte ER because administered synthetic peptides will likely be rapidly metabolized.[50] Finally, the multiple manner by which the degradation systems can apparently operate might even allow for the eventual discovery of novel diagnostic markers and/or prognostic indicators for both the lung and liver diseases.

546 R.N. Sifers

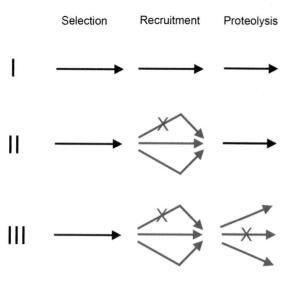

FIGURE 50.4. Three proposed series of requisite events are presented. Type I depicts a single, nondivergent, degradation pathway. Type II depicts a pathway that diverges at the level of substrate recruitment. Type III depicts a pathway that diverges at the level of substrate recruitment and proteolysis. The latter is representative of how Z variant molecules are thought to be degraded. The Xs depict sites of therapeutic intervention that might be selective for a minor class of glycoproteins.

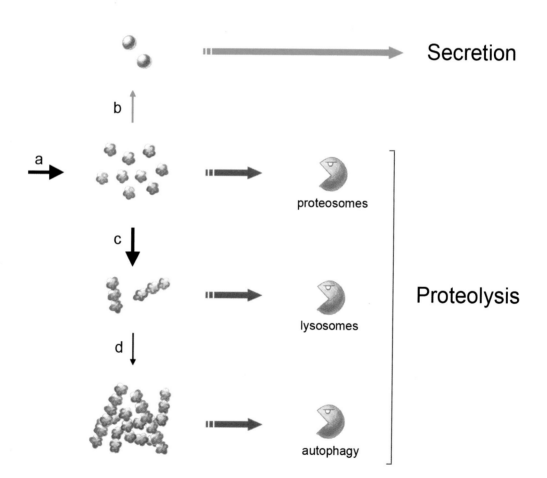

FIGURE 50.5. A small fraction of the newly synthesized Z variant (step a) capable of achieving conformational maturation (step b) is productively released from the endoplasmic reticulum for eventual secretion (green arrow). In contrast, unfolded mono- mers eventually form soluble loop-sheet polymers (step c). These can elongate to form insoluble material (d). The proteo- lytic activities considered to degrade each population are depicted.

References

1. Carrell RW, Pemberton PA, Boswell DR. The serpins: evolution and adaptation in a family of protease inhibitors. Cold Spring Harb Symp Quant Biol 1987;52:527–535.

2. Bao JJ, Sifers RN, Kidd VJ, et al. Molecular evolution of serpins: homologous structure of the human alpha 1-antichymotrypsin and alpha 1-antitrypsin genes. Biochemistry 1987;26(24):7755–7759.

3. Crowther DC, Belorgey D, Miranda E, et al. Practical genetics: alpha-1-antitrypsin deficiency and the serpinopathies. Eur J Hum Genet 2004;12(3):167–172.

4. Sifers RN, Finegold MJ, Woo SL. Molecular biology and genetics of alpha 1-antitrypsin deficiency. Semin Liver Dis 1992;12(3):301–310.

5. Eriksson, S. Studies in alpha 1-antitrypsin deficiency. Acta Med Scand Suppl 1965;432:1–85.

6. Lomas, DA. Chronic obstructive pulmonary disease. Introduction. Thorax 2002;57(8):735.

7. Carrell R, Lomas D, Stein P, et al. Dysfunctional variants and the structural biology of the serpins. Adv Exp Med Biol 1997;425:207–22.

8. Parmar JS, Mahadeva R, Reed BJ, et al. Polymers of alpha(1)-antitrypsin are chemotactic for human neutrophils: a new paradigm for the pathogenesis of emphysema. Am J Respir Cell Mol Biol 2002;26(6):723–730.

9. Graham KS, Le A, Sifers RN. Accumulation of the insoluble PiZ variant of human alpha 1-antitrypsin within the hepatic endoplasmic reticulum does not elevate the steady-state level of grp78/BiP. J Biol Chem 1990;265(33):20463–8.

10. Carlson JA, Rogers BB, Sifers RN, et al. Accumulation of PiZ alpha 1-antitrypsin causes liver damage in transgenic mice. J Clin Invest 1989;83(4):1183–1190.

11. Perlmutter DH. Liver disease associated with alpha 1-antitrypsin deficiency. Prog Liver Dis 1993;11:139–165.

12. Perlmutter DH. Pathogenesis of chronic liver injury and hepatocellular carcinoma in alpha-1-antitrypsin deficiency. Pediatr Res 2006;60(2):233–238.

13. Carrell RW, Whisstock J, Lomas DA. Conformational changes in serpins and the mechanism of alpha 1-antitrypsin deficiency. Am J Respir Crit Care Med 1994;150(6 Pt 2):S171–S175.

14. Lomas DA. Loop-sheet polymerization: the structural basis of Z alpha 1-antitrypsin accumulation in the liver. Clin Sci (Lond) 1994;86(5):489–495.

15. Lomas DA, Evans DL, Finch JT, et al. The mechanism of Z alpha 1-antitrypsin accumulation in the liver. Nature 1992;357(6379):605–607.

16. Lomas DA, Mahadeva R, Alpha1-antitrypsin polymerization and the serpinopathies: pathobiology and prospects for therapy. J Clin Invest 2002;110(11):1585–1590.

17. Mahadeva R, Atkinson C, Li Z, et al. Polymers of Z alpha1-antitrypsin co-localize with neutrophils in emphysematous alveoli and are chemotactic in vivo. Am J Pathol 2005;166(2):377–386.

18. Le A, Graham KS, Sifers RN. Intracellular degradation of the transport-impaired human PiZ alpha 1-antitrypsin variant. Biochemical mapping of the degradative event among compartments of the secretory pathway. J Biol Chem 1990;265(23):14001–14007.

19. Sifers RN, Brashears-Macatee S, Kidd VJ, et al. A frameshift mutation results in a truncated alpha 1-antitrypsin that is retained within the rough endoplasmic reticulum. J Biol Chem 1988;263(15):7330–7335.

20. Teckman JH, Perlmutter DH. The endoplasmic reticulum degradation pathway for mutant secretory proteins alpha1-antitrypsin Z and S is distinct from that for an unassembled membrane protein. J Biol Chem 1996;271(22):13215–13220.

21. Qu D, Teckman JH, Perlmutter DH. Review: alpha 1-antitrypsin deficiency associated liver disease. J Gastroenterol Hepatol 1997;12(5):404–416.

22. Perlmutter DH. Liver injury in alpha 1-antitrypsin deficiency. Clin Liver Dis 2000;4(2):387–408.

23. Wu Y, Whitman I, Molmenti E, et al. A lag in intracellular degradation of mutant alpha 1-antitrypsin correlates with the liver disease phenotype in homozygous PiZZ alpha 1-antitrypsin deficiency. Proc Natl Acad Sci USA 1994;91(19): 9014–9018.

24. Perlmutter DH. The cellular basis for liver injury in alpha 1-antitrypsin deficiency. Hepatology 1991;13(1):172–185.

25. Perlmutter DH. Misfolded proteins in the endoplasmic reticulum. Lab Invest 1999;79(6):623–638.

26. Le A, Ferrell GA, Dishon DS, et al. Soluble aggregates of the human PiZ alpha 1-antitrypsin variant are degraded within the endoplasmic reticulum by a mechanism sensitive to inhibitors of protein synthesis. J Biol Chem 1992;267(2): 1072–1080.

27. Ellgaard L, Helenius A. ER quality control: towards an understanding at the molecular level. Curr Opin Cell Biol 2001;13(4):431–437.

28. Cabral CM, Liu Y, Sifers RN. Dissecting glycoprotein quality control in the secretory pathway. Trends Biochem Sci 2001;26(10):619–624.

29. Hammond C, Helenius A. Quality control in the secretory pathway. Curr Opin Cell Biol 1995;7(4):523–529.

30. Helenius A. Quality control in the secretory assembly line. Philos Trans R Soc Lond B Biol Sci 2001;356(1406): 147–150.

31. Sifers RN. Insights into checkpoint capacity. Nat Struct Mol Biol 2004;11(2):108–109.

32. Helenius A, Marquardt T, Braakman I. The endoplasmic reticulum as a protein-folding compartment. Trends Cell Biol 1992;2(8):227–231.

33. Liu Y, Choudhury P, Cabral CM, et al. Intracellular disposal of incompletely folded human alpha1-antitrypsin involves release from calnexin and post-translational trimming of asparagine-linked oligosaccharides. J Biol Chem 1997;272(12):7946–7951.

34. Cabral CM, Choudhury P, Liu Y, et al. Processing by endoplasmic reticulum mannosidases partitions a secretion-impaired glycoprotein into distinct disposal pathways. J Biol Chem 2000;275(32):25015–25022.

35. Termine D, Wu Y, Liu Y, et al. Alpha1-antitrypsin as model to assess glycan function in endoplasmic reticulum. Methods 2005;35(4):348–353.

36. Helenius A. How N-linked oligosaccharides affect glycoprotein folding in the endoplasmic reticulum. Mol Biol Cell 1994;5(3):253–265.

37. Helenius A, Aebi M. Roles of N-linked glycans in the endoplasmic reticulum. Annu Rev Biochem 2004;73:1019–1049.
38. Cannon KS, Helenius A. Trimming and readdition of glucose to N-linked oligosaccharides determines calnexin association of a substrate glycoprotein in living cells. J Biol Chem 1999;274(11):7537–7544.
39. Hebert DN, Foellmer B, Helenius A. Calnexin and calreticulin promote folding, delay oligomerization and suppress degradation of influenza hemagglutinin in microsomes. EMBO J 1996;15(12):2961–2968.
40. Hammond C, Braakman I, Helenius A. Role of N-linked oligosaccharide recognition, glucose trimming, and calnexin in glycoprotein folding and quality control. Proc Natl Acad Sci USA 1994;91(3):913–917.
41. Hebert DN, Foellmer B, Helenius A. Glucose trimming and reglucosylation determine glycoprotein association with calnexin in the endoplasmic reticulum. Cell 1995;81(3):425–433.
42. Trombetta ES, Helenius A. Conformational requirements for glycoprotein reglucosylation in the endoplasmic reticulum. J Cell Biol 2000;148(6):1123–1129.
43. Sifers RN, Finegold MJ, Woo SL. Alpha-1-antitrypsin deficiency: accumulation or degradation of mutant variants within the hepatic endoplasmic reticulum. Am J Respir Cell Mol Biol 1989;1(5):341–345.
44. Le A, Steiner JL, Ferrell GA, et al. Association between calnexin and a secretion-incompetent variant of human alpha 1-antitrypsin. J Biol Chem 1994;269(10):7514–7519.
45. Wu Y, Swulius MT, Moremen KW, et al. Elucidation of the molecular logic by which misfolded alpha 1-antitrypsin is preferentially selected for degradation. Proc Natl Acad Sci USA 2003;100(14):8229–8234.
46. Lederkremer GZ, Glickman MH. A window of opportunity: timing protein degradation by trimming of sugars and ubiquitins. Trends Biochem Sci 2005;30(6):297–303.
47. Kamhi-Nesher S, Shenkman M, Tolchinsky S, et al. A novel quality control compartment derived from the endoplasmic reticulum. Mol Biol Cell 2001;12(6):1711–1723.
48. Cabral CM, Liu Y, Moremen KW, et al. Organizational diversity among distinct glycoprotein endoplasmic reticulum–associated degradation programs. Mol Biol Cell 2002;13(8):2639–2650.
49. Teckman JH, Burrows J, Hidvegi T, et al. The proteasome participates in degradation of mutant alpha 1-antitrypsin Z in the endoplasmic reticulum of hepatoma-derived hepatocytes. J Biol Chem 2001;276(48):44865–44872.
50. Zhou A, Stein PE, Huntington JA, et al. How small peptides block and reverse serpin polymerisation. J Mol Biol 2004;342(3):931–941.

51
Asthma

David B. Corry and Farrah Kheradmand

Introduction

Asthma is an inflammatory disease of the airways in which patients suffer from episodic dyspnea, cough, and related symptoms accompanied by characteristic abnormalities of the airways that include the presence of eosinophil-predominant allergic inflammation and airway hyperresponsiveness to provocative challenge. The latter abnormality reflects the exaggerated tendency of the asthmatic airway to constrict in response to a broad range of provocative stimuli. Enhanced constrictive responses to especially histamine and cholinergic agonists are used in the bronchial provocation test as a diagnostic aid where disease status remains uncertain based on clinical grounds alone. Additional highly characteristic histologic features of asthma include a metaplastic response of the airway epithelium involving the appearance of mucous-secreting goblet cells with enhanced secretion into the airway of mucin gene products and subepithelial airway fibrosis (Figure 51.1). Both of these abnormalities contribute to airway obstruction acutely and chronically, with airway mucous impaction strongly linked to asphyxiation and death in severe asthma.[1-3]

Although many clinical variants of asthma have been identified, a consistent link to allergic inflammation nonetheless unifies these putatively distinct entities through a common underlying immunopathologic mechanism. Typical evidence of allergic inflammation in asthma patients, irrespective of clinical subtype, includes elevated total or antigen-specific immunoglobulin E (IgE) levels, T helper type 2 (Th2) cells, terminally differentiated CD4+ T cells that secrete a restricted repertoire of cytokines including interleukin 4 (IL-4), IL-5, IL-6, IL-10 and IL-13, and the presence in the blood or airways of eosinophils. Enhanced recruitment of neutrophils to the airways has also been linked to severe asthma.

The contribution of the many molecules and signaling pathways to asthma is best understood in the context of the major immunologic paradigms shown to underlie asthma pathogenesis as established through human, animal, and cell culture studies (see Figure 51.1). For many years, the major theory for the pathogenesis of asthma was the type I hypersensitivity mechanism, which derived from the study of IgE and its ability to activate immune cells such as mast cells that express a high affinity receptor for IgE, FcεRI.[4-7] Studies conducted much later established that the cytokine IL-4 was the major secreted factor regulating B-cell secretion of IgE.[8-10] Furthermore, growth and development of mast cells and eosinophils was shown to be under the control of additional cytokines, especially IL-3, IL-5, and IL-9. Although these cytokines derive from diverse cellular sources, Th2 cells are a major source during established allergic inflammation, suggesting that Th2 cells were likely essential mediators of allergic airway inflammation in asthma.[11] This concept has received abundant experimental validation, largely through study of rodents.[12-15]

An important additional advance regarding the pathogenesis of asthma as derived from experimental systems was the discovery that Th2 cells directly mediate airway disease independent of immunoglobulins.[12,16] Major disease obstructive features such as airway hyperresponsiveness, goblet cell metaplasia, and glycoprotein hypersecretion are mediated by IL-4 and IL-13 acting directly on lung cells through a receptor complex that includes the α-chain of the IL-4 receptor (IL-4Rα).[17,18] Interleukin-4 and IL-13 ultimately induce these highly characteristic lung abnormalities through a receptor that includes IL-4Rα and the transcription factor signal transducer and activator of transcription 6 (STAT6).[19-24] Figure 51.1 provides an overview of the major immune mechanisms relevant to asthma and some of the major molecules through which these mechanisms are coordinated.

The relevance of many additional molecules implicated, either through human or animal studies or both, to the pathogenesis of asthma can be understood in terms of the major physiologic checkpoints regulating disease expression (Figure 51.2). The earliest inflammatory

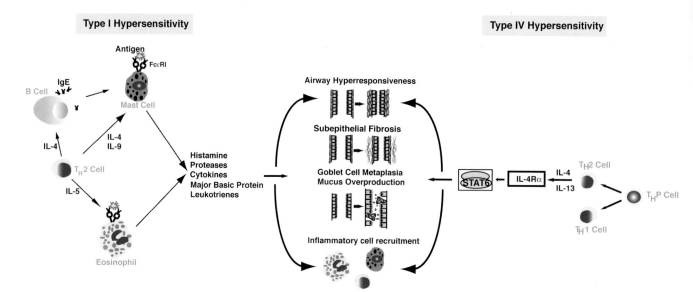

FIGURE 51.1. The major immune mechanisms underlying asthma pathogenesis. Two major mechanisms, type I hypersensitivity and type IV hypersensitivity, are thought to contribute to the major structural and physiologic changes associated with asthma, including airway hyperresponsiveness, goblet cell metaplasia with mucous hypersecretion, subepithelial airway fibrosis, and recruitment to the lungs of diverse inflammatory cells. During type I hypersensitivity, immunoglobulin (Ig) E secreted by B cells is captured by high-affinity receptors (FcεRI) present on mast cells and eosinophils. Cross-linking of surface-associated IgE induced by exposure to cognate antigen results in activation of FcεRI-bearing cells and the release of a large number of potentially toxic molecules that together contribute to the asthma phenotype. In contrast, type I hypersensitivity involves predominantly T lymphocytes and is immunoglobulin independent. The cytokines interleukin (IL)-4 and IL-13, secreted predominantly by Th2 cells, act directly on target tissues of the airway to elicit the asthma phenotype. Note that Th2 cells, through the cytokines that they secrete, are critical mediators of both disease mechanisms and provide the factors necessary for the growth and differentiation of asthma-associated inflammatory cells. STAT, signal transducer and activator of transcription.

events in asthma are not directly tied to Th2 cells but rather begin through innate inflammatory pathways initiated by allergens that are only now beginning to be understood (stage I). Among many effects, innate inflammatory mechanisms likely initiate the developmental programs governing maturation of Th2 cells, eosinophils, and other allergic effector cells while simultaneously initiating the recruitment of these cells to the lungs through additional signaling programs (stages II and III). Once allergic inflammatory cells become established in the lung, their effector mechanisms begin the process of lung remodeling that results in acute and chronic airway obstruction (stage IV). Finally, the asthmatic lung can turn in one of two distinct directions. For reasons that are currently obscure, asthma can evolve into more complex clinical syndromes that include allergic bronchopulmonary mycosis, Churg-Strauss syndrome, chronic eosinophilic pneumonia, and possibly others (stage V). Conversely, and at any point in disease, allergic inflammation can resolve and the lung remodeling, if any, can, at least to some degree, attenuate to a more normal pathologic and physiologic state (stage VI).

In this chapter, we review the contribution of the many molecules implicated in asthma pathogenesis, emphasizing the genetic studies that have linked specific polymorphisms to disease. It should be noted that for most of these studies, little insight yet exists as to why specific polymorphisms associate with asthma, although it is clear that other mutations modulate in significant ways the most important allergic signaling pathways controlling disease expression.

Molecular Pathogenesis of Asthma

For ease of presentation, molecules are considered in the context of closely related members that share key characteristics. Occasionally, molecules closely related based on structure will have markedly different functions in asthma, creating the potential for confusion. Cross-referencing to Figure 51.2, which regroups the same molecules according to the major checkpoint(s) in which they participate, will minimize such confusion.

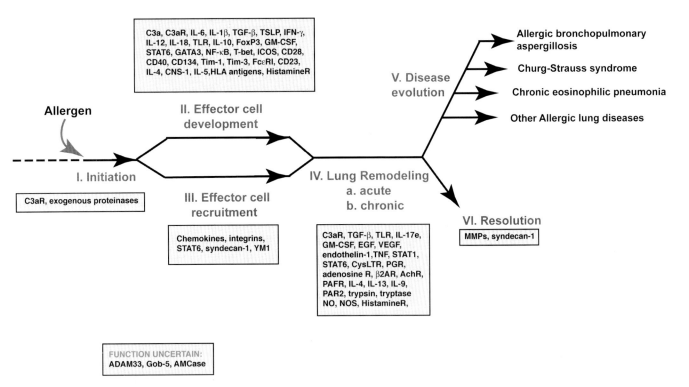

FIGURE 51.2. The major checkpoints in the evolution of asthma and related allergic lung syndromes. Following initiation of allergic lung inflammation by inhaled allergens, distinct genetic programs are activated that direct the development and recruitment of allergic effector cells to the lung. Recruited inflammatory cells, through their secreted products, then begin the process of lung remodeling, acute and chronic structural changes that ultimately cause airway obstruction and reduced lung function. From this point, disease can either resolve or progress to a variety of more complex clinical forms. The molecules regulating each checkpoint, where known, are indicated in the highlighted boxes. Ach, acetylcholine; ADAM33, a disintegrin and metalloprotease domain 33; AMCase, acidic mammalian chitin- ase; C3a, complement 3a; C3aR, complement 3a receptor; CNS, conserved noncoding sequence; CysLTR, cysteinyl leukotriene receptor; EGF, epidermal growth factor; GM-CSF, granulo- cyte–macrophage colony-stimulating factor; ICOS, inducible costimulator; IFN, interferon; IL, interleukin; MMP, matrix metalloproteinase; NF, nuclear factor; NO, nitric oxide; NOS, nitric oxide synthase; PAFR, platelet-activating factor receptor; PGR, prostaglandin receptor; R, receptor; STAT, signal trans- ducer and activator of transcription; T-bet, T-box expressed in T cells; TGF, transforming growth factor; TIM, T-cell immuno- globulin and mucin domain protein molecule; TNF, tumor necrosis factor; TLR, Toll-like receptor; TSLP, thymic stromal lymphopoietin.

Cytokines, Growth Factors, and Related Regulatory DNA

Interleukin-4 and Interleukin-13

Cytokines are the currency through which immune cells mediate physiologic change in the lungs and elsewhere and contribute, positively and negatively, to the regulation of allergic inflammation in asthma. As discussed previously, IL-4 and IL-13 are related cytokines critical to the induction of allergic inflammation and for lung remodeling leading to airway obstruction. Despite sharing the same receptor signaling subunit (IL-4Rα) and activating the same major transcription factor (STAT6), IL-4 and IL-13 have unique functions, although some overlap in their activities can be detected (Figure 51.3). Thus, the function of IL-4 is confined largely to the immune compartment, where it serves as the most important factor regulating the growth and differentiation of Th2 cells and IgE-secreting B cells. In contrast, IL-13 is the most important Th2 factor mediating physiologic change within the airways (airway hyperresponsiveness, goblet cell metaplasia, eosinophil recruitment), and therefore its effects are primarily extraimmune. Because of the similarity in their signaling functions, it is inevitable that IL-13 will have some effect on IgE production and, similarly, that IL-4 can contribute directly to airway disease, but these latter effects are probably dispensable in comparison with the contribution of the other cytokine.[25]

Within the *IL-4* gene exist several polymorphisms that have been linked to asthma, including cytosine to thymidine mutations at position −34 and −589 that occur in

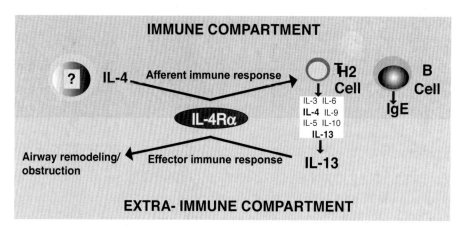

FIGURE 51.3. Interleukin (IL)-4 and IL-13 in asthma pathogenesis. Despite sharing the IL-4Rα receptor signaling subunit, IL-4 and IL-13 play distinct but equally critical roles. The effects of IL-4, the original source of which is uncertain, are confined largely to the immune compartment where IL-4 determines the growth and development of Th2 cells and immunoglobulin E (IgE)–secreting B cells. In contrast, IL-13, which is produced predominantly by mature Th2 cells, acts largely on extraimmune target tissues of the lung to induce the remodeling changes linked to airway obstruction.

diverse populations.[26–29] A cytosine to thymidine exchange occurring at position −1055 of the IL-13 promoter was also linked to asthma, and additional data suggested that this polymorphism enhanced expression of IL-13 transcriptionally.[30,31] The *IL-13* gene contains a nonconservative mutation involving an arginine to glutamine substitution at position 110 (or 130 if the signal peptide is included) that was linked to asthma in British and Japanese patients[32] but not in a United States cohort.[33] Additional studies have shown that this mutation enhances STAT6-dependent signaling in vitro and that the R130Q mutant is less susceptible to inhibition by soluble IL-13Rα2, an IL-13-inhibiting agent.[34] These findings together indicate that the R130Q *IL-13* mutant may be substantially more active in vivo than other isoforms.

Interleukin-4 Receptor α-Subunit

The principal component of the IL-4 and IL-13 receptors, IL-4Rα, is linked to asthma through several mutations, including an isoleucine to valine polymorphism at position 50,[35,36] an arginine mutation at position 576,[37] and several others in Hutterites.[38] Additional mutations, although not significant individually, in combination produce an IL-4 receptor that is more sensitive to IL-4 signaling and a haplotype with significant linkage to atopic asthma.[29,39] However, the strongest genetic linkages with asthma are associated with more complex haplotypes involving combinatorial mutations in the genes for IL-4, IL-13, IL-4Rα, and STAT6.[40–42] Thus, analysis of the IL-4/IL-13 signaling pathway indicates that individual polymorphisms can have an additive effect that dramatically enhances the expression and/or severity of asthma, a

finding that agrees well with the overall importance of this pathway as shown in experimental systems.[17]

Conserved Noncoding Sequence 1

Within the short region spanning the *IL-4* and *IL-13* genes exists a highly conserved noncoding sequence, CNS-1, that coordinately regulates the expression of these two cytokines and is required for optimal Th2-cell development.[43] Mutations in this region, although uncommon, are also associated with asthma.[28] Presumably, these mutations affect Th2-cell development, but this has yet to be formally proven.

Interleukin-5 and Interleukin-9

The cytokines IL-5 and IL-9 are located within the distal arm of chromosome 5 near the IL-4 and IL-13 loci and are Th2 cytokines as well. The overall importance of IL-5 in asthma remains unclear. Interleukin-5 is indisputably important as a growth and differentiation factor for eosinophils,[44] but various experimental strategies have failed to resolve the overall importance of either IL-5 or eosinophils in asthma.[13,45–47] Human clinical trials have shown that neutralization of IL-5 has little effect during established asthma,[48,49] but, because this treatment failed to completely remove lung eosinophils, a role for these cells in perpetuating disease remains possible.[50] Despite initial interest in IL-9 as an important factor in asthma, newer studies have demonstrated its dispensable role in experimental asthma.[51] No polymorphisms are known from the *IL-5* and *IL-9* genes that show clear linkage to asthma, but two noncoding polymorphisms within the

IL-5Rα gene, which is required for IL-5 signaling, have shown linkage to asthma in Korean patients.[52]

Transforming Growth Factor-β1

Transforming growth factor (TGF)-β1 is a highly pleiotropic cytokine secreted from diverse sources that is implicated in two phenomena relevant to asthma: enhancement of airway fibrosis and suppression of inflammation. Transforming growth factor-β expression by airway epithelial cells is upregulated by IL-13,[53] suggesting that it may enhance the airway fibrosis that is seen especially during chronic allergen challenge[54,55] and that is believed to contribute to fixed decline in lung function with long-standing asthma. Despite these observations, overall airway TGF-β expression does not vary between patients with asthma and other obstructive diseases, nor do expression levels of TGF-β distinguish asthma patients with different degrees of severity.[56,57]

Conversely, TGF-β is also highly immunosuppressive. Mice lacking this cytokine succumb to a lethal immune proliferative state marked by massive infiltration of most tissues with inflammatory cells. Transforming growth factor-β specifically coordinates the activation of CD4+CD25+CD62L+ T regulatory cells that suppress the development of allergic lung inflammation by activating the transcription factor Foxp3.[58] T regulatory cells secrete IL-10 and/or TGF-β itself to inhibit activation of Th2 cells, secretion of proinflammatory cytokines, and experimental asthma.[58,59]

Several polymorphisms in the TGF-β1 gene have been linked to asthma.[60] The threonine allele at position −509 (T509) of the TGF-β1 promoter, which may encode for a new transcription factor binding site, was significantly linked to allergy and greater asthma severity, particularly when homozygous,[60–62] although subsequent studies have failed to confirm this finding in Caucasian patients.[63] A second TGF-β1 polymorphism (T869C) has also been linked to increased asthma susceptibility in Chinese atopic patients.[64] How these polymorphisms affect the expression of allergic disease has not been defined.

Interleukin-1α and Interleukin-1β

Interleukin-1α and -1β are macrophage and epithelial cytokines with potent T-cell–activating potential that signal through the same receptor (IL-1R1). Under some, but not all, experimental conditions, both IL-1 isoforms and IL-1R1 are required for normal Th2-cell proliferation and cytokine secretion and therefore allergic lung inflammation, but, paradoxically, lack of IL-1α alone results in enhanced allergic lung responses and Th2-cell activity.[65,66] Although a link between IL-1 polymorphisms and asthma has yet to be clearly established,[67,68] several polymorphisms encompassing many distinct haplotypes

of the IL-1 receptor antagonist gene (IL-1RA), which encodes for a soluble protein that inhibits IL-1 signaling, are associated with asthma susceptibility.[69]

Interleukin-6

Interleukin-6 is a cytokine that is thought to primarily regulate T-cell, especially Th2-cell, responses and IgE secretion.[70] Although originally thought to be a requisite factor in Th2 differentiation,[71] it is now clear that IL-6 is not required for murine allergic responses.[72] Indeed, there exists evidence to support an antiinflammatory role for IL-6 in allergic responses of the lung and other organs.[73–76] No polymorphisms in the IL-6 and related genes have yet been linked to asthma.

Thymic Stromal Lymphopoietin

Thymic stromal lymphopoietin (TSLP) is related to IL-7 and was originally described as a B-cell growth and differentiation factor.[77] More recent studies have, however, revealed that TSLP is produced outside of the thymus, especially in the airways of asthmatic humans and epithelial cells to promote allergic responses.[78,79] Thymic stromal lymphopoietin signaling is required for optimal Th2 development from naïve precursor cells and allergic lung inflammation.[80,81] At least for human T cells, TSLP promotes Th2 differentiation by inducing expression of OX-40 ligand.[82] Thymic stromal lymphopoietin signaling–deficient mice further show enhanced Th1 responses,[80] suggesting that TSLP might be a master regulator of Th2 responses.[83]

Interleukin-10

Interleukin-10 was originally described as a Th2 cytokine but is now known to be secreted by diverse cells, including T cells, macrophages, monocytes, and epithelial cells. Interleukin-10 is readily detected in the lungs and airways of asthmatic patients where it is thought to exert an immunosuppressive role. Although IL-10 can promote IgE and IgG1 responses under some conditions,[84] studies of IL-10–deficient mice in asthma and asthma-like inflammation models consistently demonstrate enhanced inflammation and disease parameters, including airway hyperresponsiveness, in its absence.[85,86] Interleukin-10, together with TGF-β1, is thought to account for much of the antiinflammatory properties of T regulatory cells.

Many polymorphisms in the IL-10 gene have been linked to asthma and IgE secretion. These include a cytosine to adenine exchange at position −571 of the IL-10 promoter, which linked to elevated total serum IgE in subjects hetero- or homozygous for the mutation,[87] and a similar cytosine to adenine mutation at position −627, which was associated with a higher risk of developing asthma.[67] A thymidine to cytosine exchange at position 4299 of the 3′ untranslated region was significantly associated with forced expiratory volume in 1 sec (FEV$_1$) percent predicted.[88] The promoter haplotype GCC, involving three distinct polymorphisms at positions −1117, −854, and −627, respectively, was positively associated with IgE levels and FEV$_1$ percent predicted, whereas the haplotype ATA involving the same loci was negatively linked to airway hyperreactivity and FEV$_1$.[88] Additional haplotypes involving the IL-10 promoter that show complex links to asthma (positive and negative associations) have also been identified in persons of Indian descent.[89] The molecular basis for these IL-10–based polymorphism associations have yet to be defined.

Interleukin-17

Interleukin-17 actually represents a family with at least six members (IL-17a–f); IL-17e is also termed IL-25. Thus far, only one member of this extended cytokine family has been shown to have relevance to asthma, although more than one isotype is found in respiratory secretions of asthma patients.[90–92] IL-17e/IL-25 promotes Th2 responses, airway eosinophilia, and airway mucin secretion as assessed in studies of mice.[92–96] No studies have demonstrated, however, whether IL-17e/IL-25 is required for either Th2 responses or allergic lung inflammation and therefore whether this cytokine represents a suitable therapeutic target. No associations were found between polymorphisms in the *IL-17f* gene and asthma.[97]

Granulocyte–Macrophage Colony-Stimulating Factor

Granulocyte–macrophage colony-stimulating factor (GM-CSF) is a product of eosinophils, T cells, and respiratory epithelium that is consistently found in the respiratory secretions of asthma patients.[11,98,99] Although known principally as a growth factor for macrophages and related cells, GM-CSF is an important survival factor for lung eosinophils in asthma.[100–102] Additional studies from rodents indicate an important role for GM-CSF in regulating the expression of allergic lung disease. Adenoviral-mediated expression of GM-CSF in the respiratory epithelium enhanced the allergic immune response to airway allergen challenge, resulting in prolonged and exaggerated allergic inflammation.[103] Granulocyte–macrophage colony-stimulating factor was also important for the expression of allergic inflammation and airway hyperresponsiveness due to ovalbumin, ragweed pollen, and diesel exhaust particles.[104–106] These findings are of particular interest because GM-CSF is able to overcome the tolerogenic (noninflammatory) reaction of the lung to inhaled antigens such as ovalbumin and ragweed pollen that otherwise require exogenous adjuvant factors and systemic immunization before intranasal challenge results in significant inflammation. Granulocyte–macrophage colony-stimulating factor may therefore serve as an important endogenous adjuvant factor that conditions the airways for subsequent allergic responses.

Epidermal Growth Factor

Epidermal growth factor (EGF) is one of many factors that affect the growth and differentiation of the epithelium and other lung tissues. Expression of both EGF and its receptor was enhanced in airway biopsy specimens from asthmatic patients, particularly on airway goblet cells, with enhanced expression correlating with disease severity.[107–109] While these studies only suggest a role for EGF in the regulation of airway remodeling during allergic inflammation, subsequent studies of rats confirmed the ability of EGF to induce goblet cell metaplasia and mucin gene expression, although this required the prior intratracheal administration of tumor necrosis factor.[110] Thus, EGF is similar to other cytokines, such as IL-4 and IL-13, that are capable of inducing airway epithelial remodeling, especially goblet cell metaplasia, but it remains unclear if EGF, like these other factors, is required for this effect.

Vascular Endothelial Growth Factor

A distinct aspect of airway remodeling is the proliferation of blood vessels (angiogenesis) that accompanies inflammation.[111] Peribronchovascular angiogenesis is believed to contribute to airway narrowing and may promote edema formation that further enhances airway obstruction in asthma. Multiple secreted factors potentially regulate this process, including vascular endothelial growth factor (VEGF), endothelin-1, angiogenin, and fibroblast growth factor (FGF). Expression of all four angiogenic factors was increased in the airways or induced sputum of asthma patients.[111–115] Overexpression of VEGF in mouse airways promoted growth of new vessels as expected but also resulted in both allergic inflammation alone and enhanced allergic inflammation in response to inhaled allergen.[116,117] Similarly, inhibition of the VEGF receptor in an allergen-dependent model of asthma resulted in a modest decrease in airway inflammation but failed to inhibit IgE responses, nor did inhibition of VEGF alter the vascularity of lung parenchyma.[118] These surprising findings indicate that VEGF in the context of allergic inflammation plays an important, but not obligatory, role in coordinating the airway inflammatory response to inhaled allergen but may not be important to the process of neovascularization at least during acute inflammation.

Endothelin-1

Endothelin-1 is a vasoactive factor secreted by endothelium and epithelium and is capable of inducing tracheobronchial constriction.[119–123] Inhibition of endothelin in allergen-challenged rodents further inhibited allergic inflammation and proinflammatory cytokine secretion,[124,125] but mice with 50% of normal endothelin expression showed no impairment in airway hyperresponsiveness following allergen challenge.[126] Asthma patients exposed to endothelin aerosol uniformly showed bronchoconstriction but no alteration in inflammatory parameters.[127] Despite these insights, further studies are required to define the importance of endothelin in asthma in relation to other proinflammatory factors.

Fibroblast Growth Factors, Angiogenin, and Platelet-Derived Growth Factor

Fibroblast growth factors, angiogenin, and platelet-derived growth factor show enhanced expression in the airways of asthma patients and could potentially contribute to disease manifestations through their ability to support fibroblast proliferation and angiogenesis. However, few functional data as yet clearly support such roles in asthma.[111,128,129]

Tumor Necrosis Factor

Tumor necrosis factor (TNF) is a potent inflammatory cytokine that is strongly implicated in T-cell–dependent inflammation underlying autoimmune diseases, but it is also detected in elevated amounts in the lungs of asthma patients, especially following allergen challenge.[130,131] Neutralization of TNF in allergen-challenged mice consistently resulted in less airway inflammation and reduced airway hyperreactivity.[132–134] Human studies of TNF inhibition in asthma have, however, been inconsistent. A phase I study of 21 patients given soluble TNF receptor showed no benefit for asthma and was terminated because of serious neurologic side effects.[135] However, the same agent given to a different patient cohort with refractory disease significantly improved airway hyperresponsiveness and other disease indices.[136] Thus, TNF is clearly expressed in the airways of asthma patients and at least for some patients appears to contribute to disease expression, but through mechanisms that remain obscure.

Genetic studies have linked a complex haplotype involving the *TNF* gene (glycine substitution for alanine at position 308) and a closely linked allele for lymphotoxin-α, a cytokine very similar to TNF, and expression of asthma in Caucasian populations in the United Kingdom, Taiwanese Asians, and North Indians.[137–139] but studies from distinct populations have failed to support this association.[27,140,141] A distinct polymorphism involving the lymphotoxin-α promoter (glycine to alanine change at position −753) was found to associate more frequently with asthmatic children from Japan. This polymorphism conferred less transcriptional activity compared with the nontransmitted allele.[142]

As with many genetic linkage studies in asthma, small population size, as well as genetic heterogeneity, might have contributed to discordant results involving TNF polymorphisms in distinct populations. The largest study of TNF and related polymorphisms in human asthma involved an analysis of 708 children for both single and multiple polymorphisms. In this analysis, no associations between single polymorphisms and asthma were found, but a complex haplotype involving both the lymphotoxin-α and TNF loci was found.[143]

Interleukin-12

Several soluble factors are important for their inhibitory role in Th2 development and allergic lung inflammation. Perhaps the best known of these is IL-12, a heterodimeric product of dendritic cells and other antigen-presenting cells (consisting of p35 and p40 subunits) that controls Th1-cell development and the secretion of interferon (IFN)-γ. Both IL-12 and IFN-γ directly inhibit the activity of Th2 cells and have been linked to the suppression of allergic lung inflammation induced by allergen.[144,145] Interleukin-18 has activity similar to that of IL-12,[146] but it also enhances IgE secretion and allergic lung inflammation under some conditions.[147,148]

Heterozygosity in IL-12B (p40 subunit) promoter polymorphisms strongly correlated with increased risk for asthma severity in atopic and nonatopic Australian children, whereas no link was established for these mutations in their homozygous state.[149] The heterozygous state was associated with less production of IL-12 by dendritic cells, suggesting a mechanism by which less production of a powerful suppressant of allergic lung inflammation might lead to more severe disease in heterozygous individuals.[149] This finding, however, was not replicated in a much larger longitudinal cohort study of similar child and adult asthmatics.[150] Additional polymorphisms in the IL-12B promoter and 3′ untranslated region correlated with transcript instability, lower transcriptional level of mature IL-12 mRNA, and protection against childhood asthma.[151] Additional polymorphisms within the *IL-12* gene have been linked to adult asthma,[152] but these preliminary studies require verification in larger and more diverse cohorts.

Toll-Like Receptors

Allergic lung inflammation can be inhibited through the endogenous release of IL-12 and related factors through the Toll-like receptor (TLR) family, which in humans includes at least 10 members. Unique products derived from bacteria, viruses, fungi, and parasites activate these cell surface- and cytoplasm-associated receptors and induce powerful type 1 immune responses especially when given in combination,[153] Evidence further suggests that endotoxin (lipopolysaccharide, a TLR4 agonist) present in homes promotes type 1 immunity and protects against asthma.[154] However, when administered individually, endotoxin and peptidoglycan, a TLR2 ligand, can paradoxically elicit Th2 activation and allergic lung inflammation in mice under some experimental conditions.[155,156]

Numerous single nucleotide polymorphisms involving TLR4 and TLR9 have been described, of which none of the common ones has been linked to asthma in diverse North American cohorts.[157–159] However, a point mutation in TLR4 (Asp299Gly) resulted in less secretion of IL-12 and IL-10 from peripheral blood mononuclear cells with lipopolysaccharide stimulation and was further linked to a fourfold higher risk for allergic asthma in Swedish school children.[160] A single mutation on *TLR2* was also linked to asthma and allergies in European children of farmers but failed to associate with disease in children not living on farms.[161]

Chemokines and Their Receptors

Studies from asthma patients have established that allergic airway inflammation is commonly, if not invariably, present with active disease. Additional studies from mice have established two fundamental findings regarding asthma pathogenesis: (1) Allergic inflammation is necessary for airway hyperresponsiveness and other physiologic changes linked to asthma, and (2) allergic inflammatory cells must be recruited to the lungs, not merely be present in the animal, to induce disease. Therefore, a critical aspect of asthma pathogenesis is the molecules regulating recruitment of allergic inflammatory cells to lung. This important molecular family includes chemokines and other chemotactic molecules and their receptors that regulate the extravasation of circulating leukocytes into the lung parenchyma.

Chemokines are small (8–10-kDa) cytokines secreted by numerous tissues that activate cells through seven transmembrane spanning, G protein–coupled receptors to coordinate the recruitment (i.e., homing) of inflammatory cells to sites of inflammation.[162,163] These molecules are classified into four subfamilies based on the N-terminal position of their cysteine residues: C, CC, CXC, and CXXXC.[163,164] The CC ligand (CCL) subfamily of chemokines currently has over 28 members in humans and 21 homologs in the mouse; all genes reside on chromosomes 17 and 11 in the human and mouse, respectively. Although all members of this large family have

been implicated in leukocyte migration, CCL subfamily members are of particular interest because they play a key role in antigen-specific Th2 activation, proliferation, and release of cytokines and as such play an important role in asthma.[164–167] Of particular interest are the chemokines CCL17 (thymus and activation related chemokine) and eotaxins1–3, which are essential for homing to lung of Th2 cells and eosinophils.[168] The receptor for CCL17, CCR4 (but not other receptors, e.g., CXCR3, that are more specific for Th1 cells), is preferentially expressed by Th2 cells[169] and T cells from lungs of asthmatics,[170] and its inhibition results in attenuation of experimental allergic lung disease.[171] The other major chemokine receptor known to be relevant to allergic lung disease is CCR3, which is important to regulating eosinophilia through eotaxin and other chemokines. The CCR3 receptor may also influence the development of airway hyperresponsiveness in animal models under some but not all experimental conditions.[172,173] Other chemokine receptors relevant to the recruitment of allergic inflammatory cells, where known, are summarized in Table 51.1.

Several polymorphisms in eotaxins and their receptor have been linked to allergic lung disease, including eotaxin 2 (negative association) and CCR3 (T51C; positive association).[174,175] A single nucleotide polymorphism in the RANTES promoter further conferred a 6.5-fold increased risk for moderate to severe airway obstruction in asthma.[176] Two additional polymorphisms encoding amino acid exchanges in one of the IL-8 receptors (CXCR1; methionine to arginine change at position 31 and an arginine to cysteine change at position 335) was significantly linked to expression of asthma in children.[177] However, the mechanism by which these polymorphisms may contribute to or ameliorate allergic disease have yet to be defined.

Integrins

The heterodimeric integrins are the principal molecules governing recruitment of allergic inflammatory cells through adhesive events and thus are functionally linked to the chemokines. Integrin subunits expressed by CD4+

TABLE 51.1. Asthma inflammatory cell-related chemokines and their receptors and agonists.

Allergic effector cell	Chemokine receptors expressed	Cognate chemokines	Chemokine agonists
Th2 cell, eosinophil	CCR3, CCR4, CCR8	CCL17, CCL7, CCL11, CCL6, CCL8	IL-13, IL-4, allergens?
Neutrophil	CXCR1,2	CXCL1, CXCL3, CXCL5	Endotoxin, many others

T cells include CD29 (β_1-integrin), CD18 (β_2-integrin), and β_7-integrin, but only CD29 and CD18 integrins have been significantly linked to human or experimental asthma. A large number of α-chain subunits may pair with these β-chains. These relationships, their counter ligands including matrix and soluble proteins and cell-associated addressins, and the complex nomenclature that has evolved to describe these molecules are listed in Table 51.2.

Chemokine receptor signaling results in the phosphorylation of integrins, which in turn changes their structure into a more adhesive conformation required for homing. The I (inserted) domain of the α-subunit is the critical domain that binds to addressins and facilitates extravasation. The α-subunit is typically the larger integrin and undergoes conformational change in response to cellular activation.

Analysis of CD29 integrins in experimental asthma has produced mixed results, with some studies indicating an absolute requirement and others indicating a relatively unimportant role.[178–180] CD29 integrins are difficult to block entirely, and the route by which the same inhibitor is given to rodents and the timing of administration dramatically affect the outcome of blockade.[181,182] Additional studies, most likely with genetically defined animals, are required to clearly establish the importance of CD29 integrins in asthma models.

In contrast, studies from humans and animal models consistently support a requisite role for CD18 integrins in allergic lung disease. Both CD54 (intercellular cell adhesion molecule-1) and lymphocyte function-associated antigen-1 (LFA-1) are essential for induction of allergic lung disease in the mouse.[183,184] Moreover, CD102 (intercellular cell adhesion molecule-2), an addressin for LFA-1, is expressed on vascular endothelium and serves to promote eosinophil egression from lung parenchyma. Lack of CD102 results in prolonged lung interstitial eosinophilia and enhanced airway hyperresponsiveness.[185] Although some reports suggested a role for LFA-1 in Th2-cell development, additional studies of CD18-deficient mice have refuted an important developmental role for this integrin but established that CD18 is selectively required for the homing of Th2 cells, but not eosinophils, to lung.[186] Two polymorphisms in the *CD54* gene, one encoding an amino acid exchange (lysine for glutamic acid at position 469) and another in the 3′ untranslated region, have, individually and in combination, been linked to asthma in German children.[187]

Transcription Factors

By controlling the expression of genes essential for allergic lung inflammation and lung physiologic changes, transcription factors are crucial elements regulating asthma pathogenesis. As intermediate factors in the signaling cascades most important to the expression of asthma, the contribution of transcription factors is coded according to their activating ligands, where known, and genes induced (Table 51.3). Most transcription factors relevant to asthma models control the development of Th2 cells but are likely to play additional roles as well. For example, STAT6 is also required in the airway epithelium for airway hyperresponsiveness and for production of chemokines necessary for allergic cell recruitment.[19,188]

Signal Transducer and Activator of Transcription 1

Signal transducer and activator of transcription 1 was found to be constitutively active in the airway epithelium of asthma patients, but the overall significance of this finding remains unclear.[189] The role of STAT1 in experimental asthma has not been tested directly, but activation of STAT1 through IFN-γ[190] or indirectly through IL-12[144] leads to resolution of allergic changes, indicating a protective effect. However, STAT1 can coordinate pulmonary chemokine expression as seen during allergic inflammation and can be activated by IL-4 and IL-13 under some in vitro conditions,[191] suggesting that a pro-allergic effect through STAT1 may be possible under some conditions.

TABLE 51.2. Integrins and their receptors. Molecules most clearly linked to asthma are shown in bold.

Name	CD Classification	Ligand
Integrin family		
β_1-integrins		
$\alpha_1\beta_1$ (VLA-1)	CD49a/CD29	Col I, Col IV, LN
$\alpha_2\beta_1$ (VLA-2)	CD49b/CD29	Col I, Col IV, LN
$\alpha_3\beta_1$ (VLA-3)	CD49c/CD29	FN, ColI, LN
$\alpha_4\beta_1$ (VLA-4)	**CD49d/CD29**	**FN, CD106, Tsp**
$\alpha_5\beta_1$ (VLA-5)	CD49e/CD29	FN, Tsp
$\alpha_6\beta_1$ (VLA-6)	CD49f/CD29	LN
β_2 integrins		
$\alpha_L\beta_2$ (LFA-1)	**CD11a/CD18**	**CD54**, ICAM-2, ICAM-3
$\alpha_M\beta_2$ (Mac-1)	CD11b/CD18	**CD54**, iC3b, FN, factor X
$\alpha_X\beta_2$ (p150, 95)	CD11c/CD18	iC3b, factor X
$\alpha_D\beta_2$	CD11d/CD18	ICAM-3
Immunoglobulin superfamily		
ICAM-1	**CD54**	LFA-1, CD11b/CD18
ICAM-2	**CD102**	LFA-1
VCAM-1	**CD106**	CD29 integrins

Col, collagen; FN, fibronectin; ICAM, intercellular adhesion molecule; LFA-1, leukocyte function associated antigen 1; LN, laminin; Tsp, thrombospondin; VCAM, vascular cell adhesion molecule; VLA, very late antigen.

TABLE 51.3. Transcription factors implicated in the regulation of asthma.

Transcription factor	Activating molecules	Genes regulated	Role in asthma models
STAT1	TLRL, interferons	Cytokines and other genes linked to type I immunity	Reduces allergic inflammation and AHR
STAT6	IL-4, IL-13	Cytokines and other genes linked to type 2 immunity	Required for Th2 cell development and recruitment; AHR
GATA3	STAT6	Th2 cytokines, IL-12Rβ2	Required for Th2 development
NF-κB	TLRLs, TNF, IL-1, many other cytokines and other factors	Proinflammatory cytokines, chemokines, many other molecules	Required for Th2 development and AHR
T-bet	?	Genes required for Th1 development	Suppresses Th2 development and AHR

Note: AHR, airway hyperresponsiveness; IL, interleukin; NF, nuclear factor; STAT, signal transducer and activator of transcription; T-bet, T-box expressed in T cells; TLRL, Toll-like receptor ligand; TNF, tumor necrosis factor.

Signal Transducer and Activator of Transcription 6

Signal transducer and activator of transcription 6 is activated by the Th2 cytokines IL-4 and IL-13. As discussed earlier, these molecules together coordinate the allergic lung response from multiple checkpoints, including Th2-cell development, Th2-cell and eosinophil recruitment to the lung, and airway remodeling changes that include airway hyperresponsiveness and goblet cell metaplasia (see Figures 51.1 and 51.2).[19,188,192,193]

GATA3

GATA3 is a transcription factor activated by STAT6 and regulates Th2-cell development by controlling the production of type 2 cytokines.[194,195] GATA3 may also activate in the absence of STAT6. This could reflect "autoactivation" or the action of nuclear factor-κB (NF-κB), which is also required for experimental asthma.[196,197] As with STAT6, GATA3 is required to produce the experimental asthma phenotype in mice.[197]

Nuclear Factor-κB

The TLRs generally signal through the transcription factor NF-κB, typically to activate type 1 immune responses that antagonize type 2 immunity. Surprisingly, however, the p50 subunit of NF-κB was shown to be essential for stable Th2, but not Th1, development, but not for maintenance of the committed Th2 phenotype. Mice deficient in p50 were further incapable of mounting allergic inflammation of the lung because of their inability produce the Th2 cytokines IL-4, IL-5, and IL-13.[197] This important finding demonstrates that the NF-κB complex is a more general regulator of inflammation than previously recognized and specifically is relevant to the expression of allergic lung disease.

T-Box Expressed in T Cells

The T-box expressed in T cells (T-bet) transcription factor is perhaps the most important factor regulating the development of type 1 responses and Th1 cells.[198] Genetic deletion of T-bet from mice results in the spontaneous expression of IL-13–dependent asthma-like disease, suggesting that T-bet suppresses allergic lung inflammation.[199,200] A mutation encoding for glutamine instead of histidine at position 33 of T-bet was linked to significant improvement in airway hyperresponsiveness in asthmatic children receiving corticosteroids and functionally encoded for greater Th1 cytokine secretion.[201] Subsequent studies of asthma patients have demonstrated additional T-bet polymorphisms that predict the presence of asthma and airway hyperresponsiveness.[202]

Costimulatory Molecules

Signals from some of the many known costimulatory molecules and their receptors are, in addition to antigen, required for stable B- and T-cell activation and effector function. They are therefore essential for expression of the experimental asthma phenotype (Table 51.4).

CD28 and CD134

Numerous studies have documented the marked requirement of the costimulatory molecules CD28 and CD134 for allergic lung inflammation.[203–211] These molecules are necessary for optimal Th2-cell development that is required for allergic inflammation, but their importance to asthma probably diminishes with chronic disease. For example, inhibition of CD28, while highly effective if initiated prior to allergic lung inflammation becoming established, had little effect at time points during which allergic lung inflammation was already established.[212]

TABLE 51.4. Costimulatory molecules in asthma pathogenesis.

Costimulatory molecules	Receptors or ligands	Roles in asthma models
ICOS	ICOS ligand, B7RP1, others	Promotes development of T regulatory cells that suppress inflammation
CD28	CD80, CD86	Required for inflammation and AHR (CD28)
CD40	CD154	Required for allergen-specific antibody secretion, but not allergic inflammation
CD134	OX-40 ligand	Required for inflammation and AHR
TIM-1, TIM-3	Hepatitis A virus, TIM-4	Promote IL-4 transcription and experimental asthma

Note: AHR, airway hyperresponsive; ICOS, inducible costimulator; IL, interleukin.

Cytotoxic T-Lymphocyte Antigen 4

Cytotoxic T-lymphocyte antigen 4 (CTLA4) is a costimulatory receptor closely related to CD28, (i.e., it shares the same ligands), but it has been more closely linked to suppression of inflammatory responses unrelated to asthma.[213] Nonetheless, a cytosine to thymidine single nucleotide polymorphism at position −1147 in the promoter for CTLA4 was linked to bronchial hyperresponsiveness and asthma. This polymorphism encoded for significantly less expression of surface CTLA4, suggesting that the expression level of this costimulatory receptor is an important factor modifying the development of allergic inflammation and asthma.[214]

CD40

CD40 is a costimulatory molecule expressed on T, B, and endothelial cells. Signaling through this molecule is critical for immunoglobulin responses, but not for Th2 cytokine secretion in asthma or in experimental allergic lung inflammation.[215,216] CD40 is thus important for regulating type 1 but not type 4 hypersensitivity responses.

T-Cell Immunoglobulin and Mucin Domain Protein Molecules

The T-cell immunoglobulin and mucin domain protein molecule (TIM) family of costimulatory molecules was originally identified as Tapr, a Mendelian trait linked to T-cell IL-13 and IL-4 production and airway hyperreactivity.[217] There are four known TIM family members that were subsequently cloned, all existing near the 5q31–33 locus. Molecule 1 (TIM-1) is the cellular receptor for the hepatitis A virus and TIM-4 and provides a costimulatory

signal for T-cell activation that promotes IL-4 transcription and experimental asthma.[218,219] Preliminary studies have linked a complex haplotype consisting of three polymorphisms in exon 4 of the *TIM-1* gene and a guanine to thymidine substitution at position −574 of the TIM-3 promoter to asthma in Korean patients.[220] Additional polymorphisms in exon 4 of *TIM-1* have been linked to asthma in persons of African descent.[221] Mutations in *TIM-1* may thus directly promote Th2 responses. In contrast, TIM-3 is expressed only on Th1 cells; mutations involving *TIM-3* may indirectly promote Th2 responses through suppression of Th1-cell function.[222]

Seven Transmembrane Spanning Receptors

The largest family of receptors in mammals, the seven transmembrane spanning receptors (STSRs) are enormously important in regulating airway inflammation and physiologic changes in asthma. Most STSRs relevant to asthma serve as receptors for small, often nonpeptidic molecules and are most frequently implicated in the regulation of lung remodeling during established inflammation (Table 51.5). Other receptors are, however, critical for effector cell development (anaphylatoxin receptors),

TABLE 51.5. Seven transmembrane spanning receptors in asthma pathogenesis.

Seven transmembrane spanning receptors	Ligands	Roles in asthma models
C3aR	C3a	Essential for establishing allergic airway inflammation and AHR
C5aR	C5a	Promotes or suppresses allergic airway inflammation and AHR
CysLTR1,2	Cysteinyl leukotrienes (LTC4, D4, E4)	Promote airway inflammation and AHR
TP, DP1-2, EP1-4, IP, FP	Prostaglandins	Promote or suppress airway inflammation and AHR
A1, A2A, A2B, A3	Adenosine	Promote airway inflammation and AHR
β2-Adrenergic	Epinephrine	Relaxes airway smooth muscle and inhibits bronchoconstriction
M2,M3	Ach	Promote bronchoconstriction/AHR
PAF-R	Platelet-activating factor	Promote bronchoconstriction/AHR

Note: A1, A2A, A2B, A3, adenosine receptors; Ach, acetylcholine; AHR, airway hyperresponsiveness; C3a, C5a, complements 3a and 5a; C3aR, C5aR, complements 3a and 5a receptors; CysLTR, cysteinyl leukotriene receptor; M2, M3, muscarinic receptors; TP, DP1-2, EP1-4, IP, FP, prostaglandin receptors; PAF-R, platelet-activating factor receptor.

cell recruitment (chemokines), and disease resolution (chemokines). Signaling through STSRs is often, but not exclusively, coupled to cytoplasmic G proteins, hence their former name of G protein–coupled receptors. All STSRs are encoded by single-exon genes producing single polypeptide products that span the surface membrane seven times. Although included among the STSRs, chemokine receptors and their ligands are discussed earlier in this chapter.

Complements 3a and 5a

Complement anaphylatoxins, especially complement 3a (C3a) and its receptor, C3aR, are required for initiating robust allergic inflammatory reactions and allergic lung disease.[223–225] Complement can be activated through several pathways, including antibodies, suggesting that anaphylatoxins may also modify allergic reactions after T- and B-cell responses have already become established. However, the anaphylatoxins (which also include C5a) can also be activated directly by agents implicated in allergic disease, such as fungi.[226] Furthermore, expression of anaphylatoxin receptors on target tissues of the lung suggests that these molecules can directly influence airway function independent of inflammatory cells.[227]

Depending on the experimental design, C5a may exacerbate[228,229] allergic lung inflammation and physiologic dysfunction. However, mice deficient in C5 show increased susceptibility to airway dysfunction during allergic inflammation, indicating a suppressive role for this complement protein. Additional studies are required to clarify the precise role of C5a in models of allergic lung inflammation.

A single study of Japanese children and adults reveals multiple single nucleotide polymorphisms in the genes controlling C3, C3aR, and C5 that are linked to asthma susceptibility. The 4896C/T allele in the *C3* gene was linked to asthma susceptibility in children and adults, as was the 912G-1692A-1836G-4896T (GAGT) haplotype. Similarly, asthma severity was linked to the 1526G/A allele of the *C3AR1* gene. In contrast, the GGCGA haplotype of the *C5* gene was linked to less susceptibility (i.e., protection) in asthma.[230]

Cysteinyl Leukotrienes

The cysteinyl leukotrienes (CysLTs), which are potent mediators of lung inflammation and bronchoconstriction, signal through two receptors, CysLT1 and CysLT2 (Figure 51.4). Cysteinyl leukotriene receptor 1 is the better characterized receptor and is found on eosinophils, monocytes, macrophages, basophils, mast cells, neutrophils, T cells, B lymphocytes, airway epithelium, and smooth muscle cells. Leukotriene receptor–modifying agents inhibit almost exclusively this receptor, with little effect

on CysLT2. Furthermore, CysLT2 has a distinct tissue distribution from that of CysLT1, suggesting that CysLT2 may also contribute importantly, perhaps in novel ways, to the expression of asthma.[231–233]

An adenine for cytosine substitution at position −1220 of the *CYSLT2* gene was linked to the development of asthma in Japanese patients, and additional complex haplotypes have been linked to aspirin intolerance in asthma patients of Korean descent.[234,235] Numerous additional molecules are implicated in asthma through their role in CysLT biosynthesis. Leukotriene C4 synthase, which is required for the synthesis of all CysLTs, exists in two major allelic variants distinguished by the presence of either an adenine or cytosine at position −444 of the promoter. The −444C allele was found to be expressed to a significantly higher degree in aspirin-intolerant asthmatics of Eastern European and Japanese descent and was linked to mild asthma in Australian patients, but no associations could be established for patients from the United States.[236–239] Although aspirin intolerant asthma is more strongly linked to leukotrienes than other asthma variants, it is nonetheless unclear how these polymorphisms relevant to leukotriene biosynthesis lead to or exacerbate disease.

Prostaglandins

The prostaglandins are derived from the same membrane lipid as the leukotrienes (arachidonic acid) but enter a separate metabolic pathway initiated by cyclooxygenases 1 and 2 (Figure 51.4). There are five major prostaglandins, each arising as a product of a distinct enzyme acting on the precursor prostaglandin PGH2 and contributing in unique ways to allergic lung disease. As documented through animal and human studies, thromboxane A2 (TxA2) is a potent bronchoconstricting agent,[240,241] but antagonists of TxA2 have, after initial promise in animals and some clinical trials,[242,243] proven to be disappointing in humans, indicating that other mediators of bronchoconstriction are of more importance in asthma.[241,242,244–249] A threonine to cysteine substitution at position 924 in the TxA2 receptor has been linked to asthma in adult Japanese and Chinese pediatric patients.[250,251]

Other prostaglandins show divergent contributions to the asthma phenotype. Prostaglandin D2 (PGD2) signals through two receptors, DP1 and DP2 (CRTh2) to mediate bronchoconstriction and potentiate airway hyperreactivity and allergic inflammation.[252–256] Prostaglandin F2 is also a significant bronchoconstricting agent.[257,258] In contrast, inhaled PGI2 relaxes bronchospasm and attenuates allergic inflammation and airway remodeling.[259–261] Because of its many receptors, the contribution of PGE2 to asthma has been the most difficult to understand. Activation of the PGE2 receptors EP2 and EP4 promotes IgE secretion from mouse B cells[262] and prolongs the survival

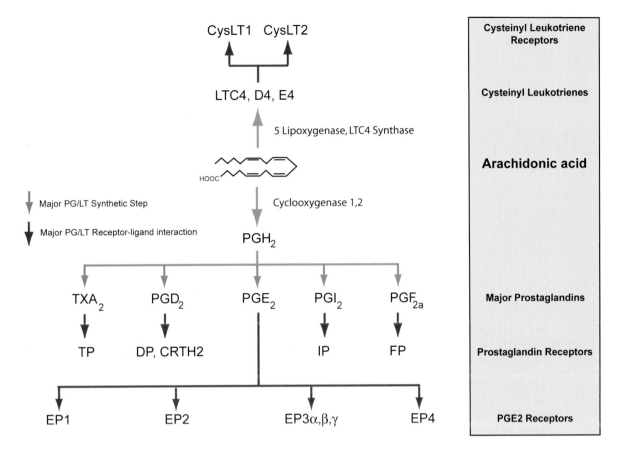

FIGURE 51.4. Major prostaglandins (PGs) and leukotrienes (LTs) linked to asthma and their biosynthetic pathways (green arrows) and receptors (red arrows). Both PGs and LTs originate from the membrane lipid arachidonic acid. Oxidation of arachidonic acid by distinct enzymes leads to PG and LT precursors, which after further modification by additional enzymes yields mature PGs and the cysteinyl LTs. Each PG has at least one unique receptor, whereas the cysteinyl LTs are all capable of activating the two known cysteinyl LT receptors. CRTH2, chemoattractant receptor-homologous molecule expressed on Th2 cells; DP, EP, FP, IP, TP, five classes of prostanoid receptors; TXA_2, thromboxane A_2.

of human eosinophils,[263] whereas activation of EP1 increases airway hyperresponsiveness in mice.[264] However, inhaled PGE2 powerfully suppresses antigen-induced allergic lung inflammation and relieves airway obstruction in rats[265] and furthermore acts as a bronchodilator when given to asthmatic patients.[257,258] The inhibitory effect of inhaled PGE2 appears to be dominant under experimental conditions most consistent with asthma and is mediated through the EP3 receptor, the major PGE2 receptor in the lung.[266]

Adenosine

Adenosine is a nucleoside found in elevated amounts in respiratory secretions of asthma patients and is a significant bronchoconstricting agent.[267] Furthermore, greatly elevated respiratory tract adenosine concentrations promote allergic lung inflammation and airway hyperreactivity in mice.[268] At least in part, the proallergic effects of adenosine are related to mast cell degranulation medi-

ated especially through the A3 receptor, although other receptors are expressed in the lung and are likely important.[269,270] Furthermore, adenosine and IL-13 reciprocally induce each other, suggesting that adenosine contributes to asthma through multiple distinct mechanisms.[271]

The β_2-Adrenergic Receptor

The β_2-adrenergic receptor (β2AR) is the principal lung catecholamine (epinephrine) receptor, activation of which relaxes airway smooth muscle and promotes bronchodilation. Pharmaceutical agonists of this receptor (albuterol and others) are among the most important and commonly prescribed asthma medications. Although β2AR antagonists (nadolol and others) are commonly thought to be hazardous in asthma by promoting bronchoconstriction, more recent studies indicate that chronic treatment with β2AR antagonists reduces allergen-induced airway hyperresponsiveness.[272] This paradoxic effect is likely mediated by a massive upregulation of airway β2ARs that become more responsive to endogenous and exogenous agonists. An arginine to glycine substitution at position 16 of the β2AR results in enhanced receptor activation-dependent downregulation and was associated with both nocturnal and severe asthma.[273,274] Downregulation of β2ARs occurs principally at night and may impair bronchorelaxation, suggesting that this polymorphism specifically contributes to both nocturnal and severe asthma.[274]

Muscarinic Acetylcholine Receptors

The major neural pathway controlling bronchoconstriction is the parasympathetic system. The principal neurotransmitter mediating parasympathetic-dependent bronchoconstriction is acetylcholine, which signals through two distinct muscarinic receptor types in the airway, M2 and M3. The M2 receptors are located on smooth muscle cells and postganglionic nerves at the neuromuscular junction. They serve as feedback inhibitory receptors, inhibiting acetylcholine release by parasympathetic nerve fibers. The M3 receptors are located exclusively on smooth muscle cells and are the principal mediators of acetylcholine-dependent smooth muscle contraction.[275] Although several mutations in the M2 and M3 receptor types have been discovered, no link between these polymorphisms and asthma has yet been shown.[276]

Platelet-Activating Factor

Platelet-activating factor (PAF) is a lipid mediator of inflammation secreted by macrophages and has long been linked to induction of bronchoconstriction.[277] Deficiency in the PAF receptor did not affect allergen-induced allergic inflammation but attenuated airway hyperresponsiveness in mice.[278] In support of its apparent proasthmatic role, deficiency in PAF acetylhydrolase, a serum enzyme that destroys PAF activity, was linked to higher asthma incidence and severity in Japanese patients.[279] Furthermore, multiple coding single nucleotide polymorphisms in PAF acetylhydrolase have been linked to asthma and are predicted to prolong the in vivo half-life of PAF and therefore worsen at least airway hyperresponsiveness.[280]

Immunoglobulin E and Its Receptors

As discussed earlier, IgE is likely to participate in asthma through type I hypersensitivity reactions in which antigen–cross-linked IgE activates FcεR1, the principal IgE receptor, present on a variety of allergic effector cells. A second, lower affinity, IgE receptor, CD23, is widely expressed and most likely serves in a complex manner to regulate IgE levels: in the presence of low levels of antigen-specific IgE, IgE–antigen complexes serve to enhance additional IgE secretion by B cells;[281–283] con-versely, in the context of high levels of antigen-specific IgE, extensive CD23 cross-linking serves to inhibit further IgE secretion.[284–286] Although not required for lower respiratory tract allergic responses and airway obstruction, type I hypersensitivity reactions probably contribute to asthma pathogenesis through their role in upper respiratory tract allergic disease. Allergic rhinitis and sinusitis are common in asthma patients and may exacerbate lower respiratory tract disease through the elaboration of inflammatory mediators (cytokines, prostaglandins, leukotrienes, etc.) that drain directly into the lower airways.[287,288] Although no genetic linkage between polymorphisms in CD23 and asthma have been identified, two polymorphisms in FcεR1, including a polymorphic microsatellite marker in the fifth inton of the β-subunit and a glutamic acid to glycine (E237G) change in the same subunit, have been linked to a diagnosis of asthma.[289,290] The latter mutation is near the critical immunotyrosine-based activation motif in the cytoplasmic portion that is critical for signaling, suggesting that this mutation affects FcεR1 signaling and therefore IgE effector function.

Both IgE and the factors that regulate its production are strong risk factors for asthma.[291] The genes for several IgE regulatory factors are located on the distal arm of human chromosome 5 (5q31–33), a region that exhibits strong genetic linkage to asthma and other atopic diseases in many,[292–297] but not all,[298–301] studies. Interestingly, even where linkage between asthma and chromosome 5q has been established, such linkage cannot be explained on the basis of IgE production alone.[301] Rather, it is likely that one or more factors in the 5q31–33 region both influence IgE production and, independently, the manifestations of asthma. The most important associations within the 5q region and asthma are the genes for the cytokines that were discussed earlier, IL-4, IL-5, IL-13, IL-9, and related but noncoding DNA sequences. Additional genes in the 5q region hold intriguing associations with asthma (e.g., the fragile X mental retardation protein–interacting protein 2 gene[302]) but through mechanisms that remain unclear.

Endogenous and Exogenous Proteinases

By cleaving endogenous substrates to either enhance or suppress their activity, endogenous proteinases potentially contribute in diverse ways to the manifestations of asthma. Proteinases are difficult to study in asthma because most, if not all, have endogenous inhibitors (secretory leukoproteinase inhibitor, α1-antitrypsin, α2-macroglobulin, aprotinin, tissue inhibitors of metalloproteinases, etc.) that critically regulate their function. Studies often do not account for the role of endogenous enzyme inhibitors (e.g., during proteinase reconstitution experiments) or the specificity (or lack thereof) of exogenously administered proteinase inhibitors, with attendant difficulties in data interpretation. Nonetheless, evidence suggests that diverse proteinases are likely to be important in regulating airway inflammation in asthma.

Matrix Metalloproteinases

Matrix metalloproteinases are a diverse family of zinc- and other cation-dependent proteolytic enzymes that have traditionally been linked to the degradation of matrix proteins (collagen, elastin). This activity may be important to the movement of recruited inflammatory cells through lung tissue. However, whereas this effect is not important for the recruitment of allergic inflammatory cells to lung, it is crucial for egression of such cells into the airways. Matrix metalloproteinases 2 and 9 are two such enzymes that coordinate cellular egression from lung without which resolution of allergic lung inflammation is delayed and mice become highly susceptible to lethal asphyxiation.[303,304] In addition to matrix proteins, matrix metalloproteinases are likely to have numerous additional substrates, modification of which is important in regulating inflammation in asthma.

Trypsin

Trypsin is a digestive enzyme that is also present in the airway epithelium that activates proteinase activated receptor 2 (PAR2). Activation of PAR2 induces release of a cyclooxygenase product, most likely PGE2, which inhibits bronchoconstriction, providing a unique airway protective effect, at least in nonallergen challenged animals.[305] In contrast, during allergic inflammation, trypsin and PAR2 promote allergic inflammation and experimental asthma through mechanisms distinct from PGE2.[306–308] Additional studies are required to understand the mechanisms by which PAR2 contributes to allergic lung inflammation.

Tryptase

Mast cells are a potent source of numerous secreted proteinases, the most abundant of which is tryptase. Studies from mice, sheep, and humans indicate that inhibition of trypsin reduces allergic inflammation, although not necessarily airway hyperreactivity.[308–311] The mechanism by which tryptase contributes to asthma is potentially through activation of PAR2, although other mechanisms are possible.[312] As with PAR2, the precise contribution of tryptase and other mast cell proteinases to asthma requires clarification.

Neutrophil Elastase

Neutrophil elastase is an elastolytic proteinase secreted by neutrophils. Secretion of neutrophil elastase into airways is dramatically enhanced during status asthmaticus, which is also marked by significantly enhanced recruitment of airway neutrophils.[131] Experimentally, neutrophil elastase promotes airway mucous secretion and therefore may contribute to airway obstruction in asthma.[313]

Other Endogenous Proteinases

In addition to these enzymes that have been studied directly, many additional enzymes are required for the production of mediators known to be important in asthma, for example, complement protein C3a (C3 convertase) and TNF (TNF-α converting enzyme). Several polymorphisms within a membrane intrinsic proteinase, a disintegrin, and metalloproteinase 33 (ADAM33), which is thought to shed various membrane proteins, was linked to asthma diagnosis and accelerated lung function in Caucasian, but not Mexican or Puerto Rican populations.[314–317] The mechanism by which this proteinase potentially contributes to asthma remains to be clarified.

Exogenous Proteinases

Finally, in addition to endogenous enzymes of importance to asthma, exogenous proteinases are of primary importance in establishing experimental allergic inflammation through intranasal challenge. Proteinases derived from a variety of sources relevant to asthma, including plants (ragweed pollen), fungi (*Aspergillus* spp.), and dust mites (*Dermatophagoides pteronyssinus*) have all been shown to induce experimental asthma-like disease.[318,319] Moreover, these enzymes induce allergic lung disease if given strictly through the airway, in contrast to ovalbumin, the most widely used experimental allergen, which must be administered remotely from the lung (intraperitoneally, subcutaneously) before airway challenge induces allergic lung inflammation. Thus, exogenous proteinases are uniquely capable of initiating Th2 responses through the airway. However, these proteinases also cleave a variety of endogenous proteins, including CD23 and tight junction proteins of airway epithelium, potentially disrupting the IgE network and facilitating antigen presentation.[320,321] *Dermatophagoides pteronyssinus* enzymes may also inhibit the production of IFN-γ to favor allergic responses.[319] Bacterial proteinases have been repeatedly implicated in outbreaks of occupational asthma and may contribute to diverse forms of asthma.[322,323]

Miscellaneous Molecules
Syndecan-1

Syndecan-1 is a heparan sulfate glycoprotein expressed on airway epithelial cells and is shed into the airway lumen under diverse inflammatory conditions. During allergic lung inflammation, shed syndecan-1 binds to and inhibits Th2-cell–specific chemokines such as CCL11 and CCL17, thereby inhibiting the recruitment of Th2 cells and eosinophils and attenuating manifestations of asthma.[324] This endogenous antiinflammatory mechanism provides a molecular explanation of the beneficial effect of aerosolized heparin, the pharmaceutical functional mimic of endogenous heparan, in asthma.[325,326]

Gob-5

Gob-5 (human CLCA1) was originally identified as a chloride channel from murine intestine but was shown later shown to be present in airway epithelium of mice and humans, especially during allergic inflammation.[327,328] Preliminary findings indicated that Gob-5 was an important regulator of airway hyperresponsiveness and mucous overproduction.[329] However, subsequent studies have shown that Gob-5 is in fact neither a chloride channel nor required for mucin gene expression, and its precise function and importance in asthma remain in doubt.[330,331] Nonetheless, a complex haplotype involving eight distinct polymorphisms all occurring in intronic DNA have been strongly linked to a diagnosis of asthma in Japanese children.[332]

Human Leukocyte Antigens

The human leukocyte antigen (HLA) family of molecules includes major histocompatibility complex antigens type I (MHC I) and MHC II genes required for antigen presentation to CD8+ (cytotoxic) and CD4+ (helper) T cells, respectively. Major histocompatibility complex II antigens are especially important for activating T helper cells, the Th2 subset of which is essential for coordinating allergic lung inflammation and airway obstruction in experimental asthma. The only MHC I locus linked to asthma is the *HLA-G* gene cluster on chromosome 6.[333] Many more associations between asthma MHC II loci are known, including the *HLA-DR* locus for soybean,[334] grass pollen,[335] and toluene diisocyanate asthma[336] and the *HLA-DQ* locus for ragweed pollen.[337] The *DP* and *DQ* loci have also been linked to toluene diisocyanate asthma.[336,338] The different HLA associations with specific antigens linked to asthma presumably reflects the greater affinity of specific HLA antigen for distinct antigens, with greater affinity correlating with enhanced ability to activate antigen-specific Th2, and possibly Th1, cells.

Nitric Oxide Synthase

Nitric oxide synthase (NOS) genes exist in three isoforms, including an inducible isoform (iNOS) expressed in airway epithelium and macrophages and neuronal and endothelial types. Interest in nitric oxide (NO), a principal product of NOS activity, as a bronchodilator in asthma began with the discovery that NO is an important vasodilator. Nitric oxide is increased in asthma,[339] and both the neuronal and inducible forms of NOS have been shown experimentally to be relevant to airway hyperresponsiveness and allergic inflammation.[340,341] Additional studies have linked a byproduct of NO metabolism, S-nitrosoglutathione, to bronchodilation in experimental asthma.[342] Polymorphisms in both the neuronal and endothelial NOS genes have been linked to asthma in Caucasian and Korean patients, although the effect of these mutations is unknown.[343,344]

Histamine and Its Receptors

Histamine, similar to acetylcholine and serotonin, is a neurotransmitter that elicits smooth muscle contraction. Endogenous release of histamine from neurons, but also mast cells, probably elicits bronchoconstriction in asthma, and histamine is widely used as a provocative agent during bronchial provocation challenge testing for asthma. In contrast to other neurotransmitters, however, histamine has important proallergic effects.

The diverse properties of histamine can be explained by the numerous receptors (H1–H4) that are expressed on diverse airway and immune tissues. The H1 receptors are present on airway smooth muscle cells and mediate bronchoconstriction. The H2 receptors are found on airway goblet cells and can contribute to goblet cell degranulation, possibly contributing to airway obstruction.[345] The H1, H2, and H3 receptors are also present on T cells; their activation has complex effects on the secretion of Th1 and Th2 cytokines and immunoglobulin production.[346] However, the H4 receptor may have the most potent proinflammatory effect through its costimulatory activity on T cells and dendritic cells.[346]

Chitinases and Related Molecules

A family of mammalian genes closely related to chitinases of bacteria and other primitive organisms exists on human chromosome 1 (mouse chromosomes 1 and 3), most of which have no enzymatic activity, and, in fact, their function remains obscure.[347–349] One of these gene products, YM1, which is found only in the mouse, is upregulated in the setting of allergic lung inflammation and has weak chemotactic activity.[350] In contrast, acidic mammalian chitinase (AMCase) retains its enzymatic activity and is found in elevated levels in lungs of both humans and mice with asthma-like disease. Neutralization of AMCase was protective in a mouse asthma model, possibly because of disruption of an IL-13–dependent mechanism regulating lung chemokine expression.[351] Two polymorphisms (a lysine to arginine change at position

17 and a noncoding adenine to guanine mutation in exon 4) in the *AMCase* gene were linked to asthma in German children, with more complex haplotypes being very strongly linked to disease. Despite the linkage of chitinase activity to asthma through diverse approaches, the relevance of chitinases to disease expression remains obscure.

Conclusion

We have combined studies based on two fundamentally different investigative approaches to understand the molecular basis of asthma. Genetic studies, which determine the statistical association between disease or disease markers and specific polymorphisms, are advantageous because they may identify candidate disease-related genes that are difficult to reveal by other approaches as well as provide unique insight into gene function as suggested through multiple allelic isoforms. However, most genetic studies also share several important limitations, including the possibility that polymorphisms relevant to one population may be irrelevant to the asthma population at large; small sample size that in many studies both limits statistical power and raises the possibility of Type II statistical error; and, generally, a lack of complimentary experiments that reveal the functional importance of specific genes and polymorphisms in disease models. In contrast, laboratory-based approaches have the power to reveal in detail how specific genes and their variants contribute to asthma pathogenesis. However, these more functional studies are performed largely in nonhuman disease models, creating the possibility that such findings may be irrelevant in human asthma.

Agreement between human genetic and laboratory-based animal studies therefore provides a more robust indication of the importance of specific molecules in the pathogenesis of asthma. Remarkably, the majority of molecules implicated in human genetic studies have been confirmed to be relevant to the expression of experimental asthma in rodents. Many of these molecules are also upregulated in the context of human asthma. Conversely, many genes shown to be important in experimental disease also show enhanced expression in asthma, even when their actual function is uncertain (e.g., *Gob-5*, *AMCase*). The unexpectedly large number of genes relevant to asthma as indicated by agreement between these diverse approaches reveals the enormous complexity of asthma pathogenesis and suggests the difficulties likely to be encountered with future therapeutic approaches based on the targeting of specific immune molecules.

Comparison of the many asthma-related molecules further suggests the existence of a hierarchy, with the most important being related to disease initiation (e.g., complement anaphylatoxin C3a) and for mediating type IV hypersensitivity (e.g., IL-13, IL-4Rα, STAT6). Equally important are the molecules required for Th2-cell development, including IL-4, GATA3, CD28, OX-40, and possibly TSLP. Confirmation that these molecules are indeed relevant in humans will require clinical trials in which asthma patients receive molecule- or at least pathway-specific pharmaceutical inhibitors.

The genes implicated in asthma pathogenesis are not equally distributed among the checkpoints regulating disease expression but rather are concentrated at the effector cell development and lung remodeling checkpoints (checkpoints II and IV in Figure 51.2). The relatively few genes implicated elsewhere in Figure 51.2 may simply reflect the asymmetric biology of asthma, but more likely this pattern is the result of the greater emphasis that the topics of effector cell development and lung remodeling have received from researchers in recent years. The complete lack of insight into the genes and mechanisms controlling the evolution of asthma into more complex clinical entities such as Churg-Strauss syndrome and allergic bronchopulmonary aspergillosis alone suggests that many additional genes of great importance to asthma pathogenesis await discovery. Future research directed at the mechanisms controlling the initiation of allergic lung inflammation through allergens, disease evolution, and disease resolution will likely speed the process of gene discovery in asthma and provide a more complete understanding of asthma pathogenesis.

References

1. Aikawa T, Shimura S, Sasaki H, et al. Marked goblet cell hyperplasia with mucus accumulation in the airways of patients who died of severe acute asthma attack. Chest 1992;101(4):916–921.
2. Flora GS, Sharma AM, Sharma OP. Asthma mortality in a metropolitan county hospital, a 38-year study. Allergy Proc 1991;12(3):169–179.
3. Lange P, Nyboe J, Appleyard M, et al. Relation of ventilatory impairment and of chronic mucus hypersecretion to mortality from obstructive lung disease and from all causes. Thorax 1990;45(8):579–585.
4. Ishizaka T, Ishizaka K, Tomioka H. Release of histamine and slow reacting substance of anaphylaxis (SRS-A) by IgE-anti-IgE reactions on monkey mast cells. J Immunol 1972;108(2):513–520.
5. Tomioka H, Ishizaka K. Mechanisms of passive sensitization. II. Presence of receptors for IgE on monkey mast cells. J Immunol 1971;107(4):971–978.
6. Ishizaka T, Tomioka H, Ishizaka K. Degranulation of human basophil leukocytes by anti-gamma E antibody. J Immunol 1971;106(3):705–710.
7. Ishizaka K, Tomioka H, Ishizaka T. Mechanisms of passive sensitization. I. Presence of IgE and IgG molecules on human leukocytes. J Immunol 1970;105(6):1459–1467.
8. Pene J, Rousset F, Briere F, et al. IgE production by normal human lymphocytes is induced by interleukin 4

and suppressed by interferons a, g and prostaglandin E2. Proc Natl Acad Sci USA 1988;85:6880.

9. Finkelman FD, Katona IM, Urban JF Jr, et al. IL-4 is required to generate and sustain in vivo IgE responses. J Immunol 1988;141(7):2335–2341.

10. Brown MA, Pierce JH, Watson CJ, et al. B cell stimulatory factor-1/interleukin-4 mRNA is expressed by normal and transformed mast cells. Cell 1987;50(5):809–818.

11. Robinson DS, Hamid Q, Ying S, et al. Predominant TH2-like bronchoalveolar T-lymphocyte population in atopic asthma. N Engl J Med 1992;326(5):298–304.

12. Corry DB, Grunig G, Hadeiba H, et al. Requirements for allergen-induced airway hyperreactivity in T and B cell-deficient mice. Mol Med 1998;4(5):344–355.

13. Corry DB, Folkesson HG, Warnock ML, et al. Interleukin 4, but not interleukin 5 or eosinophils, is required in a murine model of acute airway hyperreactivity. J Exp Med 1996;183(1):109–117.

14. Watanabe A, Mishima H, Renzi PM, et al. Transfer of allergic airway responses with antigen-primed CD4+ but not CD8+ T cells in brown Norway rats. J Clin Invest 1995;96(3):1303–1310.

15. Van Loveren H, Garssen J, Nijkamp FP. T cell–mediated airway hyperreactivity in mice. Eur Respir J 1991;13:16s–26s.

16. MacLean JA, Sauty A, Luster AD, et al. Antigen-induced airway hyperresponsiveness, pulmonary eosinophilia, and chemokine expression in B cell-deficient mice. Am J Respir Cell Mol Biol 1999;20(3):379–387.

17. Grunig G, Warnock M, Wakil AE, et al. Requirement for IL-13 independently of IL-4 in experimental asthma. Science 1998;282(5397):2261–2263.

18. Wills-Karp M, Luyimbazi J, Xu X, et al. Interleukin-13: central mediator of allergic asthma. Science 1998;282(5397):2258–2261.

19. Kuperman D, Schofield B, Wills-Karp M, et al. Signal transducer and activator of transcription factor 6 (Stat6)-deficient mice are protected from antigen-induced airway hyperresponsiveness and mucus production. J Exp Med 1998;187(6):939–948.

20. Akimoto T, Numata F, Tamura M, et al. Abrogation of bronchial eosinophilic inflammation and airway hyperreactivity in signal transducers and activators of transcription (STAT)6-deficient mice. J Exp Med 1998; 187:1537–1542.

21. Wang HY, Zamorano J, Keegan AD. A role for the insulin-interleukin (IL)-4 receptor motif of the IL-4 receptor alpha-chain in regulating activation of the insulin receptor substrate 2 and signal transducer and activator of transcription 6 pathways. Analysis by mutagenesis. J Biol Chem 1998;273(16):9898–9905.

22. Murata T, Noguchi PD, Puri RK. IL-13 induces phosphorylation and activation of JAK2 Janus kinase in human colon carcinoma cell lines: similarities between IL-4 and IL-13 signaling. J Immunol 1996;156(8):2972–2978.

23. Hou J, Schindler U, Henzel WJ, et al. An interleukin-4-induced transcription factor: IL-4 Stat. Science 1994; 265(5179):1701–1706.

24. Fenghao X, Saxon A, Nguyen A, et al. Interleukin 4 activates a signal transducer and activator of transcription (Stat) protein which interacts with an interferon-gamma activation site-like sequence upstream of the I epsilon exon in a human B cell line. Evidence for the involvement of Janus kinase 3 and interleukin-4 Stat. J Clin Invest 1995;96(2):907–914.

25. Corry DB. IL-13 in allergy: home at last. Curr Opin Immunol 1999;11(6):610–614.

26. Noguchi E, Shibasaki M, Arinami T, et al. Association of asthma and the interleukin-4 promoter gene in Japanese. Clin Exp Allergy 1998;28(4):449–453.

27. Zhu S, Chan-Yeung M, Becker AB, et al. Polymorphisms of the IL-4, TNF-alpha, and Fcepsilon RIbeta genes and the risk of allergic disorders in at-risk infants. Am J Respir Crit Care Med 2000;161(5):1655–1659.

28. Noguchi E, Nukaga-Nishio Y, Jian Z, et al. Haplotypes of the 5′ region of the IL-4 gene and SNPs in the intergene sequence between the IL-4 and IL-13 genes are associated with atopic asthma. Hum Immunol 2001;62(11):1251–1257.

29. Beghe B, Barton S, Rorke S, et al. Polymorphisms in the interleukin-4 and interleukin-4 receptor alpha chain genes confer susceptibility to asthma and atopy in a Caucasian population. Clin Exp Allergy 2003;33(8):1111 1117.

30. Moissidis I, Chinoy B, Yanamandra K, et al. Association of IL-13, RANTES, and leukotriene C4 synthase gene promoter polymorphisms with asthma and/or atopy in African Americans. Genet Med 2005;7(6):406–410.

31. van der Pouw Kraan TC, van Veen A, Boeije LC, et al. An IL-13 promoter polymorphism associated with increased risk of allergic asthma. Genes Immun 1999;1(1):61–65.

32. Heinzmann A, Mao XQ, Akaiwa M, et al. Genetic variants of IL-13 signalling and human asthma and atopy. Hum Mol Genet 2000;9(4):549–559.

33. DeMeo DL, Lange C, Silverman EK, et al. Univariate and multivariate family-based association analysis of the IL-13 ARG130GLN polymorphism in the Childhood Asthma Management Program. Genet Epidemiol 2002;23(4):335–348.

34. Vladich FD, Brazille SM, Stern D, et al. IL-13 R130Q, a common variant associated with allergy and asthma, enhances effector mechanisms essential for human allergic inflammation. J Clin Invest 2005;115(3):747–754.

35. Izuhara K, Shirakawa T. Signal transduction via the interleukin-4 receptor and its correlation with atopy. Int J Mol Med 1999;3(1):3–10.

36. Takabayashi A, Ihara K, Sasaki Y, et al. Childhood atopic asthma: positive association with a polymorphism of IL-4 receptor alpha gene but not with that of IL-4 promoter or Fc epsilon receptor I beta gene. Exp Clin Immunogenet 2000;17(2):63–70.

37. Rosa-Rosa L, Zimmermann N, Bernstein JA, et al. The R576 IL-4 receptor alpha allele correlates with asthma severity. J Allergy Clin Immunol 1999;104(5):1008–1014.

38. Ober C, Leavitt SA, Tsalenko A, et al. Variation in the interleukin 4-receptor alpha gene confers susceptibility to asthma and atopy in ethnically diverse populations. Am J Hum Genet 2000;66(2):517–526.

39. Risma KA, Wang N, Andrews RP, et al. V75R576 IL-4 receptor alpha is associated with allergic asthma and enhanced IL-4 receptor function. J Immunol 2002;169(3): 1604–1610.

40. Hytonen AM, Lowhagen O, Arvidsson M, et al. Haplo-types of the interleukin-4 receptor alpha chain gene associate with susceptibility to and severity of atopic asthma. Clin Exp Allergy 2004;34(10):1570–1575.

41. Lee SG, Kim BS, Kim JH, et al. Gene–gene interaction between interleukin-4 and interleukin-4 receptor alpha in Korean children with asthma. Clin Exp Allergy 2004;34(8):1202–1208.

42. Kabesch M, Schedel M, Carr D, et al. IL-4/IL-13 pathway genetics strongly influence serum IgE levels and childhood asthma. J Allergy Clin Immunol 2006;117(2):269–274.

43. Mohrs M, Blankespoor CM, Wang ZE, et al. Deletion of a coordinate regulator of type 2 cytokine expression in mice. Nat Immunol 2001;2(9):842–847.

44. Coffman RL, Seymour BW, Hudak S, et al. Antibody to interleukin-5 inhibits helminth-induced eosinophilia in mice. Science 1989;245(4915):308–310.

45. Foster PS, Hogan SP, Ramsay AJ, et al. Interleukin 5 deficiency abolishes eosinophilia, airways hyperreactivity, and lung damage in a mouse asthma model. J Exp Med 1996;183(1):195–201.

46. Lee JJ, Dimina D, Macias MP, et al. Defining a link with asthma in mice congenitally deficient in eosinophils. Science 2005;305:1773–1776.

47. Humbles AA, Lloyd CM, McMillan SJ, et al. A critical role for eosinophils in allergic airways remodeling. Science 2005;305:1776–1779.

48. Leckie MJ, ten Brinke A, Khan J, et al. Effects of an interleukin-5 blocking monoclonal antibody on eosinophils, airway hyper-responsiveness, and the late asthmatic response. Lancet 2000;356(9248):2144–2148.

49. Kips JC, O'Connor BJ, Langley SJ, et al. Effect of SCH55700, a humanized anti-human interleukin-5 antibody, in severe persistent asthma: a pilot study. Am J Respir Crit Care Med 2003;167(12):1655–1659.

50. Flood-Page PT, Menzies-Gow AN, Kay AB, et al. Eosinophil's role remains uncertain as anti-interleukin-5 only partially depletes numbers in asthmatic airway. Am J Respir Crit Care Med 2003;167(2):199–204.

51. McMillan SJ, Bishop B, Townsend MJ, et al. The absence of interleukin 9 does not affect the development of allergen-induced pulmonary inflammation nor airway hyperreactivity. J Exp Med 2002;195(1):51–57.

52. Cheong HS, Kim LH, Park BL, et al. Association analysis of interleukin 5 receptor alpha subunit (IL5RA) polymorphisms and asthma. J Hum Genet 2005;50(12):628–634.

53. Kumar RK, Herbert C, Foster PS. Expression of growth factors by airway epithelial cells in a model of chronic asthma: regulation and relationship to subepithelial fibrosis. Clin Exp Allergy 2004;34(4):567–575.

54. McMillan SJ, Lloyd CM. Prolonged allergen challenge in mice leads to persistent airway remodelling. Clin Exp Allergy 2004;34(3):497–507.

55. Kenyon NJ, Ward RW, McGrew G, et al. TGF-beta1 causes airway fibrosis and increased collagen I and III mRNA in mice. Thorax 2003;58(9):772–777.

56. Chu HW, Halliday JL, Martin RJ, et al. Collagen deposition in large airways may not differentiate severe asthma from milder forms of the disease. Am J Respir Crit Care Med 1998;158(6):1936–1944.

57. Aubert JD, Dalal BI, Bai TR, et al. Transforming growth factor beta 1 gene expression in human airways. Thorax 1994;49(3):225–232.

58. Chen W, Jin W, Hardegen N, et al. Conversion of peripheral CD4+CD25− naive T cells to CD4+CD25+ regulatory T cells by TGF-beta induction of transcription factor Foxp3. J Exp Med 2003;198(12):1875–1886.

59. Hansen G, McIntire JJ, Yeung VP, et al. CD4(+) T helper cells engineered to produce latent TGF-beta1 reverse allergen-induced airway hyperreactivity and inflammation. J Clin Invest 2000;105(1):61–70.

60. Pulleyn LJ, Newton R, Adcock IM, et al. TGFbeta1 allele association with asthma severity. Hum Genet 2001;109(6):623–627.

61. Silverman ES, Palmer LJ, Subramaniam V, et al. Transforming growth factor-beta1 promoter polymorphism C-509T is associated with asthma. Am J Respir Crit Care Med 2004;169(2):214–219.

62. Meng J, Thongngarm T, Nakajima M, et al. Association of transforming growth factor-beta1 single nucleotide polymorphism C-509T with allergy and immunological activities. Int Arch Allergy Immunol 2005;138(2):151–160.

63. Heinzmann A, Bauer E, Ganter K, et al. Polymorphisms of the TGF-beta1 gene are not associated with bronchial asthma in Caucasian children. Pediatr Allergy Immunol 2005;16(4):310–314.

64. Mak JCW, Leung HCM, Ho SP, et al. Analysis of TGF-beta(1) gene polymorphisms in Hong Kong Chinese patients with asthma. J Allergy Clin Immunol 2006;117(1):92–96.

65. Nakae S, Komiyama Y, Yokoyama H, et al. IL-1 is required for allergen-specific Th2 cell activation and the development of airway hypersensitivity response. Int Immunol 2003;15(4):483–490.

66. Schmitz N, Kurrer M, Kopf M. The IL-1 receptor 1 is critical for Th2 cell type airway immune responses in a mild but not in a more severe asthma model. Eur J Immunol 2003;33(4):991–1000.

67. Hang LW, Hsia TC, Chen WC, et al. Interleukin-10 gene – 627 allele variants, not interleukin-I beta gene and receptor antagonist gene polymorphisms, are associated with atopic bronchial asthma. J Clin Lab Anal 2003;17(5):168–173.

68. Karjalainen J, Nieminen MM, Aromaa A, et al. The IL-1beta genotype carries asthma susceptibility only in men. J Allergy Clin Immunol 2002;109(3):514–516.

69. Gohlke H, Illig T, Bahnweg M, et al. Association of the interleukin-1 receptor antagonist gene with asthma. Am J Respir Crit Care Med 2004;169(11):1217–23.

70. Sanchez-Guerrero IM, Herrero N, Muro M, et al. Co-stimulation of cultured peripheral blood mononuclear cells from intrinsic asthmatics with exogenous recombinant IL-6 produce high levels of IL-4-dependent IgE. Eur Respir J 1997;10(9):2091–2096.

71. Rincon M, Anguita J, Nakamura T, et al. Interleukin (IL)-6 directs the differentiation of IL-4–producing CD4+ T cells. J Exp Med 1997;185(3):461–469.

72. La Flamme AC, Pearce EJ. The absence of IL-6 does not affect Th2 cell development in vivo, but does lead to

impaired proliferation, IL-2 receptor expression, and B cell responses. J Immunol 1999;162(10):5829–5837.

73. Qiu Z, Fujimura M, Kurashima K, et al. Enhanced airway inflammation and decreased subepithelial fibrosis in interleukin 6-deficient mice following chronic exposure to aerosolized antigen. Clin Exp Allergy 2004;34(8):1321–1328.

74. Tanaka T, Katada Y, Higa S, et al. Enhancement of T helper2 response in the absence of interleukin (IL-)6; an inhibition of IL-4-mediated T helper2 cell differentiation by IL-6. Cytokine 2001;13(4):193–201.

75. Wang J, Homer RJ, Chen Q, et al. Endogenous and exogenous IL-6 inhibit aeroallergen-induced Th2 inflammation. J Immunol 2000;165(7):4051–4061.

76. Kuhn C 3rd, Homer RJ, Zhu Z, et al. Airway hyperresponsiveness and airway obstruction in transgenic mice. Morphologic correlates in mice overexpressing interleukin (IL)-11 and IL-6 in the lung. Am J Respir Cell Mol Biol 2000;22(3):289–295.

77. Ray RJ, Furlonger C, Williams DE, et al. Characterization of thymic stromal-derived lymphopoietin (TSLP) in murine B cell development in vitro. Eur J Immunol 1996;26(1):10–16.

78. Ying S, O'Connor B, Ratoff J, et al. Thymic stromal lymphopoietin expression is increased in asthmatic airways and correlates with expression of Th2-attracting chemokines and disease severity. J Immunol 2005;174(12):8183–8190.

79. Soumelis V, Reche PA, Kanzler H, et al. Human epithelial cells trigger dendritic cell mediated allergic inflammation by producing TSLP. Nat Immunol 2002;3(7):673–680.

80. Al-Shami A, Spolski R, Kelly J, et al. A role for TSLP in the development of inflammation in an asthma model. J Exp Med 2005;202(6):829–839.

81. Zhou B, Comeau MR, De Smedt T, et al. Thymic stromal lymphopoietin as a key initiator of allergic airway inflammation in mice. Nat Immunol 2005;6(10):1047–1053.

82. Ito T, Wang YH, Duramad O, et al. TSLP-activated dendritic cells induce an inflammatory T helper type 2 cell response through OX40 ligand. J Exp Med 2005;202(9):1213–1223.

83. Liu Y-J. Thymic stromal lymphopoietin: master switch for allergic inflammation. J Exp Med 2006;203(2):269–273.

84. Jeannin P, Lecoanet S, Delneste Y, et al. IgE versus IgG4 production can be differentially regulated by IL-10. J Immunol 1998;160(7):3555–3561.

85. Grunig G, Corry DB, Leach MW, et al. Interleukin-10 is a natural suppressor of cytokine production and inflammation in a murine model of allergic bronchopulmonary aspergillosis. J Exp Med 1997;185(6):1089–1099.

86. Akbari O, DeKruyff RH, Umetsu DT. Pulmonary dendritic cells producing IL-10 mediate tolerance induced by respiratory exposure to antigen. Nat Immunol 2001;2(8):725–731.

87. Hobbs K, Negri J, Klinnert M, et al. Interleukin-10 and transforming growth factor-beta promoter polymorphisms in allergies and asthma. Am J Respir Crit Care Med 1998;158(6):1958–1962.

88. Lyon H, Lange C, Lake S, et al. IL10 gene polymorphisms are associated with asthma phenotypes in children. Genet Epidemiol 2004;26(2):155–165.

89. Chatterjee R, Batra J, Kumar A, et al. Interleukin-10 promoter polymorphisms and atopic asthma in North Indians. Clin Exp Allergy 2005;35(7):914–919.

90. Molet S, Hamid Q, Davoine F, et al. IL-17 is increased in asthmatic airways and induces human bronchial fibroblasts to produce cytokines. J Allergy Clin Immunol 2001;108(3):430–438.

91. Kawaguchi M, Onuchic LF, Li XD, et al. Identification of a novel cytokine, ML-1, and its expression in subjects with asthma. J Immunol 2001;167(8):4430–4435.

92. Barczyk A, Pierzchala W, Sozanska E. Interleukin-17 in sputum correlates with airway hyperresponsiveness to methacholine. Respir Med 2003;97(6):726–733.

93. Pan G, French D, Mao W, et al. Forced expression of murine IL-17E induces growth retardation, jaundice, a Th2-biased response, and multiorgan inflammation in mice. J Immunol 2001;167(11):6559–6567.

94. Hurst SD, Muchamuel T, Gorman DM, et al. New IL-17 family members promote Th1 or Th2 responses in the lung: in vivo function of the novel cytokine IL-25. J Immunol 2002;169(1):443–453.

95. Kim MR, Manoukian R, Yeh R, et al. Transgenic overexpression of human IL-17E results in eosinophilia, B-lymphocyte hyperplasia, and altered antibody production. Blood 2002;100(7):2330–2340.

96. Chen Y, Thai P, Zhao YH, et al. Stimulation of airway mucin gene expression by interleukin (IL)-17 through IL-6 paracrine/autocrine loop. J Biol Chem 2003;278(19):17036–1743.

97. Ramsey CD, Lazarus R, Camargo CA Jr, et al. Polymorphisms in the interleukin 17F gene (IL17F) and asthma. Genes Immun 2005;6(3):236–241.

98. Broide DH, Paine MM, Firestein GS. Eosinophils express interleukin 5 and granulocyte macrophage-colony-stimulating factor mRNA at sites of allergic inflammation in asthmatics. J Clin Invest 1992;90(4):1414–1424.

99. Woolley KL, Adelroth E, Woolley MJ, et al. Granulocyte-macrophage colony-stimulating factor, eosinophils and eosinophil cationic protein in subjects with and without mild, stable, atopic asthma. Eur Respir J 1994;7(9):1576–1584.

100. Park CS, Choi YS, Ki SY, et al. Granulocyte macrophage colony-stimulating factor is the main cytokine enhancing survival of eosinophils in asthmatic airways. Eur Respir J 1998;12(4):872–878.

101. Adachi T, Motojima S, Hirata A, et al. Eosinophil viability-enhancing activity in sputum from patients with bronchial asthma, Contributions of interleukin-5 and granulocyte/macrophage colony-stimulating factor. Am J of Respir Crit Care Med 1995;151(3 Pt 1):618–623.

102. Soloperto M, Mattoso VL, Fasoli A, et al. A bronchial epithelial cell-derived facto in asthma that promotes eosinophil activation and survival as GM-CSF. Am J of Physiol 1991;260(6 Pt 1):L530–L538.

103. Lei XF, Ohkawara Y, Stampfli MR, et al. Compartmentalized transgene expression of granulocyte–macrophage colony-stimulating factor (GM-CSF) in mouse lung enhances allergic airways inflammation. Clin Exp Immunol 1998;113(2):157–165.

104. Ohta K, Yamashita N, Tajima M, et al. Diesel exhaust particulate induces airway hyperresponsiveness in a murine

model: essential role of GM-CSF. J Allergy Clin Immunol 1999;104(5):1024–1030.

105. Yamashita N, Tashimo H, Ishida H, et al. Attenuation of airway hyperresponsiveness in a murine asthma model by neutralization of granulocyte–macrophage colony-stimulating factor (GM-CSF). Cell Immunol 2002;219(2): 92–97.

106. Cates EC, Gajewska BU, Goncharova S, et al. Effect of GM-CSF on immune, inflammatory, and clinical responses to ragweed in a novel mouse model of mucosal sensitization. J Allergy Clin Immunol 2003;111(5):1076–1086.

107. Amishima M, Munakata M, Nasuhara Y, et al. Expression of epidermal growth factor and epidermal growth factor receptor immunoreactivity in the asthmatic human airway. Am J Respir Crit Care Med 1998;157(6 Pt 1):1907–1912.

108. Puddicombe SM, Polosa R, Richter A, et al. Involvement of the epidermal growth factor receptor in epithelial repair in asthma. FASEB J 2000;14(10):1362–1374.

109. Takeyama K, Fahy JV, Nadel JA. Relationship of epidermal growth factor receptors to goblet cell production in human bronchi. Am J Respir Crit Care Med 2001;163(2): 511–516.

110. Takeyama K, Dabbagh K, Lee HM, et al. Epidermal growth factor system regulates mucin production in airways. Proc Natl Acad Sci USA 1999;96(6):3081–3086.

111. Hoshino M, Takahashi M, Aoike N. Expression of vascular endothelial growth factor, basic fibroblast growth factor, and angiogenin immunoreactivity in asthmatic airways and its relationship to angiogenesis. J Allergy Clin Immunol 2001;107(2):295–301.

112. Hoshino M, Nakamura Y, Hamid QA. Gene expression of vascular endothelial growth factor and its receptors and angiogenesis in bronchial asthma. J Allergy Clin Immunol 2001;107(6):1034–1038.

113. Kanazawa H, Hirata K, Yoshikawa J. Involvement of vascular endothelial growth factor in exercise induced bronchoconstriction in asthmatic patients. Thorax 2002; 57(10):885–888.

114. Feltis BN, Wignarajah D, Zheng L, et al. Increased vascular endothelial growth factor and receptors: relationship to angiogenesis in asthma. Am J Respir Crit Care Med 2006;173(11):1201–1207.

115. Abdel-Rahman AMO, el-Sahrigy SAF, Bakr SI. A comparative study of two angiogenic factors: vascular endothelial growth factor and angiogenin in induced sputum from asthmatic children in acute attack. Chest 2006;129(2): 266–271.

116. Lee CG, Link H, Baluk P, et al. Vascular endothelial growth factor (VEGF) induces remodeling and enhances TH2-mediated sensitization and inflammation in the lung. Nat Med 2004;10(10):1095–1103.

117. Baluk P, Lee CG, Link H, et al. Regulated angiogenesis and vascular regression in miceoverexpressing vascular endothelial growth factor in airways. Am J Pathol 2004;165(4):1071–1085.

118. Suzaki Y, Hamada K, Sho M, et al. A potent antiangiogenic factor, endostatin prevents the development of asthma in a murine model. J Allergy Clin Immunol 2005;116(6): 1220–1227.

119. Chalmers GW, Little SA, Patel KR, et al. Endothelin-1-induced bronchoconstriction in asthma. Am J Respir Crit Care Med 1997;156(2 Pt 1):382–388.

120. Springall DR, Howarth PH, Counihan H, et al. Endothelin immunoreactivity of airway epithelium in asthmatic patients. Lancet 1991;337(8743):697–701.

121. Goldie RG, Henry PJ, Paterson JW, et al. Contractile effects and receptor distributions for endothelin-1 (ET-1) in human and animal airways. Agents Actions Suppl 1990;31:229–232.

122. Mattoli S, Soloperto M, Marini M, et al. Levels of endothelin in the bronchoalveolar lavage fluid of patients with symptomatic asthma and reversible airflow obstruction. J Allergy Clin Immunol 1991;88(3 Pt 1):376–384.

123. Aoki T, Kojima T, Ono A, et al. Circulating endothelin-1 levels in patients with bronchial asthma. Ann Allergy 1994;73(4):365–369.

124. Finsnes F, Lyberg T, Christensen G, et al. Effect of endothelin antagonism on the production of cytokines in eosinophilic airway inflammation. Am J Physiol Lung Cell Mol Physiol 2001;280(4):L659–L665.

125. Fujitani Y, Trifilieff A, Tsuyuki S, et al. Endothelin receptor antagonists inhibit antigen-induced lung inflammation in mice. Am J Respir Crit Care Med 1997;155(6):1890–1894.

126. Nagase T, Kurihara H, Kurihara Y, et al. Airway hyperresponsiveness to methacholine in mutant mice deficient in endothelin-1. Am J Respir Crit Care Med 1998;157(2): 560–564.

127. Chalmers GW, MacLeod KJ, Thomson LJ, et al. Sputum cellular and cytokine responses to inhaled endothelin-1 in asthma. Clin Exp Allergy 1999;29(11):1526–1531.

128. Redington AE, Roche WR, Madden J, et al. Basic fibroblast growth factor in asthma: measurement in bronchoalveolar lavage fluid basally and following allergen challenge. J Allergy Clin Immunol 2001;107(2):384–387.

129. Ohno I, Nitta Y, Yamauchi K, et al. Eosinophils as a potential source of platelet-derived growth factor B-chain (PDGF-B) in nasal polyposis and bronchial asthma. Am J Respir Cell Mol Biol 1995;13(6):639–647.

130. Gosset P, Tsicopoulos A, Wallaert B, et al. Increased secretion of tumor necrosis factor alpha and interleukin-6 by alveolar macrophages consecutive to the development of the late asthmatic reaction. J Allergy Clin Immunol 1991;88(4):561–571.

131. Tonnel AB, Gosset P, Tillie-Leblond I. Characteristics of the inflammatory response in bronchial lavage fluids from patients with status asthmaticus. Int Arch Allergy Immunol 2001;124(1–3):267–271.

132. Kim J, McKinley L, Natarajan S, et al. Anti-tumor necrosis factor-alpha antibody treatment reduces pulmonary inflammation and methacholine hyper-responsiveness in a murine asthma model induced by house dust. Clin Exp Allergy 2006;36(1):122–132.

133. Choi IW, Sun-Kim, Kim YS, et al. TNF-alpha induces the late-phase airway hyperresponsiveness and airway inflammation through cytosolic phospholipase A(2) activation. J Allergy Clin Immunol 2005;116(3):537–543.

134. Zuany-Amorim C, Manlius C, Dalum I, et al. Induction of TNF-alpha autoantibody production by AutoVac TNF106: a novel therapeutic approach for the treatment

of allergic diseases. Int Arch Allergy Immunol 2004;133(2): 154–163.

135. Rouhani FN, Meitin CA, Kaler M, et al. Effect of tumor necrosis factor antagonism on allergen-mediated asthmatic airway inflammation. Respir Med 2005;99(9): 1175–1182.

136. Berry MA, Hargadon B, Shelley M, et al. Evidence of a role of tumor necrosis factor alpha in refractory asthma. N Engl J Med 2006;354(7):697–708.

137. Shin HD, Park BL, Kim LH, et al. Association of tumor necrosis factor polymorphisms with asthma and serum total IgE. Hum Mol Genet 2004;13(4):397–403.

138. Winchester EC, Millwood IY, Rand L, et al. Association of the TNF-alpha-308 (G→A) polymorphism with self-reported history of childhood asthma. Hum Genet 2000;107(6):591–596.

139. Moffatt MF, Cookson WO. Tumour necrosis factor haplotypes and asthma. Hum Mol Genet 1997;6(4):551–554.

140. Lin YC, Lu CC, Su HJ, et al. The association between tumor necrosis factor, HLA-DR alleles, and IgE-mediated asthma in Taiwanese adolescents. Allergy 2002;57(9): 831–834.

141. Buckova D, Holla LI, Vasku A, et al. Lack of association between atopic asthma and the tumor necrosis factor alpha-308 gene polymorphism in a Czech population. J Invest Allergol Clin Immunol 2002;12(3):192–197.

142. Migita O, Noguchi E, Koga M, et al. Haplotype analysis of a 100 kb region spanning TNF-LTA identifies a polymorphism in the LTA promoter region that is associated with atopic asthma susceptibility in Japan. Clin Exp Allergy 2005;35(6):790–796.

143. Randolph AG, Lange C, Silverman EK, et al. Extended haplotype in the tumor necrosis factor gene cluster is associated with asthma and asthma-related phenotypes. Am J Respir Crit Care Med 2005;172(6):687–692.

144. Gavett SH, O'Hearn DJ, Li X, et al. Interleukin 12 inhibits antigen-induced airway hyperresponsiveness, inflammation, and Th2 cytokine expression in mice. J Exp Med 1995;182(5):1527–1536.

145. Hofstra CL, Van Ark I, Hofman G, et al. Differential effects of endogenous and exogenous interferon-gamma on immunoglobulin E, cellular infiltration, and airway responsiveness in a murine model of allergic asthma. Am J Respir Cell Mol Biol 1998;19(5):826–835.

146. Walter DM, Wong CP, DeKruyff RH, et al. Il-18 gene transfer by adenovirus prevents the development of and reverses established allergen-induced airway hyperreactivity. J Immunol 2001;166:6392–6398.

147. Yoshimoto T, Min B, Sugimoto T, et al. Nonredundant roles for CD1d-restricted natural killer T cells and conventional CD4+ T cells in the induction of immunoglobulin E antibodies in response to interleukin 18 treatment of mice. J Exp Med 2003;197(8):997–1005.

148. Yoshimoto T, Mizutani H, Tsutsui H, et al. IL-18 induction of IgE: dependence on CD4+ T cells, IL-4 and STAT6. Nat Immunol 2000;1:132–137.

149. Morahan G, Huang D, Wu M, et al. Association of IL12B promoter polymorphism with severity of atopic and non-atopic asthma in children. Lancet 2002;360(9331):455–459.

150. Khoo SK, Hayden CM, Roberts M, et al. Associations of the IL12B promoter polymorphism in longitudinal data from asthmatic patients 7 to 42 years of age. J Allergy Clin Immunol 2004;113(3):475–481.

151. Hirota T, Suzuki Y, Hasegawa K, et al. Functional haplotypes of IL-12B are associated with childhood atopic asthma. J Allergy Clin Immunol 2005;116(4):789–795.

152. Randolph AG, Lange C, Silverman EK, et al. The IL12B gene is associated with asthma. Am J Hum Genet 2004;75(4):709–715.

153. Napolitani G, Rinaldi A, Bertoni F, et al. Selected Toll-like receptor agonist combinations synergistically trigger a T helper type 1-polarizing program in dendritic cells. Nat Immunol 2005;6(8):769–776.

154. Gereda JE, Leung DY, Thatayatikom A, et al. Relation between house-dust endotoxin exposure, type 1 T-cell development, and allergen sensitisation in infants at high risk of asthma. Lancet 2000;355(9216):1680–1683.

155. Redecke V, Hacker H, Datta SK, et al. Cutting edge: activation of Toll-like receptor 2 induces a Th2 immune response and promotes experimental asthma. J Immunol 2004;172(5):2739–2743.

156. Eisenbarth SC, Piggott DA, Huleatt JW, et al. Lipopolysaccharide-enhanced, toll-like receptor 4-dependent T helper cell type 2 responses to inhaled antigen. J Exp Med 2002;196(12):1645–1651.

157. Raby BA, Klimecki WT, Laprise C, et al. Polymorphisms in toll-like receptor 4 are not associated with asthma or atopy-related phenotypes. Am J Respir Crit Care Med 2002;166(11):1449–1456.

158. Berghofer B, Frommer T, Konig IR, et al. Common human Toll-like receptor 9 polymorphisms and haplotypes: association with atopy and functional relevance. Clin Exp Allergy 2005;35(9):1147–1154.

159. Lazarus R, Klimecki WT, Raby BA, et al. Single-nucleotide polymorphisms in the Toll-like receptor 9 gene (TLR9): frequencies, pairwise linkage disequilibrium, and haplotypes in three U.S. ethnic groups and exploratory case-control disease association studies. Genomics 2003;81(1): 85–91.

160. Fageras Bottcher M, Hmani-Aifa M, Lindstrom A, et al. A TLR4 polymorphism is associated with asthma and reduced lipopolysaccharide-induced interleukin-12(p70) responses in Swedish children. J Allergy Clin Immunol 2004;114(3):561–567.

161. Eder W, Klimecki W, Yu L, et al. Toll-like receptor 2 as a major gene for asthma in children of European farmers. J Allergy Clin Immunol 2004;113(3):482–488.

162. Rossi D, Zlotnik A. The biology of chemokines and their receptors. Annu Rev Immunol 2000;18:217–242.

163. Zlotnik A, Yoshie O. Chemokines: a new classification system and their role in immunity. Immunity 2000;12(2): 121–127.

164. D'Ambrosio D, Mariani M, Panina-Bordignon P, et al. Chemokines and their receptors guiding T lymphocyte recruitment in lung inflammation. Am J Respir Crit Care Med 2001;164(7):1266–1275.

165. Chensue SW, Lukacs NW, Yang TY, et al. Aberrant in vivo T helper type 2 cell response and impaired eosinophil

recruitment in CC chemokine receptor 8 knockout mice. J Exp Med 2001;193(5):573–584.

166. Homey B, Zlotnik A. Chemokines in allergy. Curr Opin Immunol 1999;11(6):626–634.

167. Teran LM. CCL chemokines and asthma. Immunol Today 2000;21(5):235–242.

168. Kawasaki S, Takizawa H, Yoneyama H, et al. Intervention of thymus and activation-regulated chemokine attenuates the development of allergic airway inflammation and hyperresponsiveness in mice. J Immunol 2001;166(3):2055–2062.

169. Yamamoto J, Adachi Y, Onoue Y, et al. Differential expression of the chemokine receptors by the Th1- and Th2-type effector populations within circulating CD4+ T cells. J Leuk Biol 2000;68(4):568–574.

170. Panina-Bordignon P, Papi A, Mariani M, et al. The C-C chemokine receptors CCR4 and CCR8 identify airway T cells of allergen-challenged atopic asthmatics. J Clin Invest 2001;107(11):1357–1364.

171. Schuh JM, Power CA, Proudfoot AE, et al. Airway hyperresponsiveness, but not airway remodeling, is attenuated during chronic pulmonary allergic responses to *Aspergillus* in CCR4–/– mice. FASEB J Online 2002;16(10):1313–1315.

172. Humbles AA, Lu B, Friend DS, et al. The murine CCR3 receptor regulates both the role of eosinophils and mast cells in allergen-induced airway inflammation and hyperresponsiveness. Proc Natl Acad Sci USA 2002;99(3):1479–1484.

173. Ma W, Bryce PJ, Humbles AA, et al. CCR3 is essential for skin eosinophilia and airway hyperresponsiveness in a murine model of allergic skin inflammation. J Clin Invest 2002;109(5):621–628.

174. Shin HD, Kim LH, Park BL, et al. Association of eotaxin gene family with asthma and serum total IgE. Hum Mol Genet 2003;12(11):1279–1285.

175. Fukunaga K, Asano K, Mao XQ, et al. Genetic polymorphisms of CC chemokine receptor 3 in Japanese and British asthmatics. Eur Respir J 2001;17(1):59–63.

176. Fryer AA, Spiteri MA, Bianco A, et al. The -403 G→A promoter polymorphism in the RANTES gene is associated with atopy and asthma. Genes Immun 2000;1(8):509–514.

177. Stemmler S, Arinir U, Klein W, et al. Association of interleukin-8 receptor alpha polymorphisms with chronic obstructive pulmonary disease and asthma. Genes Immun 2005;6(3):225–230.

178. Milne AA, Piper PJ. Role of the VLA-4 integrin in leucocyte recruitment and bronchial hyperresponsiveness in the guinea-pig. Eur J Pharmacol 1995;282(1–3):243–249.

179. Borchers MT, Crosby J, Farmer S, et al. Blockade of CD49d inhibits allergic airway pathologies independent of effects on leukocyte recruitment. Am J Physiol Lung Cell Mol Physiol 2001;280(4):L813–L821.

180. Lobb RR, Abraham WM, Burkly LC, et al. Pathophysiologic role of alpha 4 integrins in the lung. Ann NY Acad Sci 1996;796:113–123.

181. Henderson WR Jr, Chi EY, Albert RK, et al. Blockade of CD49d (alpha4 integrin) on intrapulmonary but not circulating leukocytes inhibits airway inflammation and hyper-

182. Kanehiro A, Takeda K, Joetham A, et al. Timing of administration of anti-VLA-4 differentiates airway hyperresponsiveness in the central and peripheral airways in mice. Am J Respir Crit Care Med 2000;162(3 Pt 1):1132–1139.

183. Wegner CD, Gundel RH, Reilly P, et al. Intercellular adhesion molecule-1 (ICAM-1) in the pathogenesis of asthma. Science 1990;247(4941):456–459.

184. Buckley TL, Bloemen PG, Henricks PA, et al. LFA-1 and ICAM-1 are crucial for the induction of hyperreactivity in the mouse airways. Ann NY Acad Sci 1996;796:149–161.

185. Gerwin N, Gonzalo JA, Lloyd C, et al. Prolonged eosinophil accumulation in allergic lung interstitium of ICAM-2 deficient mice results in extended hyperresponsiveness. Immunity 1999;10(1):9–19.

186. Lee SH, Prince JE, Rais M, et al. Differential requirement for CD18 in T helper effector homing. Nat Med 2003;9(10):1281–1286.

187. Puthothu B, Krueger M, Bernhardt M, et al. ICAM1 amino-acid variant K469E is associated with paediatric bronchial asthma and elevated sICAM1 levels. Genes Immun 2006;7(4):322–326.

188. Mathew A, MacLean JA, DeHaan E, et al. Signal transducer and activator of transcription 6 controls chemokine production and T helper cell type 2 cell trafficking in allergic pulmonary inflammation. J Exp Med 2001;193(9):1087–1096.

189. Sampath D, Castro M, Look DC, et al. Constitutive activation of an epithelial signal transducer and activator of transcription (STAT) pathway in asthma. J Clin Invest 1999;103(9):1353–1361.

190. Shi ZOQ, Fischer MJ, De Sanctis GT, et al. IFN-gamma, but not Fas, mediates reduction of allergen-induced mucous cell metaplasia by inducing apoptosis. J Immunol 2002;168(9):4764–4771.

191. Wang IM, Lin H, Goldman SJ, et al. STAT-1 is activated by IL-4 and IL-13 in multiple cell types. Mol Immunol 2004;41(9):873–884.

192. Venkayya R, Lam M, Willkom M, et al. The Th2 lymphocyte products IL-4 and IL-13 rapidly induce airway hyperresponsiveness through direct effects on resident airway cells. Am J Respir Cell Mol Biol 2002;26(2):202–208.

193. Kuperman DA, Huang X, Koth LL, et al. Direct effects of interleukin-13 on epithelial cells cause airway hyperreactivity and mucus overproduction in asthma. Nat Med 2002;8(8):885–889.

194. Zheng W, Flavell RA. The transcription factor GATA-3 is necessary and sufficient for Th2 cytokine gene expression in CD4 T cells. Cell 1997;89(4):587–596.

195. Zhang DH, Cohn L, Ray P, et al. Transcription factor GATA-3 is differentially expressed in murine Th1 and Th2 cells and controls Th2-specific expression of the interleukin-5 gene. J Biol Chem 1997;272(34):21597–21603.

196. Ouyang W, Lohning M, Gao Z, et al. Stat6-independent GATA-3 autoactivation directs IL-4-independent Th2 development and commitment. Immunity 2000;12(1):27–37.

197. Das J, Chen CH, Yang L, et al. A critical role for NF-kappa B in GATA3 expression and TH2 differentiation in

allergic airway inflammation. Nat Immunol 2001;2(1):45–50.

198. Szabo SJ, Kim ST, Costa GL, et al. A novel transcription factor, T-bet, directs Th1 lineage commitment. Cell 2000;100(6):655–669.

199. Finotto S, Neurath MF, Glickman JN, et al. Development of spontaneous airway changes consistent with human asthma in mice lacking T-bet. Science 2002;295(5553): 336–338.

200. Finotto S, Hausding M, Doganci A, et al. Asthmatic changes in mice lacking T-bet are mediated by IL-13. Int Immunol 2005;17(8):993–1007.

201. Tantisira KG, Hwang ES, Raby BA, et al. TBX21: a functional variant predicts improvement in asthma with the use of inhaled corticosteroids. Proc Natl Acad Sci USA 2004;101(52):18099–18104.

202. Raby BA, Hwang ES, Van Steen K, et al. T-bet polymorphisms are associated with asthma and airway hyperresponsiveness. Am J Respir Crit Care Med 2006;173(1): 64–70.

203. Deurloo DT, van Berkel MAT, van Esch BCAM, et al. CD28/CTLA4 double deficient mice demonstrate crucial role for B7 co-stimulation in the induction of allergic lower airways disease. Clin Exp Allergy 2003;33(9):1297–304.

204. Mathur M, Herrmann K, Qin Y, et al. CD28 interactions with either CD80 or CD86 are sufficient to induce allergic airway inflammation in mice. Am J Respir Cell Mol Biol 1999;21(4):498–509.

205. Padrid PA, Mathur M, Li X, et al. CTLA4Ig inhibits airway eosinophilia and hyperresponsiveness by regulating the development of Th1/Th2 subsets in a murine model of asthma. Am J Respir Cell Mol Biol 1998;18(4):453–462.

206. Keane-Myers A, Gause WC, Linsley PS, et al. B7-CD28/CTLA-4 costimulatory pathways are required for the development of T helper cell 2-mediated allergic airway responses to inhaled antigens. J Immunol 1997;158(5): 2042–2049.

207. Krinzman SJ, De Sanctis GT, Cernadas M, et al. Inhibition of T cell costimulation abrogates airway hyperresponsiveness in a murine model. J Clin Invest 1996;98(12):2693–2699.

208. Salek-Ardakani S, Song J, Halteman BS, et al. OX40 (CD134) controls memory T helper 2 cells that drive lung inflammation. J Exp Med 2003;198(2):315–324.

209. Hoshino A, Tanaka Y, Akiba H, et al. Critical role for OX40 ligand in the development of pathogenic Th2 cells in a murine model of asthma. Eur J Immunol 2003;33(4): 861–869.

210. Arestides RSS, He H, Westlake RM, et al. Costimulatory molecule OX40L is critical for both Th1 and Th2 responses in allergic inflammation. Eur J Immunol 2002;32(10): 2874–2880.

211. Jember AG, Zuberi R, Liu FT, et al. Development of allergic inflammation in a murine model of asthma is dependent on the costimulatory receptor OX40. J Exp Med 2001;193(3):387–392.

212. Deurloo DT, van Esch BC, Hofstra CL, et al. CTLA4-IgG reverses asthma manifestations in a mild but not in a more "severe" ongoing murine model. Am J Respir Cell Mol Biol 2001;25(6):751–760.

213. Tivol EA, Borriello F, Schweitzer AN, et al. Loss of CTLA-4 leads to massive lymphoproliferation and fatal multiorgan tissue destruction, revealing a critical negative regulatory role of CTLA-4. Immunity 1995;3(5):541–547.

214. Howard TD, Postma DS, Hawkins GA, et al. Fine mapping of an IgE-controlling gene on chromosome 2q: Analysis of CTLA4 and CD28. J Allergy Clin Immunol 2002;110(5): 743–751.

215. Jaffar ZH, Stanciu L, Pandit A, et al. Essential role for both CD80 and CD86 costimulation, but not CD40 interactions, in allergen-induced Th2 cytokine production from asthmatic bronchial tissue: role for alphabeta, but not gammadelta, T cells. J Immunol 1999;163(11):6283–6291.

216. Hogan SP, Mould A, Kikutani H, et al. Aeroallergen-induced eosinophilic inflammation, lung damage, and airways hyperreactivity in mice can occur independently of IL-4 and allergen-specific immunoglobulins. J Clin Invest 1997;99(6):1329–1339.

217. McIntire JJ, Umetsu SE, Akbari O, et al. Identification of Tapr (an airway hyperreactivity regulatory locus) and the linked Tim gene family. Nat Immunol 2001;2(12):1109–1116.

218. de Souza AJ, Oriss TB, O'Malley KJ, et al. T cell Ig and mucin 1 (TIM-1) is expressed on in vivo-activated T cells and provides a costimulatory signal for T cell activation. Proc Natl Acad Sci USA 2005;102(47):17113–17118.

219. Meyers JH, Chakravarti S, Schlesinger D, et al. TIM-4 is the ligand for TIM-1, and the TIM-1-TIM-4 interaction regulates T cell proliferation. Nat Immunol 2005;6(5):455–464.

220. Chae SC, Song JH, Heo JC, et al. Molecular variations in the promoter and coding regions of human Tim-1 gene and their association in Koreans with asthma. Hum Immunol 2003;64(12):1177–1182.

221. Gao PS, Mathias RA, Plunkett B, et al. Genetic variants of the T-cell immunoglobulin mucin 1 but not the T-cell immunoglobulin mucin 3 gene are associated with asthma in an African American population. J Allergy Clin Immunol 2005;115(5):982–988.

222. Monney L, Sabatos CA, Gaglia JL, et al. Th1-specific cell surface protein Tim-3 regulates macrophage activation and severity of an autoimmune disease. Nature 2002; 415(6871):536–541.

223. Drouin SM, Corry DB, Hollman TJ, et al. Absence of the complement anaphylatoxin C3a receptor suppresses Th2 effector functions in a murine model of pulmonary allergy. J Immunol 2002;169(10):5926–5933.

224. Drouin SM, Corry DB, Kildsgaard J, et al. Cutting edge: the absence of C3 demonstrates a role for complement in Th2 effector functions in a murine model of pulmonary allergy. J Immunol 2001;167(8):4141–4145.

225. Humbles AA, Lu B, Nilsson CA, et al. A role for the C3a anaphylatoxin receptor in the effector phase of asthma. Nature 2000;406(6799):998–1001.

226. Kozel TR, Wilson MA, Farrell TP, et al. Activation of C3 and binding to *Aspergillus fumigatus* conidia and hyphae. Infect Immun 1989;57(11):3412–3417.

227. Drouin SM, Kildsgaard J, Haviland J, et al. Expression of the complement anaphylatoxin C3a and C5a receptors

on bronchial epithelial and smooth muscle cells in models of sepsis and asthma. J Immunol 2001;166(3): 2025–2032.

228. Abe M, Shibata K, Akatsu H, et al. Contribution of anaphylatoxin C5a to late airway responses after repeated exposure of antigen to allergic rats. J Immunol 2001;167(8): 4651–4660.

229. Peng T, Hao L, Madri JA, et al. Role of C5 in the development of airway inflammation, airway hyperresponsiveness, and ongoing airway response. J Clin Invest 2005;115(6): 1590–1600.

230. Hasegawa K, Tamari M, Shao C, et al. Variations in the C3, C3a receptor, and C5 genes affect susceptibility to bronchial asthma. Hum Genet 2004;115(4):295–301.

231. Heise CE, O'Dowd BF, Figueroa DJ, et al. Characterization of the human cysteinyl leukotriene 2 receptor. J Biol Chem 2000;275(39):30531–30536.

232. Lynch KR, O'Neill GP, Liu Q, et al. Characterization of the human cysteinyl leukotriene CysLT1 receptor. Nature 1999;399(6738):789–793.

233. Hui Y, Yang G, Galczenski H, et al. The murine cysteinyl leukotriene 2 (CysLT2) receptor. cDNA and genomic cloning, alternative splicing, and in vitro characterization. J Biol Chem 2001;276(50):47489–47495.

234. Fukai H, Ogasawara Y, Migita O, et al. Association between a polymorphism in cysteinyl leukotriene receptor 2 on chromosome 13q14 and atopic asthma. Pharmacogenetics 2004;14(10):683–690.

235. Park JS, Chang HS, Park CS, et al. Association analysis of cysteinyl-leukotriene receptor 2 (CYSLTR2) polymorphisms with aspirin intolerance in asthmatics. Pharmacogenet Genomics 2005;15(7):483–492.

236. Kawagishi Y, Mita H, Taniguchi M, et al. Leukotriene C4 synthase promoter polymorphism in Japanese patients with aspirin-induced asthma. J Allergy Clin Immunol 2002;109(6):936–942.

237. Van Sambeek R, Stevenson DD, Baldasaro M, et al. 5′ Flanking region polymorphism of the gene encoding leukotriene C4 synthase does not correlate with the aspirin-intolerant asthma phenotype in the United States. J Allergy Clin Immunol 2000;106(1 Pt 1):72–76.

238. Sanak M, Pierzchalska M, Bazan-Socha S, et al. Enhanced expression of the leukotriene C(4) synthase due to overactive transcription of an allelic variant associated with aspirin-intolerant asthma. Am J Respir Cell Mol Biol 2000;23(3):290–296.

239. Sanak M, Simon HU, Szczeklik A. Leukotriene C4 synthase promoter polymorphism and risk of aspirin-induced asthma. Lancet 1997;350(9091):1599–1600.

240. Jones GL, Saroea HG, Watson RM, et al. Effect of an inhaled thromboxane mimetic (U46619) on airway function in human subjects. Am Rev Respir Dis 1992;145(6): 1270–1274.

241. Fujimura M, Saito M, Kurashima K, et al. Bronchoconstrictive properties and potentiating effect on bronchial responsiveness of inhaled thromboxane A2 analogue (STA2) in guinea pigs. J Asthma 1989;26(4):237–242.

242. Fujimura M, Sasaki F, Nakatsumi Y, et al. Effects of a thromboxane synthetase inhibitor (OKY-046) and a lipoxygenase inhibitor (AA-861) on bronchial responsiveness to acetylcholine in asthmatic subjects. Thorax 1986;41(12): 955–959.

243. Arimura A, Asanuma F, Kurosawa A, et al. Antiasthmatic activity of a novel thromboxane A2 antagonist, S-1452, in guinea pigs. Int Arch Allergy Appl Immunol 1992;98(3): 239–246.

244. Nagai H, Yakuo I, Togawa M, et al. Effect of OKY-046, a new thromboxane A2 synthetase inhibitor, on experimental asthma in guinea pigs. Prostaglandins Leukot Med 1987;30(2–3):111–121.

245. Beasley RC, Featherstone RL, Church MK, et al. Effect of a thromboxane receptor antagonist on PGD2- and allergen-induced bronchoconstriction. J Appl Physiol 1989; 66(4):1685–1693.

246. Finnerty JP, Twentyman OP, Harris A, et al. Effect of GR32191, a potent thromboxane receptor antagonist, on exercise induced bronchoconstriction in asthma. Thorax 1991;46(3):190–192.

247. Manning PJ, Stevens WH, Cockcroft DW, et al. The role of thromboxane in allergen-induced asthmatic responses. Eur Respir J 1991;4(6):667–672.

248. Stenton SC, Young CA, Harris A, et al. The effect of GR32191 (a thromboxane receptor antagonist) on airway responsiveness in asthma. Pulm Pharmacol 1992;5(3): 199–202.

249. Gardiner PV, Young CL, Holmes K, et al. Lack of short-term effect of the thromboxane synthetase inhibitor UK-38,485 on airway reactivity to methacholine in asthmatic subjects. Eur Respir J 1993;6(7):1027–1030.

250. Leung TF, Tang NLS, Lam CWK, et al. Thromboxane A2 receptor gene polymorphism is associated with the serum concentration of cat-specific immunoglobulin E as well as the development and severity of asthma in Chinese children. Pediatr Allergy Immunol 2002;13(1):10–17.

251. Unoki M, Furuta S, Onouchi Y, et al. Association studies of 33 single nucleotide polymorphisms (SNPs) in 29 candidate genes for bronchial asthma: positive association a T924C polymorphism in the thromboxane A2 receptor gene. Hum Genet 2000;106(4):440–446.

252. Hardy CC, Robinson C, Tattersfield AE, et al. The bronchoconstrictor effect of inhaled prostaglandin D2 in normal and asthmatic men. N Engl J Med 1984;311(4):209–213.

253. Fuller RW, Dixon CM, Dollery CT, et al. Prostaglandin D2 potentiates airway responsiveness to histamine and methacholine. Am Rev Respir Dis 1986;133(2):252–254.

254. Matsuoka T, Hirata M, Tanaka H, et al. Prostaglandin D2 as a mediator of allergic asthma. Science 2000;287(5460): 2013–2017.

255. Hirai H, Tanaka K, Yoshie O, et al. Prostaglandin D2 selectively induces chemotaxis in T helper type 2 cells, eosinophils, and basophils via seven-transmembrane receptor CRTH2. J Exp Med 2001;193(2):255–261.

256. Spik I, Brenuchon C, Angeli V, et al. Activation of the prostaglandin D2 receptor DP2/CRTH2 increases allergic inflammation in mouse. J Immunol 2005;174(6):3703–3708.

257. Smith AP, Cuthbert MF, Dunlop LS. Effects of inhaled prostaglandins E1, E2, and F2alpha on the airway resistance of healthy and asthmatic man. Clin Sci Mol Med 1975;48(5):421–430.

258. Mathe AA, Hedqvist P. Effect of prostaglandins F2 alpha and E2 on airway conductance in healthy subjects and asthmatic patients. Am Rev Respir Dis 1975;111(3):313–320.

259. Nagao K, Tanaka H, Komai M, et al. Role of prostaglandin I2 in airway remodeling induced by repeated allergen challenge in mice. Am Respir Cell Mol Biol 2003;29(3 Pt 1):314–320.

260. Takahashi Y, Tokuoka S, Masuda T, et al. Augmentation of allergic inflammation in prostanoid IP receptor deficient mice. Br J Pharmacol 2002;137(3):315–322.

261. Bianco S, Robuschi M, Ceserani R, et al. Prevention of a specifically induced bronchoconstriction by PGI2 and 20-methyl-PGI2 in asthmatic patients. Pharmacol Res Commun 1978;10(7):657–674.

262. Fedyk ER, Phipps RP. Prostaglandin E2 receptors of the EP2 and EP4 subtypes regulate activation and differentiation of mouse B lymphocytes to IgE-secreting cells. Proc Natl Acad Sci USA 1996;93(20):10978–10983.

263. Profita M, Sala A, Bonanno A, et al. Increased prostaglandin E2 concentrations and cyclooxygenase-2 expression in asthmatic subjects with sputum eosinophilia. J Allergy Clin Immunol 2003;112(4):709–716.

264. Tilley SL, Hartney JM, Erikson CJ, et al. Receptors and pathways mediating the effects of prostaglandin E2 on airway tone. Am J Physiol Lung Cell Mol Physiol 2003;284(4):L599–L606.

265. Martin JG, Suzuki M, Maghni K, et al. The immunomodulatory actions of prostaglandin E2 on allergic airway responses in the rat. J Immunol 2002;169(7):3963–3969.

266. Kunikata T, Yamane H, Segi E, et al. Suppression of allergic inflammation by the prostaglandin E receptor subtype EP3. Nat Immunol 2005;6(5):524–531.

267. Cushley MJ, Tattersfield AE, Holgate ST. Inhaled adenosine and guanosine on airway resistance in normal and asthmatic subjects. Br J Clin Pharmacol 1983;15(2):161–165.

268. Chunn JL, Young HW, Banerjee SK, et al. Adenosine-dependent airway inflammation and hyperresponsiveness in partially adenosine deaminase-deficient mice. J Immunol 2001;167:4676–4685.

269. Zhong H, Shlykov SG, Molina JG, et al. Activation of murine lung mast cells by the adenosine A3 receptor. J Immunol 2003;171(1):338–345.

270. Tilley SL, Tsai M, Williams CM, et al. Identification of A3 receptor- and mast cell-dependent and -independent components of adenosine-mediated airway responsiveness in mice. J Immunol 2003;171(1):331–337.

271. Blackburn MR, Lee CG, Young HW, et al. Adenosine mediates IL-13-induced inflammation and remodeling in the lung and interacts in an IL-13-adenosine amplification pathway. J Clin Invest 2003;112(3):332–344.

272. Callaerts-Vegh Z, Evans KLJ, Dudekula N, et al. Effects of acute and chronic administration of beta-adrenoceptor ligands on airway function in a murine model of asthma. Proc Natl Acad Sci USA 2004;101(14):4948–4953.

273. Holloway JW, Dunbar PR, Riley GA, et al. Association of beta2-adrenergic receptor polymorphisms with severe asthma. Clin Exp Allergy 2000;30(8):1097–1103.

274. Turki J, Pak J, Green SA, et al. Genetic polymorphisms of the beta 2-adrenergic receptor in nocturnal and non-nocturnal asthma. Evidence that Gly16 correlates with the nocturnal phenotype. J Clin Invest 1995;95(4):1635–1641.

275. Roux E, Molimard M, Savineau JP, et al. Muscarinic stimulation of airway smooth muscle cells. Gen Pharmacol 1998;31(3):349–356.

276. Fenech AG, Ebejer MJ, Felice AE, et al. Mutation screening of the muscarinic M(2) and M(3) receptor genes in normal and asthmatic subjects. Br J Pharmacol 2001;133(1):43–48.

277. Denjean A, Arnoux B, Benveniste J, et al. Bronchoconstriction induced by intratracheal administration of platelet-activating factor (PAF-acether) in baboons. Agents Actions 1981;11(6–7):567–568.

278. Ishii S, Nagase T, Shindou H, et al. Platelet-activating factor receptor develops airway hyperresponsiveness independently of airway inflammation in a murine asthma model. J Immunol 2004;172(11):7095–7102.

279. Stafforini DM, Numao T, Tsodikov A, et al. Deficiency of platelet-activating factor acetylhydrolase is a severity factor for asthma. J Clin Invest 1999;103(7):989–997.

280. Kruse S, Mao XQ, Heinzmann A, et al. The Ile198Thr and Ala379Val variants of plasmatic PAF-acetylhydrolase impair catalytical activities and are associated with atopy and asthma. Am J Hum Genet 2000;66(5):1522–1530.

281. Campbell KA, Lees A, Finkelman FD, et al. Co-crosslinking Fc epsilon RII/CD23 and B cell surface immunoglobulin modulates B cell activation. Eur J Immunol 1992;22(8):2107–2112.

282. Squire CM, Studer EJ, Lees A, et al. Antigen presentation is enhanced by targeting antigen to the Fc epsilon RII by antigen-anti-Fc epsilon RII conjugates. J Immunol 1994;152(9):4388–4396.

283. Fujiwara H, Kikutani H, Suematsu S, et al. The absence of IgE antibody-mediated augmentation of immune responses in CD23-deficient mice. Proc Natl Acad Sci USA 1994;91(15):6835–6839.

284. Gustavsson S, Hjulstrom S, Liu T, et al. CD23/IgE-mediated regulation of the specific antibody response in vivo. J Immunol 1994;152(10):4793–4800.

285. Stief A, Texido G, Sansig G, et al. Mice deficient in CD23 reveal its modulatory role in IgE production but no role in T and B cell development. J Immunol 1994;152(7):3378–3390.

286. Yu P, Kosco-Vilbois M, Richards M, et al. Negative feedback regulation of IgE synthesis by murine CD23. Nature 1994;369(6483):753–756.

287. Tsao CH, Chen LC, Yeh KW, et al. Concomitant chronic sinusitis treatment in children with mild asthma: the effect on bronchial hyperresponsiveness. Chest 2003;123(3):757–764.

288. Guerra S, Sherrill DL, Martinez FD, et al. Rhinitis as an independent risk factor for adult-onset asthma. J Allergy Clin Immunol 2002;109(3):419–425.

289. Hill MR, Cookson WO. A new variant of the beta subunit of the high-affinity receptor for immunoglobulin E (Fc epsilon RI-beta E237G): associations with measures of atopy and bronchial hyper-responsiveness. Hum Mol Genet 1996;5(7):959–962.

290. van Herwerden L, Harrap SB, Wong ZY, et al. Linkage of high-affinity IgE receptor gene with bronchial hyperreactivity, even in absence of atopy. Lancet 1995;346(8985): 1262–1265.

291. Burrows B, Martinez FD, Halonen M, et al. Association of asthma with serum IgE levels and skin-test reactivity to allergens. N Engl J Med 1989;320(5):271–277.

292. Postma DS, Bleecker ER, Amelung PJ, et al. Genetic susceptibility to asthma—bronchial hyperresponsiveness coinherited with a major gene for atopy. N Engl J Med 1995;333(14):894–900.

293. Amelung PJ, Postma D, Panhuysen CI, et al. Susceptibility loci regulating total serum IgE levels, bronchial hyperresponsiveness, and clinical asthma map to chromosome 5q. Chest 1997;111(6 Suppl):77S–78S.

294. Noguchi E, Shibasaki M, Arinami T, et al. Evidence for linkage between asthma/atopy in childhood and chromosome 5q31–q33 in a Japanese population. Am J Respir Crit Care Med 1997;156(5):1390–1393.

295. Palmer LJ, Daniels SE, Rye PJ, et al. Linkage of chromosome 5q and 11q gene markers to asthma-associated quantitative traits in Australian children. Am J Respir Crit Care Med 1998;158(6):1825–1830.

296. Lonjou C, Barnes K, Chen H, et al. A first trial of retrospective collaboration for positional cloning in complex inheritance: assay of the cytokine region on chromosome 5 by the consortium on asthma genetics (COAG). Proc Natl Acad Sci USA 2000;97(20):10942–10947.

297. Donfack J, Schneider DH, Tan Z, et al. Variation in conserved non-coding sequences on chromosome 5q and susceptibility to asthma and atopy. Respir Res 2005;6(1):145.

298. Kamitani A, Wong ZY, Dickson P, et al. Absence of genetic linkage of chromosome 5q31 with asthma and atopy in the general population. Thorax 1997;52(9):816–817.

299. Laitinen T, Kauppi P, Ignatius J, et al. Genetic control of serum IgE levels and asthma: linkage and linkage disequilibrium studies in an isolated population. Hum Mol Genet 1997;6(12):2069–2076.

300. Mansur AH, Bishop DT, Markham AF, et al. Association study of asthma and atopy traits and chromosome 5q cytokine cluster markers. Clin Exp Allergy 1998;28(2):141–150.

301. Jacobs KB, Burton PR, Iyengar SK, et al. Pooling data and linkage analysis in the chromosome 5q candidate region for asthma. Genet Epidemiol 2001;21(Suppl 1):S103–S108.

302. Noguchi E, Yokouchi Y, Zhang J, et al. Positional identification of an asthma susceptibility gene on human chromosome 5q33. Am J Respir Crit Care Med 2005;172(2): 183–188.

303. Corry DB, Kiss A, Song LZ, et al. Overlapping and independent contributions of MMP2 and MMP9 to lung allergic inflammatory cell egression through decreased CC chemokines. FASEB J 2004;18(9):995–997.

304. Corry DB, Rishi K, Kanellis J, et al. Decreased allergic lung inflammatory cell egression and increased susceptibility to asphyxiation in MMP2-deficiency. Nat Immunol 2002;3(4): 347–353.

305. Cocks TM, Fong B, Chow JM, et al. A protective role for protease-activated receptors in the airways. Nature 1999; 398(6723):156–160.

306. Ebeling C, Forsythe P, Ng J, et al. Proteinase-activated receptor 2 activation in the airways enhances antigen-mediated airway inflammation and airway hyperresponsiveness through different pathways. J Allergy Clin Immunol 2005;115(3):623–630.

307. Schmidlin F, Amadesi S, Dabbagh K, et al. Protease-activated receptor 2 mediates eosinophil infiltration and hyperreactivity in allergic inflammation of the airway. J Immunol 2002;169(9):5315–5321.

308. Oh SW, Pae CI, Lee DK, et al. Tryptase inhibition blocks airway inflammation in a mouse asthma model. J Immunol 2002;168(4):1992–2000.

309. Krishna MT, Chauhan A, Little L, et al. Inhibition of mast cell tryptase by inhaled APC 366 attenuates allergen-induced late-phase airway obstruction in asthma. J Allergy Clin Immunol 2001;107(6):1039–1045.

310. Wright CD, Havill AM, Middleton SC, et al. Inhibition of allergen-induced pulmonary responses by the selective tryptase inhibitor 1,5-bis-[4-[(3-carbamimidoyl-benzenesulfonylamino)-methyl]-phenoxy]-pentane (AMG-126737). Biochem Pharmacol 1999;58(12):1989–1996.

311. Elrod KC, Moore WR, Abraham WM, et al. Lactoferrin, a potent tryptase inhibitor, abolishes late-phase airway responses in allergic sheep. Am J Respir Crit Care Med 1997;156(2 Pt 1):375–381.

312. Fiorucci L, Ascoli F. Mast cell tryptase, a still enigmatic enzyme. Cell Mol Life Sci 2004;61(11):1278–1295.

313. Nadel JA, Takeyama K, Agusti C. Role of neutrophil elastase in hypersecretion in asthma. Eur Respir J 1999;13(1): 190–196.

314. Werner M, Herbon N, Gohlke H, et al. Asthma is associated with single-nucleotide polymorphisms in ADAM33. Clin Exp Allergy 2004;34(1):26–31.

315. Jongepier H, Boezen HM, Dijkstra A, et al. Polymorphisms of the ADAM33 gene are associated with accelerated lung function decline in asthma. Clin Exp Allergy 2004;34(5): 757–760.

316. Lind DL, Choudhry S, Ung N, et al. ADAM33 is not associated with asthma in Puerto Rican or Mexican populations. Am J Respir Crit Care Med 2003;168(11):1312–1316.

317. Van Eerdewegh P, Little RD, Dupuis J, et al. Association of the ADAM33 gene with asthma and bronchial hyper-responsiveness. Nature 2002;418(6896):426–430.

318. Kheradmand F, Kiss A, Xu J, et al. A protease-activated pathway underlying Th cell type 2 activation and allergic lung disease. J Immunol 2002;169(10):5904–5911.

319. Comoy EE, Pestel J, Duez C, et al. The house dust mite allergen, *Dermatophagoides pteronyssinus*, promotes type 2 responses by modulating the balance between IL-4 and IFN-gamma. J Immunol 1998;160(5):2456–2462.

320. Wan H, Winton HL, Soeller C, et al. Der p 1 facilitates transepithelial allergen delivery by disruption of tight junctions. J Clin Invest 1999;104(1):123–133.

321. Hewitt CR, Brown AP, Hart BJ, et al. A major house dust mite allergen disrupts the immunoglobulin E network by selectively cleaving CD23: innate protection by antiproteases. J Exp Med 1995;182(5):1537–1544.

322. Pepys J, Longbottom JL, Hargreave FE, et al. Allergic reactions of the lungs to enzymes of *Bacillus subtilis*. Lancet 1969;1(7607):1181–1184.

323. Cullinan P, Harris JM, Newman Taylor AJ, et al. An outbreak of asthma in a modern detergent factory. Lancet 2000;356(9245):1899–1900.

324. Xu J, Park PW, Kheradmand F, et al. Endogenous attenuation of allergic lung inflammation by syndecan-1. J Immunol 2005;174(9):5758–5765.

325. Diamant Z, Timmers MC, van der Veen H, et al. Effect of inhaled heparin on allergen-induced early and late asthmatic responses in patients with atopic asthma. Am J Respir Crit Care Med 1996;153(6 Pt 1):1790–1795.

326. Ahmed T, Garrigo J, Danta I. Preventing bronchoconstriction in exercise-induced asthma with inhaled heparin. N Engl J Med 1993;329(2):90–95.

327. Hoshino M, Morita S, Iwashita H, et al. Increased expression of the human Ca2$^+$-activated Cl$^-$ channel 1 (CaCC1) gene in the asthmatic airway. Am J Respir Crit Care Med 2002;165(8):1132–1136.

328. Komiya T, Tanigawa Y, Hirohashi S. Cloning and identification of the gene gob-5, which is expressed in intestinal goblet cells in mice. Biochem Biophys Res Commun 1999; 255(2):347–351.

329. Nakanishi A, Morita S, Iwashita H, et al. Role of gob-5 in mucus overproduction and airway hyperresponsiveness in asthma. Proc Natl Acad Sci USA 2001;98(9):5175–5180.

330. Robichaud A, Tuck SA, Kargman S, et al. Gob-5 is not essential for mucus overproduction in preclinical murine models of allergic asthma. Am J Respir Cell Mol Biol 2005;33(3):303–314.

331. Gibson A, Lewis AP, Affleck K, et al. hCLCA1 and mCLCA3 are secreted non-integral membrane proteins and therefore are not ion channels. J Biol Chem 2005; 280(29):27205–27212.

332. Kamada F, Suzuki Y, Shao C, et al. Association of the hCLCA1 gene with childhood and adult asthma. Genes Immun 2004;5(7):540–547.

333. Nicolae D, Cox NJ, Lester LA, et al. Fine mapping and positional candidate studies identify HLA-G as an asthma susceptibility gene on chromosome 6p21. Am J Hum Genet 2005;76(2):349–357.

334. Soriano JB, Ercilla G, Sunyer J, et al. HLA class II genes in soybean epidemic asthma patients. Am J Respir Crit Care Med 1997;156(5):1394–1398.

335. Woszczek G, Kowalski ML, Borowiec M. Association of asthma and total IgE levels with human leucocyte antigen-DR in patients with grass allergy. Eur Respir J 2002;20(1): 79–85.

336. Kim SH, Oh HB, Lee KW, et al. HLA DRB1*15-DPB1*05 haplotype: a susceptible gene marker for isocyanate-induced occupational asthma? Allergy 2006;61(7):891–894.

337. Torio A, Sanchez-Guerrero I, Muro M, et al. HLA class II genotypic frequencies in atopic asthma: association of DRB1*01-DQB1*0501 genotype with *Artemisia vulgaris* allergic asthma. Hum Immunol 2003;64(8):811–815.

338. Mapp CE, Beghe B, Balboni A, et al. Association between HLA genes and susceptibility to toluene diisocyanate-induced asthma. Clin Exp Allergy 2000;30(5):651–656.

339. Kharitonov SA, O'Connor BJ, Evans DJ, et al. Allergen-induced late asthmatic reactions are associated with elevation of exhaled nitric oxide. Am J Respir Crit Care Med 1995;151(6):1894–1899.

340. Xiong Y, Karupiah G, Hogan SP, et al. Inhibition of allergic airway inflammation in mice lacking nitric oxide synthase 2. J Immunol 1999;162(1):445–452.

341. De Sanctis GT, MacLean JA, Hamada K, et al. Contribution of nitric oxide synthases 1, 2, and 3 to airway hyperresponsiveness and inflammation in a murine model of asthma. J Exp Med 1999;189(10):1621–1630.

342. Que LG, Liu L, Yan Y, et al. Protection from experimental asthma by an endogenous bronchodilator. Science 2005;308(5728):1618–1621.

343. Grasemann H, Yandava CN, Drazen JM. Neuronal NO synthase (NOS1) is a major candidate gene for asthma. Clin Exp Allergy 1999;29(Suppl 4):39–41.

344. Lee YC, Cheon KT, Lee HB, et al. Gene polymorphisms of endothelial nitric oxide synthase and angiotensin-converting enzyme in patients with asthma. Allergy 2000; 55(10):959–963.

345. Tamaoki J, Nakata J, Takeyama K, et al. Histamine H2 receptor-mediated airway goblet cell secretion and its modulation by histamine-degrading enzymes. J Allergy Clin Immunol 1997;99(2):233–238.

346. Jutel M, Watanabe T, Klunker S, et al. Histamine regulates T-cell and antibody responses by differential expression of H1 and H2 receptors. Nature 2001;413(6854): 420–425.

347. Boot RG, Blommaart EF, Swart E, et al. Identification of a novel acidic mammalian chitinase distinct from chitotriosidase. J Biol Chem 2001;276(9):6770–6778.

348. Jin HM, Copeland NG, Gilbert DJ, et al. Genetic characterization of the murine Ym1 gene and identification of a cluster of highly homologous genes. Genomics 1998;54 (2):316–322.

349. Hu B, Trinh K, Figueira WF, et al. Isolation and sequence of a novel human chondrocyte protein related to mammalian members of the chitinase protein family. J Biol Chem 1996;271(32):19415–19420.

350. Webb DC, McKenzie AN, Foster PS. Expression of the Ym2 lectin-binding protein is dependent on interleukin (IL)-4 and IL-13 signal transduction: identification of a novel allergy-associated protein. J Biol Chem 2001;276 (45):41969–41676.

351. Zhu Z, Zheng T, Homer RJ, et al. Acidic mammalian chitinase in asthmatic Th2 inflammation and IL-13 pathway activation. Science 2004;304(5677):1678–1682.

52
Cystic Fibrosis

Annick Clement, Harriet Corvol, and Brigitte Fauroux

Introduction

Cystic fibrosis (CF) is the most common lethal inherited disease of Caucasians. It is a disease of exocrine gland function involving many tissues and leading to a diverse range of pathologic and clinical problems. Although most patients have multiple organ involvement, pulmonary disease is the principal cause of both morbidity and mortality in more than 90% of patients surviving the neonatal period.[1,2]

Genetics

Cystic fibrosis segregates as an autosomal recessive disorder. Although primarily a disease of Caucasians, CF has been described in virtually every race, with an approximate incidence of 1 per 17,000 in blacks and 1 per 90,000 in Orientals. In Caucasians, the carrier incidence is around 4%. Cystic fibrosis results from mutations in the CF transmembrane conductance regulator *(CFTR)* gene.[3] This gene, located on the long arm of chromosome 7, was identified by using chromosome "jumping" and chromosome "walking" techniques in 1989 in a large-scale multinational research effort. The *CFTR* gene has been characterized as a segment, approximately 250 kilobases (kb) in length, located in the 7q31 region and consists of 27 exons. The gene is transcribed into a 6.5 kb of mRNA that encodes a 1,480 amino acid membrane protein. Soon after the identification of the gene, the molecule encoded was found to be a cyclic adenosine monophosphate–activated chloride (Cl⁻) ion channel.[4]

Thus far, more than 1,400 *CFTR* mutant alleles and over 300 DNA sequence polymorphisms have been reported to the CF Genetic Analysis Consortium and are listed in the CF Mutation Database (www.genet.sickkids.on.ca/cftr/). More than 70% of CF patients have homozygous deletion of the three base pairs encoding phenylalanine at position 508 (F508del). A useful framework for considering genotype–phenotype relationships is the grouping of mutations into classes based on the primary mechanism responsible for reduced CFTR function.[5] Five major classes are currently individualized. Class I mutations, such as G542X and R553X, are those in which stop codons or frame shift mutations lead to premature termination of mRNA translation and thus essentially no protein production. In class II mutations, CFTR protein fails to mature properly in the biosynthetic pathway, with degradation of translated protein before it can progress past the endoplasmic reticulum. In the F508del mutation, the prototypic class II mutation, mutant CFTR protein is misfolded, leading to rapid ubiquitinylation and degradation, with little or no mature protein detectable at the plasma membrane. Like the F508del mutation, several other clinically important mutations, such as N1303K, G85E, and G91R, lead to misfolded protein that is prematurely degraded. Thus, class I and II mutations prevent sufficient CFTR expression at the cell surface and are associated with typical multiorgan diseases including progressive obstructive pulmonary disease, pancreatic insufficiency, and male infertility with congenital bilateral absence of vas deferens (CBAVD).

In contrast, class III and IV mutations allow protein production and transit to the apical surface, but they result in channels that are insensitive to activation or display altered chloride conductance. Class III mutations, such as G551D, are regulatory mutations in which single amino acid substitutions or deletions result in a properly processed protein that is virtually insensitive to channel activation. Class IV mutations, such as R117H and R347P, respond to activation by cyclic adenosine monophosphate (cAMP) agonists but exhibit reduced chloride channel conductance or channel opening probability. As such, these mutations would be expected to result in mild disease manifestations, and several reports have confirmed that this is the case for pancreatic disease.

Class V mutations include promoter abnormalities and splice site mutations, which affect the efficiency of normal mRNA splicing and thereby alter the abundance of normally processed and functional CFTR at the cell membrane. The prototype of this class is the 3,849 + 10 kb C to T mutation, in which a nucleotide substitution at a splice site reduces but does not preclude correct mRNA splicing. Consequently, this mutation yields at least some mRNA capable of producing functional protein that would be expected to be associated with mild disease. Other new classes are proposed such as class VI mutations, which are associated with defective CFTR stability at the cell surface and accelerated turnover.

Several polymorphisms within the *CFTR* gene have been identified and found to influence the penetrance of some CFTR mutations.[6] An example is variations in the length of the polypyrimidine tract in the intron 8 splice acceptor site. Three length variants were reported to be associated with varying efficiencies of exon 9 splicing. The lower number of thymidine (T), 5T, results in less efficient splicing of CFTR transcripts and therefore a lower amount of functional CFTR protein. In the general white ethnic population, the 5T polymorphism is found on about 5% of the *CFTR* gene and on about 21% of the *CFTR* genes derived from patients with CBAVD. Other polymorphisms such as the polymorphic TGm locus (11, 12, or 13 TG repeats) in front of the Tn locus were demonstrated to contribute to the variable penetrance of the 5T allele. A higher number of TG repeats results in less efficient splicing of the CFTR transcripts. There is therefore strong evidence that such polymorphisms may contribute to heterogeneity in both CFTR chloride channel and disease phenotype among individuals with the same *CFTR* mutation.

Structure and Function of the Cystic Fibrosis Transmembrane Conductance Regulator

The CFTR protein has 1,480 amino acids and is a member of the adenosine triphosphate (ATP) binding cassette (ABC) transport protein superfamily, which uses ATP as an energy source to move substrates against a concentration gradient.[7] The NH_2 and COOH terminal halves of CFTR both contain a transmembrane domain comprising six putative membrane spanning α-helices followed by a nucleotide-binding domain (NBD), and the two halves are linked by a cytoplasmic regulatory (R) domain that incorporates multiple sites for phosphorylation by cAMP protein kinase A and protein kinase C. Both the NBDs and the R domain reside intracellularly (Figure 52.1). In the ABC transporter family, the NBDs are the site of ATP hydrolysis. When the R domain channel blockade is relieved by phosphorylation, and binding and hydrolysis take place at the first NBD, the channel opens. Binding

and hydrolysis at the second NBD closes the channel. Thus, conformational changes brought about by NBD1 and NBD2 result in chloride conductance. The closed state of the molecule can be secured by dephosphorylation of the R domain. The F508del mutation results in an in-frame deletion within NBD1.

Cystic fibrosis transmembrane conductance regulator is primarily a membrane protein and is expressed in epithelial cells. Besides its function as a chloride channel, CFTR also regulates other apical membrane conductance pathways. It is involved in the activity of the epithelial sodium channel (ENaC). Amiloride-sensitive sodium absorption is an important function of epithelial cells and is controlled by ENaC. Regulation of Cl^- and Na^+ transport affects the homeostasis of the airway surface liquid. In CF, there is excess Na^+ absorption across the respiratory epithelium. In vitro experiments have shown that the absence of CFTR results in increased Na^+ conductance. The interaction between CFTR and ENaC is probably regulated by cAMP, although the details are as yet uncertain. Cystic fibrosis transmembrane conductance regulator is also important in the regulation of the outwardly rectifying chloride channel, a second chloride channel found in epithelial cells. The activity of outwardly rectifying chloride channels is reduced in the presence of *CFTR* mutations. Potassium channels help regulate Cl^- transport, and their function may be disturbed by *CFTR* mutations. Finally, CFTR also interacts with Na^+/hydrogen and chloride bicarbonate exchangers in epithelial cells, but the significance of this has yet to be confirmed.

From many reports, it is established that CFTR function is not restricted to ion transport.[7] It is involved in transport of other molecules, for example, glutathione.[8,9] It plays a role in intracellular enzyme distribution, glycolipid sulfation, and thus the density of cell surface bacterial receptors. It may have prenatal effects on cell differentiation and maturity. It serves important roles in exocytosis and the formation of molecular complexes at the plasma membrane. At the cell surface, CFTR is part

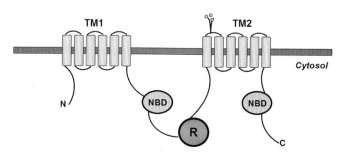

FIGURE 52.1. Diagram of the cystic fibrosis transmembrane conductance regulator. NBD, nucleotide binding domain; R, regulatory domain; TM, transmembrane domain; N, normal halve; C, C terminal halve.

of a multiprotein complex. The final three amino acids (threonine, arginine, and leucine) anchor the protein to PDZ-type of receptors in close proximity to a number of membrane receptors and cytoskeleton. Consequently, CFTR is likely to interfere with the expression of a number of gene products, including proteins of the signaling pathways of the inflammatory response.[6]

Pathophysiologic Features of Lung Disease in Cystic Fibrosis

Abnormalities of salt and fluid metabolism represent key factors of the progression of airway obstruction in the CF lung and are considered as chief contributors to morbidity and mortality of the patients.[5,6,10] Water loss increases mucous viscosity.[11,12] The levels of CFTR in airways serous glandular cells are among the highest of any cell type in the body. The submucosal glands are progressively obstructed by thick, and viscous mucus, and glandular hyperplasia is observed in submucosal regions surrounded by peribronchiolar inflammation and scar tissue. In the small airways, where surface epithelial cells also contribute to the production of mucus, the defect in Cl⁻ and fluid secretion results in decreased airway surface liquid and mucosal obstruction.[13,14] Luminal dilatation is one of the earliest changes in the lungs of young patients with CF and is the consequence of the plastering of airway surfaces by neutrophil-dominated mucopurulent debris. Desiccated secretions lead to trapping of bacteria in the lung and reduced mucociliary clearance, allowing bacterial infection to become established. Pathogens such as *Staphylococcus aureus*, *Haemophilus influenzae*, and *Pseudomonas aeruginosa* are not effectively eradicated because of the retention of mucus, which is thought to favor bacterial overgrowth and then triggers a cycle of repeated or chronic infections associated with intense neutrophilic airway inflammation. It is also suggested that altered pH leads to reduced sialysation of glycoconjugates on CF epithelial cells. Increasing numbers of asialoGM1 molecules, a receptor for many bacterial respiratory pathogens, result in an increased concentration of bacteria in the airways. In addition, pathogens such as *P. aeruginosa* specifically adapt to the pulmonary environment in the CF airways through the formation of macrocolonies (or biofilms) and the production of a capsular polysaccharide (an alginate product) that inhibits penetration by antimicrobial agents and confers the mucoid phenotype. This cascade of events is also favored by the inactivation of endogenous antimicrobial peptides, which is thought to be in part caused by altered salt concentrations in the airway surface liquid.[13,14]

A pathologic feature of lung disease in CF is the presence of an early and excessive inflammatory response.[15–17]

The sequence of events at the onset of pulmonary infection and inflammation has been addressed in a number of studies. Indeed, the origin of airway inflammation has been the subject of debate following the finding of neutrophil-dominated inflammation in the absence of bacterial or viral pathogens on bronchial lavage in some studies of CF infants.[18–20] Elevated levels of interleukin (IL)-8, IL-6, and leukotriene B4 have been found in the airways of patients with CF.[21,22] Also, an elevated ratio of arachidonic acid to docosahexaenoic acid was found in mucosal scrapings from patients with CF. Consequently, these findings have led to the proposal that inflammation, or alternatively the failure to downregulate inflammation, is intrinsic to CF and relates to the molecular defect of the disease.[23] However, in vitro and ex vivo cell cultures and model systems yield conflicting data, with results seemingly more dependent on experimental conditions than on intrinsic differences in CFTR function. It is more likely that infection and inflammation are intimately linked early in the course of CF lung disease and that infection from a few weeks of age is accompanied by a significantly increased inflammatory response, which may display some features of an altered regulation.[24] As such, bronchoalveolar lavage fluids in CF have been reported to contain low concentrations of the antiinflammatory cytokine IL-10.[25]

It is reasonable to suggest that several pathophysiologic processes result in lung disease in CF. These processes most likely influence the development of the CF phenotype in different ways and at various ages and stages of the disease. Impaired mucociliary clearance and reduced innate defenses may set the scene for early infection. Later on, abnormalities in the inflammatory response may be more critical in the progression of lung disease.

It is also not surprising that some patients have a CF-like syndrome ("variant CF") reflecting environmental and genetic influences other than mutations in *CFTR*. There have been several reports of mutations in different genes that produce similar phenotypes, including disorders with clinical features that overlap those of CF.[26,27] The diversity of CF manifestations also needs to take into account the concept that other genetic factors modify the phenotypic appearance of the disease. These modifier genes, which include genes that could affect CFTR function, innate and adopted immune response, airway inflammation, and progression of chronic lung disease, as well as genes involved in defense mechanisms against pathogens, may also modulate the phenotypic outcome.[28–33] Therefore, clinical variability in CF, within the range from classic or typical CF to nonclassic or atypical CF, is certainly linked not only to the type of *CFTR* mutations but also the influence of other non–disease-causing genes that can alter the course of CF.

Diagnosis

Cystic fibrosis is characterized by a tremendous heterogeneity in its clinical manifestations. Classic or typical CF reflects two loss-of-function mutations in the *CFTR* gene and is characterized by elevated concentrations of chloride in sweat (>60 mmol/L), chronic obstructive pulmonary disease with bacterial infection, exocrine pancreatic insufficiency, and infertility in males due to obstructive azoospermia.[34,35] Nonclassic or atypical CF includes patients with a dysfunction of at least one organ system and a normal (<30 mmol/L) or a borderline (30–60 mmol/l) chloride concentration in sweat. Most of these patients have a milder lung disease and exocrine pancreatic sufficiency.[36–38]

To cope with the diagnostic challenges, consensus about terminology and diagnosis is being proposed. Definition of CF relies on the presence of a coherent clinical syndrome plus either evidence of CFTR dysfunction (based on abnormal values for sweat chloride or nasal potential difference) or confirmation of CF-causing mutations on both alleles. Patients who have disease linked to mutant *CFTR* with residual protein function but do not meet the diagnostic criteria are considered to have CFTR-related disease.[37]

Clinical Manifestations

Clinical signs for the diagnosis of CF include pulmonary manifestations with airway obstruction and chronic productive cough, airway colonization with pathogens (*S. aureus*, *P. aeruginosa*), persistent abnormalities on chest imaging with bronchiectasis, and altered lung function with air trapping and obstructive ventilatory defect. Gastrointestinal manifestations include meconium ileus, pancreatic insufficiency, distal intestinal obstruction syndrome, rectal prolapse, pancreatitis, biliary cirrhosis, failure to thrive, and deficiency in fat-soluble vitamins. Other manifestations include nasal polyps, pansinusitis, and infertility due to obstructive azoospermia.[34,39]

Clinical tests that do not directly assess the *CFTR* defect can also aid diagnosis. Almost 90% of patients with CF have pancreatic insufficiency, and a reduced fecal concentration of pancreas-specific elastase can confirm this disorder. Bacterial pathogens typical for CF such as *P. aeruginosa* can be detected by analysis of sputum or throat swab samples.

Cystic fibrosis is nearly always a clinical diagnosis. However, in a neonatal screening program or in a sibling of a known patient, the diagnosis of CF may come before the child has shown any symptoms. Neonatal screening programs have been introduced in many countries.[40–44] They are based on the immunoreactive trypsinogen (IRT) assay, which is adaptable to large numbers of subjects.

Increased IRT concentrations at birth are observed in newborns affected by CF but can also be found in healthy children. To improve the specificity of neonatal screening, a second measurement of IRT is performed, and only infants with confirmed raised IRT values progress to a sweat test. In most screening programs, the sweat test is performed after analysis of a panel of CF-causing mutations in the neonatal blood samples.

Another situation pertinent to CF diagnosis is family history. As indicated earlier, because of the extreme clinical heterogeneity of the disease, siblings of affected CF children should be investigated, as lack of symptoms is insufficient to exclude the diagnosis of CF. The test to be performed first in this situation is the sweat test.

Function Assays

Sweat Test

Since the 1950s, demonstration of elevated sweat chloride levels has been the principal method of confirming the diagnosis of CF. The quantitative pilocarpine iontophoresis sweat test developed by Gilson and Cookes is currently the only uniformly accepted method.[45] Errors in the collection of sweat samples may affect the results, and it is important to have the test performed in an experienced laboratory. A sweat chloride level >6 mmol/L is consistent with the diagnosis of CF. Normal sweat chloride levels are <30 mmol/L. A minimum of 50 mg of sweat is required, although a quantity greater than 100 mg is preferable for accurate analysis. A positive test should be confirmed, and negative tests should be repeated if clinically indicated. The test can be performed on subjects of any age; however, it may be difficult to induce adequate sweating in infants younger than 1 month. In practice, testing can be carried out after the first 3 weeks of life in infants weighing more than 3 kg who are normally hydrated and without significant illness.

Borderline sweat chloride levels represent a difficult problem. Sweat chloride concentrations of 30–60 mmol/L are seen in about 4% of sweat tests, with 23% of these patients subsequently be found to have two *CFTR* mutations. Several studies have discussed the value of the cut-off level. Recent reports indicate that CF-affected patients occur with similar frequency in the 30–40 mmol/L range as in the 40–60 mmol/L range. Therefore, in most CF centers, a chloride cut-off level of 30 mmol/L is now used.

Transepithelial Nasal Potential Difference

Measurement of ion transport across the proximal epithelia in the nose is the most widely used test.[46] Nasal potential difference (PD) is measured between a fluid-filled exploring bridge on the nasal mucosa and a reference bridge on the skin of the forearm. The active transport of charged ions across the electrically tight respiratory epithelia results in a voltage termed potential difference. Absorption of Na^+ is the main ion transport of the airway. The basal PD gives an indication of Na^+ transport via the amiloride-sensitive epithelial Na^+ channel. The nasal PD of a patient with classic CF is remarkably different from that of controls. In this situation, Na^+ hyperabsorption and Cl^- impermeability result in a high negative baseline PD, a magnitude of voltage that falls precipitously following perfusion with a solution that blocks Na^+ absorption (amiloride) and a lack of response to solutions that stimulates Cl^- secretion. In a significant number of individuals with an equivocal sweat test, nasal PD measurement can provide useful information toward making or refuting the diagnosis of CF. However, in nonclassic CF, the nasal PD may be borderline, and there is not yet a consensus as to what exactly constitutes an abnormal result. To date, the nasal PD measurements can be used as an outcome measure in therapeutic trials.

Treatment Approaches

Current treatment approaches aim to improve airway clearance, eradicate or suppress the growth of bacterial pathogens, and attenuate airway inflammation. The constant improvement of treatment strategies since the description of the disease has considerably increased the life expectancy from approximately 6 months to 35 years. Treatment of airway infections and obstruction by antibiotics and physiotherapy, nutritional repletion, and the use of pancreatic enzymes, antiinflammatory therapy, and lung transplantation have tremendously contributed to improve quality of life and survival outcomes.[35]

Gene therapy, despite initial hopes and focused efforts of several groups worldwide, remains a challenge, as a gene therapy product with proven clinical efficacy still does not exist.[47] Consequently, a tremendous amount of work has been oriented toward a CFTR pharmacologic approach aimed at correcting the CFTR primary defects caused by CF mutations.[48] In recent years, important advances have improved our understanding of the pathophysiology of CF and the role of CFTR in lung disease. These discoveries open a new era of translational research that incorporates specific therapeutic targets and new cellular pathways. Therapies aimed at correcting specific CFTR defects are currently being investigated. For example, compounds that correct the F508del abnormality (class II mutations) have been identified by robotic drug screening. Curcumin, a nontoxic compound and the major constituent of the spice tumeric, has been shown to correct F508del protein processing in a number of in vitro model systems and prolong the lives of mice that are homozygous for this mutation.[49]

Pharmacologic correction of stop codon mutations is an important area of investigation and targets class I mutations. Aminoglycosides have been shown in vitro and in vivo to allow for the read through of stop codon mutations leading to the synthesis of an almost normal CFTR protein. The proposed mechanism is based on the alteration of a ribosomal complex involved in protein translation with misreading of the stop codon and the insertion of another amino acid with a codon similar to the termination codon. The same concept has been applied to other diseases cause by premature stop codons, such as Duchenne's muscular dystrophy.

High-throughput screening programs specifically designed to identify drugs that activate residual CFTR activity (class III and IV mutations) are also in progress. To date, a series of compounds belonging to different chemical scaffolds have been found to increase the activity of mutant CFTR. These activators are potentially useful for the development of drugs targeting CFTR channels with gating defects. Also a number of molecules based on strategies allowing identification of molecular targets important in CFTR trafficking by new tools, such as proteomics or gene silencing with siRNA libraries, will rapidly increase the list of drugs that may be of clinical interest. Consequently, in the near future, it will be critical to develop novel assays to evaluate candidate drugs for CFTR pharmacotherapy.

Conclusion

Important advances have been made in understanding the mechanisms underlying lung disease in CF, the sequelae stemming from the absence of a functional CFTR gene, and the therapeutic strategies devised to correct these abnormalities. It will soon be imperative to undertake randomized trials with young CF patients at an early stage of the disease. Translating clinical research into clinical practice is an important challenge. In the CF field, this will be achieved only by the development of an international infrastructure to assist with the recruitment and coordination of pediatric trials

Another important challenge emerging with the tremendous increased knowledge regarding CFTR gene structure and function and the introduction of neonatal screening programs is the definition and diagnosis of atypical CF and, consequently, the management of patients who do not meet the classic CF diagnostic criteria.[50,51] These patients should be considered to have CFTR-related disease and should benefit from appropriate intensive supportive treatment and follow-up.

References

1. Ratjen F, Doring G. Cystic fibrosis. Lancet 2003;361:681–689.
2. Robinson P. Cystic fibrosis. Thorax 2001;56:237–241.
3. Riordan JR, Rommens JM, Kerem B, et al. Identification of the cystic fibrosis gene: cloning and characterization of complementary DNA. Science 1989;245:1066–1073.
4. Akabas MH. Cystic fibrosis transmembrane conductance regulator. Structure and function of an epithelial chloride channel. J Biol Chem 2000;275:3729–3732.
5. McAuley DF, Elborn JS. Cystic fibrosis: basic science. Paediatr Respir Rev 2000;1:93–100.
6. Rowe SM, Miller S, Sorscher EJ. Cystic fibrosis. N Engl J Med 2005;352:1992–2001.
7. Sheppard DN, Welsh MJ. Structure and function of the CFTR chloride channel. Physiol Rev 1999;79:S23–S45.
8. Gao L, Kim KJ, Yankaskas JR, Forman HJ. Abnormal glutathione transport in cystic fibrosis airway epithelia. Am J Physiol 1999;277:L113–L118.
9. Gao L, Broughman JR, Iwamoto T, Tomich JM, et al. Synthetic chloride channel restores glutathione secretion in cystic fibrosis airway epithelia. Am J Physiol Lung Cell Mol Physiol 2001;281:L24–L30.
10. Pilewski J, Frizzell R. Role of CFTR in airway disease. Physiol Rev 1999;79:S215–S255.
11. Tarran R, Grubb BR, Parsons D, et al. The CF salt controversy: in vivo observations and therapeutic approaches. 2001;8:149–158.
12. Tarran R, Boucher RC. Thin-film measurements of airway surface liquid volume/composition and mucus transport rates in vitro. Methods Mol Med 2002;70:479–492.
13. Jayaraman S, Joo NS, Reitz B, et al. Submucosal gland secretions in airways from cystic fibrosis patients have normal [Na(+)] and pH but elevated viscosity. Proc Natl Acad Sci 2001;98:8119–8123.
14. Jayaraman S, Song Y, Vetrivel L, et al. Noninvasive in vivo fluorescence measurement of airway-surface liquid depth, salt concentration, and pH. 2001;107:317–324.
15. Aldallal N, McNaughton EE, Manzel LJ, et al. Inflammatory response in airway epithelial cells isolated from patients with cystic fibrosis. Am J Respir Crit Care Med 2002;166:1248–1256.
16. Stecenko A, King G, Torii K, et al. Dysregulated cytokine production in human cystic fibrosis bronchial epithelial cells. Inflammation 2001;25:145–155.
17. Velsor LW, van Heeckeren A, Day BJ. Antioxidant imbalance in the lungs of cystic fibrosis transmembrane conductance regulator protein mutant mice. 2001;281:L31–L38.
18. Accurso FJ. Early pulmonary disease in cystic fibrosis. Curr Opin Pulm Med 1997;3:400–403.
19. Armstrong DS, Grimwood K, Carlin JB, et al. Lower airway inflammation in infants and young children with cystic fibrosis. Am J Respir Crit Care Med 1997;156:1197–1204.
20. Khan TZ, Wagener JS, Bost T, et al. Early pulmonary inflammation in infants with cystic fibrosis. Am J Respir Crit care Med 1995;151:1075–1082.
21. Corvol H, Fitting C, Chadelat K, et al. Distinct cytokine production by lung and blood neutrophils from children with cystic fibrosis. Am J Physiol Lung Cell Mol Physiol 2003;284:L997–L1003.
22. Osika E, Cavaillon JM, Chadelat K, et al. Distinct sputum cytokine profiles in cystic fibrosis and other chronic inflammatory airway disease. Eur Respir J 1999;14:339–346.
23. Tirouvanziam R, Khazaal I, Peault B. Primary inflammation in human cystic fibrosis small airways. 2002;283:L445–L451.
24. Scheid P, Kempster L, Griesenbach U, et al. Inflammation in cystic fibrosis airways: relationship to increased bacterial adherence. Eur Respir J 2001;17:27–35.
25. Armstrong DS, Hook SM, Jamsen KM, et al. Lower airway inflammation in infants with cystic fibrosis detected by newborn screening. Pediatr Pulmonol 2005;40:500–510.
26. Kerem E, Kerem B. Genotype-phenotype correlations in cystic fibrosis. Pediatr Pulmonol 1996;22:387–395.
27. Kerem E, Kerem B. The relationship between genotype and phenotype in cystic fibrosis. Curr Opin Pulm Med 1995;1:450–456.
28. Drumm ML. Modifier genes and variation in cystic fibrosis. Respir Res 2001;2:125–128.
29. Drumm ML, Konstan MW, Schluchter MD, et al. Genetic modifiers of lung disease in cystic fibrosis. N Engl J Med 2005;353:1443–1453.
30. Flamant C, Henrion-Caude A, Boelle P, et al. Glutathione-S-transferase, M1, M3, P1, and T1 polymorphisms and severity of lung disease in children with cystic fibrosis. Pharmacogenetics 2004;14:295–301.
31. Hull J, Thomson AH. Contribution of genetic factors other than CFTR to disease severity in cystic fibrosis. Thorax 1998;53:1018–1021.
32. Salvatore F, Scudiero O, Castaldo G. Genotype–phenotype correlation in cystic fibrosis: the role of modifier genes. Am J Med Genet 2002;111:88–95.
33. Zielenski J. Genotype and phenotype in cystic fibrosis. Respiration 2000;67:117–133.
34. Davis PB, Drumm M, Konstan MW. Cystic fibrosis. 1996;154:1229–1256.
35. Bush A, Accurso F, Macnee W, et al. Cystic fibrosis, pediatrics, control of breathing, pulmonary physiology and anatomy, and surfactant biology in AJRCCM in 2004. Am J Respir Crit Care Med 2005;171:545–553.
36. Stern S. The diagnosis of cystic fibrosis. N Engl J Med 1997;336:487–491.
37. De Boeck K, Wilschanski M, Castellani C, et al. Cystic fibrosis: terminology and diagnostic algorithms. Thorax 2006;61:627–635.
38. De Braekeleer M, Allard C, Leblanc JP, et al. Genotype–phenotype correlation in cystic fibrosis patients compound heterozygous for the A455E mutation. Hum Genet 1997;101:208–211.
39. Marshall B. Pulmonary exacerbations in cystic fibrosis. Am J Respir Crit Care Med 2004;169:781–782.
40. Dezateux C. Screening newborn infants for cystic fibrosis. J Med Screen 2001;8:57–58.
41. Doull IJ, Ryley HC, Weller P, Goodchild MC. Cystic fibrosis–related deaths in infancy and the effect of newborn screening. Pediatr Pulmonol 2001;31:363–366.

42. Larsson A. Neonatal screening for metabolic, endocrine, infectious, and genetic disorders. Current and future directions. Clin Perinatol 2001;28:449–461.

43. McCormick J, Green MW, Mehta G, et al. Demographics of the UK cystic fibrosis population: implications for neonatal screening. Eur J Hum Genet 2002;10:583–590.

44. Young SS, Kharrazi M, Pearl M, Cunningham G. Cystic fibrosis screening in newborns: results from existing programs. Curr Opin Pulm Med 2001;7:427–433.

45. Baumer JH. Evidence based guidelines for the performance of the sweat test for the investigation of cystic fibrosis in the UK. Arch Dis Child 2003;88:1126–1127.

46. Wallace HL, Barker PM, Southern KW. Nasal airway ion transport and lung function in young people with cystic fibrosis. Am J Respir Crit Care Med 2003;168:594–600.

47. Griesenbach U, Geddes DM, Alton EW. Gene therapy progress and prospects: cystic fibrosis. Gene Ther 2006;13:1061–1067.

48. Verkman AS, Lukacs GL, Galietta LJ. CFTR chloride channel drug discovery—inhibitors as antidiarrheals and activators for therapy of cystic fibrosis. Curr Pharm Des 2006;12:2235–2247.

49. Jobin C, Bradhman CA, Russo Maria P, et al. Curcumin blocks cytokine-mediated NF-kB Activation and proinflammatory gene expression by inhibiting inhibitory factor I-kB kinase activity. J Immunol 1999;163:3474–3483.

50. Havermans T, De Boeck K. Cystic fibrosis: a balancing act? J Cyst Fibros 2007;6(2):161–162.

51. Knowles MR, Durie PR. What is cystic fibrosis? N Engl J Med 2002;347:439–442.

53
Pulmonary Organogenesis and Developmental Abnormalities

Timothy Craig Allen and Philip T. Cagle

Lung Organogenesis

Introduction

Lung organogenesis involves the emergence of the lung anlage from the anterior foregut, laryngeal and tracheo-esophageal morphogenesis and septation, tracheal bifurcation, patterning of the major bronchi, lobation of the lungs, branching morphogenesis of approximately 23 generations of airways, and formation of alveoli.[1] In the third week of gestation, the lung begins to develop as a ventral outpouching on the floor of the primitive foregut.[2] The lung's development may be divided into five phases: the embryonic, pseudoglandular, acinar or canalicular, saccular, and alveolar phases.[2–4] A variety of factors influence normal lung development, including normal fetal breathing movements, adequate intrathoracic space, appropriate volumes of extra- and intrapulmonary fluid, pulmonary blood flow, as well as maternal factors such as nutrition and smoking.[3] The foregut endoderm differentiates into epithelial cell types that line the developing lung and trachea, whereas lung mesenchyme originates from the lateral plate mesoderm and develops into several lung components, including connective tissue, smooth muscle surrounding airways and medium- and small-sized blood vessels, endothelial cell precursors, lymphatics, tracheal cartilage, and pleura.[5] Some authors have shown a role for blood vessels as a source of inductive signals to epithelium, but such roles have not been completely elucidated.[5–7]

Control of fetal lung development and growth is tightly orchestrated and regulated. Development of the lung occurs in three segments—specification of lung primordium via septation from the esophagus and tracheal formation, branching morphogenesis, and alveologenesis and distal epithelial cell type differentiation. On approxi-

mately embryonal day 25, epithelial cells "bud," or grow into mesenchymal cells off of the ventral foregut, and develop into the trachea and bilateral primary bronchi, giving rise to lung primordium. Branching morphogenesis describes the development of the lungs that occurs through sequential rounds of branching. The primary bronchi grow and elongate, followed by "branching," the development of secondary bronchi, which then elongate and divide to form tertiary bronchi, and so forth for approximately 22–24 generations.[1,5,8]

The first approximately 16 generations of this process of branching are highly stereotyped and under strict genetic control.[8] Such genetically controlled stereotypical development has been described as *hard wired*.[8] Branching morphogenesis is carefully organized with cell growth and differentiation, proliferation, and apoptosis in a spatially and temporally dependent manner.[1] Some of the signals and pathways mediating these events have recently been uncovered, but much remains unknown.[1–5,8] This genomically encoded, hard-wired emergence of the laryngotracheal groove and early lung branching morphogenesis is mediated by highly regulated, interactive growth factor signaling mechanisms that influence the automaticity of branching, interbranch length, stereotypy of branching, left–right asymmetry, and gas diffusion surface area.[8] The extracellular matrix is an important regulator as well as a target for growth factor signaling in both branching morphogenesis and alveologenesis.[1,8] Coordination not only of epithelial but also endothelial branching morphogenesis determines bronchial branching and the eventual alveolar–capillary interface.[1,4,8] Finally, alveologenesis occurs, beginning in the canalicular stage, with branching of distal airway saccules into immature alveoli, primitive airspace formation, and apposition of capillaries to form a potential air–blood interface for future gas exchange. Mesenchymal cells adjacent to airways undergo apoptosis, allowing formation of thin interstitial septae.[1,3]

Signaling Pathways

Several signaling pathways have thus far been identified to be involved in lung organogenesis, including Notch, transforming growth factor (TGF)-β/bone morphogenic protein 4 (BMP4), Wingless (Wnt), Sonic Hedgehog, fibroblast growth factor (FGF), and epithelial growth factor (RGF) (see Chapter 2 for detailed discussion of these pathways).[9]

Wingless Signaling Pathway

The Wnt growth family of secreted glycoproteins consists of 19 different ligands that interact with 10 known Frizzled (Fzd) receptors and two low-density-lipoprotein–related protein-5 and -6 coreceptors.[10,11] Wingless signaling controls several developmental processes, including proliferation and migration.[9,10] Wingless signaling, through both canonical and noncanonical pathways, has been found to be critical for embryonic lung development.[9–24] Canonical Wnt signaling, necessary for the regulation of branching morphogenesis and mesenchymal differentiation, has been identified throughout mouse embryonic lung development.[9,11,12] β-Catenin, a critical component of canonical Wnt signaling, localizes in the cytoplasm and sometimes the nuclei of undifferentiated primordial epithelial cells, differentiating alveolar epithelial cells, and associated mesenchymal cells.[9,13] Activation of the Wnt canonical pathway results in β-catenin nuclear localization and its interactions with transcription factors of the T-cell factor/lymphoid enhancer-binding factor family that regulate target gene transcription.[10,14] Other studies have identified Wnt2 expression predominantly within mesenchyme, Wnt7b expression exclusively in lung epithelium, and Wnt11 and Wnt5a expression within both epithelium and mesenchyme.[9,11,16–19] The noncanonical pathway involves activation of c-Jun kinase or regulation of calcium flux.[11,16]

Sonic Hedgehog

Sonic Hedgehog (Shh) is one of several factors derived from lung endoderm that is critical for lung epithelial branching morphogenesis and peribronchial smooth muscle development.[10,11,25–35] Sonic Hedgehog, the mammalian ortholog of *Drosophila* hedgehog, is highly expressed in lung epithelium.[10,27] Sonic Hedgehog signaling occurs with the binding of Shh to its receptor, Patched, resulting in the loss of Patched-mediated inhibition of Smoothened protein, which in turn causes transduction of Shh signaling to the Gli proteins, which translocate into the nucleus and bind Shh-responsive elements.[10,11,25,26,28] Sonic Hedgehog is important for normal peribronchial smooth muscle development as well as for branching morphogenesis.[11] It has also been proposed that Shh may be important in lung stem cell maintenance, given the findings of increased cell proliferation and changes of cellular differentiation caused by Shh overexpression.[10,35] Transient Shh activation has been identified in adult lung airway epithelium during repopulation of injured airways after acute proximal injury, suggesting that Shh activation might drive epithelial cell proliferation during lung epithelial repair.[10]

Fibroblast Growth Factor

Fibroblast growth factor-10 has been found to be a signaling pathway critical for normal lung branching morphogenesis.[11,27,36–43] Fibroblast growth factor signaling is required at specific times during lung organogenesis for normal peripheral lung formation.[25,39,40] Other FGF family members, including FGF-1, FGF-7, and FGF-18, are expressed in lung organogenesis.[25] Targeted deletion of FGF-9 has been found to cause lung hypoplasia in mice.[25,42]

Notch

Notch is a transmembrane signaling protein initially identified for its involvement in *Drosophila* neurogenesis, and complete loss of Notch causes massive neuronal hyperplasia.[44] Notch-1, Notch-2, and Notch-3 are members of the Notch family, and Notch ligands include Jagged-1 and Jagged-2.[44]

Epithelial Growth Factor

Epithelial growth factor (EGF) is involved in regulating the growth and development of fetal lung.[45] It induces gender-specific and development-specific changes in fetal lung surfactant synthesis (see Chapter 54).[45] Villanueva et al., studying fetal rabbit lung culture cells, found that EGF affected the expression of EGF receptor on EGF-specific binding in fetal lung.[45]

Transforming Growth Factor-β/Bone Morphogenic Protein 4

Bone morphogenic protein 4, a member of the TGF-β family, is induced in epithelial cells in the distal epithelial tips as a response to FGF-10 in the mesenchyme.[11,27,38,46] This protein is expressed in lung mesenchyme also, with its highest expression adjacent to proximal epithelium.[11] Bone morphogenic protein 4 is also expressed in peribronchial smooth muscle cells.[11,38] Its receptors are identified throughout lung epithelium, including distal mesenchyme, suggesting that the BMP-4 signaling pathways relevant to lung development are found in the distal mesenchyme and proximal epithelium.[11]

Branching

Canonical Wnt signaling represses lung branching morphogenesis.[11] Using cultured lung explants, Dean et al. found that depletion of β-catenin in both epithelium and mesenchyme increased mesenchymal FGF-10 expression and increased branching morphogenesis.[11,21] De Langhe et al., however, studying lung explants, found that Wnt signaling inhibition impaired branching morphogenesis, including failed cleft formation and reduced parabronchial smooth muscle differentiation.[11,22] These discrepant findings underscore the complex nature of Wnt signaling pathways in lung organogenesis.[11]

Sonic Hedgehog is secreted by epithelial cells in embryonic lung buds.[25] Clinical syndromes that include pulmonary malformations, such as Pallister-Hall syndrome, VACTERL, and Smith-Lemli-Opitz syndrome, have been linked to Shh signaling pathways.[25,29,30] Mice with a targeted *SHH* gene null mutation have hypoplastic lungs with impaired branching.[11] Diffuse FGF-10 expression hinders directed lung epithelial cell growth, and loss of *SHH*, with resultant delocalized FGF-10 expression, may be the cause of impaired branching morphogenesis in *SHH* null lungs.[11] Mice research has emphasized the importance of FGF-10 in initiating airway branching, demonstrating that null mutations of FGF-10 and misexpression of a dominant negative FGF receptor prevent airway branching distal to the trachea.[11,37] Deletion of FGF-R2IIIb or inhibition of FGF signaling via Sprouty expression, an intracellular FGF signaling inhibitor, or via FGF mutant receptors inhibiting receptor signaling blocks lung branching morphogenesis.[25,39,40] Retinoic acid downregulates expression of FGF-10 and inhibits lung epithelial branching morphogenesis via a mechanism of action not presently understood.[11,43]

Examining mouse fetal lung, Kong et al. identified Notch-1, Notch-2, Notch-3, Jagged-1, and Jagged-2 expression in embryonic mouse lung and identified increased branching morphogenesis in lung buds cultured with antisense to Notch-1, increased neuroendocrine cell differentiation with Notch-1 and Jagged-1 antisense, and increased neural tissue with Notch-3 antisense.[44] The authors concluded that Notch-1 plays a role in the regulation of branching in developing lung.[44] The authors speculated that Notch signaling effects might be mediated by altered cell adhesion to other cells or to extracellular matrix components or to altered cell motility.[44] The authors noted that the absence of changes in cell proliferation or apoptosis suggests that altered cell adhesion or migration

is the mechanism for altered branching with Notch family antisense oligonucleotides.[44] Although the role of BMP-4 is not well-defined, Shannon and Hyatt propose that BMP-4 helps regulate epithelial proliferation and proximal–distal patterning in lung epithelium.[11,46] Bone morphogenic protein 4 may regulate lung branching by induction of peribronchial smooth muscle cell differentiation.[11,46]

Airway

Wingless plays a role in lymphoid enhancer-binding factor-1 expression in submucosal gland buds, potential stem cells for submucosal gland, and airway surface epithelium regeneration, suggesting that the Wnt/β-catenin pathway may play a role in stem cell maintenance of airway epithelium.[10,23,24]

Peripheral Airway

Mucenski et al. have shown β-catenin to be important for peripheral airway formation but dispensable for proximal airway formation.[9,15]

Alveoli

Thyroid transcription factor-1 (TTF-1), essential for lung epithelium differentiation, was shown by Minoo et al. to regulate Wnt7b promoter activity, and *TTF-1* null mice were found to have a lethal lung phenotype with increased mesenchymal and epithelial proliferation without functional alveoli.[9,20] These findings suggest that dysregulated Wnt7b signaling leads to the absence of functional alveoli.[9,19]

Mesenchyme

Investigators propose that Shh is a negative feedback signal downregulating FGF-10 expression in lung mesenchyme.[11,27,31,32] Sonic Hedgehog overexpression in distal lung epithelium causes increased epithelial cell and mesenchymal cell proliferation and reduced expression of FGF-10, whereas loss of expression of Shh causes lung hypoplasia along with increased cell death, decreased mesenchymal proliferation, and ectopic FGF-10 expression in both proximal and distal mesenchyme.[11,33] As Shh expression is high at the distal epithelial tips where mesenchymal FGF-10 expression occurs, Shh expression may not correlate with Shh activity.[11] Authors propose that Shh activity may depend on a balance among Shh modulators, including hedgehog interacting protein and Patched; alternatively, Shh activity might be spatially restricted so that Shh expression in the distal epithelial tips only represses FGF-10 expression in the immediately adjacent lung mesenchyme.[11,34]

The identification of delocalized FGF-10 expression and the absence of peribronchial smooth muscle in Shh null lungs suggests that peribronchial smooth muscle cells may mediate FGF-10 expression inhibition by Shh.[11] Such a possibility could explain the association of high Shh expression in the distal epithelial tips along with high FGF-10 expression in adjacent lung mesenchyme.[11] Fibroblast growth factor-10 may function by promoting growth of distal epithelial buds toward it, as FGF-10 expression is localized to distal lung mesenchyme surrounding the tip of extending epithelial buds.[11] Fibroblast growth factor-10 receptors are identified throughout lung epithelium, and studies suggest that proximal as well as distal lung epithelial cells have the capacity to respond to FGF-10.[11] Signals arising from proximal lung mesenchyme have been considered as possible suppressors of proximal FGF-10 function.[11] Fibroblast growth factor-10 also plays a role in regulating development of peribronchial smooth muscle.[11,41]

Vascular Factors

It is important to remember that the pulmonary circulation involves duel blood supplies from both bronchial and pulmonary arteries. The pulmonary arteries arise from the right ventricle and divide into left and right mainstem pulmonary arteries, further dividing into lobar arteries, and upon entering the lung follow and divide with bronchi and bronchioles. The bronchial artery typically arises near the descending portion of the aortic arch and follows and nourishes the bronchial tree to the level of the respiratory bronchiole. Within the periphery a capillary network is established early, which most probably is stepwise connected to the central arterial branches as the bronchial buds are developed.

To ensure optimal gas exchange, vascularization must precisely match epithelial morphogenesis.[8] A variety of vascular epithelial growth factor (VEGF) isoforms are expressed in the developing lung epithelium, whereas their cognate receptors are expressed in, and direct the emergence of, developing vascular and lymphatic capillary networks within the mesenchyme.[8] Vascular epithelial growth factor signaling may possibly occur downstream of FGF signaling, as in vivo abrogation of FGF signaling severely affects both epithelial and endothelial morphogenesis.[8] When the lung buds evaginate from the foregut, vasculogenesis begins.[8] Vascular epithelial growth factor is critical for branching morphogenesis, and the loss of even a single VEGF allele causes embryonic lethality in mice.[8] Vascular epithelial growth factor is diffusely dis-tributed in pulmonary epithelial and mesenchymal cells and is important for controlling endothelial proliferation and vascular structure maintenance.[8]

Vascular epithelial growth factor-120, VEGF-164, and VEGF-188 are expressed in mice during development, and the VEGF-164 isoform is most highly expressed and active during embryogenesis. Vascular epithelial growth factor signals through the cognate receptors fetal liver kinase-1 (FLK-1 or VEGFR2) and fetal liver tyrosinase-1 (FLT-1 or VEGFR1).[8] Vascular epithelial growth factor signaling is critical for embryonic mesenchymal cell differentiation into endothelial cells.[8] Epithelial and mesenchymal cell interactions contribute to lung neo-vascularization, crucial in normal lung formation, and epithelial cells in the airways are positive for VEGF, especially at the budding regions of the distal airway.[8] Vascular epithelial growth factor–misexpressing trans-genic mice, with the *Vegf* transgene under the control of the *surfactant protein C (SP-C)* promoter, show gross abnormalities in lung morphogenesis associated with a decrease in acinar tubules and mesenchyme.[8] VEGF-treated human lung explant tissue shows an increase in distal airway epithelial cell proliferation with up-regulation of the mRNA expression of surfactant protein A (SP-A) and C (SP-C) but not SP-B.[8] Vascular epithelial growth factor also helps maintain alveolar structure.[8] Lungs from newborn mice treated with antibodies to FLT-1 are reduced in size and display significant immaturity with a less complex alveolar pattern, whereas VEGF accumulation in the alveoli makes *Vegf* trans-genic mice more resistant to hypoxic injury.[8] Vascular epithelial growth factor is a target of hypoxia-inducible transcription factor (HIF)-2α, and HIF-2α–deficient newborn mice die from respiratory distress syndrome.[8] Vascular epithelial growth factor expression in *HIF-2α* null mice is greatly reduced in alveolar epithelial type 2 cells.[8] Furthermore, VEGF signaling may be required for matching the epithelial–capillary interface during lung morphogenesis.[8]

Specific Genes and Developmental Abnormalities

Several pathways have been discussed that are involved in lung organogenesis and are likely involved in developmental abnormalities. A summary of specific genes associated with specific syndromes and pulmonary developmental abnormalities is provided in Table 53.1.[25] Surfactant abnormalities are discussed in Chapter 54. Other specific inherited lung diseases, such as α$_1$-antitrypsin deficiency (Chapter 50) and cystic fibrosis (Chapter 52), are discussed in their respective chapters.

TABLE 53.1. Pathways and genes associated with specific pulmonary developmental abnormalities.

Pathway	Gene	Syndrome	Findings
Signaling			
Shh	*SHH/Gli*	Pallister–Hall, VACTERL	Tracheoesophageal (TE) fistula, tracheal malformations
	DHCR7	Smith-Lemli-Opitz	Pulmonary hypoplasia
Fibroblast growth factor (FGF) signaling	FGF receptors	Apert, Pfeiffer, Crouzon, Carpenter	Tracheal cartilage abnormalities, pulmonary hyperplasia
Transcription factors			
	RARα/β	Mouse	Lung agenesis, hypoplasia
	TTF-1	Pulmonary hypoplasia/dysplasia; human and mouse	TE fistula Hypothyroidism, chorea, pulmonary dysfunction
	Hox-b5	Human	Bronchopulmonary sequestration
	Lfty-1/Gdf-1 Nodal	Left–right symmetry; mouse	Disruption of left–right lobulation
	Foxj1	Mouse	Absent cilia and situs inversus

Source: Adapted from Whitsett et al.,[25] with permission of Oxford University Press.

Conclusion

Continuing investigation into the molecular genetics of lung organogenesis might provide therapeutic targets for treatment of abnormalities of lung morphogenesis, possibly via the activation of systemic or pulmonary stem cells.[1,27] As well, such continuing research will provide increased knowledge of the molecular genetics of lung repair and neoplasia.

References

1. Warburton D, Belusci S. The molecular genetics of lung morphogenesis and injury repair. Pediatr Respir Rev 2004; 5(Suppl A):S283–S287.
2. Mendeloff EN. Sequestrations, congenital cystic adenomatoid malformations, and congenital lobar emphysema. Semin Thorac Cardiovasc Surg 2004;16:209–214.
3. Kotecha S. Lung growth for beginners. Pediatr Resp Rev 2000;1:308–313.
4. Barnes NA, Pilling DW. Bronchopulmonary foregut malformations: embryology, radiology and quandary. Eur Radiol 2003;13:2659–2673.
5. Cardoso WV, Lu J. Regulation of early lung morphogenesis: questions, facts and controversies. Development 2006; 1611–1624.
6. Lammert E, Cleaver O, Melton D. Induction of pancreatic differentiation by signals from blood vessels. Science 2001; 294:564–567.
7. Matsumoto K, Yoshitomi H, Rossant J, Zaret KS. Liver organogenesis promoted by endothelial cells prior to vascular function. Science 2001;294:559–563.
8. Warburton D, Bellusci S, De Langhe S, et al. Molecular mechanisms of early lung specification and branching morphogenesis. Pediatr Res 2005;57:26R–37R.
9. Pongracz JE, Stockley RA. Wnt signaling in lung development and diseases. Respir Res 2006;26:15.
10. Borok Z, Li C, Liebler J, et al. Developmental pathways and specification of intrapulmonary stem cells. Pediatr Res 2006;59:84R–93R.
11. Kim N, Vu TH. Parabronchial smooth muscle cells and alveolar myofibroblasts in lung development. Birth Defects Res (Part C) 2006;78:80–89.
12. Okubo T, Hogan BLM. Hyperactive Wnt signaling changes the developmental potential of embryonic lung endoderm. J Biol 2004;3:11.
13. Tebar M, Destree O, de Vree WJ, et al. Expression of Tcf/Lef and sFrp and localization of beta-catenin in the developing mouse lung. Mech Dev 2001;109:437–440.
14. Duan D, Yue Y, Zhou W, et al. Submucosal gland development in the airway is controlled by lymphoid enhancer binding factor 1 (LEF1). Development 1999;126:4441–4453.
15. Mucenski ML, Wert SE, Nation JM, et al. Beta-catenin is required for specification of proximal/distal cell fate during lung morphogenesis. J Biol Chem 2003;278:40231–40238.
16. Wang Z, Shu W, Lu MM, et al. Wnt7b activates canonical signaling in epithelial and vascular smooth muscle cells through interactions with Fzd1, Fzd10, and LRPS. Mol Cell Biol 2005;25(12):5022–5030.
17. Monkley SJ, Delaney SJ, Pennisi DJ, et al. Targeted disruption of the Wnt2 gene results in placentation defects. Development 1996;122:3343–3353.
18. Lako M, Strachan T, Bullen P, et al. Isolation, characterization and embryonic expression of WNTII, a gene which maps to IIq13.5 and has possible roles in the development of skeleton, kidney and lung. Gene 1998;219:101–110.
19. Weidenfeld J, Shu W, Zhang I, et al. The Wnt7b promoter is regulated by TTF-1, GATA6, and Foxa2 in lung epithelium. J Biol Chem 2002;277:21061–21070.
20. Minoo P, Hamdan H, Bu D, et al. TTF-1 regulates lung epithelial morphogenesis. Dev Biol 1995;172:694–68.
21. Dean CH, Miller LA, Smith AN, et al. Canonical Wnt signaling negatively regulates branching morphogenesis of the lung and lacrimal gland. Dev Biol 2005;286:270–286.

22. De Langhe SP, Sala FG, Del Moral PM, et al. Dickkopf-1 (DKK-1) reveals that fibronectin is a major target of Wnt signaling in branching morphogenesis of the mouse embryonic lung. Dev Biol 2005;277:316–331.

23. Driskell RR, Liu X, Luo M, et al. Wnt-responsive element controls Lef-1 promoter expression during submucosal gland morphogenesis. Am J Physiol Lung Cell Mol Physiol 2004;287:L752–L763.

24. Filali M, Cheng N, Abbott D, et al. Wnt-3A/beta-catenin signaling induces transcription from the LEF-1 promoter. J Biol Chem 2002;277:33398–33410.

25. Whitsett JA, Wert SE, Trapnell BC. Genetic disorders influencing lung formation and function at birth. Hum Mol Genet 2004;13:R207–R215.

26. Li Y, Zhang H, Choi SC, et al. Sonic hedgehog signaling regulates Gli3 processing, mesenchymal proliferation, and differentiation during mouse lung organogenesis. Dev Biol 2004;270:214–231.

27. Bellusci S, Furuta Y, Rush MG, et al. Involvement of Sonic hedgehog (Shh) in mouse embryonic lung growth and morphogenesis. Development 1997;124:53–63.

28. McMahon AP. More surprises in the Hedgehog signaling pathway. Cell 2000;100:185–188.

29. Okdak M, Grzela T, Lazarczyk M, et al. Clinical aspects of disrupted hedgehog signaling. Int J Mol Med 2001;8: 445–452.

30. Ming JE, Roessler E, Muenke M. Human developmental disorders and the sonic hedgehog pathway. Mol Med Today 1998;4:343–349.

31. Bitgood MJ, McMahon AP. Hedgehog and Bmp genes are coexpressed at many diverse sites of cell–cell interaction in the mouse embryo. Dev Biol 1995;172:126–138.

32. Urase K, Mukasa T, Igarashi H, et al. Spatial expression of Sonic hedgehog in the lung epithelium during branching morphogenesis. Biochem Biophys Res Commun 1996; 225:161–166.

33. Pepicelli CV, Lewis PM, McMahon AP. Sonic hedgehog regulates branching morphogenesis in mammalian lung. Curr Biol 1998;8:1083–1086.

34. Chuang PT, McMahon AP. Branching morphogenesis of the lung: new molecular insights into an old problem. Trends Cell Biol 2003;13:86–91.

35. Watkins DN, Berman DM, Burkholder SG, et al. Hedgehog signaling within airway epithelial progenitors and in small-cell lung cancer. Nature 2003;422:313–317.

36. Min H, Danilenko DM, Scully SA, et al. Fgf-10 is required for both limb and lung development and exhibits striking functional similarity to Drosophila branchless. Genes Dev 1998;12:3156–3161.

37. Sekine K, Ohuchi H, Fujiwara M, et al. Fgf10 is essential for limb and lung formation. Nat Genet 1999;21:138–141.

38. Weaver M, Dunn NR, Hogan BL. Bmp4 and Fgf10 play opposing roles during lung bud morphogenesis. Development 2000;127:2695–2704.

39. Perl AK, Hokuto I, Impagnatiello MA, et al. Temporal effects of sprouty on lung morphogenesis. Dev Biol 2003;258:154–168.

40. Hokuto I, Perl AK, Whitsett JA. Prenatal, but not postnatal, inhibition of fibroblast growth factor receptor signaling causes emphysema. J Biol Chem 2003;278:415–421.

41. Mailleux AA, Kelly R, Veltmaat JM, et al. Fgf10 expression identifies parabronchial smooth muscle cell progenitors and is required for their entry into the smooth muscle cell lineage. Development 2005;132:2157–2166.

42. Colvin JS, White AC, Pratt SJ, et al. Lung hypoplasia and neonatal death in Fgf9-null mice identify this gene as an essential regulator of lung mesenchyme. Development 2001;128:2095–2106.

43. Mendelsohn C, Lohnes D, Decimo D, et al. Function of the retinoic acid receptors (RARs) during development (II). Multiple abnormalities at various stages of organogenesis in RAR double mutants. Development 1994;120:2749–2771.

44. Kong V, Glickman J, Subramaniam M, et al. Functional diversity of notch family genes in fetal lung development. Am J Physiol Lung Cell Mol Physiol 2004;286:L1075–L1083.

45. Villanueva D, McCants D, Nielsen HC. Effects of epidermal growth factor (EGF) on the development of EGF-receptor (EGF-R) binding in fetal rabbit lung organ culture. Pediatr Pulmonol 2000;29:27–33.

46. Shannon JM, Hyatt BA. Epithelial–mesenchymal interactions in the developing lung. Annu Rev Physiol 2004;66: 625–645.

54
Genetic Abnormalities of Surfactant Metabolism

Lawrence M. Nogee and Susan E. Wert

Introduction

Pulmonary surfactant is the complex mixture of lipids and proteins needed to reduce alveolar surface tension at the air–liquid interface and prevent alveolar collapse at the end of expiration. It has been recognized for almost 50 years that a deficiency in surfactant production due to pulmonary immaturity is the principal cause of the respiratory distress syndrome (RDS) observed in prematurely born infants.[1] Secondary surfactant deficiency due to injury to the cells involved in its production and functional inactivation of surfactant is also important in the pathophysiology of acute respiratory distress syndrome (ARDS) observed in older children and adults.[2,3] In the past 15 years, it has been recognized that surfactant deficiency may result from genetic mechanisms involving mutations in genes encoding critical components of the surfactant system or proteins involved in surfactant metabolism.[4,5] Although rare, these single gene disorders provide important insights into normal surfactant metabolism and into the genes in which frequently occurring allelic variants may be important in more common pulmonary diseases.

Overview of Pulmonary Surfactant

Pulmonary surfactant is synthesized, stored, and secreted by alveolar type II cells. Alveolar type II cells contain a specialized, lysosomally derived organelle, the lamellar body, in which surfactant lipids and proteins are stored.[6] Surfactant phospholipids, particularly disaturated or dipalmitoyl phosphatidylcholine, are critical for its ability to effectively lower alveolar surface tension.[7] A large number of enzymes are involved in surfactant lipid synthesis, but in general these enzymes are found in many tissues and are not specific for type II cells. Only a few, such as fatty acid synthase and CTP:phosphocholine cytidylyltransferase (CCTα), the rate-limiting enzyme in PC synthesis, are developmentally regulated.[8–11] In contrast, member A3 of the adenosine triphosphate (ATP) binding cassette family of proteins (ABCA3) is highly expressed in type II cells, where it is localized to the limiting membrane of the lamellar body, and appears to have an essential role in lamellar body biogenesis and likely in surfactant lipid metabolism.[12,13] Surfactant is secreted by exocytosis of the lamellar body contents, where it unravels into an intermediate known as tubular myelin before adsorbing to the air–liquid interface. Surfactant lipids and proteins are both recycled by the type II cell through an endocytic pathway, as well as being catabolized by alveolar macrophages, which are dependent on granulocyte-macrophage colony stimulating factor (GM-CSF) for their appropriate maturation.

About 10% of mammalian surfactants by weight is composed of protein, and, while the majority of protein in surfactant is derived from serum, specific proteins found primarily or largely in surfactant have been identified that have important roles in its function and metabolism. Surfactant proteins A and D (SP-A, SP-D) are hydrophilic proteins that are part of the collectin family, having both a collagenous domain and a carbohydrate binding or lectin domain. In their native forms in the airspaces, both are composed of high-order multimers. Both are encoded on chromosome 10, with two genes (*SFTPA1, SFTPA2*) contributing to the SP-A protein and a single gene (*SFTPD*) for SP-D.[14] The principal roles for SP-A and SP-D appear to be in innate immunity and regulation of local pulmonary inflammation.[15,16] Although both are highly expressed in the lung, SP-A and, even more so, SP-D are also expressed in extrapulmonary tissues.[17–21] Multiple allelic variants of *SFTPA1*, *SFTPA2*, and *SFTPD* that alter their encoded protein sequences have been identified, and genetic association studies have linked certain *SFTPA* and *SFPTD* alleles to susceptibility to a variety of pulmonary diseases, ranging from RDS in premature newborns and viral infection in children to chronic obstructive pulmonary disease and lung cancer in adults.[22–28] However, the functional significance of these variants is uncertain. Currently, no human diseases due to genetic mechanisms disrupting either SP-A or SP-D production or structure have been reported. It may be that deficiencies of these two proteins do not result in human lung disease or that the phenotype associated with deficiencies of these proteins has not yet been determined. Mice genetically engineered to be deficient in SP-A have been generated, and, although more susceptible to a number of different pathogens, they do not have respiratory distress at birth or spontaneously develop lung disease with age.[29–34] Moreover, as there are two SP-A genes, complete deficiency of SP-A will likely have to result from a major deletion involving their loci. In contrast, SP-D null mice develop a pulmonary lipoidosis and emphysema with age, and thus SP-D remains a candidate gene for pulmonary disease.[35–37] As both SP-A and SP-D contain collagenous domains and form higher order multimers in the airway, it is possible that mutations introducing structural changes in the collagenous domains or elsewhere could prevent oligomerization and thus result in deficiency of SP-A or SP-D by a dominant negative mechanism.

Surfactant proteins B and C (SP-B, SP-C) are small, hydrophobic proteins that have essential roles in surfactant's ability to lower surface tension. Both SP-B and SP-C when combined with surfactant lipids yield a surfactant that effectively lowers surface tension in vitro and is effective in treating animal models of RDS. Both are found in varying amounts in mammalian derived exogenous surfactant preparations used clinically to treat human infants with RDS.[38,39] Abnormalities in both SP-B and SP-C expression and structure due to mutations in the genes encoding these proteins have been associated with acute and chronic human lung disease and are discussed in more detail later. While regulation of expression of both SP-B and SP-C is distinct, both are increased with glucocorticoids.[40–42] The promoter regions of both genes have been extensively studied, and numerous transcription factors are involved in their expression as well as that of other key components of the surfactant system, with thyroid transcription factor 1 (TTF-1, also known as Nkx2.1), forkhead box A2 (Foxa2), and CCAAT/enhancer binding protein α (C/EBPα) of particular importance in determining tissue specificity and developmentally regulated expression.[43–51] Selective inactivation of these transcription factors in the distal respiratory epithelium of experimental animals results in perinatal lethality with decreased production of surfactant proteins and lipids.

Respiratory Distress Syndrome

The primary lung disease related to surfactant is RDS caused by deficient production of surfactant due to pulmonary immaturity. The primary pathologic changes observed in the lungs of infants dying from RDS are diffuse atelectasis and the formation of hyaline membranes lining small airways. Although a great deal of effort initially focused on the role of the hyaline membranes in the pathophysiology of RDS, the seminal observations of Avery and Mead in 1959 demonstrated the functional absence of surfactant and its ability to lower surface tension as the primary cause of the disease.[1,52]

Respiratory distress syndrome results not from the selective production of one surfactant component but from global decreases in surfactant lipid and protein production. Immature type II cells do not contain well-developed lamellar bodies but are instead rich in glycogen, which disappears as lamellar bodies appear.[8,53] The expression of SP-A, SP-B, and SP-C, as well as other proteins involved in surfactant lipid production and homeostasis such as ABCA3, fatty acid synthase, and CCTα, are developmentally regulated, with their expression increasing with advancing gestation.[11,12,54–61] Decreased expression of SP-A and SP-B has been observed in lung tissue from newborns that died from RDS compared with controls.[62] Measurements of surfactant lipids in amniotic fluid, including PC (also known as lecithin), disaturated phosphatidylcholine, and phosphatidylglycerol (PG), as well as assessments of lamellar body counts, can be used to predict maturity of the surfactant system in the fetus. Clinical testing for fetal lung maturity introduced in the 1970s resulted in a reduction in iatrogenic RDS.[63,64]

Along with technical advances in neonatal mechanical ventilation, RDS is now very effectively treated with exogenous surfactant preparations that have substantially reduced mortality from RDS in premature infants.[65–67] Respiratory distress syndrome is principally a disease of premature infants, with the risk for RDS primarily dependent on gestational age, although it may also be observed in full-term or near-term infants. As many more infants are born at >35 weeks, RDS in larger infants represents a considerable cause of neonatal morbidity, although mortality in such infants is low.[68,69] With the effectiveness of modern therapies for RDS in reducing mortality, the phenotype of severe RDS unresponsive to current treatment strategies is one that suggests another etiology for lung disease, particularly a genetic or developmental mechanism disrupting lung development or impairing surfactant metabolism.

Surfactant Protein B

Surfactant protein B is encoded by a single gene (called *SFTPB*) located on the short arm of chromosome 2, spanning approximately 10 kb.[70,71] The gene contains 11 exons, of which the last is untranslated. The gene is transcribed into an approximate 2 kb mRNA, which is translated into a 381 amino acid preproprotein.[72] After cotranslational cleavage of a signal peptide, the proprotein (pro-SP-B) undergoes several proteolytic processing steps at both the amino- and carboxy-terminal ends to yield the 79 amino acid mature SP-B protein that is secreted into the airspaces. Proprotein SP-B has homology to the saposins, proteins that bind to and interact with a number of lipids, and contains three saposin domains. Mature SP-B is encoded in exons 6 and 7 of the gene, which corresponds to the middle domain.[73,74] Proprotein SP-B contains one potential site for N-linked glycosylation in the carboxy-terminal domain and a possible second site in the amino-terminal domain depending on which variant of a commonly occurring single nucleotide polymorphism (SNP) is present in codon 131.[75] Alternative splicing at the beginning of exon 8 yields a small percentage of transcripts lacking four amino acids from the carboxy-terminal domain. The functional consequences of this alternative splicing are unknown, although this transcript may be overrepresented in RNA from diseased lung tissues.[76] Surfactant protein B is expressed in both non-ciliated bronchiolar epithelium in the lung and alveolar type II epithelial cells, although only alveolar type II cells fully process pro-SP-B to mature SP-B.[60,77] Hereditary SP-B deficiency was the first recognized inborn error of surfactant metabolism, with the first report in 1993.[78] The index patient was a full-term infant with diffuse lung disease clinically and radiographically suggestive of surfactant deficiency. Unlike premature infants with surfactant deficiency, who generally improve toward the end of the first week of life, this child had persistent hypoxemic respiratory failure and eventually died at age 5 months. The family history was notable for a previous child born to the same parents who also died from neonatal lung disease. Lung biopsy findings included changes similar to those of alveolar proteinosis in adults, with distal airspaces filled with granular eosinophilic material. This pathology had also been observed rarely in newborns with clinically similar lung disease, often with a positive family history.[79,80] A selective absence of SP-B in lung tissue from this infant was demonstrated by immunologic assays, and SP-B deficiency was established as the basis for the lung disease with the demonstration of a frame shift mutation that precluded SP-B production on both SP-B alleles in affected infants.[81]

Surfactant protein B deficiency is an extremely rare disorder. Approximately 50 cases have been reported in the literature, and extrapolations from estimates of the population frequency of the most frequently encountered *SFTPB* mutation yields an expected disease incidence of about 1 in 1 million live births in the United States.[82–84] Although the disease is almost always fatal, affected infants can survive for months with aggressive support, and it is thus important to establish the diagnosis so as to avoid futile therapy or provide timely referral for lung transplantation, as well as for proper counseling regarding recurrence risk.

Over 40 different mutations in *SFTPB* have been identified. The first identified mutation consists of a substitution of GAA for C in codon 121 of the SP-B mRNA and has been termed 121ins2.[81] This mutation has accounted for 60%–70% of the mutant alleles in patients of Northern European descent, and the finding of a common mutation likely is the result of a common ancestral origin or "founder" effect.[85] Other mutations have been found in more than one unrelated family in specific ethnic groups. Although some mutations allow for the production of pro-SP-B, processing to mature SP-B is impaired such that all known mutations lead to an absence or severe reduction in the amount of mature SP-B and can thus be viewed as loss-of-function mutations.[86] The disease is inherited as an autosomal recessive condition, with mutations needed on both alleles to manifest disease.

The usual clinical presentation is that of a full-term infant without risk factors for lung disease or infection who presents with symptoms of respiratory distress, hypoxemia, and diffuse, homogenous infiltrates on chest radiographs. Although many of the initial reports of infants with this condition involved children with very severe lung disease who often required extracorporeal membrane oxygenation for support, it is clear that some affected infants may have milder disease initially and may not require mechanical ventilation for days to weeks.[87,88] The disease is progressive, and the diagnosis should thus be considered in full-term infants with a history of neonatal lung disease that is progressive after the first week of life, especially if there is a family history of neonatal lung disease.

The pathophysiology of the lung disease due to SP-B deficiency is incompletely understood. Certainly the lack of mature SP-B could contribute to poorly functioning surfactant and thus accounts for some of the initial clinical symptoms consistent with severe surfactant deficiency. In addition, deficiency of SP-B results in a block in processing of pro-SP-C to mature SP-C. This results in both deficiency of mature SP-C as well as an accumulation of partially processed SP-C-related peptides that are secreted into the airspaces but are not very surface-active and contribute to the pathophysiology of the lung injury.[89,90] Type II cells in SP-B-deficient lung do not contain normally form lamellar bodies, indicating a fundamental intracellular role for SP-B or pro-SP-B, and the lack of normal lamellar bodies may explain the impaired processing of pro-SP-C, as the final processing steps for pro-SP-C take place in a distal cellular compartment.[6,91,92]

Genetically engineered SP-B knockout mice have been generated and have a phenotype that recapitulates the human disease, with homozygous null mice dying at birth from respiratory failure.[93] The lung pathology of mice dying in the neonatal period is notable principally for atelectasis and does not have many of the histopathology features observed in lung tissue from human infants with SP-B deficiency (described in detail later). Potential reasons for the differences in histopathology findings include the inherent variations between species, the fact that some changes may take time to develop after birth or are a result of the treatments used to sustain life in human infants with SP-B deficiency, or some combination of these factors. Homozygous SP-B null mice are completely lacking in mature SP-B protein and also have abnormal lamellar bodies and aberrant processing of pro-SP-C to SP-C, indicating that these are due to the primary deficiency of SP-B and are not secondary to other post-natal factors.[94]

Mice that conditionally express SP-B under the control of a tetracycline responsive promoter have also been generated and bred with knockout mice in order to generate animals that can survive the neonatal period and then have SP-B production shut off when the antibiotic is removed from their diet. These animals develop lung disease when SP-B levels fall below 20%–25% of the levels in control mice, indicating that there is a critical level of SP-B needed for proper lung function.[95] This concept is supported by the observation that human patients with SP-B mutations allowing for some SP-B production survive longer than those with null mutations.[87,88] Mice heterozygous for one SP-B null allele survive and have only mild abnormalities in lung function but are more susceptible to pulmonary oxygen toxicity.[96,97] Genetic control of SP-B levels could thus be an important determinant of risk for lung disease, with individuals who have a lower capacity for SP-B production being at risk for lung disease should additional environmental factors (premature birth, inflammation) further reduce SP-B levels.

Multiple polymorphic variants have been identified within the SFTPB locus, including an SNP in codon 131 that alters a potential site for N-linked glycosylation, several SNPs in the promoter region that could affect gene transcription, and a variable tandem nucleotide repeat sequence in intron 4.[26,98–102] This latter variant in intron 4 has been associated with increased risk for several pulmonary diseases, ranging from RDS and bronchopulmonary dysplasia in premature infants to lung cancer in adults.[101,103–107] The mechanisms by which this variant affects SP-B expression are unknown, although effects on gene transcription based on potential transcription factor binding sites and on mRNA splicing have been proposed.[104,108] The codon 131 SNP has been associated with both risk for RDS in premature infants as well as acute and chronic lung injury in adults.[99,109,110] The observed associations have been relatively weak, however, and often in combination with other risk factors or genetic variants at other loci. Additional studies will be needed to fully address the question of whether and which SFTPB alleles may predispose to different disease conditions.

Currently there is no specific effective therapy for SP-B deficiency other than lung transplantation. Children with SP-B deficiency have been transplanted in early infancy, with short- and long-term outcomes comparable to those for lung transplantation for other disorders in infancy.[111] As lung transplantation carries with it significant burdens for the family as well as long-term morbidity and mortality risks, compassionate care is also an appropriate option once the diagnosis is established. Identification of the responsible mutations allows for proper genetic counseling and the option for prenatal or even preimplantation diagnosis for future pregnancies.

Surfactant Protein C

Surfactant protein C is encoded by a single gene (SFTPC) on the short arm of chromosome 8. The gene is relatively small, spanning some 3,500 bases, and contains 6 exons, of which the last is untranslated.[112] The gene is transcribed into an approximately 0.9 kb mRNA, which directs the synthesis of a 191 or 197 proprotein (pro-SP-C), depending on alternative splicing at the beginning of exon 5.[38,72] Proprotein SP-C does not contain a signal peptide but is a transmembrane protein in which the domain corresponding to mature SP-C acts as the membrane anchoring domain, with the amino-terminus oriented toward the cytoplasm.[113,114] Proprotein SP-C undergoes a number of posttranslational modifications, including palmitoylation of cysteine residues within the mature peptide domain, such that SP-C is a proteolipid.[115,116] Like SP-B, pro-SP-C is proteolytically processed at both the carboxy and amino termini, to yield the 34 or 35 amino acid mature SP-C, whose protein sequence is encoded within exon 2 of the gene and is secreted into the airspaces along with SP-B and surfactant lipids. The carboxy-terminal domain of pro-SP-C has homology with a group of proteins linked to forms of familial dementia and cancer (BRICHOS domain), with their common pathogenesis hypothesized as being related to abnormal protein folding and hence conformational diseases.[117,118] Surfactant protein C expression is confined to type II cells within the lung, and the SP-C human and mouse promoter sequences have been widely used in animal experiments to drive lung-specific gene expression.[47,119–121]

Lung disease due to SFTPC mutations is rare, although the incidence and prevalence are unknown as population-based studies have not been performed. The majority of reported cases have involved single cases or families or small series of cases, and patients have been evaluated primarily by phenotype. The typical presentation in infancy is with symptoms and signs of diffuse lung disease, including tachypnea, retractions, and hypoxemia in room air; digital clubbing and failure to thrive may also occur.[84,122] Most affected infants do not have symptoms at birth, although neonatal lung disease similar to that of RDS has been observed and may prove fatal in the neonatal period.[123] A family history of interstitial lung disease or pulmonary fibrosis may provide a clue to the diagnosis, although sporadic disease may result from de novo germline mutations, or family members may be asymptomatic.[124–127] Of reported patients, the majority have presented in the pediatric age group. In one study of adults with idiopathic pulmonary fibrosis (n = 89) or nonspecific interstitial pneumonia (n = 46) evaluated for *SFTPC* mutations, only one patient was found to have an *SFTPC* mutation likely related to lung disease.[128] Two commonly occurring SNPs that alter the pro-SP-C coding sequence in codons 138 (threonine [T] or asparagine [N]) and 186 (serine [S] or asparagine) have been identified. These two variants are in strong linkage disequilibrium with one another, and the 186N variant was found with increased frequency in patients with RDS compared with controls in one study.[129] This variant is of particular interest, as 186S has been strongly conserved during evolution, and several *SFTPC* mutations associated with lung disease have been identified in nearby codons. An additional preliminary study noted an association with pulmonary fibrosis in adults.[130] Further studies are needed to confirm or refute these interesting preliminary observations.

As opposed to SP-B deficiency in which all known mutations would be predicted to preclude or reduce the amount of mature SP-B, all known mutations in *SFTPC* associated with human disease have been missense mutations, small insertions or deletions, splicing mutations that would maintain the reading frame, or frame shifts in the fourth or fifth exons that are likely to be associated with stable transcripts.[84,122–127,131–133] Almost all of the mutations have mapped to the carboxy-terminal domain of pro-SP-C. Thus the mutations are ones that would be predicted to result in the production of an abnormal form of pro-SP-C. Furthermore, mutations have generally been found on only one allele. When familial, the lung disease associated with *SFTPC* mutations is inherited in an autosomal dominant pattern, with a variable age of onset of lung disease, ranging from early infancy to the fifth or sixth decade of life.[102,125] Whether there is complete penetrance of the lung disease associated with *SFTPC* mutations is uncertain. Individuals with mutations who do not have lung disease have been reported, but in general these individuals have not been formally evaluated for lung disease and may simply have a later onset of disease.

The exact mechanisms whereby *SFTPC* mutations result in lung disease are unclear. The abnormal pro-SP-C resulting from the mutation may be targeted for degradation, and as pro-SP-C self-associates in the secretory pathway, this may result in degradation of wild-type pro-SP-C as well, leading to SP-C deficiency due to a dominant negative mechanism.[113,134,135] In support of this,

reduced pro-SP-C and mature SP-C have been demonstrated in lung tissue associated with an SP-C mutation that resulted in the skipping of the fourth exon (Δexon 4), and expression of this mutation in vitro resulted in its rapid degradation that was prevented by inhibitors of proteasome-mediated degradation.[131,134,136] Surfactant protein C null mice also develop lung disease in a strain-dependent fashion, with progressive interstitial lung disease and aging.[137,138] Thus SP-C deficiency may be involved in the pathogenesis of lung disease in some patients with *SFTPC* mutations, although precisely how deficiency of mature SP-C results in chronic lung disease is not known. Although complete SP-C deficiency does not result in RDS at birth, SP-C-deficient surfactant may not be as effective at maintaining low surface tension at low lung volumes and may be particularly important if SP-B levels are also decreased, and thus relative deficiency of SP-C may lead to intermittent alveolar atelectasis over time.[137,139] In addition, SP-C binds lipopolysaccharide, and SP-C deficiency may therefore lead to an increased inflammatory response.[140–142]

A second mechanism whereby SP-C mutations may result in lung disease is direct toxicity due to the effects of mutated pro-SP-C. Proprotein SP-C contains the extremely hydrophobic epitopes of mature SP-C, and mutations in pro-SP-C may allow exposure of these epitopes with secondary deleterious effects. Transfection of a construct expressing an SP-C missense mutation (L188Q) into lung epithelial lines in vitro resulted in cytotoxicity as demonstrated by lactate dehydrogenase release.[102] Abnormally folded pro-SP-C due to mutations could also form aggregates, and abnormal accumulation of pro-SP-C containing the SP-C Δexon 4 mutation has been demonstrated in vitro and in lung tissue from at least one infant with a small in-frame deletion in *SFTPC*.[126,136] Pro-SP-C molecules containing mutations are likely to be misfolded and hence trigger the unfolded protein response in the endoplasmic reticulum with resultant endoplasmic reticulum stress. Transfection of constructs expressing the SP-C Δexon 4 mutation identified in index patients has been shown to be associated with induction of the unfolded protein response and with secondary apoptosis of alveolar epithelial cells.[134,143] In addition, cells stably transfected in vitro with constructs expressing the SP-C Δexon 4 mutation that induced a state of chronic endoplasmic reticulum stress were more vulnerable to viral infection, thus suggesting a mechanism by which environmental insults could trigger or exacerbate lung disease primarily due to a genetic mechanism.[144] The potential toxic effects of abnormal pro-SP-C have also been demonstrated in vivo in that transgenic mice expressing the human SP-C Δexon 4 mutation had markedly disrupted lung development that correlated with amount of transgene expression.[134] Although there are currently no specific treatments for the lung disease due to *SFTPC* mutations, agents that facilitate trafficking through the secretory pathway that are currently under evaluation for other genetic lung diseases may also be of benefit for SP-C-related lung disease.[136,145,146]

Member A3 of the Adenosine Triphosphate Binding Cassette Family of Proteins

ABCA3 is a member of the ATP binding cassette family of proteins, transmembrane proteins that hydrolyze ATP in order to translocate a wide variety of substrates across biologic membranes.[147] The gene encoding ABCA3 (*ABCA3*) is located on the short arm of chromosome 16 and spans over 80 kb, containing 33 exons.[148] The gene directs the synthesis of a 1,704 amino acid protein and is considered a full transporter with 12 membrane spanning domains and 2 nucleotide binding domains. A number of tissues express ABCA3, but it is highly expressed in lung tissue where it is localized to the limiting membrane of lamellar bodies.[12,57] As the ABCA subfamily is often involved in transport of lipids, this localization for ABCA3 is consistent with a role for ABCA3 in importing lipids needed for surfactant function into lamellar bodies.[149,150]

The importance of ABCA3 in surfactant metabolism has been demonstrated by the observation that mutations on both *ABCA3* alleles resulted in severe lung disease in full-term newborns who had clinical and radiographic features of surfactant deficiency.[13,151-153] In addition, surfactant isolated from bronchoalveolar lavage specimens of children who required lung transplantation for ABCA3 deficiency was shown to have markedly reduced ability to lower surface tension and an abnormal composition, with a particular reduction in phosphatidylcholine content observed.[152] In an in vitro study, downregulation of ABCA3 expression was associated with decreased lipid uptake into lamellar bodies of alveolar type II cells, and cells transfected with constructs expressing forms of ABCA3 containing mutations identified in patients had reduced uptake of lipids into lysosomes compared with cells transfected with wild-type ABCA3.[154] Collectively these observations support a fundamental role for ABCA3 importing surfactant lipids into lamellar bodies, although the exact substrates remain to be determined. Thus quantitative and functional deficiencies of surfactant components likely contribute to the symptoms of surfactant deficiency observed in ABCA3-deficient infants. As lamellar body biogenesis is interfered with, processing of pro-SP-B and pro-SP-C to their mature forms may also be hindered in this condition, leading to deficiencies of these surfactant components as well.[151]

Although ABCA3 deficiency is the most recently identified inborn error of surfactant metabolism, it is likely a more common cause of disease than *SFTPB* or *SFTPC* mutations. *ABCA3* mutations accounted for a combined 24 of 35 cases of unexplained respiratory failure in two reports[13,151] and for 8 of 12 infants who underwent lung transplantation in the first year of life for severe lung disease of unknown etiology.[152] Well over 100 different *ABCA3* mutations have been identified[13,151-153] (and L. Nogee, unpublished observations) and markedly reduced or absent ABCA3 expression has been demonstrated in the lung tissue of affected infants consistent with disease resulting from a loss-of-function mechanism.[151] Aside from mutations that completely preclude ABCA3 expression, mutations may also result in abnormal intracellular routing of ABCA3 or decreased functional activity.[154,155] Although initial studies focused on children with fatal or very severe lung disease, survival with chronic interstitial lung disease is possible.[153] Because identified patients with interstitial lung disease shared one particular *ABCA3* mutation, this may be a result of partial deficiency, and genotype may thus be important in predicting phenotype in this disease. Additional studies are needed to evaluate this hypothesis.

Detailed studies of the clinical features associated with *ABCA3* mutations have not yet been published. From the initial reports, the phenotype of patients with ABCA3 deficiency often resembles that of infants with SP-B deficiency, with severe neonatal lung disease resembling RDS in premature infants.[13,151] As with SP-B deficiency, however, some infants may have considerably milder neonatal lung disease, and yet others may not have symptoms in the neonatal period.[153] The initial lung disease may also improve with time such that affected infants are able to be discharged. The clinical picture associated with ABCA3 deficiency thus overlaps that associated with SP-B deficiency and SP-C mutations.

The incidence and prevalence of lung disease due to ABCA3 deficiency are unknown. Population studies have not yet been done on the frequency of *ABCA3* mutations in the general population. It is likely that the disease is rare, but, particularly if milder variants contribute to chronic lung disease, it may prove to be more common than has initially been appreciated.

Lung Pathology Associated with Inborn Errors of Surfactant Metabolism

The lung pathology changes associated with all three single gene disorders disrupting surfactant metabolism are similar and overlapping (Figure 54.1) These include marked alveolar type II cell hyperplasia, interstitial

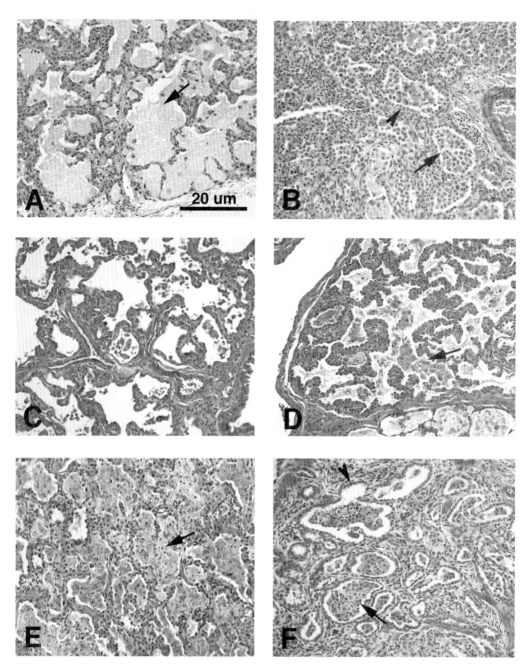

FIGURE 54.1. Lung histopathology of inborn errors of surfactant metabolism. **(A,B)** Representative histopathology of two children with *SFTPB* mutations. Features of pulmonary alveolar proteinosis (PAP) with eosinophilic, proteinaceous material filling the alveoli (arrow) are shown in A. Features of desquamative interstitial pneumonitis with accumulation of foamy alveolar macrophages in the alveoli (arrow) are shown in B. **(C,D)** Representative histopathology of two children with *SFTPC* mutations. Features of nonspecific interstitial pneumonitis with thickened alveolar septa are shown in C. An example of chronic pneumonitis of infancy with both macrophages and granular, eosinophilic material in the alveoli (arrow) is shown in D. **(E,F)** Representative histopathology of two children with *ABCA3* mutations. Features of PAP (arrow) are shown in E. Features of desquamative interstitial pneumonitis (arrow) are shown in F. Features of alveolar proteinosis with eosinophilic material and/or foamy macrophages and prominent type II cell hyperplasia (arrowheads) are highlighted in B and F, and thickened alveolar septa are variably present in all three types of disorders. (Hematoxylin and eosin stains. All original magnifications, ×10; bar = 20 μm.)

thickening with variable amounts of fibrosis, and numerous foamy macrophages in the airspaces. A prominent feature can be the accumulation of granular, eosinophilic material filling distal airspaces that stains positively with periodic acid–Schiff reagent or alveolar proteinosis material. Although findings of alveolar proteinosis were prominent in the index patient with SP-B deficiency and provided an important clue to the mechanism, similar findings may be seen with other inborn errors of surfactant metabolism due to mutations in the *SFTPC* or *ABCA3* genes. The composition of this material is also likely different in the different disorders and differs from the proteinosis material observed in older children and adults who have alveolar proteinosis due to an immune mechanism.[156] The proteinosis material may be minimal in appearance and the sensitivity and specificity of this finding for each of the disorders has not been critically examined. The term *congenital alveolar proteinosis* is thus probably best avoided in describing these conditions.

In older children with the clinical picture of interstitial lung disease histopathologic diagnoses associated with *SFTPC* and *ABCA3* mutations have included chronic pneumonitis of infancy, nonspecific interstitial pneumonia, and idiopathic pulmonary fibrosis.[124,125,131,133] Usual interstitial pneumonia has also been reported in older individuals in association with an *SFTPC* mutation.[127] Desquamative interstitial pneumonia has also been reported as the histologic diagnoses in children with *ABCA3* and *SFTPC* mutations, although the course is much more severe than with desquamative interstitial pneumonia observed in adults.[153,157,158] The majority of these children were given this diagnosis before the description of chronic pneumonitis of infancy.[159] Although it has not been formally studied, it is likely that histology findings will be unable to discriminate between the three known conditions. Recently the term *surfactant dysfunction mutation* has been used to encompass the changes found in all three disorders, and it is also likely that other genetic mechanisms leading to disruption of surfactant metabolism will yield similar pathology.[160]

Specific immunostaining of the lung may be helpful in establishing the specific diagnosis of SP-B deficiency (Figure 54.2) With *SFTPB* mutations, absent or markedly reduced staining for both pro-SP-B and SP-B may be observed, although, depending on the genotype, some staining for both may be detected.[86] Reduced staining for SP-B may also be seen in association with *ABCA3* mutations, and hence absent staining for SP-B is not sufficient for a specific diagnosis.[151] However, because of the presence of large amounts of secreted aberrantly processed SP-C peptides, the extracellular material in SP-B-deficient lung stains intensely with antibodies directed against pro-SP-C and appear to be a specific marker for this disorder.[86] Specific staining for the surfactant proteins has not revealed a consistent pattern associated with *SFTPC* mutations. Proprotein SP-C may be readily detected in alveolar epithelial cells or may be markedly reduced or absent.[125,131] Markedly reduced staining for pro-SP-C has also been observed with familial lung disease in which, however, no *SFTPC* mutations could be identified.[161]

Ultrastructural studies may be very helpful in establishing a specific diagnosis. Electron microscopy of lung tissue from SP-B-deficient children demonstrates specific changes within the lamellar bodies within type II cells. Instead of normally formed lamellar bodies with well-organized layers and lamellae, the type II cells contain intracellular inclusions with poorly formed lamellae and vesicles of varying size (Figure 54.3).[162,163] These observations are consistent with a function for SP-B in membrane fusion and indicate a fundamental intracellular role for SP-B in lamellar body biogenesis. These abnormal lamellar bodies appear characteristic for SP-B deficiency.

ABCA3 is localized to the limiting membrane of lamellar bodies, and specific ultrastructural changes have also been observed in the type II cells of ABCA3-deficient infants.[13,151,163–165] Normal-appearing lamellar bodies may appear to be absent, and instead the cytoplasm of alveolar type II cells contains many small, dense bodies that on higher magnification may be seen to contain tightly packed membrane. An eccentrically placed electron-dense core in these small bodies may give them a "fried egg" appearance.[165] Although only a limited number of studies are available, the finding of these bodies has had a very high correlation with the identification of mutations in the *ABCA3* gene, and they have not yet been reported in other conditions. However, the exact sensitivity and specificity of this finding remain unknown. Anecdotal experience indicates that some type II cells in infants with *ABCA3* mutations may have more normal-appearing lamellar bodies, and there are few data on the ultrastructural findings in children with milder lung disease due to *ABCA3* mutations. Currently, no consistent ultrastructural abnormalities in association with *SFTPC* mutations have been identified. Some abnormally formed lamellar bodies were observed both in vitro and in vivo in association with two *SFTPC* mutations, but normal lamellar bodies were also observed[126,127] and additional study is needed. However, the ultrastructural findings associated with SP-B and ABCA3 deficiencies are so striking that the preparation of tissue for electron microscopy should be included in autopsies of children dying from neonatal respiratory disease or in biopsies of young infants with diffuse lung disease.[166]

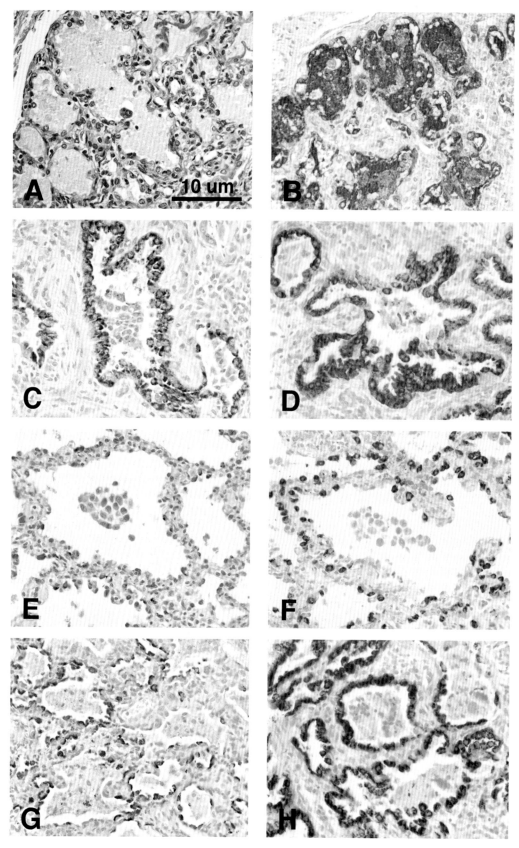

FIGURE 54.2. Immunohistochemical staining for mature surfactant protein B (SP-B) and proprotein surfactant protein C (pro-SP-C). **(A,B)** Specimens from a child with SP-B deficiency showing absent staining for mature SP-B (A) and intense staining for pro-SP-C (B) of both alveolar epithelium and the intra-alveolar material. **(C,D)** Specimens from a child with an *SFTPC* mutation showing robust staining for both mature SP-B (C) and pro-SP-C (D) that is confined to the epithelium. **(E–H)** Specimens from two subjects with ABCA3 deficiency. In one subject, staining for mature SP-B is severely reduced (E), whereas in the other there is robust staining for mature SP-B (G). Proprotein SP-C staining is robust in both subjects (F and H) and is confined to the alveolar epithelium. (All original magnifications, ×20; bar = 10 μm.)

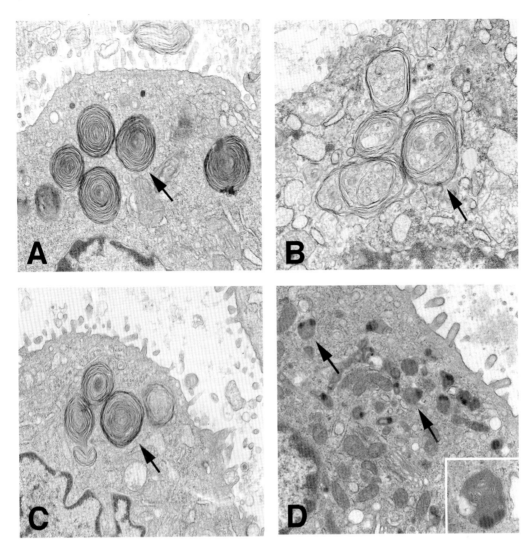

FIGURE 54.3. Electron micrographs of alveolar type II cells. **(A)** Normal lung, showing well-developed lamellar bodies (arrow) within alveolar type II cells. **(B)** Child with surfactant protein B deficiency, demonstrating disorganized, large multivesicular bodies (arrow) in lieu of lamellar bodies. **(C)** Child with an *SFTPC* mutation, showing well-formed lamellar bodies (arrow) similar to those observed in normal lung (A). **(D)** Child with ABCA3 deficiency, demonstrating small, dense bodies (arrows) with eccentrically placed electron-dense inclusions and tightly packed phospholipid lamellae (inset). (A–C, original magnifications, ×5,000; D, original magnification, ×10,000; inset in D, ×30,000.)

Genetic Testing

The identification of single gene defects that cause both acute neonatal respiratory failure and chronic interstitial lung disease allows for potential diagnostic testing through analysis of genomic DNA for potential mutations in these genes. Such testing has the advantage that it is noninvasive, potentially obviating the need for biopsy in an unstable patient, and can yield a specific diagnosis. Clinical testing is now available through Clinical Laboratory Improvement Amendments–certified laboratories. The sensitivity of such testing in different clinical situations is unknown, the testing is not inexpensive and costs may not be covered by insurance, and results may take weeks to months to receive. The interpretation of such testing can be potentially problematic. It may not be possible to distinguish rare yet benign *SFTPC* variants from mutations responsible for disease, and it is apparent that not all *ABCA3* mutations are detected by current methods. In the case of a child with lung disease of unclear etiology in whom only one *ABCA3* mutation is found, it may be difficult to determine whether such an individual is affected with an unknown mutation on the second allele or whether is simply a carrier for an *ABCA3* genetic variant that is unrelated to the cause of the lung disease.

Other Proteins Important in Surfactant Metabolism Linked to Genetic Diseases

Alterations in two other proteins resulting in abnormalities of surfactant expression have been reported in association with human lung disease. A single report associated infantile alveolar proteinosis and interstitial lung disease with abnormalities of the common β-chain of the GM-CSF/IL-3/IL-5 receptors.[167] The rationale for examining this protein was based on observations in genetically engineered mice that targeted disruption of either the ligand (GM-CSF) or common beta chain (βc) of the receptor resulted in a phenotype of alveolar proteinosis as the mice aged.[168–171] In four infants examined, defective expression of the receptor was demonstrated on peripheral blood leukocytes, as well as decreased signaling for GM-CSF, but not G-CSF in vitro. Thus, these infants appeared to have a clear functional defect in this receptor. However, in only one infant was an abnormality in the gene encoding βc identified: a substitution of threonine for proline in codon 602, which was found on only one allele and may well have represented a polymorphism. To date, no clear disease-causing mutations in this gene have been identified, and no subsequent reports have appeared to confirm these initial observations.

Thyroid transcription factor 1 (also known as Nkx2.1) is a homeodomain transcription factor that has been shown to be critical for pulmonary development and expression of SP-A, SP-B, and SP-C. Several reports have linked genetic causes of reduced amounts of TTF-1 due to either deletion of a region containing the gene or loss-of-function mutations on one copy of the gene with neonatal respiratory disease with symptoms and signs of surfactant deficiency.[172–175] As TTF-1 is also expressed in extrapulmonary sites, not surprisingly these patients have had abnormalities in other organ systems, specifically transient neonatal hypothyroidism and central nervous system abnormalities. In general these patients have recovered from the neonatal lung disease, and lung pathology information is not available for these patients. Hypothyroidism and central nervous system abnormalities have also been observed without any respiratory symptoms.[176] Some have had recurrent pulmonary infections, possibly related to the reduced amounts of SP-A, although other explanations are also possible. The incidence and prevalence of this disorder are unknown; only five families have been reported in the literature.

Pulmonary Alveolar Proteinosis

Pulmonary alveolar proteinosis is a lung disease of insidious onset due to an accumulation of surfactant in the airspaces and was first described in 1958.[177] The accumulation of material in the airspaces results in a restrictive lung defect with resultant hypoxemia and pulmonary symptoms. The disease is primarily seen in adults and may occur either in a primary form or secondary to a number of pulmonary insults, including infection and toxic inhalation.[156,178] The material accumulating in the lungs of patients with pulmonary alveolar proteinosis is rich in surfactant lipids and proteins, and lung lavage material from such patients was often the starting material for the purification of the surfactant proteins.[179,180] The surfactant material accumulates as the result of the decreased catabolism rather than increased production. Primary pulmonary alveolar proteinosis in adults is now known to largely (if not entirely) be an autoimmune disease due to neutralizing autoantibodies to GM-CSF.[181–183] Such antibodies have been found in both serum and bronchoalveolar lavage fluid of affected patients. The absence of functional GM-CSF interferes with alveolar macrophage function, leading to defective catabolism of surfactant and accumulation of the pulmonary alveolar proteinosis material in the airspaces.

Similar pathology can be seen in newborns and young infants with severe respiratory failure and has been termed *congenital alveolar proteinosis*. Although aspects of the pathology in these infants may be similar to that seen in adults with pulmonary alveolar proteinosis, the underlying causes are different; specifically, in young infants the disease is more likely due to the inborn errors of lung cell metabolism described earlier. As a result, the material accumulating in the lungs of these infants differs from that observed in adults, and the course of the disease differs, with a more rapid downhill course in young infants that is refractory to therapy. Alveolar proteinosis in young infants and children may also occur in children with lysinuric protein intolerance, a disorder of cationic amino acid transport due to mutations in the gene encoding the solute transporter SLC7A7.[184,185] Children affected with lysinuric protein intolerance usually have other systemic symptoms, such as recurrent vomiting and failure to thrive, but the pulmonary disease may be the most prominent feature and may prove fatal.

Conclusion

An intact pulmonary surfactant system is essential for normal respiratory function. Too little or too much surfactant can lead to profound lung disease, such as surfactant deficiency due to decreased production as a result of developmental immaturity causing RDS in newborn infants, and accumulation of pulmonary surfactant from decreased catabolism as a result of inactivation of GM-CSF due to neutralizing antibodies leading to alveolar proteinosis in adults. The identification of rare genetic variants in genes important in surfactant metabolism and correlation with the resulting phenotypes provides potential insights into the role of their gene products in surfactant function and support for polymorphic variants in these genes as having a role in more common pulmonary diseases.

Acknowledgments. This work was supported by grants from the National Institutes of Health, HL 56387 (S.E.W., L.M.N.) and HL-54703 (L.M.N.) and the Eudowood Foundation (L.M.N.). The authors are grateful for the continued collaboration of Drs. Jeffrey Whitsett, Timothy Weaver, Stephan Glasser, Michael Dean, Aaron Hamvas. and F. Sessions Cole.

References

1. Avery ME, Mead J. Surface properties in relation to atelectasis and hyaline membrane disease. AMA J Dis Child 1959;97(5, Part 1):517–523.
2. Gregory TJ, Longmore WJ, Moxley MA, et al. Surfactant chemical composition and biophysical activity in acute respiratory distress syndrome. J Clin Invest 1991;88(6): 1976–1981.
3. Greene KE, Wright JR, Steinberg KP, et al. Serial changes in surfactant-associated proteins in lung and serum before and after onset of ARDS. Am J Respir Crit Care Med 1999;160(6):1843–1850.
4. Nogee LM. Genetic mechanisms of surfactant deficiency. Biol Neonate 2004;85(4):314–318.
5. Whitsett JA, Wert SE, Xu Y. Genetic disorders of surfactant homeostasis. Biol Neonate 2005;87(4):283–287.
6. Weaver TE, Na CL, Stahlman M. Biogenesis of lamellar bodies, lysosome-related organelles involved in storage and secretion of pulmonary surfactant. Semin Cell Dev Biol 2002;13(4):263–270.
7. Goerke J. Pulmonary surfactant: functions and molecular composition. Biochim Biophys Acta 1998;1408(2–3): 79–89.
8. Ridsdale R, Post M. Surfactant lipid synthesis and lamellar body formation in glycogen-laden type II cells. Am J Physiol Lung Cell Mol Physiol 2004;287(4):L743–L751.
9. Ridsdale R, Tseu I, Wang J, et al. CTP:phosphocholine cytidylyltransferase alpha is a cytosolic protein in pulmonary epithelial cells and tissues. J Biol Chem 2001;276(52): 49148–49155.
10. Rooney SA, Young SL, Mendelson CR. Molecular and cellular processing of lung surfactant. FASEB J 1994; 8(12):957–967.
11. McCoy DM, Fisher K, Robichaud J, et al. Transcriptional regulation of lung cytidylyltransferase in developing transgenic mice. Am J Respir Cell Mol Biol 2006;35(3): 394–402.
12. Mulugeta S, Gray JM, Notarfrancesco KL, et al. Identification of LBM180, a lamellar body limiting membrane protein of alveolar type II cells, as the ABC transporter protein ABCA3. J Biol Chem 2002;277(25):22147–22155.
13. Shulenin S, Nogee LM, Annilo T, et al. ABCA3 gene mutations in newborns with fatal surfactant deficiency. N Engl J Med 2004;350(13):1296–1303.

14. Floros J, Hoover RR. Genetics of the hydrophilic surfactant proteins A and D. Biochim Biophys Acta 1998; 1408(2–3):312–322.
15. Crouch E, Wright JR. Surfactant proteins a and d and pulmonary host defense. Annu Rev Physiol 2001;63: 521–554.
16. Hawgood S, Poulain FR. The pulmonary collectins and surfactant metabolism. Annu Rev Physiol 2001;63:495–519.
17. Akiyama J, Hoffman A, Brown C, et al. Tissue distribution of surfactant proteins A and D in the mouse. J Histochem Cytochem 2002;50(7):993–996.
18. Lin Z, deMello D, Phelps DS, et al. Both human SP-A1 and SP-A2 genes are expressed in small and large intestine. Pediatr Pathol Mol Med 2001;20(5):367–386.
19. Paananen R, Postle AD, Clark G, et al. Eustachian tube surfactant is different from alveolar surfactant: determination of phospholipid composition of porcine eustachian tube lavage fluid. J Lipid Res 2002;43(1):99–106.
20. Leth-Larsen R, Floridon C, Nielsen O, et al. Surfactant protein D in the female genital tract. Mol Hum Reprod 2004;10(3):149–154.
21. Madsen J, Kliem A, Tornoe I, et al. Localization of lung surfactant protein D on mucosal surfaces in human tissues. J Immunol 2000;164(11):5866–5870.
22. Seifart C, Lin HM, Seifart U, et al. Rare SP-A alleles and the SP-A1–6A(4) allele associate with risk for lung carcinoma. Clin Genet 2005;68(2):128–136.
23. Kala P, Ten Have T, Nielsen H, et al. Association of pulmonary surfactant protein A (SP-A) gene and respiratory distress syndrome: interaction with SP-B. Pediatr Res 1998;43(2):169–177.
24. Floros J, Fan R, Matthews A, et al. Family-based transmission disequilibrium test (TDT) and case-control association studies reveal surfactant protein A (SP-A) susceptibility alleles for respiratory distress syndrome (RDS) and possible race differences. Clin Genet 2001;60(3):178–187.
25. Lahti M, Lofgren J, Marttila R, et al. Surfactant protein D gene polymorphism associated with severe respiratory syncytial virus infection. Pediatr Res 2002;51(6):696–699.
26. Guo X, Lin HM, Lin Z, et al. Surfactant protein gene A, B, and D marker alleles in chronic obstructive pulmonary disease of a Mexican population. Eur Respir J 2001;18(3): 482–490.
27. Ramet M, Haataja R, Marttila R, et al. Association between the surfactant protein A (SP-A) gene locus and respiratory-distress syndrome in the Finnish population. Am J Hum Genet 2000;66(5):1569–1579.
28. Lofgren J, Ramet M, Renko M, et al. Association between surfactant protein A gene locus and severe respiratory syncytial virus infection in infants. J Infect Dis 2002; 185(3):283–289.
29. Korfhagen TR, Bruno MD, Ross GF, et al. Altered surfactant function and structure in SP-A gene targeted mice. Proc Natl Acad Sci USA 1996;93(18):9594–9599.
30. Korfhagen TR, LeVine AM, Whitsett JA. Surfactant protein A (SP-A) gene targeted mice. Biochim Biophys Acta 1998;1408(2–3):296–302.
31. LeVine AM, Gwozdz J, Stark J, et al. Surfactant protein-A enhances respiratory syncytial virus clearance in vivo. J Clin Invest 1999;103(7):1015–1021.

32. LeVine AM, Hartshorn K, Elliott J, et al. Absence of SP-A modulates innate and adaptive defense responses to pulmonary influenza infection. Am J Physiol Lung Cell Mol Physiol 2002;282(3):L563–L572.

33. LeVine AM, Kurak KE, Bruno MD, et al. Surfactant protein-A–deficient mice are susceptible to *Pseudomonas aeruginosa* infection. Am J Respir Cell Mol Biol 1998; 19(4):700–708.

34. LeVine AM, Kurak KE, Wright JR, et al. Surfactant protein-A binds group B *Streptococcus* enhancing phagocytosis and clearance from lungs of surfactant protein-A–deficient mice. Am J Respir Cell Mol Biol 1999;20(2): 279–286.

35. Botas C, Poulain F, Akiyama J, et al. Altered surfactant homeostasis and alveolar type II cell morphology in mice lacking surfactant protein D. Proc Natl Acad Sci USA 1998;95(20):11869–11874.

36. Korfhagen TR, Sheftelyevich V, Burhans MS, et al. Surfactant protein-D regulates surfactant phospholipid homeostasis in vivo. J Biol Chem 1998;273(43):28438–28443.

37. Wert S, Jones T, Korfhagen T, et al. Spontaneous emphysema in surfactant protein D gene-targeted mice. Chest 2000;117(5 Suppl 1):248S.

38. Weaver TE, Conkright JJ. Function of surfactant proteins B and C. Annu Rev Physiol 2001;63:555–578.

39. Whitsett JA, Ohning BL, Ross G, et al. Hydrophobic surfactant-associated protein in whole lung surfactant and its importance for biophysical activity in lung surfactant extracts used for replacement therapy. Pediatr Res 1986;20(5):460–467.

40. Whitsett JA, Weaver TE, Clark JC, et al. Glucocorticoid enhances surfactant proteolipid Phe and pVal synthesis and RNA in fetal lung. J Biol Chem 1987;262(32):15618–15623.

41. Ballard PL, Ertsey R, Gonzales LW, et al. Transcriptional regulation of human pulmonary surfactant proteins SP-B and SP-C by glucocorticoids. Am J Respir Cell Mol Biol 1996;14(6):599–607.

42. Venkatesh VC, Iannuzzi DM, Ertsey R, et al. Differential glucocorticoid regulation of the pulmonary hydrophobic surfactant proteins SP-B and SP-C. Am J Respir Cell Mol Biol 1993;8(2):222–228.

43. Bohinski RJ, Di Lauro R, Whitsett JA. The lung-specific surfactant protein B gene promoter is a target for thyroid transcription factor 1 and hepatocyte nuclear factor 3, indicating common factors for organ-specific gene expression along the foregut axis. Mol Cell Biol 1994;14(9):5671–5681.

44. Margana R, Berhane K, Alam MN, et al. Identification of functional TTF-1 and Sp1/Sp3 sites in the upstream promoter region of rabbit SP-B gene. Am J Physiol Lung Cell Mol Physiol 2000;278(3):L477–L484.

45. Margana RK, Boggaram V. Functional analysis of surfactant protein B (SP-B) promoter. Sp1, Sp3, TTF-1, and HNF-3alpha transcription factors are necessary for lung cell- specific activation of SP-B gene transcription. J Biol Chem 1997;272(5):3083–3090.

46. DeFelice M, Silberschmidt D, DiLauro R, et al. TTF-1 phosphorylation is required for peripheral lung morpho-

genesis, perinatal survival, and tissue-specific gene expression. J Biol Chem 2003;278(37):35574–35583.

47. Wan H, Xu Y, Ikegami M, et al. Foxa2 is required for transition to air breathing at birth. Proc Natl Acad Sci USA 2004;101(40):14449–14454.

48. Lin S, Perl AK, Shannon JM. Erm/thyroid transcription factor 1 interactions modulate surfactant protein C transcription. J Biol Chem 2006;281(24):16716–16726.

49. Yang MC, Guo Y, Liu CC, et al. The TTF-1/TAP26 complex differentially modulates surfactant protein-B (SP-B) and -C (SP-C) promoters in lung cells. Biochem Biophys Res Commun 2006;344(2):484–490.

50. Whitsett JA. Genes and transcriptional programs regulating alveolar homeostasis. Respirology 2006;11(Suppl 1): S11.

51. Martis PC, Whitsett JA, Xu Y, et al. C/EBPalpha is required for lung maturation at birth. Development 2006; 133(6):1155–11564.

52. Farrell PM, Avery ME. Hyaline membrane disease. Am Rev Respir Dis 1975;111(5):657–688.

53. Brehier A, Rooney SA. Phosphatidylcholine synthesis and glycogen depletion in fetal mouse lung: developmental changes and the effects of dexamethasone. Exp Lung Res 1981;2(4):273–287.

54. Pryhuber GS, Hull WM, Fink I, et al. Ontogeny of surfactant proteins A and B in human amniotic fluid as indices of fetal lung maturity. Pediatr Res 1991;30(6):597–605.

55. Ross GF, Ikegami M, Steinhilber W, et al. Surfactant protein C in fetal and ventilated preterm rabbit lungs. Am J Physiol 1999;277(6 Pt 1):L1104–L1108.

56. Yoshida I, Ban N, Inagaki N. Expression of ABCA3, a causative gene for fatal surfactant deficiency, is up-regulated by glucocorticoids in lung alveolar type II cells. Biochem Biophys Res Commun 2004;323(2):547–555.

57. Yamano G, Funahashi H, Kawanami O, et al. ABCA3 is a lamellar body membrane protein in human lung alveolar type II cells. FEBS Lett 2001;508(2):221–225.

58. Zen K, Notarfrancesco K, Oorschot V, et al. Generation and characterization of monoclonal antibodies to alveolar type II cell lamellar body membrane. Am J Physiol 1998;275(1 Pt 1):L172–L183.

59. Khoor A, Gray ME, Hull WM, et al. Developmental expression of SP-A and SP-A mRNA in the proximal and distal respiratory epithelium in the human fetus and newborn. J Histochem Cytochem 1993;41(9):1311–1319.

60. Khoor A, Stahlman MT, Gray ME, et al. Temporal-spatial distribution of SP-B and SP-C proteins and mRNAs in developing respiratory epithelium of human lung. J Histochem Cytochem 1994;42(9):1187–1199.

61. Ballard PL, Merrill JD, Godinez RI, et al. Surfactant protein profile of pulmonary surfactant in premature infants. Am J Respir Crit Care Med 2003;168(9):1123–1128.

62. deMello DE, Phelps DS, Patel G, et al. Expression of the 35 kDa and low molecular weight surfactant-associated proteins in the lungs of infants dying with respiratory distress syndrome. Am J Pathol 1989;134(6):1285–1293.

63. Karcher R, Sykes E, Batton D, et al. Gestational age-specific predicted risk of neonatal respiratory distress

syndrome using lamellar body count and surfactant-to-albumin ratio in amniotic fluid. Am J Obstet Gynecol 2005;193(5):1680–1684.

64. Berkowitz GS, Chang K, Chervenak FA, et al. Decreasing frequency of iatrogenic neonatal respiratory distress syndrome. Am J Perinatol 1986;3(3):205–208.

65. Hamvas A, Wise PH, Yang RK, et al. The influence of the wider use of surfactant therapy on neonatal mortality among blacks and whites. N Engl J Med 1996;334(25): 1635–1640.

66. Malloy MH, Freeman DH. Respiratory distress syndrome mortality in the United States, 1987 to 1995. J Perinatol 2000;20(7):414–420.

67. Schwartz RM, Luby AM, Scanlon JW, et al. Effect of surfactant on morbidity, mortality, and resource use in newborn infants weighing 500 to 1500 g. N Engl J Med 1994;330(21):1476–1480.

68. Clark RH. The epidemiology of respiratory failure in neonates born at an estimated gestational age of 34 weeks or more. J Perinatol 2005;25(4):251–257.

69. Angus DC, Linde-Zwirble WT, Clermont G, et al. Epidemiology of neonatal respiratory failure in the United States: projections from California and New York. Am J Respir Crit Care Med 2001;164(7):1154–1160.

70. Pilot-Matias TJ, Kister SE, Fox JL, et al. Structure and organization of the gene encoding human pulmonary surfactant proteolipid SP-B. DNA 1989;8(2):75–86.

71. Vamvakopoulos NC, Modi WS, Floros J. Mapping the human pulmonary surfactant-associated protein B gene (SFTP3) to chromosome 2p12 → p11.2. Cytogenet Cell Genet 1995;68(1–2):8–10.

72. Weaver TE. Synthesis, processing and secretion of surfactant proteins B and C. Biochim Biophys Acta 1998; 1408(2–3):173–179.

73. Hawgood S. Surfactant protein B: structure and function. Biol Neonate 2004;85(4):285–289.

74. Patthy L. Homology of the precursor of pulmonary surfactant-associated protein SP-B with prosaposin and sulfated glycoprotein 1. J Biol Chem 1991;266(10):6035–6037.

75. Wang G, Christensen ND, Wigdahl B, et al. Differences in N-linked glycosylation between human surfactant protein-B variants of the C or T allele at the single-nucleotide polymorphism at position 1580: implications for disease. Biochem J 2003;369(Pt 1):179–184.

76. Lin Z, Wang G, Demello DE, et al. An alternatively spliced surfactant protein B mRNA in normal human lung: disease implication. Biochem J 1999;343 Pt 1:145–149.

77. Hawgood S, Latham D, Borchelt J, et al. Cell-specific posttranslational processing of the surfactant-associated protein SP-B. Am J Physiol 1993;264(3 Pt 1):L290–L299.

78. Nogee LM, de Mello DE, Dehner LP, et al. Brief report: deficiency of pulmonary surfactant protein B in congenital alveolar proteinosis. N Engl J Med 1993;328(6):406–410.

79. Schumacher RE, Marrogi AJ, Heidelberger KP. Pulmonary alveolar proteinosis in a newborn. Pediatr Pulmonol 1989;7(3):178–182.

80. Moulton SL, Krous HF, Merritt TA, et al. Congenital pulmonary alveolar proteinosis: failure of treatment with extracorporeal life support. J Pediatr 1992;120(2 Pt 1): 297–302.

81. Nogee LM, Garnier G, Dietz HC, et al. A mutation in the surfactant protein B gene responsible for fatal neonatal respiratory disease in multiple kindreds. J Clin Invest 1994;93(4):1860–1863.

82. Cole FS, Hamvas A, Rubinstein P, et al. Population-based estimates of surfactant protein B deficiency. Pediatrics 2000;105(3 Pt 1):538–541.

83. Hamvas A, Trusgnich M, Brice H, et al. Population-based screening for rare mutations: high-throughput DNA extraction and molecular amplification from Guthrie cards. Pediatr Res 2001;50(5):666–668.

84. Nogee LM. Alterations in SP-B and SP-C expression in neonatal lung disease. Annu Rev Physiol 2004;66:601–623.

85. Tredano M, Cooper DN, Stuhrmann M, et al. Origin of the prevalent SFTPB indel g.1549C > GAA (121ins2) mutation causing surfactant protein B (SP-B) deficiency. Am J Med Genet A 2006;140(1):62–69.

86. Nogee LM, Wert SE, Proffit SA, et al. Allelic heterogeneity in hereditary surfactant protein B (SP-B) deficiency. Am J Respir Crit Care Med 2000;161(3 Pt 1):973–981.

87. Ballard PL, Nogee LM, Beers MF, et al. Partial deficiency of surfactant protein B in an infant with chronic lung disease. Pediatrics 1995;96(6):1046–1052.

88. Dunbar AE, 3rd, Wert SE, Ikegami M, et al. Prolonged survival in hereditary surfactant protein B (SP-B) deficiency associated with a novel splicing mutation. Pediatr Res 2000;48(3):275–282.

89. Li J, Ikegami M, Na CL, et al. N-terminally extended surfactant protein (SP) C isolated from SP-B-deficient children has reduced surface activity and inhibited lipopolysaccharide binding. Biochemistry 2004;43(13):3891–3898.

90. Vorbroker DK, Profitt SA, Nogee LM, et al. Aberrant processing of surfactant protein C in hereditary SP-B deficiency. Am J Physiol 1995;268(4 Pt 1):L647–L656.

91. Brasch F, Ochs M, Kahne T, et al. Involvement of napsin A in the C- and N-terminal processing of surfactant protein B in type-II pneumocytes of the human lung. J Biol Chem 2003;278(49):49006–49014.

92. Ueno T, Linder S, Na CL, et al. Processing of pulmonary surfactant protein B by napsin and cathepsin H. J Biol Chem 2004;279(16):16178–16184.

93. Clark JC, Wert SE, Bachurski CJ, et al. Targeted disruption of the surfactant protein B gene disrupts surfactant homeostasis, causing respiratory failure in newborn mice. Proc Natl Acad Sci USA 1995;92(17):7794–7798.

94. Stahlman MT, Gray MP, Falconieri MW, et al. Lamellar body formation in normal and surfactant protein B–deficient fetal mice. Lab Invest 2000;80(3):395–403.

95. Melton KR, Nesslein LL, Ikegami M, et al. SP-B deficiency causes respiratory failure in adult mice. Am J Physiol Lung Cell Mol Physiol 2003;285(3):L543–L549.

96. Clark JC, Weaver TE, Iwamoto HS, et al. Decreased lung compliance and air trapping in heterozygous SP-B–deficient mice. Am J Respir Cell Mol Biol 1997;16(1): 46–52.

97. Tokieda K, Iwamoto HS, Bachurski C, et al. Surfactant protein-B–deficient mice are susceptible to hyperoxic lung injury. Am J Respir Cell Mol Biol 1999;21(4):463–472.

98. Liu W, Bentley CM, Floros J. Study of human SP-A, SP-B and SP-D loci: allele frequencies, linkage disequilibrium and heterozygosity in different races and ethnic groups. BMC Genet 2003;4(1):13.

99. Lin Z, Pearson C, Chinchilli V, et al. Polymorphisms of human SP-A, SP-B, and SP-D genes: association of SP-B Thr131Ile with ARDS. Clin Genet 2000;58(3):181–191.

100. Guo X, Lin HM, Lin Z, et al. Polymorphisms of surfactant protein gene A, B, D, and of SP-B-linked microsatellite markers in COPD of a Mexican population. Chest 2000;117(5 Suppl 1):249S–2450S.

101. Floros J, Veletza SV, Kotikalapudi P, et al. Dinucleotide repeats in the human surfactant protein-B gene and respiratory-distress syndrome. Biochem J 1995;305(Pt 2): 583–590.

102. Thomas KH, Meyn P, Suttorp N. Single nucleotide polymorphism in 5′-flanking region reduces transcription of surfactant protein B gene in H441 cells. Am J Physiol Lung Cell Mol Physiol 2006;291(3):L386–L390.

103. Floros J, Fan R, Diangelo S, et al. Surfactant protein (SP) B associations and interactions with SP-A in white and black subjects with respiratory distress syndrome. Pediatr Int 2001;43(6):567–576.

104. Rova M, Haataja R, Marttila R, et al. Data mining and multiparameter analysis of lung surfactant protein genes in bronchopulmonary dysplasia. Hum Mol Genet 2004;13(11):1095–1104.

105. Haataja R, Ramet M, Marttila R, et al. Surfactant proteins A and B as interactive genetic determinants of neonatal respiratory distress syndrome. Hum Mol Genet 2000;9(18): 2751–2760.

106. Ewis AA, Kondo K, Dang F, et al. Surfactant protein B gene variations and susceptibility to lung cancer in chromate workers. Am J Ind Med 2006;49(5):367–373.

107. Seifart C, Seifart U, Plagens A, et al. Surfactant protein B gene variations enhance susceptibility to squamous cell carcinoma of the lung in German patients. Br J Cancer 2002;87(2):212–217.

108. Lin Z, Thomas NJ, Wang Y, et al. Deletions within a CA-repeat–rich region of intron 4 of the human SP-B gene affect mRNA splicing. Biochem J 2005;389(Pt 2):403–412.

109. Marttila R, Haataja R, Ramet M, et al. Surfactant protein B polymorphism and respiratory distress syndrome in premature twins. Hum Genet 2003;112(1):18–23.

110. Selman M, Lin HM, Montano M, et al. Surfactant protein A and B genetic variants predispose to idiopathic pulmonary fibrosis. Hum Genet 2003;113(6):542–550.

111. Hamvas A, Nogee LM, Mallory GB, Jr., et al. Lung transplantation for treatment of infants with surfactant protein B deficiency. J Pediatr 1997;130(2):231–239.

112. Glasser SW, Korfhagen TR, Weaver TE, et al. cDNA, deduced polypeptide structure and chromosomal assignment of human pulmonary surfactant proteolipid, SPL(pVal). J Biol Chem 1988;263(1):9–12.

113. Conkright JJ, Bridges JP, Na CL, et al. Secretion of surfactant protein C, an integral membrane protein, requires the N-terminal propeptide. J Biol Chem 2001;276(18): 14658–14664.

114. Keller A, Eistetter HR, Voss T, et al. The pulmonary surfactant protein C (SP-C) precursor is a type II transmembrane protein. Biochem J 1991;277(Pt 2):493–499.

115. Curstedt T, Johansson J, Persson P, et al. Hydrophobic surfactant-associated polypeptides: SP-C is a lipopeptide with two palmitoylated cysteine residues, whereas SP-B lacks covalently linked fatty acyl groups. Proc Natl Acad Sci USA 1990;87(8):2985–2989.

116. Vorbroker DK, Dey C, Weaver TE, et al. Surfactant protein C precursor is palmitoylated and associates with subcellular membranes. Biochim Biophys Acta 1992;1105(1):161–169.

117. Sanchez-Pulido L, Devos D, Valencia A. BRICHOS: a conserved domain in proteins associated with dementia, respiratory distress and cancer. Trends Biochem Sci 2002; 27(7):329–332.

118. Beers MF, Mulugeta S. Surfactant protein C biosynthesis and its emerging role in conformational lung disease. Annu Rev Physiol 2005;67:663–696.

119. Glasser SW, Burhans MS, Eszterhas SK, et al. Human SP-C gene sequences that confer lung epithelium-specific expression in transgenic mice. Am J Physiol Lung Cell Mol Physiol 2000;278(5):L933–L9345.

120. Glasser SW, Eszterhas SK, Detmer EA, et al. The murine SP-C promoter directs type II cell-specific expression in transgenic mice. Am J Physiol Lung Cell Mol Physiol 2005;288(4):L625–L632.

121. Whitsett JA, Glasser SW, Tichelaar JW, et al. Transgenic models for study of lung morphogenesis and repair: Parker B. Francis lecture. Chest 2001;120(1 Suppl):27S–30S.

122. Nogee LM, Dunbar AE, 3rd, Wert S, et al. Mutations in the surfactant protein C gene associated with interstitial lung disease. Chest 2002;121(3 Suppl):20S–21S.

123. Soraisham AS, Tierney AJ, Amin HJ. Neonatal respiratory failure associated with mutation in the surfactant protein C gene. J Perinatol 2006;26(1):67–70.

124. Brasch F, Griese M, Tredano M, et al. Interstitial lung disease in a baby with a de novo mutation in the SFTPC gene. Eur Respir J 2004;24(1):30–39.

125. Cameron HS, Somaschini M, Carrera P, et al. A common mutation in the surfactant protein C gene associated with lung disease. J Pediatr 2005;146(3):370–375.

126. Hamvas A, Nogee LM, White FV, et al. Progressive lung disease and surfactant dysfunction with a deletion in surfactant protein C gene. Am J Respir Cell Mol Biol 2004;30(6):771–776.

127. Thomas AQ, Lane K, Phillips J, 3rd, et al. Heterozygosity for a surfactant protein C gene mutation associated with usual interstitial pneumonitis and cellular nonspecific interstitial pneumonitis in one kindred. Am J Respir Crit Care Med 2002;165(9):1322–1328.

128. Lawson WE, Grant SW, Ambrosini V, et al. Genetic mutations in surfactant protein C are a rare cause of sporadic cases of IPF. Thorax 2004;59(11):977–980.

129. Lahti M, Marttila R, Hallman M. Surfactant protein C gene variation in the Finnish population—association with perinatal respiratory disease. Eur J Hum Genet 2004; 12(4):312–320.

130. Setoguchi Y, Ikeda T, Fukuchi Y. Clinical features and genetic analysis of surfactant protein C in adult-onset familial interstitial pneumonia. Respirology 2006;11 (Suppl 1):S41–S45.

131. Nogee LM, Dunbar AE, 3rd, Wert SE, et al. A mutation in the surfactant protein C gene associated with familial interstitial lung disease. N Engl J Med 2001;344(8):573–579.

132. Tredano M, Griese M, Brasch F, et al. Mutation of SFTPC in infantile pulmonary alveolar proteinosis with or without fibrosing lung disease. Am J Med Genet A 2004;126(1):18–26.

133. Stevens PA, Pettenazzo A, Brasch F, et al. Nonspecific interstitial pneumonia, alveolar proteinosis, and abnormal proprotein trafficking resulting from a spontaneous mutation in the surfactant protein C gene. Pediatr Res 2005;57(1):89–98.

134. Bridges JP, Wert SE, Nogee LM, et al. Expression of a human surfactant protein C mutation associated with interstitial lung disease disrupts lung development in transgenic mice. J Biol Chem 2003;278(52):52739–52746.

135. Wang WJ, Russo SJ, Mulugeta S, et al. Biosynthesis of surfactant protein C (SP-C). Sorting of SP-C proprotein involves homomeric association via a signal anchor domain. J Biol Chem 2002;277(22):19929–199937.

136. Wang WJ, Mulugeta S, Russo SJ, et al. Deletion of exon 4 from human surfactant protein C results in aggresome formation and generation of a dominant negative. J Cell Sci 2003;116(Pt 4):683–692.

137. Glasser SW, Burhans MS, Korfhagen TR, et al. Altered stability of pulmonary surfactant in SP-C-deficient mice. Proc Natl Acad Sci USA 2001;98(11):6366–6371.

138. Glasser SW, Detmer EA, Ikegami M, et al. Pneumonitis and emphysema in sp-C gene targeted mice. J Biol Chem 2003;278(16):14291–14298.

139. Ikegami M, Weaver TE, Conkright JJ, et al. Deficiency of SP-B reveals protective role of SP-C during oxygen lung injury. J Appl Physiol 2002;92(2):519–526.

140. Augusto L, Le Blay K, Auger G, et al. Interaction of bacterial lipopolysaccharide with mouse surfactant protein C inserted into lipid vesicles. Am J Physiol Lung Cell Mol Physiol 2001;281(4):L776–L785.

141. Augusto LA, Li J, Synguelakis M, et al. Structural basis for interactions between lung surfactant protein C and bacterial lipopolysaccharide. J Biol Chem 2002;277(26):23484–23492.

142. Chaby R, Garcia-Verdugo I, Espinassous Q, et al. Interactions between LPS and lung surfactant proteins. J Endotoxin Res 2005;11(3):181–185.

143. Mulugeta S, Nguyen V, Russo SJ, et al. A surfactant protein C precursor protein BRICHOS domain mutation causes endoplasmic reticulum stress, proteasome dysfunction, and caspase 3 activation. Am J Respir Cell Mol Biol 2005;32(6):521–530.

144. Bridges JP, Xu Y, Na CL, et al. Adaptation and increased susceptibility to infection associated with constitutive expression of misfolded SP-C. J Cell Biol 2006;172(3):395–407.

145. Perlmutter DH. Chemical chaperones: a pharmacological strategy for disorders of protein folding and trafficking. Pediatr Res 2002;52(6):832–836.

146. Zeitlin PL, Gail DB, Banks-Schlegel S. Protein processing and degradation in pulmonary health and disease. Am J Respir Cell Mol Biol 2003;29(5):642–645.

147. Dean M, Hamon Y, Chimini G. The human ATP-binding cassette (ABC) transporter superfamily. J Lipid Res 2001;42(7):1007–1017.

148. Connors TD, Van Raay TJ, Petry LR, et al. The cloning of a human ABC gene (ABC3) mapping to chromosome 16p13.3. Genomics 1997;39(2):231–234.

149. Stefkova J, Poledne R, Hubacek JA. ATP-binding cassette (ABC) transporters in human metabolism and diseases. Physiol Res 2004;53(3):235–243.

150. Knight BL. ATP-binding cassette transporter A1: regulation of cholesterol efflux. Biochem Soc Trans 2004;32(Pt 1):124–127.

151. Brasch F, Schimanski S, Muhlfeld C, et al. Alteration of the pulmonary surfactant system in full-term infants with hereditary ABCA3 deficiency. Am J Respir Crit Care Med 2006;174(5):571–580.

152. Garmany TH, Moxley MA, White FV, et al. Surfactant composition and function in patients with ABCA3 mutations. Pediatr Res 2006;59(6):801–805.

153. Bullard JE, Wert SE, Whitsett JA, et al. ABCA3 Mutations Associated with Pediatric Interstitial Lung Disease. Am J Respir Crit Care Med 2005;172(8):1026–1031.

154. Cheong N, Madesh M, Gonzales LW, et al. Functional and trafficking defects in ATP binding cassette A3 mutants associated with respiratory distress syndrome. J Biol Chem 2006;281(14):9791–9800.

155. Matsumura Y, Ban N, Ueda K, Inagaki N. Characterization and classification of ATP-binding cassette transporter ABCA3 mutants in fatal surfactant deficiency. J Biol Chem 2006;281(45):34503–34514.

156. Trapnell BC, Whitsett JA, Nakata K. Pulmonary alveolar proteinosis. N Engl J Med 2003;349(26):2527–2539.

157. Dinwiddie R, Sharief N, Crawford O. Idiopathic interstitial pneumonitis in children: a national survey in the United Kingdom and Ireland. Pediatr Pulmonol 2002;34(1):23–29.

158. Sharief N, Crawford OF, Dinwiddie R. Fibrosing alveolitis and desquamative interstitial pneumonitis. Pediatr Pulmonol 1994;17(6):359–365.

159. Katzenstein AL, Gordon LP, Oliphant M, et al. Chronic pneumonitis of infancy. A unique form of interstitial lung disease occurring in early childhood. Am J Surg Pathol 1995;19(4):439–447.

160. Deterding R, Fan LL. Surfactant dysfunction mutations in children's interstitial lung disease and beyond. Am J Respir Crit Care Med 2005;172(8):940–941.

161. Amin RS, Wert SE, Baughman RP, et al. Surfactant protein deficiency in familial interstitial lung disease. J Pediatr 2001;139(1):85–92.

162. deMello DE, Heyman S, Phelps DS, et al. Ultrastructure of lung in surfactant protein B deficiency. Am J Respir Cell Mol Biol 1994;11(2):230–239.

163. Edwards V, Cutz E, Viero S, et al. Ultrastructure of lamellar bodies in congenital surfactant deficiency. Ultrastruct Pathol 2005;29(6):503–509.

164. Cutz E, Wert SE, Nogee LM, et al. Deficiency of lamellar bodies in alveolar type II cells associated with fatal respiratory disease in a full-term infant. Am J Respir Crit Care Med 2000;161(2 Pt 1):608–614.

165. Tryka AF, Wert SE, Mazursky JE, et al. Absence of lamellar bodies with accumulation of dense bodies characterizes a novel form of congenital surfactant defect. Pediatr Dev Pathol 2000;3(4):335–345.

166. Langston C, Patterson K, Dishop MK, et al. A protocol for the handling of tissue obtained by operative lung biopsy: recommendations of the chILD pathology cooperative group. Pediatr Dev Pathol 2006;9(3):173–180.

167. Dirksen U, Nishinakamura R, Groneck P, et al. Human pulmonary alveolar proteinosis associated with a defect in GM-CSF/IL-3/IL-5 receptor common beta chain expression. J Clin Invest 1997;100(9):2211–2217.

168. Robb L, Drinkwater CC, Metcalf D, et al. Hematopoietic and lung abnormalities in mice with a null mutation of the common beta subunit of the receptors for granulocyte-macrophage colony-stimulating factor and interleukins 3 and 5. Proc Natl Acad Sci USA 1995;92(21):9565–9569.

169. Nishinakamura R, Nakayama N, Hirabayashi Y, et al. Mice deficient for the IL-3/GM-CSF/IL-5 beta c receptor exhibit lung pathology and impaired immune response, while beta IL3 receptor-deficient mice are normal. Immunity 1995;2(3):211–222.

170. Stanley E, Lieschke GJ, Grail D, et al. Granulocyte/macrophage colony-stimulating factor–deficient mice show no major perturbation of hematopoiesis but develop a characteristic pulmonary pathology. Proc Natl Acad Sci USA 1994;91(12):5592–5596.

171. Dranoff G, Crawford AD, Sadelain M, et al. Involvement of granulocyte-macrophage colony-stimulating factor in pulmonary homeostasis. Science 1994;264(5159):713–716.

172. Krude H, Schutz B, Biebermann H, et al. Choreoathetosis, hypothyroidism, and pulmonary alterations due to human NKX2-1 haploinsufficiency. J Clin Invest 2002;109(4):475–480.

173. Pohlenz J, Dumitrescu A, Zundel D, et al. Partial deficiency of thyroid transcription factor 1 produces predominantly neurological defects in humans and mice. J Clin Invest 2002;109(4):469–473.

174. Iwatani N, Mabe H, Devriendt K, et al. Deletion of NKX2.1 gene encoding thyroid transcription factor-1 in two siblings with hypothyroidism and respiratory failure. J Pediatr 2000;137(2):272–276.

175. Devriendt K, Vanhole C, Matthijs G, et al. Deletion of thyroid transcription factor-1 gene in an infant with neonatal thyroid dysfunction and respiratory failure. N Engl J Med 1998;338(18):1317–1318.

176. Moya CM, Perez de Nanclares G, Castano L, et al. Functional study of a novel single deletion in the TITF1/NKX2.1 homeobox gene that produces congenital hypothyroidism and benign chorea but not pulmonary distress. J Clin Endocrinol Metab 2006;91(5):1832–1841.

177. Rosen SH, Castleman B, Liebow AA. Pulmonary alveolar proteinosis. N Engl J Med 1958;258(23):1123–1142.

178. Seymour JF, Presneill JJ. Pulmonary alveolar proteinosis: progress in the first 44 years. Am J Respir Crit Care Med 2002;166(2):215–235.

179. Kogishi K, Kurozumi M, Fujita Y, et al. Isolation and partial characterization of human low molecular weight protein associated with pulmonary surfactant. Am Rev Respir Dis 1988;137(6):1426–1431.

180. Strong P, Kishore U, Morgan C, et al. A novel method of purifying lung surfactant proteins A and D from the lung lavage of alveolar proteinosis patients and from pooled amniotic fluid. J Immunol Methods 1998;220(1–2):139–149.

181. Bonfield TL, Russell D, Burgess S, et al. Autoantibodies against granulocyte macrophage colony-stimulating factor are diagnostic for pulmonary alveolar proteinosis. Am J Respir Cell Mol Biol 2002;27(4):481–486.

182. Kitamura T, Uchida K, Tanaka N, et al. Serological diagnosis of idiopathic pulmonary alveolar proteinosis. Am J Respir Crit Care Med 2000;162(2 Pt 1):658–662.

183. Kitamura T, Tanaka N, Watanabe J, et al. Idiopathic pulmonary alveolar proteinosis as an autoimmune disease with neutralizing antibody against granulocyte/macrophage colony-stimulating factor. J Exp Med 1999;190(6):875–880.

184. Borsani G, Bassi MT, Sperandeo MP, et al. SLC7A7, encoding a putative permease-related protein, is mutated in patients with lysinuric protein intolerance. Nat Genet 1999;21(3):297–301.

185. Sperandeo MP, Bassi MT, Riboni M, et al. Structure of the SLC7A7 gene and mutational analysis of patients affected by lysinuric protein intolerance. Am J Hum Genet 2000;66(1):92–99.

55
Usual Interstitial Pneumonia

Marco Chilosi, Bruno Murer, and Venerino Poletti

Introduction

Idiopathic pulmonary fibrosis (IPF), the most common and severe among idiopathic interstitial pneumonias, has now been definitively recognized as a distinct clinical entity, defined in the American Thoracic Society/European Respiratory Society (ATS/ERS) consensus statement as a specific form of chronic fibrosing interstitial pneumonia limited to the lung and associated with the histologic appearance of usual interstitial pneumonia (UIP) in surgical lung biopsy material.[1–3] Thus, the precise definition of the "UIP" pattern is crucial for the diagnosis of IPF when histology is available and also for the understanding of the specific changes characterizing this devastating disease. The morphologic criteria for defining the UIP pattern have been progressively refined, from the seminal studies of Liebow to the recent ATS/ERS classification. It is worth noting that the different morphologic patterns that characterize the idiopathic interstitial pneumonias—UIP, nonspecific interstitial pneumonia (NSIP), acute interstitial pneumonia (AIP), cryptogenic organizing pneumonia (COP), lymphocytic interstitial pneumonia (LIP), desquamative interstitial pneumonia (DIP), and respiratory bronchiolitis–combined interstitial lung disease (RB-ILD)—have been progressively defined following a process of matching the clinical, radiologic, and morphologic features, using varying terms and criteria, in the absence of a precise knowledge of the etiology and pathogenesis of the different diseases.

Because this complex process is still ongoing, it is reasonable to think that diagnostic criteria should be constantly reevaluated in the light of the knowledge provided by new technologies. In fact, although the classic morphologic criteria are widely applied, and in most cases can provide correct diagnostic evaluations in interstitial lung diseases, problems still remain in a substantial number of cases. The principal areas of diagnostic uncertainty occur in the differential diagnosis of the UIP pattern versus other chronic lung diseases, including NSIP (especially

fibrosing NSIP), fibrosis associated with collagen-vascular diseases (CVD), and more rarely, COP, chronic hypersensitivity pneumonitis, and pulmonary Langerhans cell histiocytosis. Although the histologic patterns among idiopathic interstitial pneumonias have been well established in consensus classifications on the basis of several notable differences, diagnostic confidence levels are variable. According to several studies, a full diagnostic agreement is not reached even among expert lung pathologists, and it is highly probable that the interobserver variabilities in pathologic interpretations among general pathologists is higher.[4] The introduction of new therapeutic strategies for IPF, a disorder that still remains a deadly disease, adds a further level of complexity and new needs in diagnostic approaches. Some data provided by the results of clinical trials using interferon (IFN)-γ for IPF suggest that this therapy can be more beneficial and less harmful when patients are treated in earlier stages of the disease.[5] This means that establishing early diagnosis could become a crucial need and that radiologists and pathologists will be requested to improve their diagnostic criteria. We hypothesize that new information regarding the pathogenesis of IIP, and in particular IPF/UIP, can potentially provide new insights into the mechanisms leading to lung tissue effacement and remodeling. New information could also be relevant for developing new therapeutic strategies and new morphologic and molecular markers for improving the diagnostic yield of histologic data.

Pathogenesis

Although the etiology of IPF still remains elusive, a growing body of evidence suggests new concepts in its biology and pathogenesis. It is now clear that inflammation does not play a major role, as previously hypothesized, and that central to the development of the disease is a sequential epithelial cell injury, followed by deranged regeneration of parenchymal tissue and abnormal activation of reparative processes.[6-10] According to this alternative pathogenic route, abnormally increased, although focally distributed, epithelial cell loss and dysfunctional epithelial repair characterize the UIP pattern in IPF at variance with other interstitial pneumonias in which inflammatory responses are the crucial pathogenic events triggering the fibrogenic process. The mechanisms leading to epithelial damage in IPF are currently unknown, as is the etiology of this disease.

Some data suggest that in IPF abnormal reepithelialization after injury can be caused by cellular defects related to either a predisposing genetic background (familial IPF is a well recognized entity) or to the aging-related accumulation of metabolic alterations (e.g., due to toxic effects of smoking, pollution, or other causes). In this scheme, IPF could be then considered within the spectrum of dysplastic/neoplastic disorders. Accordingly, IPF is typically a disease of advanced age, there is increased risk for IPF in smokers and in people exposed to other toxic substances, IPF is complicated at exceeding frequency by epithelial malignancies, and molecular abnormalities at loci associated to lung cancer are frequent.[11-16] Surfactant protein A and B genetic variants predispose to pulmonary fibrosis, and an association with surfactant protein C has been found in familial IPF that is not common in sporadic cases.[17-19] Oncogenic viruses are very appealing as causative agents, because they may provide both direct and indirect mechanisms of abnormal cell behavior. Among these, Epstein-Barr and human herpesvirus 8 viruses have been investigated as possible causative agents of IPF/UIP with contrasting results.[20-22]

DNA Microarray Studies

Microarray technology allows the simultaneous evaluation of the expression of thousands of genes, thus providing a widespread molecular profile of pathologic tissue samples. A large number of tumors have been investigated with this technique, defining distinct aberrant profiles of neoplastic cells. The same approach has recently been applied to a few seminal studies aimed at defining the expression profile of IPF compared with normal lung and other interstitial lung diseases.[23-25] This powerful approach is extremely promising for understanding the pathogenesis of IPF and for detecting new diagnostic markers.

As elegantly shown in these studies, gene expression patterns can in fact clearly distinguish between IPF/UIP and normal samples. Among the genes that are increased in fibrotic lungs, matrilysin (matrix metalloproteinase-7 [MMP-7]) was the most informative increased gene; this was confirmed in situ by immunohistochemistry in UIP samples.[26] Selman and coworkers have clearly demon-

strated that the gene expression signatures of UIP and hypersensitivity pneumonitis are significantly different.[24] The IPF signature was characterized by the absence of proinflammatory genes and by the expression of a series of genes involved in active tissue remodeling, and it was fully consistent with the pathogenic model based on an epithelial/fibroblastic pathway. Accordingly, several epithelial-related genes were among those upregulated in IPF, including genes related to epithelial cell growth, differentiation, and adhesion/migration (those for keratins 6 and 8, mucin 6, stratifin, N-cadherin, as well as a number of target genes of the canonical Wingless (Wnt)/β-catenin pathway such as *MMP-7* and that for osteopontin). Genes related to tissue fibrogenesis were also upregulated in IPF, including various collagen peptides, tenascin, versican, and asporin. On the other hand, the hypersensitivity pneumonitis signature was enriched for genes related to inflammation, T-cell activation, and immune response. Interestingly, hypersensitivity pneumonitis and IPF gene expression signatures were able to identify subgroups of NSIP, thus potentially providing a more consistent basis to classify interstitial lung diseases and to improve the diagnostic assignment of difficult cases.

Molecular Pathways Involved in Alveolar Damage and Reepithelialization

Alveolar epithelium is generally considered to represent a major target of injury in UIP, where alveolar gas exchange units are progressively substituted by dense fibrosis. Occurrence of pneumocyte apoptosis and increased expression of molecular pathways involved in cell death and apoptosis have been demonstrated in IPF/UIP.[27-29] Nevertheless, evidence of alveolar damage and repair is typically focal in UIP samples, and the presence of normal or minimally affected alveolar tissue is a major morphologic feature of the UIP pattern.[2,3] On the other hand, pneumocyte loss following alveolar damage is a common feature in most, if not all, interstitial lung diseases, and the limited involvement of alveolar epithelium that gives the patchy appearance characterizing UIP can hardly explain by itself the rapid and irreversible evolution of IPF.

The damage and regeneration of alveolar epithelium involves a variety of complex molecular and cellular mechanisms, including programmed-cell death (apoptosis), cell proliferation, cell migration, and also epithelial–mesenchymal transition (EMT).[30] The presence of microscopic areas of epithelial cell dropout, typically observed in IPF, is considered as a consequence of focal pneumocyte death, and activation of the proapoptotic p53 pathway has been involved in this finding. Increased expressions of p53 and regulatory proteins p21[WAF1] and MDM2 are in fact observed in IPF at sites of pneumocyte hyperplasia cannot be considered as specific features of IPF because similar findings occur in AIP/diffuse alveolar damage (DAD), NSIP, organizing pneumonia (OP), and asbestosis.[16,31–33] A direct confirmation is further provided by global analysis of gene expression on experimental pulmonary fibrosis where *GADD45* and *p21[WAF1]* are among the few genes induced early by bleomycin.[34]

The Wnt/β-catenin pathway is activated in pneumocytes in IPF samples as evidenced by the nuclear localization of β-catenin (Figure 55.1) and up-modulation of target genes such as *cyclin D1*, *MMP-7*, osteopontin *(SPP1)*, *c-Myc*, and others.[23,26] Nevertheless, nuclear localization of β-catenin in pneumocytes is a feature that can be observed in a variety of lung diseases, including AIP/DAD (see Figure 55.1), COP/OP, and NSIP, and cannot be considered a specific pathogenic mechanism

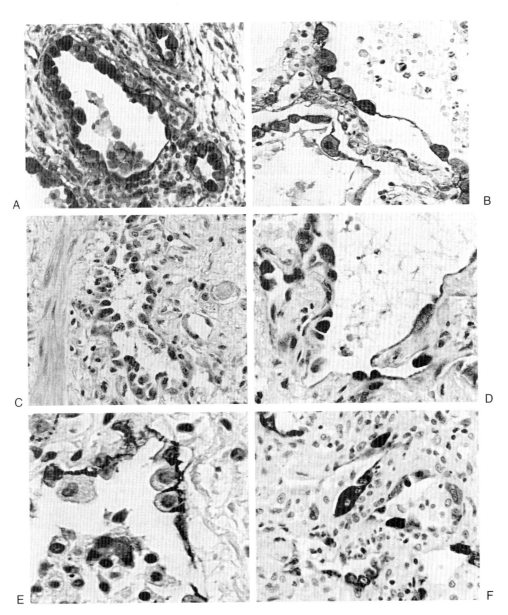

FIGURE 55.1. Hyperplastic pneumocytes in both idiopathic pulmonary fibrosis (IPF) and diffuse alveolar damage (DAD) are characterized by molecular changes suggestive of Wnt pathway activation and epithelial–mesenchymal transition (EMT), including β-catenin nuclear localization (**A**, IPF; **B**, DAD) and high levels of slug, a transcription factor involved in EMT (**C**, IPF; **D**, DAD). Hyperplastic pneumocytes in DAD also express decreased levels of E-cadherin (**E**) and increased levels of laminin-5 γ₂-chain (**F**).

for IPF/UIP. The activation of the Wnt signaling pathway is in fact involved in physiologic repair mechanisms of damaged alveoli, and activation of the Wnt pathway is crucial in the regulation of the proximal–distal patterning in the lung during embryonal life, where it is central for the correct formation of alveolar tissue but not for bronchiolar development and branching.[35] The precise tuning of the Wnt/β-catenin pathway is so crucial that when aberrantly expressed it severely modifies the histogenetic program of pulmonary epithelial development. In fact, high levels of Wnt pathway activity in embryonic lung progenitor cells expressing a lung-specific gene (SFTPC) lead to the generation of intestinal progenitors that subsequently give rise to multiple intestinal and gut cell types.[36] Epithelial mesenchymal transition is one of the most intriguing functions triggered by β-catenin transactivation,[37] and evidence has been recently provided of EMT involvement in fibrosis related to regeneration of alveolar tissue in IPF.[38] The pathogenic specificity of this phenomenon is nevertheless questionable, because EMT activation may represent an intrinsic mechanism involved in alveolar regeneration, as suggested by different experimental studies.[30,39] In line with this view are the recent data of our group, demonstrating that hyperplastic pneumocytes in AIP/DAD, IPF/UIP, and NSIP are able to express an EMT phenotype, as defined by the down-modulation of E-cadherin, as well as by the up-modulation of slug, a transcription factor involved in EMT triggering (Chilosi et al., unpublished data; see also Figure 55.1).[40,41]

A potential molecular trigger of progressive pneumocyte depletion that can be taken into account in this scheme is c-Myc, a downstream target of Wnt/β-catenin activation. The β-catenin/T-cell factor complex is the master switch that controls proliferation versus differentiation, and c-Myc is one of its most relevant mediators.[42,43] It is possible to speculate that in IPF/UIP, at sites where abnormal levels of β-catenin, and hence c-Myc, are expressed, migrating bronchiolar cells could behave as supercompetitors.[43]

Molecular Characterization of Fibroblast Foci

If the molecular mechanisms involved in pneumocyte regeneration are not apparently aberrant, the peculiarity of the alveolar loss in IPF/UIP may be more likely centered on the overwhelming fibrotic process. Damaged epithelial cells can produce factors stimulating fibroblast migration, proliferation, and differentiation into contractile myofibroblasts. Evidence of this tissue reaction is observed in a variety of diseases, in particular in AIP/ DAD, where myofibroblast accumulate along interstitial alveolar walls, and in COP/OP, where polypoid aggregates of myofibroblasts obliterate the alveolar lumina. In IPF/UIP the fibrotic reaction is distinctive, because discrete collections of myofibroblasts, generally known as *fibroblast foci*, are scattered at the borders between normal and dense scar tissue. Fibroblast foci are considered a key element for defining the UIP pattern, because they give the appearance of *temporal* heterogeneity and represent the leading edge of ongoing lung injury and abnormal repair. The fibroblast foci in UIP are similar to those observed in organizing pneumonia (the so-called Masson's body) but have a different location (interstitial/ intramural versus intraalveolar) and biologic features, such as the absence of blood vessels and inflammatory cells.[44] Fibroblast foci occur in the majority of UIP samples, and their frequency seems to be related to disease severity and prognosis.[11,45]

A number of studies have focused on the molecular characterization of myofibroblasts in UIP FF, searching for abnormalities justifying the increased proliferation and/or decreased apoptotic clearance of these cells. Accordingly, increased numbers of proliferating cells, as defined by Ki-67 immunostaining, occur in FF of UIP, together with elevated expression of TIMP-2, a member of tissue inhibitors of metalloproteinases.[46] Abnormal nuclear accumulation of β-catenin is observed in FF of UIP, at variance with OP.[26] This finding is part of the activation of the Wnt pathway in UIP described before, and transactivation of antiapoptotic and/or proproliferative β-catenin target genes could be implicated in the abnormal persistence of FF in UIP.

Another recent finding characterizing the myofibroblasts forming FF in patients with IPF is the lack of Thy-1 expression, at variance with normal lung fibroblasts, which are predominantly Thy-1 positive.[47] Further information can be obtained from in vitro studies investigating the molecular features of lung fibroblasts. A recent study comparing normal lung fibroblasts and fibroblasts obtained from patients with IPF showed a switch in responsiveness to interleukin-6, corresponding to a shift from signal transducer and activator of transcription 3–dependent to extracellular signal-regulated kinase (ERK)–dependent signaling in IPF [48]. Interestingly, the ERK-pathway is activated by the Wnt/β-catenin pathway in fibroblasts, providing for them a significant proliferative advantage.[49] Functional abnormalities of IPF fibroblasts can be involved in the abnormal regeneration of pneumocytes, thus contributing to the progressive alveolar loss observed in this disease, as elegantly shown in a recent study demonstrating that the basal hepatocyte growth factor secretion by IPF fibroblasts is decreased by 50% when compared with control fibroblasts.[50]

Molecular Pathways Involved in Bronchiolar Reepithelialization

The epithelial cells overlying fibroblast foci of UIP have been described as "cuboidal" epithelial cells of undetermined nature. These epithelial cells, which likely represent target cells in the injury–repair sequence occurring in IPF, have been recognized as either alveolar or bronchiolar in different studies.[2] As determined with immunophenotypic analysis, the majority of FF are covered by bronchiolar epithelium,[26,33,51] and honeycomb cysts frequently have myofibroblast collections resembling FF in their wall (Figure 55.2).

Honeycombing is a major feature of the UIP pattern, although it is not specific for this disease. The cysts as

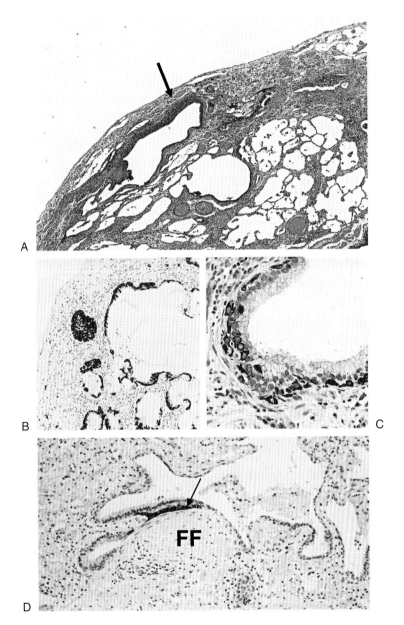

FIGURE 55.2. Evidence of bronchiolar involvement and molecular abnormalities characterizing bronchiolar lesions in idiopathic pulmonary fibrosis/usual interstitial pneumonia. **(A)** Areas of dense fibrosis, large portions of spared alveolated tissue, and honeycomb cysts lined by bronchiolar epithelium are present. (Hematoxylin and eosin stain.) Note a peripheral dilated bronchiolar honeycomb lesion with a large fibroblast focus in its wall (arrow). **(B)** Cytokeratin-5 highlights the basal cell proliferation in a honeycomb zone. **(C)** Abnormally elevated expression of matrix metalloproteinase-7/matrilysin in an enlarged bronchiole. **(D)** A sandwich focus, characterized by strong expression of laminin-5 γ_2-chain, in basal cells overlying a fibroblast focus (FF) within an area of microscopic honeycombing (arrow).

recognized on high-resolution computed tomography slides correspond to lesions of different types when observed at the microscopic level, where three different types of honeycomb lesions can be recognized: (1) those formed by large emphysematous spaces (lined by alveolar epithelium) surrounded by dense collagen scarring; (2) cysts formed by large dilated bronchiolar structures; and (3) areas of dense fibrosis including irregular bronchiolar structures, frequently filled by mucus, and showing features of hyperplasia and bronchiolization (so-called microscopic honeycombing). The latter type of honeycomb cyst is in most instances peripheral and appears early in the evolution of the disease. These lesions are in our view the most typical type of honeycombing observed in IPF/UIP.

In a pathogenic model of IPF, we hypothesized that bronchiolar epithelium is a major target of injury and abnormal repair and that this abnormal bronchiolar regeneration can play a central role in triggering abnormal mesenchymal accumulation and tissue remodeling that progressively obliterate contiguous alveolar parenchyma.[51] This view is in line with the frequent occurrence of bronchiolar lesions, encompassing basal cell hyperplasia, bronchiolization, squamous metaplasia and atypia.[33,51] In a proportion of cases of IPF/UIP, the bronchiolar changes are so prominent that they mimic an epithelial neoplasm. In IPF/UIP, aberrant accumulation of mesenchymal tissue, including smooth muscle cells, newly formed blood vessels, and dense fibrous tissue, are spa-

tially related to bronchiolar proliferative lesions and honeycombing.[51] Interestingly, the molecular abnormalities occurring in bronchiolar proliferative lesions are all centered on basal cells, which are characterized by abnormal activation of the Wnt/β-catenin pathway, as evidenced by the expression of nuclear β-catenin, cyclin D1, and MMP-7/matrilysin (Figure 55.2).[26] This observation is relevant because basal cells are stem cells involved in the renewal of airway epithelium,[52] and in physiologic conditions they do not express significant levels of these molecules.[26]

As for other stratified epithelia, basal cells express a defined molecular repertoire, involved in the anchorage and survival within their stem cell niches, including the antiapoptotic ΔN-p63 truncated isoform of the p63 gene [53]. This interesting molecular species is able to antagonize the transactivating functions of p53, and p63 gene amplification is involved in the pathogenesis of squamous carcinomas.[54,55] In addition, ΔN-p63 represents an highly specific marker of bronchiolar basal cells, thus allowing the precise detection of these cells on tissue.

Molecular Characterization of Epithelial Cells in Fibroblast Foci

In a recent study we investigated the functional profile of bronchiolar lesions of IPF/UIP by analyzing the expression of molecules involved in cell motility and invasiveness, including laminin-5 γ2-chain (LAM5γ2), fascin, and

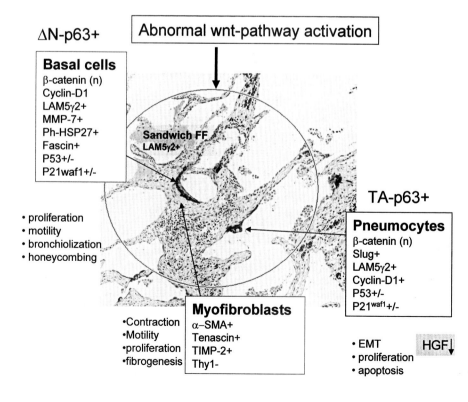

FIGURE 55.3. Hypothetical pathogenic model focused on the abnormal "field" expression of the Wingless (Wnt) signaling pathway centered on bronchoalveolar junctions. A sandwich fibroblast focus (FF) is shown in the center, characterized by abnormal expression of laminin-5 γ2-chain (LAMγ2) in basal cells. The various molecular species described in this review are assigned to different cell compartments, with special emphasis on target molecules of the Wnt pathway involved in cell proliferation and motility. EMT, epithelial–mesenchymal transition; HGF, hepatocyte growth factor; MMP, matrix metalloproteinase; SMA, smooth muscle actin; TIMP, tissue inhibitor of matrix metalloproteinase.

phosphorylated heat shock protein 27 (Hsp27).[56] These molecules were expressed in bronchiolar basal cells overlying fibroblast foci in virtually all investigated UIP samples (28/30 cases). The relevance of this finding is related to the specific functions of the investigated molecules, as well as the peculiar tissue localization of their abnormal expression. Heat shock protein 27 is a small molecule rapidly induced and phosphorylated by heat shock and other stressing agents and behaves as an actin-capping protein interfering with its polymerization, thus regulating cell adhesion and motility under the control of p38 mitogen-activated protein kinase. In addition, Hsp27 can mediate resistance against cell death induced by stress and differentiation, preventing apoptosis by blocking interactions of Daxx with Ask-1 and Fas.[57] The trimeric protein laminin-5 ($\alpha_3\beta_3\gamma_2$-chain) is an integral part of the basal lamina of stratified epithelia where it plays a crucial role in the organization of the basal stem cell niche by providing epithelial–mesenchymal connections by interacting with $\alpha_6\beta_4$-integrin.[58] These interactions are critical for regulating cell migration, an event required in different processes, such as wound healing, embryogenesis, and metastatic dissemination.[59,60]

The γ_2-chain of laminin-5 is induced by β-catenin and acts as a soluble cell motility factor in a variety of conditions after its cleaving by metalloproteinases.[61,62] The enhanced expression of LAM5γ_2 is considered one of the best markers of invasiveness in different carcinomas.[62,63] Laminin-5 γ_2-chain, is considered a reliable marker of reepithelialization, and type II hyperplastic pneumocytes focally express this molecule in all diseases where in which regeneration takes place, including COP/OP and IPF/UIP[64] and especially AIP/DAD (see Figure 55.1).[56] Within the fibroblast foci, the LAM5γ_2-positive cells appeared as wedged between luminal epithelial cells and myofibroblasts, forming peculiar negative-positive-negative three-layered lesions (which we named *sandwich fibroblast foci*; see Figures 55.2 and 55.3). According to this study, the "sandwich foci" appear specific for IPF/UIP, because similar lesions were extremely rare in a large variety of control samples, including NSIP, DIP, CVD, hypersensitivity pneumonia, Langerhans cell histiocytosis, COP, AIP, acute eosinophilic pneumonia, airway-centered interstitial fibrosis, and others. Interestingly, these fibroblast foci were often located at the bronchoalveolar junction. This microenvironmental compartment represents a complex stem cell niche homing different multipotent progenitors,[52] and aberrant stimulation of this compartment in IPF could be involved in the abnormal remodeling process.

References

1. American Thoracic Society/European Respiratory Society International Multidisciplinary Consensus Classification of the Idiopathic Interstitial Pneumonias. This joint statement of the American Thoracic Society (ATS), and the European Respiratory Society (ERS) was adopted by the ATS board of directors, June 2001 and by the ERS Executive Committee, June 2001. Am J Respir Crit Care Med 2002;165:277–304.

2. Katzenstein AL, Myers JL. Idiopathic pulmonary fibrosis: clinical relevance of pathologic classification. Am J Respir Crit Care Med 1998;157:1301–1315.

3. American Thoracic Society. Idiopathic pulmonary fibrosis: diagnosis and treatment. International consensus statement. American Thoracic Society (ATS), and the European Respiratory Society (ERS). Am J Respir Crit Care Med 2000;161:646–664.

4. Nicholson AG, Addis BJ, Bharucha H, et al. Inter-observer variation between pathologists in diffuse parenchymal lung disease. Thorax 2004;59:500–505.

5. Selman M. A dark side of interferon-gamma in the treatment of idiopathic pulmonary fibrosis? Am J Respir Crit Care Med 2003;167:945–946.

6. Selman M, King TE, Pardo A. Idiopathic pulmonary fibrosis: prevailing and evolving hypotheses about its pathogenesis and implications for therapy. Ann Intern Med 2001;134:136–151.

7. Selman M, Pardo A. Idiopathic pulmonary fibrosis: misunderstandings between epithelial cells and fibroblasts? Sarcoidosis Vasc Diffuse Lung Dis 2004;21:165–172.

8. Selman M, Pardo A. The epithelial/fibroblastic pathway in the pathogenesis of idiopathic pulmonary fibrosis. Am J Respir Cell Mol Biol 2003;29(3 Suppl):S93–S97.

9. Gauldie J, Kolb M, Sime PJ. A new direction in the pathogenesis of idiopathic pulmonary fibrosis? Respir Res 2002; 3:1.

10. Noble PW, Homer RJ. Back to the future: historical perspective on the pathogenesis of idiopathic pulmonary fibrosis. Am J Respir Cell Mol Biol 2005;33:113–120.

11. King TE Jr. Clinical advances in the diagnosis and therapy of the interstitial lung diseases. Am J Respir Crit Care Med 2005;172:268–279.

12. Baumgartner KB, Samet JM, Stidley CA, et al. Cigarette smoking: a risk factor for idiopathic pulmonary fibrosis. Am J Respir Crit Care Med 1997;155:242–248.

13. Aubry MC, Myers JL, Douglas WW, et al. Primary pulmonary carcinoma in patients with idiopathic pulmonary fibrosis. Mayo Clin Proc 2002;77:763–770.

14. Mori M, Kida H, Morishita H, et al. Microsatellite instability in transforming growth factor-beta 1 type II receptor gene in alveolar lining epithelial cells of idiopathic pulmonary fibrosis. Am J Respir Cell Mol Biol 2001;24:398–404.

15. Kawasaki H, Ogura T, Yokose T, et al. p53 gene alteration in atypical epithelial lesions and carcinoma in patients with idiopathic pulmonary fibrosis. Hum Pathol 2001;32:1043–1049.

16. Kuwano K, Kunitake R, Kawasaki M, et al. P21Waf1/Cip1/Sdi1 and p53 expression in association with DNA strand breaks in idiopathic pulmonary fibrosis. Am J Respir Crit Care Med 1996;154:477–483.

17. Selman M, Lin HM, Montano M, et al. Surfactant protein A and B genetic variants predispose to IPF. Hum Genet 2003;113:542–550.

18. Chibbar R, Shih F, Baga M, et al. Nonspecific interstitial pneumonia and usual interstitial pneumonia with mutation in surfactant protein C in familial pulmonary fibrosis. Mod Pathol 2004;17:973–980.

19. Lawson WE, Grant SW, Ambrosini V, et al. Genetic mutations in surfactant protein C are a rare cause of sporadic cases of IPF. Thorax 2004;59:977–980.

20. Tang YW, Johnson JE, Browning PJ, et al. Herpesvirus DNA is consistently detected in lungs of patients with IPF. J Clin Microbiol 2003;41:2633–2640.

21. Vergnon JM, Vincent M, de The G, et al. Cryptogenic fibrosing alveolitis and Epstein-Barr virus: an association? Lancet 1984;2:768–771.

22. Zamo A, Poletti V, Reghellin D, et al. HHV-8 and EBV are not commonly found in IPF. Sarcoidosis Vasc Diffuse Lung Dis 2005;22:123–128.

23. Zuo F, Kaminski N, Eugui E, et al. Gene expression analysis reveals matrilysin as a key regulator of pulmonary fibrosis in mice and humans. Proc Natl Acad Sci USA 2002;99:6292–6297.

24. Selman M, Pardo A, Barrera L, et al. Gene expression profiles distinguish idiopathic pulmonary fibrosis from hypersensitivity pneumonitis. Am J Respir Crit Care Med 2006;173:188–198.

25. Pardo A, Gibson K, Cisneros J, et al. Up-regulation and profibrotic role of osteopontin in human IPF. PLoS Med 2005;2:e251.

26. Chilosi M, Poletti V, Zamo A, et al. Aberrant Wnt/beta-catenin pathway activation in IPF. Am J Pathol 2003;162:1495–1502.

27. Maeyama T, Kuwano K, Kawasaki M, et al. Upregulation of Fas-signalling molecules in lung epithelial cells from patients with idiopathic pulmonary fibrosis. Eur Respir J 2001;17:180–189.

28. Kuwano K, Hagimoto N, Maeyama T, et al. Mitochondria-mediated apoptosis of lung epithelial cells in idiopathic interstitial pneumonias. Lab Invest 2002;82:1695–1706.

29. Plataki M, Koutsopoulos AV, Darivianaki K, et al. Expression of apoptotic and antiapoptotic markers in epithelial cells in idiopathic pulmonary fibrosis. Chest 2005;127:266–274.

30. Kasai H, Allen JT, Mason RM, et al. TGF-beta1 induces human alveolar epithelial to mesenchymal cell transition (EMT). Respir Res 2005;6:56.

31. Nakashima N, Kuwano K, Maeyama T, et al. The p53-Mdm2 association in epithelial cells in idiopathic pulmonary fibrosis and non-specific interstitial pneumonia. J Clin Pathol 2005;58:583–589.

32. Panduri V, Surapureddi S, Soberanes S, et al. P53 mediates amosite asbestos-induced alveolar epithelial cell mitochondria-regulated apoptosis. Am J Respir Cell Mol Biol 2006;34:443–452.

33. Chilosi M, Poletti V, Murer B, et al. Abnormal re-epithelialization and lung remodeling in idiopathic pulmonary fibrosis: the role of deltaN-p63. Lab Invest. 2002;82:1335–1345.

34. Kaminski N, Allard JD, Pittet JF, et al. Global analysis of gene expression in pulmonary fibrosis reveals distinct programs regulating lung inflammation and fibrosis. Proc Natl Acad Sci USA 2000;97:1778–1783.

35. Mucenski ML, Wert SE, Nation JM, et al. beta-Catenin is required for specification of proximal/distal cell fate during lung morphogenesis. J Biol Chem 2003;278:40231–40238.

36. Okubo T, Hogan BL. Hyperactive Wnt signaling changes the developmental potential of embryonic lung endoderm. J Biol 2004;3:11.

37. Kim K, Lu Z, Hay ED. Direct evidence for a role of beta-catenin/LEF-1 signaling pathway in induction of EMT. Cell Biol Int 2002;26:463–476.

38. Willis BC, Liebler JM, Luby-Phelps K, et al. Induction of epithelial–mesenchymal transition in alveolar epithelial cells by transforming growth factor-beta1: potential role in idiopathic pulmonary fibrosis. Am J Pathol 2005;166:1321–1332.

39. Yao HW, Xie QM, Chen JQ, et al. TGF-beta1 induces alveolar epithelial to mesenchymal transition in vitro. Life Sci 2004;76:29–37.

40. Savagner P, Yamada KM, Thiery JP. The zinc-finger protein slug causes desmosome dissociation, an initial and necessary step for growth factor-induced epithelial–mesenchymal transition. J Cell Biol 1997;137:1403–1419.

41. Conacci-Sorrell M, Simcha I, Ben-Yedidia T, et al. Autoregulation of E-cadherin expression by cadherin–cadherin interactions: the roles of beta-catenin signaling, Slug, and MAPK. J Cell Biol. 2003;163:847–857.

42. He TC, Sparks AB, Rago C, et al. Identification of c-MYC as a target of the APC pathway. Science 1998;281:1509–1512.

43. Donaldson TD, Duronio RJ. Cancer cell biology: Myc wins the competition. Curr Biol 2004;14:R425–R427.

44. Lappi-Blanco E, Kaarteenaho-Wiik R, Soini Y, et al. Intraluminal fibromyxoid lesions in bronchiolitis obliterans organizing pneumonia are highly capillarized. Hum Pathol 1999;30:1192–1196.

45. Nicholson AG, Fulford LG, Colby TV, et al. The relationship between individual histologic features and disease progression in idiopathic pulmonary fibrosis. Am J Respir Crit Care Med 2002;166:173–177.

46. Selman M, Ruiz V, Cabrera S, et al. TIMP-1, -2, -3, and -4 in idiopathic pulmonary fibrosis. A prevailing nondegradative lung microenvironment? Am J Physiol Lung Cell Mol Physiol 2000;279:L562–L574.

47. Hagood JS, Prabhakaran P, Kumbla P, et al. Loss of fibroblast Thy-1 expression correlates with lung fibrogenesis. Am J Pathol 2005;167:365–379.

48. Moodley YP, Scaffidi AK, Misso NL, et al. Fibroblasts isolated from normal lungs and those with idiopathic pulmonary fibrosis differ in interleukin-6/gp130-mediated cell signaling and proliferation. Am J Pathol 2003;163:345–354.

49. Yun MS, Kim SE, Jeon SH, et al. Both ERK and Wnt/beta-catenin pathways are involved in Wnt3a-induced proliferation. J Cell Sci 2005;118:313–322.

50. Marchand-Adam S, Marchal J, Cohen M, et al. Defect of hepatocyte growth factor secretion by fibroblasts in idiopathic pulmonary fibrosis. Am J Respir Crit Care Med 2003;168:1156–1161.

51. Chilosi M, Poletti V, Murer B, et al. Bronchiolar epithelium in idiopathic pulmonary fibrosis/usual interstitial pneumonia. In Lynch JPI, ed. Lung Biology in Health and Disease. New York: Marcel Dekker; 2004:631–664.

52. Hong KU, Reynolds SD, Watkins S, et al. Basal cells are a multipotent progenitor capable of renewing the bronchial epithelium. Am J Pathol 2004;164:577–588.

53. Chilosi M, Doglioni C. Constitutive p63 expression in airway basal cells. A molecular target in diffuse lung diseases. Sarcoidosis Vasc Diffuse Lung Dis 2001;18:23–26.

54. Hibi K, Trink B, Patturajan M, et al. AIS is an oncogene amplified in squamous cell carcinoma. Proc Natl Acad Sci USA 2000;97:5462–5467.

55. Massion PP, Taflan PM, Jamshedur Rahman SM, et al. Significance of p63 amplification and overexpression in lung cancer development and prognosis. Cancer Res 2003;63: 7113–7121.

56. Chilosi M, Zamò A, Doglioni C, et al. Migratory marker expression in fibroblast foci of idiopathic pulmonary fibrosis. Respir Res 2006;7:95.

57. Charette SJ, Landry J. The interaction of HSP27 with Daxx identifies a potential regulatory role of HSP27 in Fas-induced apoptosis. Ann NY Acad Sci 2000;926:126–131.

58. Niessen CM, Hogervorst F, Jaspars LH, et al. The alpha 6 beta 4 integrin is a receptor for both laminin and kalinin. Exp Cell Res 1994;211:360–367.

59. Hintermann E, Quaranta V. Epithelial cell motility on laminin-5: regulation by matrix assembly, proteolysis, integrins and erbB receptors. Matrix Biol 2004;23:75–85.

60. Coraux C, Meneguzzi G, Rousselle P, et al. Distribution of laminin 5, integrin receptors, and branching morphogenesis during human fetal lung development. Dev Dyn 2002;225: 176–185.

61. Kariya Y, Miyazaki K. The basement membrane protein laminin-5 acts as a soluble cell motility factor. Exp Cell Res 2004;297:508–520.

62. Hlubek F, Jung A, Kotzor N, et al. Expression of the invasion factor laminin gamma2 in colorectal carcinomas is regulated by beta-catenin. Cancer Res 2001;61:8089–8093.

63. Pyke C, Romer J, Kallunki P, et al. The gamma 2 chain of kalinin/laminin 5 is preferentially expressed in invading malignant cells in human cancers. Am J Pathol 1994;145: 782–791.

64. Lappi-Blanco E, Kaarteenaho-Wiik R, Salo S, et al. Laminin-5 gamma2 chain in cryptogenic organizing pneumonia and idiopathic pulmonary fibrosis. Am J Respir Crit Care Med 2004;169:27–33.

56
Sarcoidosis: Are There Sarcoidosis Genes?

Helmut H. Popper

Introduction

More than 100 years have passed since the first description of sarcoidosis by Hutchinson[1] and the identification of sarcoid granulomas by Besnier,[2] Boeck,[3] and Schaumann,[4] but the causative agent or agents of sarcoidosis still have not been identified. However, in these intervening years, considerable knowledge has accumulated about the pathogenesis and the molecular events that lead to the granulomatous reaction. Clinical evaluation has shed some light on this systemic disease; pathology and immunology have contributed to our understanding of the inflammatory process. More recently, genetics and molecular biology have opened new avenues of research for this still enigmatic disease. There is some hope that new techniques provided by molecular biology, employing samples from bronchoalveolar lavage and biopsies, might elucidate the causative agents behind this disease and define the genetic modifications that make some people prone to developing sarcoidosis.

Morphology and Its Implications

Sarcoidosis begins with local infiltration of alveolar septa and bronchial mucosa by alveolar macrophages and lymphocytes, predominantly of the T helper phenotype. This early infiltration is centered on blood and lymphatic vessels (Figure 56.1). It is most probable that the antigens, which induce the accumulation of these cells, enter or reenter the lung via the blood stream and the lymphatic system. This is in contrast to airway epithelium-centered granulomas as seen in infectious granulomatosis. At these early stages of sarcoidosis the granulomas have ill-defined borders and abundant lymphocytes. As the granulomas mature, lymphocytes are less numerous and the granulomas organize with central epithelioid histiocytes and Langerhans giant cells surrounded by a smaller rim of lymphocytes (Figure 56.2). Within this outer rim of lym-

phocytes, T-helper lymphocytes (CD4[+]) predominate, whereas CD8[+] T cells and B lymphocytes are found outside the granulomas. This suggests a functional relationship: Within the granulomas the secretion of cytokines and chemokines from CD4[+] lymphocytes and epithelioid cells is necessary to maintain the immune reaction toward the antigen(s), develop the granulomas, and stimulate the differentiation of epithelioid and giant cells out of the macrophage/monocyte cell pool. The function of the CD8[+] lymphocytes outside the granulomas is still not understood; maybe they are downregulating inflammatory signals or are involved in limiting the immune reaction and inflammation.

Variants of Sarcoidosis

Löfgren's Disease/Acute Sarcoidosis

The Swedish physician Sven Halvar Löfgren described acute sarcoidosis as a variant of sarcoidosis presenting with erythema nodosum and hilar lymphadenopathy,[5] and this disease now bears his name. Pulmonary involvement in Löfgren's disease is usually also present but radiographically not always detectable. As in the classic form of sarcoidosis, there is a lymphocytic infiltration and also early granuloma formation. However, the granulomas are usually smaller (500 μm in diameter) and less numerous. The course of acute sarcoidosis most often is benign with an acute onset, a short duration, and a spontaneous resolution. Muscular pain and joint swelling may be present and are probably caused by a granulomatous inflammation (unpublished personal observation), but most often no biopsies are performed.

Nodular Sarcoidosis

Romer[6] and later Churg[7] described nodular sarcoidosis as a variant of sarcoidosis. The main features are confluent sarcoid granulomas, absence of necrosis, and ischemic infarcts. The nodules are usually in the range of 1–7 cm, but usually 1–3 cm prevails. Besides the lung, several other organs can be involved. Most often the macronodular pattern is accompanied by conventional microscopic granulomas as well. There is no known cause for nodular sarcoidosis. Treatment follows the same regimen as for sarcoidosis.

Necrotizing Sarcoid Granulomatosis

Necrotizing sarcoid granulomatosis (NSG) was originally described by Averill Liebow as a separate entity.[8] For Liebow, NSG shared a mixture of patterns of sarcoidosis and Wegener's granulomatosis, showing sarcoid granulomas, most often a macronodular pattern, and ischemic necrosis and vasculitis as in Wegener's granulomatosis. All of Liebow's original NSG cases presented in the lungs and hilar lymph nodes. In cases published subsequently by Andrew Churg and colleagues, extrapulmonary involvement was found in some cases, and the separation of NSG from sarcoidosis was questioned.[9] In the largest series published so far, Popper et al. demonstrated that NSG has features of sarcoidosis: sarcoid granulomas, nodular sarcoid aggregates, and epithelioid cell granulomatous vasculitis.[10] The only difference was vascular occlusion by the vasculitis and subsequent ischemic infarcts.

All these variants of classic sarcoidosis might be caused by the same mechanisms, but disease modifiers might influence the reaction pattern. Some genetic differences from classic sarcoidosis are recognized in Löfgren's disease (see subsequent paragraphs); however, nodular sarcoidosis and NSG have not been investigated thus far.

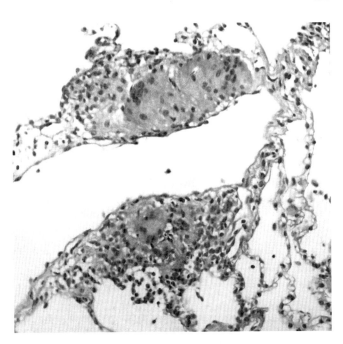

FIGURE 56.2. Epithelioid cell granulomas in sarcoidosis. Note the intimate location of the granulomas to this dilated lymphatic, whereas there is a distance to the alveolar side. This is a typical finding in sarcoidosis and might be caused by antigens entering via bloodstream and lymphatics. (Hematoxylin and eosin stain; ×200.)

What Is the Meaning of Indistinguishable Differentials?

Chronic allergic metal disease, such as chronic berylliosis and zirkoniosis, and so-called sarcoid-like reactions in the lung and lymph nodes are indistinguishable histopathologically from sarcoidosis. Both present with nonnecrotizing epithelioid cell granulomas, and there are no organisms detectable within the granulomas. In sarcoid-like reaction, granulomas are distributed along lymphatics and blood vessels within the lung and in pulmonary and mediastinal lymph nodes in patients with primary pulmonary carcinomas and other malignancies in the lung. The mechanism of granuloma formation in this condition is not fully explored, but release of various cytokines and chemokines, like interleukin (IL)-1β, IL-2, interferon (IFN)-γ, granulocyte–macrophage colony stimulating factor (GM-CSF), and tumor necrosis factor (TNF)-α from tumor cells might be responsible for this reaction.[11–14]

Genetic susceptibility to chronic berylliosis has been associated with human leukocyte antigen (HLA)-DP alleles, possessing a glutamic acid at the 69th position of the β-chain. These HLA-DP molecules bind and present beryllium to pathogenic CD4[+] T cells. These helper T cells secrete Th1-type cytokines upon beryllium recognition. The presence of circulating beryllium-specific CD4[+]

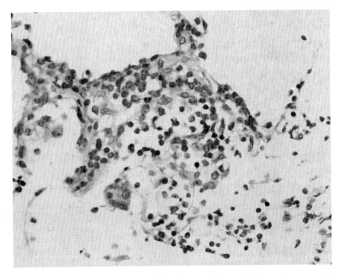

FIGURE 56.1. Early epithelioid cell granuloma. Macrophages and a few developing epithelioid cells are infiltrating the lung together with lymphocytes. (Hematoxylin and eosin stain; ×200.)

T cells directly correlates with the severity of lymphocytic alveolitis.[15] In addition to *HLA-DP*-Glu69, *HLA-DR*-Glu71 is capable of inducing beryllium-specific proliferation and IFN-γ expression by lung CD4+ T cells.[16] The metal oxide acts as a hapten, associates with *HLA-DP* and *HLA-DR* to form an allergen, and then induces a type IV immune reaction.[17–19] In both berylliosis and sarcoidosis CD4+ helper cells are the major immune cell population within the granulomas. CD8+ and B cells can be found outside the granulomas in much lesser quantity.

Other granulomatous diseases caused by infectious organisms can also mimic sarcoidosis. Good examples are granulomas caused by slow growing mycobacteria such as *Mycobacterium avium* and *Mycobacterium intracellulare*.

These granulomatous reactions demonstrate that there can be different causes but one mechanism to induce nonnecrotizing sarcoid granulomas. This is primarily because many of these antigens, such as mycobacterial capsules, are of low solubility and are minimally degradable. Other antigens, such as BeO by its association with HLA molecules, can directly stimulate CD4+ T lymphocytes. Probably many of these antigens are processed similarly by the dendritic cells and stimulate similar subpopulations of helper T cells by a selection of T-cell receptors and costimulatory molecules of the HLA system. The analysis of costimulatory molecules by comparing different types of epithelioid cell granulomas and their immune cells is also a focus of research. A few important findings in this field are emerging such as the butyrophilin-like 2 gene and Toll-like receptor 4 (TLR4; see later discussion).

The Cells in Sarcoidosis

The first cells to appear in a granuloma are alveolar macrophages followed by T lymphocytes. Not much is known about the phenotype and function of the macrophages. What morphologically appears as a macrophage might not always be a classic phagocytic cell. Antigen-presenting dendritic or Langerhans cells may resemble macrophages histologically. Even among CD68+ macrophages there are phagocytic cells, as well as cells capable of antigen processing and stimulating an immune reaction. In experimental assays, immunostaining of multiple surface markers can easily define these cells, but in formalin-fixed tissue sections or in cytologic specimens, immunopositivity of many of these markers is lost. Given that alveolar macrophages are the primary cells, which induce a lymphocytic influx in sarcoidosis, these cells most probably have the capability to process antigens and present them to lymphocytes. A better characterization of the cellular compartments in this early granulo-

matous reaction is warranted. In addition, the participation of dendritic cells and Langerhans cells needs to be elucidated. Because macrophages and lymphocytes induce the differentiation of macrophages/monocytes into epithelioid cells and giant cells, and release chemokines to maintain the granulomas, this granulomatous reaction is most likely not the primary antigen contact but recognition of antigens to which the patient has been previously sensitized.

T Lymphocytes

The major cell population in sarcoidosis is helper T cells. Most of these express the αβ receptor, produce/secrete IFN-γ and IL-2, and therefore belong to the Th1 subset of helper cells.[20] The selection of a Th1-dominated reaction can be facilitated by a release of various chemokines/cytokines or by the presence of antigens and costimulatory molecules. Interleukin-18 expressed by airway epithelial cells and macrophages drive a Th1 reaction with an increase of IFN-γ–producing cells.[21] Interleukin-27 induces the expression of the major Th1-specific transcription factor T-bet (T-box expressed in T cells) and its downstream target IL-12Rβ2. Interleukin-27 suppresses expression of GATA-3, the Th2-specific transcription factor. Interleukin-27 induces phosphorylation of signal transducer and activator of transcription (STAT) 1, STAT3, STAT4, and STAT5. STAT1 is required for suppression of GATA3.[22] Another mechanism for selecting a Th1 or Th2 response is by activation of the aryl hydrocarbon receptor. Aryl hydrocarbon receptor activation by the addition of representative ligands suppresses naive helper T-cell differentiation into Th2 cells.[23] A further mechanism that suppresses Th2 differentiation and thus the balance of Th1/2 is by the Src kinase homology domain 2.[24] A Th2 cell differentiation can also be achieved by the ras/extracellular signal-regulated kinase/mitogen-activated protein kinase system, which facilitates GATA3 protein stability and GATA3-mediated chromatin remodeling at Th2 cytokine gene loci.[25]

Some conflicting reports exist on the role of TNF-α: overexpression of TNF-α and IFN-γ together leads to persistence and progression in sarcoidosis,[26] whereas in animal models TNF-α is required for Th1 accumulation, granuloma formation, and antigen clearance, which should lead to a downregulation of inflammation.[27]

Epithelioid Cells

Epithelioid cells are the secretory cells within the granulomas. Epithelioid cells secrete many different chemokines and cytokines, such as migration inhibitory factor and various interleukins. Their major role is the maintenance of the granulomas and the immune reaction. In part they support the helper T lymphocytes functionally.

Giant Cells (Foreign Body and Langerhans Type)

Giant cells form by fusion of macrophages as well as by nuclear division without concomitant cell division. Giant cells are specialized in phagocytosis and have large lysosomes capable of digesting poorly soluble and slowly degradable material. In tuberculosis and other infectious diseases, these cells are directed against the resistant capsules of mycobacteria and similar organisms. However, the reason for giant cell formation in sarcoidosis is not clear. A comparison with rheumatoid arthritis might shed some light on this phenomenon. Antigen–antibody complexes, sometimes combined with additional idiotypic and antiidiotypic antibodies, form very robust complexes deposited in the synovial membrane in rheumatoid arthritis. In these usually seropositive cases, histiocytic granulomas with giant cells develop. One might speculate that antigen–antibody complexes in sarcoidosis are also insoluble and thus induce a giant cell reaction.

Mycobacteria and Other Trigger Mechanisms—Is Sarcoidosis an Infectious Disease?

Because of the close resemblance of granulomas in sarcoidosis to those in mycobacterial diseases, an infection caused by *Mycobacterium tuberculosis* or other mycobacteria has been proposed in sarcoidosis. Culture of mycobacteria from sarcoidosis granulomas of the skin has been reported,[28] but this finding was not confirmed in other investigations.[28–30] Several investigators have reported mycobacterial DNA and RNA in sarcoidosis.[31–37] However, other investigators have reported negative results for mycobacterial DNA or RNA.[38–40] It has been speculated that cell wall–deficient mycobacteria, unable to grow in culture, might induce sarcoidosis.[31,41,42] In some cases, DNA insertion sequences characteristic for *M. avium* were reported to be amplified from granulomas.[43] In three cases of recurrent sarcoidosis in lung transplant patients, mycobacterial DNA other than tuberculosis complex could be demonstrated in the explanted native lungs and in the transplanted lungs with recurrent sarcoidosis.[36] Other recent reports have shown that naked mycobacterial DNA is capable of inducing a strong immune response.[44,45] It is known that mycobacteria can persist preferentially in macrophages. In accordance with these observations, heat shock protein 90 is upregulated in sarcoidosis, which is part of the initial immunologic response mechanism in mycobacterial infections. Heat shock protein together with TLR4 expression is one of the mechanisms by which the selection of HLA types and costimulatory molecules is facilitated in mycobacterial infections (unpublished observation).[46–49]

In a working hypothesis, we assume that slow-growing mycobacteria or even breakdown products thereof might elicit an allergic reaction in the background of a host's hyperergic predisposition. These allergens could be distributed to different organ systems via the circulation, eliciting the well-known perivascular granulomatous reaction.[35,50]

Other investigators demonstrated *Propionibacterium acnes* DNA in sarcoidosis. A scenario similar to that with mycobacteria was reported. Propionibacteria DNA or RNA could be amplified from tissue sections of sarcoidosis granulomas, and in experimental settings these bacteria can elicit a granulomatous reaction.[51–53] Many other agents have been discussed as probable causes or trigger mechanisms of sarcoidosis, including herpesvirus and Chlamydia.[54,55] None of these has attracted as much attention and controversy as mycobacteria and propionibacteria.

Risk Factors

The course of sarcoidosis remains unpredictable. Approximately two thirds of patients will recover from the disease. However, in one third the disease progresses. The most serious complication is lung fibrosis, starting with fibrosis of the granulomas and extending into the surrounding lung parenchyma. Many studies have focused on factors predicting fibrosis, because these patients should be treated with corticosteroids.

The combination *DQB1*0602/DRB1*150101* haplotype was found to be positively associated with severe pulmonary sarcoidosis indicated by radiographic stages II–IV. However, there was no association with fibrosis.[56,57] In the study by Kruit et al. an association of the *TGF-β3 17369C* allele was demonstrated more frequently in patients with fibrotic lung than in patients with acute/self-remitting and chronic sarcoidosis.[58] The *TGF-β2 59941G* allele also was more abundant in fibrosis combined with sarcoidosis. *TGFβ1* gene polymorphisms were not associated with fibrosis.[58]

Prostaglandin-endoperoxide synthase 2 (PTGS2) is a key regulatory enzyme for the synthesis of the antifibrotic prostaglandin E_2 and is reduced in sarcoidosis lung. A promoter polymorphism −765G > C in *PTGS2* identified individuals who are susceptible to sarcoidosis and, more importantly, at risk of pulmonary fibrosis. An altered Sp1/Sp3 binding to the −765 region may reduce *PTGS2* expression.[59]

In Löfgren's syndrome, which usually presents with sudden onset, short duration, and quick resolution of the disease, other genetic variations have been demonstrated that could be responsible for this disease modification. In Löfgren's syndrome significantly increased frequency of the *CCR2* haplotype 2 was observed compared with controls.[60] A prevalence of *DRB1*03*, HSP (+2437)-C and (+2763)-G was observed in patients with Löfgren's syndrome and might confer a susceptibility toward this variant of sarcoidosis.[61]

The Steps of an Immune Reaction and What Might Happen in Sarcoidosis

If we suppose a working hypothesis that is based on the induction of the disease by different immunogenic agents, such as mycobacteria, propionibacteria, chlamydia, and even viruses or other unknown antigens, there are several steps within the immune reaction that might bear a gene modification or mutation conferring susceptibility to sarcoidosis (Figure 56.3):

Antigen recognition and take up by macrophages or dendritic cells

Antigen handover and antigen processing usually within dendritic cells and/or macrophages

Antigen presentation to effector cells together with preselected costimulatory molecules

Finally, the immune reaction by a concerted action of T and B cells[46]

An upregulated allergic or hyperimmune reaction could be buried within each of these steps and might be responsible for the heterogeneity of clinical courses in sarcoidosis. Allergic reaction may have already been induced at the antigen presentation site. For example, antigen presented in association with costimulatory molecules could induce prolonged stimulation of lymphocytes as a result of phenotypic variations or point mutations in these molecules, resulting in increased susceptibility to sarcoidosis. Other possible explanations for a hyperimmune reaction include a hyperreactive effector cell system that has an exaggerated response to antigen stimulation or impairment of a counterbalance system such as apoptosis.

Antigen Uptake and Processing

It is reasonable to assume that the susceptible individual has had previous exposure to the antigen(s) that cause sarcoidosis. Otherwise, a short onset reaction as in Löfgren's disease would not be possible. It is well known that the tertiary antigen structure preselects the type of immune reaction. Selection of Toll-like receptors (TLRs), heat shock proteins, and so forth, determines the type of immune reaction toward an antigen as well as the cells for response: CD4 (Th1, Th2), CD8, or B cells.[62] Antigens within the mycobacteria family, for example, dictate a Th1 reaction via an upregulation of various cytokines.[63,64]

A failure in this selection process, or prolongation of the immune cell stimulation, could be one of the possible

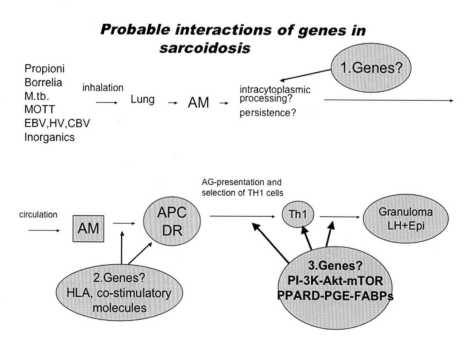

FIGURE 56.3. Possible steps where in the pathogenesis of sarcoidosis genes might interact (probably the reason why this disease is so multifaceted). **(1)** Genes might be responsible for an inability to degrade invading organisms, thus leading to persistence of these organisms. The organisms might produce proteins and induce an autoimmune reaction. **(2)** The immune reaction might be altered by a predisposition in the organism to select improper costimulatory molecules, thus inducing an adverse immune reaction. Here also an alteration of antigen-presenting cells (APC) might come into play. **(3)** There might be a genetically abnormal and prolonged type IV immune reaction determined by genetic modification or mutations.

mechanisms of susceptibility to sarcoidosis. As noted previously, little is known about the regulatory mechanisms of activation and deactivation of the antigen-presenting cells.

Not much is known about the processing of antigens within macrophages or dendritic cells, although this might be another factor that influences disease susceptibility. If the antigens that cause sarcoidosis are not degraded within a given time, they might persist intracellularly, resulting in protein transcription eliciting an allergic reaction.

Antigen Presentation, Costimulatory Molecules, and Gene Polymorphisms and Where They Come Into Play

Antigen presentation is another potential step where an allergic or hyperimmune reaction could occur. Processed antigens are presented to T cells in association with costimulatory molecules. This combination can exert opposite effects on the T cells. For example, CD28 activates phosphatidylinositol-3 kinase (PI3K) and Akt1 kinase, causing downstream impaired recruitment of procaspase-8 to the death-inducing signaling complex, inhibiting apoptosis.[65] Inducible costimulator (ICOS), another costimulatory molecule, augments PI3K levels, whereas only CD28 costimulation activates c-Jun N-terminal kinase. However, only CD28 induces high levels of IL-2 and Bcl-xL, which also prevent apoptosis.[66]

Tripartite motif-containing genes (TRIMs) are costimulatory molecules and are able to stimulate proliferation of lymphocytes via an activation of the PI3K pathway. The TRIMs 5, 16, and 22 are upregulated in sarcoidosis and in Löfgren's disease.[50] This pathway might also contribute to inhibition of apoptosis in sarcoidosis.

Toll-like receptors might play a role in the development of sarcoidosis. Toll-like receptor 4 is usually upregulated in response to certain substances present in the capsules of bacteria.[52,67] An association of a TLR4 phenotypic mutation with chronic sarcoidosis has been found recently.[68] Toll-like receptors are an important mechanism for maintenance of a balanced immune system. Toll-like receptors induce an upregulation of IL-12, IL-1 receptor associated kinase-M, and suppressor of cytokine signaling-1. Normally an excess of these proinflammatory action proteins is limited by PI3K, which suppress IL-12.[69] An imbalance in this gate-keeping system might be another facet in the sarcoidosis mosaic.

Valentonyte et al. have identified the butyrophilin-like 2 gene (BTNL2) as strongly associated with sarcoidosis.[70] The authors demonstrated a truncated protein whose function is impaired in sarcoidosis. In a subsequent study, a strong association with sarcoidosis susceptibility was shown for Caucasians but was weaker for African-Americans.[71] BTNL2 is a member of the immunoglobulin superfamily of genes and is a homolog to B7-1. Recently it was shown that BTNL2 is a receptor expressed on activated B and T lymphocytes. It inhibits T-cell proliferation and T-cell receptor mediated activation of nuclear factor of activated T cells (NFAT), nuclear factor (NF)-κB, and activator protein-1 (AP1) signaling pathways.[72]

Members of the HLA system, located on chromosome 6, are strongly associated with immune reactions as well as with autoimmune disorders. However, it can be concluded that HLA molecules associated with sarcoidosis have most often been identified as disease modifiers and, thus far, not as disease-causing agents. Polymorphisms have been identified in many of the HLA genes, and these are responsible for stimulation of the immune reaction and also for organotypic involvement.

Human Leukocyte Antigen Class I Genes

Human leukocyte antigen B8 (HLA-B8) has been found in sarcoidosis patients with acute onset and short duration of the disease.[73] HLA-B*07 and HLA-B*08 have been associated with higher risk of developing sarcoidosis.[74] An association with persistent disease was conferred by a combination of the HLA alleles A*03, B*07, and DRB1*15 (see also later discussion).

Human Leukocyte Antigen Class II Genes

In a genetic linkage study using 122 affected siblings from 55 families Schürmann et al. have defined a locus close to major histocompatibility complex (MHC) II and III frequently altered in these affected persons.[75] In a follow-up study analyzing 63 families with affected siblings, this observation was expanded, and a peak was identified again at the D6S1666 marker.[76] In addition, other peaks were identified, including genes for chemokine receptor 2 (CCR2) and 5 (CCR5), T cell receptor B, TGF-β receptor 1, and IL-2 receptor. In a subsequent study focusing on CCR2, an association with sarcoidosis could not be confirmed.[77]

In the ACCESS study, HLA-DRB1 alleles were associated with sarcoidosis in Caucasians as well as African Americans. The DRB1*1101 allele confers risk in both ethnic populations, whereas the allele DRB1*1501 was differently distributed among the tested patients and controls.[78] Another class II gene DQB1, namely, the allele *0602, was significantly associated with progressive disease.[56] This was confirmed in a subsequent study within a European population.[79] HLA-DR1 and HLA-DR4 have been shown to be protective in Scandinavian, Japanese, Italian, English, Polish, and Czech populations.[80] A major problem with most of these studies is that they do not attempt to investigate the function of these HLA alleles, and thus the importance of mutations or phenotypic variations remains obscure.

Tumor necrosis factor genes are located on chromosome 6, in close proximity to most genes of the MHC complex. Tumor necrosis factor-α is a proinflammatory mediator found in most inflammatory conditions and also early in sarcoidosis.[11] A genetic variation within the TNF-α gene at positions 308 (G to A mutation, *TNFA*) has been shown to be associated with high TNF-α production and was found in Löfgren's disease,[81] but an 857 T mutation was observed in sarcoidosis and not in Löfgren's disease.[82] This point mutation was associated with higher promoter activity and thus resulted in increased TNF-α release. Another variation in the first intron of the TNF-β gene *(TNFB)* was associated with prolonged disease but not with severity.[83]

Effector Mechanisms, the Lymphocyte– Macrophage Network, and Gene Expression in Sarcoidosis

Once an immune reaction has been started, it is regulated through activation and deactivation. Regulatory T cells might be responsible for this fine tuning. However, as

earlier, the susceptibility of patients to elicit a type IV granulomatous immune reaction might also be based on a hyperreactive T-cell system. Recently it was shown that in bronchoalveolar lavage cells from sarcoidosis patients, predominantly composed of T-helper cells and macrophages, there was an upregulated signaling cascade for proliferation and a downregulation of apoptosis. Conflicting reports have been published on the upregulation of apoptosis-associated ligands and receptors.[84–86] Fas is highly expressed in sarcoidosis T lymphocytes, and high levels of soluble Fas ligand (FasL) are found,[87,88] favoring apoptosis. However, once Fas and FasL are associated, they activate downstream death receptors, which subsequently cleave and activate caspase-8. Caspase-8 either cleaves Bid and thus activates the mitochondria-mediated pathway or cleaves caspase-9 and activates the direct apoptosis pathway finally leading to the activation of caspase-3. Petzmann et al. found that the extracellular concentration of FasL or other proapoptotic molecules might have no effect, because the apoptosis signaling in sarcoidosis is blocked at the intracellular level of the mitochondria-mediated and the direct apoptotic pathways (Figure 56. 4).[50] This was also confirmed in another study.[89] p21[WAF1] is highly expressed in sarcoidosis[90] and

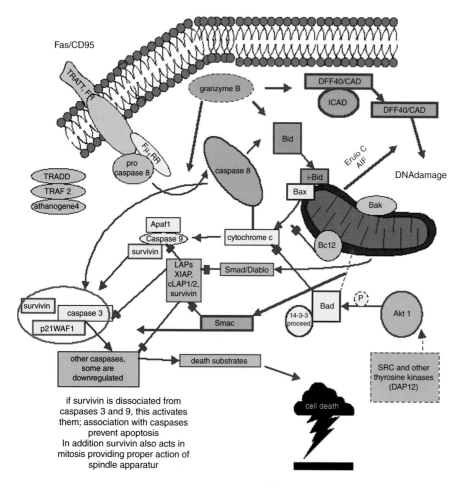

if survivin is dissociated from caspases 3 and 9, this activates them; association with caspases prevent apoptosis
In addition survivin also acts in mitosis providing proper action of spindle apparatur

FIGURE 56.4. Antiapoptotic mechanisms might prolong the lifetime of sarcoidosis lymphocytes. Independent of the concentration of outside proapoptotic ligands there is a downregulation of key molecules within the mitochondrial apoptosis pathway (tumor necrosis factor receptor–associated death domain, tumor necrosis factor receptor–associated factors, athanogene4, Bid), upregulation of antiapoptotic molecules (14-3-3, Bad, Akt), and upregulation of molecules that act antiapoptotic for the mitochondrial as well as intrinsic apoptosis pathways (surviving).

FIGURE 56.5. Probable activation of proliferation pathways in sarcoidosis CD4⁺ lymphocytes and CD68⁺ macrophages. Tripartite motif molecules might be the main receptor type signaling into the phosphoinositol-3 kinase pathway and activating Akt and signal transducer and activator of transcription 3 downstream. Other receptors such as CD28 and inducible costimulator and the T-cell receptor system might interplay here, because Crk is also upregulated. In Löfgrens disease (acute sarcoidosis) an additional proliferation pathway is turned on by prostaglandins and fatty acid binding proteins 4 and 5, which associate with peroxisome proliferator-activated receptor and again activate Akt.

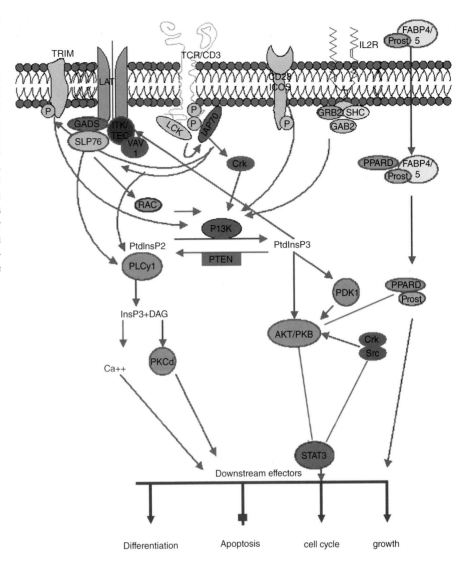

inhibits apoptosis in alveolar macrophages and lymphocytes. p21 is predominantly regulated by IFN-γ and might be another mechanism by which macrophages and lymphocytes in sarcoidosis can escape apoptosis.

In addition to prolonged survival of CD4⁺ lymphocytes and macrophages in sarcoidosis, there is also an enhanced stimulation of proliferation by an activation of the PI3K/Akt2 kinase/mTOR/STAT3 pathway. The antagonist PTEN, which can interrupt the PI3K activation system, was downregulated in sarcoidosis.[50] Moreover, in lavage cells of patients with Löfgren's, an additional stimulatory signal for proliferation was found. The mRNA for peroxisome proliferator-activated receptor (PPARD) and its shuffle proteins fatty acid binding proteins 4 and 5 (FABP4/5) were all upregulated. The PPARD needs FABPs for a translocation into the nucleus. If shuffled into the nuclei, PPARD associates with E-type prosta-

glandins or leukotrienes and stimulate cell proliferation.[50] This additional proliferation signal might be responsible for the rapid increase of macrophages and lymphocytes in this variant of sarcoidosis (Figure 56.5).

Disease Modifier Genes and Aspects of Organ Involvement in Sarcoidosis

A switch from Th1 to Th2 cells occurs in progressive sarcoidosis. There is an increase of IL-4, which can stimulate fibroblast proliferation. Interleukin-1 stimulates granuloma formation, fibroblast proliferation, and collagen deposition. Insulin-like growth factor I, TGF-β, and platelet-derived growth factor, produced and secreted by macrophages and epithelioid cells, might also be responsible for fibrosis.[91,92]

Organs other than the lungs may be involved in sarcoidosis. It has long been recognized that organ involvement does not occur randomly. For example, sarcoid myocarditis is common in Japan,[93] whereas skin involvement is common in other ethnic groups.[94] This has prompted research for factors responsible for the distribution of specific organ involvement. Although at an early stage, several observations have been reported. Cardiac sarcoidosis probably is mediated by an *HLA-DQB1*0601* allele in addition to an unusual A2-allele of the *TNF* gene.[95,96]

Cytotoxic T-lymphocyte antigen 4 (*CTLA-4*) with a phenotypic CC mutation at 318 and AG or GG mutation at position 49 was significantly associated with ocular involvement in association with involvement of three or more organs.[97] Cytotoxic T-lymphocyte antigen 4 is another costimulatory molecule that counterbalances T cell activation, serving as an antagonist to CD28.[98] Thus far, nothing is known about an impaired function as a result of phenotypic point mutations of the *CTLA-4* gene. No molecular genetic data are available regarding most other organ involvement in sarcoidosis, probably because these cases are rare and can only be investigated by multicenter studies to acquire sufficient numbers of patients for the study.

References

1. Hutchinson J. Mortimer's malady: a form of lupus pernio. Arch Surg 1898;9:307–315.
2. Besnier E. Lupus pernio de la face. Ann Dermatol Syphiligr 1889;10:33–36.
3. Boeck C. Multiple benign sarcoid of the skin. Norsk Mag Laegevid 1899;14:1321–1345.
4. Schaumann J. Lymphogranuloma benigna in the light of prolonged clinical observations and autopsy findings. Br J Dermatol 1936;48:346–399.
5. Löfgren S. Primary pulmonary sarcoidosis. I Early signs and symptoms. Acta Med Scand 1953;145:424–431.
6. Romer FK. Sarcoidosis with large nodular lesions simulating pulmonary metastases. An analysis of 126 cases of intrathoracic sarcoidosis. Scand J Respir Dis 1977;58:11–16.
7. Churg A. Pulmonary angiitis and granulomatosis revisited. Hum Pathol 1983;14:868–883.
8. Liebow AA. The J. Burns Amberson lecture—pulmonary angiitis and granulomatosis. Am Rev Respir Dis 1973;108:1–18.
9. Churg A, Carrington CB, Gupta R. Necrotizing sarcoid granulomatosis. Chest 1979;76:406–413.
10. Popper HH KH, Churg A, Colby TV. Necrotizing sarcoid granulomatosis—is it different from nodular sarcoidosis? Pneumology 2003;57:268–271.
11. Ishioka S, Saito T, Hiyama K, et al. Increased expression of tumor necrosis factor-alpha, interleukin-6, platelet-derived growth factor-B and granulocyte–macrophage colony-stimulating factor mRNA in cells of bronchoalveolar lavage fluids from patients with sarcoidosis. Sarcoidosis Vasc Diffuse Lung Dis 1996;13:139–145.

12. Llombart A, Jr., Escudero JM. The incidence and significance of epithelioid and sarcoid-like cellular reaction in the stromata of malignant tumours. A morphological and experimental study. Eur J Cancer 1970;6:545–551.
13. Bassler R, Birke F. Histopathology of tumour associated sarcoid-like stromal reaction in breast cancer. An analysis of 5 cases with immunohistochemical investigations. Virchows Arch A Pathol Anat Histopathol 1988;412:231–239.
14. Parra ER, Canzian M, Saber AM, et al. Pulmonary and mediastinal "sarcoidosis" following surgical resection of cancer. Pathol Res Pract 2004;200:701–705.
15. Amicosante M, Fontenot AP. T cell recognition in chronic beryllium disease. Clin Immunol 2006;121(2):134–143.
16. Bill JR, Mack DG, Falta MT, et al. Beryllium presentation to CD4+ T cells is dependent on a single amino acid residue of the MHC class II beta-chain, J Immunol 2005;175:7029–7037.
17. Saltini C, Amicosante M. Beryllium disease. Am J Med Sci 2001;321:89–98
18. Fontenot AP, Torres M, Marshall WH, et al. Beryllium presentation to CD4+ T cells underlies disease-susceptibility HLA-DP alleles in chronic beryllium disease. Proc Natl Acad Sci USA 2000;97:12717–12722.
19. Gaede KI, Amicosante M, Schurmann M, et al. Function associated transforming growth factor-beta gene polymorphism in chronic beryllium disease. J Mol Med 2005;83:397–405.
20. Shigehara K, Shijubo N, Ohmichi M, et al. Enhanced mRNA expression of Th1 cytokines and IL-12 in active pulmonary sarcoidosis. Sarcoidosis Vasc Diffuse Lung Dis 2000;17:151–157.
21. Cameron LA, Taha RA, Tsicopoulos A, et al. Airway epithelium expresses interleukin-18. Eur Respir J 1999;14:553–559.
22. Lucas S, Ghilardi N, Li J, et al. IL-27 regulates IL-12 responsiveness of naive CD4+ T cells through Stat1-dependent and -independent mechanisms. Proc Natl Acad Sci USA 2003;100:15047–15052.
23. Negishi T, Kato Y, Ooneda O, et al. Effects of aryl hydrocarbon receptor signaling on the modulation of TH1/TH2 balance. J Immunol 2005;175:7348–7356.
24. Salmond RJ, Huyer G, Kotsoni A, et al. The src homology 2 domain-containing tyrosine phosphatase 2 regulates primary T-dependent immune responses and Th cell differentiation. J Immunol 2005;175:6498–6508.
25. Yamashita M, Shinnakasu R, Asou H, et al. Ras-ERK MAPK cascade regulates GATA3 stability and Th2 differentiation through ubiquitin-proteasome pathway. J Biol Chem 2005;280:29409–29419.
26. Ziegenhagen MW, Benner UK, Zissel G, et al. Sarcoidosis: TNF-alpha release from alveolar macrophages and serum level of sIL-2R are prognostic markers. Am J Respir Crit Care Med 1997;156:1586–1592.
27. Kunkel SL, Lukacs NW, Strieter RM, et al. Th1 and Th2 responses regulate experimental lung granuloma development. Sarcoidosis Vasc Diffuse Lung Dis 1996;13:120–128.
28. Graham DY MD, Kalter DC, Yoshimura HH. Isolation of cell wall defective acid fast bacteria from skin lesions in patients with sarcoidosis. In Grassi C, Rizzato G, Pozzi E, eds. Sarcoidosis and Other Granulomatous Disorders. 1988:161–164.

29. Ikonomopoulos JA, Gorgoulis VG, Kastrinakis NG, et al. Experimental inoculation of laboratory animals with samples collected from sarcoidal patients and molecular diagnostic evaluation of the results. In Vivo 2000;14:761–765.

30. Milman N, Lisby G, Friis S, et al. Prolonged culture for mycobacteria in mediastinal lymph nodes from patients with pulmonary sarcoidosis. A negative study. Sarcoidosis Vasc Diffuse Lung Dis 2004;21:25–28.

31. el-Zaatari FA, Naser SA, Markesich DC, et al. Identification of *Mycobacterium avium* complex in sarcoidosis. J Clin Microbiol 1996;34:2240–2245.

32. Fidler H, Rook GA, Johnson NM, et al. Search for mycobacterial DNA in granulomatous tissues from patients with sarcoidosis using the polymerase chain reaction. Am Rev Respir Dis 1993;147:777–778.

33. Gudit VS, Campbell SM, Gould D, et al. Activation of cutaneous sarcoidosis following Mycobacterium marinum infection of skin. J Eur Acad Dermatol Venereol 2000;14:296–297.

34. Mitchell IC, Turk JL, Mitchell DN. Detection of mycobacterial rRNA in sarcoidosis with liquid-phase hybridisation. Lancet 1992;339:1015–1017.

35. Popper HH, Klemen H, Hoefler G, et al. Presence of mycobacterial DNA in sarcoidosis. Hum Pathol 1997;28:796–800.

36. Klemen H, Husain AN, Cagle PT, et al. Mycobacterial DNA in recurrent sarcoidosis in the transplanted lung—a PCR-based study on four cases. Virchows Arch 2000;436:365–369.

37. Saboor SA, Johnson NM, McFadden J. Detection of mycobacterial DNA in sarcoidosis and tuberculosis with polymerase chain reaction. Lancet 1992;339:1012–1015.

38. Ghossein RA, Ross DG, Salomon RN, et al. A search for mycobacterial DNA in sarcoidosis using the polymerase chain reaction. Am J Clin Pathol 1994;101:733–737.

39. Richter E, Greinert U, Kirsten D, et al. Assessment of mycobacterial DNA in cells and tissues of mycobacterial and sarcoid lesions. Am J Respir Crit Care Med 1996;153:375–380.

40. Vokurka M, Lecossier D, du Bois RM, et al. Absence of DNA from mycobacteria of the *M. tuberculosis* complex in sarcoidosis. Am J Respir Crit Care Med 1997;156:1000–1003.

41. Alavi HA, Moscovic EA. Immunolocalization of cell-wall-deficient forms of *Mycobacterium tuberculosis* complex in sarcoidosis and in sinus histiocytosis of lymph nodes draining carcinoma. Histol Histopathol 1996;11:683–694.

42. Graham DY, Markesich DC, Kalter DC, et al. Mycobacterial aetiology of sarcoidosis. Lancet 1992;340:52–53.

43. Popper HH, Klemen H, Hoefler G, et al. Presence of mycobacterial DNA in sarcoidosis. Hum Pathol 1997;28:796–800.

44. Ragno S CM, Lowrie DB, Winrow VR, et al. Protection of rats from adjuvant arthritis by immunization with naked DNA encoding for mycobacterial heat shock protein 65. Arthritis Rheum 1997;40:277–283.

45. Huygen K CJ, Denis O, Montgomery DL, et al. Immunogenicity and protective efficacy of a tuberculosis DNA vaccine. Nat Med 1996;2:893–898.

46. Thonhofer R, Maercker C, Popper HH. Expression of sarcoidosis related genes in lung lavage cells. Sarcoidosis Vasc Diffuse Lung Dis 2002;19:59–65.

47. Vabulas RM, Ahmad-Nejad P, da Costa C, et al. Endocytosed HSP60s use toll-like receptor 2 (TLR2) and TLR4 to activate the toll/interleukin-1 receptor signaling pathway in innate immune cells. J Biol Chem 2001;276:31332–31339.

48. Kirschning CJ, Schumann RR. TLR2: cellular sensor for microbial and endogenous molecular patterns. Curr Top Microbiol Immunol 2002;270:121–144.

49. Rha YH, Taube C, Haczku A, et al. Effect of microbial heat shock proteins on airway inflammation and hyperresponsiveness. J Immunol 2002;169:5300–5307.

50. Petzmann SCM, Markert E, Kern I, et al. Enhanced proliferation and decreased apoptosis in lung lavage cells of sarcoidosis patients. Sarcoidosis Vasc Diffuse Lung Dis 2007 (in press.)

51. Ishige I, Usui Y, Takemura T, et al. Quantitative PCR of mycobacterial and propionibacterial DNA in lymph nodes of Japanese patients with sarcoidosis. Lancet 1999;354:120–123.

52. McCaskill JG, Chason KD, Hua X, et al. Pulmonary immune responses to *Propionibacterium acnes* in C57BL/6 and BALB/c mice. Am J Respir Cell Mol Biol 2006;35(3):347–356.

53. Minami J, Eishi Y, Ishige Y, et al. Pulmonary granulomas caused experimentally in mice by a recombinant trigger-factor protein of *Propionibacterium acnes*. J Med Dent Sci 2003;50:265–274.

54. Costabel U, Hunninghake GW. ATS/ERS/WASOG statement on sarcoidosis. Sarcoidosis Statement Committee. American Thoracic Society. European Respiratory Society. World Association for Sarcoidosis and Other Granulomatous Disorders. Eur Respir J 1999;14:735–737.

55. McGrath DS, Goh N, Foley PJ, et al. Sarcoidosis: genes and microbes—soil or seed? Sarcoidosis Vasc Diffuse Lung Dis 2001;18:149–164.

56. Iannuzzi MC, Maliarik MJ, Poisson LM, et al. Sarcoidosis susceptibility and resistance HLA-DQB1 alleles in African Americans. Am J Respir Crit Care Med 2003;167:1225–1231.

57. Voorter CE, Drent M, van den Berg-Loonen EM. Severe pulmonary sarcoidosis is strongly associated with the haplotype HLA-DQB1*0602-DRB1*150101. Hum Immunol 2005;66:826–835.

58. Kruit A, Grutters JC, Ruven HJ, et al. Transforming growth factor-beta gene polymorphisms in sarcoidosis patients with and without fibrosis. Chest 2006;129:1584–1591.

59. Hill MR, Papafili A, Booth H, et al. Functional prostaglandin-endoperoxide synthase 2 polymorphism predicts poor outcome in sarcoidosis. Am J Respir Crit Care Med 2006;174(8):915–922.

60. Spagnolo P, Renzoni EA, Wells AU, et al. C-C chemokine receptor 2 and sarcoidosis: association with Lofgren's syndrome. Am J Respir Crit Care Med 2003;168:1162–1166.

61. Bogunia-Kubik K, Koscinska K, Suchnicki K, et al. HSP70-hom gene single nucleotide (+2763 G/A and +2437 C/T) polymorphisms in sarcoidosis. Int J Immunogenet 2006;33:135–140.

62. Akira S, Takeda K. Toll-like receptor signalling. Nat Rev Immunol 2004;4:499–511.

63. Leung TF, Tang NL, Wong GW, et al. CD14 and toll-like receptors: potential contribution of genetic factors and mechanisms to inflammation and allergy, Curr Drug Targets Inflamm Allergy 2005;4:169–175.

64. Vabulas RM, Ahmad-Nejad P, Ghose S, et al. HSP70 as endogenous stimulus of the Toll/interleukin-1 receptor signal pathway. J Biol Chem 2002;277:15107–15112.

65. Jones RG, Elford AR, Parsons MJ, et al. CD28-dependent activation of protein kinase B/Akt blocks Fas-mediated apoptosis by preventing death-inducing signaling complex assembly. J Exp Med 2002;196:335–348.

66. Parry RV, Rumbley CA, Vandenberghe LH, et al. CD28 and inducible costimulatory protein Src homology 2 binding domains show distinct regulation of phosphatidylinositol 3-kinase, Bcl-xL, and IL-2 expression in primary human CD4 T lymphocytes. J Immunol 2003;171:166–174.

67. Beutler B. Inferences, questions and possibilities in Toll-like receptor signalling. Nature 2004;430:257–263.

68. Pabst S, Baumgarten G, Stremmel A, et al. Toll-like receptor (TLR) 4 polymorphisms are associated with a chronic course of sarcoidosis. Clin Exp Immunol 2006;143:420–426.

69. Fukao T, Koyasu S. PI3K and negative regulation of TLR signaling. Trends Immunol 2003;24:358–363.

70. Valentonyte R, Hampe J, Huse K, et al. Sarcoidosis is associated with a truncating splice site mutation in BTNL2. Nat Genet 2005;37:357–364.

71. Rybicki BA, Walewski JL, Maliarik MJ, et al. The BTNL2 gene and sarcoidosis susceptibility in African Americans and Whites. Am J Hum Genet 2005;77:491–499.

72. Nguyen T, Liu XK, Zhang Y, et al. BTNL2, a butyrophilin-like molecule that functions to inhibit T cell activation. J Immunol 2006;176:7354–7360.

73. Martinetti M, Tinelli C, Kolek V, et al. "The sarcoidosis map": a joint survey of clinical and immunogenetic findings in two European countries. Am J Respir Crit Care Med 1995;152:557–564.

74. Grunewald J, Eklund A, Olerup O. Human leukocyte antigen class I alleles and the disease course in sarcoidosis patients. Am J Respir Crit Care Med 2004;169:696–702.

75. Schürmann M, Lympany PA, Reichel P, et al. Familial sarcoidosis is linked to the major histocompatibility complex region. Am J Respir Crit Care Med 2000;162:861–864.

76. Schurmann M, Reichel P, Muller-Myhsok B, et al. Results from a genome-wide search for predisposing genes in sarcoidosis. Am J Respir Crit Care Med 2001;164:840–846.

77. Valentonyte R, Hampe J, Croucher PJ, et al. Study of C-C chemokine receptor 2 alleles in sarcoidosis, with emphasis on family-based analysis. Am J Respir Crit Care Med 2005;171:1136–1141.

78. Rossman MD, Thompson B, Frederick M, et al. HLA-DRB1*1101: a significant risk factor for sarcoidosis in blacks and whites. Am J Hum Genet 2003;73:720–735.

79. Sato H, Grutters JC, Pantelidis P, et al. HLA-DQB1*0201: a marker for good prognosis in British and Dutch patients with sarcoidosis. Am J Respir Cell Mol Biol 2002;27:406–412.

80. Foley PJ, McGrath DS, Puscinska E, et al. Human leukocyte antigen-DRB1 position 11 residues are a common protective marker for sarcoidosis. Am J Respir Cell Mol Biol 2001;25:272–277.

81. Seitzer U, Swider C, Stuber F, et al. Tumour necrosis factor alpha promoter gene polymorphism in sarcoidosis. Cytokine 1997;9:787–790.

82. Grutters JC, Sato H, Pantelidis P, et al. Increased frequency of the uncommon tumor necrosis factor −857T allele in British and Dutch patients with sarcoidosis. Am J Respir Crit Care Med 2002;165:1119–1124.

83. Yamaguchi E, Itoh A, Hizawa N, et al. The gene polymorphism of tumor necrosis factor-beta, but not that of tumor necrosis factor-alpha, is associated with the prognosis of sarcoidosis. Chest 2001;119:753–761.

84. Herry I, Bonay M, Bouchonnet F, et al. Extensive apoptosis of lung T-lymphocytes maintained in vitro. Am J Respir Cell Mol Biol 1996;15:339–347.

85. Kunitake R, Kuwano K, Miyazaki H, et al. Apoptosis in the course of granulomatous inflammation in pulmonary sarcoidosis. Eur Respir J 1999;13:1329–1337.

86. Stridh H, Planck A, Gigliotti D, et al. Apoptosis resistant bronchoalveolar lavage (BAL) fluid lymphocytes in sarcoidosis. Thorax 2002;57:897–901.

87. Dai H, Guzman J, Costabel U. Increased expression of apoptosis signalling receptors by alveolar macrophages in sarcoidosis. Eur Respir J 1999;13:1451–1454.

88. Shikuwa C, Kadota J, Mukae H, et al. High concentrations of soluble Fas ligand in bronchoalveolar lavage fluid of patients with pulmonary sarcoidosis. Respiration 2002;69:242–246.

89. Rutherford RM, Staedtler F, Kehren J, et al. Functional genomics and prognosis in sarcoidosis—the critical role of antigen presentation. Sarcoidosis Vasc Diffuse Lung Dis 2004;21:10–18.

90. Xaus J, Besalduch N, Comalada M, et al. High expression of p21 Waf1 in sarcoid granulomas: a putative role for long-lasting inflammation. J Leukoc Biol 2003;74:295–301.

91. Daniels CE, Wilkes MC, Edens M, et al. Imatinib mesylate inhibits the profibrogenic activity of TGF-beta and prevents bleomycin-mediated lung fibrosis. J Clin Invest 2004;114:1308–1316.

92. Homma S, Nagaoka I, Abe H, et al. Localization of platelet-derived growth factor and insulin-like growth factor I in the fibrotic lung. Am J Respir Crit Care Med 1995;152:2084–2089.

93. Yoshida Y, Morimoto S, Hiramitsu S, et al. Incidence of cardiac sarcoidosis in Japanese patients with high-degree atrioventricular block. Am Heart J 1997;134:382–386.

94. Baughman RP, Teirstein AS, Judson MA, et al. Clinical characteristics of patients in a case control study of sarcoidosis. Am J Respir Crit Care Med 2001;164:1885–1889.

95. Naruse TK, Matsuzawa Y, Ota M, et al. HLA-DQB1*0601 is primarily associated with the susceptibility to cardiac sarcoidosis. Tissue Antigens 2000;56:52–57.

96. Takashige N, Naruse TK, Matsumori A, et al. Genetic polymorphisms at the tumour necrosis factor loci (TNFA and TNFB) in cardiac sarcoidosis. Tissue Antigens 1999;54:191–193.

97. Hattori N, Niimi T, Sato S, et al. Cytotoxic T-lymphocyte antigen 4 gene polymorphisms in sarcoidosis patients. Sarcoidosis Vasc Diffuse Lung Dis 2005;22:27–32.

98. Sharpe AH, Freeman GJ. The B7-CD28 superfamily. Nat Rev Immunol 2002;2:116–126.

57
Histiocytic Diseases of the Lung

Carol Farver and Tracey L. Bonfield

Introduction

Histiocytic lesions of the lung are a group of diseases that arise out of defects in the lung's macrophage population. Although histiocytes play a major role in many diseases of the lung, including granulomatous diseases (mycobacterial and fungal infections, sarcoidosis)[1] and other interstitial lung disease,[2] we discuss only those lesions with the primary defect in the lung histiocyte or those systemic diseases with notable lung involvement. These include pulmonary Langerhans cell histiocytosis, Erdheim-Chester disease, Niemann-Pick disease, Gaucher's disease, and Hermansky-Pudlak syndrome.

Pulmonary Histiocytosis X

Clinical Disease

Pulmonary Langerhans cell histiocytosis (PLCH) is a disease of the dendritic cells of the lung referred to as *Langerhans cells*. The Langerhans cell histiocytoses are a heterogeneous group of diseases that are characterized by a proliferation of Langerhans cells in organs throughout the body that range from a malignant systemic disease as is seen in children[3] to the more benign pulmonary variant that is seen in adolescents and adults. This pulmonary form is usually the result of inflammatory or neoplastic stimuli in lungs of smokers or in lungs involved by some neoplasms.[4] The disease usually presents with bilateral nodules on chest radiographs, suspicious for metastatic disease. Treatment is smoking cessation and steroid therapy, but, predominantly, the disease undergoes spontaneous regression. Approximately 15%–20% of patients will progress to irreversible end-stage fibrosis.[5]

Pathologic Features

Pulmonary Langerhans cell histiocytosis is characterized by airway-based lesions that consist of a proliferation of Langerhans cells. The early cellular lesions are, on average, 1–5 mm in greatest dimension and consist of Langerhans cells, lymphocytes, plasma cells, and eosinophils. Although previously referred to as *eosinophilic granuloma*, eosinophils are not the major cell type present, and the lesion is, at best, a loosely formed granuloma, consisting of dendritic cells and not the epithelioid histiocytes seen in other granulomatous diseases. Immunohistochemistry reveals the Langerhans cells to be diffusely, strongly immunoreactive to S100 protein and CD1a.[6] Ultrastructural analysis reveals intracytoplasmic organelles called *Birbeck granules*, a normal constituent of Langerhans cells, in greater numbers in PLCH.[7]

Cellular and Molecular Biology

The pathogenetic mechanisms involved in the development of PLCH center on the homeostasis of dendritic cells in the lungs of smokers and the possibility of tobacco smoke as a trigger that disturbs this steady state and induces the proliferation of these cells.[8] Increased numbers of Langerhans cells in the bronchoalveolar lavage fluid in heavy smokers and the abnormal T-cell response to tobacco antigens by Langerhans cells supports a smoking theory.[9] In addition, the presence of the lesion around airways and the upper lobe distribution argues for an inhaled etiology.

The mechanism by which tobacco smoke stimulates the proliferation of Langerhans cells is not known. The role of cytokines in the pathogenesis of this disease has, not surprisingly, received significant attention. Some studies suggest that stimulation of alveolar macrophages near the airway results in secretion of such cytokines as granulocyte–macrophage colony-stimulating factor, transforming growth factor (TGF)-β and tumor necrosis factor (TNF)-α.[10] Excess granulocyte–macrophage colony-stimulating factor in transgenic mice can cause accumulation of dendritic cells around airways.[11] In addition, other cytokines, such as TGF-β, interleukin (IL)-1, and IL-4 have been localized to PLCH lesions, and it is thought that IL-4 may be responsible for the eosinophilic infiltrate in the lesions.[12] Other theories speculate that cigarette smoke stimulates the secretion of bombesin-like peptide by the neuroendocrine cells in the bronchiolar epithelium and leads to a similar stimulation of alveolar macrophages and a cytokine milieu that promotes the proinflammatory proliferative changes.[13]

Because PLCH occurs in only a small percentage of all smokers, some suggest that factors in addition to tobacco smoke are needed to produce the uncontrollable proliferation of Langerhans cells that occurs. Studies have established that, at least in some cases, the Langerhans cells in PLCH are clonal, suggesting that cellular abnormalities must play some part in the pathogenesis of the diseases.[14] Molecular evidence for this theory includes studies that show genetic predisposition, mutations, and allelic loss of tumor suppressor genes.[15] Also, other environmental exposures such as viral infections have been proposed to increase the susceptibility of some smokers to this disease.[16] However, studies have failed to identify viral DNA in PLCH.[17]

The final area of research in this enigmatic disease is the mechanism by which Langerhans cells destroy the bronchiolar epithelium, leading to the pathology that is seen. Although Langerhans cells in normal lungs have little ability to interact with T cells or act as effective antigen-presenting cells, the Langerhans cells of PLCH have a mature immunophenotype, expressing B7–1 and B7–2, the costimulatory molecules needed for lymphostimulatory activity.[18] This may allow the initiation of an "uncontrolled" local immune response that results in the tissue destruction that is seen. Furthermore, these bronchiolar epithelial cells may provoke the expression of this mature phenotype that leads to their own destruction either by secreting cytokines in response to environmental stimulants such as cigarette smoke or viral infections or by the development of hyperplastic or dysplastic lesions that express new "foreign" antigens.[18] Considerable research into the molecular and cellular events of this disease is needed to substantiate these theories.

Erdheim-Chester Disease

Clinical Disease

Erdheim-Chester disease (ECD) is a systemic non–Langerhans cell histiocytosis that usually affects adults and most commonly involves the long bones. Involvement of other organs, including the lung, has been reported. Lung involvement occurs in approximately 20%–35% of the cases,[19–25] and the symptoms are those of interstitial lung disease with cough, dyspnea, rhonchi, and pleuritic pain. Radiographically, the lungs reveal infiltrates in a lymphatic distribution, predominantly upper lobe, with prominent interstitial septal markings that can mimic sarcoidosis.

Pulmonary involvement by ECD may have an unfavorable prognosis, and the fibrosis that ensues is one of the most frequently reported causes of death.[19,20] The treatment of ECD is variable with corticosteroids, chemotherapy, surgical resection, and radiation therapy reported.[24]

Pathologic Features

The infiltrate in ECD consists of non–Langerhans cell histiocytes of dendritic cell phenotype.[13] The infiltrate is a histiocytic proliferation that contains large, foamy histiocytes with scattered giant cells, a scant number of lymphocytes or plasma cells, and some fibroblasts. The histiocytes express CD68 (macrophage antigen) and factor XIIIa (dendritic cell antigen) but express S100 protein weakly or not at all and do not express CD1a. Ultrastructural analysis reveals phagolysosomes, but no Birbeck granules are present.[26] This infiltrate involves the lung in a lymphangitic distribution (i.e., expanding the pleura and subpleura) in the interlobular septa and around the bronchovascular structures. The adjacent lung is usually essentially normal, although paracicatricial emphysema may be present if the fibrosis that can be sequelae of the infiltrate develops.

Cellular and Molecular Biology

Erdheim-Chester disease is a nonfamilial histiocytosis. The etiology of ECD is not known, but this rare disease has been established as primarily a macrophage disorder.[27] The lack of CD1a expression in these cells and the abundant phagolysosomes are consistent with a phagocytic cell, most likely closely related to alveolar macrophages. The peripheral monocytosis and the proinflammatory cytokine profile that are found in these patients might suggest that the histiocytic infiltrate is a result of systemic monocytic activation and invasion of circulating monocytes into the tissues throughout the body.[28] A recent publication documenting the successful treatment of an ECD patient by an agent toxic to monocytes supports a role for these cells in the disease.[28] Alternatively, end-organ cytokine production by local inflammatory cells resulting in proliferation and differentiation of resident immature histiocyte populations may produce a similar picture. Indeed, its coexistence with Langerhans cell histiocytosis[21] suggests that it may represent a disease in which macrophages transition between two different phenotypes along the differentiation spectrum of tissue dendritic cells.[29] Whether this is a benign or malignant proliferation has not been established. Of five patients studied, clonality has been demonstrated in three by polymerase chain reaction.[30]

Lysosomal Storage Disorders

Gaucher's Disease

Clinical Disease

Gaucher's disease (GD) is an autosomal recessive inherited lipid storage disease with an accumulation of glucosylceramide in the phagocytic cells due to a deficiency in the enzyme lysosomal hydrolase acid β-glucosidase.[31] There are three types of clinical diseases that are usually distinguished by their central nervous system involvement. Type I, the most common form, spares the central nervous system and is common in Ashkenazi Jews. Type II involves the central nervous system and usually leads to death before the age of 3 years. Type III involves the central nervous system later in life and usually has a more chronic clinical course.[32] Pulmonary involvement is found in both type I and type II GD but is most common in the latter. In both types, bronchopneumonia and increasing dyspnea are the most common complaints. Imaging studies can show consolidation, reticulonodular infiltrates, or interstitial thickening.[33]

Pathologic Disease

The pathologic picture of pulmonary involvement by GD is that of foamy macrophages, or Gaucher cells, infiltrating the alveolar or interstitial spaces and the peribronchial or vascular walls, including the septal capillaries. This vascular involvement may produce pulmonary hypertensive changes, especially in type I GD.[32] The Gaucher cells are macrophages with abundant cytoplasm that have a "crumpled silk" appearance. When infiltration of the Gaucher cells is diffuse, pulmonary fibrosis may occur.[31]

Cellular and Molecular Biology

The gene for GD is located on chromosome 1q21 and encodes for acid β-glucosidase. Two major haplotypes have been defined at this locus, *N370S* and *c84 ins G* alleles, and two minor haplotypes, *L444P* and *IVS 2*. The relationship of these alleles to the clinical phenotype has not been clearly elucidated, although Type I GD may be associated with the *NS70S* allele.[34] The allele frequency depends on the ethnic group, with Ashkenazi Jews containing a relatively small number of mutations. However, in the overall population, there may be many rare alleles, limiting an accurate diagnosis by DNA.[31]

The pulmonary injury in GD may be a result of macrophage activation by the accumulation of the undigested material due to the lysosomal enzyme dysfunction and surrounding lung parenchymal damage by proinflammatory cytokines secreted. Gaucher's disease patients have higher levels of circulating IL-6, IL-10, and IL-1β mRNA and TNF-α.[35] These cytokines also increased with disease severity, suggesting an etiologic link.[34]

Niemann-Pick Disease

Clinical Disease

Niemann-Pick disease (NPD) is one of several lysosomal storage diseases that can involve the lungs. It is a rare, autosomal recessive inherited lipid storage disease with accumulation of sphingomyelin due to a deficiency of the lysosomal enzyme acid sphingomyelinase, which degrades sphingomyelin into ceramide and phosphocholine.[36] Six clinical types of NPD have been described as NPD-A through NPD-F. In patients with NPD-B, lung involvement is the most important clinical symptom and prognostic factor. Patients with NPD-C have predominantly neurodegenerative disease, but a rare subtype of these patients with the *NPC2* gene mutation may also have some pulmonary involvement. Clinically, the NPD-B patients have recurrent pneumonias starting early in life, usually around 40 years of age, and imaging studies usually demonstrate a ground-glass infiltrate with interlobular septal thickening anywhere in the lungs.[37] Progression of the lung disease can cause significant morbidity and mortality, and treatment is difficult. However, a case of successful treatment by whole-lung lavage has been reported.[38] Despite this, compared with other NPD patients, those with NPD-B have a more favorable prognosis.[39]

Pathologic Disease

The usual pathology in the lungs is an endogenous lipoid pneumonia with abundant foamy "sea blue" histiocytes, usually referred to as *Pick cells* (Figure 57.1). These macrophages are present within both the alveolar spaces and the interstitium. Other inflammation is minimal, and there is only mild fibrosis with little, if any, loss of the underlying lung architecture.[40] Irregular emphysema has been reported in one case of a patient with NPD-C type2 disease.[41] Ultrastructural analysis of the alveolar macrophages in patients with pulmonary involvement reveals an abundance of lysosomes with lamellar bodies, the same structures found in other tissues.

Cellular and Molecular Disease

Like all lysosomal storage diseases, Niemann-Pick disease is a single gene disorder. The gene for acid sphingomyelinase is on chromosome 11p15.1. However, the molecular nature of the genetic heterogeneity underlying the

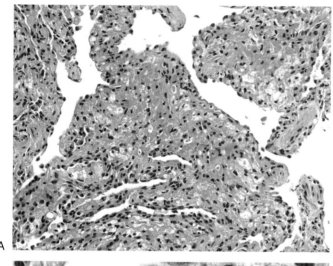

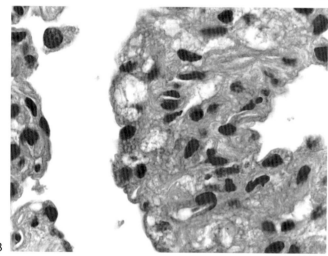

FIGURE 57.1. **(A)** Foamy macrophages present in the lung of patient with Niemann-Pick disease type B. (Hematoxylin and eosin; ×200.) **(B)** The macrophages are present within the interstitium and have grey-blue cytoplasm with lipid vacuoles that indent the nuclei.

clinical phenotypes is not well understood. In general, the cell injury in this disease is due to the accumulated sphingomyelin, stored as lamellar bodies in the lysosomes. In the lung, the focus is on the macrophages, where abundant sphingomyelin is stored. The mechanism by which this induces cell injury is not known. Unlike GD, there is no evidence in NPD for an increase in proinflammatory cytokines or macrophage activation in the lungs of these patients.[42] However, there is evidence of increased chemokine levels in lungs of the NPD-B patients, perhaps due to an increase in overall number of macrophages.

Studies from an acid sphingomyelinase knockout mouse model reveal elevated levels of macrophage inflammatory protein-1α, a monocyte chemoattractant in the bronchoalveolar lavage fluid. In addition, the macrophages present have a more mature phenotype when compared with mice of similar age. This suggests an increased number of monocytes are being recruited into the lungs from the periphery, and a slower rate of turnover of mature macrophages may be occurring in the lungs, leading to an increase in numbers of macrophages. The stimuli for the increased macrophage inflammatory protein-1α is unclear, but some speculate that the sphingomyelin–ceramide signal transduction pathway may be involved in the stimulation of this chemokine production.[42]

In addition to macrophage dysfunction, some have speculated that the recurrent infections in these patients may be due to an aberrant surfactant composition. Some NPD-B patients have pulmonary alveolar proteinosis-like pathology due to an accumulation of surfactant material in the alveolar space. This accumulation may be due to decreased catabolism by macrophages, and the increased amount of surfactant, especially surfactant protein A, may inhibit the macrophage response to infection and lead to the recurrent pneumonias that are seen clinically.[43]

Hermansky-Pudlak Syndrome

Clinical Disease

Hermansky-Pudlak syndrome (HPS) is a triad of oculocutaneous albinism, a bleeding defect due to a platelet storage pool deficiency and ceroid lipofuscin lysosomal storage disease.[44] Some patients have granulomatous colitis and pulmonary fibrosis.[45] The pulmonary fibrosis, found in approximately 50% of patients, develops during the third and fourth decades and is secondary to abnormal ceroid deposition in the lung. Chest imaging studies usually show a homogeneous distribution of reticulonodular infiltrates and fibrosis in the upper or lower lobes. The only effective treatment to date is lung transplantation, which is quite risky given the bleeding diathesis associated with the disease.[45]

Pathologic Disease

Hermansky-Pudlak syndrome–associated lung pathology consists of pulmonary fibrosis with characteristic type II pneumocytes with a foamy cytoplasm, sometimes referred to as giant lamellar body degeneration, foamy alveolar macrophages, probably containing ceroid-like material, patchy airway-centered fibrosis, and honeycomb changes without a predilection for any particular lobe.[46] Hermansky-Pudlak syndrome can even simulate a usual interstitial pneumonia pattern; however, the foamy alveolar macrophages will always help in the differential diagnosis. A lymphocytic infiltration usually accompanies the fibrosis. On bronchoalveolar lavage, the alveolar macrophages contain the granular ceroid pigment, which is positive with PAS and Sudan black histochemical staining. The origin of this ceroid-like material is not known; however, it may be a result of defective catabolism of lipids.[47]

Cellular and Molecular Biology

Hermansky-Pudlak syndrome is a group of eight related autosomal recessive disorders (HPS-1 through HPS-8). The common cellular defect is an abnormal intracellular trafficking that results in a dysfunction of specialized secretory organelles such as melanosomes. Other organelles are also involved as in platelets, T cells, and type II pneumocytes. The primary defect in all of the cells is found in the lysosome-related organelles.[48] Of the eight HPS diseases, HPS-1 and HPS-4 are the major causes of pulmonary fibrosis. This is thought to be the result of defects in the protein BLOC-3 complex in these two groups of patients. This complex regulates the function of the lung lamellar body.[49] Studies in both human and mouse models support the hypothesis that the primary organelle defect is in the production and secretion of this lamellar body, which leads to its accumulation in the type II pneumocytes.[46] Because the lamellar bodies store the surfactant lipids, the presence of these giant lamellar bodies indicates formation of cellular degeneration and accumulation of surfactant.[50] This initiates a cycle of cell injury, inflammation, and fibrosis. In addition, a ceroid lipofuscin substance that consists of a lipid–protein complex accumulates in the cellular lysosomes.[51] Phagocytosis of the excess lipid, surfactant, or ceroid-like material by alveolar macrophages may lead to alveolar macrophage activation and increased superoxide production and release, contributing to the parenchymal damage and fibrosis.[44]

The *HPS1* gene is located on chromosome 10[52] and encodes for a protein that contains two transmembrane domains.[44] Twenty-three disease-causing mutations have been found in the *HPS1* gene, although one variant accounts for the overwhelming majority of the cases, most found in Puerto Rico.[53] In Puerto Rican HSP-1 patients, homozygous 16-bp duplication in the *HPS1* gene is present and results in a clinical picture of restrictive lung disease, hemorrhage, and granulomatous colitis.[54,55] Fifteen patients have been reported with HPS-4, with 10 mutations documented on the *HPS4* gene present on chromosome 22.[49] Most mutations result in a loss of amino acids from a carboxyl terminus. Severe pulmonary fibrosis has been reported in these patients and HPS-4 RNA isolated from fibroblasts.[56]

References

1. Perez RL, Rivera-Marrero CA, Roman J. Pulmonary granulomatous inflammation: from sarcoidosis to tuberculosis. Semin Respir Infect 2003;18(1):23–32.
2. Popper HH. Epithelioid cell granulomatosis of the lung: new insights and concepts. Sarcoidosis Vasc Diffuse Lung Dis 1999;16(1):32–46.
3. Favara BE, Feller AC, Pauli M, et al. Contemporary classification of histiocytic disorders. The WHO Committee on Histiocytic/Reticulum Cell Proliferations. Reclassification Working Group of the Histiocyte Society. Med Pediatr Oncol 1997;29(3):157–166.
4. Tazi A. Cells of the dendritic cell lineage in human lung carcinomas and pulmonary histiocytosis X. In Lipscomb M, Russell S, eds. Lung Macrophages and Dendritic Cells in Health and Disease. New York: Marcel Dekker; 1997: 725–757.
5. Vassallo R, Limper AH. Pulmonary Langerhans' cell histiocytosis. Semin Respir Crit Care Med 2002;23(2):93–101.
6. Flint A, Lloyd RV, Colby TV, Wilson BW. Pulmonary histiocytosis X. Immunoperoxidase staining for HLA-DR antigen and S100 protein. Arch Pathol Lab Med 1986;110(10):930–933.
7. Tazi A, Bonay M, Grandsaigne M, et al. Surface phenotype of Langerhans cells and lymphocytes in granulomatous lesions from patients with pulmonary histiocytosis X. Am Rev Respir Dis 1993;147(6 Pt 1):1531–1536.
8. Vermaelen K, Pauwels R. Pulmonary dendritic cells. Am J Respir Crit Care Med 2005;172(5):530–551.
9. Sundar KM, Gosselin MV, Chung HL, Cahill BC. Pulmonary Langerhans cell histiocytosis: emerging concepts in pathobiology, radiology, and clinical evolution of disease. Chest 2003;123(5):1673–1683.
10. Annels NE, Da Costa CE, Prins FA, et al. Aberrant chemokine receptor expression and chemokine production by Langerhans cells underlies the pathogenesis of Langerhans cell histiocytosis. J Exp Med 2003;197(10):1385–1390.
11. Wang J, Snider DP, Hewlett BR, et al. Transgenic expression of granulocyte–macrophage colony-stimulating factor induces the differentiation and activation of a novel dendritic cell population in the lung. Blood 2000;95(7):2337–2345.
12. de Graaf JH, Tamminga RY, Dam-Meiring A, et al. The presence of cytokines in Langerhans' cell histiocytosis. J Pathol 1996;180(4):400–406.
13. Tazi A, Moreau J, Bergeron A, et al. Evidence that Langerhans cells in adult pulmonary Langerhans cell histiocytosis are mature dendritic cells: importance of the cytokine microenvironment. J Immunol 1999;163(6):3511–3515.
14. Yousem SA, Colby TV, Chen YY, et al. Pulmonary Langerhans' cell histiocytosis: molecular analysis of clonality. Am J Surg Pathol 2001;25(5):630–636.
15. Dacic S, Trusky C, Bakker A, et al. Genotypic analysis of pulmonary Langerhans cell histiocytosis. Hum Pathol 2003;34(12):1345–1349.
16. Casolaro MA, Bernaudin JF, Saltini C, et al. Accumulation of Langerhans' cells on the epithelial surface of the lower respiratory tract in normal subjects in association with cigarette smoking. Am Rev Respir Dis 1988;137(2):406–411.

17. Willman CL, McClain KL. An update on clonality, cytokines, and viral etiology in Langerhans cell histiocytosis. Hematol Oncol Clin North Am 1998;12(2):407–416.

18. Tazi A, Soler P, Hance AJ. Adult pulmonary Langerhans' cell histiocytosis. Thorax 2000;55(5):405–416.

19. Egan AJ, Boardman LA, Tazelaar HD, et al. Erdheim-Chester disease: clinical, radiologic, and histopathologic findings in five patients with interstitial lung disease. Am J Surg Pathol 1999;23(1):17–26.

20. Veyssier-Belot C, Cacoub P, Caparros-Lefebvre D, et al. Erdheim-Chester disease. Clinical and radiologic characteristics of 59 cases. Medicine (Baltimore) 1996;75(3):157–169.

21. Kambouchner M, Colby TV, Domenge C, et al. Erdheim-Chester disease with prominent pulmonary involvement associated with eosinophilic granuloma of mandibular bone. Histopathology 1997;30(4):353–358.

22. Madroszyk A, Wallaert B, Remy M, et al. [Diffuse interstitial pneumonia revealing Erdheim-Chester's disease.] Rev Mal Respir 1994;11(3):304–307.

23. Murray D, Marshall M, England E, et al. Erdheim-Chester disease. Clin Radiol 2001;56(6):481–484.

24. Shamburek RD, Brewer HB Jr, Gochuico BR. Erdheim-Chester disease: a rare multisystem histiocytic disorder associated with interstitial lung disease. Am J Med Sci 2001;321(1):66–75.

25. Rao RN, Chang CC, Uysal N, et al. Fulminant multisystem non-Langerhans cell histiocytic proliferation with hemophagocytosis: a variant form of Erdheim-Chester disease. Arch Pathol Lab Med 2005;129(2):e39–e43.

26. Rush WL, Andriko JA, Galateau-Salle F, et al. Pulmonary pathology of Erdheim-Chester disease. Mod Pathol 2000;13(7):747–754.

27. Devouassoux G, Lantuejoul S, Chatelain P, et al. Erdheim-Chester disease: a primary macrophage cell disorder. Am J Respir Crit Care Med 1998;157(2):650–653.

28. Myra C, Sloper L, Tighe PJ, et al. Treatment of Erdheim-Chester disease with cladribine: a rational approach. Br J Ophthalmol 2004;88(6):844–847.

29. Wittenberg KH, Swensen SJ, Myers JL. Pulmonary involvement with Erdheim-Chester disease: radiographic and CT findings. AJR Am J Roentgenol 2000;174(5):1327–1331.

30. Chetritt J, Paradis V, Dargere D, et al. Chester-Erdheim disease: a neoplastic disorder. Hum Pathol 1999;30(9):1093–1096.

31. Germain DP. Gaucher's disease: a paradigm for interventional genetics. Clin Genet 2004;65(2):77–86.

32. Amir G, Ron N. Pulmonary pathology in Gaucher's disease. Hum Pathol 1999;30(6):666–670.

33. Goitein O, Elstein D, Abrahamov A, et al. Lung involvement and enzyme replacement therapy in Gaucher's disease. Q J Med 2001;94(8):407–415.

34. Zhao H, Grabowski GA. Gaucher disease: perspectives on a prototype lysosomal disease. Cell Mol Life Sci 2002;59(4):694–707.

35. Lichtenstein M, Zimran A, Horowitz M. Cytokine mRNA in Gaucher disease. Blood Cells Mol Dis 1997;23(3):395–401.

36. Vellodi A. Lysosomal storage disorders. Br J Haematol 2005;128(4):413–431.

37. Mendelson DS, Wasserstein MP, Desnick RJ, et al. Type B Niemann-Pick disease: findings at chest radiography, thin-section CT, and pulmonary function testing. Radiology 2006;238(1):339 345.

38. Nicholson AG, Wells AU, Hooper J, et al. Successful treatment of endogenous lipoid pneumonia due to Niemann-Pick type B disease with whole-lung lavage. Am J Respir Crit Care Med 2002;165(1):128–131.

39. Minai OA, Sullivan EJ, Stoller JK. Pulmonary involvement in Niemann-Pick disease: case report and literature review. Respir Med 2000;94(12):1241–1251.

40. Nicholson AG, Florio R, Hansell DM, et al. Pulmonary involvement by Niemann-Pick disease. A report of six cases. Histopathology 2006;48(5):596–603.

41. Elleder M, Houstkova H, Zeman J, et al. Pulmonary storage with emphysema as a sign of Niemann-Pick type C2 disease (second complementation group). Report of a case. Virchows Arch 2001;439(2):206–211.

42. Dhami R, He X, Gordon RE, Schuchman EH. Analysis of the lung pathology and alveolar macrophage function in the acid sphingomyelinase—deficient mouse model of Niemann-Pick disease. Lab Invest 2001;81(7):987–999.

43. Ikegami M, Dhami R, Schuchman EH. Alveolar lipoproteinosis in an acid sphingomyelinase-deficient mouse model of Niemann-Pick disease. Am J Physiol Lung Cell Mol Physiol 2003;284(3):L518–L525.

44. Kobashi Y, Yoshida K, Miyashita N, et al. Hermansky-Pudlak syndrome with interstitial pneumonia without mutation of HSP1 gene. Intern Med 2005;44(6):616–621.

45. Lederer DJ, Kawut SM, Sonett JR, et al. Successful bilateral lung transplantation for pulmonary fibrosis associated with the Hermansky-Pudlak syndrome. J Heart Lung Transplant 2005;24(10):1697–1699.

46. Tang X, Yamanaka S, Miyagi Y, et al. Lung pathology of pale ear mouse (model of Hermansky-Pudlak syndrome 1) and beige mouse (model of Chediak-Higashi syndrome): severity of giant lamellar body degeneration of type II pneumocytes correlates with interstitial inflammation. Pathol Int 2005;55(3):137–143.

47. Witkop CJ Jr, White JG, Gerritsen SM, et al. Hermansky-Pudlak syndrome (HPS): a proposed block in glutathione peroxidase. Oral Surg Oral Med Oral Pathol 1973;35(6):790–806.

48. Li W, Rusiniak ME, Chintala S, et al. Murine Hermansky-Pudlak syndrome genes: regulators of lysosome-related organelles. Bioessays 2004;26(6):616–628.

49. Wei ML. Hermansky-Pudlak syndrome: a disease of protein trafficking and organelle function. Pigment Cell Res 2006;19(1):19–42.

50. Nakatani Y, Nakamura N, Sano J, et al. Interstitial pneumonia in Hermansky-Pudlak syndrome: significance of florid foamy swelling/degeneration (giant lamellar body degeneration) of type-2 pneumocytes. Virchows Arch 2000;437(3):304–313.

51. Brantly M, Avila NA, Shotelersuk V, et al. Pulmonary function and high-resolution CT findings in patients with an

inherited form of pulmonary fibrosis, Hermansky-Pudlak syndrome, due to mutations in HPS-1. Chest 2000;117(1): 129–136.

52. Oh J, Bailin T, Fukai K, et al. Positional cloning of a gene for Hermansky-Pudlak syndrome, a disorder of cytoplasmic organelles. Nat Genet 1996;14(3):300–306.

53. Lyerla TA, Rusiniak ME, Borchers M, et al. Aberrant lung structure, composition, and function in a murine model of Hermansky-Pudlak syndrome. Am J Physiol Lung Cell Mol Physiol 2003;285(3):L643–L653.

54. Gahl WA, Brantly M, Kaiser-Kupfer MI, et al. Genetic defects and clinical characteristics of patients with a form of oculocutaneous albinism (Hermansky-Pudlak syndrome). N Engl J Med 1998;338(18):1258–1264.

55. Pierson DM, Ionescu D, Qing G, et al. Pulmonary fibrosis in Hermansky-Pudlak syndrome. A case report and review. Respiration 2006;73(3):382–395.

56. Anderson PD, Huizing M, Claassen DA, et al. Hermansky-Pudlak syndrome type 4 (HPS-4): clinical and molecular characteristics. Hum Genet 2003;113(1):10–17.

58
Pulmonary Arterial Hypertension

Wim Timens

Introduction

Pulmonary arterial hypertension is and has often been classified into two separate categories: primary pulmonary (arterial) hypertension, presently more often called idiopathic pulmonary arterial hypertension (iPAH), and secondary pulmonary arterial hypertension.[1] As in many other diseases, the secondary form was defined by presence of proven causes or risk factors, whereas the diagnosis of the primary form could be made only after excluding other causes of pulmonary arterial hypertension. In 1998, a clinical classification of pulmonary arterial hypertension was put forth, the so-called Evian classification.[2] In a recent conference in Venice a revised clinical classification of pulmonary arterial hypertension was proposed (Table 58.1).[3] Both the original and the revised classification was based on a clinical subdivision aimed at separating different categories within each category based on pathophysiology, clinical presentation, and therapeutic options. The clinical classifications were more or less based on assumptions that subsets of pulmonary arterial hypertension have a comparable spectrum of pathologic changes. However, it became clear that in the different categories different segments of the pulmonary vascular tree are involved in more or less specific combinations of pathologic changes to arteries and to veins. In an attempt to better document the types of vascular changes and to standardize the pathologic reporting and description of background and extent of vascular pathology, a descriptive histopathologic system of classification was put forward at the Venice conference (Table 58.2).[4]

In the clinical and pathologic classifications of the plexiform pulmonary arterial hypertension, arteriopathies as well as venopathies were included. However, in this chapter the attention is focused on the arterial changes in pulmonary arterial hypertension either or not having an identifiable cause.

Pathology

In all forms of pulmonary arterial hypertension common pathologic features can be observed. These changes comprise medial hypertrophy of muscular and elastic arteries, dilation lesions and intimal thickening of elastic pulmonary arteries, and right ventricular hypertrophy. As these changes are found in all forms of severity of pulmonary arterial hypertension, it is obvious that these aspects of pulmonary vascular remodeling have limited diagnostic value. In addition, medial and intimal thickening of pulmonary arteries can be found incidentally in certain areas of the lung without a clear association to pulmonary arterial hypertension. Pulmonary arterial hypertension is, however, characterized by a specific set of changes to pulmonary arteries of which a comprehensive overview has been given by Pietra et al.[4] The main features are discussed, and present knowledge of the possible pathogenetic mechanisms that play a major role in development of these pathologic features are reviewed.

Constrictive changes are present in all parts of the arterial wall resulting from medial hypertrophy and thickening of intimal adventitia (Figure 58.1). At present the main opinion is that these changes result from imbalance between increased proliferation and reduced apoptosis of the different cell types that are present in the vessel wall. With respect to hemodynamics, these changes may have different consequences. On the one hand, vasorelaxant or vasoconstrictive properties of certain cells may be lost, with or without associated loss of ability to respond to external stimulants. On the other hand, the number and volume of the different cell types may be changed, resulting in actual thickening of the vascular wall with loss of available lumen.

Hypertrophy of the media results in an increase in the actual number of smooth muscle cells in the media, which leads to an increase in the cross-sectional area in pre- and

634

TABLE 58.1. World Health Organization's clinical classification of pulmonary hypertension (Venice 2003).

Pulmonary arterial hypertension
  Idiopathic
  Familial
  Associated with
    Collagen vascular disease
    Congenital systemic-to-pulmonary shunts
    Portal hypertension
    Human immunodeficiency virus infection
    Drugs and toxins
    Other (thyroid disorders, glycogen storage disease, Gaucher's disease, hereditary hemorrhagic telangiectasia, hemoglobinopathies, myeloproliferative disorders, splenectomy)
  Associated with significant venous or capillary involvement
    Pulmonary venoocclusive disease
    Pulmonary capillary hemangiomatosis
  Persistent pulmonary hypertension of the newborn
Pulmonary venous hypertension (with left heart disease)
  Left-sided atrial or ventricular heart disease
  Left-sided valvular heart disease
Pulmonary hypertension associated with lung diseases and/or hypoxemia
  Chronic obstructive pulmonary disease
  Interstitial lung disease
  Sleep-disordered breathing
  Alveolar hypoventilation disorders
  Chronic exposure to high altitude
  Developmental abnormalities
Pulmonary hypertension due to chronic thrombotic and/or embolic disease
  Thromboembolic obstruction of proximal pulmonary arteries
  Thromboembolic obstruction of distal pulmonary arteries
  Nonthrombotic pulmonary embolism (tumor, parasites, foreign material)
Miscellaneous
  Sarcoidosis
  Histiocytosis X
  Lymphangiomatosis
  Compression of pulmonary vessels (adenopathy, tumor, fibrosing mediastinitis)

Source: Simonneau et al.[3]

intraacinar pulmonary arteries. In general, not only the number but also the volume of the smooth muscle cells increases, thus leading to both hypertrophy and hyperplasia. Furthermore, in general also an increase in connective tissue matrix is observed. As a seeming contradiction, atrophy of the media also occurs in developing dilation lesions and in arteries with marked intimal thickening.

The increase in the intima can be concentric laminar or eccentric or concentric nonlaminar. The intimal thickening can be cellular and fibrous, each to a variable extent. Apart from endothelial cells, in the intima cells with features of fibroblasts and myofibroblasts are observed. In the so-called pulmonary plexogenic arteriopathy, concentric laminar thickening is a characteristic feature. Eccentric and nonlaminar changes contain mainly connective tissue matrix and fibroblasts and are in general associated with thromboembolic arteriopathy (Figure 58.2). Such thromboembolic arteriopathy can, apart from a primary presentation also be observed secondary to pulmonary arterial hypertension, most likely due to endothelial damage and perhaps shear stress phenomena. As in pulmonary arterial hypertension cells in both media and intima produce many growth factors, it can be envisaged that these growth factors also affect the changes associated with secondary thromboembolic arteriopathy. Therefore, further research should sort out these effects that may lead to identification of phenotypic changes that

TABLE 58.2. Pathologic classification of vasculopathies of pulmonary hypertension.

Pulmonary arteriopathy (pre- and intraacinar arteries) and subsets
  Pulmonary arteriopathy with isolated medial hypertrophy
  Pulmonary arteriopathy with medial hypertrophy and intimal thickening (cellular, fibrotic)
    Concentric laminar
    Eccentric, concentric nonlaminar
  Pulmonary arteriopathy with plexiform and/or dilation lesions or arteritis
  Pulmonary arteriopathy with isolated arteritis

As above, but with coexisting venous–venular changes (cellular and/or fibrotic intimal thickening, muscularization). The presence of the following changes should be noted: adventitial thickening; thrombotic lesions (fresh, organized, recanalized, colander lesion); necrotizing or lymphomonocytic arteritis; elastic artery changes (fibrotic or atheromatous intimal plaques, elastic laminae degeneration); bronchial vessel changes, ferruginous incrustation, calcifications, foreign body emboli, organized infarct; perivascular lymphocytic infiltrates

Pulmonary occlusive venopathy (veins of various size and venules) with or without coexisting arteriopathy. Histopathologic features:
  Venous changes: intimal thickening/obstruction (cellular, fibrotic); obstructive fibrous luminal septa (recanalization)
  Adventitial thickening (fibrotic); muscularization; iron and calcium incrustation with foreign body reaction
  Capillary changes: dilated, congested capillaries; angioma-like lesions
  Interstitial changes: edema; fibrosis; hemosiderosis; lymphocytic infiltrates
  Others: dilated lymphatic; alveoli with hemosiderin-laden macrophages; type II cell hyperplasia

Pulmonary microvasculopathy with or without coexisting arteriopathy and/or venopathy
  Histopathologic features
    Microvessel changes: localized capillary proliferations within pulmonary interstitium; obstructive capillary proliferation in veins and venular walls
    Venous-venular intimal fibrosis
    Interstitial changes: edema, fibrosis, hemosiderosis
    Others: dilated lymphatics: alveoli with hemosiderin-laden macrophages; type II cell hyperplasia
  Unclassifiable

Source: Pietra et al.[4]

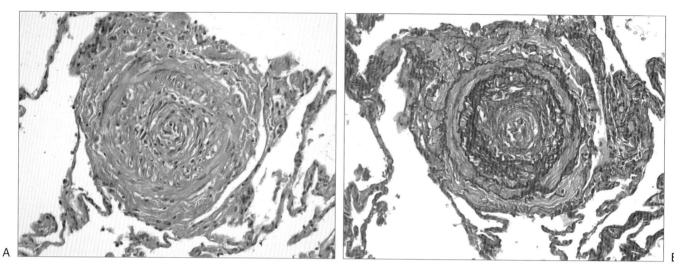

Figure 58.1. Small arteriole in pulmonary hypertension with medial hypertrophy and thickening of intimal adventitia. (A) Hematoxylin and eosin stain. (B) Verhoeff's elastin stain (original magnification, ×200).

may allow distinction between primary and secondary thromboembolic arteriopathies. The latter may be of interest as this may help to better identify the etiology of disease in patients who present with pulmonary arterial hypertension as well as thromboembolic pathology.

Adventitial thickening seems to be of less importance in adults, as in most cases involvement of the adventitia is not readily apparent. Whereas the above-described constrictive changes are mostly seen in early or relatively mild cases of pulmonary arterial hypertension, the more advanced or severe cases have additional hallmarks that are taken together as complex lesions in the recently proposed pathologic classification.[4] Pietra et al.[4] put forth

that the plexiform lesions, dilation lesions, and arteritis represent important focal changes that can be considered markers of severity and/or rapid progression of pulmonary arterial hypertension.

The plexiform lesion (Figure 58.3) consists of many vascular channels that are interconnected but are lined with endothelial cells. The tissue strands intertwining the vascular spaces are occupied by myofibroblasts with smooth muscle cells and extracellular matrix (Figure 58.4). This lesion is mainly found in the pre- and intraacinar pulmonary arteries, expanding into the arterial walls with extension into the perivascular connective tissue. Such plexiform lesions are hardly ever seen in pulmonary

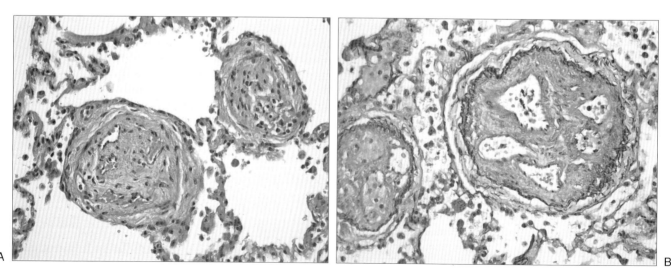

Figure 58.2. Postthrombotic vasculopathy: recanalized obstructed vessels (multiple lumina) (A) Hematoxylin and eosin stain. (B) Verhoeff's elastin stain (original magnification, ×200).

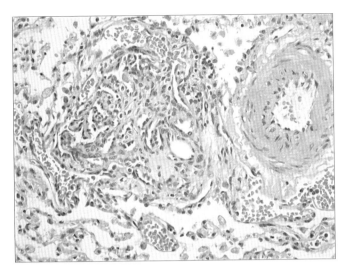

FIGURE 58.3. Complex lesion with thickened arteriole at the left and plexiform lesion at the right, with small dilation lesion at the edges. (Hematoxylin and eosin stain; original magnification, ×100.)

arterial hypertension in connective tissue disease or in pulmonary arterial hypertension associated with persistent fetal circulation. Arguments have been made that plexiform lesions are mainly based on proliferation of endothelial cells that are likely to be intrinsically abnormal,[5] even considered of a neoplastic nature by some authors, as these endothelial cells have been found to be monoclonal.[6] The endothelial cells express vascular endothelial growth factor (VEGF) and its receptors. The plexiform lesions are considered to result from this neoangiogenesis. Although an association between the vas-

culotropic human herpesvirus type 8 (HHV-8) and plexiform lesions of pulmonary arterial hypertension has been reported by some authors,[7] this could not be confirmed by several other studies performed later,[8] even with very sensitive molecular detection methods.[9]

Dilation lesions are in general found in association with plexiform lesions. Dilation lesions are very thin walled and are therefore considered vulnerable and possibly the origin of pulmonary hemorrhage.

Arteritis is considered to occur as a secondary phenomenon in pulmonary arterial hypertension, associated with the lesions described earlier. The morphologic presentation is that of a necrotizing arteritis with fibrinoid changes and infiltrates of chronic and acute inflammatory cells in the vessel wall.

Furthermore, in the histopathologic classification of changes associated with pulmonary arterial hypertension venous changes have been described,[4] now termed pulmonary occlusive venopathy, and pulmonary microvasculopathy, which are proposed to replace the previous terms of pulmonary venoocclusive disease and pulmonary capillary hemangiomatosis. These venous changes are not further described in this chapter.

Genetics

Bone Morphogenetic Protein Receptor Gene Mutations

Although there is a genetic basis for all forms of pulmonary arterial hypertension, much knowledge has been gained from studies of familial primary pulmonary

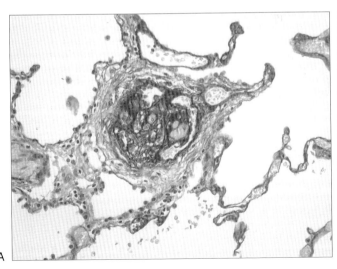

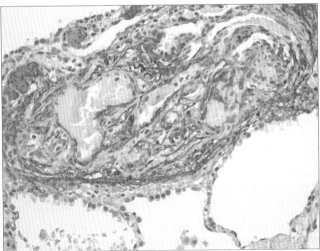

FIGURE 58.4. (A) Actin immunostaining of smooth muscle cells and myofibroblasts in plexiform lesion. (B) Collagen IV immunostaining in plexiform lesion. (A) Immunoperoxidase (original magnification, ×100). (B) Immunoperoxidase (original magnification, ×200).

arterial hypertension (fPAH).[10–14] This is an autosomal dominant inherited disease with great variation in expression within families, sometimes incomplete, and is predominantly found in females. The clinical course is similar to that of nonfamilial pulmonary arterial hypertension. Within fPAH, a strong association was found with mutations in bone morphogenetic protein receptor type II (BMPR2) and in activin-like kinase type I (ALK1).[10,11,15] Both of these molecules are receptors belonging to the transforming growth factor (TGF)-β family. In contrast to the BMPR2 gene mutations, the ALK1 receptor mutations were in particular found in some persons with the rare disease hereditary hemorrhagic telangiectasia (HHT). In HHT patients a mutation in the ALK1 receptor was associated with susceptibility to pulmonary arterial hypertension, in addition to the HHT lesions. As both BMPR2 and ALK1 belong to the TGF-β family, it is supposed that these mutated molecules share signaling modalities.[15]

The BMPR2 gene is located on chromosome 2q33, and this gene has 13 exons. The mutations have been reported in many of these exons (except for 5 and 13), with polymorphisms in some exons.[11] In general, each specific family is associated with a unique mutation that cosegregates with the disease.[16] All mutations are supposed to lead to an altered BMPR2 function.

Also in sporadic cases of pulmonary arterial hypertension BMPR2 mutations have been demonstrated in about 10%.[17] Initially this percentage was thought to be higher, but part of these were demonstrated to be associated to a first detected case of inheritable pulmonary arterial hypertension and therefore in fact should be considered a family case.[11] Until now the majority of sporadic cases of pulmonary arterial hypertension have not been associated with a major genetic abnormality. In addition it is clear that the mutation in BMPR2 itself is not sufficient to cause the disease, as several human subjects in whom mutations are found do not develop the disease.[10,11] It is clear that additional modifiers or effectors are needed[13] and that in an individual patient the effects of all these components together determine the outcome and severity of pulmonary arterial hypertension in that subject.

Serotonin Transporter Gene Overexpression

A second important molecule with abnormal expression in pulmonary arterial hypertension that can be associated with pathophysiology is the serotonin transporter (5-HTT) that is overexpressed in pulmonary arterial hypertension due to a functional polymorphism of the 5-HTT gene promoter with homozygosity for the L/L genotype.[12,14] This overexpression has been demonstrated in cultured pulmonary artery smooth muscle cells (PASMCs) from patients with pulmonary arterial hypertension to lead to abnormally strong proliferative responses to sero-

tonin or serum. This 5-HTT gene polymorphism has been shown to be related to the severity of pulmonary arterial hypertension in case of hypoxia in patients with chronic lung disease, indicating that 5-HTT overexpression in this particular L/L genotype is related to the pathophysiology of the different forms of pulmonary arterial hypertension.[18,19]

Pathogenesis

Role of Bone Morphogenic Protein and Its Receptor

Similar to TGF-β, signal transduction of BMP-mediated pathways involves two types of transmembrane receptors, BMP receptor types I and II. These receptors associate to form homo- or heteromeric proteins.[20] The binding of different ligands to one of these receptors results in activation of a downstream signaling cascade involving among others the Smad protein pathway. This Smad pathway is involved in different activities. It is one of the main pathways involved in TGF-β–induced extracellular matrix regulation and in antiapoptotic protein regulation. When BMPR1 is activated, the R-Smad protein phosphorylation needed for transcription to Smad-responsive genes, of which some encode for proapoptotic or antiproliferative genes, is induced.[20] Similar to that found in extracellular matrix regulation,[21] also in this pathway antagonistic Smads, such as Smad6 and Smad7, have a negative feedback role. Mutations in the BMPR2 gene may lead to a hampered binding of BMP ligands to either of its receptors because of diminished BMPR2 protein expression or by production of proteins that are structurally inadequate. This will lead to a diminished formation of proapoptotic Smad complexes.[20,22] A more extensive review of the possible mechanisms of this intracellular pathway in relation to the role of apoptosis in pulmonary arterial hypertension, including cellular and biochemical pathophysiology, is given by Mandegar et al.[20] and illustrated in Figure 58.5.

In iPAH a mutation in the BMPR gene would lead to reduced apoptosis, thereby counteracting the body's natural solution to counterbalance superfluous vascular smooth muscle cell hyperplasia. Furthermore, it has been demonstrated that BMP4, which constitutes another ligand for BMPR2, inhibits proliferation of arterial muscle cells from proximal pulmonary arteries but stimulates proliferation of PASMCs from peripheral arteries.[22] Further studies by this group show that patients with mutations in the BMPR2 gene show a defect in Smad1 activation and also a loss of growth suppressive response to BMP4.[22,23] Moreover, findings in animal models indicate that hypoxia induces production of endothelium-derived BMP4 associated with increased proliferation

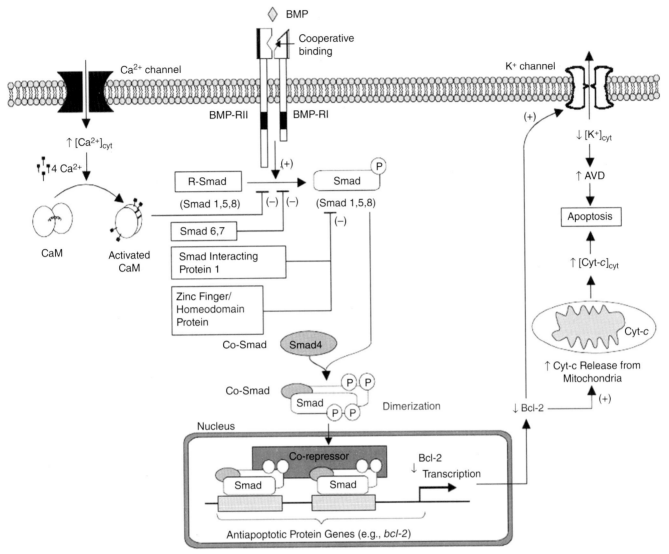

FIGURE 58.5. Schematic diagram depicting the proposed role of bone morphogenic protein (BMP)-mediated apoptosis in human pulmonary artery smooth muscle cells (PASMCs). There are two types of BMP receptors (BMP-RI and BMP-RII) that dimerize with one another and form a BMP ligand–receptor complex. The activated BMP-RI phosphorylates and activates the receptor-activated Smads (R-Smad), which then form dimerized complexes with co-Smads and enter the nucleus. The R-Smad/co-Smad interact with DNA in the nucleus and regulate the transcription of various target genes whose primers contain the Smad binding sequence (5′-AGAC-3′). In the nucleus, Smad1 (an R-Smad) and Smad4 (a co-Smad) in association with different corepressors appear to be involved in downregulating the expression of Bcl-2, an antiapoptotic protein that blocks the release of cytochrome c (Cyt-c) from the mitochondrial intermembrane space to the cytosol. Bcl-2 also downregulates the mRNA expression and inhibits the function of sarcolemmal K⁺ channels in PASMCs. Downregulation of Bcl-2 via the BMP/BMP-R/Smad1 pathway thus leads to an increase in K⁺ efflux and a decrease in cytoplasmic [K⁺] ([K⁺]cyt), which subsequently accelerate apoptotic volume decrease (AVD) and promote apoptosis; and an increase in cytosolic Cyt-c ([Cyt-c]cyt), which induces cell apoptosis by activating caspases. P, phosphorylation. (From Mandegar et al.,[20] with permission of Elsevier.)

and migration of vascular smooth muscle cells.[24] Therefore, BMP4 has a suppressive effect on arterial smooth muscle cells from normal subjects but not iPAH patients, in whom, in cases of hypoxia, it may even have a stimulating effect. In addition, BMP2 and BMP7 are able to induce more apoptosis in normal than in iPAH PASMCs.[25]

The role of apoptosis may be somewhat more complex than initially supposed.[25,26] A hypothesis was put forward[25] that in an early phase there may be increased cell death of arterial endothelial cells with loss of small capillaries, which may lead to survival of apoptosis-resistant endothelial cells possibly leading to proliferation in intimal and plexogenic lesions. At that time, the initial loss of endothelial cells would expose medial smooth muscle cells to circulating growth factors in a way that normally would not happen, except as a temporary phenomenon as in local vascular injury. It is suggested that in this process the so-called survivin pathway may play a main role in providing a positive feedback loop contributing to resistance to apoptosis.[27] Thus, in the above hypothesis early pulmonary arterial hypertension would be characterized by increased apoptosis in endothelial cells, whereas in a late phase reduced apoptosis and increased proliferation would be found in both intima and media.

With respect to therapeutic options, it has been suggested that modulation of apoptosis may provide new options but that the choice for either antiapoptotic or proapoptotic approaches should depend on the stage of disease. Considering the stage variation in different areas of the lung with respect to vascular changes in an individual patient, it remains to be determined whether such strategies will be feasible. New molecular imaging techniques or in vivo assessment of apoptosis in humans may provide new possibilities to evaluate such new therapeutic possibilities in this respect.

Role of Serotonin and Serotonin Transporters

Serotonin plays an important role in smooth muscle cell hyperplasia in pulmonary arterial hypertension by its interaction with specific receptors and internalization by a specific plasma membrane transporter. In pulmonary arterial hypertension an increased expression of 5-HTT has been found partly explained by polymorphism of the 5-HTT gene promoter.[14,28] This 5-HTT overexpression is proposed to represent a common pathogenetic mechanism in various forms of pulmonary arterial hypertension.[29] Expression of the different receptors is predominantly observed in the media of the pulmonary arteries with some weak staining in the endothelium. Immunoreactivity for 5-HTT was much stronger in lungs from patients with pulmonary arterial hypertension, especially in arteries with extensive medial hypertrophy. This intensity was in addition found to be expressed more in primary/idiopathic pulmonary arterial hypertension than in the secondary forms. Furthermore, recent findings indicate that the BMPR2 agonists BMP4 and BMP6 may be able to inhibit 5-HTT expression.[30] It can easily be envisaged that loss of BMPR2 together with increased serotonin exposition provides a direct interaction, synergistically contributing to pulmonary arterial hypertension.

Next to many other factors such as hypoxia and inflammatory cytokines, several drugs are known to affect 5-HTT expression. In particular the long-term use of certain appetite suppressants has been shown to be associated with an up to 30-fold risk of pulmonary arterial hypertension.[31–33] These appetite suppressant drugs belong to a class of drugs that interact with the monoamine system of the brain with potent inhibition of the neuronal 5-HT reuptake by inhibition of 5-HTT. This leads to a consistent increase in the availability of extracellular 5-HT.[20] Despite the association, not all subjects who use these appetite suppressants get pulmonary arterial hypertension, and in addition it is surprising that the use of these drugs is only associated with vascular remodeling in the lung but not in any other organ system. This strongly suggests that likely there is a genetic predisposition in some individuals that make these subjects vulnerable to developing this pulmonary arterial hypertension only after use of an additional factor, in this case these drugs.

Role of the Endothelium

Damage of the endothelium may allow arterial smooth muscle cells to be exposed to several mediators and factors, and in addition endothelial cells themselves are potent producers of various vasoactive mediators, such as endothelin-1 (ET-1), nitric oxide (NO), serotonin, thromboxane, and prostacyclins, as well as several inflammatory mediators. In pulmonary arterial hypertension, in late stages, excessive endothelial cell proliferation is observed in relation to neoangiogenesis resulting in formation of plexiform lesions. Although mediators produced by endothelial cells may contribute to development of these lesions, once established, the locally prominent presence of endothelial cells is likely to contribute further to arterial pathology.

Nitric oxide is an important molecule involved in vascular tone. Local vascular presence of NO is mainly regulated by different NO synthases (NOS) of which three distinctive isoforms can be discerned.[34,35] Two constitutional forms are recognized: the neuronal NOS (nNOS; also called NOS-I as expressed in neuronal cells) and endothelial NOS (eNOS; also called NOS-III and expressed in vascular endothelial cells). In addition, an inducible form of NOS (iNOS; also called NOS-II) is expressed in a variety of cells. In particular, iNOS is found in inflammatory cells and cells that are located at interfaces of different areas of the bodies (i.e., epithelia and endothelia). In pulmonary arteries of patients with pulmonary arterial hypertension in particular diminished eNOS is observed.[36]

One peptide produced by endothelial cells is ET-1. Endothelin-1 is a mitogen involved in vasoconstriction but also promotes inflammation and proliferation in smooth muscle cells. Pulmonary arteries with smooth muscle cells have specific receptors for ET-1, the ETA receptors, which are responsible for the vasoconstrictor effect, and the ETB receptors on endothelial cells, which are involved in vasodilatation, autocrine synthesis of ET-1, and clearing of circulating ET-1.[37,38] The vasodilative affects of ET-1 mediated through ETB-R in fact has been demonstrated to result from ETB-R–induced release of NO. With respect to angiogenic factors in pulmonary arterial hypertension, TGF-β and VEGF play a main role for which in particular the VEGF-A variant has been suggested to be involved in pulmonary arterial hypertension.[20] This has been demonstrated in animal models in which chronic hypoxia was shown to increase the expression of VEGF-A and its receptors VEGFR-1 and VEGR-2.[39] Circumstantial evidence of the role of VEGF is the fact that prostaglandins used in the treatment of pulmonary arterial hypertension promote VEGF production and prevent progression of the disease.[16]

Another important contributor to vascular remodeling associated with iPAH is thromboxane A_2 (TxA_2), which functions as a vasoconstrictor and a mitogen for vascular smooth muscle and is in addition an agonist for platelet aggregation.[20] Also for this molecule circumstantial support for a role in pathogenesis of iPAH is hypothesized based on finding an increased total TxA_2 synthesis in addition to elevated levels of urinary metabolites of TxA_2 in patients with iPAH.

Extracellular Matrix Remodeling

In addition to cellular changes in pulmonary arterial hypertension, remodeling of the vascular ECM component is also observed. The normal turnover of extracellular matrix is mainly regulated by matrix metalloproteinases (MMPs) and their natural counterpart, the tissue inhibitors of metalloproteinases (TIMPs). In pulmonary arterial hypertension, increases in extracellular matrix components, such as collagen, fibronectin, and elastin, is observed in intima, media, and adventitia. In an early phase, the initial endothelial damage is supposed to allow serum factors to accumulate and to activate smooth muscle serine elastase.[40] Despite the overall observation of increased extracellular matrix, in this early phase this would lead to elastolysis, in this way to local destruction of elastic lamina in arteries and arterioles, and thus contribute to vascular remodeling.[41]

In animal models[28] studying toxic or hypoxic pulmonary arterial hypertension, increased MMPs have been found, apparently insufficient to counterbalance the superfluous matrix production. Even so, inhibition of MMPs leads to pulmonary arterial hypertension exacerbations and enhanced vascular remodeling.[28] In iPAH in humans, this seems to be quite different, with decreased MMP-3 and increased MMP-2 and TIMP-1.[42] Considering the fact that extracellular matrix changes in pulmonary arterial hypertension contribute to changes in arterial wall caliber as well as loss of elasticity, it seems obvious to aim at use and further development of selective protease modulators as therapeutic tool in pulmonary arterial hypertension. However, as MMPs and TIMPs not only play a role in ECM remodeling but also can have profound effects on cell proliferation (like the stimulating effect of MMP-2 on smooth muscle cell migration and proliferation), it is not readily clear what the exact meaning is of observed abnormal levels in different forms of pulmonary arterial hypertension. This, together with the conflicting findings from animal and human studies, indicates the need of further human studies to provide the basis for therapeutic extracellular matrix and protease modulators.

The Thrombotic System

In pulmonary arterial hypertension, pulmonary artery thrombosis is often considered a phenomenon secondary to endothelial damage in advanced stages. However, intravascular coagulation has been shown to be a continuous process in pulmonary arterial hypertension and other forms of pulmonary hypertension, with altered procoagulant activity and fibrinolytic function.[15,43] Shear stress and endothelial injury are supposed to lead to a vulnerable thrombogenic intravascular surface. In the thrombotic process platelets are involved that release many mediators that also have vasoactive and proliferative capacities. For most of the (pro)thrombotic events it is unclear whether these are a cause or a consequence (or both), but taking the produced mediators into consideration, these events will likely enhance arterial wall remodeling. This is further supported by the demonstration of a thrombin-responsive kinase, serum- and glucocorticoid-inducible kinase 1 (Sgk-1), in the media of remodeled pulmonary arteries.[44]

Inflammatory Mechanisms

In addition to the intrinsic molecular genetic features linked to the pathogenesis of pulmonary arterial hypertension, inflammatory mechanisms also appear to play a significant role in some types of pulmonary arterial hypertension, such as those associated with connective tissue diseases. Circumstantial evidence for this role of inflammation is found by improvement of the hypertension with immune suppressive therapy. Some immunologic abnormalities were also found in primary pulmonary arterial hypertension with demonstration of circulating autoantibodies as well as decreased levels in the circulation of the proinflammatory cytokines interleukin-1 and interleukin-6. Furthermore, in histology inflammatory infiltrates have been found related to plexiform lesions in severe pulmonary arterial hypertension together with increased expression of RANTES and fractalkine.[45,46] Several questions remain related to the described inflammatory features. Changes in flow and circulation in the lung may result in inflammatory events in different lung areas, in particular in connective tissue diseases. It is not always clear whether there is a causal relationship between the inflammation and the pulmonary arterial hypertension or whether this may be a coincidental presence related to the underlying systemic disease.[47]

Conclusion

Several aspects of the development of vascular changes in pulmonary arterial hypertension and the possible role these vascular changes play in manifestation and pathogenesis of the disease are now clearer. The BMPR2 and similar receptors, together with changes in the serotonin-mediated effects on pulmonary arteries, have been shown to be main components in the pathogenesis of this disease. Furthermore, it is likely that several completely different factors play additional roles leading to the heterogeneity and also variable severity of the disease in individual patients and families.

Many of the presently advocated therapeutic modalities in pulmonary arterial hypertension reflect the recent advances in knowledge of the underlying genetic background and pathogenetic mechanisms.[48–50] Prostanoids prevent platelet aggregation and provide potent vasodilation; phosphodiesterase-5 inhibitors enhance NO-mediated vascular effects; and endothelin receptor antagonists are supposed to reduce vascular tone and inhibit vascular smooth muscle cell proliferation. Some of the used therapies are mainly symptomatic or adjunctive, such as anticoagulants, diuretics, supplemental oxygen, sometimes inotropics, and ultimately of course lung transplantation. Consistent with the heterogeneity in disease pathogenesis, the response to the different therapeutic modalities can vary considerably among individual patients. Promising new therapeutic horizons are formed by the serotonin-transporter inhibitors, ion channel blockers such as dichloroacetate, and statins such as simvastatin.[49]

Not yet clear is the relative contribution of the different pathologic changes and the way the different changes in the pathways cooperate in determining the outcome in individual patients. Therefore, although in recent years several important steps were made in unraveling the central molecular disease mechanisms of pulmonary arterial hypertension, this knowledge has to be integrated to further unravel the molecular interactions between different pathways. This will enable development of new therapeutic modalities and just as important, will allow better phenotyping of individual pulmonary arterial hypertension patients, providing opportunities for better tailoring of the present array of therapeutic options.

References

1. Newman JH. Pulmonary hypertension. Am J Respir Crit Care Med 2005;172:1072–1077.
2. Fishman AP. Clinical classification of pulmonary hypertension. Clin Chest Med 2001;22:385–391.
3. Simonneau G, Galie N, Rubin LJ, et al. Clinical classification of pulmonary hypertension. J Am Coll Cardiol 2004;43:5S–12S.
4. Pietra GG, Capron F, Stewart S, et al. Pathologic assessment of vasculopathies in pulmonary hypertension. J Am Coll Cardiol 2004;43:25S–32S.
5. Fishman AP. Changing concepts of the pulmonary plexiform lesion. Physiol Res 2000;49:485–492.
6. Lee SD, Shroyer KR, Markham NE, et al. Monoclonal endothelial cell proliferation is present in primary but not secondary pulmonary hypertension. J Clin Invest 1998;101:927–934.
7. Cool CD, Rai PR, Yeager ME, et al. Expression of human herpesvirus 8 in primary pulmonary hypertension. N Engl J Med 2003;349:1113–1122.
8. Katano H, Hogaboam CM. Herpesvirus-associated pulmonary hypertension? Am J Respir Crit Care Med 2005;172:1485–1486.
9. Henke-Gendo C, Mengel M, Hoeper MM, et al. Absence of Kaposi's sarcoma–associated herpesvirus in patients with pulmonary arterial hypertension. Am J Respir Crit Care Med 2005;172:1581–1585.
10. Humbert M, Trembath RC. Genetics of pulmonary hypertension: from bench to bedside. Eur Respir J 2002;20:741–749.
11. Newman JH, Trembath RC, Morse JA, et al. Genetic basis of pulmonary arterial hypertension: current understanding and future directions. J Am Coll Cardiol 2004;43:33S–39S.
12. Machado RD, Koehler R, Glissmeyer E, et al. Genetic association of the serotonin transporter in pulmonary arterial hypertension. Am J Respir Crit Care Med 2006;173:793–797.
13. Machado RD, James V, Southwood M, et al. Investigation of second genetic hits at the BMPR2 locus as a modulator of disease progression in familial pulmonary arterial hypertension. Circulation 2005;111:607–613.
14. Eddahibi S, Adnot S. From functional to genetic studies of a candidate gene for pulmonary hypertension: any point? Am J Respir Crit Care Med 2006;173:693–694.
15. Humbert M, Morrell NW, Archer SL, et al. Cellular and molecular pathobiology of pulmonary arterial hypertension. J Am Coll Cardiol 2004;43:13S–24S.
16. Machado RD, Pauciulo MW, Thomson JR, et al. BMPR2 haploinsufficiency as the inherited molecular mechanism for primary pulmonary hypertension. Am J Hum Genet 2001;68:92–102.
17. Thomson JR, Machado RD, Pauciulo MW, et al. Sporadic primary pulmonary hypertension is associated with germline mutations of the gene encoding BMPR-II, a receptor member of the TGF-beta family. J Med Genet 2000;37:741–745.
18. Eddahibi S, Humbert M, Fadel E, et al. Serotonin transporter overexpression is responsible for pulmonary artery

smooth muscle hyperplasia in primary pulmonary hypertension. J Clin Invest 2001;108:1141–1150.

19. Eddahibi S, Chaouat A, Morrell N, et al. Polymorphism of the serotonin transporter gene and pulmonary hypertension in chronic obstructive pulmonary disease. Circulation 2003;108:1839–1844.

20. Mandegar M, Fung YC, Huang W, et al. Cellular and molecular mechanisms of pulmonary vascular remodeling: role in the development of pulmonary hypertension. Microvasc Res 2004;68:75–103.

21. Zandvoort A, Postma DS, Jonker MR, et al. Altered expression of the Smad signalling pathway: implications for COPD pathogenesis. Eur Respir J 2006;8(3):533–541.

22. Yang X, Long L, Southwood M, et al. Dysfunctional Smad signaling contributes to abnormal smooth muscle cell proliferation in familial pulmonary arterial hypertension. Circ Res 2005;96:1053–1063.

23. Stewart DJ. Bone morphogenetic protein receptor-2 and pulmonary arterial hypertension: unraveling a riddle inside an enigma? Circ Res 2005;96:1033–1035.

24. Frank DB, Abtahi A, Yamaguchi DJ, et al. Bone morphogenetic protein 4 promotes pulmonary vascular remodeling in hypoxic pulmonary hypertension. Circ Res 2005;97:496–504.

25. Michelakis ED. Spatio-temporal diversity of apoptosis within the vascular wall in pulmonary arterial hypertension: heterogeneous BMP signaling may have therapeutic implications. Circ Res 2006;98:172–175.

26. Teichert-Kuliszewska K, Kutryk MJ, Kuliszewski MA, et al. Bone morphogenetic protein receptor-2 signaling promotes pulmonary arterial endothelial cell survival: implications for loss-of-function mutations in the pathogenesis of pulmonary hypertension. Circ Res 2006;98:209–217.

27. Sakao S, Taraseviciene-Stewart L, Lee JD, et al. Initial apoptosis is followed by increased proliferation of apoptosis-resistant endothelial cells. FASEB J 2005;19:1178–1180.

28. Eddahibi S, Morrell N, d'Ortho MP, et al. Pathobiology of pulmonary arterial hypertension. Eur Respir J 2002;20:1559–1572.

29. Marcos E, Fadel E, Sanchez O, et al. Serotonin-induced smooth muscle hyperplasia in various forms of human pulmonary hypertension. Circ Res 2004;94:1263–1270.

30. Marcos E, Fadel E, Sanchez O, et al. Serotonin transporter and receptors in various forms of human pulmonary hypertension. Chest 2005;128:552S–553S.

31. Eddahibi S, Adnot S, Frisdal E, et al. Dexfenfluramine-associated changes in 5-hydroxytryptamine transporter expression and development of hypoxic pulmonary hypertension in rats. J Pharmacol Exp Ther 2001;297:148–154.

32. Eddahibi S, Adnot S. Anorexigen-induced pulmonary hypertension and the serotonin (5-HT) hypothesis: lessons for the future in pathogenesis. Respir Res 2002;3:9.

33. Abenhaim L, Moride Y, Brenot F, et al. Appetite-suppressant drugs and the risk of primary pulmonary hypertension. International Primary Pulmonary Hypertension Study Group. N Engl J Med 1996;335:609–616.

34. Coers W, Timens W, Kempinga C, et al. Specificity of antibodies to nitric oxide synthase isoforms in human, guinea pig, rat, and mouse tissues. J Histochem Cytochem 1998;46:1385–1392.

35. Wolf G. Nitric oxide and nitric oxide synthase: biology, pathology, localization. Histol Histopathol 1997;12:251–261.

36. Giaid A, Saleh D. Reduced expression of endothelial nitric oxide synthase in the lungs of patients with pulmonary hypertension. N Engl J Med 1995;333:214–221.

37. Goldie RG, Henry PJ, Rigby PJ, et al. Influence of respiratory tract viral infection on endothelin-1–induced modulation of cholinergic nerve-mediated contractions in murine airway smooth muscle. J Cardiovasc Pharmacol 1998;31 (Suppl 1):S219–S221.

38. Davie N, Haleen SJ, Upton PD, et al. ET(A) and ET(B) receptors modulate the proliferation of human pulmonary artery smooth muscle cells. Am J Respir Crit Care Med 2002;165:398–405.

39. Tuder RM, Flook BE, Voelkel NF. Increased gene expression for VEGF and the VEGF receptors KDR/Flk and Flt in lungs exposed to acute or to chronic hypoxia. Modulation of gene expression by nitric oxide. J Clin Invest 1995;95:1798–1807.

40. Cowan KN, Jones PL, Rabinovitch M. Elastase and matrix metalloproteinase inhibitors induce regression, and tenascin-C antisense prevents progression, of vascular disease. J Clin Invest 2000;105:21–34.

41. Hassoun PM. Deciphering the "matrix" in pulmonary vascular remodelling. Eur Respir J 2005;25:778–779.

42. Lepetit H, Eddahibi S, Fadel E, et al. Smooth muscle cell matrix metalloproteinases in idiopathic pulmonary arterial hypertension. Eur Respir J 2005;25:834–842.

43. Herve P, Humbert M, Sitbon O, et al. Pathobiology of pulmonary hypertension. The role of platelets and thrombosis. Clin Chest Med 2001;22:451–458.

44. BelAiba RS, Djordjevic T, Bonello S, et al. The serum- and glucocorticoid-inducible kinase Sgk-1 is involved in pulmonary vascular remodeling: role in redox-sensitive regulation of tissue factor by thrombin. Circ Res 2006;98:828–836.

45. Balabanian K, Foussat A, Dorfmuller P, et al. CX(3)C chemokine fractalkine in pulmonary arterial hypertension. Am J Respir Crit Care Med 2002;165:1419–1425.

46. Dorfmuller P, Zarka V, Durand-Gasselin I, et al. Chemokine RANTES in severe pulmonary arterial hypertension. Am J Respir Crit Care Med 2002;165:534–539.

47. Dorfmuller P, Perros F, Balabanian K, et al. Inflammation in pulmonary arterial hypertension. Eur Respir J 2003;22:358–363.

48. Rubin LJ. Pulmonary arterial hypertension. Proc Am Thorac Soc 2006;3:111–115.

49. Martin KB, Klinger JR, Rounds SIS. Pulmonary arterial hypertension: new insights and new hope. Respirology 2006;11:6–17.

50. Dandel M, Lehmkuhl HB, Hetzer R. Advances in the medical treatment of pulmonary hypertension. Kidney Blood Press Res 2005;28:311–324.

59
Immunopathology of Pulmonary Vasculitides

Steven N. Emancipator, Philip T. Cagle, and Abida K. Haque

Introduction

Vasculitis refers to a number of distinct disease entities characterized by cellular inflammation within and adjacent to the blood vessel wall.[1] Typically, there is destruction of the vessel but leukocytoclastic vasculitis exhibits only leukocytic infiltrates within the vessel wall. Multiple classification schemes have been proposed to categorize this group of diseases (Table 59.1). Lung involvement is most common in primary idiopathic, small vessel, or anti-neutrophil cytoplasmic antibody (ANCA)–associated vasculitides of Wegener's granulomatosis, microscopic polyangiitis, and Churg-Strauss syndrome.[2] However, medium vessel vasculitis of classic polyarteritis nodosa, large and medium vessel vasculitis of Takayasu's arteritis (causing associated pulmonary hypertension), primary immune complex–mediated vasculitis of Goodpasture's syndrome, and lupus erythematosus can all affect the lungs. The pulmonary circulation is characterized by low perfusion pressure, and large- and medium-sized pulmonary arteries are shorter in length and contain less elastin than in the systemic circulation; these factors apparently limit involvement of the larger pulmonary vessels by vasculitis. Takayasu's arteritis, polyarteritis nodosa and its variants, Cogan's syndrome, thromboangiitis obliterans (Buerger's disease), and primary angiitis of the central nervous system do not affect the pulmonary parenchyma. Although pulmonary artery involvement occurs in giant cell arteritis (and in the associated polymyalgia rheumatica), extension beyond the main branches of the pulmonary artery are rare, or questionable. Behçet's disease and Kawasaki's disease, themselves uncommon, only infrequently (≈5% of patients) include a component of pulmonary vasculitis. Pulmonary involvement in these processes closely resembles that in other sites and is not discussed in this chapter. Pulmonary vasculitis may be seen in infections, with or without direct invasion of vessels by bacteria, fungi, viruses, and rickettsiae, and these are not discussed in this chapter either. The remaining noninfectious, immunologically mediated vasculitides that involve the lungs primarily affect arterioles, capillaries and venules, and perhaps small arteries and veins. Thus, by the Chapel Hill Consensus Classification, they are "small vessel" diseases.[1]

The immunologically mediated pulmonary vasculitides may be divided into three categories that derive from their apparent pathogenesis. Most common are those typically associated with detectable levels of ANCAs: Wegener's granulomatosis (WG), microscopic polyangiitis (MPA), Churg-Strauss Syndrome (CSS; also referred to as allergic granulomatosis and angiitis), and drug-induced vasculitis. Some include the anti-glomerular basement membrane (anti-GBM) antibody associated Goodpasture's syndrome in this category.[2] There is a voluminous literature on each of these diseases, collectively referred to as *ANCA-associated vasculitis* (AAV) notwithstanding the fact that not all patients with any of these conditions have positive serum titers of ANCA at all times during their course. From this literature, collections of clinical and/or pathologic descriptions that are especially comprehensive or insightful stand out. Those relevant to WG,[3–14] MPA,[15–22] and CSS[12,23–29] are cited here and then summarized in the following discussions on clinical and pathologic features without further citation.

The second category of anti-GBM disease is caused by antibodies specific for basement membranes. Again, these patients need not have sustained titers of specific antibody throughout the course of their disease. However, some evidence of autoimmune specificity for a basement membrane antigen at some time is required for this diagnosis. This subgroup of patients is considerably smaller than the combined population with AAV but has also been the subject of intense scrutiny in the literature. Compilations of patients with anti-GBM disease are also cited here.[30–34] The third category of pulmonary vasculitis represents lung involvement in a variety of "connective tissue" diseases. Because of the association of these processes with immune complexes, conditions such as

TABLE 59.1. Classification of pulmonary vasculitides based on size of the vessel involved.

Large vessel vasculitis
  Takayasu's arteritis
  Giant cell arteritis
Medium vessel vasculitis
  Polyarteritis nodosa
  Kawasaki's disease
  Isolated central nervous system vasculitis
  Temporal arteritis
Small vessel vasculitis
  Wegener's granulomatosis
  Churg-Strauss syndrome
  Henoch-Schönlein purpura
  Hypersensitivity vasculitis
  Cryoglobulinemia
  Goodpasture's syndrome due to anti GBM antibody
  Microscopic polyangiitis
  Other diseases (rheumatoid arthritis, systemic lupus erythematosus, polymyositis, dermatomyositis, Sjögren's syndrome)

Henoch-Schönlein purpura (HSP),[35–38] systemic lupus erythematosus,[39–41] rheumatoid arthritis,[42–46] Sjögren's syndrome,[47,48] mixed connective tissue disease,[49–53] polymyositis/dermatomyositis,[54–56] primary biliary cirrhosis,[57,58] and cryoglobulinemia[59] are presented herein as a group immune complex mediated vasculitides (ICMV). Curiously, other rheumatic diseases such as progressive systemic sclerosis (scleroderma), relapsing polychondritis, ankylosing spondylitis, and Marfan's disease do not elicit vasculitis. These latter diseases are not considered here, even though they may involve pulmonary parenchyma by other processes.

These three broad categories, AAV, anti-GBM disease, and ICMV, have significant commonalities. One such commonality is the clinical association of lung involvement with collateral renal involvement. In fact, these entities represent the vast majority of diseases characterized as pulmonary–renal syndrome. Of course, many of these diseases also have clinical, pathologic, and/or molecular features that distinguish them from the others and from other forms of systemic vasculitis in which pulmonary involvement is exceptional or unrecognized. Throughout this chapter, the common elements will be presented, followed by discussion of the distinctive features for the specific diseases, as applicable.

The diseases that elicit pulmonary vasculitis with regularity underlie the pulmonary–renal syndrome first reported by Goodpasture. Certainly, other organ systems are involved and may predominate in WG and CSS. The unifying elements of all the diseases discussed in this chapter, in terms of molecular pathogenesis and focal points for therapy, are pulmonary and renal involvement. For example, disease in both the lung and kidney is present in 85%–95% of patients with WG, the most common among these conditions. Many of the clinical and pathologic aspects of disease outside the lung and glomerulus represent important discriminators among these otherwise heavily overlapping conditions.

Pathologic Features

The common histologic expression of the pulmonary parenchymal involvement in all the diseases under consideration is capillaritis: neutrophils, and a varying minor component of monocytes, marginate and infiltrate into subendothelial and interstitial sites within the alveolar walls. There is often extension to adjacent portions of the alveolar space, but restriction of the intraalveolar infiltrate to elliptical or crescent-shaped zones immediately adjacent to interstitial foci of dense neutrophilic infiltrate represents an important feature distinguishing these foci from bacterial pneumonia (Figure 59.1). To a variable extent, fibrinoid necrosis, an admixture of monocytes, plasma cells, or lymphocytes, and/or capillary thrombosis may be present. Usually, but not inevitably, focal or diffuse intraalveolar hemorrhage is evident as erythrocytes accumulate in or fill alveoli. Later, erythrocytes are seen as phagocytic particles within macrophages. Ultimately, variable numbers of hemosiderin-laden macrophages, in numbers far exceeding those observed in chronic passive congestion or chronic infectious pneumonia, are evident.

In MPA, anti-GBM disease, and the ICMV, capillaritis, with irregular involvement of arterioles and venules, and perhaps limited extension to small arteries and veins, represents the sum total histologic expression. Relatively pure capillaritis (including alveolar hemorrhage) is most frequent in anti-GBM disease and ICMV. In MPA, inflammation in arterioles, venules, and small arteries and veins often complicates the pure capillaritis, and

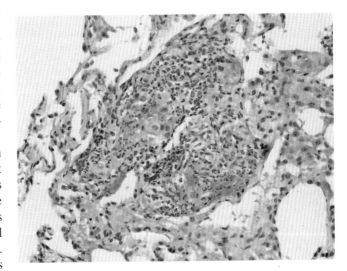

FIGURE 59.1. Microscopic polyangiitis showing neutrophil infiltrate of alveolar capillary walls. No destruction of the vessel wall is seen. (Hematoxylin and eosin; ×200.)

hyperplasia of type II pneumocytes is detected. However, involvement of medium-sized arteries or veins in anti-GBM, disease or ICMV is quite unusual. Light microscopy cannot reliably discriminate among MPA, anti-GBM disease, and ICMV. Immunohistochemical techniques, preferably immunofluorescence performed on cryostat sections, show linear or granular accumulations of immunoglobulins complement components in the alveolar wall in anti-GBM disease and ICMV, respectively. Until complicated by necrotic injury, lung tissue in lesions from AAV lack immune deposits. HSP is particularly distinctive among the ICMVs, because IgA and C3 are the exclusive or predominant components of the granular immune deposits. However, not all cases offer clear-cut findings. On the other hand, several histologic features in addition to capillaritis and small vessel vasculitis distinguish WG and CSS from MPA, anti-GBM disease and ICMV, and from each other.

The overall process of WG exhibits three cardinal components: vasculitis, granulomatous necrosis, and an inflammatory background. These elements combine in varying proportions in the multiple sites of active disease. Small biopsy specimens, and even specimens obtained during open biopsies of lung, might lack one or even two of these elements. In fact, all of the features are seldom present in a single histologic sample. The seminal vasculitic component in WG is capillaritis, as mentioned earlier. However, medium-sized arteries and veins are also typically affected in WG; such lesions evolve as neutrophil endothelialitis (with exudates confined to the intima) and progress to transmural inflammation with microabscess formation. Wegener's granulomatosis may present as diffuse pulmonary hemorrhage, and in a series by Travis et al.[34] WG was the most frequent specific diagnosis in a series of 34 cases of diffuse pulmonary hemorrhage for which lung biopsy was performed.

Granulomatous necrosis arises in alveolar walls as macrophages palisade around the clusters of neutrophils, typically in association with liquefactive necrosis (Figure 59.2). Similar, but somewhat larger lesions develop in small- to medium-sized arteries and veins, wherein widely distributed transmural neutrophil-rich infiltrates give rise to eccentrically placed microabscesses that develop into necrotizing intramural granulomata. These latter focal lesions in the larger vessels represent the closest approximation within the highly vascularized lung to the evolution of extra-pulmonary granulomata around foci of necrosis and microabscesses. Unlike the granulomata in many other processes, the formation of granulomata remote from zones of necrosis is unusual in WG, and the necrosis cannot be ascribed to ischemia of tissue perfused by involved vessels. Rather, in WG, necrosis and granuloma formation occur pari passu. The appearance of non-necrotizing granulomata apart from foci of necrosis is distinctly unusual in WG. Both within and beyond the lung, foci of granulomatous necrosis often coalesce to form confluent regions of irregular densely basophilic necrosis, as so-called geographic necrosis. Occasionally, microthrombi and/or foci of fibrinoid necrosis are also present, but such foci are not prominent. Careful examination shows necrosis beyond and independent of vasculitis, underscoring the principle that granulomatous necrosis is a process separate from vasculitis rather than a complication of vasculitis.

The inflammatory background in WG is highly variable, but potentially widespread. Acute foci of alveolar

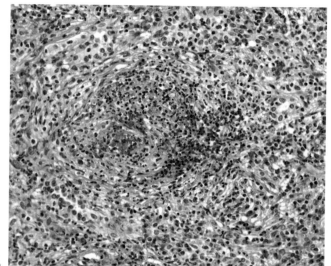
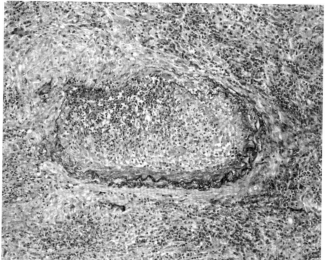

FIGURE 59.2. Wegener's granulomatosis. **(A)** Granulomatous and acute inflammatory infiltration and destruction of a small blood vessel. (Hematoxylin and eosin; ×150.) **(B)** Destruction of elastic lamina of the vessel. (Verhoeff-Van Gieson elastic stain; ×300.)

hemorrhage, hyaline membranes, edema, fibrinopurulent exudates, bronchiolitis obliterans and/or organizing pneumonitis, and foci of lymphohistiocytic or lymphoplasmacytic infiltrate, fibrosis, and hemosiderin macrophages can be encountered in virtually any combination and distribution. Particularly in zones of granulomatous necrosis, but also within the inflammatory background, multinucleate giant cells are often conspicuous and numerous. Although eosinophils are present in the infiltrates in WG, they do not represent a major component.

The lesions of CSS include eosinophil-dominant inflammation, extravascular necrotizing granulomata, and vasculitis. In the early phase of pulmonary involvement, CSS resembles eosinophilic pneumonia and is characterized by interstitial accumulation of eosinophils, with varying numbers of lymphocytes, plasma cells, and macrophages. In addition to tissue infiltration by eosinophils, a so-called eosinophilic capillaritis can be encountered. As disease progresses, alveoli become filled with eosinophils and histiocytes, and eosinophilic microabscesses may be detected in alveolar walls and air spaces (Figure 59.3). Histiocytes palisade around eosinophilic debris to form extravascular necrotizing granulomata that differ sharply from the basophilic granulomatous necrosis, often within the vessel wall, that is so characteristic of WG.

Some patients with CSS have well-developed nonnecrotizing granulomata, generally remote from but occasionally within blood vessels. The vasculitis in CSS is generally low grade compared with that in WG and even in MPA. Vasculitis in CSS, which often involves medium-sized arteries and veins as well as smaller vessels, ranges from an eosinophilic leukocytoclastic vasculitis to cir-

cumferential fibrinoid necrosis. Vascular granulomata are unusual and, if present, are small; they may be necrotizing or nonnecrotizing. In the later phases, changes associated with healing, such as granulation tissue and/or fibrosis, are encountered. Finally, in the majority of CSS patients, who have suffered chronically from asthma, goblet cell hyperplasia and smooth muscle hypertrophy is demonstrable in the airways.

Molecular Pathology

Only a small fraction of the aggregate evidence implicating particular gene products in the genesis and/or evolution of the diseases considered herein are derived from evaluation of the sequence or levels of nucleic acid. Therefore, the levels of molecules such as proteins and oligosaccharides in the circulation and diseased tissues are considered herein in conjunction with the levels of mRNA and genetic polymorphisms. Similarly, the functional effects of such molecules, as disclosed by the effects of pharmacologic antagonists, recombinant molecules, or their analogs, are evaluated alongside those from cell culture and/or animal models that incorporate targeted deletions of the relevant biomolecules.

Another potential departure in this chapter is inclusion of data derived from extrapulmonary disease. Involvement of multiple organs or systems is an intrinsic element in the vasculitides. As such, data derived from many organs and from patients with minor or no pulmonary disease are included in this chapter, because the central properties of injury are applicable broadly. Indeed, these diseases are frequently distinguished from one another by extrapulmonary clinical signs or symptoms. Particularly, renal and cutaneous involvement is common in these diseases, and their mechanisms are more widely studied than, yet highly pertinent to, lung disease.

In this section, an overarching conceptualization of the molecular pathogenesis common to these diseases will be followed by a summary of current information supporting the roles of particular molecules or classes of molecules. This approach should promote an appreciation of the complexity of interaction among a panoply of cells and molecules, of the similarities in the processes, of modifying features that shape each disease as a unique entity, and finally of the state of the art at present.

Overwhelmingly, pulmonary vasculitis is not only immune mediated but autoimmune in nature. Anti-GBM disease affects only a small minority of such patients but nonetheless is well accepted as disease instigated by a response to a self-protein, specifically, the noncollagen domain I of the α3 chain of type IV collagen, the isoform of collagen characteristic of and essentially confined to

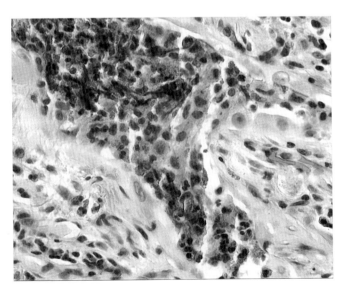

FIGURE 59.3. Eosinophilic and histiocytic infiltrate in Churg-Strauss syndrome. (Hematoxylin and eosin; ×600.)

basement membranes. The AAVs, which collectively account for the vast majority of pulmonary vasculitides, are increasingly recognized as autoimmune diseases as well.

Antineutrophil Cytoplasmic Antibody–Associated Vasculitides

In a literature too voluminous to cite here, growing evidence indicates that the characteristic ANCA autoantibodies specific for neutrophil proteins are not simply markers but actively contribute to and perhaps wholly underlie disease onset.[60] The ANCAs are autoantibodies directed against the components of primary granules of neutrophils and the peroxidase-positive lysosomes of monocytes. The primary antigenic targets are proteinase 3 (PR3 or PRTN3), a 29-kD neutral serine protease, and myeloperoxidase (MPO), a 140-kD enzyme involved in oxidative cell injury.[2,61–63]

The inducers of ANCA are not known; however, it is postulated that ANCA is part of a preexisting autoimmune repertoire that is activated by environmental factors such as exposure to silica and infectious agents.[2] Arbovirus and *Staphylococcus aureus* infections and subacute bacterial endocarditis are reportedly associated with ANCA. Molecular similarity between ANCA antigens and infectious pathogens can trigger ANCA induction in susceptible subjects; however, evidence for similarities to infectious agents is limited. Recent studies suggest that the initial trigger for the autoimmune response to PR3 is a protein with an amino acid sequence complementary to PR3, with induction of an idiotypic antibody (anti-cPR3) that induces a second immune response.[64] The resulting antiidiotypic antibodies react with PR3. Table 59.2 outlines the current understanding of pathogenesis of ANCA-associated vasculitis. There is experimental evidence that both PR3-ANCA, and MPO-ANCA contribute to vasculitis. Antineutrophil cytoplasmic antibody immunoglobulin G (IgG) can activate neutrophils and monocytes, the cells containing ANCA antigens, resulting in release of reactive oxygen species and enzymes. Furthermore, coincubation of ANCA-activated neutrophils and endothelial cells induces neutrophil adherence and endothelial cell necrosis. The ANCA-mediated activation of neutrophils and monocytes can also induce proinflammatory cytokines and chemokines such as interleukin (IL)-1, IL-6, IL-8, and tumor necrosis factor (TNF). These mediators can contribute to the propagation of vascular inflammation. The mechanisms that underlie the ANCA-mediated activation of neutrophils and monocytes are still under investigation; however, it has been shown that neutrophil activation requires priming with proinflammatory factors, especially TNF. Tumor necrosis factor priming induces the translocation of the ANCA antigens PR3 and MPO

TABLE 59.2. Pathogenesis of antineutrophil cytoplasmic antibody (ANCA)–associated vasculitis.

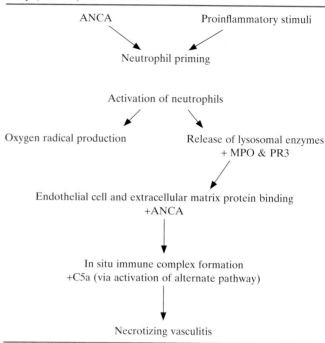

Note: C5a, complement 5a; MPO, myeloperoxidase; PR3, proteinase 3.

to the cell surface, making them accessible for interaction with ANCA. It is thought that the simultaneous engagement of the F (ab′)$_2$ portion of ANCA with ANCA antigens on the cell surface and interaction of the Fc part of antibody with Fcγ receptors is the trigger that initiates the signaling cascade for neutrophil activation.

T Cells in Antineutrophil Cytoplasmic Antibody–Mediated Vasculitis

IgG1 and IgG4 predominate in the ANCA mediated autoantibody response, implying isotype switching dependent on repeated antigenic stimulation and factors secreted by antigen-specific T lymphocytes. Several markers of T-cell activation are increased in ANCA-associated vasculitides, such as soluble IL-2 receptor, soluble CD4, and soluble CD8. Additionally, activated CD4$^+$ and CD8$^+$ T cells are increased in patients with active WG compared with healthy adults. The majority of cells in ANCA-associated vasculitis are CD4$^+$, T cells that recognize major histocompatibility class II molecules, and secrete cytokines upon activation. Furthermore, the cytokine profile points to a predominance of T-cell helper 1 (Th1) cells, with significant interferon (IFN)-γ production, although it is not clear whether this is a specific response to ANCA antigens or a nonspecific response to injury.

Leukocyte–Endothelial Cell Interaction

Two aspects surrounding the activation of and interaction among leukocytes and endothelial cells distinguish the evolution of vasculitic lesions from the inflammatory process in general. First, whereas leukocyte diapedesis is nearly totally confined to postcapillary venules in general inflammation, leukocytes adhere to and penetrate the endothelial lining of arteries, arterioles, capillaries, and veins in the vasculitides. Moreover, leukocytes remain within or immediately adjacent to the vessel wall in vasculitis, whereas the infiltrate in other inflammatory processes (e.g., pneumonia) is much more widely dispersed. These variations from more common situations have ramifications for pathogenesis and pathophysiology. Particularly, the activation of endothelium for leukocyte recruitment at sites that rarely participate in diapedesis implies a distinct mode of stimulation. In the vasculitides, the cytokines, chemokines, and adhesion molecules that typically orchestrate the exodus of leukocytes from the bloodstream into the tissues must be sufficiently proximate and powerful to involve endothelial cells that do not generally instigate leukocyte diapedesis. Moreover, at least some of these stimuli likely arise within the vessel wall itself if the inflammatory infiltrate is to remain around the vessel.

Alveolar capillary endothelium in the normal human lung does not express any of the major adhesion molecules considered integral to leukocyte diapedesis[65] and yet are the nexus for pulmonary vasculitis. Approximately half of the endothelial cells in the larger intrapulmonary vessels bear immunohistochemically demonstrable E-selectin and vascular cell adhesion molecule-1 (VCAM-1), but very few express intercellular cell adhesion molecule-1 (ICAM-1). In the vasculitides, up-regulation of adhesion molecules on the endothelium is the linchpin; circulating neutrophils, although activated, do not increase surface expression of adhesion molecules.[66] This situation is distinct from that in sepsis and other conditions, wherein fully activated circulating neutrophils regularly bear increased levels of adhesion molecules on their surface.[66]

Cytokines in Vasculitides

Among the cytokines TNF-α, IL-1 (in α or β isoforms), and IL-6 emerge as particularly pivotal modulators of inflammation, active on both endothelial cells and leukocytes. Generally, cytokines act locally, but significant increases in circulating TNF-α (relative to healthy volunteers) are reported in WG, CSS, MPA and ICMV.[67–72] Higher levels are recorded during disease exacerbation compared with remission. Often, patients also have abnormally low levels of endogenous receptor antagonists; such so-called decoy receptors could reduce the biologic effects of the cytokine itself.[69,73] An increase in bioavailable TNF-α present in serum from patients with ICMV[74] was not observed by another group,[75] although this latter group did observe higher levels of bioavailable TNF-α in the serum of patients with active lupus vasculitis. Fluids from affected organs (e.g., bronchial lavage from CSS patients or urine from ICMV patients) are also reportedly enriched in TNF-α content.[70,76] Increased serum or plasma levels of IL-6 are recognized in WG, CSS and other AAV as well as ICMV,[67–69,71,72,74,77–82] but were not observed in one study of ICMV patients.[76] Evaluation of circulating IL-1 levels in AAV and ICMV have proved less satisfying, with highly variable results.[79,83–85] However, more severe disease in both AAV and ICMV was correlated with a "secretory phenotype" of relatively high amounts of IL-1b in relation to the IL-1 receptor antagonist.[79,84,85]

Incubation of human (umbilical vein) endothelial cells with TNF-α promotes binding of antiendothelial cell antibodies in vitro.[86] Intraarterial infusion of TNF-α (but not IL-6 or endotoxin) into human volunteers evoked massive increases in plasma tissue plasminogen activator and IL-6 levels and impaired endothelial-dependent vasodilation.[87] Therefore, TNF-α exerts both salutary and deleterious effects on the microcirculation.

By immunohistochemistry, local production of TNF-α in granulomatous lesions from patients with WG appears to arise principally from CD4+CD28− T cells, which also are the primary source of IFN-γ in tissue.[88] Circulating CD4+CD28− T cells are increased in WG patients and produce copious amounts of these cytokines spontaneously.[88] Both TNF-α and IFN-γ are very potent activators of monocytes and macrophages. In WG, progression from capillaritis to granulomatous vasculitis likely requires the effects of these cytokines. In turn, lung biopsy specimens from patients with WG revealed that the majority of lymphocytes in lesions are memory phenotype T cells (CD45RO+), with few or no B cells or natural killer cells. Concordant with this observation, the chemokine regulated upon activation, normal T-cell expressed and secreted (RANTES) was expressed at very high levels in lung biopsy specimens from WG patients compared with normal controls by reverse transcription–polymerase chain reaction (RT-PCR), and in situ hybridization and immunohistochemistry disclosed activated macrophages as the source of RANTES.[89] Thus, a positive feedback whereby memory/effector T cells recruit and activate a macrophage population, and in turn are recruited themselves by macrophage production of RANTES (and probably other chemokines), likely elicits the granulomatous vasculitis in WG. Presumably, these circuits operate less robustly in MPA, in which granulomatous vasculitis is unusual.

Genetic Polymorphism

Recently, a genetic polymorphism in the promoter region of TNF-α showed significant association with WG, with an odds ratio of 5.01 compared with healthy controls.[90] Earlier studies failed to detect polymorphisms in the genes encoding TNF-α[91–93] or its receptors,[91] but the specific allelic variation at position −238 in the affirmative report was not evaluated in these negative studies. In ICMV, no association with the TNF-α variation at −308 was observed.[94] To date, no polymorphisms in IL-6 or IL-1 have been associated with AAV.[91,92] Therapy of AAV with a monoclonal antibody that blocks TNF-α (infliximab) appears effective, with the widest experience with patients with WG.[73,81,95–98] On the other hand, etanercept did not exhibit efficacy in several studies that included a large randomized prospective trial.[96,99,100] In some cases (often arising in the course of treatment of rheumatoid arthritis), evolution of leukocytoclastic vasculitis has been associated with either of these drugs.[101–103] Overall, TNF-α antagonists show appreciable promise, but their use is by no means well established or straightforward.[96,104]

Interleukin-10

A Swedish group reported an association of polymorphism in a tandem repeat in the IL-10 gene with risk for WG.[105] This particular allele, IL-10.G, had previously been associated with a proclivity for abundant production of autoantibodies and hence with humorally mediated autoimmune disease. Another group reported a significant difference in genotype frequency in the IL-10 promoter region (at position −1082) in WG and later in a larger series that included both WG and MPA patients.[106,107] A different group did not observe the shift to the AA homozygous genotype at this locus in a smaller cohort of WG patients but did note that the G/A heterozygotes were more frequent among patients who did not progress to end-stage renal disease.[90] In another study, although circulating levels of IL-10 were abnormally high in patients with AAV, the serum IL-10 level in each patient was far higher during remission than during disease flares.[80] Yet another study reported that the levels of IL-10 mRNA and IL-10 protein were significantly higher in frozen nasal biopsy tissue and peripheral blood mononuclear cells from WG patients with disease confined to the upper respiratory tract compared to those with generalized disease (or healthy controls).[108] Among patients with AAV, those with CSS, characterized by generally less severe disease, had higher levels of circulating IL-10 than patients with WG or MPA[109]; this investigative group did not observe higher serum IL-10 levels in patients with localized as opposed to generalized WG. Conversely, mice bearing a targeted deletion of IL-10 exhibited significant increases in endothelial injury and

oxidative stress in a model of vascular inflammation when compared with wild-type mice.[110] Collectively, these observations support the principle that the higher expression of IL-10 (and lower levels of secretion of proinflammatory cytokines associated with the AA homozygotic state) favors either reduced risk for disease or a less severe involvement. Indeed, IL-10 is known to interfere with nuclear factor (NF)-κB transcriptional activation and might interfere with activator protein-1 transactivation as well. Transactivation by NF-κB and activator protein-1, of course, synergize to dramatically intensify inflammation. Indeed, incubation of peripheral blood mononuclear cells from WG patients with exogenous IL-10 markedly inhibited the abnormally high production of the proinflammatory pair of cytokines IL-12 and IFN-γ otherwise observed.[111] Perhaps IL-10, or an analog, would prove salutary in the therapy of AAV and other vasculitides.

Transforming Growth Factor-β

Transforming growth factor (TGF)-β has many effects, some good and some bad. In addition to potential suppression of immune responses, under some circumstances TGF-β can exhibit significant antiinflammatory effects. Recently, the major intracellular signal transducers of TGF-β, Smads, have been implicated.[112] Specifically, Smad3 acts favorably by decreasing activator protein-1 activation and chemokine expression (see below)[113] Although an early report indicated a trend toward a decrease in the CG genotype in codon 25 of the gene encoding TGF-β among WG patients,[107] no significant differences in the polymorphisms within codons 10 or 25 were detected in patients with WG or MPA compared with controls in a larger cohort by the same investigators or in another study.[90,106] In ICMV, the TT genotype in the promoter (at position −509) was more common and associated with increased disease severity.[94]

Other Cytokines

Interferon-α

Chronic hepatitis is often effectively treated with administration of IFN-α, which reduces viral load and often leads to diminished cryoglobulinemia. Therefore, it is not surprising that IFN-α ameliorates vasculitic complications of chronic hepatitis.[114–120] The mechanism(s) whereby IFN-α acts is not clear, and vasculitis in the context of CSS and in association with hairy cell leukemia has also improved upon treatment with IFN-α.[121–123] However, therapeutic use of IFN-α can instigate, or is apparently related to, onset of leukocytoclastic vasculitis.[124–135] Leukoencephalopathy, presumably secondary to vasculitis, is also reportedly associated with IFN-α therapy.[136] Moreover, IFN-α is not always effective in chronic hepatitis C, as exemplified by a case of fatal pulmonary vasculitis refractory to IFN-α treatment.[137] The administration of granulocyte colony-stimulating factor, generally to expand marrow or stem cells in severely ill patients, has also been associated with onset of vasculitis, sometimes severe.[138–143]

Chemokines

The chemokines are low-molecular-weight proteins that fall into the CC, CXC, and CXXXC families. Many of the chemokines are chemotactic or chemokinetic for leukocytes. Interleukin-8 is a CXC chemokine that is a potent neutrophil chemotaxin. Serum levels of IL-8 are elevated in AAV, and particularly in WG, as well as in ICMV.[80,144,145] Moreover, sera from patients with active ICMV evoke IL-8 synthesis from human endothelium if applied to the cells in culture.[145] Allelic polymorphism of the A genotype of IL-8 occurs significantly more frequently in ICMV patients with renal disease as opposed to those without, even though there was no difference between ICMV patients as a whole and healthy controls.[146]

Monocyte chemoattractant protein 1, a CC chemokine, is best characterized as a chemotactic agent for monocytes, but it is also active upon primed neutrophils and, perhaps, macrophages. Circulating levels of MCP-1 are elevated in patients with WG and in the urine of AAV patients with active glomerulonephritis.[144,147,148] Moreover, MCP-1 is histologically demonstrable in lesional glomeruli in patients with AAV but not in normal glomeruli.[148] Although serum levels of MCP-1 were not increased significantly among patients with retinal vasculitis compared with healthy controls, the levels of MCP-1 did correlate with disease activity in most individuals.[149] Transfection of a natural MCP-1 antagonist into (MRL/lpr) mice that spontaneously develop a lupus-like multisystem vasculitic disease reduced the severity of glomerulonephritis and vasculitis.[150] Several cytokines elicit MCP-1 from endothelial cells, whereas NO, itself a product of activated leukocytes (and especially monocytes) inhibits MCP-1 production, in part by reducing activation of NF-kB.[147] Conversely, superoxide quenches NO (to form peroxynitrite) and promotes NF-kB activation. Therefore, the balance between pro- and antiinflammatory effects of leukocyte activation can vary widely. As already noted, activation of Smad 3 in response to TGF-β decreases MCP expression, thereby diminishing inflammation.[112]

The CC chemokine RANTES recruits T cells, B cells, and monocytes toward its concentration peak. Among patients with WG, and perhaps other AAV, increased levels of RANTES are present in the blood,[144] and histologically detectable RANTES mRNA and protein have been demonstrated.[89] Other chemokines, such as fractalkine, macrophage migration inhibitory factor[151] macrophage inflammatory protein-1α and perhaps macrophage inflammatory protein-1β levels are increased in patients with WG, ICMV and retinal vasculitis compared with normal controls.[149,151–153]

Adhesion Molecules

Leukocytes and endothelial cells constitutively express complementary pairs of adhesion molecules; additional quantities of these constitutive molecules and additional adhesion partners can be induced upon stimulation. Relatively weak leukocyte–endothelial interaction is supported by the expression of endothelial (E) selectin and leukocyte (L) selectin. These proteins have affinity for glycoconjugates (sialyl-Lewis X and mucin-like glycoproteins such as GlyCam-1 and CD34) expressed on the reciprocal cell type. The numerous but individually weak attachments produce a rolling motion, whereby a leukocyte is propelled by the bloodstream along the endothelial surface in a motion likened to a tank track. Eventually, retention of leukocytes in a particular spot can be supported by additional ligand pairs; notably, the β_2-integrins (CD18 family members) on leukocytes bind ICAM-1 expressed by endothelial cells. The β_1-integrins (CD29 family) on leukocytes can similarly bind endothelial proteins, exemplified by VCAM-1. Upon simple binding to ligand, the integrins transduce intracellular signals that recruit additional adhesion molecules to the region and modify the properties of the cell. The recruitment of additional adhesion molecules initiates expression of CD31 (platelet endothelial cell adhesion molecule-1); ultimately the leukocytes insinuate themselves among the endothelial cells and transmigrate.

Increased circulating levels of ICAM-1,[154–158] often in association with VCAM-1,[66,79,159] E-selectin,[160–162] or both[67,163–165] are documented in the AAV. Others reported elevated levels of E-selectin in serum, but did not evaluate the other adhesion molecules.[77,166] However, the concentrations of adhesion molecules in serum or plasma are not always correlated closely to disease activity,[67,161,164,165,167] and caution must be applied to their interpretation, just as is the case in other small vessel vasculitides in which heightened soluble adhesion molecules are reported.[78,168–172] Perhaps more cogently, histologic demonstration of increased expression of these various adhesion molecules is reported in AAV[173,174] and ICMV,[173] albeit in renal rather than lung tissue, rheumatic, and hypersensitivity diseases.[175–177]

Apoptosis in Wegener's Granulomatosis

Wegener's granulomatosis may be influenced by polymorphisms in the apoptosis-related gene *receptor (TNFRSF)-interacting serine-threonine kinase 1* or *Ripk1*. Ripk1 interacts with TNF receptor-associated protein with death domain (TRADD) in the process of apoptosis (see Chapter 4). The recruiting of RIPK1 to TNFR1 results in apoptosis and activation of nuclear factor κ light chain gene enhancer in B cells.[171,172]

References

1. Jennette JC, Falk RJ, Andrassy K, et al. Nomenclature of systemic vasculitides. Proposal of an international consensus conference. Arthritis Rheum 1994;37(2):187–192.

2. Heeringa P, Schreiber A, Falk RJ, et al. Pathogenesis of pulmonary vasculitis. Semin Respir Crit Care Med 2004;25:465–474.

3. Abdou NI, Kullman GJ, Hoffman GS, et al. Wegener's granulomatosis: survey of 701 patients in North America. Changes in outcome in the 1990s. J Rheumatol 2002;29(2): 309–316.

4. Anderson G, Coles ET, Crane M, et al. Wegener's granuloma. A series of 265 British cases seen between 1975 and 1985. A report by a sub-committee of the British Thoracic Society Research Committee. Q J Med 1992;83(302): 427–438.

5. Colby TV, Specks U. Wegener's granulomatosis in the 1990s—a pulmonary pathologist's perspective. Monogr Pathol 1993(36):195–218.

6. Cordier JF, Valeyre D, Guillevin L, et al. Pulmonary Wegener's granulomatosis. A clinical and imaging study of 77 cases. Chest 1990;97(4):906–912.

7. Galateau F, Loire R, Capron F, et al. [Pulmonary lesions in Wegener's disease. Report of the French Anatomo-clinical Research Group. Study of 40 pulmonary biopsies.] Rev Mal Respir 1992;9(4):431–442.

8. Hoffman GS, Kerr GS, Leavitt RY, et al. Wegener granulomatosis: an analysis of 158 patients. Ann Intern Med 1992;116(6):488–498.

9. Lombard CM, Duncan SR, Rizk NW,et al. The diagnosis of Wegener's granulomatosis from transbronchial biopsy specimens. Hum Pathol 1990;21(8):838–842.

10. Mark EJ, Matsubara O, Tan-Liu NS, et al. The pulmonary biopsy in the early diagnosis of Wegener's (pathergic) granulomatosis: a study based on 35 open lung biopsies. Hum Pathol 1988;19(9):1065–1071.

11. Mark EJ, Ramirez JF. Pulmonary capillaritis and hemorrhage in patients with systemic vasculitis. Arch Pathol Lab Med 1985;109(5):413–418.

12. Travis WD, Hoffman GS, Leavitt RY, et al. Surgical pathology of the lung in Wegener's granulomatosis. Review of 87 open lung biopsies from 67 patients. Am J Surg Pathol 1991;15(4):315–333.

13. Yousem SA. Bronchocentric injury in Wegener's granulomatosis: a report of five cases. Hum Pathol 1991;22(6): 535–540.

14. Yousem SA, Lombard CM. The eosinophilic variant of Wegener's granulomatosis. Hum Pathol 1988;19(6):682–688.

15. Adu D, Howie AJ, Scott DG, et al. Polyarteritis and the kidney. Q J Med 1987;62(239):221–237.

16. D'Agati V, Chander P, Nash M, et al. Idiopathic microscopic polyarteritis nodosa: ultrastructural observations on the renal vascular and glomerular lesions. Am J Kidney Dis 1986;7(1):95–110.

17. Guillevin L, Durand-Gasselin B, Cevallos R, et al. Microscopic polyangiitis: clinical and laboratory findings in eighty-five patients. Arthritis Rheum 1999;42(3):421–430.

18. Jennings CA, King TE Jr, Tuder R, et al. Diffuse alveolar hemorrhage with underlying isolated, pauciimmune pulmonary capillaritis. Am J Respir Crit Care Med 1997; 155(3):1101–1109.

19. Lhote F, Cohen P, Guillevin L. Polyarteritis nodosa, microscopic polyangiitis and Churg-Strauss syndrome. Lupus 1998;7(4):238–258.

20. Saltzman PW, West M, Chomet B. Pulmonary hemosiderosis and glomerulonephritis. Ann Intern Med 1962;56:409–421.

21. Savage CO, Winearls CG, Evans DJ, et al. Microscopic polyarteritis: presentation, pathology and prognosis. Q J Med 1985;56(220):467–483.

22. Serra A, Cameron JS, Turner DR, et al. Vasculitis affecting the kidney: presentation, histopathology and long-term outcome. Q J Med 1984;53(210):181–207.

23. Chumbley LC, Harrison EG J., DeRemee RA. Allergic granulomatosis and angiitis (Churg-Strauss syndrome). Report and analysis of 30 cases. Mayo Clin Proc 1977;52(8): 477–484.

24. Churg A. Recent advances in the diagnosis of Churg-Strauss syndrome. Mod Pathol 2001;14(12):1284–1293.

25. Churg J, Strauss L. Allergic granulomatosis, allergic angiitis, and periarteritis nodosa. Am J Pathol 1951;27(2): 277–301.

26. Clutterbuck EJ, Pusey CD. Severe alveolar haemorrhage in Churg-Strauss syndrome. Eur J Respir Dis 1987;71(3): 158–163.

27. Koss MN, Antonovych T, Hochholzer L. Allergic granulomatosis (Churg-Strauss syndrome): pulmonary and renal morphologic findings. Am J Surg Pathol 1981;5(1):21–28.

28. Lanham JG, Elkon KB, Pusey CD, et al. Systemic vasculitis with asthma and eosinophilia: a clinical approach to the Churg-Strauss syndrome. Medicine (Baltimore) 1984;63(2):65–81.

29. Reid AJ, Harrison BD, Watts RA, et al. Churg-Strauss syndrome in a district hospital. Q J Med 1998;91(3): 219–229.

30. Abboud RT, Chase WH, Ballon HS, et al. Goodpasture's syndrome: diagnosis by transbronchial lung biopsy. Ann Intern Med 1978;89(5 Pt 1):635–638.

31. Beechler CR, Enquist RW, Hunt KK, et al. Immunofluorescence of transbronchial biopsies in Goodpasture's syndrome. Am Rev Respir Dis 1980;121(5):869–872.

32. Lombard CM, Colby TV, Elliott CG. Surgical pathology of the lung in anti-basement membrane antibody-associated Goodpasture's syndrome. Hum Pathol 1989;20(5): 445–451.

33. Tobler A, Schurch E, Altermatt HJ, et al. Anti-basement membrane antibody disease with severe pulmonary haemorrhage and normal renal function. Thorax 1991;46(1): 68–70.

34. Travis WD, Colby TV, Lombard C, et al. A clinicopathologic study of 34 cases of diffuse pulmonary hemorrhage with lung biopsy confirmation. Am J Surg Pathol 1990; 14(12):1112–1125.

35. Kathuria S, Cheifec G. Fatal pulmonary Henoch-Schönlein syndrome. Chest 1982;82(5):654–656.

36. Markus HS, Clark JV. Pulmonary haemorrhage in Henoch-Schönlein purpura. Thorax 1989;44(6):525–526.

37. Rusby NL, Wilson C. Lung Purpura with Nephritis. Annu Rev Med 1965;16:301–308.

38. Weiss VF, Naidu S. Fatal pulmonary hemorrhage in Henoch-Schönlein purpura. Cutis 1979;23(5):687–688.

39. Fayemi AO. Pulmonary vascular disease in systemic lupus erythematosus. Am J Clin Pathol 1976;65(3):284–290.

40. Roncoroni AJ, Alvarez C, Molinas F. Plexogenic arteriopathy associated with pulmonary vasculitis in systemic lupus erythematosus. Respiration 1992;59(1):52–56.

41. Wisnieski JJ, Emancipator SN, Korman NJ, et al. Hypocomplementemic urticarial vasculitis syndrome in identical twins. Arthritis Rheum 1994;37(7):1105–1111.

42. Armstrong JG, Steele RH. Localised pulmonary arteritis in rheumatoid disease. Thorax 1982;37(4):313–314.

43. Baydur A, Mongan ES, Slager UT. Acute respiratory failure and pulmonary arteritis without parenchymal involvement: demonstration in a patient with rheumatoid arthritis. Chest 1979;75(4):518–520.

44. Kay JM, Banik S. Unexplained pulmonary hypertension with pulmonary arteritis in rheumatoid disease. Br J Dis Chest 1977;71(1):53–59.

45. Vollertsen RS, Conn DL, Ballard DJ, et al. Rheumatoid vasculitis: survival and associated risk factors. Medicine (Baltimore) 1986;65(6):365–375.

46. Yousem SA, Colby TV, Carrington CB. Lung biopsy in rheumatoid arthritis. Am Rev Respir Dis 1985;131(5):770–777.

47. Bucher UG, Reid L. Sjögren's syndrome: report of a fatal case with pulmonary and renal lesions. Br J Dis Chest 1959;53:237–252.

48. Fox RI, Howell FV, Bone RC, et al. Primary Sjogren syndrome: clinical and immunopathologic features. Semin Arthritis Rheum 1984;14(2):77–105.

49. Germain MJ, Davidman M. Pulmonary hemorrhage and acute renal failure in a patient with mixed connective tissue disease. Am J Kidney Dis 1984;3(6):420–424.

50. Jones MB, Osterholm RK, Wilson RB, et al. Fatal pulmonary hypertension and resolving immune-complex glomerulonephritis in mixed connective tissue disease. A case report and review of the literature. Am J Med 1978;65(5):855–863.

51. Prakash UB. Lungs in mixed connective tissue disease. J Thorac Imaging 1992;7(2):55–61.

52. Sanchez-Guerrero J, Cesarman G, Alarcon-Segovia D. Massive pulmonary hemorrhage in mixed connective tissue diseases. J Rheumatol 1989;16(8):1132–1134.

53. Wiener-Kronish JP, Solinger AM, Warnock ML, et al. Severe pulmonary involvement in mixed connective tissue disease. Am Rev Respir Dis 1981;124(4):499–503.

54. Lakhanpal S, Lie JT, Conn DL, et al. Pulmonary disease in polymyositis/dermatomyositis: a clinicopathological analysis of 65 autopsy cases. Ann Rheum Dis 1987;46(1):23–9.

55. Mino M, Noma S, Taguchi Y, et al. Pulmonary involvement in polymyositis and dermatomyositis: sequential evaluation with CT. Am J Roentgenol 1997;169(1):83–87.

56. Schwarz MI, Sutarik JM, Nick JA, et al. Pulmonary capillaritis and diffuse alveolar hemorrhage. A primary manifestation of polymyositis. Am J Respir Crit Care Med 1995;151(6):2037–2040.

57. Bissuel F, Bizollon T, Dijoud F, et al. Pulmonary hemorrhage and glomerulonephritis in primary biliary cirrhosis. Hepatology 1992;16(6):1357–1361.

58. Conn DL, Dickson ER, Carpenter HA. The association of Churg-Strauss vasculitis with temporal artery involvement, primary biliary cirrhosis, and polychondritis in a single patient. J Rheumatol 1982;9(5):744–748.

59. Martinez JS, Kohler PF. Variant "Goodpasture's syndrome"? The need for immunologic criteria in rapidly progressive glomerulonephritis and hemorrhagic pneumonitis. Ann Intern Med 1971;75(1):67–76.

60. van Passen P, Tervaert JWC, Heeringa P. Mechanisms of vasculitis: How pauci-immune is ANCA-associated renal vasculitis? Nephron Exp Nephrol 2007;105:e10–e16.

61. Jagiello P, Gross WL, Epplen JT. Complex genetics of Wegener granulomatosis. Autoimmun Rev 2005;4(1):42–47.

62. Jennette JC, Xiao H, Falk RJ. Pathogenesis of vascular inflammation by anti-neutrophil cytoplasmic antibodies. J Am Soc Nephrol 2006;17(5):1235–1242.

63. Falk RJ, Jennette JC. Anti-neutrophil cytoplasmic autoantibodies with specificity for myeloperoxidase in patients with systemic vasculitis and idiopathic necrotizing and crescentic glomerulonephritis. N Engl J Med 1988;318:1651–1657.

64. Pendergraft WF, Preston GA, Shah RR, et al. Autoimmunity is triggered by cPR-3 (105–201), a protein complementary to human autoantigen proteinase-3. Nat Med 2004;10:72–79.

65. Feuerhake F, Fuchsl G, Bals R, et al. Expression of inducible cell adhesion molecules in the normal human lung: immunohistochemical study of their distribution in pulmonary blood vessels. Histochem Cell Biol 1998;110(4):387–394.

66. Muller Kobold AC, Mesander G, Stegeman CA, et al. Are circulating neutrophils intravascularly activated in patients with anti-neutrophil cytoplasmic antibody (ANCA)–associated vasculitides? Clin Exp Immunol 1998;114(3):491–499.

67. Ohta N, Fukase S, Aoyagi M. Serum levels of soluble adhesion molecules ICAM-1, VCAM-1 and E-selectin in patients with Wegener's granulomatosis. Auris Nasus Larynx 2001;28(4):311–314.

68. Papi M, Didona B, De Pita O, et al. Livedo vasculopathy vs small vessel cutaneous vasculitis: cytokine and platelet P-selectin studies. Arch Dermatol 1998;134(4):447–452.

69. Tesar V, Jirsa M, Jr., Zima T, et al. Soluble cytokine receptors in renal vasculitis and lupus nephritis. Med Sci Monit 2002;8(1):BR24–BR29.

70. Tsukadaira A, Okubo Y, Kitano K, et al. Eosinophil active cytokines and surface analysis of eosinophils in Churg-Strauss syndrome. Allergy Asthma Proc 1999;20(1):39–44.

71. Kuryliszyn-Moskal A. Cytokines and soluble CD4 and CD8 molecules in rheumatoid arthritis: relationship to systematic vasculitis and microvascular capillaroscopic abnormalities. Clin Rheumatol 1998;17(6):489–495.

72. Besbas N, Saatci U, Ruacan S, et al. The role of cytokines in Henoch Schonlein purpura. Scand J Rheumatol 1997;26(6):456–460.

73. Booth A, Harper L, Hammad T, et al. Prospective study of TNFalpha blockade with infliximab in anti-neutrophil cytoplasmic antibody-associated systemic vasculitis. J Am Soc Nephrol 2004;15(3):717–721.

74. Rostoker G, Rymer JC, Bagnard G, et al. Imbalances in serum proinflammatory cytokines and their soluble receptors: a putative role in the progression of idiopathic IgA nephropathy (IgAN) and Henoch-Schonlein purpura nephritis, and a potential target of immunoglobulin therapy? Clin Exp Immunol 1998;114(3):468–476.

75. Gattorno M, Picco P, Barbano G, et al. Differences in tumor necrosis factor-alpha soluble receptor serum concentrations between patients with Henoch-Schonlein purpura and pediatric systemic lupus erythematosus: pathogenetic implications. J Rheumatol 1998;25(2):361–365.

76. Wu TH, Wu SC, Huang TP, et al. Increased excretion of tumor necrosis factor alpha and interleukin 1 beta in urine from patients with IgA nephropathy and Schonlein-Henoch purpura. Nephron 1996;74(1):79–88.

77. Muller Kobold AC, van Wijk RT, Franssen CF, et al. In vitro up-regulation of E-selectin and induction of interleukin-6 in endothelial cells by autoantibodies in Wegener's granulomatosis and microscopic polyangiitis. Clin Exp Rheumatol 1999;17(4):433–440.

78. Alecu M, Coman G, Galatescu E. Serological level of ICAM and ELAM adhesion molecules in allergic vascularitis. Rom J Intern Med 1997;35(1–4):83–88.

79. Tesar V, Jelinkova E, Masek Z, et al. Influence of plasma exchange on serum levels of cytokines and adhesion molecules in ANCA-positive renal vasculitis. Blood Purif 1998;16(2):72–80.

80. Ohlsson S, Wieslander J, Segelmark M. Circulating cytokine profile in anti-neutrophilic cytoplasmatic autoantibody-associated vasculitis: prediction of outcome? Mediators Inflamm 2004;13(4):275–283.

81. Booth AD, Jayne DR, Kharbanda RK, et al. Infliximab improves endothelial dysfunction in systemic vasculitis: a model of vascular inflammation. Circulation 2004;109(14):1718–1723.

82. Yokoyama A, Kohno N, Fujino S, et al. IgG and IgM rheumatoid factor levels parallel interleukin-6 during the vasculitic phase in a patient with Churg-Strauss syndrome. Intern Med 1995;34(7):646–648.

83. Amoli MM, Calvino MC, Garcia-Porrua C, et al. Interleukin 1beta gene polymorphism association with severe renal manifestations and renal sequelae in Henoch-Schonlein purpura. J Rheumatol 2004;31(2):295–298.

84. Rauta V, Teppo AM, Tornroth T, et al. Lower urinary-interleukin-1 receptor-antagonist excretion in IgA nephropathy than in Henoch-Schonlein nephritis. Nephrol Dial Transplant 2003;18(9):1785–1791.

85. Borgmann S, Endisch G, Hacker UT, et al. Proinflammatory genotype of interleukin-1 and interleukin-1 receptor antagonist is associated with ESRD in proteinase 3-ANCA vasculitis patients. Am J Kidney Dis 2003;41(5):933–942.

86. Yang YH, Wang SJ, Chuang YH, et al. The level of IgA antibodies to human umbilical vein endothelial cells can be enhanced by TNF-alpha treatment in children with Henoch-Schonlein purpura. Clin Exp Immunol 2002;130(2):352–357.

87. Chia S, Qadan M, Newton R, et al. Intra-arterial tumor necrosis factor-alpha impairs endothelium-dependent vasodilatation and stimulates local tissue plasminogen activator release in humans. Arterioscler Thromb Vasc Biol 2003;23(4):695–701.

88. Komocsi A, Lamprecht P, Csernok E, et al. Peripheral blood and granuloma CD4(+)CD28(−) T cells are a major source of interferon-gamma and tumor necrosis factor-alpha in Wegener's granulomatosis. Am J Pathol 2002;160(5):1717–1724.

89. Coulomb-L'Hermine A, Capron F, Zou W, et al. Expression of the chemokine RANTES in pulmonary Wegener's granulomatosis. Hum Pathol 2001;32(3):320–326.

90. Spriewald BM, Witzke O, Wassmuth R, et al. Distinct tumour necrosis factor alpha, interferon gamma, interleukin 10, and cytotoxic T cell antigen 4 gene polymorphisms in disease occurrence and end stage renal disease in Wegener's granulomatosis. Ann Rheum Dis 2005;64(3):457–461.

91. Zhou Y, Huang D, Paris PL, et al. An analysis of CTLA-4 and proinflammatory cytokine genes in Wegener's granulomatosis. Arthritis Rheum 2004;50(8):2645–2650.

92. Huang D, Giscombe R, Zhou Y, et al. Polymorphisms in CTLA-4 but not tumor necrosis factor-alpha or interleukin 1beta genes are associated with Wegener's granulomatosis. J Rheumatol 2000;27(2):397–401.

93. Mascher B, Schmitt W, Csernok E, et al. Polymorphisms in the tumor necrosis factor genes in Wegener's granulomatosis. Exp Clin Immunogenet 1997;14(3):226–233.

94. Yang YH, Lai HJ, Kao CK, et al. The association between transforming growth factor-beta gene promoter C-509T polymorphism and Chinese children with Henoch-Schonlein purpura. Pediatr Nephrol 2004;19(9):972–975.

95. Kleinert J, Lorenz M, Kostler W, et al. Refractory Wegener's granulomatosis responds to tumor necrosis factor blockade. Wien Klin Wochenschr 2004;116(9–10):334–338.

96. Gause A, Arbach O, Lamprecht P. [Treatment of primary systemic vasculitis with TNF alpha-antagonists.] Z Rheumatol 2003;62(3):228–234.

97. Arbach O, Gross WL, Gause A. Treatment of refractory Churg-Strauss syndrome (CSS) by TNF-alpha blockade. Immunobiology 2002;206(5):496–501.

98. Lamprecht P, Voswinkel J, Lilienthal T, et al. Effectiveness of TNF-alpha blockade with infliximab in refractory Wegener's granulomatosis. Rheumatology (Oxford) 2002;41(11):1303–1307.

99. Mukhtyar C, Luqmani R. Current state of tumour necrosis factor {alpha} blockade in Wegener's granulomatosis. Ann Rheum Dis 2005;64(Suppl 4):iv31–iv36.

100. Wegener's Granulomatosis Etanercept Trial (WGET) Research Group. Etanercept plus standard therapy for Wegener's granulomatosis. N Engl J Med 2005;352(4):351–361.

101. Uthman IW, Touma Z, Sayyad J, et al. Response of deep cutaneous vasculitis to infliximab. J Am Acad Dermatol 2005;53(2):353–354.

102. Mohan N, Edwards ET, Cupps TR, et al. Leukocytoclastic vasculitis associated with tumor necrosis factor-alpha blocking agents. J Rheumatol 2004;31(10):1955–1958.

103. Jarrett SJ, Cunnane G, Conaghan PG, et al. Anti-tumor necrosis factor-alpha therapy-induced vasculitis: case series. J Rheumatol 2003;30(10):2287–2291.

104. Lamprecht P. TNF-alpha inhibitors in systemic vasculitides and connective tissue diseases. Autoimmun Rev 2005; 4(1):28–34.

105. Zhou Y, Giscombe R, Huang D, et al. Novel genetic association of Wegener's granulomatosis with the interleukin 10 gene. J Rheumatol 2002;29(2):317–320.

106. Bartfai Z, Gaede KI, Russell KA, et al. Different gender-associated genotype risks of Wegener's granulomatosis and microscopic polyangiitis. Clin Immunol 2003;109(3): 330–337.

107. Murakozy G, Gaede KI, Ruprecht B, et al. Gene polymorphisms of immunoregulatory cytokines and angiotensin-converting enzyme in Wegener's granulomatosis. J Mol Med 2001;79(11):665–670.

108. Muller A, Trabandt A, Gloeckner-Hofmann K, et al. Localized Wegener's granulomatosis: predominance of CD26 and IFN-gamma expression. J Pathol 2000;192(1):113–120.

109. Schonermarck U, Csernok E, Trabandt A, et al. Circulating cytokines and soluble CD23, CD26 and CD30 in ANCA-associated vasculitides. Clin Exp Rheumatol 2000;18(4):457–463.

110. Gunnett CA, Heistad DD, Berg DJ, et al. IL-10 deficiency increases superoxide and endothelial dysfunction during inflammation. Am J Physiol Heart Circ Physiol 2000; 279(4):H1555–H1562.

111. Ludviksson BR, Sneller MC, Chua KS, et al. Active Wegener's granulomatosis is associated with HLA-DR+ CD4+ T cells exhibiting an unbalanced Th1-type T cell cytokine pattern: reversal with IL-10. J Immunol 1998; 160(7):3602–3609.

112. Feinberg MW, Jain MK. Role of transforming growth factor-beta1/Smads in regulating vascular inflammation and atherogenesis. Panminerva Med 2005;47(3):169–186.

113. Feinberg MW, Shimizu K, Lebedeva M, et al. Essential role for Smad3 in regulating MCP-1 expression and vascular inflammation. Circ Res 2004;94(5):601–608.

114. Cacoub P, Saadoun D, Limal N, et al. PEGylated interferon alfa-2b and ribavirin treatment in patients with hepatitis C virus-related systemic vasculitis. Arthritis Rheum 2005;52(3):911–915.

115. Cacoub P, Lidove O, Maisonobe T, et al. Interferon-alpha and ribavirin treatment in patients with hepatitis C virus-related systemic vasculitis. Arthritis Rheum 2002;46(12):3317–3326.

116. Willson RA. The benefit of long-term interferon alfa therapy for symptomatic mixed cryoglobulinemia (cutaneous vasculitis/membranoproliferative glomerulonephritis) associated with chronic hepatitis C infection. J Clin Gastroenterol 2001;33(2):137–140.

117. Erhardt A, Sagir A, Guillevin L, et al. Successful treatment of hepatitis B virus associated polyarteritis nodosa with a combination of prednisolone, alpha-interferon and lamivudine. J Hepatol 2000;33(4):677–683.

118. Avsar E, Savas B, Tozun N, et al. Successful treatment of polyarteritis nodosa related to hepatitis B virus with interferon alpha as first-line therapy. J Hepatol 1998;28(3): 525–526.

119. Schirren CA, Zachoval R, Schirren CG, et al. A role for chronic hepatitis C virus infection in a patient with cutaneous vasculitis, cryoglobulinemia, and chronic liver disease. Effective therapy with interferon-alpha. Dig Dis Sci 1995;40(6):1221–1225.

120. Sepp NT, Umlauft F, Illersperger B, et al. Necrotizing vasculitis associated with hepatitis C virus infection: successful treatment of vasculitis with interferon-alpha despite persistence of mixed cryoglobulinemia. Dermatology 1995;191(1):43–45.

121. Reissig A, Forster M, Mock B, et al. [Interferon-alpha treatment of the Churg-Strauss syndrome.] Dtsch Med Wochenschr 2003;128(27):1475–1478.

122. Tatsis E, Schnabel A, Gross WL. Interferon-alpha treatment of four patients with the Churg-Strauss syndrome. Ann Intern Med 1998;129(5):370–374.

123. Carpenter MT, West SG. Polyarteritis nodosa in hairy cell leukemia: treatment with interferon-alpha. J Rheumatol 1994;21(6):1150–1152.

124. Debat Zoguereh D, Boucraut J, Beau-Salinas F, et al. [Cutaneous vasculitis with renal impairment complicating interferon-beta 1a therapy for multiple sclerosis.] Rev Neurol (Paris) 2004;160(11):1081–1084.

125. Batisse D, Karmochkine M, Jacquot C, et al. Sustained exacerbation of cryoglobulinaemia-related vasculitis following treatment of hepatitis C with peginterferon alfa. Eur J Gastroenterol Hepatol 2004;16(7):701–703.

126. Pinto JM, Marques MS, Correia TE. Lichen planus and leukocytoclastic vasculitis induced by interferon alpha-2b in a subject with HCV-related chronic active hepatitis. J Eur Acad Dermatol Venereol 2003;17(2): 193–195.

127. Gupta G, Holmes SC, Spence E, et al. Capillaritis associated with interferon-alfa treatment of chronic hepatitis C infection. J Am Acad Dermatol 2000;43(5 Pt 2):937–938.

128. Gordon AC, Edgar JD, Finch RG. Acute exacerbation of vasculitis during interferon-alpha therapy for hepatitis C–associated cryoglobulinaemia. J Infect 1998;36(2):229–230.

129. Krainick U, Kantarjian H, Broussard S, et al. Local cutaneous necrotizing lesions associated with interferon injections. J Interferon Cytokine Res 1998;18(10):823–827.

130. Hamid S, Cruz PD, Jr., Lee WM. Urticarial vasculitis caused by hepatitis C virus infection: response to interferon alfa therapy. J Am Acad Dermatol 1998;39(2 Pt 1):278–280.

131. Christian MM, Diven DG, Sanchez RL, et al. Injection site vasculitis in a patient receiving interferon alfa for chronic hepatitis C. J Am Acad Dermatol 1997;37(1):118–120.

132. Kruger M, Boker KH, Zeidler H, et al. Treatment of hepatitis B–related polyarteritis nodosa with famciclovir and interferon alfa-2b. J Hepatol 1997;26(4):935–939.

133. Pateron D, Fain O, Sehonnou J, et al. Severe necrotizing vasculitis in a patient with hepatitis C virus infection treated by interferon. Clin Exp Rheumatol 1996;14(1):79–81.

134. Beuthien W, Mellinghoff HU, Kempis J. Vasculitic complications of interferon-alpha treatment for chronic hepatitis C virus infection: case report and review of the literature. Clin Rheumatol 2005;24(5):507–515.

135. Niewold TB, Swedler WI. Systemic lupus erythematosus arising during interferon-alpha therapy for cryoglobulinemic vasculitis associated with hepatitis C. Clin Rheumatol 2005;24(2):178–181.

136. Metzler C, Lamprecht P, Hellmich B, et al. Leucoencephalopathy after treatment of Churg-Strauss syndrome with interferon {alpha}. Ann Rheum Dis 2005;64(8):1242–1243.

137. Roithinger FX, Allinger S, Kirchgatterer A, et al. A lethal course of chronic hepatitis C, glomerulonephritis, and pulmonary vasculitis unresponsive to interferon treatment. Am J Gastroenterol 1995;90(6):1006–1008.

138. Iking-Konert C, Ostendorf B, Foede M, et al. Granulocyte colony-stimulating factor induces disease flare in patients with antineutrophil cytoplasmic antibody-associated vasculitis. J Rheumatol 2004;31(8):1655–1658.

139. Hill PA. Gastrointestinal small vessel vasculitis in a patient with crescentic glomerulonephritis and longstanding idiopathic neutropaenia treated with G-CSF. Pathology 2003;35(2):179–183.

140. Farhey YD, Herman JH. Vasculitis complicating granulocyte colony stimulating factor treatment of leukopenia and infection in Felty's syndrome. J Rheumatol 1995;22(6):1179–1182.

141. Vidarsson B, Geirsson AJ, Onundarson PT. Reactivation of rheumatoid arthritis and development of leukocytoclastic vasculitis in a patient receiving granulocyte colony-stimulating factor for Felty's syndrome. Am J Med 1995;98(6):589–591.

142. Couderc LJ, Philippe B, Franck N, et al. Necrotizing vasculitis and exacerbation of psoriasis after granulocyte colony-stimulating factor for small cell lung carcinoma. Respir Med 1995;89(3):237–238.

143. Jain KK. Cutaneous vasculitis associated with granulocyte colony-stimulating factor. J Am Acad Dermatol 1994;31(2 Pt 1):213–215.

144. Torheim EA, Yndestad A, Bjerkeli V, et al. Increased expression of chemokines in patients with Wegener's granulomatosis—modulating effects of methylprednisolone in vitro. Clin Exp Immunol 2005;140(2):376–383.

145. Yang YH, Lai HJ, Huang CM, et al. Sera from children with active Henoch-Schonlein purpura can enhance the production of interleukin 8 by human umbilical venous endothelial cells. Ann Rheum Dis 2004;63(11):1511–1513.

146. Amoli MM, Thomson W, Hajeer AH, et al. Interleukin 8 gene polymorphism is associated with increased risk of nephritis in cutaneous vasculitis. J Rheumatol 2002;29(11):2367–2370.

147. Desai A, Miller MJ, Huang X, et al. Nitric oxide modulates MCP-1 expression in endothelial cells: implications for the pathogenesis of pulmonary granulomatous vasculitis. Inflammation 2003;27(4):213–223.

148. Tam FW, Sanders JS, George A, et al. Urinary monocyte chemoattractant protein-1 (MCP-1) is a marker of active renal vasculitis. Nephrol Dial Transplant 2004;19(11):2761–2768.

149. Wallace GR, Farmer I, Church A, et al. Serum levels of chemokines correlate with disease activity in patients with retinal vasculitis. Immunol Lett 2003;90(1):59–64.

150. Hasegawa H, Kohno M, Sasaki M, et al. Antagonist of monocyte chemoattractant protein 1 ameliorates the initiation and progression of lupus nephritis and renal vasculitis in MRL/lpr mice. Arthritis Rheum 2003;48(9):2555–2566.

151. Ohwatari R, Fukuda S, Iwabuchi K, et al. Serum level of macrophage migration inhibitory factor as a useful parameter of clinical course in patients with Wegener's granulomatosis and relapsing polychondritis. Ann Otol Rhinol Laryngol 2001;110(11):1035–1040.

152. Cockwell P, Chakravorty SJ, Girdlestone J, et al. Fractalkine expression in human renal inflammation. J Pathol 2002;196(1):85–90.

153. Kinoshita M, Okada M, Hara M, et al. Mast cell tryptase in mast cell granules enhances MCP-1 and interleukin-8 production in human endothelial cells. Arterioscler Thromb Vasc Biol 2005;25(9):1858–1863.

154. Gutfleisch J, Baumert E, Wolff-Vorbeck G, et al. Increased expression of CD25 and adhesion molecules on peripheral blood lymphocytes of patients with Wegener's granulomatosis (WG) and ANCA positve vasculitides. Adv Exp Med Biol 1993;336:397–404.

155. John S, Neumayer HH, Weber M. Serum circulating ICAM-1 levels are not useful to indicate active vasculitis or early renal allograft rejection. Clin Nephrol 1994;42(6):369–375.

156. Pall AA, Adu D, Drayson M, et al. Circulating soluble adhesion molecules in systemic vasculitis. Nephrol Dial Transplant 1994;9(7):770–774.

157. Wang CR, Liu MF, Tsai RT, et al. Circulating intercellular adhesion molecules-1 and autoantibodies including anti-endothelial cell, anti-cardiolipin, and anti-neutrophil cytoplasma antibodies in patients with vasculitis. Clin Rheumatol 1993;12(3):375–380.

158. Hauschild S, Schmitt WH, Kekow J, et al. [Elevated serum levels of ICAM-1 in Wegener's granulomatosis.] Immun Infekt 1992;20(3):84–85.

159. Mrowka C, Sieberth HG. Circulating adhesion molecules ICAM-1, VCAM-1 and E-selectin in systemic vasculitis: marked differences between Wegener's granulomatosis and systemic lupus erythematosus. Clin Invest 1994;72(10):762–768.

160. Di Lorenzo G, Pacor ML, Mansueto P, et al. Circulating levels of soluble adhesion molecules in patients with ANCA-associated vasculitis. J Nephrol 2004;17(6):800–807.

161. Takizawa M, Maguchi S, Nakamaru Y, et al. Correlation between the levels of circulating adhesion molecules and

PR3-ANCA in Wegener's granulomatosis. Auris Nasus Larynx 2001;28(Suppl):S59–S62.

162. Blann AD, Herrick A, Jayson MI. Altered levels of soluble adhesion molecules in rheumatoid arthritis, vasculitis and systemic sclerosis. Br J Rheumatol 1995;34(9)814–819.

163. Ara J, Mirapeix E, Arrizabalaga P, et al. Circulating soluble adhesion molecules in ANCA-associated vasculitis. Nephrol Dial Transplant 2001;16(2):276–285.

164. Mrowka C, Sieberth HG. Detection of circulating adhesion molecules ICAM-1, VCAM-1 and E-selectin in Wegener's granulomatosis, systemic lupus erythematosus and chronic renal failure. Clin Nephrol 1995;43(5):288–296.

165. Stegeman CA, Tervaert JW, Huitema MG, et al. Serum levels of soluble adhesion molecules intercellular adhesion molecule 1, vascular cell adhesion molecule 1, and E-selectin in patients with Wegener's granulomatosis. Relationship to disease activity and relevance during follow up. Arthritis Rheum 1994;37(8):1228–1235.

166. Yaqoob M, West DC, McDicken I, Bell GM. Monitoring of endothelial leucocyte adhesion molecule-1 in antineutrophil-cytoplasmic-antibody-positive vasculitis. Am J Nephrol 1996;16(2):106–113.

167. Boehme MW, Schmitt WH, Youinou P, et al. Clinical relevance of elevated serum thrombomodulin and soluble E-selectin in patients with Wegener's granulomatosis and other systemic vasculitides. Am J Med 1996;101(4):387–394.

168. Witkowska AM, Kuryliszyn-Moskal A, Borawska MH, et al. A study on soluble intercellular adhesion molecule-1 and selenium in patients with rheumatoid arthritis complicated by vasculitis. Clin Rheumatol 2003;22(6):414–419.

169. Sais G, Vidaller A, Jucgla A, et al. Adhesion molecule expression and endothelial cell activation in cutaneous leukocytoclastic vasculitis. An immunohistologic and clinical study in 42 patients. Arch Dermatol 1997;133(4):443–450.

170. Voskuyl AE, Martin S, Melchers L, et al. Levels of circulating intercellular adhesion molecule-1 and -3 but not circulating endothelial leucocyte adhesion molecule are increased in patients with rheumatoid vasculitis. Br J Rheumatol 1995;34(4):311–315.

171. Kaplanski G, Maisonobe T, Marin V, et al. Vascular cell adhesion molecule-1 (VCAM-1) plays a central role in the pathogenesis of severe forms of vasculitis due to hepatitis C-associated mixed cryoglobulinemia. J Hepatol 2005;42(3):334–340.

172. Soylemezoglu O, Sultan N, Gursel T, et al. Circulating adhesion molecules ICAM-1 E-selectin, and von Willebrand factor in Henoch-Schonlein purpura. Arch Dis Child 1996;75(6)507–511.

173. Pall AA, Howie AJ, Adu D, et al. Glomerular vascular cell adhesion molecule-1 expression in renal vasculitis. J Clin Pathol 1996;49(3):238–242.

174. Rastaldi MP, Ferrario F, Tunesi S, et al. Intraglomerular and interstitial leukocyte infiltration, adhesion molecules, and interleukin-1 alpha expression in 15 cases of antineutrophil cytoplasmic autoantibody-associated renal vasculitis. Am J Kidney Dis 1996;27(1):48–57.

175. Turkcapar N, Sak SD, Saatci M, et al. Vasculitis and expression of vascular cell adhesion molecule-1, intercellular adhesion molecule-1, and E-selectin in salivary glands of patients with Sjogren's syndrome. J Rheumatol 2005;32(6):1063–1070.

176. Flipo RM, Cardon T, Copin MC, et al. ICAM-1, E-selectin, and TNF alpha expression in labial salivary glands of patients with rheumatoid vasculitis. Ann Rheum Dis 1997;56(1):41–44.

177. Burrows NP, Molina FA, Terenghi G, et al. Comparison of cell adhesion molecule expression in cutaneous leucocytoclastic and lymphocytic vasculitis. J Clin Pathol 1994;47(10):939–944.

178. Hsu H, Huang J, Shu HB, et al. TNF-dependent recruitment of the protein kinase RIP to the TNF receptor-1 signaling complex. Immunity 1996;4:387–396.

179. Jagiello P, Gencik M, Arning L, et al. New genomic region for Wegener's granulomatosis as revealed by an extended association screen with 202 apoptosis-related genes. Hum Genet 2004;114:468–477.

60
Asbestosis and Silicosis

Philip T. Cagle and Timothy Craig Allen

Introduction

Many of the lung diseases discussed in this book are the result of exposures to environmental substances, including infections, malignancies, immune reactions, and chronic interstitial diseases. Individual sections and chapters discuss lung cancer and mesothelioma (Sections 3 and 4), infections (Section 5), asthma (Chapter 51), and nonneoplastic smoking-related diseases (Chapter 49). This chapter focuses on those exposures that occur in the occupational environment and produce nonneoplastic lung disease. Although occupational exposures may produce asthma, small airways disease, acute lung injury, and hypersensitivity pneumonitis, this chapter discusses the pneumoconioses.

The pneumoconioses are caused by inhalation of mineral dusts that are used for specific purposes, such as in building materials, or are contaminants of materials used in an occupational setting. These dusts are derived from the earth, and background exposures to them may occur from the general ambient air, usually in lesser amounts than in occupational settings but in comparatively large amounts in some locales.[1] Among the more frequently encountered pneumoconioses are asbestosis[1,2] and silicosis,[1,3] and these have been investigated the most in terms of molecular mechanisms.

An observation among the pneumoconioses is that the generation of reactive oxygen species (ROS) and reactive nitrogen species (RNS) leading to subsequent chronic inflammation and fibrosis are a common denominator in the development and progression of these diseases. The production of ROS and RNS has two sources in the pneumoconioses: direct chemical reactions on the surface of the dust itself and generation of ROS and RNS by macrophages or other cells that have ingested the dust.

Asbestosis

Asbestos is a fibrous silicate derived from the earth that has been used in more than 2,000 industrial products because of its resistance to heat and chemicals.[1,2] The asbestos fibers are categorized as serpentine type (chrysotile) and amphibole type (amosite, crocidolite, and others) based on differing chemical compositions, shapes, and physiochemical properties. Asbestos fibers of appropriate size that have shed into the air as dust particles can be inhaled into the lungs.

Asbestos fibers are clear, but a percentage of inhaled fibers will be coated with iron and protein, creating an asbestos body that can be seen on routine cytology and histology sections. Asbestos bodies are one type of iron-coated or ferruginous bodies that are found in the lung. Iron stains highlight the iron coatings of asbestos bodies as bright blue against a pale pink background, making them more readily identifiable. A count of asbestos bodies by light microscopy or asbestos fibers by electron microscopy can be performed after digestion of a known weight of lung tissue to give a concentration in the person's lung tissue.[1,2]

Because asbestos is present in the ambient air, everyone has asbestos fibers and asbestos bodies in their lungs. Although asbestos is now mostly banned in the developed countries, a wide variety of occupations have had a potential for exposure to asbestos at levels above background, including miners, millers, insulators, boilermakers, and those involved in the manufacture of asbestos products or removal of asbestos materials. High levels of asbestos exposure may produce asbestosis, a distinctive type of pulmonary fibrosis, in susceptible individuals after a latency of many years. Asbestosis begins as fibrosis in the first tiers of alveolar septa in respiratory bronchioles and in some cases may progress, producing more extensive fibrosis that is most prominent in the periphery and lower zones of both lungs. In some cases, the amount of interstitial fibrosis may increase until there is end-stage fibrosis or honeycomb lung.[1,2] In addition to causing asbestosis, high levels of asbestos exposure may potentially increase the risk of lung cancer above that of tobacco smoking in some individuals with asbestosis, and, even in the absence of asbestosis, asbestos exposure is a major risk factor for diffuse malignant mesothelioma (see Chapters 23 and 34).

Investigations of the mechanisms by which asbestosis is initiated and progresses include studies of human tissues but have also relied on studies of animal models (see Chapter 14) in which the animals are exposed to asbestos through inhalation or instillation and on in vitro studies of cell lines, cell cultures, and tracheal explants (see Chapter 15). In the latter studies, cells such as macrophages, bronchial epithelial cells, or fibroblasts are often cultured in association with asbestos fibers. Inhalation of asbestos fibers causes epithelial cell proliferation in rodent lungs that is believed to be a probable factor in lung injury and repair in asbestosis. Alveolar epithelial cell apoptosis is believed to be an early event in the pathogenesis of asbestosis.[4–6] In animal models, the asbestos fibers initially deposit and accumulate at the alveolar duct junctions, and fibrotic lesions first appear in these foci.[7–10]

The mediators that initiate and cause progression of asbestosis are either generated directly from asbestos fibers or produced by cells exposed to asbestos fibers.[4–6,11–20] Oxidants as the cause of DNA damage, and their association with signaling pathways and mediators such as cytokines and growth factors, are discussed in detail in Chapter 44. Asbestos fibers often contain iron, and crocidolite ($Na_2[Fe^{3+}]_2[Fe^{2+}]_3Si_8O_{22}[OH]_2$) is especially rich in iron. Oxidants can be generated directly from the surfaces of asbestos fibers, especially crocidolite, by redox reactions, beginning with reduction of oxygen to superoxide by surface or leachable iron. This leads to the production of hydrogen peroxide and eventually the hydroxyl radical in a Fenton-like reaction in the presence of iron.[4–6,11–20]

In addition to the direct generation of oxidants on fiber surfaces, asbestos fibers may stimulate a variety of target cells, many of which may phagocytize the fibers, including pulmonary macrophages (both alveolar and interstitial), alveolar and airway epithelial cells, and fibroblasts. Phagocytosis of asbestos fibers by macrophages produces ROS and RNS. Macrophages and bronchiolar epithelial cells in asbestos-exposed rats produce peroxynitrite from RNS and reactive oxygen and nitrotyrosine residues as a result of peroxynitrite formation. Both the extracellular and intracellular generation of ROS and RNS cause DNA damage, modification of enzymes in signaling pathways, and release of cytokines. Among the cytokines that inves-

tigators have associated with the development of asbestosis are tumor necrosis factor (TNF), interleukin (IL)-8, IL-6, IL-1, macrophage inflammatory protein 2, and cytokine-induced neutrophil chemoattractant.[21–26]

In vitro studies have shown that asbestos fibers cause macrophages to increase TNF production.[27,28] Transgenic mice that overexpress TNF in alveolar epithelial cells spontaneously develop pulmonary fibrosis that resembles asbestosis.[29] Tumor necrosis factor receptor knockout mice fail to develop fibrosis even after increases in TNF following exposure to asbestos.

Growth factors and growth factor receptors are also believed to potentially play a role in the development of asbestosis. Upregulation of tumor growth factor-α (TGF-α) and upregulation of tumor growth factor-β (TGF-β) have been observed in developing fibrotic lesions of asbestos-exposed rats.[30,31] Jagirdar et al.[32] reported that TGF-β isoforms are upregulated in the fibrotic lungs of asbestos-exposed workers. Increased expression of the extracellular domain of the epidermal growth factor receptor was observed in the serum of patients with asbestosis by Partanen et al.[33] In 1998, Lasky et al.[34] reported that asbestos exposure upregulated PDGF-α receptor expression in rats.

A number of signaling pathways are activated by asbestos exposure and are likely to play a role in asbestosis. Asbestos fibers and TGF-α activate the extracellular signal-related kinases (ERKs), proteins of the mitogen-activated protein kinase (MAPK) pathways, through epidermal growth factor receptor. Timblin et al.[35] have shown that asbestos activates the ERK MAPK pathway and increases mRNA levels of c-fos through phosphorylation of epidermal growth factor receptor, resulting in early apoptosis and subsequent compensatory proliferation. Robledo et al.[36] reported increased phosphorylation of ERK in epithelial cells at sites of developing fibrotic lesions, and Cummins et al.[37] demonstrated increased expression and phosphorylation of ERKs in epithelial cells in mouse models of asbestos-induced fibrosis.

Multiple studies indicate that nuclear factor κ-B (NF-κB) activity is induced by asbestos through cytokines and oxidants. In addition, a variety of investigations have shown increased activity of activator protein-1 (AP-1), c-Jun and c-Fos in response to asbestos exposure.[38–40]

Increased p53 expression occurs in alveolar epithelial cells and macrophages at the alveolar duct junction in rats exposed to asbestos.[41] In an investigation using both in vitro and animal models, Panduri et al.[42] reported that asbestos-induced mitochondrial dysfunction and apoptosis are mediated by p53-dependent transcription, in part as a result of iron-derived ROS from the mitochondria and due to Bax and p53 mitochondrial translocation.

Virag[43] speculated that activation of poly(ADP-ribose) polymerase-1 in response to oxidative stress might have a role in asbestosis. Iakhiaev and Idell[44] reported that crocidolite induced tissue factor expression in cultured airway epithelial cells, probably involving the phosphatidylinositol 3-kinase/protein kinase C zeta signaling pathway, potentially contributing to lung remodeling.

Silicosis

Silicosis is a type of pulmonary fibrosis that occurs in susceptible individuals after exposure to large amounts of crystalline silica. Crystalline silica consists of silicon and oxygen (SiO_2) with trace amounts of aluminum, iron, and magnesium. Types of crystalline silica that can cause disease are coesite, cristobalite, melanophlogite, moganite, quartz, stishovite, and tridymite. Exposure to high levels of silica can potentially occur in coal and other miners, sandblasters, glass manufacturers, and stone and quarry workers.[1,3]

Similar to asbestosis, classic nodular silicosis is a chronic fibrotic disease that becomes manifest many years, usually decades, after initial exposure. Rare forms of silicosis have a more rapid course: accelerated silicosis may develop in less than 10 years, and acute silicosis results from a massive, overwhelming exposure and is clinically and pathologically very different from classic silicosis.[1,3]

Silicosis is characterized by accumulation of distinctive silicotic nodules composed of dust-laden macrophages in their early stages and dense whorls of hyalinized collagen with a rim of dust-laden macrophages in later stages. The nodules are in a lymphangitic distribution. Silica particles appear as tiny 2 μm weakly birefringent crystals on polarized light. Patients with silicosis have an associated susceptibility to infection with *Mycobacterium tuberculosis*, atypical mycobacteria, and fungus. Antinuclear antibodies, immune complexes, and scleroderma are seen with increased frequency in patients with silicosis.[1,3]

Similar to the development of asbestosis, ROS and RNS are generated in silicosis both from reactions on the surface of the silica particles and from products produced by macrophages that have phagocytized silica particles. Development of silicosis is believed to be related to the redox potential of the silica surface, which is increased with fractured silica that is produced during sandblasting. The surface is reactive with hydrogen, oxygen, carbon, and nitrogen. Alveolar macrophages ingest silica, which causes their death. This leads to release of the intracellular silica that is subsequently ingested by other macrophages in a cycle of ingestion and macrophage death.[45–48]

Freshly fractured silica is more toxic to alveolar macrophages than older silica particles. Crystalline silica produces a respiratory burst in macrophages with production of O^-, H_2O_2, and nitric oxide. The damaged macrophages release oxidants, proteolytic enzymes, and cytokines, including TNF-α and IL-1, which recruit inflammatory cells to alveolar surfaces and walls. Expression of IL-10 is also believed to contribute to silica-induced lung fibrosis by inducing T helper type 2 cytokines and cytokines IL-4 and IL-13. Additional oxidants and proteases are released by the inflammatory cells recruited to the parenchymal tissues.[49–53] Reactive oxygen species production due to silica activates MEK, ERK, NF-κB, and AP-1. Ding et al.[54] demonstrated that freshly fractured silica induces AP-1 activation, which may be mediated through p38 MAPK and ERK pathways.

Crystalline silica induces macrophage apoptosis. Silica induces Fas ligand (FasL) expression in macrophages in vitro and in vivo, stimulating FasL-dependent apoptosis of macrophages. FasL-deficient gld mice are resistant to the development of silicosis in association with a lack of macrophage apoptosis. Anti-FasL antibody blocks the development of silicosis in vivo.[55–57] On the other hand, anti-Fas autoantibodies have been identified in patients with silicosis, as well as in patients with autoimmune diseases associated with silicosis such as systemic sclerosis and systemic lupus erythematosis, and these autoantibodies stimulate Fas-related apoptosis.[57] Similar observations were reported for caspase-8.[58] Delgado et al.[59] analyzed 23 lung biopsy specimens from silicotic patients and five controls using immunohistochemistry and morphometry to evaluate the amount of FasL and Bcl-2. They concluded that the stage or extent of the silicosis was significantly related to FasL, mast cell, and extracellular matrix remodeling, with an inverse relationship to FasL expression. Therefore, induction of apoptosis and death receptors is an important mechanism in the development of silicosis.

It also appears that p53 plays an important role in the signaling pathways of silica-induced apoptosis. Wang et al.[60] observed that silica stimulates p53 transactivation with induction of p53 protein expression and phosphorylation of p53 protein.

Conclusion

Investigations have disclosed key roles for oxidative injury, cytokine pathways, and apoptosis in asbestosis and silicosis. These and future studies may yield a basis for molecular-targeted therapies for these diseases.

References

1. Churg AM, Green FHY. Occupational lung disease. In Churg AM, Myers JL, Tazelaar HD, Wright JL, eds. Pathology of the Lung, 3rd ed. New York: Thieme Medical Publishers; 2005:769–862.
2. Laga AC, Allen T, Cagle PT. Asbestosis. In Cagle PT, ed. The Color Atlas and Text of Pulmonary Pathology. New York: Lippincott Williams & Wilkins; 2005:393–396.

3. Laga AC, Allen T, Cagle PT. Silicosis. In Cagle PT, ed. The Color Atlas and Text of Pulmonary Pathology. New York: Lippincott Williams & Wilkins; 2005:397–399.

4. Kamp DW, Weitzman SA. The molecular basis of asbestos induced lung injury. Thorax 1999;54(7):638–652.

5. Manning CB, Vallyathan V, Mossman BT. Diseases caused by asbestos: mechanisms of injury and disease development. Int Immunopharmacol 2002;2(2–3):191–200.

6. Upadhyay D, Kamp DW. Asbestos-induced pulmonary toxicity: role of DNA damage and apoptosis. Exp Biol Med (Maywood) 2003;228(6):650–659.

7. Adamson IYR, Bowden DH. Response of mouse lung to crocidolite asbestos. I. Mineral fibrosis reaction to short fibres. J Pathol 1987;152:99–107.

8. Adamson IYR, Bowden DH. Response of mouse lung to crocidolite asbestos. II. Pulmonary fibrosis after long fibres. J Pathol 1987;152:109–117.

9. Dixon D, Bowser AD, Badgett A, et al. Incorporation of bromodeoxyuridine (BrdU) in the bronchiolar-alveolar regions of the lungs following two inhalation exposures to chrysotile asbestos in strain A/J mice. J Environ Pathol Toxicol Oncol 1995;14:205–213.

10. BeruBe KA, Quinlan TR, Moulton G, et al. Comparative proliferative and histopathologic changes in rat lungs after inhalation of chrysotile or crocidolite asbestos. Toxicol Appl Pharmacol 1996;137:67–74.

11. Weitzman SA, Graceffa P. Asbestos catalyzes hydroxyl and superoxide radical generation from hydrogen peroxide. Arch Biochem Biophys 1984;228:373–376.

12. Holley JA, Janssen YMW, Mossman BT, et al. Increased manganese superoxide dismutase protein in type II epithelial cells of rat lungs after inhalation of crocidolite asbestos or cristobalite silica. Am J Pathol 1992;141:475–485.

13. Janssen YMW, Marsh JP, Absher MP, et al. Expression of antioxidant enzymes in rat lungs after inhalation of asbestos or silica. J Biol Chem 1992;267:10625–10630.

14. Lund LG, Aust AE. Iron mobilization from crocidolite asbestos greatly enhances crocidolite-dependent formation of DNA single-strand breaks in phi X174 RFI DNA. Carcinogenesis 1992;13:637–642.

15. Kamp DW, Israbian VA, Yeldandi AV, et al. Phytic acid, an iron chelator, attenuates pulmonary inflammation and fibrosis in rats after intratracheal instillation of asbestos. Toxicol Pathol 1995;23:689–695.

16. Chao CC, Park SH, Aust AE. Participation of nitric oxide and iron in the oxidation of DNA in asbestos-treated human lung epithelial cells. Arch Biochem Biophys 1996;326:152–157.

17. Gilmour PS, Brown DM, Beswick PH, et al. Free radical activity of industrial fibers: role of iron in oxidative stress and activation of transcription factors. Environ Health Perspect 1997;105(Suppl 5):1313–1317.

18. Park SH, Aust AE. Regulation of nitric oxide synthase induction by iron and glutathione in asbestos-treated human lung epithelial cells. Arch Biochem Biophys 1998;360:47–52.

19. Quinlan TR, Hacker MP, Taatjes D, et al. Mechanisms of asbestos-induced nitric oxide production by rat alveolar macrophages in inhalation and in vitro models. Free Radic Biol Med 1998;24:778–788.

20. Tanaka S, Choe N, Hemenway DR, et al. Asbestos inhalation induces reactive nitrogen species and nitrotyrosine formation in the lungs and pleura of the rat. J Clin Invest 1998;102:445–454.

21. Driscoll KE, Hassenbein DG, Carter JM, et al. TNF-alpha and increased chemokine expression in rat lung after particle exposure. Toxicol Lett 1995;82/83:483–489.

22. Driscoll KE, Maurer JK, Higgins J, et al. Alveolar macrophage cytokine and growth factor production in a rat model of crocidolite-induced pulmonary inflammation and fibrosis. J Toxicol Environ Health 1995;46:155–169.

23. Broser M, Zhang Y, Aston C, et al. Elevated interleukin-8 in the alveolitis of individuals with asbestos exposure. Int Arch Occup Environ Health 1996;68:109–114.

24. Lemaire I, Ouellet S. Distinctive profile of alveolar macrophage-derived cytokine release induced by fibrogenic and nonfibrogenic mineral dusts. J Toxicol Environ Health 1996;47:465–478.

25. Dai J, Gilks B, Price K, et al. Mineral dusts directly induce epithelial and interstitial fibrogenic mediators and matrix components in the airway wall. Am J Respir Crit Care Med 1998;158:1907–1913.

26. Driscoll KE, Carter JM, Howard BW, et al. Crocidolite activates NF-kB and MIP-2 gene expression in rat alveolar epithelial cells. Role of mitochondrial-derived oxidants. Environ Health Perspect 1998;106(Suppl 5):1171–1174.

27. Simeonova PP, Luster MI. Iron and reactive oxygen species in the asbestos-induced tumor necrosis factor-alpha response from alveolar macrophages. Am J Respir Cell Mol Biol 1995;12:676–683.

28. Driscoll KE, Carter JM, Hassenbein DG, et al. Cytokines and particle-induced inflammatory cell recruitment. Environ Health Perspect 1997;105(Suppl 5):1159–1164.

29. Miyazaki Y, Araki K, Vesin C, et al. Expression of a tumor necrosis factor-alpha transgene in murine lung causes lymphocytic and fibrosing alveolitis. J Clin Invest 1995;96:250–259.

30. Perdue TD, Brody AR. Distribution of transforming growth factor-beta1, fibronectin, and smooth muscle actin in asbestos-induced pulmonary fibrosis in rats. J Histochem Cytochem 1994;42:1061–1070.

31. Liu J-Y, Morris GF, Lei W-H, et al. Up-regulated expression of transforming growth factor-alpha in the bronchiolar-alveolar duct regions of asbestos-exposed rats. Am J Pathol 1996;149:205–217.

32. Jagirdar J, Lee TC, Reibman J, et al. Immunological localization of transforming growth factor beta isoforms in asbestos-related disease. Environ Health Perspect 1997;105(Suppl 5):1197–1203.

33. Partanen R, Hemminki K, Koskinen H, et al. The detection of increased amounts of the extracellular domain of the epidermal growth factor receptor in serum during carcinogenesis in asbestosis patients. J Med 1994;36:1324–1328.

34. Lasky JA, Coin PG, Lindroos PM, et al. Chrysotile asbestos stimulates platelet-derived growth factor-AA production by fat lung fibroblasts in vitro: evidence for an autocrine loop. Am J Respir Crit Care 1995;Med 12:162–170.

35. Timblin C, Robledo R, Rincon M, et al. Transgenic mouse models to determine the role of epidermal growth factor

receptor in epithelial cell proliferation, apoptosis, and asbestosis. Chest 2001;120(1 Suppl):22S–24S.

36. Robledo RF, Buder-Hoffmann SA, Cummins AB, et al. Increased phosphorylated extracellular signal-regulated kinase immunoreactivity associated with proliferative and morphologic lung alterations after chrysotile asbestos inhalation in mice. Am J Pathol 2000;156(4):1307–1316.

37. Cummins AB, Palmer C, Mossman BT, et al. Persistent localization of activated extracellular signal-regulated kinases (ERK1/2) is epithelial cell-specific in an inhalation model of asbestosis. Am J Pathol 2003;162(3):713–720.

38. Janssen YMW, Barchowsky A, Treadwell M, et al. Asbestos induces nuclear factor-kappa B (NF-kB) DNA-binding activity and NF-kB–dependent gene expression in tracheal epithelial cells. Proc Natl Acad Sci USA 1995;92:8458–8462.

39. Cheng N, Shi X, Ye J, et al. Role of transcription factor NF-kappaB in asbestos-induced TNFalpha response from macrophages. Exp Mol Pathol 1999;66(3):201–210.

40. Janssen YMW, Heintz NH, Mossman BT. Induction of c-fos and c-jun protooncogene expression by asbestos is ameliorated by N-acetyl-L-cysteine in mesothelial cells. Cancer Res 1995;55:2065–2089.

41. Mishra A, Liu J-Y, Brody AR, et al. Inhaled asbestos fibers induce p53 expression in the rat lung. Am J Respir Cell Mol Biol 1997;16:479–485.

42. Panduri V, Surapureddi S, Soberanes S, et al. P53 mediates amosite asbestos-induced alveolar epithelial cell mitochondria-regulated apoptosis. Am J Respir Cell Mol Biol 2006;34(4):443–452.

43. Virag L. Poly(ADP-ribosyl)ation in asthma and other lung diseases. Pharmacol Res 2005;52(1):83–92

44. Iakhiaev A, Idell S. Asbestos induces tissue factor in Beas-2B cells via PI3 kinase-PKC-mediated signaling. J Toxicol Environ Health A 2004;67(19):1537–1547.

45. Shi X, Mao Y, Daniel LN. Generation of reactive oxygen species by quartz particles and its implication for cellular damage. Appl Occup Environ Hyg 1995;10:1138–1144.

46. Mossman BT, Churg A. Mechanisms in the pathogenesis of asbestosis and silicosis. Am J Respir Crit Care Med 1998;157:1666–1680.

47. Fubini B, Hubbard A. Reactive oxygen species (ROS) and reactive nitrogen species (RNS) generation by silica in inflammation and fibrosis. Free Radic Biol Med 2003;34: 1507–1516.

48. Rimal B, Greenberg AK, Rom WN. Basic pathogenetic mechanisms in silicosis: current understanding. Curr Opin Pulm Med 2005;11(2):169–173.

49. Piguet PF, Collart MA, Grau GE, et al. Requirement of tumour necrosis factor for development of silica-induced pulmonary fibrosis. Nature 1990;344:245–247.

50. Gossart S, Cambon C, Orfila C, et al. Reactive oxygen intermediates as regulators of TNF production in rat lung inflammation induced by silica. J Immunol 1996;156:1540–1548.

51. Davis GS, Pfeiffer LM, Hemenway D. Persistent overexpression of interleukin-1beta and tumor necrosis factor-alpha in murine silicosis. J Environ Pathol Toxicol Oncol 1998;17:99–114.

52. Barbarin V, Arras M, Huax F. Characterization of the effect of Interleukin 10 on silica induced lung fibrosis in mice. Am J Respir Crit Care Med 2004;31:78–85.

53. Barbarin V, Xing Z, Delos M, et al. Pulmonary overexpression of IL-10 augments lung fibrosis and Th2 responses induced by silica particles. Am J Physiol Lung Cell Mol Physiol 2005;288(5):L841–L848.

54. Ding M, Chen F, Shi X, et al. Diseases caused by silica: mechanisms of injury and disease development. Int Immunopharmacol 2002;2(2-3):173–182.

55. Dosreis GA, Borges VM, Zin WA. The central role of Fas-ligand cell signaling in inflammatory lung diseases. J Cell Mol Med 2004;8(3):285–293.

56. Takata-Tomokuni A, Ueki A, Shiwa M, et al. Detection, epitope-mapping and function of anti-Fas autoantibody in patients with silicosis. Immunology 2005;116(1):21–29.

57. Otsuki T, Miura Y, Nishimura Y, et al. Alterations of Fas and Fas-related molecules in patients with silicosis. Exp Biol Med (Maywood) 2006;231(5):522–533.

58. Ueki A, Isozaki Y, Kusaka M. Anti-caspase-8 autoantibody response in silicosis patients is associated with HLA-DRB1, DQB1 and DPB1 alleles. J Occup Health 2005;47(1):61–67.

59. Delgado L, Parra ER, Capelozzi VL. Apoptosis and extracellular matrix remodeling in human silicosis. Histopathology 2006;49:283–289.

60. Wang L, Bowman L, Lu Y, et al. Essential role of p53 in silica-induced apoptosis. Am J Physiol Lung Cell Mol Physiol 2005;288(3):L488–L496.

Index